Encyclopedia of COVID-19

Encyclopedia of COVID-19

Collection Editor

Stephen Bustin

MDPI

Basel • Beijing • Wuhan • Barcelona • Belgrade • Novi Sad • Cluj • Manchester

Collection Editor
Stephen Bustin
Medical Technology Research
Institute
Anglia Ruskin University
Chelmsford
UK

Editorial Office
MDPI AG
Grosspeteranlage 5
4052 Basel, Switzerland

This is a reprint of the Topical Collection, published open access by the journal *Encyclopedia* (ISSN 2673-8392), freely accessible at: https://www.mdpi.com/journal/encyclopedia/topical_collections/ency_covid_19.

For citation purposes, cite each article independently as indicated on the article page online and as indicated below:

Lastname, A.A.; Lastname, B.B. Article Title. *Journal Name* **Year**, *Volume Number*, Page Range.

ISBN 978-3-7258-3555-3 (Hbk)
ISBN 978-3-7258-3556-0 (PDF)
https://doi.org/10.3390/books978-3-7258-3556-0

Contents

About the Editor

Stephen Bustin

Stephen Bustin is Professor of Molecular Medicine at Anglia Ruskin University in the United Kingdom. His research focuses on developing novel approaches for the early diagnosis of infectious diseases. Professor Bustin's testimony as an expert witness at the 2007 Washington DC autism/MMR trial was pivotal in disproving the alleged linked between the MMR vaccine and childhood autism. He has authored numerous papers, review articles, and book chapters aimed at improving the reproducibility and robustness of molecular methods, particularly those involving reverse transcription and quantitative real-time PCR (qPCR), and he has presented hundreds of talks and workshops across the USA, Canada, Europe, Asia (most notably North Korea), and Australia. He has published three books, the "A-Z of quantitative PCR" (2004), universally known as the "qPCR Bible"; "The PCR Revolution" (2011); and "PCR Technology" (2013). He led an international consortium developing the MIQE guidelines for the use and reporting of real-time PCR (2009) and digital PCR (2013). Professor Bustin is the Editor-in Chief of Gene Expression, International Journal of Molecular Sciences and serves on the editorial boards of several peer-reviewed journals. During the COVID-19 pandemic, he published several papers highlighting the importance of accurate testing for SARS-CoV-2 and developed a novel five-plex assay targeting the virus. Professor Bustin is a Fellow of the Royal Society of Biology (FRSB) and a Member of the Academia Europaea (MAE).

Preface

The COVID-19 pandemic has had a profound impact on global health, economies, and daily life, prompting an unprecedented surge in scientific research and collaboration. This collection of articles, published in MDPI's *Encyclopedia*, captures a diverse range of perspectives on the pandemic, offering insights into its multifaceted effects and the innovative responses it has elicited. This compendium begins by exploring the pandemic's influence on mental health, including the rise of digital mental health solutions and the dynamics of romantic relationships during periods of social distancing. It further delves into the environmental consequences of lockdown measures, such as notable improvements in air quality.

In the realm of medical advances, the rapid development of mRNA vaccines, facilitated by nanotechnology, is examined. The collection also addresses the challenges faced by various sectors, including dentistry and self-service restaurants, highlighting the adaptive strategies employed to mitigate risks. Additionally, the compendium reflects on broader societal implications, such as health disparities exacerbated by the pandemic, and underscores the importance of learning from this global crisis to enhance future pandemic preparedness.

Collectively, these articles provide a comprehensive overview of the challenges and innovations that have emerged during the COVID-19 pandemic, serving as a testament to human resilience and the relentless pursuit of knowledge in the face of adversity.

Stephen Bustin
Collection Editor

encyclopedia

MDPI

Editorial

Reflections on a Global Crisis: From Response to Readiness—A Multidisciplinary Perspective on COVID-19

Stephen A. Bustin

Medical Technology Research Centre, Faculty of Health, Education, Medicine and Social Care, Anglia Ruskin University Chelmsford, Chelmsford CM1 1SQ, UK; stephen.bustin@aru.ac.uk

Received: 4 June 2025
Accepted: 12 June 2025
Published: 3 July 2025

Citation: Bustin, S.A. Reflections on a Global Crisis: From Response to Readiness—A Multidisciplinary Perspective on COVID-19. *Encyclopedia* **2025**, *5*, 94. https://doi.org/10.3390/encyclopedia5030094

The COVID-19 pandemic has had a profound impact on global health, economies, and daily life, prompting an unprecedented surge in scientific research and collaboration. This collection of articles published in MDPI's *Encyclopedia* captures a diverse range of perspectives on the pandemic and provides a multidisciplinary perspective on the COVID-19 pandemic, illustrating its biological, social, cultural, and institutional dimensions. Together, these contributions form a coherent and enduring resource for understanding arguably the most transformative public health events of the 21st century. The contributions can be grouped into a number of categories:

1. Medical Mechanisms and Pathophysiology

These papers provide an essential biomedical context by examining the direct biological impacts of SARS-CoV-2 and help clarify how SARS-CoV-2 disrupts physiological systems. Topics include analyses of vascular dysfunction via the Angiopoietin/Tie axis (Contribution 2); renal complications across SARS, MERS, and COVID-19 (Contributions 3 and 11); and organ-specific pathology in the lungs (Contribution 12), brain (Contributions 9 and 29), and kidneys. Contribution 17 reviews the auditory and vestibular symptoms, such as tinnitus, vertigo, and hearing loss, associated with SARS-CoV-2 infection and considers the underlying pathophysiological mechanisms. Other contributions detail gross pathology (Contribution 8), Bell's palsy (Contribution 6), the importance of detecting asymptomatic individuals to prevent the spread of the disease (Contribution 27), and the molecular interaction between spike protein and ACE2 (Contribution 28), offering insights into mechanisms of infection and damage. Understanding these mechanisms is vital for clinical treatment, risk stratification, and the development of targeted interventions.

2. Clinical Management and Public Health Responses

These studies document the rapid reconfiguration of healthcare and public service systems during the pandemic, revealing both resilience and emergent practices that may endure beyond the immediate crisis. Contribution 22 reviews adverse events associated with COVID-19 preventative strategies, particularly vaccines, drawing on early surveillance data. It highlights rare but serious complications and calls for prospective studies in high-risk groups. While affirming that benefits outweigh risks, the article adopts a measured tone, reflecting limited data and the need for clinical discretion. Other contributions discuss innovations in protective equipment, such as the small but significant use of barrier sheets during intubation (Contribution 33), and examine how information and communication technologies supported mental health services (Contribution 34). Contribution 4 underscores barriers to access across age, gender, race, socioeconomic status, language, and culture, which limit the uptake of these services in diverse populations. Adaptations in everyday settings are explored in studies of self-service restaurants (Contribution 41) and secondary education (Contribution 24). Alongside Contribution 10, which assesses the pedagogical, technological, and logistical challenges of hybrid learning, these studies illustrate how pandemic-driven responses may continue to shape healthcare, public services, and education in the future.

3. Reproductive and Developmental Impacts

The study in Contribution 5 assesses the impact of in utero SARS-CoV-2 exposure, emphasising the need for continued monitoring of maternal and foetal health during pandemics. This contribution is particularly significant in addressing long-term developmental risks, where data remain sparse and the implications for future generations are potentially profound.

4. Mental Health and Social Well-Being

This section highlights the human cost of the pandemic, beyond physical illness, and offers a persuasive view of how creative, cultural, and spiritual practices provided comfort and continuity in disrupted lives. Contribution 25 illustrates the challenges facing national mental health systems due to the increase in psychological symptoms both in the general population and healthcare workers, with the additional complication of the pandemic's toll on substance and behavioural addiction (Contribution 30). Its complex and not always obvious influence on romantic relationships, including intimate partner violence, is explored in Contribution 35. Hopefully, however, Contribution 1 discusses how community responses such as participatory music-making, defined as any music-making activity in which individuals engage for the sake of the activity itself, worship, and group singing, mitigate isolation and sustain social bonds. Contribution 7 describes how academic libraries serving art and architecture disciplines rapidly adapted to COVID-19 disruptions by introducing innovations in digital service delivery, especially the rise in controlled digital lending. These contributions demonstrate how the pandemic's human cost extended far beyond infection, affecting emotional well-being and community cohesion.

5. Technology, Communication, and Trust

These contributions address the critical links between science, communication, and perception, highlighting how both accurate information and technological innovation can shape public behaviour in powerful ways. Innovation has enabled real-time data modelling (Contribution 20) and breakthroughs such as mRNA vaccine delivery using nanotechnology (Contribution 36), exemplifying science's capacity to respond rapidly to global threats. At the same time, the same digital ecosystems that support rapid communication have also facilitated the spread of misinformation (Contribution 31) and fake news (Contribution 32), eroding trust in science (Contribution 21) and undermining public health compliance. Cross-cultural differences in response (Contribution 16) further underscore the importance of contextually sensitive communication. Together, these contributions demonstrate that while innovation can offer critical solutions, its benefits depend on the integrity of the information environment in which it operates.

6. Inequality and Structural Disparities

By exposing the uneven distribution of risk and access, these contributions deepen our understanding of how social structures influence vulnerability and resilience during global emergencies. Inequities are addressed through examinations of gender differences in both incidence and outcomes (Contribution 18), domestic violence (Contribution 23), health disparities (Contribution 37), and the pandemic's disproportionate burden on conflict-affected regions (Contribution 13). These issues are often under-discussed in mainstream scientific discourse, yet they are essential for any meaningful preparedness strategy. The term "health disparities" itself is broad and variably applied across disciplines and settings; these contributions highlight the real-world implications of health disparities, moving beyond abstract definitions to show who was most affected and why.

7. Environmental and Occupational Change

This final collection reflects on how public health crises reconfigure daily environments and labour conditions and offers valuable perspectives on unintended environmental benefits and structural transformations in work culture. These are lessons that are highly relevant not just for sustainable recovery but for any future planning of societal change. The pandemic's indirect effects are considered through changes in air quality (Contribution 38), challenges in the construction sector (Contribution 19), and the shift to telework (Contribution 15). Contribution 14 applies transition theory, a conceptual framework used to understand how individuals or systems adapt to significant changes or disruptions in their lives or environments, to frame the pandemic as a global turning point. Contribution 39 reviews the immediate impact of COVID-19 on dental practice, including infection control measures, procedural adaptations, and ethical concerns around aerosol-generating procedures. It also considers longer-term implications for dental education and workforce sustainability. This is complemented by contribution 26, which discusses dental care adaptations from the patients' standpoint. Finally, Contribution 40 emphasises that future prevention efforts are essential for global health security and calls for improved surveillance, strengthened public health infrastructure, greater international cooperation, and, crucially, transparent communication to build community trust.

This collection offers more than a retrospective account of the COVID-19 pandemic. It provides a lens to understand how biological mechanisms, human behaviour, institutional systems, and scientific knowledge interact under crisis conditions. The contributions examine not only immediate responses to the pandemic but also the structural conditions that shaped its course across a wide range of contexts. These range from the reconfiguration of clinical services and the emergence of new scientific practices to the psychological and social consequences of prolonged disruption.

While many sections highlight innovation and resilience, they also expose persistent vulnerabilities: the fragmentation of health infrastructures, the uneven burden of risk and access, and the fragile relationship between scientific expertise and public confidence. It brings home the realisation that although the pandemic was a calamitous biomedical crisis, its impact was also shaped by failures in communication and erosion of public trust. Several contributions underline that future pandemics are not speculative threats but expected events. Many conditions that facilitated the spread of SARS-CoV-2, such as global travel, the climate crisis, inequitable healthcare systems and vaccine hesitancy, continue unabated. Effective preparation will require not only investment in surveillance, diagnostics, and international coordination but also a cultural shift in how science engages with society. The information combined in this volume illustrates that future preparedness depends on a collective willingness to engage with the uncomfortable truths that prevention requires sustained investment and that trust, once lost, is difficult to regain. This collection provides the arguments for that conversation.

Conflicts of Interest: The author declares no conflict of interest.

List of Contributions:

1. Morgan-Ellis, E.M. COVID-19 and Participatory Music-Making. *Encyclopedia* **2024**, *4*, 709–719.
2. Janchivlamdan, D.; Shivkumar, M.; Singh, H. The Effects of SARS-CoV-2 on the Angiopoietin/Tie Axis and the Vascular Endothelium. *Encyclopedia* **2024**, *4*, 544–557.
3. Dousdampanis, P.; Mouzaki, A.; Trigka, K.; Stefanidis, I.; Galanopoulos, K.-E.; Siavelis, I.-S.; Stathopoulou, D.; Assimakopoulos, S.F. Kidney Issues Associated with COVID-19 Disease. *Encyclopedia* **2023**, *3*, 1085–1104.
4. Yu, J.; Bekerian, D.A. Telemental Health and Diverse Populations amid COVID-19. *Encyclopedia* **2023**, *3*, 267–278.
5. Kyle, M.H.; Dumitriu, D. Effects of in Utero SARS-CoV-2 Exposure on Newborn Health Outcomes. *Encyclopedia* **2022**, *3*, 15–27.
6. Tranchito, E.N.; Goslawski, A.; Cabrera, C.I.; Rabbani, C.C.; Fowler, N.M.; Li, S.; Thuener, J.E.; Lavertu, P.; Rezaee, R.P.; Teknos, T.N.; et al. COVID-19 and Bell's Palsy. *Encyclopedia* **2022**, *2*, 1935–1942.
7. Orcutt, R.; Campbell, L.; Gervits, M.; Opar, B. The Post-Pandemic Transformation of Art and Architecture Libraries. *Encyclopedia* **2022**, *2*, 1893–1901.
8. Zhang, B. Gross Pathology in COVID-19. *Encyclopedia* **2022**, *2*, 1790–1802.
9. Stoyanov, G.S.; Stoyanov, D.; Ivanov, M.; Tonchev, A.B.; Popov, H.; Petkova, L. COVID-19-Associated Encephalopathy (COVEP): Basic Aspects of Neuropathology. *Encyclopedia* **2022**, *2*, 1773–1789.
10. Batista-Toledo, S.; Gavilan, D. Implementation of Blended Learning During COVID-19. *Encyclopedia* **2022**, *2*, 1763–1772.
11. Popov, H.; Stoyanov, G.S.; Petkova, L.; Stoyanov, D.; Ivanov, M.; Tonchev, A.B. SARS, MERS and COVID-19-Associated Renal Pathology. *Encyclopedia* **2022**, *2*, 1710–1721.
12. Stoyanov, G.S.; Popov, H.; Petkova, L.; Stoyanov, D.; Ivanov, M.; Tonchev, A.B. SARS-CoV-2 Associated Pulmonary Pathology. *Encyclopedia* **2022**, *2*, 1698–1709.
13. Ossai, E.C. COVID-19 and Peace in Conflict-Affected Areas. *Encyclopedia* **2022**, *2*, 1678–1687.
14. Heanoy, E.Z.; Uzer, T.; Brown, N.R. COVID-19 Pandemic as a Transitional Event: From the Perspective of the Transition Theory. *Encyclopedia* **2022**, *2*, 1602–1610.
15. Türkes, M.C.; Vutá, D.R. Telework: Before and After COVID-19. *Encyclopedia* **2022**, *2*, 1370–1383.
16. Nair, N.; Selvaraj, P.; Nambudiri, R. Culture and COVID-19: Impact of Cross-Cultural Dimensions on Behavioral Responses. *Encyclopedia* **2022**, *2*, 1210–1224.
17. Cherchi, M. Otovestibular Symptoms of COVID-19 and Its Vaccines/Treatments. *Encyclopedia* **2022**, *2*, 1200–1209.
18. Ilardi, A. COVID-19: Gender and Outcomes. *Encyclopedia* **2022**, *2*, 864–872.
19. Elizalde, R.R. COVID-19 in the Construction Sector. *Encyclopedia* **2022**, *2*, 717–728.
20. Fokas, A.S.; Dikaios, N.; Tsiodras, S.; Kastis, G.A. Simple Formulae, Deep Learning and Elaborate Modelling for the COVID-19 Pandemic. *Encyclopedia* **2022**, *2*, 679–689.
21. Mousoulidou, M.; Christodoulou, A.; Argyrides, M.; Siakalli, M.; Constantinou, L. Trust in Science and COVID-19. *Encyclopedia* **2022**, *2*, 602–616.
22. Ajmera, K.M. Adverse Events Profile of COVID-19 Preventative Strategies. *Encyclopedia* **2022**, *2*, 457–465.
23. Zamba, C.; Mousoulidou, M.; Christodoulou, A. Domestic Violence Against Women and COVID-19. *Encyclopedia* **2022**, *2*, 441–456.
24. Siakalli, M.; Mousoulidou, M.; Christodoulou, A.; Savvidou, A.; Kouppa, K. Secondary Education and COVID-19. *Encyclopedia* **2022**, *2*, 409–427.
25. Bueno-Guerra, N. COVID-19 and Psychological Impact. *Encyclopedia* **2022**, *2*, 400–408.
26. Salgarello, S.; Audino, E.; Bertoletti, P.; Salvadori, M.; Garo, M.L. Dental Patients' Perspective on COVID-19: A Systematic Review. *Encyclopedia* **2022**, *2*, 365–382.
27. Veronese, S.; Sbarbati, A. Asymptomatic Patients and Immune Subjects. *Encyclopedia* **2022**, *2*, 109–126.
28. De Masi, L.; Argenio, M.A.; Giordano, D.; Facchiano, A. Molecular Aspects of Spike–ACE2 Interaction. *Encyclopedia* **2022**, *2*, 96–108.

29. Shnayder, N.A.; Sirbiladze, T.K.; Demko, I.V.; Petrova, M.M.; Nasyrova, R.F. Encephalitis Associated with COVID-19. *Encyclopedia* **2021**, *2*, 26–35.
30. Daglis, T. The Increase in Addiction During COVID-19. *Encyclopedia* **2021**, *1*, 1257–1266.
31. Anastasiades, E.; Argyrides, M.; Mousoulidou, M. Misinformation About COVID-19: Psychological Insights. *Encyclopedia* **2021**, *1*, 1200–1214.
32. Bustos Díaz, J.; Nicolas-Sans, R. COVID-19 and Fake News. *Encyclopedia* **2021**, *1*, 1175–1181.
33. Tsai, P.B.; Luk, H.-N. Sheet Barrier and Intubating Stylet. *Encyclopedia* **2021**, *1*, 1058–1075.
34. Balcombe, L.; De Leo, D. Digital Mental Health Amid COVID-19. *Encyclopedia* **2021**, *1*, 1047–1057
35. Candel, O.-S.; Jitaru, M. COVID-19 and Romantic Relationships. *Encyclopedia* **2021**, *1*,1038–1046.
36. Gao, Y.; Yang, K.; Shelling, A.N.; Wu, Z. Nanotechnology-Enabled COVID-19 mRNA Vaccines. *Encyclopedia* **2021**, *1*, 773–780.
37. Iyanda, A.; Boakye, K.; Lu, Y. COVID-19: Evidenced Health Disparity. *Encyclopedia* **2021**, *1*, 744–763.
38. Donzelli, G.; Cioni, L.; Cancellieri, M.; Llopis-Morales, A.; Morales-Suarez-Varela, M. Air Quality during Covid-19 Lockdown. *Encyclopedia* **2021**, *1*, 519–526.
39. Devlin, H.; Soltani, P. COVID-19 and Dentistry. *Encyclopedia* **2021**, *1*, 496–504.
40. Coccia, M. Pandemic Prevention: Lessons from COVID-19. *Encyclopedia* **2021**, *1*, 36.
41. Zandonadi, R.P.; Botelho, R.B.A.; Maynard, D.d.C.; Akutsu, R.d.C.C.d.A. Self-Service Restaurants in SARS-CoV-2 Pandemic. *Encyclopedia* **2021**, *1*, 401–408.

encyclopedia

Entry

COVID-19 and Participatory Music-Making

Esther M. Morgan-Ellis

Music Department, College of Arts and Letters, University of North Georgia, Dahlonega, GA 30597, USA; esther.morgan-ellis@ung.edu

Definition: Participatory music-making is any music-making activity in which individuals engage for the sake of the activity itself. It can be contrasted with presentational music-making, which takes the production of a performance or recording for consumption by an audience as a principal objective. During the COVID-19 pandemic, participatory musicians adopted a variety of technological means by which to make music together online. While virtual activities allowed these individuals to sustain their communities and grow as musicians, they did not satisfy all the needs met by in-person music-making. Additionally, online music-making increased access for some but posed barriers to access for others. Virtual participatory music-making remains relevant following the relaxation of pandemic restrictions, and it will likely grow in significance as communications technologies and internet access improve.

Keywords: online music-making; virtual music-making; participatory performance; Irish traditional music; old-time music; shape-note singing; congregational singing; community singing

1. Introduction

Social distancing measures that were mandated or voluntarily adopted during the COVID-19 pandemic inevitably impacted the activities of all musicians, especially those who perform for live audiences and those who gather in groups to make music. Early in the pandemic, music ensembles made headlines following several "superspreader events" that took place at choir rehearsals [1,2]. The risk undertaken by singers was scrutinized most closely, given their reliance on breath for sound production and their habit of performing in close proximity to one another using resonant indoor spaces [3,4]. Emphasis was placed on the dispersal of aerosols and droplets, which also accompanies sound production in wind instruments [5,6]. While various in-person mitigation strategies were proposed [7,8], most choral ensembles ultimately adopted virtual approaches to rehearsing and performing [9]. Other collaborative and performing musicians likewise turned to the internet as the most viable means of sustaining their practices. This entry will consider the full range of pandemic impacts on participatory musicians in particular, focusing on their uses of the internet to play and sing together.

Citation: Morgan-Ellis, E.M. COVID-19 and Participatory Music-Making. *Encyclopedia* **2024**, *4*, 709–719. https://doi.org/10.3390/encyclopedia4020044

Academic Editor: Stephen Bustin

Received: 15 March 2024
Revised: 23 April 2024
Accepted: 25 April 2024
Published: 27 April 2024

2. Defining and Categorizing Participatory Music-Making

This entry is uniquely concerned with participatory music-making, which can involve singers and/or instrumentalists. Turino has described participatory music-making as a practice in which "there are no artist-audience distinctions, only participants and potential participants", and during which "one's primary attention is on the activity, on the doing, and on the other participants, rather than on an end product that results from the activity" [10] (p. 28). While it is sometimes a simple task to identify whether a musical occasion is participatory (e.g., a sea shanty singalong in a tavern) or presentational (e.g., a choir concert in a performance hall), most collaborative music-making takes place somewhere on a spectrum between the two extremes. For example, participants in college a cappella groups rehearse and perform, which are hallmarks of presentational music-making, but they are likely to train their focus "on the activity, on the doing, and on the other participants", and the act of participation is often valued more highly than presentational accomplishments [11]. While participatory values are present in many performing ensembles, this entry will center on non-presenting collaborative musicians. During the pandemic, these individuals pursued virtual music-making for reasons that were not related to presentational performance (e.g., maintaining social connections, continuing to develop skills, and remaining immersed in a repertoire). Their needs and practices were, therefore, different from those of musicians looking to perform and reach audiences. As the pandemic recedes, these musicians have maintained many of their virtual music-making practices, which—while frustrating or valueless for presentational musicians [12]—often meet the needs of participatory communities.

In-person participatory music-making activities can be divided into two types: those in which musical participation is the purpose for convening and those in which it is secondary. The first of these categories is strongly, although not exclusively, associated with vernacular or "folk" traditions. Most of these descend from community music practices associated with a traditional culture and are accessible to participants with a low skill level yet still immersive for high-skill participants. Some communities, such as the Kaluli people of Papua New Guinea [13] or the Aymara in Southern Peru [14], collectively engage with instrumental and/or vocal music-making as a part of daily life. In Westernized contexts, participatory music-making is more likely to be a discrete activity that occurs at a scheduled time and in a specific place. Examples of participatory music communities that have been well documented in the scholarly literature include Irish traditional musicians (ITM), who play and/or sing Irish music collectively in the context of sessions [15]; old-time (OTM) and bluegrass musicians, who play American tunes at jams [16]; hip-hop rappers, beatboxers, and breakers, who exchange verses and dance moves in the context of cyphers [17]; shape-note singers, who participate in a collective hymn-singing tradition rooted in the US South [18]; English carolers, who gather in public spaces to sing traditional carols during the Christmas season [19]; and drum circle participants, who engage with a range of culturally specific drumming practices [20]. Each of these traditions is characterized by a unique repertoire and distinctive practices. However, participatory music-making is not the purview of the vernacular realm. The field also includes, for example, karaoke singers, who visit public establishments to sing popular songs—often in groups—with prerecorded accompaniment [21], and various community singing groups that adopt repertoire reflective of their shared interests or values [22]. While classical music is strongly associated with presentational performance, it too might become participatory when, for example, a group of string players gather in a domestic space to sightread string quartets [23]. What all these examples share in common is the fact that auditors are either absent or of no concern to the musicians, who participate for themselves and one another.

When participatory music-making takes place as an adjunct to a non-musical gathering, it almost always involves singing. Examples include singing in the context of worship [24], singing or chanting at sporting events [25,26], singing at protests or other political events [27], and singing for icebreakers or group bonding purposes as part of a social gathering [28]. Although these contexts decenter music-making, musical activity plays an important role in regulating participants' emotions, confirming group identity, and enhancing feelings of interpersonal connectedness [29,30]. The power of participatory music-making to accomplish these ends means that it is often employed for therapeutic reasons [31]. In this context, a Registered Music Therapist (RMT) designs and administers a participatory-music-based intervention for the purpose of improving the physical or mental health of subjects [32].

3. Participatory Music-Making and the Internet before the Pandemic

When musical participation is translated to the digital realm, there is a further distinction to be drawn between in-person communities that use the internet as an extension of their activities and online communities that convene only in digital spaces. Both types of communities have attracted scholarly attention in the past two decades, especially from music education researchers. Waldron and her collaborators have examined the formation of on- and offline convergent community [33,34] and online community [35,36] among ITM, OTM, and bluegrass musicians. Their focus has been on communities of practice [37], defined by the framework's architects as "groups of people who share a concern or a passion for something they do and learn how to do it better as they interact regularly" [38], and teaching and learning in digital spaces [39,40]. Other researchers have also considered the role of the internet in facilitating music learning in these same communities [41,42]. As this body of research demonstrates, the internet—especially YouTube and community-specific websites (e.g., Banjo Hangout, Online Academy of Irish Music)—played an important role in the activities of participatory musicians before the pandemic. Until 2020, however, online tutorials and message boards served only to supplement in-person music-making, which was the primary focus of all participants. It was only during the pandemic that these communities took the act of participatory music-making itself online.

The lack of interest in virtual music-making before 2020 was due in part to the fact that latency concerns make it difficult, if not in many cases impossible, to make music collaboratively over the internet in real time. Latency is the delay introduced as an audiovisual signal travels from one device to another. Researchers in the field of networked music performance have documented the many factors that contribute to latency and have also measured latency tolerance on behalf of musicians engaging in virtual music-making, finding the threshold to be anywhere between 20 and 50 ms [43]. These studies, however, have focused on classical and popular genres, and it might be the case that participatory musicians diverge from other populations in terms of latency tolerance. High-latency teleconferencing platforms like Zoom cannot be used to perform synchronized speech or music. Teleconferencing platforms also attempt to filter non-speech sounds and prioritize the audio of one participant at a time, further limiting their usefulness for collaborative musicians. While low-latency communication platforms are available, they demand a high degree of technical ability and benefit from high-speed internet, specialized equipment, carefully tuned settings, and hardwired connections, making them inaccessible to many [44]. In addition, the communities described here place a high value on in-person, unmediated music-making, and as a result, the online platforms did not attract their interest prior to the pandemic.

However, another community of musicians—choral singers—did adopt a virtual participatory practice before the pandemic, if only in limited numbers. The virtual choir (VC) was developed by choral composer and conductor Eric Whitacre in 2009 [45,46]. In this format, individual participants record videos of themselves singing along with a guide video or audio track, which is listened to using headphones. The videos are then compiled into a digital "performance" by a video editor [47]. Although the VC was originally developed to imitate presentational choral singing, this approach was adopted by many participatory communities during the pandemic. These included groups of both singers and instrumentalists, so the resulting products will be referred to as "VC-style" videos. VC participation has been associated with intense emotional experiences, a strong sense of community, profound feelings of connection, and a sense of presence exceeding that experienced by in-person choral singers [45,48]. This suggests that VC-style participation might meet some of the social needs of participatory musicians. In recent years, apps have also been developed that allow users to create VC-style videos without specialized editing software or expertise. These include the iOS app Acappella and the social media app TikTok [49].

4. Participatory Music-Making Communities in the COVID-19 Literature

The music-making communities studied during the COVID-19 pandemic were, for the most part, the same communities that have long attracted the attention of researchers. This section will survey the practices documented during the pandemic, summarizing the activities of each community and the outcomes for participants.

4.1. Irish Traditional Music (ITM)

Several related ITM communities transitioned to online music-making during the pandemic. Irish traditional singers found videoconferencing platforms to suit their activities particularly well since the songs are rendered by a solo singer with participation only on refrains and choruses. A number of geographically situated singing sessions moved to Zoom and continued to convene on a weekly basis, some growing to attract enormous international crowds. Facebook served as an important space in which sessions were organized and advertised. While singers appreciated the opportunity to sustain their community and the increased access provided by Zoom, they lamented the loss of encouraging comments, laughter, and sung participation [50].

Many instrumental sessions convened in Zoom, while others utilized Facebook Live (FBL) or YouTube Live (YTL). The most common format, possible only in Zoom, was the "round robin" gathering, in which musicians took turns leading a tune while others played on mute. Other sessions were led by a single player throughout, sometimes using a backing track to reproduce the sound of a session, while some made use of video recordings or combined various formats. Session musicians also experimented with chained Zoom rooms by incorporating the audio from another musician playing live over Zoom into their own Zoom broadcast. This technique requires operating two Zoom meetings on two devices at the same time. On at least one occasion, in an example of what has been termed "compounded mediation", a session host invited participants to submit recordings for assembly into a VC-style audio track that was then used to facilitate participation at a subsequent jam [51,52].

Virtual sessions maintained a strong sense of geographic location, even though participants were able to join from around the world [52]. This can be observed in the case of Mary O's Irish Music Session, which was held in person at a New York venue before the pandemic and reimagined as a YTL broadcast in March 2020. The session convened 81 times—first as Mary O's Virtual Session and later as Tune Supply's Common Tunes at Reasonable Speeds—before concluding in February 2022. The session was hosted by a local fiddler, Caitlin Warbelow, who led familiar tunes at a slow pace and broadcast video contributions from a parade of guest musicians. Although Warbelow created the virtual session to sustain local community and musical development among her fiddle students, it soon attracted global participation. Setlists were usually posted in advance, and participants were provided with links to pedagogical materials. Sessions were archived on YouTube so that players could participate asynchronously [53].

4.2. Old-Time Music (OTM)

Approaches to online jamming were similar in the OTM community, although different formats were favored. Facebook played an important role, both as a site for streaming jams and concerts and as a virtual space for discussion and community building during the pandemic [54]. Online jams were hosted by individuals (e.g., Rachel Eddy's Thursday Night Old-Time Jam) and organizations (e.g., the Berkley Old Time Music Convention's Slow Jam Fizz series), and they took place on both a weekly and an ad hoc basis. While a handful of musicians made use of low-latency communication platforms, the vast majority turned to Zoom, FBL, and YTL. In Zoom, players sometimes used a "round robin" approach, taking turns leading a tune while others joined on mute, but it was much more common for a pair of (often professional) musicians, either cohabitating or able to broadcast from an outdoor space, to lead throughout. Because each jam usually had a single leader or pair of leaders, FBL and YTL offered the same functionality as Zoom, with the added benefit that the jam was automatically recorded and archived, thereby making it available to participants after the live event had concluded. Participants reported a range of positive learning outcomes from online jamming, including the opportunity to clearly see and hear skilled leaders and to play without disturbing others while developing skills on an instrument [55].

4.3. Shape-Note Singing

Shape-note singers were quick to adapt a variety of digital media to suit their needs. By the end of March 2020, singers were using Zoom and FBL to convene in virtual spaces, and by June, a large number were using the low-latency platform Jamulus as well, often in combination with Zoom. The singers used Zoom in one of two ways: (1) a host would play audio or video recordings of songs requested by participants; (2) participants would take turns unmuting to sing the tenor (melody) line of a chosen song while others sang along on mute. As in the ITM community, Zoom singing retained a strong sense of local identity even as singers joined from around the world [56]. FBL was also used to facilitate singing but in a unique way. While singers would sometimes broadcast solo over FBL with the intention that others would sing complementary parts from their homes, more frequently, several singers would coordinate to produce a chain of FBL videos. In this procedure, a singer would use a second device to broadcast themselves as they sang along with an FBL broadcast. If enough broadcasters participated, this could ultimately produce a stream in which all four parts of the choral texture were audible [57]. Shape-note singers also contributed to VC-style videos. Some of these, such as a video made to open the Minnesota State Sacred Harp Singing Convention, were intended to facilitate participation in the context of Zoom singings [51], while others—most notably a series of videos created by the group Dispersed Harmonies—were produced for the enjoyment of participants and posted online [56]. Many of these activities were coordinated using Facebook, which had already served an important role in facilitating communication before the pandemic [58]. While online singing served to sustain the activities of the shape-note community and was valued deeply by many singers, it was not accessible or appealing to everyone. Some singers were not able to participate because they did not have a suitable domestic space in which to sing, while others found virtual singing unpleasant [59]. At the same time, online singing increased access for singers who could not easily leave home, including disabled singers and those with care responsibilities [12].

4.4. Worship

Participatory singing is an important element of worship across many traditions, although scholarship on singing during the COVID-19 pandemic was limited to a few practices. As religious services moved to digital platforms, participatory singing was facilitated in various ways. Early in the pandemic, a Lutheran church in Norway posted service videos on Vimeo with hymn texts displayed on screen to facilitate participation in sung worship. In November 2020, the congregation transitioned to Zoom, and while texts were still provided on screen, diminished sound and video quality meant that hymn singing attracted fewer participants and became less fulfilling. When the congregation returned to in-person worship in May 2021, they were required to wear masks and sit in silence throughout the service [60]. Singing was similarly prohibited for the few congregants permitted to worship in-person at Baptist and Methodist churches in the US South, although those joining online were provided with PDF leaflets and encouraged to sing. Participants in a study reported that singing from home was a poor substitute for in-person congregational singing, which they valued as a mode of community bonding and an expression of collective faith [61]. When members of the Shadhili Sufi order in Singapore were forced online, they faced additional challenges because synchronized breathing, movement, physical touch, and sonic immersion were integral to their worship. Participants quickly discovered that it was impossible to sing or chant communally in Zoom, yet they found the practice of having a single individual recite and sing all the texts to be deeply inadequate. Beginning in June 2020, groups of five were permitted to congregate, and it became possible to include the sounds of communal singing in Zoom broadcasts, making them more satisfying to participants. All the same, worshipping from home remained difficult due to domestic limitations on sound volume and the use of incense [62].

While most churches made use of videoconferencing or livestreaming platforms, a Congregational church in Massachusetts adopted an alternative approach because poor internet coverage made live broadcasting impossible. Instead, the music director assembled a weekly podcast service. Members of the congregation, as well as other singers known to the director, were invited to submit recordings of themselves singing hymns that were assembled into a VC-style product for inclusion in the podcast—an undertaking that came to be known as the "Hymn Singing in Isolation Project". The result replicated the sound of in-person hymn singing, and congregants were invited to sing along with the podcast when it was released each Sunday morning. Participants in a study reported experiencing widely varying levels of interpersonal connectivity and immersion while creating and consuming the hymn recordings [63].

4.5. Community Singing

While some of the practices described above might be categorized as "community singing", the term is used here to connote group singing activity that does not conform to any particular repertoire or historical tradition. Community singing of this type often makes use of popular or folk songs and is usually (although not necessarily) directed by a song leader [22,64]. Community singing made headlines in the early weeks of the pandemic as quarantined residents of Italian and Spanish cities took to their balconies to sing and otherwise engage in collective musicking [65,66]. Although most studies emphasized technological mediation, outdoor community singing was presumably practiced throughout the pandemic. In England, for example, community musician Hugh Nankivell led a singalong at a care home by sitting in the courtyard and inviting residents to open their windows [67].

Later in the pandemic, community singing was sustained using broadcast media. On 2 April 2020, the BBC broadcast a singalong program of listener-selected songs simultaneously across five radio stations [67]. Participants took to social media to share videos of their own singing and dancing. Beginning on 4 April 2020, Danish citizens were invited to join in with a singalong broadcast daily for fifteen minutes on Danish National TV, *Morgensang Med Phillip Faber*. The host led viewers in vocal warmups and then accompanied himself at the piano, singing two familiar songs [68]. The US-based Disney Company broadcast three singalongs in 2020, all featuring celebrity performances of songs from their catalog: *The Disney Family Singalong* (16 April), *The Disney Family Singalong: Volume II* (10 May), and *The Disney Holiday Singalong* (30 November). Viewers could join in synchronously with the broadcast or later using YouTube videos [69]. On 10 April, Bachfest Leipzig broadcast a singalong *St. John Passion* on FBL, led by three distanced performers and a small on-site choir. In another example of compounded mediation, participation took two forms: choral singers around the world submitted videos of themselves singing the chorales for inclusion in the broadcast, while home viewers sang along with the chorales using provided sheet music. Home participants were invited to film their own singing, and submitted videos were integrated into a rebroadcast on 14 June [51].

Local community singing groups also took their activities online. Participants in the Irish World Music Café, located in Limerick, sustained virtual participation both by convening in Zoom and by posting performance videos to a Facebook page. While the facilitators continued to lead community singing across three synchronous Zoom gatherings (20 June, 3 October, and 10 December 2020), the fact that they could not connect physically with participants—most of whom were immigrants seeking familiarity with local language and culture—posed significant challenges [70]. Conveners of community singing groups for dementia patients in Ireland and the UK utilized Zoom, FBL, WhatsApp, and small in-person music therapy sessions to sustain their participatory singing practices. They also created YouTube videos and facilitated virtual choirs. While these activities were successful in fostering social connections and improved access for some, not all patients were able to participate due to technological and health barriers [71,72]. Skype, SoundCloud, and Microsoft Teams were also occasionally used to facilitate virtual community singing across populations, and in general, it was found that online singing contributed to the well-being of participants during the pandemic, increased interest in in-person singing, and demonstrated potential for expanding access to community singing after the pandemic [73].

Online community singing also took place independent of in-person communities or activities. This entry will pass over the countless virtual choirs that provided a musical outlet for presentational choral singers [74], but it must address participatory singing on the social media app TikTok, which became a significant locus for music-making during the pandemic. This type of participatory musicking is not necessarily rooted in an offline community, and it engages a range of otherwise unconnected individuals. Singers in Japan—many of whom were likely karaoke enthusiasts deprived of a valued musical and social outlet—used a variety of hashtags to identify themselves as part of a community on TikTok, engaging with prerecorded material as both singers and dancers [75]. TikTok made headlines in early 2021 after Nathan Evans's recording of "The Wellerman", posted on 27 December 2020, went viral both within the app and across platforms [76]. The video inspired countless "duets" and remixes under the hashtag #shantytok (although "The Wellerman" is not technically a sea shanty, a category limited to work songs sung onboard sailing vessels). While shanty singers constitute an offline music-making community, "The Wellerman" in particular and #shantytok in general appear to have been popular with singers who had no previous knowledge of or experience with the tradition. Instead, they were social media users with a general interest in virtual participation.

5. Benefits and Drawbacks of Online Participatory Music-Making

While the practices documented above are diverse, conclusions drawn across these studies were remarkably consistent. Participants in all music-making traditions keenly felt the loss of gathering in a physical space. They commented not only on the inability to hear all the other participants but also on the elimination of opportunities for informal chatting, the loss of the physical sensation of vibrations created by a roomful of musicians, and the absence of tastes and smells associated with a shared meal or burning incense. Participatory music-making is an embodied practice sustained within a social framework, and none of the virtual approaches met all the participants' physical or social needs. This loss was most keenly felt by worshippers, who largely found that online singing did not meet their needs as participants in spiritual communities.

The various forms of online music-making adopted by each community illuminate differences in social and aesthetic values. Shape-note singers preferred to sing along with recordings, which captured the rich texture of in-person singing and indexed events and individuals of significance to the community [56]. ITM and OTM players, on the other hand, strongly preferred live performance. This was possible because each tradition requires only a single melody player and chording accompanist to fully represent the music, and live performance brought the added advantage of allowing participants to see and hear skilled performers [55]. In shape-note singing, skill is not valued in the same way, and there is no role for "professional" singers. Instead, when utilized, live-leading was valued because it allowed singers to hear one another's unique voices [56]. Additionally, while ITM and OTM leaders frequently broadcast over FBL or YTL, and players often revisited recorded sessions and jams, shape-note singers primarily met in Zoom and seldom recorded their singings.

In every category, some musicians were so displeased with online music-making that they withdrew altogether. At the same time, many participants were able to find immense value in online activity, which facilitated at least some degree of interpersonal connection and sustenance of community practice during a time of isolation and disruption. All the platforms used facilitated text-based chat, which played an important role in maintaining social connections and allowing participants to feel as if they were engaging in a communal activity. Musicians were generally delighted to see participants from around the world join their "local" activities, and many new relationships were forged. Some musicians thrived in the online environment, especially those seeking to develop their skills and those with limited or no ability to attend in-person gatherings. For these reasons, participants in studies often expressed the desire for virtual music-making to be sustained after the pandemic.

6. Conclusions

This entry has by no means addressed participatory music-making during the COVID-19 pandemic in all its breadth and diversity. While this entry has necessarily been limited to practices described in the literature, the vast majority of music-making activities pursued during the pandemic have gone unremarked upon by scholars, or else have been mentioned only in passing. For example, Crooke et al. note that one of their informants conducted online beat-making cyphers but provide no details about these gatherings, instead focusing their analysis on the circulation of social capital [77]. It also must be noted that the practices surveyed in this entry disproportionately involved socioeconomically privileged participants in Western music-making contexts. Likewise, the narrow view of participation adopted here has resulted in the omission of research into the virtual communities that formed around practices such as Mexican música huasteca [78] or the global network of brass bands that participate in HONK! Festivals [79]—communities in which participatory engagement is essential, even as it takes forms other than collaborative musical performance. It has also passed over uses of digital communication platforms and social media by presentational musicians pursuing remote creative collaborations [80–82]. The narrow approach taken in this entry, however, has allowed for the intersections and divergences among music-making communities to be starkly illuminated. While some of the practices described here have come to an end, others have remained in place, and the ways in which many members of these communities engage with participatory music-making have been fundamentally transformed.

As of the publication of this entry in mid-2024, at least three groups of shape-note singers convene weekly on Jamulus to sing together, and one still holds regular Zoom singings [83]. Virtual singing persists because it allows geographically dispersed individuals to sing in community without traveling great distances or even leaving the house. The individuals who participate in these singings know and care for one another, and they prefer to sing together online over not singing at all. It has also become typical to stream in-person singings to facilitate remote access. Virtual singing will not replace in-person singing, but it is a welcome adjunct in the shape-note and other communities. Virtual jamming has likewise found a permanent place in the OTM, ITM, and other traditional music communities. Organizations such as Phoenix Folk and the San Francisco Folk Music Club now host regular virtual sessions [84,85], while individual musicians lead virtual jams and sessions over FBL and host Zoom gatherings [86,87]. These often serve to maintain connections between professional musicians and the broader community, and they also produce income for performers through voluntary donations. Since online jamming has proven especially beneficial to learners, many of the ongoing virtual jams cater explicitly to their needs [55,88]. While the technologies that support virtual participatory music-making continue to develop and the role of these activities in specific communities remains in negotiation, it is evident that the COVID-19 pandemic greatly accelerated engagement with online music-making and permanently altered its role in participatory communities.

Funding: This research received no external funding.

Institutional Review Board Statement: Not applicable.

Informed Consent Statement: Not applicable.

Data Availability Statement: No new data were created or analyzed in this study. Data sharing is not applicable to this article.

Conflicts of Interest: The authors declare no conflicts of interest.

References

1. Miller, S.L.; Nazaroff, W.W.; Jimenez, J.L.; Boerstra, A.; Buonanno, G.; Dancer, S.J.; Kurnitski, J.; Marr, L.C.; Morawska, L.; Noakes, C. Transmission of SARS-CoV-2 by inhalation of respiratory aerosol in the Skagit Valley Chorale superspreading event. *Indoor Air* **2021**, *31*, 314–323. [CrossRef]

2. Charlotte, N. High Rate of SARS-CoV-2 Transmission Due to Choir Practice in France at the Beginning of the COVID-19 Pandemic. *J. Voice* **2023**, *37*, 292.e9–292.e14. [CrossRef]
3. O'Keeffe, J.; COVID-19 Risks and Precautions for Choirs. National Collaborating Centre for Environmental Health 2020. Available online: https://ncceh.ca/resources/evidence-reviews/covid-19-risks-and-precautions-choirs (accessed on 8 February 2024).
4. Bahl, P.; de Silva, C.; Bhattacharjee, S.; Stone, H.; Doolan, C.; Chughtai, A.A.; MacIntyre, C.R. Droplets and Aerosols Generated by Singing and the Risk of Coronavirus Disease 2019 for Choirs. *Clin. Infect. Dis.* **2021**, *72*, e639–e641. [CrossRef]
5. Alsved, M.; Matamis, A.; Bohlin, R.; Richter, M.; Bengtsson, P.E.; Fraenkel, C.J.; Medstrande, P.; Löndahl, J. Exhaled respiratory particles during singing and talking. *Aerosol. Sci. Technol.* **2020**, *54*, 1245–1248. [CrossRef]
6. Becher, L.; Gena, A.W.; Alsaad, H.; Richter, B.; Spahn, C.; Voelker, C. The spread of breathing air from wind instruments and singers using schlieren techniques. *Indoor Air* **2021**, *31*, 1798–1814. [CrossRef]
7. Nix, J.; Jers, H.; Ternström, S. Acoustical, Psychoacoustical, and Pedagogical Considerations for Choral Singing with COVID-19 Health Measures. *Choral J.* **2020**, *61*, 30–38.
8. Naunheim, M.R.; Bock, J.; Doucette, P.A.; Hoch, M.; Howell, I.; Johns, M.M.; Johnson, A.M.; Krishna, P.; Meyer, D.; Milstein, C.F.; et al. Safer Singing During the SARS-CoV-2 Pandemic: What We Know and What We Don't. *J. Voice* **2021**, *35*, 765–771. [CrossRef]
9. Daffern, H.; Balmer, K.; Brereton, J. Singing Together, Yet Apart: The Experience of UK Choir Members and Facilitators During the Covid-19 Pandemic. *Front. Psychol.* **2021**, *12*, 624474. [CrossRef]
10. Turino, T. *Music as Social Life: The Politics of Participation*; University of Chicago Press: Chicago, IL, USA, 2008.
11. Duchan, J. Community Singing in the Age of Coronavirus: The Case of Collegiate A Cappella. In *The Oxford Handbook of Community Singing*; Morgan-Ellis, E.M., Norton, K., Eds.; Oxford University Press: New York, NY, USA, 2024; pp. 106–120.
12. Norton, K. What the Pandemic Couldn't Take Away: Group Singing Benefits That Survived Going Online. In *The Oxford Handbook of Community Singing*; Morgan-Ellis, E.M., Norton, K., Eds.; Oxford University Press: New York, NY, USA, 2024; pp. 63–85.
13. Feld, S. Aesthetics and Iconicity of Style (uptown title); or, (downtown title) "Lift-up-over Sounding": Getting into the Kaluli Groove. In *Music Grooves*; Charles, K., Feld, S., Eds.; University of Chicago Press: Chicago, IL, USA, 1994; pp. 109–150.
14. Turino, T. The Coherence of Social Style and Musical Creation among the Aymara in Southern Peru. *Ethnomusicology* **1989**, *33*, 1–30. [CrossRef]
15. O'Shea, H. Getting to the Heart of the Music: Idealizing Musical Community and Irish Traditional Music Sessions. *J. Soc. Musicol. Irel.* **2007**, *2*, 1–18. [CrossRef]
16. Williams, E.E. "Pull Up a Chair!": Accommodation, Participation, and Disability in Old-Time and Bluegrass Jam Sessions. Master's Thesis, University of Tennessee, Knoxville, TN, USA, 2020.
17. Watkins, P.; Caines, R. Cyphers: Hip-Hop and Improvisation. *Stud. Improv./Études Crit. Improv.* **2014**, *10*, 1–5. [CrossRef]
18. Clawson, L. *I Belong to This Band, Hallelujah! Community, Spirituality, and Tradition Among Sacred Harp Singers*; University of Chicago Press: Chicago, IL, USA, 2011.
19. Russell, I. Vernacular Christmas Carol Singing in the Southern Pennines of England. In *The Oxford Handbook of Community Singing*; Morgan-Ellis, E.M., Norton, K., Eds.; Oxford University Press: New York, NY, USA, 2024; pp. 161–182.
20. Laurila, K.; Willingham, L. Drum circles and community music: Reconciling the difference. *Int. J. Community Music* **2017**, *10*, 139–156. [CrossRef]
21. Brown, K. *Karaoke Idols: Popular Music and the Performance of Identity*; Intellect: Bristol, UK, 2015.
22. McPherson, E. Brigadoon in the Heights: Fostering Intimacy, Community, and Activism through Secular Leftist Hymnody. In *The Oxford Handbook of Community Singing*; Morgan-Ellis, E.M., Norton, K., Eds.; Oxford University Press: New York, NY, USA, 2024; pp. 218–237.
23. Hunter, M. Amateur Chamber Music: Repertoire and Experience. In *The Chamber Musician in the Twenty-First Century*; Doğantan-Dack, M., Ed.; MDPI: Basel, Switzerland, 2022; pp. 287–307.
24. Adelstein, R. Calling Each Other To Prayer: Group Song in British Reform Synagogues. *Ethnomusicol. Rev.* **2022**, *23*, 20–37.
25. Herrera, E. Masculinity, Violence, and Deindividuation in Argentine Soccer Chants: The Sonic Potentials of Participatory Sounding-in-Synchrony. *Ethnomusicology* **2018**, *62*, 470–499. [CrossRef]
26. Mihalka, M.W. "Take Me Out" to "Sweet Caroline": Collective Singing in the Ballpark. In *The Oxford Handbook of Community Singing*; Morgan-Ellis, E.M., Norton, K., Eds.; Oxford University Press: New York, NY, USA, 2024; pp. 183–197.
27. Payerhin, M. New Firebombs in Old Bottles: Social Mobilization and Cultural Resonance of Protest Songs. In *The Oxford Handbook of Community Singing*; Morgan-Ellis, E.M., Norton, K., Eds.; Oxford University Press: New York, NY, USA, 2024; pp. 735–754.
28. Wright, T. "Scare Away the Dark": The Promotion of Singing to Create Post-Secondary Academic Communities. In *The Oxford Handbook of Community Singing*; Morgan-Ellis, E.M., Norton, K., Eds.; Oxford University Press: New York, NY, USA, 2024; pp. 315–329.
29. Borčak, L.W.; Baunvig, K.F. Medial Conditions for Social Bonding in Singing. *Int. Rev. Aesthet. Sociol. Music* **2021**, *52*, 391–416.
30. Theorell, T. Theorell, T. The Effects and Benefits of Singing Individually and in a Group. In *The Oxford Handbook of Singing*; Welch, G.F., Howard, D.M., Nix, J., Eds.; Oxford University Press: New York, NY, USA, 2019; pp. 919–933.
31. Densley, B.; Andrews, K. How participation in group singing in the community impacts on emotional wellbeing: A qualitative study on the perspectives of group singing participants. *Aust. J. Music Ther.* **2021**, *32*, 39–56.

32. Steele, M.E. How Can Music Build Community? Insight from Theories and Practice of Community Music Therapy. *Voices World Forum Music Ther.* **2016**, *16*. Available online: https://voices.no/index.php/voices/article/view/2317/2072 (accessed on 15 March 2024). [CrossRef]
33. Waldron, J. YouTube, fanvids, forums, vlogs and blogs: Informal music learning in a convergent on- and offline music community. *Int. J. Music Educ.* **2013**, *31*, 91–105. [CrossRef]
34. Bayley, J.G.; Waldron, J. "It's never too late": Adult students and music learning in one online and offline convergent community music school. *Int. J. Music Educ.* **2020**, *38*, 36–51. [CrossRef]
35. Waldron, J.L.; Veblen, K.K. The medium is the message: Cyberspace, community, and music learning in the Irish traditional music virtual community. *J. Music Technol. Educ.* **2008**, *1*, 99–111.
36. Waldron, J. User-generated content, YouTube and participatory culture on the Web: Music learning and teaching in two contrasting online communities. *Music Educ. Res.* **2013**, *15*, 257–274. [CrossRef]
37. Waldron, J. Exploring a virtual music 'community of practice': Informal music learning on the Internet. *J. Music Technol. Educ.* **2009**, *2*, 97–112. [CrossRef]
38. Wenger-Trayner, E.; Wenger-Trayner, B. Communities of Practice: A Brief Introduction. Wenger-Trayner 2015. Available online: http://wenger-trayner.com/wp-content/uploads/2015/04/07-Brief-introductionto-communities-of-practice.pdf (accessed on 8 February 2024).
39. Waldron, J.; Mantie, R.; Partti, H.; Tobias, E.S. A brave new world: Theory to practice in participatory culture and music learning and teaching. *Music Educ. Res.* **2018**, *20*, 289–304. [CrossRef]
40. Waldron, J. The Convergence of Networked Technologies in Music Teaching and Learning. In *The Oxford Handbook of Technology and Music Education*; Ruthmann, S.A., Mantie, R., Eds.; Oxford University Press: Oxford, UK, 2020; pp. 475–485.
41. Ward, F. Technology and the transmission of tradition. An exploration of the virtual pedagogies in the Online Academy of Irish Music. *J. Music Technol. Educ.* **2019**, *12*, 5–23. [CrossRef]
42. Morgan-Ellis, E.M. Learning Habits and Attitudes in the Revivalist Old-Time Community of Practice. *Bull. Counc. Res. Music Educ.* **2019**, *221*, 29–57. [CrossRef]
43. Rottondi, C.; Chafe, C.; Allocchio, C.; Sarti, A. An Overview on Networked Music Performance Technologies. *IEEE Access* **2016**, *4*, 8823–8843. [CrossRef]
44. Morgan-Ellis, E.M. Virtual Community Singing During the COVID-19 Pandemic. *Am. Sci.* **2022**, *110*, 28–36. [CrossRef]
45. Armstrong, M. Musicking in Cyberspace: Creating Music and Fostering Global Community through a Virtual Choir. Master's Thesis, Tufts University, Medford, MA, USA, 2012.
46. Carvalho, L.; Goodyear, P. Virtual Choir: Sharing Experiences of Singing Together Apart. In *Architecture of Learning Networks*; Carvalho, L., Goodyear, P., Eds.; Routledge: New York, NY, USA, 2014; pp. 209–224.
47. Bendall, C. Defining the Virtual Choir. *Choral J.* **2020**, *61*, 69–75.
48. Fancourt, D.; Steptoe, A. Present in body or just in mind: Differences in social presence and emotion regulation in live vs. virtual singing experiences. *Front. Psychol.* **2019**, *10*, 451931. [CrossRef]
49. McDaniel, B. Singing into a Smartphone: The Persuasive Affordances of Collaboration on Karaoke and Lip-Syncing Apps. In *The Oxford Handbook of Community Singing*; Morgan-Ellis, E.M., Norton, K., Eds.; Oxford University Press: New York, NY, USA, 2024; pp. 50–62.
50. Thompson, C.; O'Brien, K.S. From hearth to hard drive: Well-being benefits of online Irish traditional singing sessions during COVID-19. *Health Promot. Int.* **2022**, *37*, i4–i17. [CrossRef]
51. Morgan-Ellis, E.M. Mediated Community Singing. In *The Oxford Handbook of Community Singing*; Morgan-Ellis, E.M., Norton, K., Eds.; Oxford University Press: New York, NY, USA, 2024; pp. 8–28.
52. Bobker, A. Keeping the Tradition Alive: Irish Traditional Music Sessions during COVID-19. Master's Thesis, Michigan State University, East Lansing, MI, USA, 2021.
53. Ward, F. Enabling Musical, Pedagogical, and Social Continuities through "Participation" in Mary O's Virtual Irish Traditional Music Session. *Action Crit. Theory Music. Educ.* **2022**, *23*, 87–130.
54. Terrell, L. "Log On In, There's a Band Tonight": Social Media and the Old Time Music Community during the Time of COVID-19. Master's Thesis, University of North Carolina, Chapel Hill, NC, USA, 2021.
55. Morgan-Ellis, E.M. Learning advantages of online old-time jams. *J. Music Technol. Educ.* **2022**, *15*, 127–146. [CrossRef]
56. Morgan-Ellis, E.M. "Like Pieces in a Puzzle": Online Sacred Harp Singing During the COVID-19 Pandemic. *Front. Psychol.* **2021**, *12*, 627038. [CrossRef]
57. Morgan-Ellis, E.M. "Your network bandwidth is low": Online Participatory Music-Making in the COVID-19 Era. *Crit. Stud. Improv./Études Crit. Improv.* **2021**, *14*, 1–7.
58. Dattilo, D. Changes and Chances in a Multipart Singing Community and Its Tradition, before and throughout the Global Isolation. *J. World Pop. Music* **2023**, *10*, 60–78. [CrossRef]
59. Morgan-Ellis, E.M. Non-participation in online Sacred Harp singing during the COVID-19 pandemic. *Int. J. Community Music* **2021**, *14*, 223–245. [CrossRef]
60. Strøm, I.T. Worshipping Musically Online During Covid-19. *J. Extrem. Anthropol.* **2023**, *7*, 1–22. [CrossRef]
61. Myrick, N.; Gessner, B.; Alvarado, J. Music and Human Flourishing in Christian Communities. In *The Oxford Handbook of Community Singing*; Morgan-Ellis, E.M., Norton, K., Eds.; Oxford University Press: New York, NY, USA, 2024; pp. 852–870.

62. Othman, M.L.B. Listening for/as presence: Religious mediation of a Sufi ritual in the time of COVID-19. *Religion* **2022**, *52*, 265–283. [CrossRef]
63. Morgan-Ellis, E.M. Virtual Hymn Singing and the Imagination of Community. *J. Music Health Wellbeing* **2021**. Available online: https://storage.googleapis.com/wzukusers/user-20563976/documents/42521696a28f40c3b22566a839e988d3/Morgan%20Ellis%20October2021.pdf (accessed on 15 March 2024).
64. Morgan-Ellis, E.M. *Everybody Sing! Community Singing in the American Picture Palace*; UGA Press: Athens, GA, USA, 2018.
65. Van Der Sandt, J.; Coppi, A. MUSICOVID-19: When the world paused but singing continued. *Int. J. Community Music* **2021**, *14*, 151–167. [CrossRef]
66. Calvo, K.; Bejarano, E. Musicking on Balconies: Resilience in Times of COVID-19. *Rev. Esp. Investig. Sociol.* **2022**, *178*, 23–38. [CrossRef]
67. Crisp, M. The response of community musicians in the United Kingdom to the COVID-19 crisis: An evaluation. *Int. J. Community Music* **2021**, *14*, 129–138. [CrossRef]
68. Borčak, L.W. Transmedia Performance in Scandinavian Singalong Shows: On the Transmediation of Liveness and Participation in Community Singing. In *Words, Music, and the Popular: Global Perspectives on Intermedial Relations*; Thomas, G., Winnett, S., Eds.; Palgrave Macmillan: London, UK, 2021; pp. 133–153.
69. Camp, G. The Disney Chorus: Singing Along to the Studio's Forging of American Musical Identity. In *The Oxford Handbook of Community Singing*; Morgan-Ellis, E.M., Norton, K., Eds.; Oxford University Press: New York, NY, USA, 2024; pp. 541–558.
70. Jaber, H.; Garry, F.; Phelan, H. 'We are all facing the same problem': Lived experiences of online participation in the Irish World Music Café community music initiative in the context of the COVID-19 pandemic. *Int. J. Community Music* **2021**, *14*, 273–293. [CrossRef]
71. Lee, S.; O'Neill, D.; Moss, H. Dementia-inclusive group-singing online during COVID-19: A qualitative exploration. *Nord. J. Music Ther.* **2022**, *31*, 308–326. [CrossRef]
72. Dowson, B.; Atkinson, R.; Barnes, J.; Barone, C.; Cutts, N.; Donnebaum, E.; Hung Hsu, M.; Lo Coco, I.; John, G.; Meadows, G.; et al. Digital Approaches to Music-Making for People With Dementia in Response to the COVID-19 Pandemic: Current Practice and Recommendations. *Front. Psychol.* **2021**, *12*, 625258. [CrossRef]
73. Price, S.; Phillips, J.; Tallent, J.; Clift, S. Singing group leaders' experiences of online singing sessions during the COVID-19 pandemic: A rapid survey. *J. Music Health Wellbeing* **2021**. Available online: https://storage.googleapis.com/wzukusers/user-20563976/documents/70a39f34e9624c13925281b002d8ddf4/Price,%20S.,%20Phillips,%20J.,%20Tallent,%20J.%20and%20Clift,%20S..pdf (accessed on 15 March 2024).
74. Bendall, C. Virtual Choirs and Issues of Community Choral Practice. In *The Oxford Handbook of Community Singing*; Morgan-Ellis, E.M., Norton, K., Eds.; Oxford University Press: New York, NY, USA, 2024; pp. 86–105.
75. Petrovic, S. From karaoke to lip-syncing: Performance communities and TikTok use in Japan. *Med. Int. Aust.* **2023**, *186*, 11–28. [CrossRef]
76. Waldron, J. YouTube, TikTok, and Online Music Learning. In *Milestones in Music Education*; Randles, C., Ed.; Routledge: New York, NY, USA, 2024; pp. 151–188.
77. Crooke, A.H.D.; Hara, M.; Davidson, J.; Fraser, T.; DeNora, T. Fractured bonds and crystal capital: Social capital among COVID-era music communities. *Int. J. Community Music* **2021**, *14*, 247–272. [CrossRef]
78. Margolies, D.S.; Strub, J.A. Music Community, Improvisation, and Social Technologies in COVID-Era Música Huasteca. *Front. Psychol.* **2021**, *12*, 648010. [CrossRef]
79. Snyder, A.; Allen, E.; Garofalo, R. HONK!United: A Virtual Global Festival of Activist Brass Bands during the COVID-19 Pandemic. *Music Politics* **2022**, *16*, 1–28. [CrossRef]
80. MacDonald, R.; Burke, R.; DeNora, T.; Sappho Donohue, M.; Birrell, R. Our Virtual Tribe: Sustaining and Enhancing Community via Online Music Improvisation. *Front. Psychol.* **2021**, *11*, 623640. [CrossRef] [PubMed]
81. Kaye, D.B.V. Please Duet This: Collaborative Music Making in Lockdown on TikTok. *Netw. Knowl.* **2022**, *15*, 59–77.
82. Manley-Muller, G. Remote Musical Collaboration during the COVID-19 Pandemic. *J. Music Health Wellbeing* **2021**. Available online: https://storage.googleapis.com/wzukusers/user-20563976/documents/c7dbd5ab8f1048c49600e2e11c761c4d/Manley-Muller%20October2021.pdf (accessed on 15 March 2024).
83. Coghlan, P. (Gridley, CA, USA); Morgan-Ellis, E.M. (University of North Georgia, Dahlonega, GA, USA). Personal communication, 2024.
84. Phoenix Folk: Online Sessions. Available online: https://phoenixfolk.co.uk/online-sessions/ (accessed on 23 April 2024).
85. San Francisco Folk Music Club. Available online: https://www.sffmc.org/ (accessed on 23 April 2024).
86. The Ould Sod Traditional Virtual Irish Session on Zoom. Available online: https://michaeleskin.com/session.html?fbclid=IwAR0UxIs64n1mvAHEPcP6P29czq7ppBB4FZcGfo74TbKBLokSa5Ggdn7M5Xs (accessed on 23 April 2024).
87. Facebook: Pam Weeks. Available online: https://www.facebook.com/pam.weeks.73 (accessed on 23 April 2024).
88. Facebook: The Learner's Session. Available online: https://www.facebook.com/groups/276330881264817/ (accessed on 23 April 2024).

encyclopedia

Review

The Effects of SARS-CoV-2 on the Angiopoietin/Tie Axis and the Vascular Endothelium

Dolgormaa Janchivlamdan [1], Maitreyi Shivkumar [2] and Harprit Singh [1,*]

[1] Leicester School of Allied Health Sciences, De Montfort University, The Gateway, Leicester LE1 9BH, UK; p2699664@my365.dmu.ac.uk

[2] Leicester School of Pharmacy, De Montfort University, The Gateway, Leicester LE1 9BH, UK; maitreyi.shivkumar@dmu.ac.uk

* Correspondence: harprit.singh@dmu.ac.uk

Abstract: Severe acute respiratory syndrome coronavirus 2 (SARS-CoV-2) infection can cause potentially life-threatening coronavirus disease (COVID-19). COVID-19 is a multisystem disease and is associated with significant respiratory distress, systemic hyperinflammation, vasculitis, and multi-organ failure. SARS-CoV-2 causes the deterioration of numerous systems, with increasing evidence implying that COVID-19 affects the endothelium and vascular function. The endothelium is important for preserving vascular tone and homeostasis. The overactivation and dysfunction of endothelial cells are significant outcomes of severity in patients with COVID-19. The Angiopoietin 1/Tie 2 pathway plays an important role in endothelium quiescence and vessel stability. The disruption of Angiopoietin/Tie balance affects the vessel contact barrier and leads to vessel leakage, and this in turn causes endothelial dysfunction. Although vascular instability through SARS-CoV-2 is associated with endothelial dysfunction, it is still not understood if the virus affects the Angiopoietin/Tie axis directly or via other mechanisms such as cytokine storm and/or immune response associated with the infection. This review provides an overview of the impact SARS-CoV-2 has on endothelial function and more specifically on the Angiopoietin/Tie pathway.

Keywords: SARS-CoV-2; endothelial cell; angiopoietin; Tie1/2; ACE2; inflammatory cytokines

Citation: Janchivlamdan, D.; Shivkumar, M.; Singh, H. The Effects of SARS-CoV-2 on the Angiopoietin/Tie Axis and the Vascular Endothelium. *Encyclopedia* **2024**, *4*, 544–557. https://doi.org/10.3390/encyclopedia4010035

Academic Editors: Stephen Bustin and Raffaele Barretta

Received: 31 January 2024
Revised: 27 February 2024
Accepted: 6 March 2024
Published: 11 March 2024

1. Introduction to Coronaviruses

Coronaviruses (CoVs) are a family of single-stranded RNA viruses that are a source of respiratory and digestive diseases in humans and animals [1]. The coronavirus family is separated into four different genera, i.e., *Alphacoronavirus* (α-CoV), *Betacoronavirus* (β-CoV), *Gammacoronavirus* (Y-CoV), and *Deltacoronavirus* (δ-CoV), which are part of the subfamily of *Orthocoronavirinae*. α-CoVs and β-CoVs cause disease in humans and other mammals, whereas Y-CoVs and δ-CoVs cause disease in avian species [2]. Human coronavirus (HCoV) OC43 and HCoV-HKU1 belong to β-CoV, whereas HCoV-229E and HCoV-NL-63 belong to α-CoV. These four human coronavirus species result in varying severity [3]. Severe acute respiratory syndrome coronavirus (SARS-CoV-1), Middle East respiratory syndrome coronavirus (MERS-CoV), and, more recently, severe acute respiratory syndrome coronavirus 2 (SARS-CoV-2) belong to β-CoV genera and all of them result in more severe symptoms like pneumonia [4].

1.1. Virion Composition of Coronaviruses

The diameter of coronaviruses is about 80–120 nm in length, and the virus is surrounded by two layers of lipid molecules with envelope (E), spike (S), nucleocapsid (N), and membrane (M) proteins within the lipid bilayer. The S protein belongs to class I transmembrane proteins and is around 128–160 kDa prior to covalently attaching to carbohydrates and 150–200 kDa following N-linked glycosylation [5,6]. S protein cleaves into three identical units of polypeptides (S1–S3) by proteases found on target cells. S1 is involved in binding to receptors and S2 for membrane fusion. The endoplasmic reticulum (ER) stress response is stimulated through the infective process of the virus by S protein, which leads to apoptosis through unfolded protein response activation [7]. The M protein has a molecular weight of 25–30 kDa and has three functional regions which span the phospholipid bilayer [8]. M protein plays a role in viral infection processes such as RNA packaging and virion formation. The E protein is a relatively small protein with a molecular weight of 8–12 kDa and is involved in the assembly and release of virions [9]. N protein has a molecular weight of 43–50 kDa and supports the packaging of RNA into ribonucleocapsids. It also plays a role in numerous activities, including regulating virus assembly by interacting with M protein and the viral genome, increasing the replication and transcription of RNA genome, and in escaping the host immune reaction. Coronaviruses have one of the largest viral RNA genomes, roughly 27–32 kilobases (kb) [10]. The 5′-end of the genome encodes non-structural proteins, including proteases and transcription factors, and the 3′-end encodes structural proteins as well as cis-acting RNA elements crucial for RNA production [11].

1.2. SARS-CoV-2 Infection

SARS-CoV-2 infection can progress into a critical and potentially fatal respiratory disorder and pulmonary damage in patients through affected upper and lower respiratory epithelial cells, including alveolar type 2 (AT2) cells. The entry of SARS-CoV-2 into the target cell is the first step in the infection process and development of disease. Entry begins with attachment of the SARS-CoV-2 S glycoprotein to the host surface angiotensin converting enzyme 2 (ACE2), followed by S protein cleavage by cell surface transmembrane serine protease 2 (TMPRSS2) into the S1 and S2 domains. The S1 subunit contains the receptor-binding domain (RBD) that recognises and binds to the ACE2 receptor, and therefore regulates virus specificity to the host cell and the infection processes that lead to disease [12]. The RBD shifts from an upright posture to connect with the ACE2 receptor to a horizontal posture to escape the immune response. After S protein binds to ACE2 on the target cell surface via its RBD, cleavage by TMPRSS2 reveals the fusion peptide on the S2 subunit to initiate the fusion process of the virus to the host cell membrane [13]. TMPRSS2 is expressed in the plasma membrane of upper airway, pulmonary, digestive, heart, prostate, and liver epithelial cells [14]. SARS-CoV-2 has also been shown to use endosomal cysteine proteases cathepsin B (Cat B) and Cat L to enter the host cell aside from TMPRSS2 [15]. Kawase M et al. (2012) implied that concurrent suppression of surface receptor TMPRSS2, Cat L, and Cat B effectively inhibits virion entry into host cells in vitro [16].

Both non-specific and virus-specific immune responses contribute towards COVID-19, with escape from the innate immune response strongly affecting viral RNA replication and progression of infection. The protein kinase B (Akt) signalling pathway, which is important for cell survival, is abnormally regulated by SARS-CoV-2 to support its survival and replication. Nuclear factor-kB (NF-kb) transcription factor has been suggested to be highly active in severe inflammation during SARS-CoV-2 infection [16]. RNA replication of the SARS-CoV-2 genome forms double-stranded RNA (dsRNA), which upregulates the cytoplasmic innate immune pathway via stimulation of melanoma differentiation-associated protein 5 (MDA5) and retinoic acid-inducible gene I (RIG-I). This in turn triggers signalling by mitochondrial antiviral-signalling protein (MAVS), leading to release of type I and type III interferons [17], resulting in the activation of antiviral interferon-stimulated genes (ISGs) in neighbouring cells via the Janus kinase/signal transducer and activator of transcription (JAK/STAT) signalling pathway [18]. However, studies have shown that SARS-CoV-2 as well as SARS-CoV and MERS-CoV have various mechanisms to inhibit interferon-related immune responses, with the non-structural open reading frame 6 (Orf6) protein being involved in immune evasion and viral structural proteins inhibiting type I interferon-regulated antiviral immune responses [19,20].

The viral proteases 3-chymotrypsin-like protease (3CLpro) and papain-like protease (PLpro) are also crucial for viral replication, with roles in hydrolysing the viral polyprotein.

PLpro also disrupts the host non-specific immune reaction by targeting various host cell proteins [21]. RNA-dependent RNA polymerase (RdRp) is important for SARS-CoV-2 virus transcription, RNA genome replication, phenotype changes, and regulation of post-transcription of host cell gene expression [22]. SARS-CoV-2 also affects the target cell through its cytocidal effect, which promotes host cell death and lysis via an immune-regulated process. The formation of syncytia by fusion of SARS-CoV-2-infected cells, via formation of replication complexes formed through the movement of vesicles and disturbance of Golgi apparatus, has also been observed [23]. Rapid and unregulated non-specific responses to viral infection lead to a rise in inflammatory cytokines and immune cell activation in the lower respiratory tract, triggering damage to cells and tissues and thus exacerbation of COVID-19 [24].

2. The Endothelium

The circulatory system contains numerous blood vessels, including arteries, veins, capillaries, and lymph vessels, which transport blood, haemocytes, oxygen, nutrients, hormones, vitamins, minerals, and lymphatic fluids, which are important to supporting the survival of the human body [25]. Endothelial cells are a thin monolayer that mainly lines the interior surface of vasculature and are commonly shielded by pericytes that promote vascular stability. These cells have various roles and are predominately surrounded by smooth muscle and connective tissue. The main function of endothelial cells is regulating haemostasis, coagulation, thrombosis, permeability, inflammatory processes, remodelling of new vessels, blood vessel tone, vasorelaxation and vasoconstriction, blood flow and pressure, and forming the barrier between vessels and tissues [26–28]. The endothelium has a capacity to respond to physical damage and chemical molecules. The stability of the endothelium depends on the regulation of vascular contractile activity of vascular smooth muscle cells, vasculitis, and cellular attachment to other cells [29]. Physiological activity of certain endothelium signalling mediators, including nitric oxide, prostacyclins, and angiopoietins, are important for all features of blood vessel stability and integrity. Therefore, the metabolic function of endothelial cells is crucial for the constant adaptation of blood vessel tone, which in turn regulates blood pressure. Additionally, endothelial cells have a key role in decreasing the formation of blood clots and blood thickness equilibrium in the blood stream, including the normal control of white blood cell transport from blood vessels to tissues [30].

2.1. *Angiopoietin Family*

Angiopoietins belong to a family of vascular growth factor glycoproteins which control the formation of new blood vessels and promote angiogenesis and foetal/adult vascular development. The four isoforms, Angiopoietin (Angpt) 1, 2, 3, 4, are structurally comparable and are ligands of the Tunica Interna endothelial cell tyrosine kinase (Tie) receptor, predominantly expressed in endothelial cells [31]. Angpt 1 and 2 are key isoforms of this glycoprotein family and have been thoroughly studied, whereas Angpt 3 and 4 are less well studied. Although Angpt 3 is expressed in mice and humans, it is not biologically active in human endothelial cells. The specific and precise equilibrium of Angpt 1 and 2 is important to controlling vascular stability [32]. The alteration of these protein level ratios is connected with multiple diseases, such as cancer, sepsis, and coronary artery diseases [33].

2.2. *The Function of Angiopoietin 1*

Angpt 1 has a molecular weight of 70 kDa and consists of 498 residues [34]. Angpt 1 is suggested to be a significant angiogenic growth factor and constitutive paracrine agonist of tyrosine kinase receptor (Tie2) and supports blood vessel stability and integrity. Witzenbichler et al. (1998) reported that binding of Angpt 1 to Tie 2 in vascular endothelial cells leads to the phosphorylation of several tyrosine residues on the carboxy terminus of the receptor, initiating various intracellular secondary messengers that contribute to endothelial function, including vessel sprouting and cell viability [35]. The absence of

Angpt 1 was shown to lead to defects in blood vessel growth and foetal blood vessel development in Angpt 1 knockout mice [36]. The upregulation of Angpt 1 in a genetically modified mouse model increased angiogenesis and decreased vascular permeability [37]. Angpt 1 does not bind to the Tie 1 receptor; however, it indirectly activates it through the transphosphorylation of active Tie 2 receptors [38]. Angpt 1-induced PI3K/Akt leads to the addition of phosphate groups and inhibition of the forkhead transcription factor Foxo1 in vascular endothelial cells [39]. This transcription factor is involved in endothelial cell death and controls the synthesis of various mediators such as Angpt 2. Angpt 1 phosphorylation of the Tie 2 receptor also facilitates adhesion to pericytes and smooth muscle cells, which in turn leads to blood vessel protection and stability [40].

2.3. *The Function of Angiopoietin 2*

Angpt 1 and 2 have 60% homology in their amino acid sequence. Like Angpt 1, Angpt 2 is capable of binding to Tie 2 receptor. Angpt 2 is stored in Weibel–Palade bodies (WPBs) in endothelial cells. The release of Angpt 2 is highly controlled and exerts an autocrine action [41]. Angpt 2 has the opposite effect from Angpt 1; it facilitates vascular permeability, obstructs endothelial barrier activity, and impairs vascular integrity [42]. Although Angpt 2 obstructs the vascular protective activity of Angpt 1 after it binds to Tie 2 receptor, in some cases, this antagonist ligand can stimulate Tie 2 signalling through an unknown mechanism. In the presence of vascular endothelial growth factor (VEGF), Angpt 2 promotes angiogenesis, blood vessel sprouting, and destabilisation [43]. Also, Angpt 2 promotes pericyte detachment by decreasing the cooperation between endothelial cells and pericytes, vascular smooth muscle cells, and the extracellular matrix [44]. Also, some studies reported that upregulation of Angpt 2 in vitro activates vascular endothelial cell movement during the reorganisation stage of angiogenesis and increases cell viability via Tie 2 interaction and PI3K/Akt stimulation [45]. In physiological conditions, Angpt 2 is generally released in regions of structural changes to bloods, vessel such as the gonads, the womb, and the placenta. Its release is rapidly activated by various stimuli including thrombin, histamine, hypoxia, and VEGF. Angpt 2 also stimulates vascular endothelial cells to release inflammatory cytokines including TNF-α [46]. Angpt 2 interacts with white blood cells, including monocytes, macrophages, and neutrophils, throughout the inflammation process [47].

2.4. *Tie Receptors*

Tie 1 and Tie 2 are members of a specific receptor tyrosine kinase (RTK) family which are expressed predominantly in endothelial and hematopoietic cells. Tie 2 receptor interacts with Angpt 1, 2, 4, whereas Tie 1 is thought to be incapable of binding to Angpts and alternative ligands of Tie 1 have not yet been discovered [48]. Tie receptors contain three epidermal growth factor (EGF) domains amidst two immunoglobulin (Ig)-like domains and three fibronectin type 3 domains. Their Ig-like domains and EGF-like domains are important and sufficient to bind Angpt 1 and Angpt 2 [49]. Tie receptors play a role in the structural change and maturation of blood vessels during embryogenesis [50]. Tie 1 orphan receptor is important for blood vessel formation, integrity, and sprouting in the embryonic stage. Tie 1 synthesis decreases in adulthood, but its levels remain the same in endothelial cells of the renal, cardiovascular, and respiratory systems [51]. Tie 2 is the main signalling receptor of the Angpt pathway and receptor clustering is important for the stimulation of this transmembrane receptor [52]. Tie 1 is capable of forming heterodimer complexes with Tie 2, which decreases the activation of Angpt 1 and supports the activity of Angpt 2, whereas Tie2/Tie2 homodimers activate Angpt 1 signalling and vascular integrity. The process of Tie 2 receptor activation is still not well understood, apart from the binding of the carboxyl terminus domain of Angpt to the ligand-binding domain of this receptor [53].

2.5. Angiopoietin 1/Tie 2 Signalling

After the binding of the five subunits of multimeric Angpt 1 to the Tie 2 receptor at the cell-to-cell junctional complex, Tie 2 transmembrane receptor is phosphorylated and starts the signalling pathway, resulting in the regulation of multiple processes, including blood vessel stability and endothelial cell survival, as illustrated in Figure 1 [53,54]. Angpt 1 activates PI3K by recruiting the regulatory p85 subunit in Tie 2, which results in the stimulation of Akt and nitric oxide synthase 3 (eNOS) to inhibit endothelial apoptosis. The stimulation of Akt by the Angpt 1/Tie 2 signalling pathway leads to the phosphorylation and obstruction of the Forkhead transcription factor (FKHR) gene to support cell survival and vessel stability [55–60]. The Angpt 1/Tie pathway is also involved in cortical actin cytoskeleton stability by regulating GTPase and decreasing inflammatory molecules through the inhibition of NFκB protein [61–66].

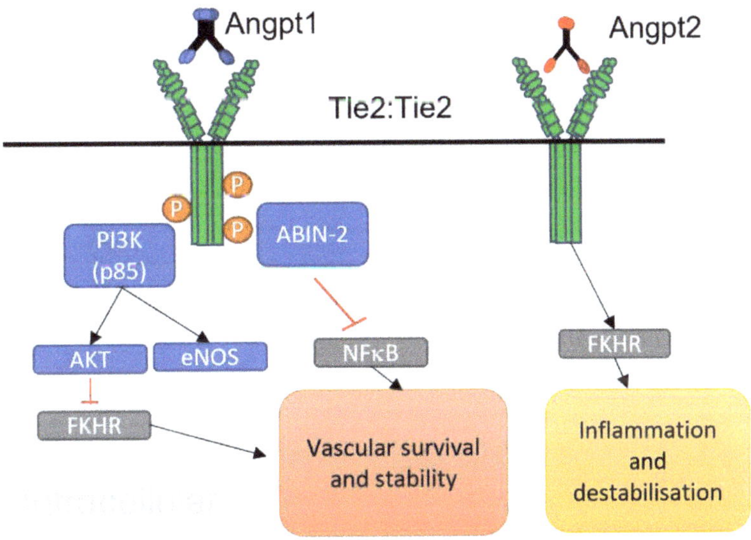

Figure 1. A schematic demonstrating Angiopoietin 1 and 2 molecular signalling in normal and abnormal vasculature. The binding of Angpt 1 to Tie 2 receptor at junctional complexes results in stimulation of PI3K/Akt, antiapoptotic protein, nitric oxide synthase 3 (eNOS), and that in turn promotes endothelial cell survival throughout normal vasculature. The inhibition of FKHR by Angpt1/Tie 2 receptor phosphorylation inhibits inflammatory molecules and supports vascular stability. In abnormal conditions, the binding of Angpt 2 and Tie 2 results in pericyte loss, increased inflammatory gene expression, and vascular destabilisation.

As discussed above, Tie 1/Tie 2 heterodimer receptors can affect Angpt 1/Tie 2 signalling. Tumour necrosis factor-α (TNF-α) is a crucial inflammatory cytokine that is able to stimulate Tie 1 ectodomain cleavage in endothelial cells. TNF-α was also shown to elevate Tie 2 expression, leading to changes in the ratio of Tie 1 to Tie 2. Similar observations have been found with VEGF, which is capable of cleaving the ectodomains of both Tie 1 and Tie 2, leading to the regulation of Angpt 1 signalling [67–71]. Tie 1 decreases the capacity of Angpt 1 to bind to Tie 2 and therefore decreases Tie 2 activation by its ectodomain. Cleavage of the extracellular domain of Tie 1 enhances the binding of Angpt 1 to Tie 2 and thus increases Angpt 1/Tie 2 activation [72]. Changes in Angpt 1 and Angpt 2 levels also regulate Tie 2 signalling. A decrease in Angpt 1 and increase in Angpt 2 promote vessel destabilisation under various disease states and have been associated with acute lung injury [73]. Some studies reported that the release of Angpt 1 changes after ischemic stroke and increased levels of this protein decrease the complications of stroke [74]. During atherosclerosis, Angpt 2 elevation promotes vessel inflammatory processes by stimulating NFκB and traffics white blood cells through the vessel to the affected regions [75]. Also, inflammation caused by infection leads to a decrease in Angpt 1 and suppression of the Angpt 1/Tie 2 pathway, leading to vascular instability and increased permeability. Several studies have mentioned that Angpt could be utilised as a molecular marker or treatment method to decrease the severity of lung inflammation and sepsis [76,77]. Some studies suggest that elevated Angpt 2 in various tumours stimulate neovascularisation in cancer mice models. Angpt 1/Tie 2 pathway therapies have been connected with recovery and survival rates in specific types of tumours, such as cervical and ovarian cancers [78–80].

3. The Impact of SARS-CoV-2 on Endothelial Cells

Post-mortem studies in COVID-19 patients have reported a procoagulant state and microvascular damage in deceased patients, demonstrating that vascular pathology caused by endothelial dysfunction is a crucial factor in the pathogenesis of SARS-CoV-2 [81–83]. Endothelial dysfunction during SARS-CoV-2 infection results in pro-inflammation and vascular permeability and leads to vascular destabilisation through the mechanisms shown in Figure 2 [84]. As mentioned above, the ACE2 receptor is one of the most important receptors that bind to the spike protein of SARS-CoV-2 and is expressed in various cells, including vascular endothelial cells. SARS-CoV-2 has been connected with substantial immune activation that directly influences endothelial cells via cytokine storm [85]. SARS-CoV-2 can infect host endothelial cells if high viral loads are used, and this leads to the activation of cell death. Infections of endothelial cells have been suggested to be less efficient compared to those of epithelial cells due to the lower expression of the ACE2 receptor and protease in endothelial cells [86].

Endothelial tissues cooperate with epithelial tissues in the respiratory tract airway barrier to control tissue stability and defend against infectious microorganisms. Epithelial cells communicate with endothelial cells during pathogenic infections to initiate immune cell activation. These two cells create a single layer bound by solid junctions that control vascular permeability, whereas adherent junctions control cell-to-cell and cell-to-matrix cooperation [87]. The endothelium in the lung contains macro- and micro-vessel endothelial cells, with the latter belonging to the epithelial and endothelial contact junction [88]. An increase in inflammatory cytokines causes local endothelial dysfunction and supports blood clotting and platelet activation [89]. The damage to endothelial cells caused by an intense immune reaction could affect the structure of blood vessel and airway junctions and cause vessel leakage, lung inflammation, white blood cell extravasation, and oxygen shortage [90]. Lung epithelial cells stimulate NOD-like receptor protein 3 (NLPR3) and inflammatory cytokines such as TNF-α and IL-6 during COVID-19 in order to start intense immune reactions; these processes result in apoptosis, cell injury, increased vessel permeability, and lung inflammation [91]. In addition, unregulated synthesis of neutrophil extracellular traps (NETs) and reactive oxygen species (ROS) impairs endothelial cells, activates platelet and blood clotting, and aids in acute respiratory distress syndrome and tissue injury. Nitric oxide and prostacyclin are vasodilators that help with vascular integrity. The levels of these hormones are reduced in SARS-CoV-2 and lead to endothelial dysfunction [92].

Intracellular adhesion molecules bind to fibrinogens and support fibrin aggregation to endothelial cells, which is involved in abnormal functioning of endothelial cells, blood clotting, and vessel narrowing [93]. Hyperactivation and dysfunction of endothelial cells are a significant hallmark of severity in patients with SARS-CoV-2. It is not clear if SARS-CoV-2 can directly and productively infect endothelial cells despite endothelial cells expressing the ACE2 receptor, which is necessary for viral entry [94–97]. Enrichment of SARS-CoV-2 RNA was found in lung endothelial cells in deceased COVID-19 patients [98], and infection was observed in in vitro-cultured endothelial cells [98,99]. On the other hand, infection of primary endothelial cells was not observed [100]. Despite this, it has been suggested that infection of neighbouring cells, such as epithelial and vascular pericyte cells, causes an elevated inflammatory response and cytokine storm and leads to endothelial dysfunction [86,100].

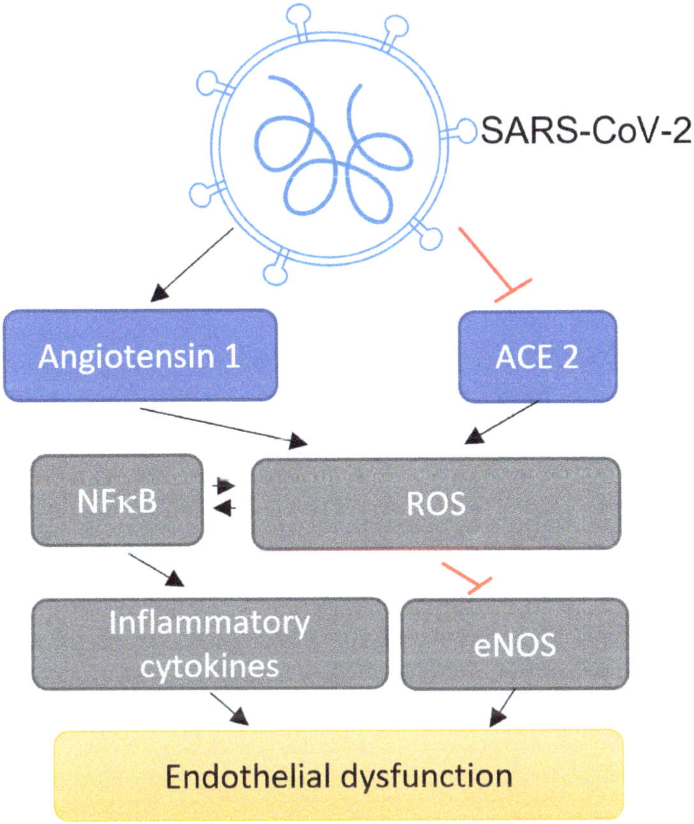

Figure 2. A schematic demonstrating the molecular mechanisms of the effect of SARS-CoV-2 infection on endothelial cells. Viral infection affects endothelial and vascular function by several pathways. The inflammation response during viral infection stimulates the renin–angiotensin system (RAS) by elevating angiotensin 1 or alternatively through decreasing the extracellular activation of angiotensin converting enzyme 2 (ACE2). SARS-CoV-2 infection elevates reactive oxygen species (ROS) and stimulates NFκB, and that in turn reduces nitric oxides and elevates inflammatory cytokines such as TNF-α and IL-6. This mechanism results in damaging the equilibrium amidst vessel relaxation and narrowing, inflammation, blood clotting in arteries and capillaries, and thrombocyte stimulation.

Some studies have speculated that SARS-CoV-2-infected epithelial cells detach at the contact barriers and that permits the virus to be transmitted from the base surfaces of epithelial cells to endothelial cells in the lungs. It has also been suggested that the virus might infect endothelial cells through the blood stream via the apical surface [101]. Also, others have suggested that ACE2 is released at high levels in small-vessel pericytes and that pericyte injury caused by SARS-CoV-2 might play a role in endothelial dysregulation. The loss or detachment of SARS-CoV-2-infected and injured pericytes causes endothelial dysfunction through declining endothelial barrier activity and endothelial activation [94,101].

It has also been reported that the SARS-CoV-2 spike protein stimulates damage to the vessel contact barrier in cerebral small-vessel endothelial cells [101]. Endothelial cells sense and respond to damage-associated molecular signals from surrounding virus-affected epithelial cells and endothelial cells. Furthermore, the vascular endothelial cell-regulated inflammatory process is an key part of the pathological mechanism of COVID-19 [52,102]. During infection, the inflammatory process activates endothelial cells, which synthesise tissue factors that result in blood clotting, hyperpermeability of small vessels, lung damage, and increased levels of cytokines such as TNF-α and IL-6, associated with amplified coagulation factor 1 or fibrinogen [102]. The extracellular activation of ACE2 is decreased and the renin–angiotensin system (RAS) is stimulated after SARS-CoV-2 entry into the host cell. ACE2 is important for supporting vessel relaxation molecules including angiotensins 1–7, preventing the activation of reactive oxygen species (ROS) through inhibition of angiotensin II type 1 receptor (AT1R), and regulates the equilibrium of the RAS [103]. Downregulation of nitric oxide and elevated vessel-narrowing molecules such as angiotensin 2 are important aspects of endothelial dysregulation during COVID-19. The reduction in nitric oxide by upregulation of NFκB leads to a reduction in endothelial nitric oxide synthase (eNOS) and to the synthesis of ROS, which are involved in disrupting endothelial function (Figure 2) [104]. During SARS-CoV-2 infection and cytokine storm, the increase in angiotensin type 2 receptor and reduction in angiotensin 1–7 are involved in decreasing vessel dilation, supporting white blood cell and thrombocyte adhesion, and therefore activate a pro-thrombotic, pro-coagulative state and inhibit the fibrinolysis process [105]. Moreover, angiotensin type 2 receptor upregulates nicotinamide adenine dinucleotide phosphate oxidase (NADPH oxidase 2), and increased expression of angiotensin type 2 receptor leads to an increase in oxidative stress and destabilisation of vascular activity [106]. People infected with SARS-CoV-2 displayed elevated amounts of fibrinogen, fibrin-dissolving fragments such as D-dimer, and blood clotting protein including factor 8, and decreased amounts of endothelial plasminogen activator inhibitor 1 [107].

3.1. Potential Impact of SARS-CoV-2 on Angpt/Tie Signalling

Angpt 2 plays an important role in elevated vascular inflammation and leakage through inactivating Angpt 1 and Tie signalling. Elevated levels of Angpt 2 have been detected in the blood serum of patients with vascular leakage, lung inflammation, and acute respiratory distress syndrome, and have been linked with complications like sepsis [108]. Lu et al. (2022) reported that SARS-CoV-2 infection impairs the structure of the vascular endothelial contact barrier due to damaging vascular endothelial cadherin barrier junctions and increasing inflammatory mediators including IL-6, IL-8, and Angpt 2 in vitro. Also, these cytokines were increased in SARS-CoV-2 infections compared to other coronaviruses such as NL63 [109]. The stimulation of phosphorylated mixed-lineage kinase domain-like protein (pMLKL), which supports necrotic apoptosis, occurred in small vessels with increased Angpt 2, connecting this to vessel damage in patients with COVID-19 [110]. Some studies suggested that thrombosis, vessel damage, and vascular endothelial cells apoptosis were observed in the tissue of deceased COVID-19 patients using pulmonary imaging mass cytometry. This result supports the speculation that COVID-19 is a vascular disorder [111]. SARS-CoV-2 uses the cellular machinery of infected cells, similar to other viruses, in order to produce proteins which are necessary for the transcription and assembly of the pathogen, resulting in atypical hyperstimulation of signalling mechanism of PI3/Akt/mTOR pathway [112]. Hypoxia caused by SARS-CoV-2 infection is also involved in angiogenesis. The lack of oxygen connected with continuing inflammation leads to hypoxia-inducible factor 1 alpha (HIF-1α) stabilisation, which interacts with molecular markers including VEGF, Angpt, and Tie 2 receptor. Also, angiopoietin-like 4 proteins (Angpt 4) are released in response to oxygen starvation and malnutrition by a HIF1-α-related mechanism. Angpt 4 is involved in several activities including controlling vessel damage, permeability, wound healing, vessel function, and cholesterol homeostasis [113]. Some studies reported that increased levels of Angpt 4 were related to acute respiratory distress syndrome and severity of SARS-CoV-2 infection [114]. SARS-CoV-2 infection activates HIF-1α, and upregulation of this factor is also involved in the pathophysiological mechanism of this pathogen, including a decrease in ACE2 receptor [115].

White blood cell endothelial adhesion molecules such as soluble E-selectin are activated by inflammatory cytokines. Elevated levels of soluble E-selectin and Angpt 2 have been reported in patients with SARS-CoV-2 infection [116]. Thrombocytes, except pericytes, produce large numbers of Angpt 1 protein. Thrombocytopenia is caused by apoptosis of thrombocytes, and build-up of thrombus aggregation leads to decline in serum Angpt 1 in patients with severe COVID-19 [117]. It has been speculated that after the first stage of SARS-CoV-2 infection, the induced expression of inflammatory cytokines and local hypoxia due to upregulated Angpt 2 results in the development of lung vessel injuries. Serum Angpt 2/Angpt 1 ratio is more substantially elevated in patients with severe symptoms or those who are critically ill than patients with less severe symptoms [118].

3.2. *Potential Clinical Implication of Angpt/Tie Signalling in COVID-19 Patients*

It is well known that endothelial dysfunction is associated with multiple organ damage [119]. Molecular imbalances of key mediators associated with ED, including decreased NO bioavailability, increase in endothelin-1 and angiotensin II, increase in intracellular adhesion molecule 1 (ICAM1) and vascular cell adhesion molecule 1 (VCAM1), and rise in plasminogen activator inhibitor 1 (PAI-1) and Angpt-2 levels, to name a few, are linked to acute kidney and liver injury, lung damage, stroke, and cardiac/peripheral vascular injury [119,120]. In vitro and early clinical evidence shows that, either by direct infection or through an indirect mechanism (cytokine storm), SARS-CoV-2 leads to ED and results in multi-organ injury [119–121]. So, it is important to explore therapeutic ways in which endothelial function and vascular integrity can be improved in the care of patients with long-term SARS-CoV-2 symptoms. Recent work on primary human umbilical vein endothelial cells (HUVECs) treated with plasma from patients with severe COVID-19 showed upregulated expression of several thromboinflammatory genes, including Angpt-2 and E-selectin [122]. Downregulation of anti-thrombotic genes, endothelial protein C receptor, and thrombomodulin was also observed in the treated cells. Interestingly, stimulating Tie2 receptor with its protective ligand Angpt1 or using a vascular endothelial protein tyrosine phosphatase (Tie2 kinase inhibitor) inhibitor (AKB-9778) significantly reduced the ability of severe COVID-19 plasma to induce procoagulant activity in HUVECs [122]. While the study had limitations in correlating the gene expression profile with clinical outcomes, this initial work indicates the Angpt/Tie2 axis as an attractive model to pursue.

4. Conclusions

Endothelial dysfunction plays a crucial role in the pathophysiology of SARS-CoV-2. The effect of SARS-CoV-2 on Tie receptor expression and Angpt 1 levels is not well studied; however, some studies indicate that infection induces changes in the levels of Angpts and Tie 2, which may potentially destabilise the vasculature and promote thrombosis, coagulation, inflammation, and permeability during severe COVID-19. It is also possible that SARS-CoV-2 may indirectly affect Angpt/Tie 2 signalling through inflammatory cytokine storm and stimulation of a pro-thrombotic state. Inflammatory cytokines such as TNF-α and IL-6 upregulate Angpt 2 by inhibition of nitric oxides and NFκB activation and thus suppress Angpt 1/Tie 2 signalling. Direct endothelial virus infection or infection of neighbouring cells may cause disruptions in Angpt 1/Tie 2 and endothelial dysfunction during immune activation against infection. As previously mentioned, SARS-CoV-2 is associated with long-term vascular pathology and endothelial injury. Therefore, based on the evidence, more research is required in order to understand the molecular impact SARS-CoV-2 has on endothelial dysfunction and the Angiopoietin/Tie axis to improve treatment and care.

Author Contributions: Wrote the main manuscript and completed conceptualization of the manuscript, D.J. and H.S.; reviewed the manuscript, D.J., M.S. and H.S.; prepared figures, D.J., M.S. and H.S. All authors have read and agreed to the published version of the manuscript.

Funding: This research received no external funding.

Data Availability Statement: No new data were created or analyzed in this study. Data sharing is not applicable to this article.

Conflicts of Interest: The authors declare no conflicts of interest.

References

1. Zhu, N.; Zhang, D.; Wang, W.; Li, X.; Yang, B.; Song, J.; Zhao, X.; Huang, B.; Shi, W.; Lu, R.; et al. A Novel Coronavirus from Patients with Pneumonia in China, 2019. *N. Engl. J. Med.* **2020**, *382*, 727–733. [CrossRef] [PubMed]
2. Banerjee, A.; Kulcsar, K.; Misra, V.; Frieman, M.; Mossman, K. Bats and Coronaviruses. *Viruses* **2019**, *11*, 41. [CrossRef]
3. V'kovski, P.; Kratzel, A.; Steiner, S.; Stalder, H.; Thiel, V. Coronavirus biology and replication: Implications for SARS-CoV-2. *Nat. Rev. Microbiol.* **2020**, *19*, 155–170. [CrossRef] [PubMed]
4. Li, Q.; Guan, X.; Wu, P.; Wang, X.; Zhou, L.; Tong, Y.; Ren, R.; Leung, K.S.M.; Lau, E.H.Y.; Wong, J.Y.; et al. Early Transmission Dynamics in Wuhan, China, of Novel Coronavirus-Infected Pneumonia. *N. Engl. J. Med.* **2020**, *382*, 1199–1207. [CrossRef]
5. Gaunt, E.R.; Hardie, A.; Claas, E.C.; Simmonds, P.; Templeton, K.E. Epidemiology and clinical presentations of the four human coronaviruses 229E, HKU1, NL63, and OC43 detected over 3 years using a novel multiplex real-time PCR method. *J. Clin. Microbiol.* **2010**, *48*, 2940–2947. [CrossRef]
6. Naskalska, A.; Dabrowska, A.; Szczepanski, A.; Milewska, A.; Jasik, K.P.; Pyrc, K. Membrane Protein of Human Coronavirus NL63 Is Responsible for Interaction with the Adhesion Receptor. *J. Virol.* **2019**, *93*, e00355-19. [CrossRef] [PubMed]
7. Corman, V.M.; Muth, D.; Niemeyer, D.; Drosten, C. Hosts and Sources of Endemic Human Coronaviruses. *Adv. Virus Res.* **2018**, *100*, 163–188.
8. Lalchhandama, K. The chronicles of coronaviruses: The bronchitis, the hepatitis and the common cold. *Sci. Vis.* **2020**, *20*, 43–53. [CrossRef]
9. Gierer, S.; Bertram, S.; Kaup, F.; Wrensch, F.; Heurich, A.; Kramer-Kuhl, A.; Welsch, K.; Winkler, M.; Meyer, B.; Drosten, C.; et al. The spike protein of the emerging betacoronavirus EMC uses a novel coronavirus receptor for entry, can be activated by TMPRSS2, and is targeted by neutralizing antibodies. *J. Virol.* **2013**, *87*, 5502–5511. [CrossRef]
10. Neuman, B.W.; Kiss, G.; Kunding, A.H.; Bhella, D.; Baksh, M.F.; Connelly, S.; Droese, B.; Klaus, J.P.; Makino, S.; Sawicki, S.G.; et al. A structural analysis of M protein in coronavirus assembly and morphology. *J. Struct. Biol.* **2011**, *174*, 11–22. [CrossRef]
11. Lamers, M.M.; Haagmans, B.L. SARS-CoV-2 pathogenesis. *Nat. Rev. Microbiol.* **2022**, *20*, 270–284. [CrossRef]
12. Letko, M.; Marzi, A.; Munster, V. Functional assessment of cell entry and receptor usage for SARS-CoV-2 and other lineage B betacoronaviruses. *Nat. Microbiol.* **2020**, *5*, 562–569. [CrossRef]
13. Wang, W.; Ye, L.; Ye, L.; Li, B.; Gao, B.; Zeng, Y.; Kong, L.; Fang, X.; Zheng, H.; Wu, Z.; et al. Up-regulation of IL-6 and TNF-α induced by SARS-coronavirus spike protein in murine macrophages via NF-κB pathway. *Virus Res.* **2007**, *128*, 1–8. [CrossRef]
14. Hoffmann, M.; Kleine-Weber, H.; Schroeder, S.; Krüger, N.; Herrler, T.; Erichsen, S.; Schiergens, T.S.; Herrler, G.; Wu, N.-H.; Nitsche, A.; et al. SARS-CoV-2 Cell Entry Depends on ACE2 and TMPRSS2 and Is Blocked by a Clinically Proven Protease Inhibitor. *Cell* **2020**, *181*, 271–280. [CrossRef] [PubMed]
15. Ou, X.; Liu, Y.; Lei, X.; Li, P.; Mi, D.; Ren, L.; Guo, L.; Guo, R.; Chen, T.; Hu, J.; et al. Characterization of spike glycoprotein of SARS-CoV-2 on virus entry and its immune cross-reactivity with SARS-CoV. *Nat. Commun.* **2020**, *11*, 1620–1629. [CrossRef] [PubMed]
16. Kawase, M.; Shirato, K.; van der Hoek, L.; Taguchi, F.; Matsuyama, S. Simultaneous treatment of human bronchial epithelial cells with serine and cysteine protease inhibitors prevents severe acute respiratory syndrome coronavirus entry. *J. Virol.* **2012**, *86*, 6537–6545. [CrossRef] [PubMed]
17. Yin, X.; Riva, L.; Pu, Y.; Martin-Sancho, L.; Kanamune, J.; Yamamoto, Y.; Sakai, K.; Gotoh, S.; Miorin, L.; Paul, D.; et al. MDA5 Governs the Innate Immune Response to SARS-CoV-2 in Lung Epithelial Cells. *Cell Rep.* **2021**, *34*, 108628. [CrossRef]
18. Lokugamage, K.G.; Hage, A.; de Vries, M.; Valero-Jimenez, A.M.; Schindewolf, C.; Dittmann, M.; Rajsbaum, R.; Menachery, V.D. Type I Interferon Susceptibility Distinguishes SARS-CoV-2 from SARS-CoV. *J. Virol.* **2020**, *94*, e01410-20. [CrossRef]
19. Reuschl, A.-K.; Thorne, L.G.; Whelan, M.V.X.; Ragazzini, R.; Furnon, W.; Cowton, V.M.; De Lorenzo, G.; Mesner, D.; Turner, J.L.E.; Dowgier, G.; et al. Evolution of enhanced innate immune suppression by SARS-CoV-2 Omicron subvariants. *Nat. Microbiol.* **2024**, *9*, 451–463. [CrossRef] [PubMed]
20. Kim, Y.; Shin, E. Type I and III interferon responses in SARS-CoV-2 infection. *Exp. Mol. Med.* **2021**, *53*, 750–760. [CrossRef]
21. Shin, D.; Mukherjee, R.; Grewe, D.; Bojkova, D.; Baek, K.; Bhattacharya, A.; Schulz, L.; Widera, M.; Mehdipour, A.R.; Tascher, G.; et al. Papain-like protease regulates SARS-CoV-2 viral spread and innate immunity. *Nature* **2020**, *587*, 657–662. [CrossRef] [PubMed]
22. Shang, J.; Ye, G.; Shi, K.; Wan, Y.; Luo, C.; Aihara, H.; Geng, Q.; Auerbach, A.; Li, F. Structural basis of receptor recognition by SARS-CoV-2. *Nature* **2020**, *581*, 221–224. [CrossRef] [PubMed]
23. Morse, J.S.; Lalonde, T.; Xu, S.; Liu, W. Learning from the Past: Possible Urgent Prevention and Treatment Options for Severe Acute Respiratory Infections Caused by 2019-nCoV. *ChemRxiv: Prepr. Serv. Chem.* **2020**, *21*, 730–738. [CrossRef] [PubMed]
24. Roberts, K.A.; Colley, L.; Agbaedeng, T.A.; Ellison-Hughes, G.M.; Ross, M.D. Vascular Manifestations of COVID-19—Thromboembolism and Microvascular Dysfunction. *Front. Cardiovasc. Med.* **2020**, *7*, 598400. [CrossRef]

25. Pugsley, M.K.; Tabrizchi, R. The vascular system. An overview of structure and function. *J. Pharmacol. Toxicol. Methods* **2000**, *44*, 333–340. [CrossRef] [PubMed]
26. Aird, W.C. Endothelium and haemostasis. *Hamostaseologie* **2015**, *35*, 11–16. [CrossRef]
27. Jia, G.; Aroor, A.R.; Jia, C.; Sowers, J.R. Endothelial cell senescence in aging-related vascular dysfunction. *Biochim. Biophys. Acta (BBA)-Mol. Basis Dis.* **2019**, *1865*, 1802–1809. [CrossRef]
28. Gullo, A.L.; Aragona, C.O.; Scuruchi, M.; Versace, A.G.; Saitta, A.; Imbalzano, E.; Loddo, S.; Campo, G.M.; Mandraffino, G. Endothelial progenitor cells and rheumatic disease modifying therapy. *Vasc. Pharmacol.* **2018**, *108*, 8. [CrossRef]
29. Deanfield, J.E.; Halcox, J.P.; Rabelink, T.J. Endothelial function and dysfunction: Testing and clinical relevance. *Circulation* **2007**, *115*, 1285–1295. [CrossRef]
30. Pearson, J.D. Normal endothelial cell function. *Lupus* **2000**, *9*, 183–188. [CrossRef] [PubMed]
31. Buhimschi, C.S.; Bhandari, V.; Dulay, A.T.; Thung, S.; Razeq, S.S.A.; Rosenberg, V.; Han, C.S.; Ali, U.A.; Zambrano, E.; Zhao, G.; et al. Amniotic fluid angiopoietin-1, angiopoietin-2, and soluble receptor tunica interna endothelial cell kinase-2 levels and regulation in normal pregnancy and intraamniotic inflammation-induced preterm birth. *J. Clin. Endocrinol. Metab.* **2010**, *95*, 3428–3436. [CrossRef]
32. Daly, C.; Eichten, A.; Castanaro, C.; Pasnikowski, E.; Adler, A.; Lalani, A.S.; Papadopoulos, N.; Kyle, A.H.; Minchinton, A.I.; Yancopoulos, G.D.; et al. Angiopoietin-2 functions as a Tie2 agonist in tumor models, where it limits the effects of VEGF inhibition. *Cancer Res.* **2013**, *73*, 108–118. [CrossRef]
33. Bilimoria, J.; Singh, H. The Angiopoietin ligands and Tie receptors: Potential diagnostic biomarkers of vascular disease. *J. Recept. Signal Transduct. Res.* **2019**, *39*, 187–193. [CrossRef] [PubMed]
34. Maisonpierre, P.C.; Suri, C.; Jones, P.F.; Bartunkova, S.; Wiegand, S.J.; Radziejewski, C.; Compton, D.; McClain, J.; Aldrich, T.H.; Papadopoulos, N.; et al. Angiopoietin-2, a natural antagonist for Tie2 that disrupts in vivo angiogenesis. *Science* **1997**, *277*, 55–60. [CrossRef] [PubMed]
35. Witzenbichler, B.; Maisonpierre, P.C.; Jones, P.; Yancopoulos, G.D.; Isner, J.M. Chemotactic properties of angiopoietin-1 and -2, ligands for the endothelial-specific receptor tyrosine kinase Tie2. *J. Biol. Chem.* **1998**, *273*, 18514–18521. [CrossRef] [PubMed]
36. Suri, C.; Jones, P.F.; Patan, S.; Bartunkova, S.; Maisonpierre, P.C.; Davis, S.; Sato, T.N.; Yancopoulos, G.D. Requisite role of angiopoietin-1, a ligand for the TIE2 receptor, during embryonic angiogenesis. *Cell* **1996**, *87*, 1171–1180. [CrossRef] [PubMed]
37. Chae, J.K.; Kim, I.; Lim, S.T.; Chung, M.J.; Kim, W.H.; Kim, H.G.; Ko, J.K.; Koh, G.Y. Coadministration of angiopoietin-1 and vascular endothelial growth factor enhances collateral vascularization. *Arterioscler. Thromb. Vasc. Biol.* **2000**, *20*, 2573–2578. [CrossRef] [PubMed]
38. Saharinen, P.; Eklund, L.; Miettinen, J.; Wirkkala, R.; Anisimov, A.; Winderlich, M.; Nottebaum, A.; Vestweber, D.; Deutsch, U.; Koh, G.Y.; et al. Angiopoietins assemble distinct Tie2 signalling complexes in endothelial cell-cell and cell-matrix contacts. *Nat. Cell Biol.* **2008**, *10*, 527–537. [CrossRef]
39. Kim, M.; Allen, B.; Korhonen, E.; Nitschke, M.; Yang, H.; Baluk, P.; Saharinen, P.; Alitalo, K.; Daly, C.; Thurston, G.; et al. Opposing actions of angiopoietin-2 on Tie2 signalling and FOXO1 activation. *J. Clin. Investig.* **2016**, *126*, 3511–3525. [CrossRef]
40. Cai, J.; Kehoe, O.; Smith, G.M.; Hykin, P.; Boulton, M.E. The angiopoietin/Tie-2 system regulates pericyte survival and recruitment in diabetic retinopathy. *Investig. Ophthalmol. Vis. Sci.* **2000**, *49*, 2163–2171. [CrossRef]
41. Stratmann, A.; Risau, W.; Plate, K.H. Cell type-specific expression of angiopoietin-1 and angiopoietin-2 suggests a role in glioblastoma angiogenesis. *Am. J. Pathol.* **1998**, *153*, 1459–1466. [CrossRef]
42. Holash, J.; Maisonpierre, P.C.; Compton, D.; Boland, P.; Alexander, C.R.; Zagzag, D.; Yancopoulos, G.D.; Wiegand, S.J. Vessel cooption, regression, and growth in tumors mediated by angiopoietins and VEGF. *Science* **1999**, *284*, 1994–1998. [CrossRef]
43. Lobov, I.B.; Brooks, P.C.; Lang, R.A. Angiopoietin-2 displays VEGF-dependent modulation of capillary structure and endothelial cell survival in vivo. *Proc. Natl. Acad. Sci. USA* **2002**, *99*, 11205–11210. [CrossRef]
44. Dumont, D.J.; Gradwohl, G.; Fong, G.H.; Puri, M.C.; Gertsenstein, M.; Auerbach, A.; Breitman, M.L. Dominant-negative and targeted null mutations in the endothelial receptor tyrosine kinase, tek, reveal a critical role in vasculogenesis of the embryo. *Genes Dev.* **1994**, *8*, 1897–1909. [CrossRef]
45. Felcht, M.; Luck, R.; Schering, A.; Seidel, P.; Srivastava, K.; Hu, J.; Bartol, A.; Kienast, Y.; Vettel, C.; Loos, E.K.; et al. Angiopoietin-2 differentially regulates angiogenesis through TIE2 and integrin signaling. *J. Clin. Investig.* **2012**, *122*, 1991–2005. [CrossRef]
46. Fiedler, U.; Scharpfenecker, M.; Koidl, S.; Hegen, A.; Grunow, V.; Schmidt, J.M.; Kriz, W.; Thurston, G.; Augustin, H.G. The Tie-2 ligand angiopoietin-2 is stored in and rapidly released upon stimulation from endothelial cell Weibel-Palade bodies. *Blood* **2004**, *103*, 4150–4156. [CrossRef] [PubMed]
47. Scholz, A.; Plate, K.H.; Reiss, Y. Angiopoietin-2: A multifaceted cytokine that functions in both angiogenesis and inflammation. *Ann. N. Y. Acad. Sci.* **2015**, *1347*, 45–51. [CrossRef] [PubMed]
48. Kontos, C.D.; Cha, E.H.; York, J.D.; Peters, K.G. The endothelial receptor tyrosine kinase Tie1 activates phosphatidylinositol 3-kinase and Akt to inhibit apoptosis. *Mol. Cell. Biol.* **2002**, *22*, 1704–1713. [CrossRef]
49. Fiedler, U.; Krissl, T.; Koidl, S.; Weiss, C.; Koblizek, T.; Deutsch, U.; Martiny-Baron, G.; Marme, D.; Augustin, H.G. Angiopoietin-1 and angiopoietin-2 share the same binding domains in the Tie-2 receptor involving the first Ig-like loop and the epidermal growth factor-like repeats. *J. Biol. Chem.* **2003**, *278*, 1721–1727. [CrossRef] [PubMed]
50. Koblizek, T.I.; Weiss, C.; Yancopoulos, G.D.; Deutsch, U.; Risau, W. Angiopoietin-1 induces sprouting angiogenesis in vitro. *Curr. Biol. CB* **1998**, *8*, 529–532. [CrossRef] [PubMed]

51. Savant, S.; Porta, S.; Budnik, A.; Busch, K.; Hu, J.; Tisch, N.; Korn, C.; Valls, A.; Benest, A.; Terhardt, D.; et al. The orphan receptor Tie1 controls Angiogenesis and vascular remodeling by differentially regulating Tie2 in Tip and Stalk cells. *Cell Rep.* **2015**, *12*, 1761–1773. [CrossRef]
52. Procopio, W.N.; Pelavin, P.I.; Lee, W.M.; Yeilding, N.M. Angiopoietin-1 and -2 coiled coil domains mediate distinct homo-oligomerization patterns, but fibrinogen-like domains mediate ligand activity. *J. Biol. Chem.* **1999**, *274*, 30196–30201. [CrossRef]
53. Leppanen, V.; Saharinen, P.; Alitalo, K. Structural basis of Tie2 activation and Tie2/Tie1 heterodimerization. *Proc. Natl. Acad. Sci. USA* **2017**, *114*, 4376–4381. [CrossRef] [PubMed]
54. Jeansson, M.; Gawlik, A.; Anderson, G.; Li, C.; Kerjaschki, D.; Henkelman, M.; Quaggin, S. Angiopoietin-1 is essential in mouse vasculature during development and in response to injury. *J. Clin. Investig.* **2011**, *121*, 2278–2289. [CrossRef]
55. Kwak, H.J.; So, J.; Lee, S.J.; Kim, I.; Koh, G.Y. Angiopoietin-1 is an apoptosis survival factor for endothelial cells. *FEBS Lett.* **1999**, *448*, 249–253. [CrossRef]
56. Kwak, H.J.; Lee, S.J.; Lee, Y.; Ryu, C.H.; Koh, K.N.; Choi, H.Y.; Koh, J.Y. Angiopoietin-1 inhibits irradiation and mannitol-induced apoptosis in endothelial cells. *Circulation* **2000**, *101*, 2317. [CrossRef]
57. Kim, I.; Kim, H.G.; So, J.; Kwak, H.J.; Koh, J.Y. Angiopoietin-1 regulates endothelial cell survival through the phosphatidylinositol 3′-kinase/Akt signal transduction pathway. *Circ. Res.* **2000**, *86*, 24–29. [CrossRef]
58. Papapetropoulos, A.; Fulton, D.; Mahboubi, K.; Kalb, R.; O'connor, D.; Li, F.; Altieri, D.; Sessa, W. Angiopoietin-1 inhibits endothelial cell apoptosis via the akt/survivin pathway. *J. Biol. Chem.* **2000**, *275*, 9102–9105. [CrossRef] [PubMed]
59. Kontos, C.D.; Stauffer, T.P.; Yang, W.; York, J.; Huang, L.; Blanar, M.; Meyer, T.; Peters, K. Tyrosine 1101 of Tie2 is the major site of association of p85 and is required for activation of phosphatidylinositol 3-kinase and Akt. *Mol. Cell Biol.* **1998**, *18*, 4131–4140. [CrossRef] [PubMed]
60. Jones, N.; Master, Z.; Jones, J.; Bouchard, D.; Gunji, Y.; Sasaki, H.; Daly, R.; Alitalo, K.; Dumont, D. Identification of tek/Tie2 binding partners. Binding to a multifunctional docking site mediates cell survival and migration. *J. Biol. Chem.* **1999**, *274*, 30896–30905. [CrossRef]
61. Jones, N.; Chen, S.H.; Sturk, C.; Master, Z.; Tran, J.; Kerbel, R.; Dumont, D. A unique autophosphorylation site on Tie2/tek mediates dok-R phosphotyrosine binding domain binding and function. *Mol. Cell Biol.* **2003**, *23*, 2658–2668. [CrossRef] [PubMed]
62. Harfouche, R.; Gratton, J.; Yancopoulos, G.D.; Noseda, M.; Karsan, A.; Hussain, S. Angiopoietin-1 activates both anti- and proapoptotic mitogen-activated protein kinases. *FASEB J.* **2003**, *17*, 1523–1525. [CrossRef] [PubMed]
63. Kichina, J.V.; Goc, A.; Al-Husein, B.; Somanath, P.; Kandel, E. PAK1 as a therapeutic target. *Expert Opin. Ther. Targets* **2010**, *14*, 703–725. [CrossRef] [PubMed]
64. David, S.; Ghosh, C.; Mukherjee, A.; Parikh, S. Angiopoietin-1 requires IQGAP1 to activate Rac1 and promote endothelial barrier defense. *Arterioscler. Thromb. Vasc. Biol.* **2011**, *31*, 2643–2652. [CrossRef] [PubMed]
65. Tadros, A.; Hughes, D.P.; Dunmore, B.J. ABIN-2 protects endothelial cells from death and has a role in the antiapoptotic effect of Angiopoietin-1. *Blood* **2003**, *102*, 4407–4409. [CrossRef]
66. Van Huffel, S.; Delaei, F.; Heyninck, K.; Valck, D.; Beyaert, R. Identification of a novel A20-binding inhibitor of nuclear factor-kappaB activation termed ABIN-2. *J. Biol. Chem.* **2001**, *276*, 30216–30223. [CrossRef]
67. Korhonen, E.A.; Lampinen, A.; Giri, H.; Anisimov, A.; Kim, M.; Allen, B.; Fang, S.; D'Amico, G.; Sipila, T.; Lohela, M.; et al. Tie1 controls angiopoietin function in vascular remodeling and inflammation. *J. Clin. Investig.* **2016**, *126*, 3495–3510. [CrossRef]
68. Inoue, M.; Itoh, H.; Ueda, M.; Naruko, T.; Kojima, A.; Komatsu, R.; Doi, K.; Ogawa, Y.; Tamura, N.; Takaya, K.; et al. Vascular endothelial growth factor (VEGF) expression in human coronary atherosclerotic lesions: Possible pathophysiological significance of VEGF in progression of atherosclerosis. *Circulation* **1998**, *98*, 2108–2116. [CrossRef]
69. Singh, H.; Hansen, T.M.; Patel, N.; Brindle, N. The molecular balance between receptor tyrosine kinases Tie1 and Tie2 is dynamically controlled by VEGF and TNFa and regulates angiopoietin signalling. *PLoS ONE* **2012**, *7*, 29319.
70. Marron, M.B.; Singh, H.; Tahir, T.A.; Kavumkal, J.; Kim, H.; Koh, J.; Brindle, N. Regulated proteolytic processing of Tie1 modulates ligand responsiveness of the receptortyrosine kinase Tie2. *J. Biol. Chem.* **2007**, *282*, 30509–30517. [CrossRef]
71. Findley, C.M.; Cudmore, M.J.; Ahmed, A.; Kontos, C. VEGF induces Tie2 shedding via a phosphoinositide 3-kinase/Akt-dependent pathway to modulate Tie2 signaling. *Arter. Thromb. Vasc. Biol.* **2007**, *27*, 2619–2626. [CrossRef]
72. Seegar, T.C.; Eller, B.; Tzvetkova-Robev, D.; Kolev, M.; Henderson, C.; Nikilov, D.; Barton, W. Tie1-Tie2 interactions mediate functional differences between angiopoietin ligands. *Mol. Cell* **2010**, *37*, 643–655. [CrossRef]
73. Schlosser, K.; Taha, M.; Deng, Y.; McIntyre, L.; Mei, S.; Stewart, D. High circulating Angiopoietin 2 levels exacerbate pulmonary inflammation but not vascular leak or mortality in endotoxin-induced lung injury in mice. *Thorax* **2018**, *73*, 248–261. [CrossRef]
74. Zhang, Z.G.; Zhang, L.; Croll, S.D.; Chopp, M. Angiopoietin-1 reduces cerebral blood vessel leakage and ischemic lesion volume after focal cerebral embolic ischemia in mice. *Neuroscience* **2002**, *113*, 683–687. [CrossRef] [PubMed]
75. Zernecke, A.; Weber, C. Inflammatory mediators in atherosclerotic vascular disease. *Basic Res. Cardiol.* **2005**, *100*, 93–101. [CrossRef] [PubMed]
76. Davis, J.S.; Yeo, T.W.; Piera, K.A.; Woodberry, T.; Celermajer, D.; Stephens, D.; Anstey, N. Angiopoietin-2 is increased in sepsis and inversely associated with nitric oxide-dependent microvascular reactivity. *Crit. Care* **2010**, *14*, R89. [CrossRef]
77. Ghosh, C.C.; Thamm, K.; Berghelli, A.V.; Schrimpf, C.; Maski, M.; Abid, T.; Milam, K.; Rajakimar, A.; Santel, A.; Kielstein, J. Drug repurposing screen identifies Foxo1-dependent Angiopoietin-2 regulation in sepsis. *Crit. Care Med.* **2015**, *43*, 230–240. [CrossRef]

78. Leow, C.C.; Coffman, K.; Inigo, I.; Breen, S.; Czapiga, M.; Soukharev, S.; Gingles, N.; Peterson, N.; Fazenbaker, C.; Woods, R., et al. MEDI3617, a human anti angiopoietin 2 monoclonal antibody, inhibits angiogenesis and tumor growth in human tumor xenograft models. *Int. J. Oncol.* **2012**, *40*, 1321–1330. [CrossRef] [PubMed]
79. White, R.R.; Shan, S.; Rusconi, C.P.; Shetty, G.; Dewhirst, M.; Kontos, C.; Sullenger, B. Inhibition of rat corneal angiogenesis by a nuclease-resistant RNA aptamer specific for Angiopoietin-2. *Proc. Natl. Acad. Sci. USA* **2003**, *100*, 5028–5033. [CrossRef]
80. Yang, P.; Chen, N.; Yang, D.; Crane, J.; Yang, S.; Wang, H.; Dong, R.; Yi, X.; Xie, L.; Jing, G.; et al. The ratio of serum Angiopoietin-1 to Angiopoietin-2 in patients with cervical cancer is a valuable diagnostic and prognostic biomarker. *PeerJ* **2017**, *5*, 3387. [CrossRef]
81. Ackermann, M.; Verleden, S.E.; Kuehnel, M.; Haverich, A.; Welte, T.; Laenger, F.; Vanstapel, A.; Werlein, C.; Stark, H.; Tzankov, A.; et al. Pulmonary vascular endothelialitis, thrombosis, and angiogenesis in Covid-19. *N. Engl. J. Med.* **2020**, *383*, 120–128. [CrossRef]
82. Goshua, G.; Pine, A.B.; Meizlish, M.L.; Chang, C.; Zhang, H.; Bahel, P.; Baluha, A.; Bar, N.; Bona, R.; Burns, A.; et al. Endotheliopathy in COVID-19-associated coagulopathy: Evidence from a single-centre, cross-sectional study. *Lancet Haematol.* **2020**, *7*, e575–e582. [CrossRef]
83. Smadja, D.M.; Mentzer, S.J.; Fontenay, M.; Laffan, M.; Ackermann, M.; Helms, J.; Jonigk, D.; Chocron, R.; Pier, G.; Gendron, N.; et al. COVID-19 is a systemic vascular hemopathy: Insight for mechanistic and clinical aspects. *Angiogenesis* **2021**, *24*, 755–788. [CrossRef]
84. Teuwen, L.A.; Geldhof, V.; Pasut, A.; Carmeliet, P. COVID-19: The vasculature unleashed. *Nat. Rev. Immunol.* **2020**, *20*, 389–391. [CrossRef]
85. Varga, Z.; Flammer, A.J.; Steiger, P.; Haberecker, M.; Andermatt, R.; Zinkernagel, A.S.; Mehra, M.R.; Schuepbach, R.A.; Ruschitzka, F.; Moch, H. Endothelial cell infection and endotheliitis in COVID-19. *Lancet* **2020**, *395*, 1417–1418. [CrossRef]
86. Schimmel, L.; Chew, K.Y.; Stocks, C.J.; Yordanov, T.E.; Essebier, P.; Kulasinghe, A.; Monkman, J.; Dos Santos Miggiolaro, A.F.R.; Cooper, C.; de Noronha, L.; et al. Endothelial cells are not productively infected by SARS-CoV-2. *Clin. Transl. Immunol.* **2021**, *10*, e1350. [CrossRef]
87. Garcia-Ponce, A.; Chanez Paredes, S.; Castro Ochoa, K.F.; Schnoor, M. Regulation of endothelial and epithelial barrier functions by peptide hormones of the adrenomedullin family. *Tissue Barriers* **2016**, *4*, e1228439. [CrossRef]
88. Millar, F.R.; Summers, C.; Griffiths, M.J.; Toshner, M.R.; Proudfoot, A.G. The pulmonary endothelium in acute respiratory distress syndrome: Insights and therapeutic opportunities. *Thorax* **2016**, *71*, 462–473. [CrossRef]
89. Noris, M.; Benigni, A.; Remuzzi, G. The case of complement activation in COVID-19 multiorgan impact. *Kidney Int.* **2020**, *98*, 314–322. [CrossRef] [PubMed]
90. Pelaia, C.; Tinello, C.; Vatrella, A.; De Sarro, G.; Pelaia, G. Lung under attack by COVID-19-induced cytokine storm: Pathogenic mechanisms and therapeutic implications. *Ther. Adv. Respir. Dis.* **2020**, *14*, 1–9. [CrossRef] [PubMed]
91. Freeman, T.L.; Swartz, T.H. Targeting the NLRP3 Inflammasome in Severe COVID-19. *Front. Immunol.* **2020**, *11*, 1518. [CrossRef]
92. Bernard, I.; Limonta, D.; Mahal, L.K.; Hobman, T.C. Endothelium Infection and Dysregulation by SARS-CoV-2: Evidence and Caveats in COVID-19. *Viruses* **2020**, *13*, 29. [CrossRef]
93. Grobler, C.; Maphumulo, S.C.; Grobbelaar, L.M.; Bredenkamp, J.C.; Laubscher, G.J.; Lourens, P.J.; Steenkamp, J.; Kell, D.B.; Pretorius, E. Covid-19: The Rollercoaster of Fibrin (Ogen), D-Dimer, Von Willebrand Factor, P-Selectin and Their Interactions with Endothelial Cells, Platelets and Erythrocytes. *Int. J. Mol. Sci.* **2020**, *21*, 5168. [CrossRef] [PubMed]
94. Nicin, L.; Abplanalp, W.T.; Mellentin, H.; Kattih, B.; Tombor, L.; John, D.; Schmitto, J.; Heineke, J.; Emrich, F.; Arsalan, M.; et al. Cell type specific expression of the putative SARS-CoV-2 receptor ACE2 in human hearts. *Eur. Heart J.* **2020**, *41*, 1804–1806. [CrossRef] [PubMed]
95. Sluimer, J.C.; Gasc, J.M.; Hamming, I.; Goor, H.; Michaud, A.; Van den Akker, L.H.; Jutten, B.; Cleutjens, J.; Bijnens, A.; Corvol, P.; et al. Angiotensin converting enzyme 2 (ACE2) expression and activity in human carotid atherosclerotic lesions. *J. Pathol.* **2008**, *215*, 273–279. [CrossRef] [PubMed]
96. Lu, R.; Zhao, X.; Li, J.; Niu, P.; Yang, B.; Wu, H.; Wang, W.; Song, H.; Huang, B.; Zhu, N.; et al. Genomic characterisation and epidemiology of 2019 novel coronavirus: Implications for virus origins and receptor binding. *Lancet* **2020**, *395*, 565–574. [CrossRef] [PubMed]
97. Hikmet, F.; Mear, L.; Edvinsson, A.; Micke, P.; Uhlen, M.; Lindskog, C. The protein expression profile of ACE2 in human tissues. *Mol. Syst. Biol.* **2020**, *16*, 9610. [CrossRef] [PubMed]
98. Delorey, T.M.; Ziegler, C.G.; Heimberg, G.; Normand, R.; Yang, Y.; Segerstolpe, Å.; Abbondanza, D.; Stephen, J.; Ayshwarya Subramanian, F.; Montoro, D.T. COVID-19 tissue atlases reveal SARS-CoV-2 pathology and cellular targets. *Nature* **2021**, *595*, 107–113. [CrossRef]
99. Wang, P.; Luo, R.; Zhang, M.; Wang, Y.; Song, T.; Tao, T.; Li, Z.; Jin, L.; Zheng, H.; Chen, W.; et al. A cross-talk between epithelium and endothelium mediates human alveolar-capillary injury during SARS-CoV-2 infection. *Cell Death Dis.* **2020**, *11*, 1042. [CrossRef]
100. Monteil, V.; Kwon, H.; Prado, P.; Hagelkrüys, A.; Wimmer, R.A.; Stahl, M.; Leopoldi, A.; Garreta, E.; Del Pozo, C.H.; Prosper, F.; et al. Inhibition of SARS-CoV-2 Infections in Engineered Human Tissues Using Clinical-Grade Soluble Human ACE2. *Cell* **2020**, *181*, 905–913. [CrossRef]

101. Andersson, M.I.; Arancibia-Carcamo, C.V.; Auckland, K.; Baillie, J.K.; Barnes, E.; Beneke, T.; Bibi, S.; Brooks, T.; Carroll, M.; Crook, D.; et al. SARS-CoV-2 RNA detected in blood products from patients with COVID-19 is not associated with infectious virus. *Wellcome Open Res.* **2020**, *5*, 181. [CrossRef] [PubMed]
102. Ranucci, M.; Ballotta, A.; Di Dedda, U.; Baryshnikova, E.; Dei Poli, M.; Resta, M.; Falco, M.; Albano, G.; Menicanti, L. The procoagulant pattern of patients with COVID-19 acute respiratory distress syndrome. *J. Thromb. Haemost. JTH* **2020**, *18*, 1747–1751. [CrossRef] [PubMed]
103. Fodor, A.; Tiperciuc, B.; Login, C.; Orasan, O.H.; Lazar, A.L.; Buchman, C.; Hanghicel, P.; Sitar-Taut, A.; Suharoschi, R.; Vulturar, R.; et al. Endothelial Dysfunction, Inflammation, and Oxidative Stress in COVID-19-Mechanisms and Therapeutic Targets. *Oxidative Med. Cell. Longev.* **2021**, 8671713. [CrossRef] [PubMed]
104. Nagele, M.; Haubner, B.; Tanner, F.; Ruschitzka, F.; Flammer, A. Endothelial dysfunction in Covid-19: Current findings and therapeutic implications. *Atherosclerosis* **2020**, *314*, 58–62. [CrossRef] [PubMed]
105. Miesbach, W.; Makris, M. COVID-19: Coagulopathy, Risk of Thrombosis, and the Rationale for Anticoagulation. *Clin. Appl. Thromb. Hemost.* **2020**, *26*, 1076029620938149. [CrossRef] [PubMed]
106. Nguyen Dinh Cat, A.; Montezano, A.C.; Burger, D.; Touyz, R.M. Angiotensin II, NADPH oxidase, and redox signaling in the vasculature. *Antioxid. Redox Signal.* **2013**, *19*, 1110–1120. [CrossRef]
107. Iba, T.; Connors, J.M.; Levy, J.H. The coagulopathy, endotheliopathy, and vasculitis of COVID-19. *Inflamm. Res.* **2020**, *69*, 1181–1189. [CrossRef]
108. Henry, B.M.; de Oliveira, M.H.S.; Cheruiyot, I.; Benoit, J.L.; Cooper, D.S.; Lippi, G.; Le Cras, T.D.; Benoit, S.W. Circulating level of Angiopoietin-2 is associated with acute kidney injury in coronavirus disease 2019 (COVID-19). *Angiogenesis* **2021**, *24*, 403–406. [CrossRef]
109. Lu, R.X.Z.; Lai, B.F.L.; Rafatian, N.; Gustafson, D.; Campbell, S.B.; Banerjee, A.; Kozak, R.; Mossman, K.; Mubareka, S.; Howe, K.L.; et al. Vasculature-on-a-chip platform with innate immunity enables identification of angiopoietin-1 derived peptide as a therapeutic for SARS-CoV-2 induced inflammation. *Lab Chip* **2022**, *22*, 1171–1186. [CrossRef]
110. Del Valle, D.M.; Kim-Schulze, S.; Huang, H.; Beckmann, N.D.; Nirenberg, S.; Wang, B.; Lavin, Y.; Swartz, T.H.; Madduri, D.; Stock, A.; et al. An inflammatory cytokine signature predicts COVID-19 severity and survival. *Nat. Med.* **2020**, *26*, 1636–1643. [CrossRef]
111. Rendeiro, A.F.; Ravichandran, H.; Bram, Y.; Chandar, V.; Kim, J.; Meydan, C.; Park, J.; Foox, J.; Hether, T.; Warren, S.; et al. The spatial landscape of lung pathology during COVID-19 progression. *Nature* **2021**, *593*, 564–569. [CrossRef]
112. Ramaiah, M.J. mTOR inhibition and p53 activation, microRNAs: The possible therapy against pandemic COVID-19. *Gene Rep.* **2020**, *20*, 100765. [CrossRef] [PubMed]
113. Lei, X.; Shi, F.; Basu, D.; Huq, A.; Routhier, S.; Day, R.; Jin, W. Proteolytic processing of angiopoietin-like protein 4 by proprotein convertases modulates its inhibitory effects on lipoprotein lipase activity. *J. Biol. Chem.* **2011**, *286*, 15747–15756. [CrossRef]
114. Bhatraju, P.K.; Morrell, E.D.; Stanaway, I.B.; Sathe, N.A.; Srivastava, A.; Postelnicu, R.; Green, R.; Andrews, A.; Gonzalez, M.; Kratochvil, C.J.; et al. Angiopoietin-Like4 Is a Novel Marker of COVID-19 Severity. *Crit. Care Explor.* **2022**, *5*, e0827. [CrossRef]
115. Reyes, A.; Corrales, N.; Galvez, N.M.S.; Bueno, S.M.; Kalergis, A.M.; Gonzalez, P.A. Contribution of hypoxia inducible factor-1 during viral infections. *Virulence* **2020**, *11*, 1482–1500. [CrossRef]
116. Hadjadj, J.; Yatim, N.; Barnabei, L.; Corneau, A.; Boussier, J.; Smith, N.; Pere, H.; Charbit, B.; Bondet, V.; Chenevier-Gobeaux, C.; et al. Impaired type I interferon activity and inflammatory responses in severe COVID-19 patients. *Science* **2020**, *369*, 718–724. [CrossRef] [PubMed]
117. Vassiliou, A.G.; Keskinidou, C.; Jahaj, E.; Gallos, P.; Dimopoulou, I.; Kotanidou, A.; Orfanos, S.E. ICU Admission Levels of Endothelial Biomarkers as Predictors of Mortality in Critically Ill COVID-19 Patients. *Cells* **2021**, *10*, 186. [CrossRef]
118. Arab, O.A.; Bennis, Y.; Gauthier, P.; Dupont, H.; Kamel, S.; Mahjoub, Y. Association between inflammation, angiopoietins, and disease severity in critically ill COVID-19 patients: A prospective study. *Br. J. Anaesth.* **2021**, *126*, 127–130. [CrossRef]
119. Xu, S.; Ilyas, I.; Weng, J. Endothelial dysfunction in COVID-19: An overview of evidence, biomarkers, mechanisms and potential therapies. *Acta Pharmacol. Sin.* **2023**, *44*, 695–709. [CrossRef]
120. Libby, P.; Lüscher, T. COVID-19 is, in the end, an endothelial disease. *Eur. Heart J.* **2020**, *41*, 3038–3044. [CrossRef] [PubMed]
121. Martínez-Salazar, B.; Holwerda, M.; Stüdle, C.; Piragyte, I.; Mercader, N.; Engelhardt, B.; Rieben, R.; Döring, Y. COVID-19 and the Vasculature: Current Aspects and LongTerm Consequences. *Front. Cell Dev. Biol.* **2022**, *10*, 824851. [CrossRef] [PubMed]
122. Schmaier, A.A.; Pajares Hurtado, G.M.; Manickas-Hill, Z.J.; Sack, K.D.; Chen, S.M.; Bhambhani, V.; Quadir, J.; Nath, A.K.; Collier, A.Y.; Ngo, D.; et al. Tie2 activation protects against prothrombotic endothelial dysfunction in COVID-19. *JCI Insight* **2021**, *6*, e151527. [CrossRef] [PubMed]

encyclopedia

MDPI

Entry

Kidney Issues Associated with COVID-19 Disease

Periklis Dousdampanis [1,*], Athanasia Mouzaki [2], Konstantina Trigka [3], Ioannis Stefanidis [4], Konstantinos-Eugenios Galanopoulos [5], Ioannis-Santo Siavelis [6], Dionysia Stathopoulou [7] and Stelios F. Assimakopoulos [8]

1. Department of Nephrology, Saint Andrews General Hospital of Patras, 26222 Patras, Greece
2. Division of Hematology, Department of Internal Medicine, Medical School, University of Patras, 26504 Patras, Greece; mouzaki@med.upatras.gr
3. Hemodialysis Unit Kyanous Stavros Patras, 26331 Patras, Greece; ktriga@gmail.com
4. Department of Nephrology, Faculty of Medicine, School of Health Sciences, University of Thessaly, 41223 Larisa, Greece; stefanid@med.uth.gr
5. Department of Nuclear Medicine, Saint Andrews General Hospital of Patras, 26222 Patras, Greece; akigalanop@yahoo.gr
6. Department of Internal Medicine, Medical School, University of Patras, 26504 Patras, Greece; jssiav@gmail.com
7. Department of Cardiology, Saint Andrews General Hospital of Patras, 26222 Patras, Greece; dinakos75@yahoo.com
8. Division of Infectious Diseases, Department of Internal Medicine, Medical School, University of Patras, 26504 Patras, Greece; sassim@upatras.gr

* Correspondence: dousdampanis@yahoo.gr

Definition: Infection with SARS-CoV-2 and the resulting COVID-19 can cause both lung and kidney damage. SARS-CoV-2 can directly infect renal cells expressing ACE2 receptors, resulting in kidney damage, and acute kidney injury (AKI) has been reported in COVID-19 hospitalized patients. The pathophysiology of COVID-19-associated AKI is multifactorial. Local and systemic inflammation, immune system dysregulation, blood coagulation disorders, and activation of the renin-angiotensin-aldosterone system (RAAS) are factors that contribute to the development of AKI in COVID 19 disease. COVID-19 patients with kidney involvement have a poor prognosis, and patients with chronic kidney disease (CKD) infected with SARS-CoV-2 have an increased mortality risk. CKD patients with COVID-19 may develop end-stage renal disease (ESRD) requiring dialysis. In particular, patients infected with SARS-CoV-2 and requiring dialysis, as well as patients who have undergone kidney transplantation, have an increased risk of mortality and require special consideration. Nephrologists and infectious disease specialists face several clinical dilemmas in the prophylaxis and treatment of CKD patients with COVID-19. This entry presents recent data showing the effects of COVID-19 on the kidneys and CKD patients and the challenges in the management of CKD patients with COVID-19, and discusses treatment strategies for these patients.

Keywords: chronic kidney disease; COVID-19; hemodialysis; kidney transplantation; peritoneal dialysis; SARS-CoV-2

Citation: Dousdampanis, P.; Mouzaki, A.; Trigka, K.; Stefanidis, I.; Galanopoulos, K.-E.; Siavelis, I.-S.; Stathopoulou, D.; Assimakopoulos, S.F. Kidney Issues Associated with COVID-19 Disease. *Encyclopedia* **2023**, 3, 1085–1104. https://doi.org/10.3390/encyclopedia3030079

Academic Editors: Stephen Bustin, José I. López and Raffaele Barretta

Received: 24 June 2023
Revised: 18 August 2023
Accepted: 25 August 2023
Published: 31 August 2023

1. Introduction

COVID-19 has a broad clinical spectrum. In the context of COVID-19 disease, the organ most commonly affected is the lung. The kidney is another organ that can be affected by SARS-CoV-2 [1].

SARS-CoV-2 invades cells by binding its spike protein to the angiotensin-converting enzyme2 (ACE2) receptor on the cell surface [1]. Therefore, SARS-CoV-2 can affect any system in which ACE-2 receptors are present, including cardiovascular, nervous, immune, gastrointestinal, and renal systems [1].

In addition to the spike protein, SARS-CoV-2 encodes several accessory proteins, including ORF3a, ORF3b, ORF6, ORF7a, ORF7b, ORF8, ORF9b, and ORF9c. These accessory proteins play various roles in viral replication, immune evasion, and pathogenesis. Studies have shown that SARS-CoV-2 can directly infect renal cells expressing ACE2 receptors, resulting in kidney damage [2]. The virus can disrupt normal kidney function and cause inflammation and injury. The presence of SARS-CoV-2 RNA was detected in kidney tissue samples from COVID-19 patients, indicating active virus replication in the kidneys. In addition, some accessory proteins of SARS-CoV-2 were found to contribute to kidney injury. The ORF3a protein, for example, has been associated with the promotion of apoptosis and inflammation in kidney cells. It can disrupt ion transport mechanisms and impair renal filtration function [2,3]. Other studies suggest that dysregulation of the Renin-Angiotensin-Aldosterone System (RAAS), which plays a critical role in regulating blood pressure and fluid balance, may also be involved in kidney complications associated with COVID-19 [4]. The interaction between the spike protein and the ACE2 receptor may disrupt the RAAS and lead to kidney dysfunction.

It should be noted that research into the specific mechanisms underlying renal problems associated with COVID-19 is ongoing and our understanding is constantly evolving. Nevertheless, the available evidence suggests that accessory proteins of SARS-CoV-2, together with the interaction between the spike protein and the ACE2 receptor, contribute to kidney complications in COVID-19 patients.

SARS-CoV-2 activates the immune system, resulting in the production of cytokines known as cytokine release syndrome [5]. This dysregulated immune response can cause systemic inflammatory syndrome, acute distress syndrome, and multi-organ damage. This inflammatory response persists even when the viral load decreases [5].

Infection of endothelial cells causes endotheliitis, which leads to vasoconstriction. Furthermore, the synergistic effect of inflammation and hypercoagulability leads to hypoperfusion, organ ischemia, and tissue damage [6].

SARS-CoV-2 is detected in the renal parenchyma [7]. Proteinuria, hematuria, and elevated BUN and creatinine levels have been noted in SARS-CoV-2 patients. Tubular damage and collapsing glomerulopathy were observed in affected patients [8,9]. Acute tubular damage characterized by mild focal acute tubular necrosis is the predominant finding in renal biopsies from COVID-19 patients with AKI [9]. In addition, peritubular erythrocyte aggregation and glomerular fibrin thrombi with ischemic collapse have been reported [9]. Moreover, collapsing glomerulopathy associated with COVID-19 is characterized by podocyte damage [10]. The collapsing glomerulopathy associated with COVID-19 has been associated with high-risk APOL1 genotypes [11]. The relationship between COVID-19 and CKD appears to be bidirectional and complicated.

The risk of dying in hospital is higher in hospitalized COVID-19 patients with acute kidney injury (AKI) or CKD (46.4%) than in hospitalized patients without AKI or CKD (7.3%) [12]. Interestingly, hospitalized patients affected with AKI or CKD require renal replacement therapy after discharge [12].

According to secondary meta-analyses [13] and nationwide analyses [14], hospitalized COVID-19 patients with CKD, including CKD stages 3–5, maintenance dialysis, and kidney transplantation, had a higher mortality rate than COVID patients without CKD [14]. An increased mortality rate of over 25–30% has been reported in hemodialyzed patients with COVID-19 [15,16]. Hemodialysis (HD) patients have several comorbidities such as diabetes and cardiovascular disease, which makes them more susceptible to SARS-CoV-2 infection [17]. In addition, HD patients have a weaker immune system, and CKD is considered a secondary immunodeficiency that increases the risk of infection and leads to increased mortality [17]. Therefore, special considerations should be made in medical management and prophylaxis.

Management of COVID-19 kidney transplant patients is another challenge. The balance between medical treatment of COVID-19 and immunosuppressive drugs to prevent graft rejection is an important clinical problem [18]. In addition, renal transplant patients usually present with atypical symptoms that complicate the diagnosis of COVID-19 [18].

CKD patients or ESRD patients on dialysis and kidney transplant patients are at increased risk of infection. Vaccination against SARS-CoV-2 has been reported to reduce severe infections and deaths in both CKD patients and renal transplant patients [18,19]. However, isolated cases of glomerulopathy have been reported after vaccination against COVID-19 [20].

The medical management of COVID-19 CKD patients is more complicated. Drug treatment includes anti-inflammatory (nonsteroidal) agents, anticoagulants, monoclonal antibodies, and multiple antiviral therapies alone or in various combinations [21].

Even after the approval of various antiviral therapies and vaccines, the mortality rate is not under control because new variants of the virus with altered genome sequences continue to emerge [21].

Long-term effects of COVID-19 on renal function have been reported [22]. Further studies are needed to explore and understand the long-term effects of the COVID-19 pandemic. Although the World Health Organization declared the end of the COVID-19 global emergency on 5 May 2023, COVID-19 remains a public health threat.

2. Acute Kidney Injury (AKI) Associated with COVID-19

AKI is a clinical syndrome characterized by abrupt deterioration of renal function. According to initial reports, COVID-19 was not associated with AKI [23–25]. In contrast, recent data reported an increased incidence of AKI in hospitalized patients with COVID-19 [12,26,27]. Interestingly, the incidence and severity of AKI vary by region. This discrepancy is due to both the different clinical conditions and the different definitions used to determine AKI. Several studies that used the Kidney Disease Improving Global Outcomes (KDIGO) consensus definition of AKI (characterized by a decrease in GFR over 7 days or a decrease in 6-hour urine output) reported an increased incidence (over 30–50%) of AKI in hospitalized COVID-19 patients. The incidence of AKI was higher in patients who required intensive care [25,27–29].

Data from a large meta-analysis that included 49,048 hospitalized COVID-19 patients reported an increased incidence of AKI (a total of 5152 patients with AKI) in the United States and Europe (over 28.6%), whereas the incidence of AKI was lower in China (over 5.5%) [30]. Interestingly, 45% of ICU patients with AKI required renal replacement therapy (RRT) [12,26,27]. According to another large retrospective study from New York City, 46% of 3993 hospitalized patients developed AKI, and 420 patients with COVID-19-associated AKI had persistent CKD [31]. Of these patients, 35% had stage 1 AKI, 19% had stage 2 AKI, and 42% had stage 3 AKI, according to the KDIGO definition and classification. Continuous renal replacement therapy, prolonged intermittent hemodialysis, conventional intermittent hemodialysis, and peritoneal dialysis have been used to treat patients with COVID-19-associated AKI [32]. It is known that the need for RRT indicates a more severe form of AKI and is an independent mortality risk factor for these patients [33]. The incidence of AKI in hospitalized US veterans ranged from 10% to 56% [34].

In-hospital mortality was 50% in patients with AKI and 8% in patients without AKI [31]. Interestingly, renal function did not recover in one-third of patients with AKI [22]. In another study from China involving 333 hospitalized patients with COVID-19, the percentage of patients who fully recovered renal function was less than 50% [8]. It should be emphasized that incomplete recovery of AKI and/or inadequate resolution of AKI may lead to long COVID-19 renal disease with poor clinical outcome. An important difference of AKI in COVID-19 patients is that renal function in other types of AKI usually recovers after 10 days in 80% of patients [8], whereas renal function in patients with COVID-19-associated AKI recovers only after 3 weeks. The impact on the development of CKD after AKI, progression of prior CKD, and end stage renal disease remains to be determined.

It should be emphasized that the incidence of AKI has decreased over time due to our better understanding of the disease process and changes in patient management [35]. In addition, increasingly lower rates of kidney replacement therapy were observed in the second and third waves of the pandemic. Increased age, male sex, and COVID-19 disease severity were independent mortality factors in hospitalized COVID-19 patients. Mortality risk was higher in patients with advanced AKI, hematuria, and proteinuria [36]. The etiology of the association between the high mortality risk and proteinuria and hematuria in COVID-19 patients with AKI is not clear. It could be hypothesized that the presence of proteinuria and/or hematuria indicates a more severe stage of AKI. In addition, more severe stages of AKI correlate with an increased mortality risk. It should be noted that proteinuria and hematuria are not specific for COVID-19-associated AKI.

Advanced age, the presence of diabetes and obesity, cardiovascular disease, persistent CKD, acute respiratory distress syndrome and mechanical ventilation, nephrotoxic drugs, and hypotension with tissue hypoxia and vasopressor recruitment are several risk factors for the development of AKI in COVID 19 patients [37].

3. Clinical Presentation of COVID-19-Associated AKI

COVID-19-associated AKI usually presents with proteinuria or/and hematuria [8,23]. According to a study that included 701 patients with COVID-19, 44% of them had proteinuria and 26% had hematuria. Of note, the severity of proteinuria and/or hematuria was associated with the risk of mortality in these patients, indicating a significant prognostic value of these two parameters [24].

Chan et al. [31] reported that 80% of 1835 patients with AKI had hematuria and proteinuria. Of note, more than half of hospitalized patients without AKI had hematuria and 70% had proteinuria. The presence of proteinuria and hematuria in COVID-19 patients who did not meet criteria for AKI suggests the presence of renal dysfunction predisposing to AKI. In accordance with the new AKI definition for stage 1S (subclinical AKI), the presence of Fanconi syndrome has been reported in COVID-19 patients before the development of AKI [38]. Interestingly, the presence of acute proximal tubular injury observed in Fanconi syndrome may predict AKI in COVID-19 patients. In addition, proteinuria, hypophosphatemia, hyperuricosuria, and glycosuria could be considered specific biomarkers of kidney injury preceding AKI in COVID-19 patients.

The severity of proteinuria correlates with tubular damage, and can be used to identify patients predisposed to the development of AKI or those with an increased risk factor for future loss of renal function. Thus, it could be used as a marker for AKI [39]. The contribution of proteinuria to the development of CKD in these patients is unknown and remains to be determined. Identification of biomarkers for AKI in COVID-19 patients is an unresolved challenge. Interestingly, functional biomarkers such as cystatin C, damage biomarkers, and stress biomarkers could be efficient for early detection of COVID-19-associated AKI. Delayed diagnosis of AKI in COVID-19 patients may increase the mortality risk. COVID-19-associated AKI biomarkers could serve as molecular phenotyping tools for risk stratification and earlier intervention, which could improve the clinical outcome of patients.

In addition, urinalysis data should be integrated and discussed with renal biopsy results to clarify the underlying mechanism. In this regard, renal biopsy results in COVID-19 patients have shown that renal injury is predominantly tubular in critically ill patients, whereas glomerulopathies have been observed in patients with mild disease [40]. To our knowledge, there are no data combining biopsy results with urinalysis to determine the underlying mechanism of COVID-19-associated AKI.

COVID-19-associated nephropathy (COVAN), which includes focal segmental glomerulosclerosis (FSGS) and collapsing glomerulopathy, frequently occurs in black patients because patients of African descent are carriers of APOL1 risk variants [10]. COVAN presents with proteinuria in the nephritic range and microscopic hematuria [10].

4. Pathophysiology of AKI in COVID-19 Patients

The pathophysiology of AKI in COVID-19 patients is multifactorial and complicated. Local and systemic inflammation, immune system activation, endothelial and coagulation disorders, and RAAS activation are involved in the underlying pathophysiology [41]. In addition, nonspecific factors such as mechanical ventilation, cardiac dysfunction, hemodynamic instability, and drug nephrotoxicity contribute to the development of AKI [41].

Data from autopsy studies have shown that acute tubular injury is the most common finding in COVID-19 patients with AKI [42–44]. Acute tubular injury with mild focal acute tubular necrosis has been observed in postmortem renal specimens from COVID-19 patients with AKI [42–44]. Acute tubular injury, collapsing glomerulopathy, endothelial damage, and thrombotic microangiopathy were noted in biopsies from patients with COVID-19-associated AKI [45]. In these studies, viral renal infection was not detected or was detected in only a fraction of biopsies. However, in other studies, direct viral tropism of the kidney was detected [46–48]. In one study [47], viral RNA was detected in the renal tissue of 23 of 32 patients with AKI compared with 3 of 7 patients without AKI. In another study [48], virus was detected in glomeruli; SARS-CoV-2 was also detected in urine samples, suggesting release of virus from infected tubular epithelial cells or increased glomerular filtration of viral fragments.

5. COVAN

Collapsing nephropathy is a variant of FSGS and is characterized by severe proteinuria, hypertension, and rapid loss of renal function. COVAN has been reported in African American patients with COVID-19, particularly those with apolipoprotein L1 allele [10,40]. COVAN has been observed in COVID-19 patients without severe respiratory disease and with isolated AKI, and in patients with proteinuria in the nephritic range [49]. Collapsing nephropathy has been described in HIV patients and in association with various viral infections caused mainly byparvovirusB19, cytomegalovirus, and Epstein-Barr virus [10,49]. In addition, collapsing nephropathy is associated with black race [10,49]. Collapsing glomerulopathy is characterized by collapse of glomerular tufts with hypertrophy and hyperplasia of podocytes. It is accompanied by acute tubular injury and inflammation of the interstitium [10,40].

The incidence, prognosis, and contribution to CKD and ESRD are unknown. In this context, the pathophysiology of COVAN is also unclear. Because collapsing nephropathy is observed in patients with HIV infection, COVAN might be thought to share the same mechanism as HIVAN nephropathy. Podocyte damage might play a crucial role in this pathophysiological mechanism.

Giannini et al. [50] reported that patients with COVAN have a poor prognosis, the majority of patients with COVAN developed advanced CKD and one third required renal replacement therapy or died after one year. A definitive treatment for COVAN remains unclear. Treatment with high-dose steroids in combination with inhibitors of the renin-angiotensin-aldosterone system may be beneficial in the treatment of COVAN, but this has not yet been proven [50].

6. Coagulation Disorders and Endothelial Dysfunction

Systemic microvascular and macrovascular thrombosis in kidneys and lungs was observed in COVID-19 patients [51]. SARS-CoV-2 affects the endothelium, and vascular endotheliitis has been reported in association with COVID-19 [51]. Several biomarkers of coagulation, fibrinolysis activation, and endothelial injury, including selectins and von Willebrand factor antigen, have been associated with poor prognosis and increased mortality risk [52]. Microvascular inflammation leads to endothelial activation and vasodilation with increased vascular permeability, resulting in prothrombotic states [53]. Furthermore, activation of the C5 complement pathway promotes inflammation and the coagulation cascade [54]. Necrotic cell-derived damage-associated molecular patterns may contribute to endothelial injury [55]. SARS-CoV-2 binds to platelets via ACE2 and induces thrombosis in this manner [56]. Interestingly, in severe COVID-19, high titers of prothrombotic autoantibodies were found to contribute to inflammation and thrombosis [57]. Thus, endothelial damage, platelet activation, and coagulation disorders may contribute to the pathophysiology of COVID-19-AKI.

Thrombotic microangiopathy has been reported in COVID-19 patients [58]. COVID-19-associated thrombotic microangiopathy is a severe complication with poor prognosis and is characterized by hemolytic anemia, thrombocytopenia, and renal failure [59].

SARS-CoV-2 can cause atypical hemolytic syndrome (aHUS) through endothelial dysfunction and direct activation of the alternative complement pathway [60].

The spike protein of SARS-CoV-2 is located in the renal tubules and activates the alternative complement pathway by competing with complement factor H [61]. In addition, complement elements were identified in the microvasculature of COVID-19 patients.

The membrane attack complex accumulates on renal tubules due to complement activation and promotes damage to microvascular epithelial cells, activation of the coagulation cascade, and deposition of fibrin, leading to tissue damage [62].

The anti-inflammatory and antithrombotic effects of nitric oxide, which are due to complement activation, are lost in aHUS associated with COVID-19 [63].

Thus, COVID-19-associated aHUS is an example of how SARS-CoV-2 can cause kidney injury by promoting inflammation, endothelial dysfunction, complement activation, and thrombotic microangiopathy. Interestingly, renal artery thrombosis with concomitant AKI has been reported in COVID-19 patients [64].

7. Involvement of the Immune System

In COVID-19, altered innate and adaptive immune responses have been reported, characterized by immunosenescence and including low-grade inflammation, contributing to organ dysfunction and ineffective T-cell response and antibody production [65,66], likely contributing to the high mortality risk observed in elderly patients [67].

Inflammation plays a critical role in the pathogenesis of AKI [41]. Increased production of inflammatory mediators such as TNF-α and FAS has been observed in COVID-19 [68]. These mediators bind to their specific receptors expressed by renal endothelial and epithelial cells, leading to direct injury [69]. Similar interactions have also been observed in animal models of sepsis with AKI [70].

SARS-CoV-2 can inhibit the release of IFN [71], a cytokine that suppresses viral replication. In the context of COVID-19-AKI, IFN has opposite effects: IFN is a mediator of glomerular injury and can lead to podocyte loss and glomerulosclerosis [72]. Activation of the IFN pathway promotes podocyte damage, leading to proteinuria [73]. In addition, APOL1 risk alleles trigger glomerular damage via the interferon signaling pathway [74]. On the other hand, administration of IFN to COVID-19 patients improves viral clearance and lowers IL-6 and C-reactive protein levels [71]. Patients with severe COVID-19 have autoantibodies against type I IFNs. In addition, patients with low INF-αlevels have a higher risk of severe COVID-19 than patients with high interferon levels, indicating a protective role of IFN against COVID-19 [75].

Uncontrolled and sustained activation of the complement cascade can lead to inflammation with accompanying tissue injury. Detection of C3c and C3d in renal arteries and glomerular capillaries, C3d in tubules, and C5b-9 in renal arterioles and tubular basement membrane has been reported [75]. According to these results, activation of the lectin pathway and the classical pathway appears to occur in peritubular capillaries and renal arteries, whereas the alternative pathway mediates tubular injury [75].

Complement activation is involved in endothelial dysfunction. More specifically, C5a binds to its endothelial receptor and promotes upregulation of tissue factor and loss of thrombomodulin with concomitant activation of coagulation and platelet adhesion and aggregation [76]. C5b-9 induces endothelial dysfunction, inflammation, and coagulation [76,77]. Interestingly, binding of C5a to its receptor C5aR contributes to cellular senescence by promoting DNA methylation of genes, and in this context, may play a role in the pathogenesis of AKI [77].

Decreased numbers of CD4+ and CD8+ T lymphocytes have been observed in COVID-19 patients [65]. In addition, the number of plasmacytoid dendritic cells, eosinophils, and natural killer cells is decreased [78].

Nuclear factor erythroid 2-related factor (NRF2), a transcription factor involved in the regulation of antioxidant activity, is suppressed in COVID-19 [79]. NRF2 binds to its inhibitor Kelch-like ECH-associated protein 1 (KEAP1) and remains inactive in the cytosol. Viral infection promotes oxidative stress, which leads to inactivation of KEAP1; consequently, NRF2 becomes active and induces the expression of genes responsible for stress-induced cell death [79]. In addition, NRF2 agonists have antiviral effects [80]. Data from experimental models of AKI showed that increased expression of NRF2 by T cells protects renal function [80]; specifically, NRF2 protects against kidney injury caused by ischemia and nephrotoxic drugs [81]. Thus, NRF2 is a promising therapeutic target for both COVID-19 and AKI.

Soluble ACE-2 or plasma ACE-2 is the ACE-2 enzyme domain derived from the cell surface. Soluble ACE-2 can bind SARS-CoV-2, and elevated levels of soluble ACE-2 were found in the plasma of critically ill COVID-19 patients [82]. The high affinity of the spike protein for ACE-2, which acts as a receptor for virus entry into cells, may promote the formation of SARS-CoV-2-soluble ACE-2 complexes and the formation of autoantibodies against ACE-2 in tissues [83,84]. Because ACE-2 has high homology (over 42%) with ACE, which is expressed on the surface of most types of leukocytes, autoantibodies against ACE-2 can cross-react with ACE and cause tissue inflammation and organ damage [84].

A cytokine storm is the result of hyperactivity of the immune system, including T cells, macrophages, and natural killer cells [85]. A high release of mediators and inflammatory cytokines, including IL-6, indicates both hyperactivation of the humoral immune system and a hyperinflammatory state [41]. In this context, a marked increase in acute-phase inflammatory markers, lymphopenia, and coagulation disorders have been reported in severe COVID-19 [41]. Of note, IL-6 mediates organ damage, including AKI [86,87]. According to a meta-analysis, elevated serum levels of IL-6 are associated with poor clinical outcome including death [88]. Interestingly, serum levels of IL-6 are lower in severe COVID-19 compared with those observed in sepsis and acute respiratory distress syndrome (ARDS) [89].

8. Other Factors Contributing to the Development of AKI

The acute hypoxemia observed in COVID-19 patients requiring mechanical ventilation may increase renal vascular resistance, which in turn contributes to renal hypoperfusion leading to acute tubular injury and AKI [90,91]. The increased concentrations of IL-6 caused by both decreased renal clearance and increased IL-6 production may contribute to respiratory failure and AKI, suggesting a lung-kidney interaction [91]. Interestingly, mechanical ventilation is a risk factor for the development of AKI in severe COVID-19 [92]. It appears that mechanical ventilation contributes to the pathophysiology of AKI via immune-mediated processes and hemodynamic factors [92]. Notably, the positive association between mechanical ventilation and AKI reflects the severity of the disease [34].

Interaction between the cardiovascular system and the kidneys contributes to the development of AKI. Cases of acute myocarditis and myocardial injury associated with COVID-19 have been reported [93,94]. The impaired cardiac function with decreased cardiac output and venous congestion seen in these pathological situations may contribute to the development of AKI by decreasing renal perfusion [95].

In the context of ARDS, cardiac output may decrease due to decreased right ventric ular preload and increased right ventricular afterload caused by the use of high positive end-expiratory pressure and/or high tidal volumes [92]. Right sided heart failure, in combination with increased venous pressure, leads to an increase in interstitial and tubular hydrostatic pressure, resulting in a decrease in glomerular filtration rate (GFR) [96].

Nephrotoxicity of drugs is another important risk factor for the development of AKI in COVID-19 patients. Vancomycin, colistin, and aminoglycosides must be used with caution because of their potential nephrotoxicity [97]. Calculation of GFR and dose adjustment according to renal function are required.

Remdesivir is a nucleotide analog with antiviral activity. It is excreted through the kidney and is potentially nephrotoxic, causing mitochondrial damage to renal tubular epithelial cells. Nephrotoxicity of remdesivir has been observed after prolonged use or at high doses [98,99].

Rhabdomyolysis is caused by skeletal muscle damage and commonly occurs after various viral infections, including COVID-19. Rhabdomyolysis is another nonimmune cause of AKI [100]. Myoglobin released into the blood after muscle injury exerts its nephrotoxic effects via renal vasoconstriction, formation of intratubular deposits, and direct action on tubular epithelial cells [100].

Patients on extracorporeal membrane oxygenation (ECMO) are at increased risk of developing AKI. Shaefi et al. [101] reported that 22% of patients with respiratory failure on ECMO required renal replacement therapy. Schmidt et al. [102] also reported that the percentage of patients on ECMO who required renal replacement therapy was higher (over 46%). Secondary infections such as cannula infections and ventilator-associated pneumonia, hemolysis, blending, venous congestion, and inflammation should be considered as possible mechanisms for AKI in these patients [102,103].

Overall, acute tubular injury occurs in association with COVID-19. Endothelial dysfunction, microvascular thrombi, local and systemic inflammation, and altered immune response contribute to AKI. Treatment and strategies to prevent progression of the disease and avoid the need for mechanical ventilation may prevent AKI. Until there is a specific treatment for AKI, the management of AKI associated with COVID-19 is no different from that in other situations; (see Figure 1.)

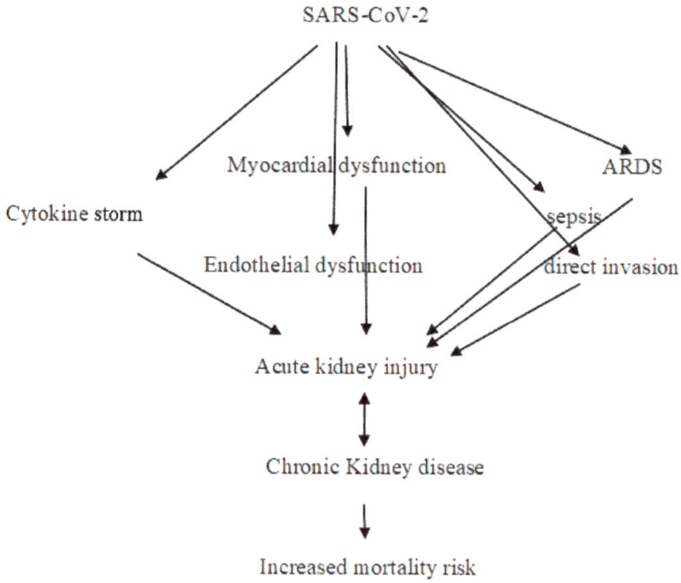

Figure 1. The interplay of SARS-CoV-2 and the kidney.

9. AKI and Progression to CKD

There is clinical evidence that AKI accelerates the progression to CKD [104]. Evidence from animal models of AKI suggests several potential mechanisms of progression to CKD, including fibrosis, microvascular rarefaction, tubular and interstitial damage, and glomerulosclerosis [105]. In addition, older age is a risk factor for COVID-19-associated AKI, and kidney aging is a risk factor for CKD. Thus, elderly patients with COVID-19 have a double risk (kidney aging +COVID-19-associated AKI) for progression to CKD.

AKI and CKD share several pathophysiological mechanisms, including glomerular and tubular cell death, local and systemic inflammation, and fibrosis [106]. In addition, several epidemiological studies reported that elderly patients with concomitant diseases such as diabetes, hypertension, heart failure, and obesity are at increased risk for COVID-19-associated AKI [103]. All of these parameters are also risk factors for CKD. Thus, there is a reciprocal relationship between AKI and CKD.

AKI causes both a decrease in the number of peritubular capillaries and a decrease in the quality of the remaining capillaries, leading to a decrease in renal blood flow [107]. At the same time, decreased renal blood flow leads to hypoxia, tubular epithelial cell damage, and apoptosis. Hypoxia triggers collagen production by fibroblasts, leading to fibrosis [108].

It must be emphasized that the long-term effects of AKI on renal function have not been fully elucidated, as most studies have focused on in-hospital outcomes, including the incidence of AKI and mortality. Therefore, there is a need for clinical studies focusing on the long-term effects of AKI on renal function.

However, two studies with 10 years of follow-up suggest that AKI is an independent risk factor for ESRD and all-cause mortality [109,110]. In addition, patients with a history of AKI had a 9-fold higher adjusted risk for CKD and a 3-fold higher adjusted risk for progression to ESRD [91].

As previously mentioned, hospitalized patients with COVID-19-associated AKI are at higher risk for renal replacement therapy, and the mortality rate was higher compared with patients without AKI [26]. Interestingly, only 30% of patients with COVID-19-associated AKI survived and recovered renal function [26].

10. COVID-19 and Cardiorenal Syndrome

Cardiac events may occur in patients with COVID-19-associated AKI, suggesting a possible role of cardiorenal syndrome [111]. As mentioned previously, in the clinical setting of COVID-19, there is an interaction between the affected organs. AKI leads to volume overload resulting in cardiac dysfunction, and conversely, cardiomyopathy caused by COVID-19 may lead to hypotension, renal hypoperfusion, and renal congestion, resulting in decreased GFR [111]. Cardiorenal syndrome carries a high risk of mortality and morbidity for COVID-19 patients and increases the healthcare costs associated with the disease [111].

SARS-CoV-2 can affect both the heart and kidneys through several mechanisms: first, a direct effect; second, a cytokine storm leading to multiorgan dysfunction; and third, induction of thrombotic microangiopathy [112]. In addition, the systemic coagulopathy associated with COVID-19 can lead to renal thrombosis and/or acute coronary syndrome [112].

Hypertension and atherosclerosis are common risk factors for CKD and cardiac dysfunction. According to the National Health Commission of China, 35% of patients with COVID-19 had hypertension, which is considered a negative prognostic factor [113]. COVID-19 patients with hypertension have higher levels of the inflammatory cytokines TNF-α and IL-6, which contributes to endothelial dysfunction and oxidative stress, which in turn promote the development of CKD and heart failure [111].

Inflammation leading to atherosclerosis has become a major problem for COVID-19 patients because it can cause cardiovascular events. Dysregulation of T cells, uncontrolled inflammation, and a cytokine storm likely contribute to the progression of atherosclerosis. Several factors involved in the pathophysiology of atherosclerosis, such as IL-1β, IL-6, IL-7, IL-8, TNF-α, IFNs, fibroblast growth factor, monocyte chemoattractant protein, macrophage inflammatory protein-1α, Von Willebrand factor antigen, and factor VIII, were significantly increased in COVID-19 patients [100,114].

In cardiorenal syndrome, angiotensin 2 promotes fibroblast proliferation, fibrosis, and hypertrophy and increases blood pressure by acting as a vasoconstrictor and causing water and salt retention. RAAS blockers have been successfully used to treat hypertension, CKD, and heart failure because of their vasodilatory, antifibrotic, and antiproteinuric effects, and they have recently been shown to have a protective effect on COVID-19 patients regardless of concomitant diseases [115].

11. COVID-19 in Dialysis Patients

The majority of patients on HD have advanced age and concomitant diseases, such as diabetes, hypertension, and cardiovascular disease. In addition, due to the immunological aging associated with uremia, these patients have a weak immune system with lower numbers of circulating CD4+ and CD8+ T cells compared with patients who are not on dialysis [116]. For these reasons, COVID-19 patients undergoing HD require more attention in their management, as they have a higher mortality risk and a worse prognosis.

The different clinical symptoms of COVID-19 in HD patients complicate their management. According to initial reports, the most common symptoms of COVID-19 patients in HD were diarrhea (80%), fever (60%), and fatigue (60%) [117]. In a study involving 65 HD centers, it was reported that 2% of HD patients tested positive for COVID-19; of these patients, 50% had fever and 20% were asymptomatic [118]. However, symptoms may vary due to infection with different SARS-CoV-2 variants. The proportion of asymptomatic SARS-CoV-2 infections in HD patients varies from 10% to 50% of patients [119]. In patients with advanced CKD infected with SARS-CoV-2, especially those on HD, viral clearance is delayed. More than two-thirds of these patients are SARS-CoV-2-positive.

The majority of COVID-19 patients on HD develop a strong antibody response. This may be due to HD patients developing more severe disease, likely associated with a stronger immune response to the virus. In addition, symptomatic HD patients had higher antibody titers to SARS-CoV-2 than asymptomatic patients [120]. Antibodies can protect against reinfection with SARS-CoV-2, but this protection is incomplete. According to a large observational study involving 2337 HD patients, serologic evidence of previous infection was associated with a greater than 45% risk of reinfection [121]. The absence of antibodies was found in 5% to 10% of HD patients. To note, these studies were conducted when the wild-type strain of the virus was prevalent. Prevention of reinfection by the delta and omicron variants of SARS-CoV-2 has not been studied in HD patients.

The mortality rate of COVID-19 patients on HD is 30% higher than in the general population with COVID-19 [118], and according to the European Dialysis and Transplantation Association Registry report, the mortality rate is over 25% [15]. The mortality of the first wave in HD patients was higher than the mortality of the subsequent viral variants, which were less pathogenic than those of the first wave in HD patients.

Another important issue is the high risk of SARS-CoV-2 infection in HD centers. According to a study in a single center in Wuhan, 20% of HD patients and 15% of staff were COVID-19-positive [122]. Hsu et al. [123] proposed guidelines to reduce the risk of SARS-CoV-2 transmission in HD centers.

Even now that the pandemic has subsided, there is still a risk of transmission. Therefore, the authors suggest that both patients and staff should continue to be educated and trained about COVID-19 prevention and management. In addition, screening strategies and education of HD patients about COVID-19 should continue. Rapid testing for SARS-CoV-2 in HD patients and personnel should continue to identify asymptomatic patients. It should be noted that patients and staff must be vaccinated against SARS-CoV-2.

According to a multicenter study from Wuhan involving 818 patients on peritoneal dialysis (PD), the incidence of symptomatic COVID-19 in PD patients was the same as in the general population [124].

PD is home dialysis, where the patient is isolated and the risk of infection is lower compared with HD patients. In addition, PD patients have been trained and educated in their method, and they follow hygiene rules and measures to prevent peritonitis. Therefore, PD patients should be more aware of the risk of infection.

Compared with HD, PD associated with COVID-19 may have some disadvantages. The introduction of intraperitoneal fluid from PD solutions may increase intraperitoneal pressure, which affects respiratory function.

Peritonitis is the most common complication of PD. It is well known that after peritonitis, the function of peritoneal membrane transport is impaired. Ultrafiltration failure due to peritonitis may lead to hypervolemia and dyspnea due to overload. Therefore, in severe COVID-19 and PD peritonitis, pulmonary function may worsen.

Gastrointestinal symptoms of COVID-19 have also been reported. Therefore, confusion of gastrointestinal symptoms of COVID-19 with those of PD peritonitis could lead to misdiagnosis of PD peritonitis.

Interestingly, Jeloka et al. [125] suggested that in the COVID-19 pandemic era, PD patients with peritonitis could be managed by video consultation to avoid hospitalization.

Data from a study of 419 hospitalized patients with ERSD, only 11 patients were on PD. PD patients had mild disease and 9 of 11 patients were discharged [126].

Data from an observational study in Turkey reported that the mortality rate was high (46.2%) in PD-hospitalized patients with COVID-19 [127]. In addition, according to the European Renal Association database, COVID-19 PD patients had a higher mortality risk than HD patients, even after accounting for patient characteristics and disease severity [15].

12. COVID-19 and Kidney Transplantation

Data from Spain and France revealed an average infection rate of 14/1000 transplants at risk [128]. Similar incidences have been reported by the Belgian Society of Nephrology and by other multicenter studies [129].

In the first wave, the hospitalization rate exceeded 80%. The mean age of transplant recipients with COVID-19 was 60 years, two-thirds were male, 80% had hypertension, and 25% had diabetes [129].

Kidney transplant patients may be at increased risk for severe disease due to immunosuppressive drugs and comorbidities. However, data are limited, and the incidence of ARDS in hospitalized kidney transplant patients varies from 12.1% to 68% [128].

The mortality risk is extremely high in hospitalized transplant patients with COVID-19. According to a meta-analysis that included 20 studies, the risk of mortality is higher in kidney transplant patients than in the general population. The risk of mortality ranges from 18% to 43% [129]. Older age, higher plasma viral load, and higher levels of proinflammatory markers were risk factors for mortality [130].

Most studies involved long-term stable recipients, and there are few data for the short-term period. However, the mortality rate in early transplant recipients with COVID-19 is high, ranging from 37% to 46%. Older age, high steroid doses, and mechanical ventilation were mortality risk factors [131].

Of note, the majority of studies were conducted in the first and second waves. Recent data from the United States report lower hospitalization rates (26% vs. 60%) and mortality rates (over 2%) during the predominance of the omicron variants. The mortality rate of transplant patients infected with the omicron variants was 4% [131]. Thus, the overall impression is that mortality is lower with omicron variants but higher than in the general population [131].

Previous recommendations for the use of immunosuppressive drugs (reduced dose and/or discontinuation) were for the first and second waves [132].

Given the prevalence of the "milder" variants, there is currently no need to change immunosuppressive therapy in asymptomatic transplant patients or in patients with mild disease. However, in severe disease with COVID-19 pneumonia, the recommendation of the DESCARTES working group of ERA-EDTA should be considered [131,132]. Current recommendations depend on disease severity and risk stratification [132].

13. Therapeutic Strategies for COVID-19 in CKD Patients

Antiviral Drugs and Monoclonal Antibodies

Remdesivir, nirmatrelvir with ritonavir and molnupiravil are currently approved for the treatment of COVID-19. Remdesivir is an intravenous antiviral agent approved for the treatment of COVID-19 in adults and paediatric patients who require hospitalization. Its nephrotoxicity and dose adjustments in CKD patients have not been well evaluated, but it is not recommended in eGFR < 30 mL/min. The excipient sulfobutylether-β-cyclodextrin accumulates in patients with reduced renal function. For eGFR ≥ 30 mL/min, no dosage adjustment is needed. Regarding the oral therapeutic options for COVID-19, for molnupiravir, there is no need for dosage adjustment in renal impairment, while nirmatrelvir with ritonavir require dosage adjustments according to eGFR level (<30, 30–60, ≥60 mL/min).

The antiviral monoclonal antibodies Sotrovimab and casirivimab + imdevimaband bamlanivimab + etesevimab are not active against Omicron variants and are not currently used (Sotrovimab has activity against Omicron BA.1 but not BA.2). No renal dose adjustments were required for these treatment options. Bebtelovimab presents activity against Omicron BA.1 and BA.2 and does not require dosage adjustment in patients with renal impairment. The tixagevimab-cilgavimab combination used for the pre-exposure prophylaxis against COVID-19 in immunosuppressed high-risk patients does not need dosage adjustments according to renal function impairment, but also possess limited activity against currently circulating SARS-CoV-2 variants.

With regard to monoclonal antibodies used for their anti-inflammatory action, tocilizumab is an IL-6 inhibitor with no need for dosage adjustments in patients with mild or moderate renal impairment, but there are only scarce data on severe renal impairment. Baricitinib and tofacitinib are JAK-inhibitors whose dose is adjusted according to eGFR. Anakinra is an anti-IL-1 factor that should not be used in patients with eGFR < 30 mL/min. Vilobelimab is an anti-complement factor with lack of adequate data in patients with renal impairment [21] (Table 1).

Table 1. Antiviral drugs and monoclonal antibodies used in COVID-19 patients.

Antiviral Drugs
(1) Intravenous
Remdesevir: no renal dosage adjustment is needed but not recommended in e-GFR ≤ 30 mL/min
(2) Oral
Molnupiravir: no renal dosage adjustement
Nirmatrelvir + Ritonavir : renal dosage adjustement
Monoclonal Antibodies
Sotrovimab: no renal dosage adjustement
Casirivimab + imdevimaband: no renal dosage adjustement
Bamlanivimab + etesevimab: no renal dosage adjustement
Bebtelovimab: no renal dosage adjustement
Tixagevimab-cilgavimab: no renal dosage adjustement
Baricitinib: renal dosage adjustement
Tofacitinib: renal dosage adjustement
Anakinra: not recommended in e-GFR ≤ 30 mL/min
Vilobelimab: no data in CKD patients

14. Vaccines

There is clinical evidence that the immunogenicity of the mRNA-1273 vaccine is better than that of the BNT162b2 vaccine in HD patients.

Anand et al. [133] reported that more than one in five HD patients had an attenuated immune response to the vaccines, suggesting that vaccination against COVID-19 is less effective in this subgroup. The authors concluded that poor health, uremia, and prolonged duration of end-stage kidney disease increase the risk of a suboptimal response.

Interestingly, the development of a serologic response is delayed in HD patients. A third dose of vaccine increases antibody titers in all HD patients, and patients with a poor initial response benefit from the third dose [17].

Antibody titers to SARS-CoV-2 were higher with the mRNA-1273 vaccine than with the BNT162b2 vaccine in patients who reached the threshold of 590 BAU/mL [17]. Accordingly, the cellular response was more intense with mRNA-1273 than with BNT162b2 vaccine [17].

Both mRNA vaccines appear to have near-maximal clinical efficacy, but these studies were conducted when wild-type virus was prevalent in healthy subjects [17]. Whether the better immunogenicity of mRNA-1273 translates into better protection for HD patients remains to be determined. In this regard, the protection of mRNA-1273 appears to be inadequate.

Limited data are available on the immunogenicity of the other vaccines in HD patients. Neutralizing antibodies to the alpha, beta, and delta variants were higher after vaccination with BNT162b2 vaccine than when AZD1222 was used.

Of note, in HD patients, antibody responses to Ad26.COV2.S vaccine were lower compared with mRNA vaccines [17].

Hsu et al. [134] reported that 67.5% ofAd26.COV2.S, 32.1%of BNT162b2, and 12.3% of mRNA-1273 recipients had no antibodies to SARS-CoV-2 four months after vaccination.

According to a recent large meta-analysis that included 5628 HD patients, the vaccines elicited an adequate immune response (immune efficiency 87.5%) and may be protective against SARS-CoV-2 despite lower immunogenicity rates compared with the general population [135]. Notably, data from a meta-analysis have shown that vaccines are effective against SARS-CoV-2 variants [136–138].

There are limited data on humoral response to vaccination in HD and PD patients. Some studies reported that antibody titers were higher in PD patients compared with HD patients, whereas in other studies, antibody titers were similar in PD and HD patients [139,140].

IgA nephropathy, minimal change disease, membranous nephropathy, and pauci-immune necrotizing glomerulonephritis have been reported after mRNA-based SARS-CoV-2 vaccination, but causality remains unproven [141]. In addition, many of the reported vaccine-associated glomerulonephritides have been associated with COVID-19 infection itself [142].

Diebolt et al. [143] reported that sporadic cases of new-onset glomerulonephritis after mRNA-based SARS-CoV-2 vaccination were due to temporal coincidence. Overall, cases of glomerulopathyhave been reported after vaccination against COVID-19, but there is no evidence for the role of the vaccines.

15. Post-COVID-19 Syndrome

At the beginning of the pandemic, there were several reports of the long-term consequences of COVID-19. Post-COVID-19 syndrome is defined as a heterogeneous clinical syndrome of new onset. Usually, it appears 3 months after COVID-19 infection and it is characterized by symptoms lasting at least 2 months, which are not explained by an alternative diagnosis. Huang et al. [144] reported the long-term consequences of COVID-19 patients after discharge. In 35% of patients with COVID-19-associated AKI, GFR had decreased after a follow-up period of 6 months [145]. A retrospective cohort study found that patients with COVID-19-associated AKI had a greater decrease in GFR than patients with other types of AKI [145]. Another large retrospective study reported that 90,000 patients had a higher incidence of AKI 30 days after the diagnosis of COVID-19 [146]. In addition, a higher incidence of ESRD was found in COVID-19. In this regard, Gu et al. [147] reported similar findings. More specifically, COVID-19 patients with stage 3 AKI had 17.8% higher deterioration of renal function compared with patients without AKI.

The long-term consequences of COVID-19 on renal function are of great concern. COVID-19 can affect the kidney through direct and indirect effects. It is likely that many of these effects will persist after COVID-19 recovery and lead to an increased risk of CKD or/and recurrent AKI. In addition, the presence of diabetes may delay recovery or exacerbate the disease. Interestingly, the decline of renal function in the post COVID-19 period is multifactorial. Chronic inflammation, tubular injury, maladaptive and delayed repair of AKI, cardiac disease, and diabetes may contribute to the pathogenesis of post-COVID-19 syndrome [148]. A nephrological follow-up at 3 months for at least 12 months after hospital discharge for AKI-associated COVID-19 patients is needed.

It should be noted, that there is no specific treatment for post-COVID-19 syndrome.

16. Conclusions

- The relationship between COVID-19 and CKD is bidirectional.
- COVID-19 causes AKI and may exacerbate persistent CKD, and CKD is a risk factor for COVID-19.
- In this context, there are several common risk factors, including advanced age, diabetes, hypertension, and cardiovascular disease.
- Therefore, it is not surprising that the coexistence of COVID-19 and CKD is associated with higher morbidity and mortality.
- Further large-scale prospective cohort studies are needed to elucidate this association.

Author Contributions: P.D., conceptualization, data collection, writing, review and editing; K.T., data collection and editing; I.S., review and editing; K.-E.G., data collection; I.-S.S., data collection; D.S., data collection; A.M., review and editing; S.F.A., review and editing. All authors have read and agreed to the published version of the manuscript.

Funding: This research received no external funding.

Conflicts of Interest: The authors declare no conflict of interest.

References

1. Jackson, C.B.; Farzan, M.; Chen, B.; Hyeryun, C. Mechanisms of SARS-CoV-2 entry into cells. *Nat. Rev. Mol. Cell Biol.* **2022**, *23*, 3–20. [CrossRef]
2. Zandi, M.; Shafaati, M.; Kalantar-Neyestanaki, D.; Pourghadamyari, H.; Fani, M.; Soltani, S.; Kaleji, H.; Abbasi, S. The role of SARS-CoV-2 accessory proteins in immune evasion. *Biomed Pharmacother* **2022**, *156*, 113889. [CrossRef]
3. Zandi, M. ORF9c and ORF10 as accessory proteins of SARS-CoV-2 in immune evasion. *Nat. Rev. Immunol.* **2022**, *22*, 331. [CrossRef]
4. Dettlaff-Pokora, A.; Swierczynski, J. Dysregulation of the Renin-Angiotensin- Aldosterone System (RAA) in Patients Infected with SARS-CoV-2-Possible Clinical Consequences. *Int. J. Mol. Sci.* **2021**, *22*, 4503. [CrossRef]
5. Hu, B.; Huang, S.; Yin, L. The cytokinestorm and COVID-19. *J. Med. Virol.* **2021**, *93*, 250–256. [CrossRef] [PubMed]
6. Kaklamanos, A.; Belogiannis, K.; Skendros, P.; Gorgoulis, V.G.; Vlachoyiannopoulos, P.G.; Tzioufas, A.G. COVID-19 Immunobiology: Lessons Learned, New Questions Arise. *Front. Immunol.* **2021**, *12*, 719023. [CrossRef] [PubMed]
7. Hassler, L.; Batlle, D. Potential SARS-CoV-2 kidney infection and paths to injury. *Nat. Rev. Nephrol.* **2022**, *18*, 275–276. [CrossRef] [PubMed]
8. Pei, G.; Zhang, Z.; Peng, J.; Liu, L.; Zhang, C.; Yu, C.; Ma, Z.; Huang, Y.; Liu, W.; Yao, Y.; et al. Renal Involvement and Early Prognosis in Patients with COVID-19 Pneumonia. *J. Am. Soc. Nephrol.* **2020**, *31*, 1157–1165. [CrossRef]
9. Kudose, S.; Batal, I.; Santoriello, D.; Xu, K.; Barasch, J.; Peleg, Y.; Canetta, P.; Ratner, L.E.; Marasa, M.; Gharavi, A.G.; et al. Kidney Biopsy Findings in Patients with COVID-19. *J. Am. Soc. Nephrol.* **2020**, *31*, 1959–1968. [CrossRef]
10. Velez, J.C.Q.; Caza, T.; Larsen, C.P. COVAN is the new HIVAN: The re-emergence of collapsing glomerulopathy with COVID-19. *Nat. Rev. Nephrol.* **2020**, *16*, 565–567. [CrossRef]
11. Wu, H.; Larsen, C.P.; Hernandez-Arroyo, C.F.; Mohamed, M.M.B.; Caza, T.; Sharshir, M.; Chughtai, A.; Xie, L.; Gimenez, J.M.; Sandow, T.A.; et al. AKI and Col-lapsing Glomerulopathy Associated with COVID-19 and APOL1 High-Risk Genotype. *J. Am. Soc. Nephrol.* **2020**, *3*, 1688–1695. [CrossRef]
12. Ng, J.H.; Hirsch, J.S.; Hazzan, A.; Wanchoo, R.; Shah, H.H.; Malieckal, D.A.; Ross, D.W.; Sharma, P.; Sakhiya, V.; Fishbane, S.; et al. Northwell Nephrology COVID-19 Research Consortium. Outcomes Among Patients Hospitalized With COVID-19 and Acute KidneyInjury. *Am. J. Kidney Dis.* **2021**, *77*, 204–215. [CrossRef]
13. Chung, E.Y.; Palmer, S.C.; Natale, P.; Krishnan, A.; Cooper, T.E.; Saglimbene, V.M.; Ruospo, M.; Au, E.; Jayanti, S.; Liang, A.; et al. Incidence and Outcomes of COVID-19 in People with CKD: A Systematic Review and Meta-analysis. *Am. J. Kidney Dis.* **2021**, *78*, 804–815. [CrossRef]
14. Ozturk, S.; Turgutalp, K.; Arici, M.; Odabas, A.R.; Altiparmak, M.R.; Aydin, Z.; Cebeci, E.; Basturk, T.; Soypacaci, Z.; Sahin, G.; et al. Mortality analysis of COVID-19 infection in chronic kidney disease, haemodialysis and renal transplant patients compared with patients without kidney disease: A nationwide analysis from Turkey. *Nephrol. Dial. Transplant.* **2020**, *35*, 2083–2095. [CrossRef] [PubMed]
15. Jager, K.J.; Kramer, A.; Chesnaye, N.C.; Couchoud, C.; Sánchez-Álvarez, J.E.; Garneata, L.; Collart, F.; Hemmelder, M.H.; Ambühl, P.; Kerschbaum, J.; et al. Results from the ERA-EDTA Registry indicate a high mortality due to COVID-19 in dialysis patients and kidney transplant recipients across Europe. *Kidney Int.* **2020**, *98*, 1540–1548. [CrossRef] [PubMed]
16. Valeri, A.M.; Robbins-Juarez, S.Y.; Stevens, J.S.; Ahn, W.; Rao, M.K.; Radhakrishnan, J.; Gharavi, A.G.; Mohan, S.; Husain, S.A. Presentation and Outcomes of Patients with ESKD and COVID-19. *J. Am. Soc. Nephrol.* **2020**, *31*, 1409–1415. [CrossRef]
17. El Karoui, K.; De Vriese, A.S. COVID-19 in dialysis: Clinical impact, immune response, prevention, and treatment. *Kidney Int.* **2022**, *101*, 883–894. [CrossRef] [PubMed]

18. Jawdeh, B.G. COVID-19 in Kidney Transplantation: Outcomes, Immunosuppression Management, and Operational Challenges. *Adv. Chronic Kidney Dis.* **2020**, *27*, 383–389. [CrossRef]
19. Tylicki, L.; Biedunkiewicz, B.; Puchalska-Reglińska, E.; Gellert, R.; Burnier, M.; Wolf, J.; Dębska-Ślizień, A. COVID-19 vac-cination reduces mortality in patients on maintenance hemodialysis. *Front. Med. (Lausanne)* **2022**, *9*, 937167. [CrossRef]
20. Klomjit, N.; Alexander, M.P.; Fervenza, F.C.; Zoghby, Z.; Garg, A.; Hogan, M.C.; Nasr, S.H.; Abu Minshar, M.; Zand, L. COVID-19 Vaccination and Glomerulonephritis. *Kidney Int. Rep.* **2021**, *6*, 2969–2978. [CrossRef]
21. Kale, A.; Shelke, V.; Dagar, N.; Anders, H.J.; Gaikwad, A.B. How to use COVID-19 antiviral drugs in patients with chronic kidney disease. *Front. Pharmacol.* **2023**, *14*, 1053814. [CrossRef]
22. Copur, S.; Berkkan, M.; Basile, C.; Tuttle, K.; Kanbay, M. Post-acute COVID 19 syndrome and kidney diseases: What do we know? *J. Nephrol.* **2022**, *35*, 795–805. [CrossRef] [PubMed]
23. Guan, W.J.; Zhong, N.S. Clinical Characteristics of COVID-19 in China. *Reply. N. Engl. J. Med.* **2020**, *382*, 1861–1862. [PubMed]
24. Batlle, D.; Soler, M.; Sparks, M.A.; Hiremath, S.; South, A.M.; Welling, P.A.; Swaminathan, S. COVID-19 and ACE2 in Cardiovascular, Lung, and Kidney Working Group. Acute Kidney Injury in COVID-19: Emerging Evidence of a Distinct Pathophysiology. *J. Am. Soc. Nephrol.* **2020**, *31*, 1380–1383. [CrossRef]
25. Cheng, Y.; Luo, R.; Wang, K.; Zhang, M.; Wang, Z.; Dong, L.; Li, J.; Yao, Y.; Ge, S.; Xu, G. Kidney disease is associated with in-hospital death of patients with COVID-19. *Kidney Int.* **2020**, *97*, 829–838. [CrossRef] [PubMed]
26. Hirsch, J.S.; Ng, J.H.; Ross, D.W.; Sharma, P.; Shah, H.H.; Barnett, R.L.; Hazzan, A.D.; Fishbane, S.; Jhaveri, K.D. Northwell COVID-19 Research Consortium; Northwell Nephrology COVID-19 Research Consortium. Acute kidney injury in patients hospitalized with COVID-19. *Kidney Int.* **2020**, *98*, 209–218. [CrossRef]
27. Cummings, M.J.; Baldwin, M.R.; Abrams, D.; Jacobson, S.D.; Meyer, B.J.; Balough, E.M.; Aaron, J.G.; Claassen, J.; Rabbani, L.E.; Hastie, J.; et al. Epidemiology, clinical course, and outcomes of critically ill adults with COVID-19 in New York City: A prospective cohort study. *Lancet* **2020**, *395*, 1763–1770. [CrossRef]
28. Gupta, S.; Coca, S.G.; Chan, L.; Melamed, M.L.; Brenner, S.K.; Hayek, S.S.; Sutherland, A.; Puri, S.; Srivastava, A.; Leonberg-Yoo, A.; et al. AKI Treated with Renal Replacement Therapy in Critically Ill Patients with COVID-19. *J. Am. Soc. Nephrol.* **2020**, *32*, 161–176. [CrossRef]
29. Peng, S.; Wang, H.Y.; Sun, X.; Li, P.; Ye, Z.; Li, Q.; Wang, J.; Shi, X.; Liu, L.; Yao, Y.; et al. Early versus late acute kidney injury among patients with COVID-19-a multicenter study from Wuhan, China. *Nephrol. Dial. Transplant.* **2020**, *35*, 2095–2102. [CrossRef]
30. Fu, E.L.; Janse, R.J.; de Jong, Y.; van der Endt, V.H.; Milders, J.; van der Willik, E.M.; de Rooij, E.N.; Dekkers, O.M.; Rotmans, J.I.; van Diepen, M. Acute kidney injury and kidney replacement therapy in COVID-19: A systematic review and metaanalysis. *Clin. Kidney J.* **2020**, *13*, 550–563. [CrossRef]
31. Chan, L.; Chaudhary, K.; Saha, A.; Chauhan, K.; Vaid, A.; Zhao, S.; Paranjpe, I.; Somani, S.; Richter, F.; Miotto, R.; et al. AKI in Hospitalized Patients with COVID-19. *J. Am. Soc. Nephrol.* **2021**, *32*, 151–160. [CrossRef] [PubMed]
32. Shemies, R.S.; Nagy, E.; Younis, D.; Sheashaa, H. Renal replacement therapy for critically ill patients with COVID-19-associated acute kidney injury: A review of current knowledge. *Ther. Apher. Dial.* **2021**, *26*, 15–23. [CrossRef] [PubMed]
33. Pecly, I.M.D.; Azevedo, R.B.; Muxfeldt, E.S.; Botelho, B.G.; Albuquerque, G.G.; Diniz, P.H.P.; Silva, R.; Rodrigues, C.I.S. COVID-19 and chronic kidney disease: A comprehensive review. *Braz. J. Nephrol.* **2021**, *43*, 383–399.
34. Bowe, B.; Cai, M.; Xie, Y.; Gibson, A.K.; Maddukuri, G.; Al-Aly, Z. Acute Kidney Injury in a National Cohort of Hospitalized US Veterans th COVID-19. *Clin. J. Am. Soc. Nephrol.* **2020**, *16*, 14–25. [CrossRef]
35. Charytan, D.M.; Parnia, S.; Khatri, M.; Petrilli, C.M.; Jones, S.; Benstein, J.; Horwitz, L.I. Decreasing Incidence of Acute Kid-ney Injury in Patients with COVID-19 Critical Illness in New York City. *Kidney Int. Rep.* **2021**, *6*, 916–927. [CrossRef]
36. Chaudhri, I.; Moffitt, R.; Taub, E.; Annadi, R.R.; Hoai, M.; Bolotova, O.; Yoo, J.; Dhaliwal, S.; Sahib, H.; Daccueil, F.; et al. Association of Proteinuria and Hematuria with Acute Kidney Injury and Mortality in Hospitalized Patients with COVID-19. *Kidney Blood Press.* **2020**, *45*, 1018–1032. [CrossRef]
37. Hidayat, A.A.; Gunawan, V.A.; Iragama, F.R.; Alfiansyah, R.; Hertanto, D.M.; Tjempakasari, A.; Thaha, M. Risk Factors and Clinical Characteristics of Acute Kidney Injury in Patients with COVID-19: A Systematic Review and Meta-Analysis. *Pathophysiology* **2023**, *30*, 233–247. [CrossRef]
38. Kormann, R.; Jacquot, A.; Alla, A.; Corbel, A.; Koszutski, M.; Voirin, P.; Parrilla, M.G.; Bevilacqua, S.; Schvoerer, E.; Gueant, J.-L.; et al. Coronavirus disease 2019: Acute Fanconi syndrome precedes acute kidney injury. *Clin. Kidney J.* **2020**, *13*, 362–370. [CrossRef]
39. Werion, A.; Belkhir, L.; Perrot, M.; Schmit, G.; Aydin, S.; Chen, Z. Cliniquesuniversitaires Saint-Luc (CUSL) COVID-19 Research Group. SARS-CoV-2 causes a specific dysfunction of the kid-ney proximal tubule. *Kidney Int.* **2020**, *98*, 1296–1307. [CrossRef]
40. Ferlicot, S.; Jamme, M.; Gaillard, F.; Oniszczuk, J.; Couturier, A.; May, O.; Grünenwald, A.; Sannier, A.; Moktefi, A.; Le Mon-nier, O.; et al. AP-HP/Universities/Inserm COVID-19 research collaboration. The spectrum of kidney bi-opsies in hospitalized patients with COVID-19, acute kidney injury, and/or proteinuria. *Nephrol. Dial. Transplant.* **2021**, *12*, gfab012.
41. Legrand, M.; Bell, S.; Forni, L.; Joannidis, M.; Koyner, J.L.; Liu, K.; Cantaluppi, V. Pathophysiology of COVID-19-associated acute kidney injury. *Nat. Rev. Nephrol.* **2021**, *17*, 751–764. [CrossRef]
42. Santoriello, D.; Khairallah, P.; Bomback, A.S.; Xu, K.; Kudose, S.; Bata, I.; Barasch, J.; Radhakrishnan, J.; D'Agati, V.; Markowitz. Postmortem Kidney Pathology Findings in Patients with COVID-19G. *J. Am. Soc. Nephrol.* **2020**, *31*, 2158–2167. [CrossRef]
43. Miller, S.E.; Brealey, J.K. Visualization of putative coronavirus in kidney. *Kidney Int.* **2020**, *98*, 231–232. [CrossRef]

44. Hanley, B.; Naresh, K.N.; Roufosse, C.; Nicholson, A.G.; Weir, J.; Cooke, G.S.; Thursz, M.; Manousou, P.; Corbett, R.; Goldin, R.; et al. Histopathological findings and viral tropism in UK patients with severe fatal COVID-19: A post-mortem study. *Lancet Microbe* **2020**, *1*, e245–e253. [CrossRef] [PubMed]
45. Akilesh, S.; Nast, C.C.; Yamashita, M.; Henriksen, K.; Charu, V.; Troxell, M.L.; Kambham, N.; Bracamonte, E.; Houghton, D.; Ahmed, N.I.; et al. Multicenter Clinicopathologic Correlation of Kidney Biopsies Performed in COVID-19 Patients Presenting With Acute Kidney Injury or Proteinuria. *Am. J. Kidney Dis.* **2021**, *77*, 82–93.e1. [CrossRef]
46. Braun, F.; Lütgehetmann, M.; Pfefferle, S.; Wong, M.N.; Carsten, A.; Lindenmeyer, M.T.; Nörz, D.; Heinrich, F.; Meißner, K.; Wichmann, D.; et al. SARS-CoV-2 renal tropism associates with acute kidney injury. *Lancet* **2020**, *396*, 597–598. [CrossRef]
47. Sun, J.; Zhu, A.; Li, H.; Zheng, K.; Zhuang, Z.; Chen, Z.; Shi, Y.; Zhang, Z.; Chen, S.B.; Liu, X.; et al. Isolation of infectious SARS-CoV-2 from urine of a COVID-19 patient. *Emerg. Microbes Infect.* **2020**, *9*, 991–993. [CrossRef]
48. Puelles, V.G.; Lütgehetmann, M.; Lindenmeyer, M.T.; Sperhake, J.P.; Wong, M.N.; Allweiss, L.; Chilla, S.; Heinemann, A.; Wanner, N.; Liu, S.; et al. Multiorgan and Renal Tropism of SARS-CoV-2. *N. Engl. J. Med.* **2020**, *6*, 590–592. [CrossRef]
49. Schwimmer, J.A.; Markowitz, G.S.; Valeri, A.; Appel, G.B. Collapsing glomerulopathy. *Semin. Nephrol.* **2003**, *23*, 209–218. [CrossRef]
50. Giannini, G.; Velez, J.C.; May, R.M.; Sharma, S.G.; Mohamed, M.M.; Cassol, C.A.; Larsen, C.P.; Caza, T.N. Renal Prognosis of COVID-19 Associated Nephropathy. *Kidney Int. Rep.* **2022**, *7*, 2722–2725. [CrossRef]
51. Ackermann, M.; Verleden, S.E.; Kuehnel, M.; Haverich, A.; Welte, T.; Laenger, F.; Vanstapel, A.; Werlein, C.; Stark, H.; Tzankov, A.; et al. Pulmonary Vascular Endothelialitis, Thrombosis, and Angiogene-sis in COVID-19. *N. Engl. J. Med.* **2020**, *9*, 120–128. [CrossRef] [PubMed]
52. Vassiliou, A.G.; Keskinidou, C.; Jahaj, E.; Gallos, P.; Dimopoulou, I.; Kotanidou, A.; Orfanos, S.E. ICU Admission Levels of Endothelial Biomarkers as Predictors of Mortality in Critically Ill COVID-19 Patients. *Cells* **2021**, *10*, 186. [CrossRef] [PubMed]
53. Iba, T.; Connors, J.M.; Levy, J.H. The coagulopathy, endotheliopathy, and vasculitis of COVID-19. *Inflamm. Res.* **2020**, *69*, 1181–1189. [CrossRef] [PubMed]
54. Macor, P.; Durigutto, P.; Mangogna, A.; Bussani, R.; De Maso, L.; D'errico, S.; Zanon, M.; Pozzi, N.; Meroni, P.L.; Tedesco, F. Multiple-Organ Complement Deposition on Vascular Endothelium in COVID-19 Patients. *Biomedicines* **2021**, *9*, 1003. [CrossRef] [PubMed]
55. Ince, C. The central role of renal microcirculatory dysfunction in the pathogenesis of acute kidney injury. *Nephron Clin. Pract.* **2014**, *127*, 124–128. [CrossRef]
56. Taha, M.; Sano, D.; Hanoudi, S.; Esber Elahi, M.; Gabali, A.; Chopra, T.; Draghici, S.; Samavat, I.L. Platelets and renal failure in the SARS-CoV-2 syndrome. *Platelets* **2021**, *32*, 130–137. [CrossRef]
57. Zuo, Y.; Estes, S.K.; Ali, R.A.; Gandhi, A.A.; Yalavarthi, S.; Shi, H.; Sule, G.; Gockman, K.; Madison, J.A.; Zuo, M.; et al. Prothrombotic autoan-tibodies in serum from patients hospitalized with COVID-19. *Sci. Med. Transl.* **2020**, *12*, eabd3876. [CrossRef] [PubMed]
58. Fox, S.E.; Lameira, F.S.; Rinke, E.B.; Vander Heide, R.S. Cardiac Endotheliitis and Multisystem Inflammatory Syndrome Af-ter COVID-19. *Ann. Intern. Med.* **2020**, *173*, 1025–1027. [CrossRef]
59. Plášek, J.; Gumulec, J.; Máca, J.; Škarda, J.; Procházka, V.; Grézl, T.; Václavík, J. COVID-19 associated coagulopathy: Mecha-nisms and host-directed treatment. *Am. J. Med. Sci.* **2022**, *363*, 465–475. [CrossRef]
60. Ville, S.; Le Bot, S.; Chapelet-Debout, A.; Blancho, G.; Fremeaux-Bacchi, V.; Deltombe, C.; Fakhouri, F. Atypical HUS relapse triggered by COVID-19. *Kidney Int.* **2020**, *99*, 267–268. [CrossRef]
61. Yu, J.; Yuan, X.; Chen, H.; Chaturvedi, S.; Braunstein, E.M.; Brodsky, R.A. Direct activation of the alternative complement pathway by SARS-CoV-2 spike proteins is blocked by factor D inhibition. *Blood* **2020**, *136*, 2080–2089. [CrossRef] [PubMed]
62. Perico, L.; Benigni, A.; Casiraghi, F.; Ng, L.F.P.; Renia, L.; Remuzzi, G. Immunity, endothelial injury and comple-ment-induced coagulopathy in COVID-19. *Nat. Rev. Nephrol.* **2021**, *17*, 46–64. [CrossRef] [PubMed]
63. Fang, W.; Jiang, J.; Su, L.; Shu, T.; Liu, H.; Lai, S.; Ghiladi, R.A.; Wang, J. The role of NO in COVID-19 and potential therapeutic strategies. *Free Radic. BiolMed.* **2021**, *163*, 153–162. [CrossRef] [PubMed]
64. El Shamy, O.; Munoz-Casablanca, N.; Coca, S.; Sharma, S.; Lookstein, R.; Uribarri, J. Bilateral Renal Artery Thrombosis in a Patient With COVID-19. *Kidney Med.* **2020**, *3*, 116–119. [CrossRef]
65. Moderbacher, C.R.; Ramirez, S.I.; Dan, J.M.; Grifoni, A.; Hastie, K.M.; Weiskopf, D.; Belanger, S.; Abbott, R.K.; Kim, C.; Choi, J.; et al. Antigen-Specific Adaptive Immunity to SARS-CoV-2 in Acute COVID-19 and Associations with Age and Disease Severity. *Cell* **2020**, *183*, 996–1012.e19. [CrossRef]
66. Pawelec, G. Age and immunity: What is "immunosenescence"? *Exp. Gerontol.* **2018**, *105*, 4–9. [CrossRef]
67. Fuentes, E.; Fuentes, M.; Alarcón, M.; Palomo, I. Immune System Dysfunction in the Elderly. *An. Da Acad. Bras. De Ciências* **2017**, *89*, 285–299. [CrossRef] [PubMed]
68. Cantaluppi, V.; Quercia, A.D.; Dellepiane, S.; Ferrario, S.; Camussi, G.; Biancone, L. Interaction between systemic inflamma-tion and renal tubular epithelial cells. *Nephrol. Dial. Transplant.* **2014**, *29*, 2004–2011. [CrossRef] [PubMed]
69. Cutuli, S.L.; Artigas, A.; Fumagalli, R.; Monti, G.; Ranieri, V.M.; Ronco, C.; Antonelli, M. The EUPHAS 2 Collaborative Group Polymyxin-B hemoperfusion in septic patients: Analysis of a multicenter registry. *Ann. Intensiv. Care* **2016**, *6*, 1–9. [CrossRef]
70. Zarbock, A.; Gomez, H.; Kellum, J.A. Sepsis-induced acute kidney injury revisited: Pathophysiology, prevention and future therapies. *CurrOpinCritCare* **2014**, *20*, 588–595. [CrossRef]

71. Buszko, M.; Nita-Lazar, A.; Park, J.-H.; Schwartzberg, P.L.; Verthelyi, D.; Young, H.A.; Rosenberg, A.S. Lessons learned: New insights on the role of cytokines in COVID-19. *Nat. Immunol.* **2021**, *22*, 404–411. [CrossRef]
72. Koning, R.; Bastard, P.; Casanova, J.-L.; Brouwer, M.C.; van de Beek, D.; van Agtmael, M.; Algera, A.G.; Appelman, B.; van Baarle, F.; Bax, D.; et al. Autoantibodies against type I interferons are associated with multi-organ failure in COVID-19 patients. *Intensiv. Care Med.* **2021**, *47*, 704–706. [CrossRef]
73. Migliorini, A.; Angelotti, M.L.; Mulay, S.R.; Kulkarni, O.O.; Demleitner, J.; Dietrich, A.; Sagrinati, C.; Ballerini, L.; Peired, A.; Shankland, S.J.; et al. The antiviral cytokines IFN-α and IFN-β modulate parietal epithelial cells and promote podocyte loss: Implications for IFN toxicity, viral glomerulonephritis, and glomerular regeneration. *Am. J. Pathol.* **2013**, *183*, 431–440. [CrossRef]
74. Beckerman, P.; Bi-Karchin, J.; Park, A.S.; Qiu, C.; Dummer, P.D.; Soomro, I.; Boustany-Kari, C.M.; Pullen, S.S.; Miner, J.H.; Hu, C.A. Transgenic expression of human APOL1 risk variants in podocytes induces kidney disease in mice. *Nat. Med.* **2017**, *23*, 429–438. [CrossRef]
75. Pfister, F.; Vonbrunn, E.; Ries, T.; Jäck, H.-M.; Überla, K.; Lochnit, G.; Sheriff, A.; Herrmann, M.; Büttner-Herold, M.; Amann, K.; et al. Complement Activation in Kidneys of Patients With COVID-19. *Front. Immunol.* **2020**, *11*, 594849. [CrossRef]
76. Vinayagam, S.; Sattu, K. SARS-CoV-2 and coagulation disorders in different organs. *Life Sci.* **2020**, *260*, 118431. [CrossRef]
77. Castellano, G.; Franzin, R.; Sallustio, F.; Stasi, A.; Banelli, B.; Romani, M.; De Palma, G.; Lucarelli, G.; Divella, C.; Battaglia, M.; et al. Complement component C5a induces aberrant epigenetic modifications in renal tubular epithelial cells accelerating se-nescence by Wnt4/βcatenin signaling after ischemia/reperfusion injury. *Aging* **2019**, *11*, 4382–4406. [CrossRef]
78. Laing, A.G.; Lorenc, A.; Del Molino Del Barrio, I.; Das, A.; Fish, M.; Monin, L.; Muñoz-Ruiz, M.; McKenzie, D.R.; Hayday, T.S.; Francos-Quijorna, I.; et al. A dynamic COVID-19 immune signature includes associations with poor prognosis. *Nat. Med.* **2020**, *26*, 1623–1635. [CrossRef]
79. Olagnier, D.; Farahani, E.; Thyrsted, J.; Blay-Cadanet, J.; Herengt, A.; Idorn, M.; Hait, A.; Hernaez, B.; Knudsen, A.; Iversen, M.B.; et al. SARS-CoV2-mediated suppression of NRF2-signaling reveals potent antiviral and anti-inflammatory activity of 4-octyl-itaconate and dimethyl fumarate. *Nat Commun.* **2020**, *2*, 4938. [CrossRef]
80. Noel, S.; Martina, M.N.; Bandapalle, S.; Racusen, L.C.; Potteti, H.R.; Hamad, A.R.; Reddy, S.P.; Rabb, H.T. Lymphocyte-Specific Activation of Nrf2 Protects from AKI. *J. Am. Soc. Nephrol.* **2015**, *26*, 2989–3000. [CrossRef]
81. Liu, M.; Grigoryev, D.N.; Crow, M.T.; Haas, M.; Yamamoto, M.; Reddy, S.P.; Rabb, H. Transcription factor Nrf2 is protective during ischemic and nephrotoxic acute kidney injury in mice. *Kidney Int.* **2009**, *76*, 277–285. [CrossRef]
82. Camargo, R.L.; Bombassaro, B.; Monfort-Pires, M.; Mansour, E.; Palma, A.C.; Ribeiro, L.C.; Ulaf, R.G.; Bernardes, A.F.; Nunes, T.A.; Agrela, M.V.; et al. Plasma Angiotensin II Is Increased in Critical Coronavirus Disease 2019. *Front. Cardiovasc. Med.* **2022**, *9*, 847809. [CrossRef]
83. Beyerstedt, S.; Casaro, E.B.; Rangel, É.B. COVID-19: Angiotensin-converting enzyme 2 (ACE2) expression and tissue suscep-tibility to SARS-CoV-2 infection. *Eur. J. Clin. Microbiol. Infect. Dis.* **2021**, *40*, 905–919. [CrossRef]
84. McMillan, P.; Dexhiemer, T.; Neubig, R.R.; Uhal, B.D. COVID-19—A Theory of Autoimmunity Against ACE-2 Explained. *Front. Immunol.* **2021**, *12*, 582166. [CrossRef]
85. Fajgenbaum, D.C.; June, C.H. Cytokine Storm. *N. Engl. J. Med.* **2020**, *3*, 2255–2273. [CrossRef]
86. Xia, P.; Wen, Y.; Duan, Y.; Su, H.; Cao, W.; Xiao, M.; Ma, J.; Zhou, Y.; Chen, G.; Jiang, W.; et al. Clinico-pathological Features and Outcomes of Acute Kidney Injury in Critically Ill COVID-19 with Prolonged Disease Course: A Retrospective Cohort. *J. Am. Soc. Nephrol.* **2020**, *31*, 2205–2221.
87. Coomes, E.A.; Haghbayan, H. Interleukin-6 in COVID-19: A systematic review and meta-analysis. *Rev. Med. Virol.* **2020**, *30*, e2141. [CrossRef]
88. Leisman, D.E.; Ronner, L.; Pinotti, R.; Taylor, M.D.; Sinha, P.; Calfee, C.S.; Hirayama, A.V.; Mastroiani, F.; Turtle, C.J.; Harhay, M.O. Cytokine elevation in severe and critical COVID-19: A rapid systematic review, meta-analysis, and comparison with other inflammatory syndromes. *Lancet Respir. Med.* **2020**, *8*, 1233–1244. [CrossRef]
89. Kox, M.; Waalders, N.J.B.; Kooistra, E.J.; Gerretsen, J.; Pickkers, P. Cytokine Levels in Critically Ill Patients With COVID-19 and Other Conditions. *JAMA* **2020**, *324*, 1565–1567. [CrossRef]
90. Legrand, M.; Mik, E.G.; Johannes, T.; Payen, D.; Ince, C. Renal Hypoxia and Dysoxia After Reperfusion of the Ischemic Kidney. *Mol. Med.* **2008**, *14*, 502–516.
91. Hall, A.; Busse, L.W.; Ostermann, M. Angiotensin in Critical Care. *Crit. Care* **2018**, *22*, 1–6. [CrossRef] [PubMed]
92. Barthélémy, R.; Beaucoté, V.; Bordier, R.; Collet, M.; Le Gall, A.; Hong, A.; de Roquetaillade, C.; Gayat, E.; Mebazaa, A.; Chousterman, B.G. Haemodynamic impact of positive end-expiratory pressure in SARS-CoV-2 acute respiratory distress syndrome: Oxygenation versus oxygen delivery. *Br. J. Anaesth.* **2021**, *126*, e70–e72. [CrossRef] [PubMed]
93. Bajaj, R.; Sinclair, H.C.; Patel, K.; Low, B.; Pericao, A.; Manisty, C.; Guttmann, O.; Zemrak, F.; Miller, O.; Longhi, P.; et al. Delayed-onset myocarditis following COVID-19. *Lancet Respir. Med.* **2021**, *9*, e32–e34. [CrossRef]
94. Kotecha, T.; Knight, D.S.; Razvi, Y.; Kumar, K.; Vimalesvaran, K.; Thornton, G.; Patel, R.; Chacko, L.; Brown, J.T.; Coyle, C.; et al. Faculty Opinions recommendation of Patterns of myocardial injury in recovered troponin-positive COVID-19 patients assessed by cardiovascular magnetic resonance. *Eur. Heart J.* **2021**, *42*, 1866–1878. [CrossRef] [PubMed]
95. Legrand, M.; Dupuis, C.; Simon, C.; Gayat, E.; Mateo, J.; Lukaszewicz, A.C.; Payen, D. Association between systemic hemodynamics and septic acute kidney injury in critically ill patients: A retrospective observational study. *Crit Care* **2013**, *29*, R278. [CrossRef]

96. Cruces, P.; Lillo, P.; Salas, C.; Salomon, T.; Lillo, F.; González, C.; Pacheco, A.; Hurtado, D.E. RenalDecapsulation Prevents Intrinsic Renal Compartment Syndrome in Ischemia-Reperfusion-Induced Acute Kidney Injury: A Physiologic Approach. *CritCareMed* **2018**, *46*, 216–222.
97. Sang, L.; Chen, S.; Zheng, X.; Guan, W.; Zhang, Z.; Liang, W.; Zhong, M.; Jiang, L.; Pan, C.; Zhang, W.; et al. The incidence, risk factors and prognosis of acute kidney injury in severe and critically ill patients with COVID-19 in mainland China: A retrospective study. *BMC Pulm. Med.* **2020**, *20*, 1–10. [CrossRef]
98. Gillenwater, S.; Rahaghi, F.; Hadeh, A. Remdesivir for the Treatment of COVID-19—Final Report. *N. Engl. J. Med.* **2020**, *5*, 1813–1826.
99. Binois, Y.; Hachad, H.; Salem, J.-E.; Charpentier, J.; Lebrun-Vignes, B.; Pène, F.; Cariou, A.; Chiche, J.-D.; Mira, J.-P.; Nguyen, L.S. Acute Kidney Injury Associated With Lopinavir/Ritonavir Combined Therapy in Patients With COVID-19. *Kidney Int. Rep.* **2020**, *5*, 1787–1790. [CrossRef]
100. Geng, Y.; Ma, Q.; Du, Y.-S.; Peng, N.; Yang, T.; Zhang, S.-Y.; Wu, F.-F.; Lin, H.-L.; Su, L. Rhabdomyolysis is Associated with In-Hospital Mortality in Patients With COVID-19. *Shock* **2021**, *56*, 360–367. [CrossRef]
101. Shaefi, S.; Brenner, S.K.; Gupta, S.; O'Gara, B.P.; Krajewski, M.L.; Charytan, D.M.; Chaudhry, S. Extracorporeal mem-brane oxygenation in patients with severe respiratory failure from COVID-19. *Intensive Care Med.* **2021**, *47*, 208–221. [CrossRef] [PubMed]
102. Schmidt, M.; Hajage, D.; Lebreton, G.; Monsel, A.; Voiriot, G.; Levy, D.; Baron, E. Extracorporeal membrane oxygena-tion for severe acute respiratory distress syndrome associated with COVID-19: A retrospective cohort study. *Lancet Respir. Med.* **2020**, *8*, 1121–1131. [CrossRef] [PubMed]
103. Cai, X.; Wu, G.; Zhang, J.; Yang, L. Risk Factors for Acute Kidney Injury in Adult Patients With COVID-19: A Systematic Re-view and Meta-Analysis. *Front. Med.* **2021**, *8*, 719472. [CrossRef] [PubMed]
104. Chawla, L.S.; Eggers, P.W.; Star, R.A.; Kimmel, P.L. Acute kidney injury and chronic kidney disease as interconnected syn-dromes. *N. Engl. J. Med.* **2014**, *371*, 58–66. [CrossRef] [PubMed]
105. Ferenbach, D.A.; Bonventre, J.V. Mechanisms of maladaptive repair after AKI leading to accelerated kidney ageing and CKD. *Nat. Rev. Nephrol.* **2015**, *11*, 264–276.
106. Coca, S.G.; Singanamala, S.; Parikh, C.R. Chronic kidney disease after acute kidney injury: A systematic review and me-ta-analysis. *Kidney Int.* **2012**, *81*, 442–448. [CrossRef]
107. Karimi, Z.; Masjedi, F.; Malekmakan, L.; Doostkam, A.; Roozbeh, J.; Ghahramani, N. Potential Mechanisms of the SARS-CoV-2-induced AKI Progression to CKD: A Forward-Looking Perspective. *Iran. J. Kidney Dis.* **2021**, *15*, 243–255.
108. Tanaka, S.; Tanaka, T.; Nangaku, M. Hypoxia as a key player in the AKI-to-CKD transition. *Am. J. Physiol. Physiol.* **2014**, *307*, F1187–F1195.
109. Newsome, B.B.; Warnock, D.G.; McClellan, W.M.; Herzog, C.A.; Kiefe, C.I.; Eggers, P.W.; Allison, J.J. Long-term risk of mortality and end-stage renal disease among the elderly after small increases in serum creatinine level during hospitaliza-tion for acute myocardial infarction. *Arch Intern. Med.* **2008**, *168*, 609–616. [CrossRef]
110. Coca, S.G.; Yusuf, B.; Shlipak, M.G.; Garg, A.X.; Parikh, C.R. Long-term Risk of Mortality and Other Adverse Outcomes After Acute Kidney Injury: A Systematic Review and Meta-analysis. *Am. J. Kidney Dis.* **2009**, *53*, 961–973. [CrossRef]
111. Sifaat, M.; Patel, P.; Sheikh, R.; Ghaffar, D.; Vaishnav, H.; Nahar, L.; Rupani, S.; Quadri, S.J. Cardiorenal Disease in COVID-19 Patients. *Renin Angiotensin Aldosterone Systtem* **2022**, *18*, 4640788. [CrossRef] [PubMed]
112. Aleksova, A.; Fluca, A.L.; Gagno, G.; Pierri, A.; Padoan, L.; Derin, A.; Moretti, R.; Noveska, E.A.; Azzalini, E.; D'Errico, S.; et al. Long-term effect of SARS-CoV-2 infection on cardiovascu-lar outcomes and all-cause mortality. *Life Sci.* **2022**, *1*, 121018. [CrossRef]
113. Zheng, Y.-Y.; Ma, Y.-T.; Zhang, J.-Y.; Xie, X. COVID-19 and the cardiovascular system. *Nat. Rev. Cardiol.* **2020**, *17*, 259–260. [CrossRef]
114. Huang, C.; Wang, Y.; Li, X.; Ren, L.; Zhao, J.; Hu, Y.; Zhang, L.; Fan, G.; Xu, J.; Gu, X.; et al. Clinical features of patients infected with 2019 Novel coronavirus in Wuhan, China. *Lancet* **2020**, *395*, 497–506. [CrossRef] [PubMed]
115. Baral, R.; Tsampasian, V.; Debski, M.; Moran, B.; Garg, P.; Clark, A.; Vassiliou, V.S. Association between renin-angiotensin-aldosterone system inhibitors and clini-cal outcomes in patients with COVID-19: A systematic review and meta-analysis. *JAMA Netw. Open* **2021**, *4*, e213594. [CrossRef] [PubMed]
116. Xiong, J.; Qiao, Y.; Yu, Z.; Huang, Y.; Yang, K.; He, T.; Zhao, J. T-Lymphocyte Subsets Alteration, Infection and Renal Outcome in Advanced Chronic Kidney Disease. *Front Med. (Lausanne)* **2021**, *9*, 742419. [CrossRef]
117. Wang, R.; Liao, C.; He, H.; Hu, C.; Wei, Z.; Hong, Z.; Zhang, C.; Liao, M.; Shui, H. COVID-19 in Hemodialysis Patients: A Report of 5 Cases. *Am. J. Kidney Dis.* **2020**, *76*, 141–143. [CrossRef]
118. Xiong, F.; Tang, H.; Liu, L.; Tu, C.; Tian, J.B.; Lei, C.T.; Liu, J.; Dong, J.W.; Chen, W.L.; Wang, X.H. Clinical characteristics of and medical interventions for COVID-19 in hemodialysis pa-tients in wuhan, China. *J. Am. Soc. Nephrol.* **2020**, *31*, 1387. [CrossRef]
119. Clarke, C.; Prendecki, M.; Dhutia, A.; Ali, M.A.; Sajjad, H.; Shivakumar, O.; Lightstone, L.; Kelleher, P.; Pickering, M.C.; Thomas, D.; et al. High Prevalence of Asymptomatic COVID-19 Infection in Hemodialysis Patients Detected Using Serologic Screening. *J. Am. Soc. Nephrol.* **2020**, *31*, 1969–1975. [CrossRef]
120. Boulanger, H.; Saksi, S.A.; Achiche, J.; Batusanski, F.; Stawiarski, N.; Diddaoui, A.; Fromentin, L.; Chawki, M. SARS-CoV-2 Antibodies in Hemodialysis Patients Six Months after Infection Compared to Healthcare Workers. *Int. J. Nephrol.* **2021**, *2021*, 4747221. [CrossRef]

121. Cohen, D.E.; Sibbel, S.; Marlowe, G.; Bludorn, K.; Miller, D.; Kelley, T.; Connaire, J.; Young, A.; Tentori, F.; Brunelli, S.M. Antibody status, disease history, and incidence of SARS-CoV-2 infection among patients on chronic dialysis. *J. Am. Soc. Nephrol.* **2021**, *32*, 1880–1886. [CrossRef]
122. Ma, Y.; Diao, B.; Lv, X.; Zhu, J.; Liang, W.; Liu, L.; Bu, W.; Cheng, H.; Zhang, S.; Yang, L.; et al. 2019 novel coronavirus disease in hemodialysis (HD) patients: Report from one HD center in Wuhan, China. *medRxiv* **2020**. [CrossRef]
123. Hsu, C.M.; Weiner, D.E. COVID-19 in dialysis patients: Outlasting and outsmarting a pandemic. *Kidney Int.* **2020**, *98*, 1402–1404. [CrossRef]
124. Jiang, H.J.; Tang, H.; Xiong, F.; Chen, W.L.; Tian, J.B.; Sun, J.; Dong, J.W.; Wang, X.H.; Jin, X.F.; Ding, Y.Q.; et al. COVID-19 in peritoneal dialysis patients. *Clin. J. Am. Soc. Nephrol.* **2020**, *31*, 121–123. [CrossRef] [PubMed]
125. Jeloka, T.; Gupta, A.; Prasad, N.; Varughese, S.; Mahajan, S.; Nayak, K.S.; Agarwal, S.K.; Abraham, G. COVID-19 Working Group of Indian Society of Nephrology. *Indian J. Nephrol.* **2020**, *30*, 171–173.
126. Sachdeva, M.; Uppal, N.N.; Hirsch, J.S.; Ng, J.H.; Malieckal, D.; Fishbane, S.; Jhaveri, K.D. Northwell COVID-19 Research Consortium and the Northwell Nephrology COVID-19 Research Consortium. COVID-19 in Hospitalized Patients on Chronic Peritoneal Dialysis: A Case Series. *Am. J. Nephrol.* **2020**, *51*, 669–674. [CrossRef] [PubMed]
127. Ozturk, S.; Gursu, M.; Arici, M.; Sahin, I.; Eren, N.; Yilmaz, M.; Koyuncu, S.; Karahisar Sirali, S. Evaluation of Out-comes of Peritoneal Dialysis Patients in the Post-COVID-19 Period: A National Multicenter Case-Control Study from Turkey. *Nephron* **2023**, *147*, 272–280. [CrossRef] [PubMed]
128. Toapanta, N.; Torres, I.B.; Sellarés, J.; Chamoun, B.; Serón, D.; Moreso, F. Kidney transplantation and COVID-19 renal and patient prognosis. *Clin. Kidney J.* **2021**, *14* (Suppl. S1), i21–i29. [CrossRef]
129. Mahalingasivam, V.; Craik, A.; Tomlinson, L.A.; Ge, L.; Hou, L.; Wang, Q.; Yang, K.; Fogarty, D.G.; Keenan, C. A systematic review of COVID-19 and kidney transplantation. *Kidney Int. Rep.* **2021**, *6*, 24–45. [CrossRef]
130. Hilbrands, L.B.; Duivenvoorden, R.; Vart, P.; Franssen, C.F.M.; Hemmelder, M.H.; Jager, K.J.; Kieneker, L.M. COVID-19-related mortality in kidney transplant and dialysis patients: Results of the ERACODA collaboration. *Nephrol. Dial. Transplant* **2020**, *35*, 1973–1983. [CrossRef]
131. Gandolfini, I.; Crespo, M.; Hellemans, R.; Maggiore, U.; Mariat, C.; Mjoen, G.; Oniscu, G.C.; Peruzzi, L.; Sever, M.S.; Watschinger, B.; et al. Issues regarding COVID-19 in kidney transplantation in the ERA of the Omicron variant: A commentary by the ERA Descartes Working Group. *Nephrol. Dial. Transplant* **2022**, *22*, 1824–1829. [CrossRef] [PubMed]
132. Maggiore, U.; Abramowicz, D.; Crespo, M.; Mariat, C.; Mjoen, G.; Peruzzi, L.; Sever, M.S.; Oniscu, G.C.; Hilbrands, L.; Watschinger, B. How should I manage immunosuppression in a kidney transplant patient with COVID-19? An ERA-EDTA DESCARTES expert opinion. *Nephrol. Dial. Transplant.* **2020**, *35*, 899–904. [CrossRef] [PubMed]
133. Anand, S.; Montez-Rath, M.E.; Han, J.; Garcia, P.; Cadden, L.; Hunsader, P.; Kerschmann, R.; Beyer, P.; Dittrich, M.; Block, G.A.; et al. Antibody Response to COVID-19 Vaccination in Patients Receiving Dialysis. *J. Am. Soc. Nephrol.* **2021**, *32*, 2435–2438. [CrossRef]
134. Hsu, C.M.; Weiner, D.E.; Manley, H.J.; Aweh, G.N.; Ladik, V.; Frament, J.; Miskulin, D.; Argyropoulos, C.; Abreo, K.; Chin, A.; et al. Seroresponse to SARS-CoV-2 Vaccines among Maintenance Dialysis Patients over 6 Months. *Clin. J. Am. Soc. Nephrol.* **2022**, *17*, 403–413. [CrossRef] [PubMed]
135. Peiyao, R.; Mengjie, Y.; Xiaogang, S.; Wenfang, H.; Danna, Z.; Yuqun, Z.; Juan, J.; Qiang, H. Immunogenicity and safety of SARS-CoV-2 vaccine in hemodialysis patients: A systematic review and meta-analysis. *Front. Public Health* **2022**, *10*, 951096. [CrossRef]
136. Fiolet, T.; Kherabi, Y.; MacDonald, C.J.; Ghosn, J.; Peiffer-Smadja, N. Comparing COVID-19 vaccines for their characteristics, efficacy and effectiveness against SARS-CoV-2 and variants of concern: A narrative review. *Clin. Microbiol. Infect.* **2022**, *28*, 202–221. [CrossRef]
137. Chenchula, S.; Karunakaran, P.; Sharma, S.; Chavan, M. Current evidence on efficacy of COVID-19 booster dose vaccination against the Omicron variant: A systematic review. *J. Med. Virol.* **2022**, *94*, 2969–2976. [CrossRef]
138. Zhou, Z.; Zhu, Y.; Chu, M. Role of COVID-19 Vaccines in SARS-CoV-2 Variants. *Front. Immunol.* **2022**, *13*, 898192. [CrossRef]
139. Zheng, Q.; Wang, M.; Cheng, Y.; Liu, J.; Feng, Z.; Ye, L. Antibody response and safety of COVID-19 vaccine in peritoneal dialysis patients. *J. Infect.* **2022**, *85*, e167–e171. [CrossRef]
140. Panizo, N.; Albert, E.; Giménez-Civera, E.; Puchades, M.J.; D'Marco, L.; Gandía-Salmerón, L.; Giménez, E.; Torre, I.; Sancho, A.; Gavela, E.; et al. Dynamics of SARS-CoV-2-Spike-reactive antibody and T-cell responses in chronic kidney disease patients within 3 months after COVID-19 full vaccination. *Clin. Kidney J.* **2022**, *15*, 1562–1573. [CrossRef]
141. ElSawi, H.A.; Elborollosy, A. Immune-mediated adverse events post-COVID vaccination and types of vaccines: A systematic review and meta-analysis. *Egypt. J. Intern. Med.* **2022**, *34*, 1–11. [CrossRef]
142. Klomjit, N.; Zand, L.; Cornell, L.D.; Alexander, M.P. COVID-19 and Glomerular Diseases. *Kidney Int. Rep.* **2023**, *8*, 1137–1150. [CrossRef]
143. Diebold, M.; Locher, E.; Boide, P.; Enzler-Tschudy, A.; Faivre, A.; Fischer, I.; Helmchen, B.; Hopfer, H.; Kim, M.J.; Moll, S.; et al. Incidence of new onset glomerulonephritis after SARS-CoV-2 mRNA vaccination is not increased. *Kidney Int.* **2022**, *102*, 1409–1419. [CrossRef]
144. Huang, C.; Huang, L.; Wang, Y.; Li, X.; Ren, L.; Gu, X.; Kang, L.; Guo, L.; Liu, M.; Zhou, X.; et al. 6-month conse-quences of COVID-19 in patients discharged from hospital: A cohort study. *Lancet.* **2023**, *401*, e21–e33. [CrossRef] [PubMed]

145. Nugent, J.; Aklilu, A.; Yamamoto, Y.; Simonov, M.; Li, F.; Biswas, A.; Ghazi, L.; Greenberg, H.; Mansour, G.; Moledina, G.; et al. Assessment of Acute Kidney Injury and Longitudinal Kidney Function After Hospital Discharge Among Patients with and Without COVID-19. *JAMA Netw. Open* **2021**, *4*, e211095. [CrossRef] [PubMed]
146. Bowe, B.; Xie, Y.; Xu, E.; Al-Aly, Z. Kidney Outcomes in Long COVID. *J. Am. Soc. Nephrol.* **2021**, *32*, 2851–2862. [CrossRef] [PubMed]
147. Gu, X.; Huang, L.; Cui, D.; Wang, Y.; Wang, Y.; Xu, J.; Shang, L.; Fan, G.; Cao, B. Association of acute kidney injury with 1-year outcome of kidney function in hospital survivors with COVID-19: A cohort study. *Ebiomedicine* **2022**, *76*, 103817. [CrossRef]
148. Schiffl, H.; Lang, S.M. Long-term interplay between COVID-19 and chronic kidney disease. *Int. Urol. Nephrol.* **2023**, *55*, 1977–1984. [CrossRef]

encyclopedia

Entry

Telemental Health and Diverse Populations amid COVID-19

Jiadong Yu * and D. A. Bekerian

California School of Professional Psychology, Alliant International University, Fresno, CA 93727, USA
* Correspondence: jyu1@alliant.edu

Definition: Telemental health is defined as the delivery of psychological and mental health services via telecommunication technologies, including telephone-delivered therapy, videoconferencing, and internet-delivered programs. Research indicates that telemental health services are as effective as in-person services, and a dramatic increase in the use of telemental health has been observed during COVID-19. However, there are still persistent challenges and concerns about mental health providers' competencies, clients' data privacy, and legal and regulatory issues during this pandemic. Additionally, disparities in the use of telemental health services with diverse populations, based on factors such as age, gender, ethnicity, socioeconomic status, language, and culture, have been identified during this pandemic.

Keywords: telemental health; telemental health disparity; diverse population; COVID-19

1. Introduction

The Novel Coronavirus 2019 Disease (COVID-19) was an outbreak of severe acute respiratory syndrome (SARS), first reported in Wuhan, China [1]. The World Health Organization (WHO) declared this outbreak as a Public Health Emergency of International Concern (PHEIC) after COVID-19 infection rates rapidly spread across the world [2]. Initially, the public had to face this imminent health risk with limited information. In response, governments across the world decided to impose movement restrictions to curb COVID-19 spread [3]. The implementation of movement restrictions on daily life brought immediate challenges across all elements of society. In particular, the restrictions required mental health providers to offer and deliver care services via distance-based services rather than in-person services.

These distance-based services are collectively referred to as telemental health services. Telemental health refers to the use of telecommunication technologies to deliver mental healthcare services remotely, such as telephone-delivered therapy, videoconferencing, and internet-delivered programs. Services that can be delivered via telemental health include providing patients with health information and direct healthcare. This allows individuals to receive care from their own homes or other locations.

Telemental health has become an increasingly important tool in providing access to healthcare for the diverse population before and during the COVID-19 pandemic. However, disparities existed in access to telemental health services across different groups [4]. This entry aims to provide a general overview of the challenges and concerns that mental health providers are likely to face while delivering telemental health services and to examine disparities in telemental health services usage among diverse populations during COVID-19. However, the scope of the entry is limited to the existing literature that pertains to the use and delivery of telemental health services, and the low publication rate of Eastern countries may result in limited geographical diversity.

Citation: Yu, J.; Bekerian, D.A. Telemental Health and Diverse Populations amid COVID-19. *Encyclopedia* **2023**, *3*, 267–278. https://doi.org/10.3390/encyclopedia3010017

Academic Editor: Stephen Bustin and Raffaele Barretta

Received: 24 December 2022
Revised: 23 February 2023
Accepted: 25 February 2023
Published: 27 February 2023

2. Telemental Health Services and COVID-19

2.1. Defining Telemental Health Services

Telemental health has a history dating back to the mid-20th century. Early forms of telemental health involved the use of telegraphs and radios to transmit medical information and provide a medical examination over distances to reduce unnecessary office visits [5]. As technologies progressed, new forms of mental health intervention delivery were discovered to improve the accessibility of mental healthcare.

Telephone, videoconferencing, and internet-delivered programs are now commonly utilized to provide mental health services [6]. Based on different types of communication, telemental health services can be categorized as synchronous and asynchronous [7]. Synchronous services refer to a mode of delivering health services where a real-time meeting occurs between the client and the health provider, such as telephone-based therapy and video-based therapy. Asynchronous services, in contrast, do not require a real-time meeting between the client and the service providers. Asynchronous services use the "store-and-forward" technique where the client's history report is sent to the mental health providers for diagnoses and treatment plans, which increase the flexibility for mental health providers to deliver the treatment [7,8]. For example, computerized or web-based assessments are the common methods of providing asynchronous telemental health services.

Telemental health services were mainly provided in rural and underserved areas to bridge the gap in mental health access in the United States [9]. Research demonstrated that Americans living in rural areas were eager to use the Internet for mental health services, especially where there were limited mental health providers available in their areas [10]. To this end, the Federal Communication Commission (FCC) in the United States commits millions of dollars each year to implement telemental health programs to help Americans keep connected to health services [11]. Several studies indicated increased satisfaction in receiving telemental health interventions across rural communities in the United States [12,13]. In Middle Eastern countries, telemental health services were increasingly used to meet the growing demands for mental healthcare, typically provided through hotlines and messaging services [14]. Telemental health was also found feasible in conflict-settings in several countries in the Eastern Mediterranean region by using low-cost technologies [15]. In Southeast Asia, telemental health also has the potential to achieve universal health coverage and has started to be implemented, such as in India, where the national telehealth network scheme has provided infrastructures for telemental health services in hospitals and remote healthcare facilities over the last two decades [16,17].

Telemental health has become increasingly important as a means of delivering mental health services [9,18]. For example, there were approximately twice as many U.S. mental health facilities offering telemental health in 2017 compared to 2010 [19]. Treatments delivered via telemental health have been found effective in addressing different mental health conditions, including substance abuse, depression, and anxiety [20–22]. Research suggests that the use of telecommunication results in higher completion rates of substance abuse treatment programs compared to in-person services; clients are also inclined to demonstrate more acceptance towards Internet-based treatment programs as it is more convenient and has more perceived confidentiality [23,24]. Multiple studies on telemental health have been conducted in different countries and demonstrated its effectiveness and efficacy, which further contributed to the increased need for telemental health services [25,26]. What is more important, as Western-developed countries have more access to care compared to developing countries, telemental health can bring evidence-based practices to the under-served and difficult-to-reach areas globally [27].

Along with the implementation of telemental health, studies have also found that telemental health services can reduce costs and overall evaluation time compared to in-person services [28,29]. For example, a longitudinal study found that the use of telemental health maintained the advantages in access and quality of mental health services with cost-efficiencies in a 2-year period [30]. Even though some studies would argue that the cost of telemental health services varied widely, there is good evidence that telemental health increases access to mental health services and is as effective as in-person interventions [31,32].

It is evident that the use of telemental health services has progressed over the years. Telemental health has been proven effective in treating mental health conditions and has helped reach clients who had limited access to mental health services prior to the COVID-19 pandemic. Although the system to provide reliable access to effective telemental health services is still developing, the advent of COVID-19 inevitably accelerated the progress.

2.2. Telemental Health Competency Concern

The movement restrictions and social distancing guidelines brought immediate challenges for mental health providers and caused a rapid transition in the delivery of mental health services. In a survey conducted by the American Psychological Association between 23 April and 6 May in 2020, 76% of clinicians only provided remote services via phone, a designated telemental health platform, or videoconferencing software. In contrast, 3% of clinicians provided only in-person services [33]. Currently, many practicing mental health providers have reduced the time of seeing their clients in person and shifted to treating clients remotely because of the COVID-19 pandemic [34,35]. As there is an exponential increase in the usage of telemental health services, it is important to consider implementing telemental health training as some mental health providers might not be familiar with new technologies [36]. It is necessary for mental health providers to be comfortable with new technologies and be competent enough to utilize new technologies to facilitate individualized treatment [37].

Maheu et al.'s review (2019) presented the development of a measurable framework: the Coalition for Technology in Behavioral Science (CTiBS) for telemental health competencies based on literature reviews, technological advances, and clinical practice [38]. For example, mental health providers need to demonstrate their understanding of making decisions regarding the choice of using technology based on their own and their client's experience with technology. Maheu et al. also argued how crucial it is for mental health providers to understand how to utilize appropriate technology. Knowing how to use the technology helps maximize the therapeutic atmosphere during the meeting and spontaneously fosters a positive therapeutic relationship [38].

This framework identified the need for telemental health competency training; other studies have considered other factors that might impact new technology-based competencies, e.g., the length of time required for mental health providers to become familiar with telemental health technologies and workflows [39,40]. However, Edirippulige and Armfield's systemic review (2016) suggested there were limited programs related to the delivery of telemental health education and training. The authors found only nine studies that reported any formal telemental health training and education from universities, and public or private organizations [41]. The teaching and learning of telemental health competencies were not widely included in the formal education and training received by mental health professionals.

In response to the rapid shift during the COVID-19 pandemic, professional organizations such as American Telemedicine Association and American Psychological Association provided free online webinars, recorded content, and other resources as basic telemental health education to guide mental health providers through the transition [42,43]. A new training program was established and implemented at Virginia Commonwealth University to offer the training needed for telemental health, and the authors found the increased use of supervision via telephone or videoconferencing is a key factor for providing the necessary support for the trainees [44]. However, in India and Saudi Arabia standard practice protocols or guidelines need to be developed for mental health providers to ensure the quality of telemental health services [45,46].

Overall, the situation during the COVID-19 pandemic highlighted concerns regarding the paucity of telemental health training and education. The available literature suggests that with such a rapid transition there was limited time for mental health providers to take educational training to develop telemental health competencies. There is also little evidence to show that short-term telemental health training programs have been adequately developed or studied for their effectiveness.

2.3. *Privacy and Confidentiality Concern*

With the pressure created by the COVID-19 pandemic, regulatory adjustments on the policy have been made by the United States government to meet the significantly increased needs for telemental health services [47]. For example, the United States Drug Enforcement Administration (DEA) has relaxed the standards for prescribing controlled substances when using telemental health services [48]. Although these adjustments can promote more access to mental health services, there are concerns about privacy and data confidentiality with the relaxation of standards.

A systemic review by Ftouni et al. (2022) suggested clients were concerned about their privacy and confidentiality regarding the use of telemental health services, which became another major barrier to telemental health visits [49]. For example, third-party commercial platforms such as Zoom, FaceTime, and Skype were commonly used for telemental health services. However, there are uncertainties about adequate encryption for these platforms for healthcare use [50]. Without adequate security and privacy protection, the mistrust from clients will impact the therapeutic relationship and impede the use of telemental health services [51]. The issues of clients' privacy and confidentiality must be studied in the future if telemental health is to be successful. With the increased use of third-party commercial platforms, technical issues became a significant barrier to accessing telemental health services.

For the purpose of promoting telemental health services during the COVID-19 pandemic, China established a trillion-dollar plan to expand digital infrastructure for stable connections, which includes developing 5G networks, industrial internet, and ultra-high-voltage (UHV) power transmission [52]. In Europe, the Netherlands, as one of the leading European countries in providing telemental health services, has been advancing the transition prior to COVID-19. In response to the pandemic, a COVID-19 online portal for sharing patient information was developed and implemented within months, and this platform further safeguards clients' privacy and was made available for free to all hospitals at launch [53]. However, in Sub-Saharan African countries, infrastructure and technical barriers, including electricity and internet, still exist during the COVID-19 pandemic [54]. Limited access to technology and poor internet connection were identified as important factors that prevented clients from engaging in telemental health services [55]. These factors can also impede the communication and interactions between the client and the mental health provider [49].

2.4. *Legal and Regulatory Issues*

In the United State, as telemental health services are often provided across state lines, mental health providers often needed to confront complex state licensure requirements [56]. With regulatory adjustments on policy, the Centers for Medicare and Medicaid Services (CMS) relaxed the restrictions for interstate telemental health services during COVID-19. However, some barriers still existed. For example, licensed professional mental health counselors were excluded from the exemptions [57]. Further, many states had not completely lifted restrictions to allow clinicians to practice across state lines; some states in the United States required health providers to submit an application for an emergency license [58]. The concerns many health providers have regarding licensure requirements across state boundaries further hinder the implementation of telemental health services.

In Middle Eastern countries, the healthcare system has been influenced by different legal and regulatory frameworks. The governmental structure in some countries was found to have a negative effect on the delivery of telemental health services, which further impacted clients' intention to use telemental health [59]. Moreover, regulatory and legislative guidelines are still in need of maneuvering the practice of telemental health services to accommodate the rapid growth of telemental health during COVID-19 in these countries [60].

Reimbursement is one of the key components in considering the use of telemental health services. In the efforts to implement telemental health services, the Centers for Medicare and Medicaid Services expanded reimbursement for telemental health services during the COVID-19 pandemic [61]. Along with the recommendations from the CMS, some insurance companies started to expand coverage for telemental health services and telemental health services reimbursement [62]. Most health providers reported that they would continue to provide telemental health services if reimbursement continues [49]. However, future reimbursement for telemental health services still remains uncertain. Moreover, telemental health services were not reimbursed in all countries across the world. For example, there is no legislation for reimbursing telemental health services in countries such as Egypt and Brazil [63,64]. In Italy, a regulatory framework for telemental health started to develop along with the implementation of telemental health services in 2012 [65]. However, during COVID-19, similar to many Middle Eastern countries, telemental health services are still not considered essential levels of care in the public health system, causing the use of these services to primarily rely on out-of-pocket payment. Without support from government institutions, the implementation of telemental health services is likely to slow down in the future [60,66].

In summary, there are numerous challenges and concerns that need to be addressed for telemental health to continue to be an effective alternative to in-person treatment. Some of these challenges and concerns have been addressed in response to the COVID-19 pandemic, leading to the rapid shift to telemental health in certain countries. However, many of these challenges and concerns still persist. It is essential that all of these challenges and concerns are taken into consideration when implementing telemental health services in the future. Understanding these concerns and challenges will also aid in preparing mental health providers in the field of telemental health.

3. Disparities in the Use of Telemental Health Services

3.1. Age Disparities

The implementation of telemental health services is a promising solution to providing healthcare for people who have difficulties meeting health providers in person. Ideally, telemental health could help reduce health disparities in access to healthcare. However, disparities in the use of telemental health services during the COVID-19 pandemic have been found among diverse populations. Age, gender, race, socioeconomic status, and language factors impact on the equity of telemental health services across different populations [4,67–70].

For example, Jaffe et al.'s study found adults aged over 45 were less likely to use telemental health services compared to adults aged 18 to 44 years. This finding may be the result of older adults not being familiar with new technologies and resisting the use of telemental health services [67,71]. In addition, Luo et al.'s study (2021) suggested older adults were less likely to be prepared for telemental health services due to inexperience with technology [72,73]. Certainly, older adults preferred telemental health services to avoid the risks of in-person during the COVID-19 pandemic. However, the struggle with new technology impeded their attempt to use telemental health services [74]. Further studies are needed in the future to understand factors that contribute to the potential difficulties in using telemental health services among the older adults group.

3.2. Gender Disparities

It is evident that disparities in using telemental health services existed between older adults and young adults. However, there is also a significant gap in using telemental health services between male adults and female adults. For example, Lou et al. (2021) found more females preferred to use telemental health services [72]. One explanation for this disparity is that female adults worried more about health concerns during the COVID-19 pandemic, while male adults were more concerned with the effects on the economy and society [75]. In contrast, Rahman et al.'s study (2022) in Bangladesh suggested the opposite finding. Their study suggested male adults more commonly used telemental health services compared to female adults. The authors argued the finding was the result of the potential gap in health awareness and literacy that existed between males and females in Bangladesh during the COVID-19 pandemic [76]. Nevertheless, these results indicated there is a disparity in using telemental health services between female adults and male adults that requires more attention.

3.3. Ethnic and Socioeconomic Disparities

Notable disparities in using telemental health services also exist in different ethnic groups and across different socioeconomic statuses. A study by Ramirez et al. (2020) suggested there was a significantly lower use of telemental health services among Hispanic clients compared to non-Hispanic White clients [77]. East and Southeast Asians also reportedly used telemental health services less often than non-Hispanic Whites [78]. In addition, African Americans represented a smaller proportion of those using telemental health services compared to non-Hispanic Whites [79]. These results indicated challenges in accessing and using telemental health services in minority communities during the COVID-19 pandemic. One of the possible explanations is the consequences of the digital divide.

The term digital divide refers to unequal access to technologies and uneven access to health information and communication among different groups [80]. There are two different levels regarding the digital divide. The first-level digital divide includes two different accesses: physical access and material access. Physical access, for example, is the access to broadband internet and smartphone devices, whereas material access refers to the ability to maintain access to the Internet over time [81]. When it comes to broadband internet, Black and Hispanic Americans reported less access compared to White Americans in Vogels's recent study (2021); a similar result was found regarding smartphone ownership, where Black and Hispanic Americans have less ownership compared to White Americans [82].

This first-level digital divide could be the potential reason for the gap in using telemental health services between different ethnic groups, where there is an evident disparity in accessing the Internet and the ownership of digital devices. Noticeably, low-income clients are likely to have similar difficulties in accessing the Internet and owning digital devices [83]. Despite the difficulty in physical access, the low-income group is also likely to struggle to maintain internet access in terms of material access. Studies indicated there is a disparity in using telemental health services among different income levels, where the low-income group was reportedly less likely to use telemental health services [84,85].

The second-level digital divide is defined as the ability to find reliable information on the Internet efficiently and effectively [86]. Additionally, it can be interpreted as a person's ability to determine the trustworthiness of information from online sources [80]. For example, Hispanics were less likely to seek internet health information compared to non-Hispanic Whites, although Hispanics agreed that health information from the Internet could be helpful [87]. The language barrier, one of the possible explanations, impeded non-English speakers' ability to find reliable information on the Internet. This language factor resulted in further disparity in using telemental health services.

3.4. Language Barrier

Language also has been identified as an important barrier to telemental health use in different ethnic groups, particularly in non-English-speaking clients [88]. For example, Asian Americans reportedly have more than 100 different languages and dialects across over 50 ethnicities [89]. There is a higher percentage of limited English proficiency found in Vietnamese, Chinese, and Korean clients [90]. The linguistic barrier could discourage Asian Americans and other minority groups with limited English proficiency from seeking telemental health services. The problem of a lack of bilingual services may account for the limited use of telemental health in these populations during the COVID-19 pandemic.

For example, unprofessional interpreters and missing bilingual services are the common causes of miscommunication between patients and health provider professionals, which further resulted in poor quality of care reported by linguistic minority groups [91]. The implementation of bilingual services has been found useful in improving the quality of healthcare and the level of satisfaction, which would further promote the use of telemental health services [92]. It is also important for policy makers and health providers to consider the implementation of bilingual services and promote linguistic equity when reducing the disparity in using telemental health services.

3.5. Cultural Stigma

Despite the consequences of the digital divide, another explanation for notable disparities that existed in different ethnic groups using telemental health services is the cultural stigma. A stigma can be defined as the implication of social disproval, which leads to discrimination and exclusion and affects an individual's self-esteem [93]. Stigmatization can be identified differently across cultures in diverse populations [94]. For example, seeking mental health services would be seen as an act of a "loss of face" in East Asian Culture, where "face" is known as a symbol of strong self-esteem [95]. What is more, Asian Americans reportedly had the lowest rate of seeking mental services compared to other ethnic groups [96] as they could be afraid of being culturally stigmatized. Therefore, seeking mental health services would incur discrimination among Asian Americans. Furthermore, there is a lack of awareness and acknowledgment of the need to seek mental health services in diverse populations [70]. For example, Asian Americans were concerned about burdening others when seeking mental health services, which led to an improper understanding of mental health [70]. Regardless of the advantages telemental health services have, it is impossible for the delivery of telemental health services to close the gap in access to healthcare under these circumstances. Future research is needed to focus on the different stigmas these populations are facing and consider cultural stigma when promoting equity in the use of telemental health services.

4. Conclusions and Prospects

The use of telemental health services has progressed over the years, and the effectiveness and efficacy of telemental health services have been proven before the COVID-19 pandemic. The COVID-19 pandemic forced an unprecedently rapid transition from in-person services to telemental health services. The transition has raised many questions.

Guiding organizations such as the American Counseling Association and the American Psychological Association have highlighted the importance of several factors for mental health providers to adopt telemental health services. For example, it is suggested that providers review the research on both efficacy and effectiveness to guide technology selection, be aware of the safety and crisis planning when using telemental health services, and be ready for the adaptations for interventions [97,98]. However, some important questions remain to be answered:

- Discussion must focus on the challenges and concerns (competency, privacy and confidentiality, legal issues, and future reimbursement) that mental health providers faced during the COVID-19 pandemic.
- Future research is needed for a reliable and valid system to address these concerns. More research will enable better solutions to the challenges and concerns that impede the implementation of telemental health services after COVID-19.
- Although the use of telemental health services can provide a solution to health disparities, the extant literature strongly argues that age, gender, race, socioeconomic status, language, and culture have prevented diverse populations from accessing and using telemental health services.
- A framework for telemental health equity incorporating individual, interpersonal, community, and societal variables is needed to address the disparities in using and accessing telemental health services among diverse populations.

We acknowledge that this entry is based on a non-systematic literature review. It may have selection bias when presenting these questions. Therefore, future research could minimize the bias by using a systematic or scoping review.

Author Contributions: Conceptualization, J.Y. and D.A.B.; writing—original draft preparation, J.Y.; writing—review and editing, J.Y. and D.A.B.; supervision, D.A.B. All authors have read and agreed to the published version of the manuscript.

Funding: This research received no external funding.

Institutional Review Board Statement: Not applicable.

Informed Consent Statement: Not applicable.

Data Availability Statement: Not applicable.

Conflicts of Interest: The authors declare no conflict of interest.

References

1. World Health Organization. Pneumonia of Unknown Cause–China. 2020. Available online: https://www.who.int/emergencies/disease-outbreak-news/item/2020-DON229 (accessed on 24 December 2022).
2. World Health Organization. Statement on the Second Meeting of the International Health Regulations (2005) Emergency Committee Regarding the Outbreak of Novel Coronavirus (2019-nCoV). 2020. Available online: https://www.who.int/news/item/30-01-2020-statement-on-the-second-meeting-of-the-international-health-regulations-(2005)-emergency-committee-regarding-the-outbreak-of-novel-coronavirus-(2019-ncov) (accessed on 24 December 2022).
3. Visual, F.T.; Team, D.J. Free to Read: Lockdowns Compared: Tracking Governments' Coronavirus Responses. 2021. Available online: https://ig.ft.com/coronavirus-lockdowns/ (accessed on 24 December 2022).
4. Pierce, R.P.; Stevermer, J.J. Disparities in use of telehealth at the onset of the COVID-19 public health emergency. *J. Telemed. Telecare* **2020**, *29*, 1357633X2096389. [CrossRef] [PubMed]
5. Nesbitt, T.S. *The Evolution of Telehealth: Where Have We Been and Where Are We Going?* National Academies: Washington, DC, USA, 2012. Available online: https://www.ncbi.nlm.nih.gov/books/NBK207141/ (accessed on 24 December 2022).
6. Pruitt, L.D.; Luxton, D.D.; Shore, P. Additional clinical benefits of home-based telemental health treatments. *Prof. Psychol. Res. Pract.* **2014**, *45*, 340–346. [CrossRef]
7. Mechanic, O.J.; Persaud, Y.; Kimball, A.B. *Telehealth Systems*; StatPearls: Tampa, FL, USA, 2021. Available online: https://pubmed.ncbi.nlm.nih.gov/29083614/ (accessed on 24 December 2022).
8. Strode, S.W.; Gustke, S.; Allen, A. Technical and Clinical Progress in Telemedicine. *JAMA* **1999**, *281*, 1066–1068. [CrossRef] [PubMed]
9. Barnett, M.L.; Huskamp, H.A. Telemedicine for Mental Health in the United States: Making Progress, Still a Long Way to Go. *Psychiatr. Serv.* **2020**, *71*, 197–198. [CrossRef] [PubMed]
10. Ruggiero, K.J.; Gros, D.F.; McCauley, J.; de Arellano, M.A.; Danielson, C.K. Rural Adults' Use of Health-Related Information Online: Data from a 2006 National Online Health Survey. *Telemed. E-Health* **2011**, *17*, 329–334. [CrossRef]
11. Federal Communications Commission. Connecting Americans to Health Care. Federal Communications Commission. 2018. Available online: https://www.fcc.gov/connecting-americans-health-care (accessed on 24 December 2022).
12. Butzner, M.; Cuffee, Y. Telehealth Interventions and Outcomes Across Rural Communities in the United States: Narrative Review. *J. Med. Internet Res.* **2021**, *23*, e29575. [CrossRef]
13. Hilty, D.M.; Nesbitt, T.S.; Kuenneth, C.A.; Cruz, G.M.; Hales, R.E. Rural Versus Suburban Primary Care Needs, Utilization, and Satisfaction with Telepsychiatric Consultation. *J. Rural Health* **2007**, *23*, 163–165. [CrossRef]
14. El Hayek, S.; Nofal, M.; Abdelrahman, D.; Adra, A.; Al Harthi, M.; Al Shamli, S.; AlNuaimi, N.; Bensid, L.; Cheaito, M.A.; Emberish, A.M.; et al. Telepsychiatry in the Arab World: A Viewpoint Before and During COVID-19. *Neuropsychiatr. Dis. Treat.* **2020**, *16*, 2805–2815. [CrossRef]
15. Parkes, P.; Pillay, T.D.; Bdaiwi, Y.; Simpson, R.; Almoshmosh, N.; Murad, L.; Abbara, A. Telemedicine interventions in six conflict-affected countries in the WHO Eastern Mediterranean region: A systematic review. *Confl. Health* **2022**, *16*, 64. [CrossRef]
16. Ministry of Health & Family Wefare. E-Health & Telemedicine. 2023. Available online: https://main.mohfw.gov.in/Organisation/departments-health-and-family-welfare/e-Health-Telemedicine (accessed on 24 December 2022).
17. Gudi, N.; Konapur, R.; John, O.; Sarbadhikari, S.; Landry, M. Telemedicine supported strengthening of primary care in WHO South East Asia region: Lessons from the COVID-19 pandemic experiences. *BMJ Innov.* **2021**, *7*, 580–585. [CrossRef]
18. Barnett, M.L.; Ray, K.N.; Souza, J.; Mehrotra, A. Trends in Telemedicine Use in a Large Commercially Insured Population, 2005–2017. *JAMA* **2018**, *320*, 2147–2149. [CrossRef] [PubMed]
19. Spivak, S.; Spivak, A.; Cullen, B.; Meuchel, J.; Johnston, D.; Chernow, R.; Green, C.; Mojtabai, R. Telepsychiatry Use in U.S. Mental Health Facilities, 2010–2017. *Psychiatr. Serv.* **2020**, *71*, 121–127. [CrossRef] [PubMed]

20. Benavides-Vaello, S.; Strode, A.; Sheeran, B.C. Using Technology in the Delivery of Mental Health and Substance Abuse Treatment in Rural Communities: A Review. *J. Behav. Health Serv. Res.* **2012**, *40*, 111–120. [CrossRef] [PubMed]
21. DelliFraine, J.L.; Dansky, K.H. Home-based telehealth: A review and meta-analysis. *J. Telemed. Telecare* **2008**, *14*, 62–66. [CrossRef] [PubMed]
22. Palylyk-Colwell, E.; Argáez, C. *Telehealth for the Assessment and Treatment of Depression, Post-Traumatic Stress Disorder, and Anxiety: Clinical Evidence*; Canadian Agency for Drugs and Technologies in Health, 2018. Available online: https://www.ncbi.nlm.nih.gov/books/NBK532701/ (accessed on 24 December 2022).
23. Copeland, J.; Martin, G. Web-based interventions for substance use disorders. *J. Subst. Abus. Treat.* **2004**, *26*, 109–116. [CrossRef]
24. King, V.L.; Stoller, K.B.; Kidorf, M.; Kindbom, K.; Hursh, S.; Brady, T.; Brooner, R.K. Assessing the effectiveness of an Internet-based videoconferencing platform for delivering intensified substance abuse counseling. *J. Subst. Abus. Treat.* **2009**, *36*, 331–338. [CrossRef] [PubMed]
25. Marchand, A.; Beaulieu-Prévost, D.; Guay, S.; Bouchard, S.; Drouin, M.S.; Germain, V. Relative Efficacy of Cognitive-Behavioral Therapy Administered by Videoconference for Posttraumatic Stress Disorder: A Six-Month Follow-Up. *J. Aggress. Maltreatment Trauma* **2011**, *20*, 304–321. [CrossRef] [PubMed]
26. Langarizadeh, M.; Tabatabaei, M.; Tavakol, K.; Naghipour, M.; Moghbeli, F. Telemental Health Care, an Effective Alternative to Conventional Mental Care: A Systematic Review. *Acta Inform. Med.* **2017**, *25*, 240. [CrossRef]
27. Augusterfer, E.F.; Mollica, R.F.; Lavelle, J. A review of telemental health in international and post-disaster settings. *Int. Rev. Psychiatry* **2015**, *27*, 540–546. [CrossRef]
28. Southard, E.P.; Neufeld, J.D.; Laws, S. Telemental Health Evaluations Enhance Access and Efficiency in a Critical Access Hospital Emergency Department. *Telemed. E-Health* **2014**, *20*, 664–668. [CrossRef]
29. Grady, B.J. A Comparative Cost Analysis of an Integrated Military Telemental Health-Care Service. *Telemed. J. E-Health* **2002**, *8*, 293–300. [CrossRef]
30. Neufeld, J.; Case, R. Walk-In Telemental Health Clinics Improve Access and Efficiency: A 2-Year Follow-Up Analysis. *Telemed. E-Health* **2013**, *19*, 938–941. [CrossRef] [PubMed]
31. Naslund, J.A.; Mitchell, L.M.; Joshi, U.; Nagda, D.; Lu, C. Economic evaluation and costs of telepsychiatry programmes: A systematic review. *J. Telemed. Telecare* **2020**, *28*, 1357633X2093891. [CrossRef] [PubMed]
32. Hassan, A.; Sharif, K. Efficacy of Telepsychiatry in Refugee Populations: A Systematic Review of the Evidence. *Cureus* **2019**, *11*, e3984. [CrossRef]
33. American Psychological Association. Psychologists Embrace Telehealth to Prevent the Spread of COVID-19. 2020. Available online: https://www.apaservices.org/practice/legal/technology/psychologists-embrace-telehealth (accessed on 24 December 2022).
34. Mazziotti, R.; Rutigliano, G. Telemental Health for Reaching out to Patients in a Time of Pandemic: Provider Survey and Systematic Review with meta-analysis of Patient Satisfaction. *JMIR Ment. Health* **2021**, *8*, e26187. [CrossRef] [PubMed]
35. Zangani, C.; Ostinelli, E.G.; Smith, K.A.; Hong, J.S.W.; Macdonald, O.; Reen, G.; Reid, K.; Vincent, C.; Sheriff, R.S.; Harrison, P.J.; et al. Impact of the COVID-19 Pandemic on the Global Delivery of Mental Health Services and Telemental Health: Systematic Review. *JMIR Mental Health.* **2022**, *9*, e38600. [CrossRef]
36. Jarvis-Selinger, S.; Chan, E.; Payne, R.; Plohman, K.; Ho, K. Clinical Telehealth Across the Disciplines: Lessons Learned. *Telemed. E-Health* **2008**, *14*, 720–725. [CrossRef]
37. Anglin, C.R.; Schaafsma, J.P.; Pantazi, S.V.; Anglin, S.; Grimm, N.A.; Moehr, J.R. Video Conferencing-based Telehealth. *Methods Inf. Med.* **2005**, *44*, 334–341. [CrossRef]
38. Maheu, M.M.; Drude, K.P.; Hertlein, K.M.; Lipschutz, R.; Wall, K.; Hilty, D.M. Correction to: An Interprofessional Framework for Telebehavioral Health Competencies. *J. Technol. Behav. Sci.* **2019**, *5*, 79–111. [CrossRef]
39. Gifford, V.; Niles, B.; Rivkin, I.; Koverola, C.; Polaha, J. Continuing education training focused on the development of behavioral telehealth competencies in behavioral healthcare providers. *Rural Remote Health* **2012**, *12*, 2108. Available online: https://pubmed.ncbi.nlm.nih.gov/23240871/ (accessed on 24 December 2022). [CrossRef]
40. Perle, J.G. Mental health providers' telehealth education prior to and following implementation: A COVID-19 rapid response survey. *Prof. Psychol. Res. Pract.* **2022**, *53*, 143–150. [CrossRef]
41. Edirippulige, S.; Armfield, N. Education and training to support the use of clinical telehealth: A review of the literature. *J. Telemed. Telecare* **2016**, *23*, 273–282. [CrossRef] [PubMed]
42. American Telemedicine Association. Webinars Archives. ATA. 2023. Available online: https://www.americantelemed.org/resource_categories/webinars/ (accessed on 10 February 2023).
43. American Psychological Association. Telehealth Continuing Education Resources. 2020. Available online: https://www.apa.org/ed/ce/telehealth (accessed on 10 February 2023).
44. Perrin, P.B.; Rybarczyk, B.D.; Pierce, B.S.; Jones, H.A.; Shaffer, C.; Islam, L. Rapid telepsychology deployment during the COVID-19 pandemic: A special issue commentary and lessons from primary care psychology training. *J. Clin. Psychol.* **2020**, *76*, 1173–1185. [CrossRef] [PubMed]
45. Sagar, R.; Singh, S. National Tele-Mental Health Program in India: A step towards mental health care for all? *Indian J. Psychiatry* **2022**, *64*, 117. [CrossRef] [PubMed]

46. Almubark, B.M.; Majrashi, N.; Alghusun, N.; Alhammad, M.; Alhthifi, F.; Alyahya, R.S.W. Telehealth Clinical Practice Guide for Occupational Therapy, Physical Therapy, and Speech and Language Pathology: A Saudi and Middle Eastern Guide. *Telemed. E-Health* **2021**, *28*, 636–642. [CrossRef]
47. Panchal, N.; Kamal, R.; Cox, C.; Garfield, R. The Implications of COVID-19 for Mental Health and Substance Use. Kaiser Family Foundation. 2021. Available online: https://www.kff.org/coronavirus-covid-19/issue-brief/the-implications-of-covid-19-for-mental-health-and-substance-use/ (accessed on 24 December 2022).
48. Drug Enforcement Administration. COVID-19 Information Page. 2022. Available online: https://www.deadiversion.usdoj.gov/coronavirus.html (accessed on 24 December 2022).
49. Ftouni, R.; AlJardali, B.; Hamdanieh, M.; Ftouni, L.; Salem, N. Challenges of Telemedicine during the COVID-19 pandemic: A systematic review. *BMC Med. Inform. Decis. Mak.* **2022**, *22*, 207. [CrossRef]
50. Sinha, V.; Malik, M.; Nugent, N.; Drake, P.; Cavale, N. The Role of Virtual Consultations in Plastic Surgery During COVID-19 Lockdown. *Aesthetic Plast. Surg.* **2020**, *45*, 777–783. [CrossRef]
51. Hall, J.L.; McGraw, D. For Telehealth To Succeed, Privacy And Security Risks Must Be Identified And Addressed. *Health Aff.* **2014**, *33*, 216–221. [CrossRef]
52. Wong, D. How Can Foreign Technology Investors Benefit from China's New Infrastructure Plan? China Briefing. 2020. Available online: https://www.china-briefing.com/news/how-foreign-technology-investors-benefit-from-chinas-new-infrastructure-plan/ (accessed on 10 February 2023).
53. Invest in Holland. How the Dutch Are Responding to Coronavirus with Digital Healthcare. Health~Holland. 2020. Available online: https://www.health-holland.com/news/2020/05/how-the-dutch-are-responding-to-coronavirus-with-digital-healthcare (accessed on 11 February 2023).
54. Dodoo, J.E.; Al-Samarraie, H.; Alzahrani, A.I. Telemedicine use in Sub-Saharan Africa: Barriers and policy recommendations for Covid-19 and beyond. *Int. J. Med. Inform.* **2021**, *151*, 104467. [CrossRef]
55. Murphy, A.A.; Karyczak, S.; Dolce, J.N.; Zechner, M.; Bates, F.; Gill, K.J.; Rothpletz-Puglia, P. Challenges Experienced by Behavioral Health Organizations in New York Resulting from COVID-19: A Qualitative Analysis. *Community Ment. Health J.* **2020**, *57*, 111–120. [CrossRef]
56. Tuckson, R.V.; Edmunds, M.; Hodgkins, M.L. Telehealth. *N. Engl. J. Med.* **2017**, *377*, 1585–1592. [CrossRef]
57. Centers for Medicare & Medicaid Services. Rural Crosswalk: CMS Flexibilities to Fight COVID-19. 2021. Available online: https://www.cms.gov/files/document/omh-rural-crosswalk-5-21-21.pdf (accessed on 24 December 2022).
58. Federation of State Medical Boards. U.S. States and Territories Modifying Requirements for Telehealth in Response to COVID-19 (Out-of-State Physicians; Preexisting Provider-Patient Relationships; Audio-Only Requirements; Etc.). 2022. Available online: https://www.fsmb.org/siteassets/advocacy/pdf/states-waiving-licensure-requirements-for-telehealth-in-response-to-covid-19.pdf (accessed on 24 December 2022).
59. Jefee-Bahloul, H.; Moustafa, M.K.; Shebl, F.M.; Barkil-Oteo, A. Pilot Assessment and Survey of Syrian Refugees' Psychological Stress and Openness to Referral for Telepsychiatry (PASSPORT Study). *Telemed. E-Health* **2014**, *20*, 977–979. [CrossRef]
60. Al-Samarraie, H.; Ghazal, S.; Alzahrani, A.I.; Moody, L. Telemedicine in Middle Eastern countries: Progress, barriers, and policy recommendations. *Int. J. Med. Inform.* **2020**, *141*, 104232. [CrossRef] [PubMed]
61. Centers for Medicare and Medicaid Services. COVID-19 Emergency Declaration Blanket Waivers for Health Care Providers. 2020. Available online: https://www.cms.gov/files/document/covid19-emergency-declaration-health-care-providers-fact-sheet.pdf (accessed on 24 December 2022).
62. Blue Cross Blue Shield. Media Statement: Blue Cross and Blue Shield Companies Announce Coverage of Telehealth Services for Members. 2020. Available online: https://www.bcbs.com/press-releases/media-statement-blue-cross-and-blue-shield-companies-announce-coverage-of-telehealth-services-for-members (accessed on 16 December 2022).
63. Caetano, R.; Silva, A.B.; Guedes, A.C.C.M.; de Paiva, C.C.N.; da Rocha Ribeiro, G.; Santos, D.L.; de Silva, R.M. Challenges and opportunities for telehealth during the COVID-19 pandemic: Ideas on spaces and initiatives in the Brazilian context. *Cad Saude Publica* **2020**, *36*, e00088920. [CrossRef]
64. Mostafa, P.I.N.; Hegazy, A.A. Dermatological Consultations in the COVID-19 Era: Is Teledermatology the Key to Social Distancing? An Egyptian Experience. *J. Dermatol. Treat.* **2022**, *33*, 910–915. [CrossRef] [PubMed]
65. Italian Ministry of Health. National Guidelines on Telemedicine. 2012. Available online: https://www.salute.gov.it/portale/ehealth/homeEHealth.jsp (accessed on 12 February 2023).
66. Omboni, S. Telemedicine during The COVID-19 in Italy: A Missed Opportunity? *Telemed. E-Health* **2020**, *26*, 973–975. [CrossRef] [PubMed]
67. Jaffe, D.H.; Lee, L.; Huynh, S.; Haskell, T.P. Health Inequalities in the Use of Telehealth in the United States in the Lens of COVID-19. *Popul. Health Manag.* **2020**, *23*, 368–377. [CrossRef]
68. Ma, K.P.K.; Bacong, A.M.; Kwon, S.C.; Yi, S.S.; Đoàn, L.N. The Impact of Structural Inequities on Older Asian Americans during COVID-19. *Front. Public Health* **2021**, *9*, 1183. [CrossRef] [PubMed]
69. Qian, F.; Hastings, J.F.; Ahmed, R. Overcoming Telemental Health Disparities During The COVID-19 Pandemic. *Int. J. Qual. Health Care* **2021**, *33*, mzab127. [CrossRef] [PubMed]
70. Augsberger, A.; Yeung, A.; Dougher, M.; Hahm, H.C. Factors influencing the underutilization of mental health services among Asian American women with a history of depression and suicide. *BMC Health Serv. Res.* **2015**, *15*, 106. [CrossRef]

71. Choi, N.G.; DiNitto, D.M.; Marti, C.N.; Choi, B.Y. Telehealth Use Among Older Adults during COVID-19: Associations with Sociodemographic and Health Characteristics, Technology Device Ownership, and Technology Learning. *J. Appl. Gerontol.* **2021**, *41*, 073346482110473. [CrossRef]
72. Luo, J.; Tong, L.; Crotty, B.H.; Somai, M.; Taylor, B.; Osinski, K.; George, B. Telemedicine Adoption during the COVID-19 Pandemic: Gaps and Inequalities. *Appl. Clin. Inform.* **2021**, *12*, 836–844. [CrossRef] [PubMed]
73. Lam, K.; Lu, A.D.; Shi, Y.; Covinsky, K.E. Assessing Telemedicine Unreadiness Among Older Adults in the United States During the COVID-19 Pandemic. *JAMA Intern. Med.* **2020**, *180*, 1389. [CrossRef] [PubMed]
74. Hsiao, V.; Chandereng, T.; Lankton, R.L.; Huebner, J.A.; Baltus, J.J.; Flood, G.E.; Dean, S.M.; Tevaarwerk, A.J.; Schneider, D.F. Disparities in Telemedicine Access: A Cross-Sectional Study of a Newly Established Infrastructure during the COVID-19 Pandemic. *Appl. Clin. Inform.* **2021**, *12*, 445–458. [CrossRef]
75. van der Vegt, I.; Kleinberg, B. Women Worry about Family, Men about the Economy: Gender Differences in Emotional Responses to COVID-19. *Lect. Notes Comput. Sci.* **2020**, *12467*, 397–409. [CrossRef]
76. Rahman, S.; Amit, S.; Kafy, A.-A. Gender disparity in telehealth usage in Bangladesh during COVID-19. *SSM-Ment. Health* **2022**, *2*, 100054. [CrossRef] [PubMed]
77. Ramirez, A.V.; Ojeaga, M.; Espinoza, V.; Hensler, B.; Honrubia, V. Telemedicine in Minority and Socioeconomically Disadvantaged Communities Amidst COVID-19 Pandemic. *Otolaryngol.–Head Neck Surg.* **2020**, *164*, 019459982094766. [CrossRef] [PubMed]
78. Zhang, D.; Shi, L.; Han, X.; Li, Y.; Jalajel, N.A.; Patel, S.; Chen, Z.; Chen, L.; Wen, M.; Li, H.; et al. Disparities in telehealth utilization during the COVID-19 pandemic: Findings from a nationally representative survey in the United States. *J. Telemed. Telecare* **2021**, 1357633X2110516. [CrossRef] [PubMed]
79. Nouri, S.N.; Khoong, E.C.; Lyles, C.R.; Karliner, L. Addressing Equity in Telemedicine for Chronic Disease Management during the COVID-19 Pandemic. *NEJM Catal. Innov. Care Deliv.* **2020**, *1*. Available online: https://catalyst.nejm.org/doi/full/10.1056/CAT.20.0123 (accessed on 24 December 2022).
80. Haynes, N.; Ezekwesili, A.; Nunes, K.; Gumbs, E.; Haynes, M.; Swain, J. "Can you see my screen?" Addressing Racial and Ethnic Disparities in Telehealth. *Curr. Cardiovasc. Risk Rep.* **2021**, *15*, 23. [CrossRef]
81. van Deursen, A.J.; van Dijk, J.A. The first-level digital divide shifts from inequalities in physical access to inequalities in material access. *New Media Soc.* **2018**, *21*, 354–375. [CrossRef]
82. Atske, S.; Perrin, A. Home Broadband Adoption, Computer Ownership Vary by Race, Ethnicity in the U.S. Pew Research Center. 2021. Available online: https://www.pewresearch.org/fact-tank/2021/07/16/home-broadband-adoption-computer-ownership-vary-by-race-ethnicity-in-the-u-s/ (accessed on 24 December 2022).
83. Vogels, E. Digital Divide Persists Even as Americans with Lower Incomes Make Gains in Tech Adoption. Pew Research Center. 2021. Available online: https://www.pewresearch.org/fact-tank/2021/06/22/digital-divide-persists-even-as-americans-with-lower-incomes-make-gains-in-tech-adoption/ (accessed on 24 December 2022).
84. Lorence, D.P.; Park, H.; Fox, S. Racial disparities in health information access: Resilience of the digital divide. *J. Med. Syst.* **2006**, *30*, 241–249. [CrossRef] [PubMed]
85. Qian, A.S.; Schiaffino, M.K.; Nalawade, V.; Aziz, L.; Pacheco, F.V.; Nguyen, B.; Vu, P.; Patel, S.P.; Martinez, M.E.; Murphy, J.D. Disparities in telemedicine during COVID-19. *Cancer Med.* **2022**, *11*, 1192–1201. [CrossRef]
86. Hargittai, E. Second-Level Digital Divide. First Monday. 2002. Available online: https://firstmonday.org/ojs/index.php/fm/article/download/942/864?inline=1 (accessed on 24 December 2022).
87. Peña-Purcell, N. Hispanics' use of Internet health information: An exploratory study. *J. Med. Libr. Assoc. JMLA* **2008**, *96*, 101–107. [CrossRef] [PubMed]
88. Rodriguez, J.A.; Saadi, A.; Schwamm, L.H.; Bates, D.W.; Samal, L. Disparities in Telehealth Use Among California Patients With Limited English Proficiency. *Health Aff.* **2021**, *40*, 487–495. [CrossRef] [PubMed]
89. National Alliance on Mental Illness. Asian American and Pacific Islander | NAMI: National Alliance on Mental Illness. 2019. Available online: https://www.nami.org/Your-Journey/Identity-and-Cultural-Dimensions/Asian-American-and-Pacific-Islander (accessed on 24 December 2022).
90. Jang, Y.; Kim, M.T. Limited English Proficiency and Health Service Use in Asian Americans. *J. Immigr. Minor. Health* **2018**, *21*, 264–270. [CrossRef]
91. de Moissac, D.; Bowen, S. Impact of Language Barriers on Quality of Care and Patient Safety for Official Language Minority Francophones in Canada. *J. Patient Exp.* **2018**, *6*, 24–32. [CrossRef] [PubMed]
92. Al Shamsi, H.; Almutairi, A.G.; Al Mashrafi, S.; Al Kalbani, T. Implications of Language Barriers for Healthcare: A Systematic Review. *Oman Med. J.* **2020**, *35*, e122. [CrossRef]
93. Borenstein, J. Stigma, Prejudice and Discrimination against People with Mental Illness. American Psychiatric Association. 2020. Available online: https://www.psychiatry.org/patients-families/stigma-and-discrimination (accessed on 24 December 2022).
94. Yang, L.H.; Kleinman, A.; Link, B.G.; Phelan, J.C.; Lee, S.; Good, B. Culture and stigma: Adding moral experience to stigma theory. *Soc. Sci. Med.* **2007**, *64*, 1524–1535. [CrossRef]
95. Zane, N.; Yeh, M. The Use of Culturally-Based Variables in Assessment: Studies on Loss of Face. *Asian Am. Ment. Health* **2002**, 123–138. [CrossRef]

96. Substance Abuse and Mental Health Services Adminstration. Racial/Ethnic Differences in Mental Health Service Use among Adults. SAMHSA; 2015. Available online: https://www.samhsa.gov/data/sites/default/files/MHServicesUseAmongAdults/MHServicesUseAmongAdults.pdf (accessed on 24 December 2022).
97. American Counseling Association. ACA Code of Ethics. 2014. Available online: https://www.counseling.org/docs/default-source/default-document-library/2014-code-of-ethics-finaladdress.pdf?sfvrsn=96b532c_2 (accessed on 24 December 2022).
98. American Psychological Association. Ethical Principles of Psychologists and Code of Conduct. American Psychological Association. 2017. Available online: https://www.apa.org/ethics/code (accessed on 24 December 2022).

encyclopedia

MDPI

Review

Effects of in Utero SARS-CoV-2 Exposure on Newborn Health Outcomes

Margaret H. Kyle [1] and Dani Dumitriu [1,2,*]

1 Division of Child and Adolescent Health, Department of Pediatrics, Columbia University Vagelos College of Physicians and Surgeons, NewYork-Presbyterian Morgan Stanley Children's Hospital, New York, NY 10032, USA
2 Division of Developmental Neuroscience, Department of Psychiatry, Columbia Vagelos College of Physicians and Surgeons, New York, NY 10032, USA
* Correspondence: dani.dumitriu@columbia.edu; Tel.: +1-646-774-6255

Abstract: The severe acute respiratory syndrome coronavirus 2 (SARS-CoV-2) has infected over 600 million people worldwide, including millions of pregnant women. While newborns exposed to other viruses in utero are sometimes at high risk for vertical transmission, a substantial body of literature since early 2020 has demonstrated that vertical transmission of SARS-CoV-2 from infected mother to neonate is rare, and that newborns who do become infected with SARS-CoV-2 generally have favorable outcomes. In this review, the authors evaluate the existing literature on vertical transmission of SARS-CoV-2 and its potential mechanisms and discuss short- and long-term health outcomes in newborns who were exposed to SARS-CoV-2 in utero. The authors conclude that vertical transmission and adverse neonatal and infant/child outcomes are unlikely, but that neonates exposed to prenatal maternal SARS-CoV-2 infection may be at slightly higher risk for preterm birth, possibly related to increased risk of severe COVID-19 disease in pregnant women, placental changes, or infection timing. Ultimately, the need for additional and longer-term follow-up data in this population is highlighted.

Keywords: COVID-19; SARS-CoV-2; pregnancy; newborn; neonatal; vertical transmission; placenta; neurodevelopment

Citation: Kyle, M.H.; Dumitriu, D. Effects of in Utero SARS-CoV-2 Exposure on Newborn Health Outcomes. *Encyclopedia* **2023**, *3*, 15–27. https://doi.org/10.3390/encyclopedia3010002

Academic Editors: Stephen Bustin and Raffaele Barretta

Received: 19 September 2022
Revised: 10 December 2022
Accepted: 23 December 2022
Published: 26 December 2022

1. Introduction

Two and a half years into the COVID-19 pandemic, the severe acute respiratory syndrome coronavirus 2 (SARS-CoV-2) continues to spread worldwide. As of this writing (12 September 2022), there have been over 600 million cases globally, with over four million new cases reported in the most recent World Health Organization report for the week of 29 August 2022 [1]. The global health burden of COVID-19 disease has affected the entire world, but certain populations, including pregnant women and newborns, have been considered particularly vulnerable to potential adverse outcomes following SARS-CoV-2 infection. One fear among researchers and clinicians early on was the possibility of vertical transmission of SARS-CoV-2 from infected pregnant women to their neonates, but a large body of literature has demonstrated that this occurs in a small proportion of neonates, generally less than 5% [2–7]. Further, rates of neonatal infection do not appear to be increased when newborns breastfeed, room-in, or partake in skin-to-skin care with their mothers [5–7]. Potential mechanisms underlying rare cases of vertical transmission remain unclear, but a prevailing theory is transplacental transmission. Additionally, SARS-CoV-2 has been linked to placental alterations with the capacity to impact newborn outcomes even in the absence of placental infection [8–10]. Available data suggest that newborns exposed to maternal SARS-CoV-2 infection in utero are generally healthy, but that they may be at increased risk of premature birth [6,11–14]. The literature on long-term outcomes in these newborns is—by definition—limited. Here, the authors review the present data on vertical transmission of SARS-CoV-2 and its potential mechanisms, consider the role of the placenta in neonatal outcomes, and survey data on short- and long-term outcomes in neonates exposed to maternal SARS-CoV-2 infection in utero (Table S1).

2. Vertical Transmission of SARS-CoV-2 from Infected Mother to Newborn

2.1. Frequency of Vertical Transmission of SARS-CoV-2

Vertical transmission is defined as the transmission of an infection from an infected woman to her newborn, and may occur during intrauterine, intrapartum, or postnatal periods [15]. Possible vertical transmission of SARS-CoV-2 from infected mothers to their neonates was a source of significant concern for clinicians and researchers early in the COVID-19 pandemic, given the immature neonatal immune system [16–18]. For several viruses, including Hepatitis viruses and HIV, vertical transmission represents the major mechanism whereby infants and children develop viral infection [15,19,20]. Fortunately, a multitude of evidence since the beginning of the COVID-19 pandemic has indicated that vertical transmission of SARS-CoV-2 from infected mother to neonate is rare. Many studies, including national registries and large systematic reviews, have shown that the prevalence of vertical transmission in neonates exposed to SARS-CoV-2 in utero is generally around 5% or lower. A meta-analysis including 10,000 women infected with SARS-CoV-2 during pregnancy found a vertical transmission rate of 5.3% in exposed newborns [3], and another systematic review on 936 neonates born to SARS-CoV-2-infected mothers detected a vertical transmission rate of 3.2% [2]. Both of these analyses included reports from a wide range of countries and regions including Asia, Europe, and the Americas [2,3]. Another analysis co-reporting on 4005 pregnant women included in the American Academy of Pediatrics Section on Neonatal-Perinatal Medicine (AAP-SONPM) or the UK and Global Pregnancy and Neonatal outcomes in COVID-19 (PAN-COVID) Registry found that vertical transmission rates were 1.8% in the US registry and 2.0% in the UK registry [4].

Vertical transmission of viruses is generally thought to occur through transplacental transmission (see Section 2.2.1 below), cervicovaginal transmission during delivery, or contact with the mother during the postnatal period [19]. In addition to the low vertical transmission rates cited above, the available evidence further demonstrates that postnatal practices like vaginal delivery, breastfeeding, and rooming-in with mothers do not appear to put neonates at increased risk of infection. A systematic review by Walker et al. reported on 666 neonates born to SARS-CoV-2-infected women, 4% of whom tested positive for the virus [7]. The authors calculated separate neonatal infection rates depending on mode of delivery and postnatal care practices and found that 2.7% of vaginally delivered neonates tested positive as opposed to 5.3% of neonates born by cesarean section, and that 4.7% of breastfed newborns tested positive, a rate similar to the 5.3% of formula-fed newborns who tested positive [7]. Newborns who were allowed to room-in with their mothers also tested positive less frequently (3.7%) than those who were isolated (13%), although isolation may have occurred as a result of positive testing so this difference should be interpreted with caution. Similarly, our group reported on 101 newborns born to women infected with SARS-CoV-2 perinatally and found that 2.0% of exposed neonates tested positive for the virus, and that there was no clinical evidence of COVID-19 disease in any neonate despite encouraging rooming-in, breastfeeding, and skin-to-skin care [5]. A national cohort study from Sweden, where rooming-in, breastfeeding, and skin-to-skin care were also encouraged, reported on over 2000 newborns born to SARS-CoV-2-infected women and determined a vertical transmission rate of just 0.9% [6]. Likewise, a cohort of 177 newborns in Spain who all exclusively breastfed had a neonatal SARS-CoV-2 infection rate of 5.1% [21]. The systematic review by Kotlyar et al. that found a vertical transmission rate of 3.2% also separated rates between studies conducted in China and studies outside of China and determined that 2.0% of the neonates studied in China tested positive, as opposed to 3.5% of neonates studied outside of China [2]. It is reassuring that these rates are similar and both low, given that China has encouraged more stringent postnatal care policies to prevent neonatal infection, such as separating exposed neonates from their mothers and prohibiting breastfeeding [22]. Overall, vertical transmission appears to be unlikely in neonates exposed to maternal SARS-CoV-2 infection, and postnatal care policies like rooming-in, breastfeeding, and skin-to-skin contact that have demonstrated benefits for newborns [23–25] do not seem to augment this low risk, and are possibly even protective.

2.2. The Role of the Placenta in Vertical Transmission of SARS-CoV-2 and Neonatal Outcomes

2.2.1. Transplacental Transmission of SARS-CoV-2

Although vertical transmission of SARS-CoV 2 from mother to neonate is demonstrably rare, it is still necessary to determine the mechanism by which it may occur in infants who do become infected. Proposed mechanisms have included cervicovaginal transmission during delivery and transplacental transmission during gestation. Researchers have tested placental tissue, amniotic fluid, cord blood, and vaginal secretions from infected mothers and their neonates and shown that viral RNA is rarely detected in any of these samples using RT-PCR. A meta-analysis including 563 neonates born to SARS-CoV-2-infected mothers showed that SARS-CoV-2 was detected in 12% of placental samples and 4–6% of amniotic fluid, cord blood, and vaginal secretions tested [3]. Similarly, the above systematic review including 936 neonates born to SARS-CoV-2-infected mothers found that 7.7% of placental samples, 0% of amniotic fluid samples, and 2.9% of cord blood samples tested positive in their analysis [2]. Infection of any of these samples appears to be rare, but, notably, both analyses found higher rates SARS-CoV-2 positivity in placental samples than other samples, suggesting that transplacental transmission is more likely than cervicovaginal transmission.

The mechanism that SARS-CoV-2 uses to infect cells further implicates transplacental transmission as a possible mechanism for rare cases of vertical transmission. SARS-CoV-2 depends on two key viral factors to enter host cells: serine protease TMPRSS2 primes viral spike protein domains, facilitating cell entry using SARS-CoV receptor angiotensin-2 converting enzyme (ACE2) [26,27]. ACE2 and TMPRSS2 are highly expressed in the respiratory and gastrointestinal tracts [28], but they have also been found in placental trophoblasts [29,30], leading to speculation that placental infection and subsequent transplacental vertical transmission of SARS-CoV-2 are possible. However, transplacental infection requires co-expression of ACE2 and TMPRSS2 in placental cells as well as maternal viremia [31]. Consistent with the aforementioned low rates of vertical transmission of SARS-CoV-2, the evidence to-date has demonstrated that this co-expression is rare in placental cells [32–34], and that viremia is uncommon in SARS-CoV-2 patients [35], particularly in pregnant women [33]. Several groups have studied placental samples from SARS-CoV-2-infected mothers and found no evidence of placental infection and no difference in placental histopathology between samples taken from infected patients and those taken from uninfected patients [33,36,37]. Interestingly, even studies that found placental infection in tissue samples failed to show evidence that it predicts actual neonatal infection and vertical transmission [38–41].

To further probe the possible role of the placenta in vertical transmission, a recent study examined co-expression of ACE2 and TMPRSS2 in the placenta and in a variety of fetal tissue samples [34]. The authors found that the placenta as well as most fetal tissues analyzed did not co-express ACE2 and TMPRSS2. Only the fetal gastrointestinal tract co-expressed both proteins, suggesting that fetal infection would require swallowing of infected amniotic fluid [34]. However, in further support of the infrequency of vertical transmission, amniotic fluid is typically only infected in cases of viremia and severe disease [42].

2.2.2. Other Placental Mechanisms Related to Maternal SARS-CoV-2 Infection

The existing evidence suggests that, despite being the most plausible mechanism of vertical transmission of SARS-CoV-2, transplacental transmission from infected mother to neonate is rare and unlikely given the cellular framework required for infection. Nonetheless, placental tissue remains an important area of study in SARS-CoV-2-infected women, and recent findings indicate that adverse placental changes with the potential to impact neonatal outcomes may occur in the absence of placental infection or vertical transmission. Early in the pandemic, a research group in Chicago examined placental histopathology in 16 patients with SARS-CoV-2 during pregnancy and found that maternal vascular malperfusion (MVM) was more common in infected women compared to historical controls [9]. MVM is a pattern of placental injury related to altered blood flow to the placenta [43], and it has been linked to increased rates of adverse maternal and neonatal outcomes including preeclampsia, fetal death, small for gestational age, and preterm delivery [44]. The same group published a recent study on placental lesions in 883 women who were infected with SARS-CoV-2 during pregnancy and 185 controls with no history of infection during pregnancy or vaccination against COVID-19 [8]. Similarly, they found that MVM was significantly more common in the infected group, with 63% of women infected during pregnancy exhibiting MVM features as opposed to 47% of uninfected women. Interestingly, the authors found that MVM frequency varied depending on the stage of the pandemic during which the infection occurred, with 82% of women infected in the Delta variant era exhibiting MVM, 65% in the Alpha/Gamma era and 55% in the Omicron era [8], suggesting that viral variants may have differing effects on placental function. All Omicron patients included in the study were infected during the third trimester of pregnancy, though, so it is also possible that infection timing during gestation impacts the frequency of MVM in pregnant patients infected with SARS-CoV-2. In contrast, two other studies with sample sizes of 65 and 101 SARS-CoV-2 infected women [36,37] have shown no differences in placental pathologic features, including MVM, between infected and uninfected mothers. Of note, all studies reporting on placental lesions included in this review used the Amsterdam Criteria [45] for placental examination, so these differing findings do not appear to be related to different standardization criteria.

Given that pregnant women seem to be more susceptible to severe COVID-19 disease (see Section 3.2.2), it is also imperative to determine whether placental pathology correlates with disease severity, potentially predisposing severely ill women and their neonates to adverse pregnancy and birth outcomes. Mourad et al. [10] studied placental samples from 66 women infected with SARS-CoV-2 late in pregnancy and found that disease severity did not predict placental histopathological features, but that placental expression of ACE2 and interferon-induced transmembrane antiviral genes was higher in severely ill women, suggesting that severe disease alters the placental response to SARS-CoV-2. Contrasting this finding, the above discussed study that found increased frequency of MVM in infected women [8] also showed that MVM frequency increased with disease severity. Overall, the existing evidence regarding effects of maternal SARS-CoV-2 infection on the placenta is limited and inconclusive, but given several studies showing an altered placental environment and, separately, increased risk of preterm delivery in pregnant women with COVID-19 disease (see Section 3.2.1), it is essential that the field continues to disentangle this relationship.

3. Clinical Outcomes in Newborns Exposed to SARS-CoV-2 In Utero

3.1. Outcomes in Infected Newborns

Although vertical transmission of SARS-CoV-2 from mother to newborn is rare, outcomes must be followed in the small proportion of newborns who do become infected perinatally. The newborn immune system is immature, and newborns are especially susceptible to respiratory infections [16–18], making them a population potentially vulnerable to severe COVID-19 disease. The current literature is conflicting, but some reports have suggested increased risk in newborns infected with SARS-CoV-2. A population-level report on neonatal infection early in the pandemic in the UK found that the rate of infection in newborns was low, at 0.05–0.06% of the newborn population, but that those who were infected required intensive care or respiratory support at a high rate of 36% [46]. However, this figure is confounded by the fact that 24% of the infected infants had been born preterm and may have required respiratory support for reasons unrelated to SARS-CoV-2 infection. A study from China found that infants under one year old had severe COVID-19 disease at a higher rate than other pediatric populations, but this proportion was still low, with 10.7% of infants classified as having severe or critical disease [47], as compared to 19% of cases in the overall Chinese population classified as severe or critical during the same period [48].

In contrast to initial reports of severe disease, several studies have described asymptomatic or mild COVID-19 disease courses in newborns [6,49–52]. Early in the pandemic, two reports from large medical centers in New York [50] and Chicago [49], respectively, found that none of the newborns seen in either hospital system who had COVID-19 disease required respiratory support. Another report from New York found that 18 of 20 symptomatic newborns infected with SARS-CoV-2 and seen in the study's hospital system from March through April 2020 had a mild disease course [52]. The remaining two newborns required supplemental oxygen, but did not require intubation or other intensive intervention [52]. The national cohort from Sweden described above found that none of the 21 infants who tested positive for SARS-CoV-2 during the neonatal period had any morbidity related to COVID-19 disease [6]. Similarly, a study in India that followed outcomes in neonates with SARS-CoV-2 infection showed that a majority of the 21 neonates were asymptomatic, with only seven being diagnosed with symptomatic COVID-19 disease [53]. Three neonates required mechanical ventilation (two non-invasive, one invasive), but these neonates were born between 30- and 33-weeks gestation, and all term infants with symptomatic COVID-19 disease required only supportive care. Follow-up of 20 of the neonates two months after discharge found that none had exhibited any further symptoms or required repeat hospitalization [53]. A recent systematic review including 1214 children under the age of five, half of whom were infants under one year old, found that over 90% of children had mild or moderate disease, while only 7% had severe disease and one child died [54]. Of note, most of the available literature on newborn outcomes has come from early in the pandemic, when the Alpha/Gamma strains were dominant. More data is needed to determine differences in risk in newborns infected with SARS-CoV-2 during later variants, especially given the increased transmissibility of the recent Omicron variant and associated increased rates of hospitalization in infants and children [55]. One recent study from Massachusetts has shown that infants and children infected during the Omicron wave of the pandemic were more likely to be diagnosed with COVID-19 associated croup, but that, as has frequently been reported with earlier viral variants, no child required invasive ventilation [56]. While more studies on outcomes in newborns infected with SARS-CoV-2 are needed, the existing data indicate that newborns seem to be at lower risk of severe COVID-19 disease and death than the general population, and that adverse outcomes in neonates can typically be attributed to prematurity or other causes unrelated to COVID-19 disease.

3.2. *Neonatal Outcomes in Uninfected Newborns Exposed to SARS-CoV-2 In Utero*

3.2.1. Increased Risk of Preterm Birth in Newborns Exposed to SARS-CoV-2 In Utero

Newborns who were exposed to SARS-CoV-2 in utero but do not become infected still could be at risk for adverse outcomes, considering the demonstrated risk of delayed growth, congenital anomalies, and preterm delivery (i.e., delivery at less than 37 weeks gestation), in pregnant women with other infections and/or elevated inflammation [57–59]. The current literature indicates that maternal SARS-CoV-2 infection during pregnancy may indeed increase the risk of preterm delivery: an early study from Spain on 503 newborns exposed to SARS-CoV-2 in utero found a preterm birth rate of 15.7%, more than double the national average in Spain of 7.5% [11]. Likewise, a co-report on national registries from the US and UK including over 4000 women infected with SARS-CoV-2 during pregnancy between January and July of 2020 [4] found a 15.7% preterm birth rate in the US registry and a 12.0% preterm birth rate in the UK registry, both of which are higher than the national average rates of 10% in the US [60] and 7.5% in the UK [61]. The report from Sweden on over 2000 newborns born to mothers infected with SARS-CoV-2 during pregnancy found that these newborns appeared to have higher rates of neonatal respiratory disorders compared to case-matched controls, but this increase was mediated by their increased prevalence of preterm birth [6]. A study on 734 women in Brazil similarly found that women infected with SARS-CoV-2, and specifically those with moderate and severe COVID-19 disease, were more likely to give birth preterm and to have neonates admitted to intensive care [13]. An 18 country, multinational cohort study found further evidence of increased risk of preterm delivery in 706 SARS-CoV-2-infected women who gave birth in 2020 as compared to 1424 uninfected women, with women with symptomatic COVID-19 disease delivering on average 0.8 weeks earlier than uninfected women [14]. More recent data collected during the Omicron variant era in New York support these findings, showing a significantly increased risk of preterm birth in 631 women who were infected with SARS-CoV-2 between December 2021 and February 2022, as compared to 4107 uninfected women [12]. Conversely, two recently published studies that used data from the Alpha/Gamma variant eras found no difference in rates of preterm birth between SARS-CoV-2-infected and uninfected pregnant women in a cohort of 116 infected women in New York [62], and a six-country cohort of 510 infected women in sub-Saharan Africa [63]. While interesting, these reports had smaller sample sizes than many of the studies from the same time period that found increased risk of preterm birth, including multiple national registries. Studies that have reported on other neonatal outcomes, including Apgar scores, congenital anomalies, and small for gestational age have found no indication of abnormalities in neonates born to SARS-CoV-2-infected mothers [4,6,11,14,62,63]. Considering the evidence together, it appears that newborns who were exposed to SARS-CoV-2 in utero are at an increased risk of premature birth, but differences in gestational age at delivery between exposed and unexposed newborns are overall small, at less than one week [14]. Encouragingly, none of these studies have indicated that newborns born to SARS-CoV-2-infected mothers show increased rates of any morbidity beyond the morbidity associated with prematurity itself.

3.2.2. Possible Mechanisms Driving Increased Risk of Preterm Birth

The cause of increased rates of preterm delivery in women with SARS-CoV-2 infection during pregnancy remains unclear. One hypothesis is that increased risk of preterm delivery is related to the increased prevalence of severe COVID-19 disease in pregnant women. This is supported by several large studies and national registries that have shown that pregnant women are at higher risk of severe COVID-19 disease and intensive care unit admission. A national registry from Mexico comparing 5183 pregnant women with SARS-CoV-2 infection to 5183 non-pregnant women with SARS-CoV-2 infection and closely matched on demographic variables and underlying risk factors such as smoking, asthma, obesity, and cardiovascular disease found that pregnant women were at a significantly higher risk for death, pneumonia, and intensive care unit admission [64]. Similarly, an analysis from the Centers for Disease Control and Prevention on 400,000 women found that pregnant women with symptomatic COVID-19 disease were at higher risk than non-pregnant women with symptomatic COVID-19 disease for receiving invasive ventilation, receiving extracorporeal membrane oxygenation, being admitted to an intensive care unit, and death [65]. This analysis also adjusted for age, race, ethnicity, and underlying conditions. The most recent version of a large, living (i.e., continuously updated) systematic review on outcomes in pregnant women with SARS-CoV-2 infection included 435 studies, over 100,000 pregnant or recently pregnant women with COVID-19 disease, and 2 million non-pregnant women of reproductive age with COVID-19 disease [66]. The authors found that pregnant women were more likely to be admitted to the intensive care unit or need invasive ventilation, and were less likely to exhibit mild to moderate symptoms like fever, cough, dyspnea, and myalgia [66].

Consistent with this hypothesis that increased rates of preterm birth in women with SARS-CoV-2 infection may be driven by increased disease severity in this population, recent studies have found that disease severity predicts preterm delivery. A study pooling data on 1219 women with SARS-CoV-2 infection who delivered at 33 US hospitals showed that severe or critical COVID-19 disease was associated with higher risk of preterm birth compared to asymptomatic COVID-19 cases, but that there was no difference in risk between asymptomatic cases and mild to moderate cases [67]. Similarly, a study on over 6000 pregnant women with SARS-CoV-2 in the US found that critical COVID-19 disease was associated with increased risk of preterm birth compared to mild disease [68]. The Brazilian study mentioned above further supports this idea, finding that women with moderate and severe COVID-19 disease, but not those with asymptomatic or mild disease, were more likely than women with no SARS-CoV-2 infection during pregnancy to deliver preterm [13]. Studies on other respiratory diseases have also shown that increased disease severity is associated with preterm delivery [69], and this relationship is thought to be driven by the medical interventions and drug treatments necessary in cases of severe illness [69]. Placental infection related to other viruses has also been associated with preterm birth [70], and, given some reports of changes in the placenta in SARS-CoV-2-infected pregnant women reviewed in Section 2.2.2, particularly in cases of severe disease, placental alterations may present a possible mechanism for the increased rates of preterm birth seen in women with COVID-19 disease.

Another emerging hypothesis is that the timing of maternal SARS-CoV-2 infection relative to gestation may predict adverse neonatal outcomes like preterm delivery. It is well-established that prenatal insults affect fetal development at insult-specific critical periods during pregnancy [71], and studies on maternal malaria and influenza infection have shown that increased rates of preterm birth and low birth weight in exposed infants are driven by first or second trimester maternal infection [72–74]. Accordingly, a recent study comparing outcomes between 19,769 SARS-CoV-2-uninfected women and 882 SARS-CoV-2-infected women separated into trimester of infection groups (85 with first trimester infection, 226 with second trimester infection, and 571 with third trimester infection) found that increases in risk of preterm delivery and stillbirth in the infected group were driven by first and second trimester infections [75]. Further, the authors showed that gestational age at the time of infection was correlated with gestational age at delivery, and that maternal disease severity did not predict gestational age at delivery [75]. Another study including 402 pregnant women with SARS-CoV-2 infection in the first or second trimester and 11,705 uninfected women likewise found that infection in the first or second trimester was associated with increased risk of preterm birth, but not increased risk of moderately to extremely preterm birth (here defined as less than 34 weeks gestation), and with a slightly increased risk of fetal or neonatal death [76]. In contrast, a larger retrospective cohort study from Israel including 2753 SARS-CoV-2-infected pregnant women (478 with first trimester infection, 943 with second trimester infection, and 1332 with third trimester infection) found that third trimester infection, but not first or second trimester infection, was associated with increased risk of preterm birth [77]. Another study followed outcomes in 16 first trimester SARS-CoV-2-infected women and found no difference compared to uninfected women [78]. Clearly, the evidence on SARS-CoV-2 infection timing during pregnancy and risk of preterm birth is limited and conflicting, but, given our knowledge of trimester-specific effects of other viruses and environmental insults, this is an area that should be further explored.

4. Long-Term Outcomes in Infants and Children Exposed to SARS-CoV-2 In Utero

While immediate neonatal outcomes are largely favorable in newborns exposed to SARS-CoV-2 in utero, there is a need for longer-term research into their child development. Studies on in utero HIV-exposed uninfected children have found that exposure is associated with higher risk for neurodevelopmental delay [79,80]. The intrauterine inflammation that may result from maternal viral infection (with any virus) has been linked to epilepsy, autism spectrum disorder, and schizophrenia in offspring [81]. To investigate early indicators of this risk, our group compared Ages and Stages Questionnaire, Third Edition (ASQ-3) scores at six months of age between 114 infants exposed to SARS-CoV-2 in utero and 141 infants not exposed, and found no significant differences on any subdomain score [82]. Interestingly, though, our group found that infants born during the pandemic, irrespective of maternal infection status, had lower ASQ-3 scores in gross motor, fine motor, and personal-social domains when compared to a historical control group born prior to the pandemic, presumably mediated through maternal stress during pregnancy [82]. Another report from our group used the Infant Behavioral Questionnaire when infants were six months old and also found no differences in temperament between infants exposed vs. unexposed to SARS-CoV-2 in utero, but an association between maternal postnatal COVID-19 pandemic-related stress and both an increase in infant negative temperament and a decrease in infant positive temperament [83]. A study from Kuwait also used the ASQ-3 at 10–12 months of age in 298 infants exposed in utero to maternal SARS-CoV-2 infection, and found that 10% of infants assessed had a score that was at least two standard deviations below the population mean, indicating a possible developmental delay [84]. This report did not have a control group, but the 10% rate of developmental delay was lower than a study from Lebanon–cited by the authors as having a similar geographical and cultural setting as Kuwait–that found a pre-pandemic rate of developmental delay of 15% in healthy infants using the ASQ-3 [85], underscoring our group's findings that in utero SARS-CoV-2 exposure does not appear to predict early neurodevelopmental deficits. An ongoing longitudinal study from Italy that has followed auxologic and neurologic outcomes in infants exposed to SARS-CoV-2 in utero after discharge has also found no abnormal findings in any exposed infants during follow-up at 3, 6, and 9 months of age [86].

In contrast to the accumulating evidence against an association between in utero exposure to maternal SARS-CoV-2 infection and adverse neurodevelopmental effects, a recent study from Boston reported that 222 infants exposed to maternal SARS-CoV-2 infection in utero were more likely than 7550 unexposed infants to have received a neurodevelopmental diagnosis in the first year of life using the International Classification of Diseases, Tenth Revision (ICD-10) [87]. However, this study suffered from several limitations. First, it should be noted that only 14 of 222 (6.3%) infants in the exposed group had received a neurodevelopmental diagnosis, compared to 227 of 7550 (3.0%) in the unexposed group [87], so the rates in both groups were low. The study used retrospective chart review and therefore was limited in its control over confounding variables, and one year of age is generally considered to be too early to diagnose most neurodevelopmental disorders, including autism spectrum disorder [88]. Importantly, the study also suffered from the additional confounder of limited SARS-CoV-2 testing in Boston during the study period, reporting a positivity rate of only 2.9% in the study sample, during a period of time when the test positivity rate was 30–40% on general testing in the Boston area [89] and 15.4% on universal testing of delivering patients in New York City [90], a city with similar pandemic course. The increase in ICD-10 codes was also not statistically significant when full-term infants were evaluated separately, suggesting that prematurity mediated their main observed effect. Finally, the lower median age when infants received their ICD-10 code in the exposed group suggests increased parental concern as a strong mediating factor. Considering these methodological concerns along with the four studies discussed above that have demonstrated no differences in developmental outcomes between in utero SARS-CoV-2 exposed and unexposed infants, the currently available data on long-term outcomes and neurodevelopment in infants exposed to SARS-CoV-2 in utero overall suggests that these infants do not seem to be at any significantly increased risk of neurodevelopmental delay. However, more studies and longer-term follow-up are necessary to conclusively determine risk in this population of infants and children. In particular, there is a paucity of data on neurodevelopmental effects in infants born to mothers with a history of severe or critical COVID-19 disease, as well as a paucity of data from women infected early in pregnancy.

5. Conclusions

In sum, the literature on neonates exposed to maternal SARS-CoV-2 infection in utero indicates that these newborns generally have favorable outcomes. Vertical transmission is rare, even when newborns are roomed-in with mothers, breastfeed, and practice skin-to-skin care. In accordance with the rarity of vertical transmission of SARS-CoV-2, the mechanism by which vertical transmission may occur remains unclear: placental infection appears to be the most plausible mechanism, but it has been reported infrequently. In the rare cases that neonates do become infected with SARS-CoV-2, they tend to fare well, with very few exhibiting severe disease or requiring intensive care. Regardless of their neonatal infection status, newborns born to SARS-CoV-2-infected women do seem to have a slightly increased risk of preterm birth, which may be related to increased risk of severe COVID-19 disease in pregnant women, alterations in the placental environment, trimester of infection, or a combination of these and other factors. However, these newborns do not appear to be at risk of extreme prematurity or any other adverse neonatal outcome. Further, the limited long-term follow-up data available on these newborns is promising and indicates that their development to-date is normal, but, notably, outcomes for these infants beyond age 12 months are not yet available. Many of the child health outcomes previously associated with maternal infection and inflammation during pregnancy, including autism spectrum disorder, schizophrenia, and asthma, do not emerge until later in childhood. With this in mind, there is a strong need for more studies on development in infants and children exposed to SARS-CoV-2 in utero in order to determine long-term outcomes in this population.

- Newborns exposed to maternal SARS-CoV-2 infection in utero rarely acquire SARS-CoV-2 infection through vertical transmission, even when rooming-in, breastfeeding, and skin-to-skin care are practiced.
- The mechanism underlying rare cases of vertical transmission is unclear: placental infection is the most plausible mechanism but it occurs infrequently.
- Infants infected with SARS-CoV-2 (whether vertically or through community transmission) tend to have favorable outcomes, and very few infants require intensive care or exhibit severe disease.
- Newborns born to SARS-CoV-2 infected women have a slight increased risk of preterm birth, with possible underlying mechanisms including but not limited to severe COVID-19 disease in pregnant women, placental alterations, or trimester of maternal infection.
- Limited long-term follow-up data on infants and children exposed to SARS-CoV-2 in utero suggest that their development is normal, but there is a strong need for longer-term follow-up in these children.

Supplementary Materials: The following supporting information can be downloaded at: https://www.mdpi.com/article/10.3390/encyclopedia3010002/s1, Table S1: Summary of Literature.

Funding: This research was supported by National Institutes of Health R01MH126531 to D.D., Centers for Disease Control contract 75D30120C08150 through Abt Associates to D.D., and gift funds from Einhorn Collaborative to the Nurture Science Program.

Acknowledgments: The authors would like to thank the COVID-19 Mother Baby Outcomes (COMBO) Initiative team at Columbia University Irving Medical Center (www.ps.columbia.edu/COMBO) (accessed on 22 December 2022), and the Maternal-Child Research Oversight (MaCRO) Committee and the Departments of Pediatrics, Psychiatry, and Obstetrics and Gynecology at Columbia University Irving Medical Center for their institutional support.

Conflicts of Interest: D.D. has pending consultation fees from Medela for work unrelated to this review.

References

1. World Health Organization. *COVID-19 Weekly Epidemiological Update*; World Health Organization: Geneva, Switzerland, 2022.
2. Kotlyar, A.M.; Grechukhina, O.; Chen, A.; Popkhadze, S.; Grimshaw, A.; Tal, O.; Taylor, H.S.; Tal, R. Vertical transmission of coronavirus disease 2019: A systematic review and meta-analysis. *Am. J. Obstet. Gynecol.* **2021**, *224*, 35–53.e33. [CrossRef] [PubMed]
3. Jafari, M.; Pormohammad, A.; Sheikh Neshin, S.A.; Ghorbani, S.; Bose, D.; Alimohammadi, S.; Basirjafari, S.; Mohammadi, M.; Rasmussen-Ivey, C.; Razizadeh, M.H.; et al. Clinical characteristics and outcomes of pregnant women with COVID-19 and comparison with control patients: A systematic review and meta-analysis. *Rev. Med. Virol.* **2021**, *31*, e2208. [CrossRef]

4. Mullins, E.; Hudak, M.L.; Banerjee, J.; Getzlaff, T.; Townson, J.; Barnette, K.; Playle, R.; Perry, A.; Bourne, T.; Lees, C.C.; et al. Pregnancy and neonatal outcomes of COVID-19: Coreporting of common outcomes from PAN-COVID and AAP-SONPM registries. *Ultrasound Obstet. Gynecol. Off. J. Int. Soc. Ultrasound Obstet. Gynecol.* **2021**, *57*, 573–581. [CrossRef] [PubMed]
5. Dumitriu, D.; Emeruwa, U.N.; Hanft, E.; Liao, G.V.; Ludwig, E.; Walzer, L.; Arditi, B.; Saslaw, M.; Andrikopoulou, M.; Scripps, T.; et al. Outcomes of Neonates Born to Mothers With Severe Acute Respiratory Syndrome Coronavirus 2 Infection at a Large Medical Center in New York City. *JAMA Pediatr.* **2021**, *175*, 157–167. [CrossRef] [PubMed]
6. Norman, M.; Navér, L.; Söderling, J.; Ahlberg, M.; Hervius Askling, H.; Aronsson, B.; Byström, E.; Jonsson, J.; Sengpiel, V.; Ludvigsson, J.F.; et al. Association of Maternal SARS-CoV-2 Infection in Pregnancy With Neonatal Outcomes. *JAMA* **2021**, *325*, 2076–2086. [CrossRef] [PubMed]
7. Walker, K.F.; O'Donoghue, K.; Grace, N.; Dorling, J.; Comeau, J.L.; Li, W.; Thornton, J.G. Maternal transmission of SARS-CoV-2 to the neonate, and possible routes for such transmission: A systematic review and critical analysis. *BJOG* **2020**, *127*, 1324–1336. [CrossRef] [PubMed]
8. Shanes, E.D.; Miller, E.S.; Otero, S.; Ebbott, R.; Aggarwal, R.; Willnow, A.S.; Ozer, E.A.; Mithal, L.B.; Goldstein, J.A. Placental Pathology After SARS-CoV-2 Infection in the Pre-Variant of Concern, Alpha / Gamma, Delta, or Omicron Eras. *Int. J. Surg. Pathol.* **2022**. [CrossRef]
9. Shanes, E.D.; Mithal, L.B.; Otero, S.; Azad, H.A.; Miller, E.S.; Goldstein, J.A. Placental Pathology in COVID-19. *Am. J. Clin. Pathol.* **2020**, *154*, 23–32. [CrossRef]
10. Mourad, M.; Jacob, T.; Sadovsky, E.; Bejerano, S.; Simone, G.S.-D.; Bagalkot, T.R.; Zucker, J.; Yin, M.T.; Chang, J.Y.; Liu, L.; et al. Placental response to maternal SARS-CoV-2 infection. *Sci. Rep.* **2021**, *11*, 14390. [CrossRef]
11. Sánchez-Luna, M.; Fernández Colomer, B.; de Alba Romero, C.; Alarcón Allen, A.; Baña Souto, A.; Camba Longueira, F.; Cernada Badía, M.; Galve Pradell, Z.; González López, M.; López Herrera, M.C.; et al. Neonates Born to Mothers With COVID-19: Data From the Spanish Society of Neonatology Registry. *Pediatrics* **2021**, *147*, e2020015065. [CrossRef]
12. Gulersen, M.; Alvarez, A.; Rochelson, B.; Blitz, M.J. Preterm birth and severe maternal morbidity associated with SARS-CoV-2 infection during the Omicron wave. *Am. J. Obstet. Gynecol. MFM* **2022**, *4*, 100712. [CrossRef] [PubMed]
13. Gomez, U.T.; Francisco, R.P.V.; Baptista, F.S.; Gibelli, M.A.B.C.; Ibidi, S.M.; Carvalho, W.B.d.; Paganoti, C.d.F.; Sabino, E.C.; Silva, L.C.d.O.d.; Jaenisch, T.; et al. Impact of SARS-CoV-2 on pregnancy and neonatal outcomes: An open prospective study of pregnant women in Brazil. *Clinics* **2022**, *77*, 100073. [CrossRef] [PubMed]
14. Villar, J.; Ariff, S.; Gunier, R.B.; Thiruvengadam, R.; Rauch, S.; Kholin, A.; Roggero, P.; Prefumo, F.; do Vale, M.S.; Cardona-Perez, J.A.; et al. Maternal and Neonatal Morbidity and Mortality Among Pregnant Women With and Without COVID-19 Infection: The INTERCOVID Multinational Cohort Study. *JAMA Pediatr.* **2021**, *175*, 817–826. [CrossRef] [PubMed]
15. Benova, L.; Mohamoud, Y.A.; Calvert, C.; Abu-Raddad, L.J. Vertical Transmission of Hepatitis C Virus: Systematic Review and Meta-analysis. *Clin. Infect. Dis.* **2014**, *59*, 765–773. [CrossRef]
16. Liu, L.; Johnson, H.L.; Cousens, S.; Perin, J.; Scott, S.; Lawn, J.E.; Rudan, I.; Campbell, H.; Cibulskis, R.; Li, M.; et al. Global, regional, and national causes of child mortality: An updated systematic analysis for 2010 with time trends since 2000. *Lancet* **2012**, *379*, 2151–2161. [CrossRef]
17. Basha, S.; Surendran, N.; Pichichero, M. Immune responses in neonates. *Expert Rev. Clin. Immunol.* **2014**, *10*, 1171–1184. [CrossRef]
18. PrabhuDas, M.; Adkins, B.; Gans, H.; King, C.; Levy, O.; Ramilo, O.; Siegrist, C.-A. Challenges in infant immunity: Implications for responses to infection and vaccines. *Nat. Immunol.* **2011**, *12*, 189–194. [CrossRef]
19. Gentile, I.; Borgia, G. Vertical transmission of hepatitis B virus: Challenges and solutions. *Int. J. Womens Health* **2014**, *6*, 605–611. [CrossRef]
20. Forbes, J.C.; Alimenti, A.M.; Singer, J.; Brophy, J.C.; Bitnun, A.; Samson, L.M.; Money, D.M.; Lee, T.C.K.; Lapointe, N.D.; Read, S.E.; et al. A national review of vertical HIV transmission. *AIDS* **2012**, *26*, 757–763. [CrossRef]
21. Vigil-Vázquez, S.; Carrasco-García, I.; Hernanz-Lobo, A.; Manzanares, Á.; Pérez-Pérez, A.; Toledano-Revenga, J.; Muñoz-Chapuli, M.; Mesones-Guerra, L.; Martínez-Lozano, A.; Pérez-Seoane, B.; et al. Impact of Gestational COVID-19 on Neonatal Outcomes: Is Vertical Infection Possible? *Pediatr. Infect. Dis. J.* **2022**, *41*, 466–472. [CrossRef]
22. Fang, F.; Chen, Y.; Zhao, D.; Liu, T.; Huang, Y.; Qiu, L.; Hao, Y.; Hu, X.; Yin, W.; Liu, Z.; et al. Recommendations for the Diagnosis, Prevention, and Control of Coronavirus Disease-19 in Children—The Chinese Perspectives. *Front. Pediatr.* **2020**, *8*, 553394. [CrossRef]
23. Bystrova, K.; Ivanova, V.; Edhborg, M.; Matthiesen, A.S.; Ransjo-Arvidson, A.B.; Mukhamedrakhimov, R.; Uvnas-Moberg, K.; Widstrom, A.M. Early contact versus separation: Effects on mother-infant interaction one year later. *Birth* **2009**, *36*, 97–109. [CrossRef]
24. Lawrence, R.M.; Lawrence, R.A. Breastfeeding: More than just good nutrition. *Pediatr. Rev.* **2011**, *32*, 267–280. [CrossRef]
25. Flacking, R.; Lehtonen, L.; Thomson, G.; Axelin, A.; Ahlqvist, S.; Moran, V.H.; Ewald, U.; Dykes, F. Closeness and separation in neonatal intensive care. *Acta Paediatr.* **2012**, *101*, 1032–1037. [CrossRef]
26. Shang, J.; Wan, Y.; Luo, C.; Ye, G.; Geng, Q.; Auerbach, A.; Li, F. Cell entry mechanisms of SARS-CoV-2. *Proc. Natl. Acad. Sci. USA* **2020**, *117*, 11727. [CrossRef]
27. Hoffmann, M.; Kleine-Weber, H.; Schroeder, S.; Krüger, N.; Herrler, T.; Erichsen, S.; Schiergens, T.S.; Herrler, G.; Wu, N.-H.; Nitsche, A.; et al. SARS-CoV-2 Cell Entry Depends on ACE2 and TMPRSS2 and Is Blocked by a Clinically Proven Protease Inhibitor. *Cell* **2020**, *181*, 271–280.e278. [CrossRef]

28. Ziegler, C.G.K.; Allon, S.J.; Nyquist, S.K.; Mbano, I.M.; Miao, V.N.; Tzouanas, C.N.; Cao, Y.; Yousif, A.S.; Bals, J.; Hauser, B.M.; et al. SARS-CoV-2 Receptor ACE2 Is an Interferon-Stimulated Gene in Human Airway Epithelial Cells and Is Detected in Specific Cell Subsets across Tissues. *Cell* **2020**, *181*, 1016–1035.e1019. [CrossRef]
29. Ashary, N.; Bhide, A.; Chakraborty, P.; Colaco, S.; Mishra, A.; Chhabria, K.; Jolly, M.K.; Modi, D. Single-Cell RNA-seq Identifies Cell Subsets in Human Placenta That Highly Expresses Factors Driving Pathogenesis of SARS-CoV-2. *Front. Cell. Dev. Biol.* **2020**, *8*, 783. [CrossRef]
30. Li, M.; Chen, L.; Zhang, J.; Xiong, C.; Li, X. The SARS-CoV-2 receptor ACE2 expression of maternal-fetal interface and fetal organs by single-cell transcriptome study. *PLoS ONE* **2020**, *15*, e0230295. [CrossRef]
31. Egloff, C.; Vauloup-Fellous, C.; Picone, O.; Mandelbrot, L.; Roques, P. Evidence and possible mechanisms of rare maternal-fetal transmission of SARS-CoV-2. *J. Clin. Virol.* **2020**, *128*, 104447. [CrossRef]
32. Pique-Regi, R.; Romero, R.; Tarca, A.L.; Luca, F.; Xu, Y.; Alazizi, A.; Leng, Y.; Hsu, C.-D.; Gomez-Lopez, N. Does the human placenta express the canonical cell entry mediators for SARS-CoV-2? *elife* **2020**, *9*, e58716. [CrossRef] [PubMed]
33. Edlow, A.G.; Li, J.Z.; Collier, A.-r.Y.; Atyeo, C.; James, K.E.; Boatin, A.A.; Gray, K.J.; Bordt, E.A.; Shook, L.L.; Yonker, L.M.; et al. Assessment of Maternal and Neonatal SARS-CoV-2 Viral Load, Transplacental Antibody Transfer, and Placental Pathology in Pregnancies During the COVID-19 Pandemic. *JAMA Netw. Open* **2020**, *3*, e2030455. [CrossRef] [PubMed]
34. Beesley, M.A.; Davidson, J.R.; Panariello, F.; Shibuya, S.; Scaglioni, D.; Jones, B.C.; Maksym, K.; Ogunbiyi, O.; Sebire, N.J.; Cacchiarelli, D.; et al. COVID-19 and vertical transmission: Assessing the expression of ACE2/TMPRSS2 in the human fetus and placenta to assess the risk of SARS-CoV-2 infection. *BJOG Int. J. Obstet. Gynaecol.* **2022**, *129*, 256–266. [CrossRef] [PubMed]
35. Li, Y.; Schneider, A.M.; Mehta, A.; Sade-Feldman, M.; Kays, K.R.; Gentili, M.; Charland, N.C.; Gonye, A.L.K.; Gushterova, I.; Khanna, H.K.; et al. SARS-CoV-2 viremia is associated with distinct proteomic pathways and predicts COVID-19 outcomes. *J. Clin. Investig.* **2021**, *131*, e148635. [CrossRef]
36. Levitan, D.; London, V.; McLaren, R.A.; Mann, J.D.; Cheng, K.; Silver, M.; Balhotra, K.S.; McCalla, S.; Loukeris, K. Histologic and Immunohistochemical Evaluation of 65 Placentas From Women With Polymerase Chain Reaction-Proven Severe Acute Respiratory Syndrome Coronavirus 2 (SARS-CoV-2) Infection. *Arch. Pathol. Lab. Med.* **2021**, *145*, 648–656. [CrossRef]
37. Zhang, P.; Heyman, T.; Greechan, M.; Dygulska, B.; Al Sayyed, F.; Narula, P.; Lederman, S. Maternal, neonatal and placental characteristics of SARS-CoV-2 positive mothers. *J. Matern. Fetal Neonatal Med.* **2021**, 1–9. [CrossRef]
38. Shook, L.L.; Brigida, S.; Regan, J.; Flynn, J.P.; Mohammadi, A.; Etemad, B.; Siegel, M.R.; Clapp, M.A.; Li, J.Z.; Roberts, D.J.; et al. SARS-CoV-2 Placentitis Associated With B.1.617.2 (Delta) Variant and Fetal Distress or Demise. *J. Infect. Dis.* **2022**, *225*, 754–758. [CrossRef]
39. Schwartz, D.A.; Avvad-Portari, E.; Babál, P.; Baldewijns, M.; Blomberg, M.; Bouachba, A.; Camacho, J.; Collardeau-Frachon, S.; Colson, A.; Dehaene, I.; et al. Placental Tissue Destruction and Insufficiency From COVID-19 Causes Stillbirth and Neonatal Death From Hypoxic-Ischemic Injury. *Arch. Pathol. Lab. Med.* **2022**, *146*, 660–676. [CrossRef]
40. Penfield, C.A.; Brubaker, S.G.; Limaye, M.A.; Lighter, J.; Ratner, A.J.; Thomas, K.M.; Meyer, J.A.; Roman, A.S. Detection of severe acute respiratory syndrome coronavirus 2 in placental and fetal membrane samples. *Am. J. Obstet. Gynecol. MFM* **2020**, *2*, 100133. [CrossRef]
41. Cribiù, F.M.; Erra, R.; Pugni, L.; Rubio-Perez, C.; Alonso, L.; Simonetti, S.; Croci, G.A.; Serna, G.; Ronchi, A.; Pietrasanta, C.; et al. Severe SARS-CoV-2 placenta infection can impact neonatal outcome in the absence of vertical transmission. *J. Clin. Investig.* **2021**, *131*. [CrossRef]
42. Maeda, M.d.F.Y.; Brizot, M.d.L.; Gibelli, M.A.B.C.; Ibidi, S.M.; Carvalho, W.B.d.; Hoshida, M.S.; Machado, C.M.; Sabino, E.C.; Oliveira da Silva, L.C.d.; Jaenisch, T.; et al. Vertical transmission of SARS-CoV2 during pregnancy: A high-risk cohort. *Prenat. Diagn.* **2021**, *41*, 998–1008. [CrossRef]
43. Ernst, L.M. Maternal vascular malperfusion of the placental bed. *APMIS* **2018**, *126*, 551–560. [CrossRef]
44. Kim, Y.M.; Chaemsaithong, P.; Romero, R.; Shaman, M.; Kim, C.J.; Kim, J.S.; Qureshi, F.; Jacques, S.M.; Ahmed, A.I.; Chaiworapongsa, T.; et al. The frequency of acute atherosis in normal pregnancy and preterm labor, preeclampsia, small-for-gestational age, fetal death and midtrimester spontaneous abortion. *J. Matern. Fetal Neonatal Med.* **2015**, *28*, 2001–2009. [CrossRef]
45. Khong, T.Y.; Mooney, E.E.; Ariel, I.; Balmus, N.C.; Boyd, T.K.; Brundler, M.A.; Derricott, H.; Evans, M.J.; Faye-Petersen, O.M.; Gillan, J.E.; et al. Sampling and Definitions of Placental Lesions: Amsterdam Placental Workshop Group Consensus Statement. *Arch. Pathol. Lab. Med.* **2016**, *140*, 698–713. [CrossRef]
46. Gale, C.; Quigley, M.A.; Placzek, A.; Knight, M.; Ladhani, S.; Draper, E.S.; Sharkey, D.; Doherty, C.; Mactier, H.; Kurinczuk, J.J. Characteristics and outcomes of neonatal SARS-CoV-2 infection in the UK: A prospective national cohort study using active surveillance. *Lancet Child Adolesc. Health* **2021**, *5*, 113–121. [CrossRef]
47. Dong, Y.; Mo, X.; Hu, Y.; Qi, X.; Jiang, F.; Jiang, Z.; Tong, S. Epidemiology of COVID-19 Among Children in China. *Pediatrics* **2020**, *145*, e20200702. [CrossRef]
48. Wu, Z.; McGoogan, J.M. Characteristics of and Important Lessons From the Coronavirus Disease 2019 (COVID-19) Outbreak in China: Summary of a Report of 72314 Cases From the Chinese Center for Disease Control and Prevention. *JAMA* **2020**, *323*, 1239–1242. [CrossRef]
49. Mithal, L.B.; Machut, K.Z.; Muller, W.J.; Kociolek, L.K. SARS-CoV-2 Infection in Infants Less than 90 Days Old. *J. Pediatr.* **2020**, *224*, 150–152. [CrossRef]

50. Hassoun, A.; Dahan, N.; Kelly, C. A Case Series of SARS-CoV-2 RT-PCR-Positive Hospitalized Infants 60 Days of Age or Younger From 2 New York City Pediatric Emergency Departments. *Clin. Pediatr.* **2021**, *60*, 247–251. [CrossRef]
51. Buonsenso, D.; Costa, S.; Sanguinetti, M.; Cattani, P.; Posteraro, B.; Marchetti, S.; Carducci, B.; Lanzone, A.; Tamburrini, E.; Vento, G.; et al. Neonatal Late Onset Infection with Severe Acute Respiratory Syndrome Coronavirus 2. *Am. J. Perinatol.* **2020**, *37*, 869–872. [CrossRef]
52. Leibowitz, J.; Krief, W.; Barone, S.; Williamson, K.A.; Goenka, P.K.; Rai, S.; Moriarty, S.; Baodhankar, P.; Rubin, L.G. Comparison of Clinical and Epidemiologic Characteristics of Young Febrile Infants with and without Severe Acute Respiratory Syndrome Coronavirus-2 Infection. *J. Pediatr.* **2021**, *229*, 41–47.e41. [CrossRef]
53. Nanavati, R.; Mascarenhas, D.; Goyal, M.; Haribalakrishna, A.; Nataraj, G. A single-center observational study on clinical features and outcomes of 21 SARS-CoV-2-infected neonates from India. *Eur. J. Pediatr.* **2021**, *180*, 1895–1906. [CrossRef]
54. Bhuiyan, M.U.; Stiboy, E.; Hassan, M.Z.; Chan, M.; Islam, M.S.; Haider, N.; Jaffe, A.; Homaira, N. Epidemiology of COVID-19 infection in young children under five years: A systematic review and meta-analysis. *Vaccine* **2021**, *39*, 667–677. [CrossRef]
55. Marks, K.J.; Whitaker, M.; Agathis, N.T.; Anglin, O.; Milucky, J.; Patel, K.; Pham, H.; Kirley, P.D.; Kawasaki, B.; Meek, J.; et al. Hospitalization of Infants and Children Aged 0–4 Years with Laboratory-Confirmed COVID-19—COVID-NET, 14 States, March 2020-February 2022. *MMWR Morb. Mortal Wkly. Rep.* **2022**, *71*, 429–436. [CrossRef]
56. Brewster, R.C.L.; Parsons, C.; Laird-Gion, J.; Hilker, S.; Irwin, M.; Sommerschield, A.; Michaelis, K.A.; Lam, M.; Parsons, A.; Mansbach, J.M. COVID-19–Associated Croup in Children. *Pediatrics* **2022**, *149*, e2022056492. [CrossRef]
57. Goldenberg, R.L.; Culhane, J.F.; Johnson, D.C. Maternal infection and adverse fetal and neonatal outcomes. *Clin. Perinatol.* **2005**, *32*, 523–559. [CrossRef]
58. Tedesco, R.P.; Galvão, R.B.; Guida, J.P.; Passini-Júnior, R.; Lajos, G.J.; Nomura, M.L.; Rehder, P.M.; Dias, T.Z.; Souza, R.T.; Cecatti, J.G. The role of maternal infection in preterm birth: Evidence from the Brazilian Multicentre Study on Preterm Birth (EMIP). *Clinics* **2020**, *75*, e1508. [CrossRef]
59. Romero, R.; Espinoza, J.; Gonçalves, L.F.; Kusanovic, J.P.; Friel, L.; Hassan, S. The role of inflammation and infection in preterm birth. *Semin. Reprod. Med.* **2007**, *25*, 21–39. [CrossRef]
60. Martin, J.A.; Hamilton, B.E.; Osterman, M.J.K.; Driscoll, A.K. Births: Final Data for 2018. *Natl. Vital Stat. Rep.* **2019**, *68*, 1–47.
61. Office for National Statistics. *Provisional Births in England and Wales: 2020*; Office for National Statistics: London, UK, 2020.
62. Molenaar, N.M.; Rommel, A.S.; de Witte, L.; Dolan, S.M.; Lieb, W.; Ibroci, E.; Ohrn, S.; Lynch, J.; Capuano, C.; Stadlbauer, D.; et al. SARS-CoV-2 during pregnancy and associated outcomes: Results from an ongoing prospective cohort. *Paediatr. Perinat Epidemiol.* **2022**, *36*, 466–475. [CrossRef]
63. Nachega, J.B.; Sam-Agudu, N.A.; Machekano, R.N.; Rosenthal, P.J.; Schell, S.; de Waard, L.; Bekker, A.; Gachuno, O.W.; Kinuthia, J.; Mwongeli, N.; et al. Severe Acute Respiratory Syndrome Coronavirus 2 (SARS-CoV-2) Infection and Pregnancy in Sub-Saharan Africa: A 6-Country Retrospective Cohort Analysis. *Clin. Infect. Dis.* **2022**, *75*, 1950–1961. [CrossRef] [PubMed]
64. Martinez-Portilla, R.J.; Sotiriadis, A.; Chatzakis, C.; Torres-Torres, J.; Espino, Y.S.S.; Sandoval-Mandujano, K.; Castro-Bernabe, D.A.; Medina-Jimenez, V.; Monarrez-Martin, J.C.; Figueras, F.; et al. Pregnant women with SARS-CoV-2 infection are at higher risk of death and pneumonia: Propensity score matched analysis of a nationwide prospective cohort (COV19Mx). *Ultrasound Obstet. Gynecol.* **2021**, *57*, 224–231. [CrossRef] [PubMed]
65. Zambrano, L.D.; Ellington, S.; Strid, P.; Galang, R.R.; Oduyebo, T.; Tong, V.T.; Woodworth, K.R.; Nahabedian, J.F., 3rd; Azziz-Baumgartner, E.; Gilboa, S.M.; et al. Update: Characteristics of Symptomatic Women of Reproductive Age with Laboratory-Confirmed SARS-CoV-2 Infection by Pregnancy Status—United States, January 22-October 3, 2020. *MMWR Morb. Mortal Wkly. Rep.* **2020**, *69*, 1641–1647. [CrossRef] [PubMed]
66. Allotey, J.; Stallings, E.; Bonet, M.; Yap, M.; Chatterjee, S.; Kew, T.; Debenham, L.; Llavall, A.C.; Dixit, A.; Zhou, D.; et al. Clinical manifestations, risk factors, and maternal and perinatal outcomes of coronavirus disease 2019 in pregnancy: Living systematic review and meta-analysis. *BMJ* **2020**, *370*, m3320. [CrossRef]
67. Metz, T.D.; Clifton, R.G.; Hughes, B.L.; Sandoval, G.; Saade, G.R.; Grobman, W.A.; Manuck, T.A.; Miodovnik, M.; Sowles, A.; Clark, K.; et al. Disease Severity and Perinatal Outcomes of Pregnant Patients With Coronavirus Disease 2019 (COVID-19). *Obstet. Gynecol.* **2021**, *137*, 571–580. [CrossRef]
68. Newton, S.M.; Reeves, E.L.; O'Malley Olsen, E.; Woodworth, K.R.; Farr, S.L.; Galang, R.R.; Reynolds, M.R.; Harvey, E.; Shi, J.; Nestoridi, E.; et al. Preterm birth among pregnant persons with severe acute respiratory syndrome Coronavirus 2 infection. *J. Perinatol.* **2022**, *42*, 1328–1337. [CrossRef]
69. Bánhidy, F.; Acs, N.; Puhó, E.H.; Czeizel, A.E. Maternal acute respiratory infectious diseases during pregnancy and birth outcomes. *Eur. J. Epidemiol.* **2008**, *23*, 29–35. [CrossRef]
70. Cardenas, I.; Means, R.E.; Aldo, P.; Koga, K.; Lang, S.M.; Booth, C.J.; Manzur, A.; Oyarzun, E.; Romero, R.; Mor, G. Viral infection of the placenta leads to fetal inflammation and sensitization to bacterial products predisposing to preterm labor. *J. Immunol.* **2010**, *185*, 1248–1257. [CrossRef]
71. Class, Q.A.; Lichtenstein, P.; Långström, N.; D'Onofrio, B.M. Timing of prenatal maternal exposure to severe life events and adverse pregnancy outcomes: A population study of 2.6 million pregnancies. *Psychosom. Med.* **2011**, *73*, 234–241. [CrossRef]
72. De Beaudrap, P.; Turyakira, E.; Nabasumba, C.; Tumwebaze, B.; Piola, P.; Boum Ii, Y.; McGready, R. Timing of malaria in pregnancy and impact on infant growth and morbidity: A cohort study in Uganda. *Malar J.* **2016**, *15*, 92. [CrossRef]

73. Dorélien, A. The Effects of In Utero Exposure to Influenza on Birth and Infant Outcomes in the US. *Popul. Dev. Rev.* **2019**, *45*, 489–523. [CrossRef] [PubMed]
74. Moore, K.A.; Simpson, J.A.; Wiladphaingern, J.; Min, A.M.; Pimanpanarak, M.; Paw, M.K.; Raksuansak, J.; Pukrittayakamee, S.; Fowkes, F.J.I.; White, N.J.; et al. Influence of the number and timing of malaria episodes during pregnancy on prematurity and small-for-gestational-age in an area of low transmission. *BMC Med.* **2017**, *15*, 117. [CrossRef] [PubMed]
75. Piekos, S.N.; Roper, R.T.; Hwang, Y.M.; Sorensen, T.; Price, N.D.; Hood, L.; Hadlock, J.J. The effect of maternal SARS-CoV-2 infection timing on birth outcomes: A retrospective multicentre cohort study. *Lancet Digit. Health* **2022**, *4*, e95–e104. [CrossRef] [PubMed]
76. Hughes, B.L.; Sandoval, G.J.; Metz, T.D.; Clifton, R.G.; Grobman, W.A.; Saade, G.R.; Manuck, T.A.; Longo, M.; Sowles, A.; Clark, K.; et al. First- or second-trimester SARS-CoV-2 infection and subsequent pregnancy outcomes. *Am. J. Obstet. Gynecol.* **2022**. [CrossRef]
77. Fallach, N.; Segal, Y.; Agassy, J.; Perez, G.; Peretz, A.; Chodick, G.; Gazit, S.; Patalon, T.; Ben Tov, A.; Goldshtein, I. Pregnancy outcomes after SARS-CoV-2 infection by trimester: A large, population-based cohort study. *PLoS ONE* **2022**, *17*, e0270893. [CrossRef] [PubMed]
78. Cosma, S.; Carosso, A.R.; Cusato, J.; Borella, F.; Bertero, L.; Bovetti, M.; Bevilacqua, F.; Mengozzi, G.; Mazzone, R.; Ghisetti, V.; et al. Obstetric and neonatal outcomes after SARS-CoV-2 infection in the first trimester of pregnancy: A prospective comparative study. *J. Obstet. Gynaecol. Res.* **2022**, *48*, 393–401. [CrossRef]
79. Boivin, M.; Maliwichi-Senganimalunje, L.; Ogwang, L.; Kawalazira, R.; Sikorskii, A.; Familiar, I.; Kuteesa, A.; Nyakato, M.; Mutebe, A.; Namukooli, J.; et al. Neurodevelopmental effects of ante-partum and post-partum antiretroviral exposure in HIV-exposed and uninfected children versus HIV-unexposed and uninfected children in Uganda and Malawi: A prospective cohort study. *Lancet HIV* **2019**, *6*, e518–e530. [CrossRef]
80. Wedderburn, C.J.; Evans, C.; Yeung, S.; Gibb, D.M.; Donald, K.A.; Prendergast, A.J. Growth and Neurodevelopment of HIV-Exposed Uninfected Children: A Conceptual Framework. *Curr. HIV/AIDS Rep.* **2019**, *16*, 501–513. [CrossRef]
81. Ganguli, S.; Chavali, P.L. Intrauterine Viral Infections: Impact of Inflammation on Fetal Neurodevelopment. *Front. Neurosci.* **2021**, *15*, 771557. [CrossRef]
82. Shuffrey, L.C.; Firestein, M.R.; Kyle, M.H.; Fields, A.; Alcántara, C.; Amso, D.; Austin, J.; Bain, J.M.; Barbosa, J.; Bence, M.; et al. Association of Birth During the COVID-19 Pandemic With Neurodevelopmental Status at 6 Months in Infants With and Without In Utero Exposure to Maternal SARS-CoV-2 Infection. *JAMA Pediatr.* **2022**, *176*, e215563. [CrossRef]
83. Bianco, C.; Sania, A.; Kyle, M.H.; Beebe, B.; Barbosa, J.; Bence, M.; Coskun, L.; Fields, A.; Firestein, M.R.; Goldman, S.; et al. Pandemic beyond the virus: Maternal COVID-related postnatal stress is associated with infant temperament. *Pediatr. Res.* **2022**, 1–7. [CrossRef]
84. Ayed, M.; Embaireeg, A.; Kartam, M.; More, K.; Alqallaf, M.; AlNafisi, A.; Alsaffar, Z.; Bahzad, Z.; Buhamad, Y.; Alsayegh, H.; et al. Neurodevelopmental outcomes of infants born to mothers with SARS-CoV-2 infections during pregnancy: A national prospective study in Kuwait. *BMC Pediatr.* **2022**, *22*, 319. [CrossRef]
85. Charafeddine, L.; Dani, A.; Badr, L.K.; Sinno, D.; Tamim, H.; Khoury, J.; Nasser, F.; Makki, M. The psychometric properties of the Ages and Stages Questionnaires-3 in Arabic: Cross-sectional observational study. *Early Hum. Dev.* **2019**, *136*, 33–38. [CrossRef]
86. Buonsenso, D.; Costa, S.; Giordano, L.; Priolo, F.; Colonna, A.T.; Morini, S.; Sbarbati, M.; Pata, D.; Acampora, A.; Conti, G.; et al. Short- and mid-term multidisciplinary outcomes of newborns exposed to SARS-CoV-2 in utero or during the perinatal period: Preliminary findings. *Eur. J. Pediatr.* **2022**, *181*, 1507–1520. [CrossRef]
87. Edlow, A.G.; Castro, V.M.; Shook, L.L.; Kaimal, A.J.; Perlis, R.H. Neurodevelopmental Outcomes at 1 Year in Infants of Mothers Who Tested Positive for SARS-CoV-2 During Pregnancy. *JAMA Netw. Open* **2022**, *5*, e2215787. [CrossRef]
88. Alonso-Esteban, Y.; Alcantud-Marín, F. Screening, Diagnosis and Early Intervention in Autism Spectrum Disorders. *Children* **2022**, *9*, 153. [CrossRef]
89. Boston Public Health Commission. Boston COVID-19 Dashboard, COVID-19 Metrics. Available online: https://www.bphc-dashboard.shinyapps.io/BPHC-dashboard/ (accessed on 16 September 2022).
90. Breslin, N.; Baptiste, C.; Gyamfi-Bannerman, C.; Miller, R.; Martinez, R.; Bernstein, K.; Ring, L.; Landau, R.; Purisch, S.; Friedman, A.M.; et al. Coronavirus disease 2019 infection among asymptomatic and symptomatic pregnant women: Two weeks of confirmed presentations to an affiliated pair of New York City hospitals. *Am. J. Obstet. Gynecol. MFM* **2020**, *2*, 100118. [CrossRef]

encyclopedia

MDPI

Entry

COVID-19 and Bell's Palsy

Eve N. Tranchito [1,2], Amanda Goslawski [1,2], Claudia I. Cabrera [1,2], Cyrus C. Rabbani [1,2], Nicole M. Fowler [1,2], Shawn Li [1,2], Jason E. Thuener [1,2], Pierre Lavertu [1,2], Rod P. Rezaee [1,2], Theodoros N. Teknos [1,2] and Akina Tamaki [1,2,*]

1 Department of Otolaryngology-Head and Neck Surgery, University Hospitals Cleveland Medical Center, Cleveland, OH 44106, USA
2 School of Medicine, Case Western Reserve University, Cleveland, OH 44106, USA
* Correspondence: akina.tamaki@uhhospitals.org; Tel.: +1-216-844-7547

Definition: There are various neurological manifestations of coronavirus disease 2019 (COVID-19). Recent data suggest a connection between hemifacial paralysis, or Bell's palsy, and COVID-19. Although the etiology of Bell's palsy is unknown, the leading proposed etiology is viral in nature. Since the onset of the pandemic, numerous studies have investigated the relationship between Bell's palsy, COVID-19 infection, and COVID-19 vaccination. The researchers studied the current literature on the topic of COVID-19 as it relates to Bell's palsy.

Keywords: coronavirus disease 2019; Bell's palsy; facial paralysis; vaccination

Citation: Tranchito, E.N.; Goslawski, A.; Cabrera, C.I.; Rabbani, C.C.; Fowler, N.M.; Li, S.; Thuener, J.E.; Lavertu, P.; Rezaee, R.P.; Teknos, T.N.; et al. COVID-19 and Bell's Palsy. *Encyclopedia* **2022**, 2, 1935–1942. https://doi.org/10.3390/encyclopedia2040133

Academic Editors: Stephen Bustin and Raffaele Barretta

Received: 29 September 2022
Accepted: 29 November 2022
Published: 6 December 2022

1. Introduction

Bell's palsy (BP) is defined as idiopathic unilateral paresis or paralysis of cranial nerve VII, the facial nerve. It clinically manifests as an acute onset weakness of the muscles that control facial expression. Patients may notice drooling from the corner of the mouth, inability to completely close the eye, or facial asymmetry. Less commonly, patients may develop facial pain, numbness, alterations in taste, or sensitivity to sound. It occurs as hemi-facial paralysis (on one side) and may be partial or complete in regard to facial nerve dysfunction. It affects about 15 to 30 out of 100,000 people per year with a peak incidence between age 15 and 40 [1]. The condition equally affects men and women, however pregnant women may be at a slightly elevated risk [2]. Although the cause of BP is yet to be determined, the leading proposed etiologies are viral, ischemic, and/or immune mediated. One proposed mechanism is re-activation of the herpes simplex virus at the geniculate ganglion of the facial nerve.

Although inconsistent, studies have demonstrated a high incidence of the herpes simplex virus in cases of BP [3]. About 70% of people will fully recover facial nerve function; however, the remaining 30% are left with varying degrees of dysfunction [2]. BP is a diagnosis of exclusion, and it is important to consider other causes of facial nerve weakness, such as parotid lesions or skull base tumors, congenital or syndromic conditions, trauma, and known associated infections, such as Lyme disease or herpes zoster.

Clinical improvement occurs within three weeks of onset in 85% of people and within three to five months in the remaining 15% [2]. The House–Brackmann scale is a numeric point system typically used to measure the degree of paresis and grades recovery; it is based on grading facial symmetry and movement. Treatment at the onset of BP includes systemic corticosteroids and antivirals. Depending on the degree of dysfunction, eye precautions may be recommended to prevent exposure keratopathy in cases of incomplete eye closure. Given the overall good prognosis within 3 months, incomplete recovery should prompt workup for alternative causes of the paralysis, including magnetic resonance imaging of the brain. Physical rehabilitation, chemodenervation, and even surgical procedures may be employed in cases of incomplete recovery.

Coronavirus disease 2019 (COVID-19) is caused by the novel virus, severe acute respiratory syndrome coronavirus-2 (SARS-CoV-2). Its clinical symptomatology is most commonly characterized by respiratory illness; however, serious complications and a wide array of less predictable side effects have challenged patients, clinicians, and scientists. Acute respiratory distress syndrome, acute heart and kidney injury, disseminated intravascular coagulation, and sepsis are some of the more consequential complications of COVID-19. Since the onset of the pandemic, there have been numerous reported neurologic manifestations of the illness; anosmia (loss of smell) and ageusia (loss of taste) were two very common symptoms of COVID-19 early on. In a systematic review of 37 articles released prior to May 20th, 2020, the most common neurologic manifestations of the disease were myalgia, headache, altered sensorium, hyposmia, and hypogeusia. Other manifestations of COVID-19 included myelitis, Guillain–Barre syndrome, encephalopathy, ischemic stroke, and intracerebral hemorrhage [4].

Another neurologic manifestation of COVID-19 with numerous reports in the literature is BP. In addition to COVID-19 infections, the association of the COVID-19 vaccine and BP has also been controversial. This manuscript explores the available literature on this topic, none of which provide definitive evidence of the presence, or lack of, an association of BP with COVID-19 infection or vaccination.

2. Bell's Palsy and Association with COVID-19 Infection

The emerging literature suggests that BP is a potential neurologic sequelae of COVID-19. There are numerous case reports published describing patients who presented with BP and were found to test positive for COVID-19 (Table 1). Iacono et al. reported a case of one child presenting with BP who tested negative for COVID-19 on a nasopharyngeal swab, but positive on serology [5]. Another patient who presented with facial paralysis had signs of COVID-19 on chest imaging and was eventually found to have positive COVID-19 serology [6]. In a case series of eight patients with BP and COVID-19, three had BP as the presenting symptom [7]. These examples raised concern that COVID-19 may cause BP, thus prompting more robust studies.

In a systematic review of the literature published between March 2020 and December 2021, there were 32 relevant publications with 46 total patients who had BP as the only major neurologic manifestation of COVID-19. In 37% of these cases, BP was the initial symptom and in 63% it developed after the onset of other COVID symptoms [8]. One prospective cross-sectional study tested all patients with BP for SARS-CoV-2 IgM and IgG. Of 41 subjects, 24.3% had positive antibodies. This is a higher seroprevalence than that seen in similar studies of asymptomatic patients, suggesting COVID-19 infection may be a risk factor for BP [9]. Another study suggested the same when they examined 38 cases of BP between February and May 2020 and found that eight patients had active or recent COVID-19 symptoms compared to only 2 of 22 the year before [10]. Furthermore, in a population-based cohort and self-controlled case series out of Spain and the United Kingdom, rates of BP were higher than expected with a standardized incidence ratio of 1.33 [11]. Tamaki et al. utilized a multi-institutional database of 41 healthcare organizations and found a higher number of patients than expected who were diagnosed with BP within eight weeks of COVID-19 infection. The study suggested a relative risk of 6.8 (95% CI: 3.5–12.2 $p < 0.001$) of BP in those diagnosed with COVID-19 [12].

The current literature on this topic is conflicting, with some reports suggesting that there is no association between BP and COVID-19 infection. Mutlu et al. examined all patients who presented to their hospital due to facial paralysis and found that only 2 of 153 had a COVID-19 diagnosis [13]. Another study in Spain studied the incidence of BP and COVID-19 during different pandemic waves by comparing background incidence to that of different "peaks" of the pandemic. They found that cases of BP did not change during times of higher COVID-19 infections, suggesting BP is not necessarily influenced by COVID-19 infection [14].

Table 1. Literature on the association between Bell's palsy and COVID-19 infection.

Title	Author	Year	Study Design	Major Findings/Conclusions
Surge of Bell's Palsy in the era of COVID-19: Systematic review [8].	Gupta et al.	2022	Systematic Review	• BP can be found as the only neurological manifestation of COVID-19 • Suggests COVID-19 as another viral etiology of BP
Facial paralysis as the only symptom of COVID-19: A prospective study [9].	Islamoglu et al.	2021	Prospective longitudinal study.	• Patients presenting with BP have a higher seropositivity rate of COVID-19 than asymptomatic patients • Facial paralysis could be the only symptom of COVID-19 infection
Facial palsy during the COVID-19 pandemic [10].	Codeluppi et al.	2021	Retrospective case-control	• Higher rate of BP during COVID-19 pandemic than year prior
Association between covid-19 vaccination, SARS-CoV-2 infection, and risk of immune mediated neurological events: population based cohort and self-controlled case series analysis [11].	Li et al.	2022	Population based cohort and self-controlled case series analysis	• Higher than expected incidence of BP after COVID-19 infection • Standardized incidence ratio for BP was 1.33 (95% CI: 1.02–1.74)
Incidence of Bell Palsy in Patients with COVID-19 [12].	Tamaki et al.	2021	Retrospective longitudinal cohort study	• Higher number of patients than expected diagnosed with BP within 8 weeks of COVID-19 infection • Relative risk of 6.8 (95% CI: 3.5–12.2, $p < 0.001$) of BP in those diagnosed with COVID-19
Does the SARS-CoV-2 pandemic really increase the frequency of peripheral facial palsy [13]?	Mutlu et al.	2021	Retrospective cohort	• Number of patients with BP during COVID-19 pandemic was similar to previous years
Data from 235 Cases of Bell's Palsy during COVID-19. Pandemic: Were There Clusters of Facial Palsy [14]?	Martin-Villares et al.	2021	Retrospective cohort	• BP incidence did not differ from background incidence throughout 4 "peaks" of COVID-19

3. Bell's Palsy and Association with COVID-19 Vaccination

In addition to COVID-19 infections, the literature has also examined whether BP can be caused by the COVID-19 vaccine. Vaccines for COVID-19 were produced at an unprecedented rate; a process that typically took 8 to 15 years was achieved in less than one full year. Additionally, the use of an mRNA vaccine was the first of its kind approved for human commercial use. Multiple factors, including these, contributed to public hesitancy surrounding the COVID-19 vaccine. The three most commonly studied COVID-19 vaccines within this entry were BNT162b2, an mRNA vaccine, the ChadOx1 nCoV-19, a viral vector vaccine, and the mRNA-1273-nCoV, another mRNA vaccine. Anecdotal reports of adverse events associated with the vaccine were followed by published reports, further instilling hesitancy in those considering vaccination against COVID-19 (Table 2).

Table 2. Literature on the association between Bell's palsy and COVID-19 vaccination.

Title	Author	Year	Study Design	Major Findings/Conclusions
Safety of COVID-19 vaccination and acute neurological events: A self-controlled case series in England using the OpenSAFELY platform [15].	Walker et al.	2022	Self-controlled case series	• Increased risk of BP after ChAdOx1 (RR: 1.39, 95% CI: 1.27–1.53) • 17.9 more cases of BP per 1 million vaccines • Absolute risk is low (<1/60,000)
Adverse events of special interest and mortality following vaccination with mRNA (BNT162b2) and inactivated (CoronaVac) SARS-CoV-2 vaccines in Hong Kong: A retrospective study [16].	Wong et al.	2022	Retrospective population-based cohort	• Higher rate of BP following the first dose of CoronaVac vs BNT162b2 (67 versus 30 per 100,000 person-years; RR: 1.95, 95% CI: 1.12–3.41, *p-value*: 0.018)
Association between vaccination with the BNT162b2 mRNA COVID-19 vaccine and Bell's palsy: a population-based study [17].	Shibli et al.	2021	Retrospective longitudinal	• Possible association between BNT162b2 mRNA vaccine and BP • Standardized incidence ratios of 1.36 (95% CI: 1.14–1.61) and 1.16 (95% CI: 0.99–1.36) for first and second dose, respectively
Association of COVID-19 Vaccination and Facial Nerve Palsy: A Case-Control Study [18].	Shemer et al.	2021	Retrospective matched case-control	• No association between BP and BNT162b2
Hospital-based observational study of neurological disorders in patients recently vaccinated with COVID-19 mRNA vaccines [19].	Koh et al.	2021	Prospective observational cohort	• No association between BP and three mRNA vaccines, BNT162b2 and mRNA-1273
Risk of serious adverse events after the BNT162b2, CoronaVac, and ChAdOx1 vaccines in Malaysia: A self-controlled case series study [20].	Ab Rahman et al.	2022	Self-controlled case series	• No increased risk of BP after BNT162b2, CoronaVac, and ChAdOx1 vaccines in Malaysia

Numerous case reports of BP following vaccine administration have been published [21–27]. In one, a 60-year-old man with Human Immunodeficiency Virus developed facial droop 42 h after receiving Pfizer/BioNTech BNT162b2 [28]. Another patient who interestingly had a history of BP developed it again after the second dose of the Pfizer vaccine [29]. In another report, a 61-year-old man developed BP within five hours of the first vaccine and then again on the contralateral side after the second dose [30]. In a PubMed and Google Scholar review of case reports and case series examining neurological manifestations of COVID-19 vaccination, Sriwastava et al. found that after Guillain–Barre syndrome, BP was the second most common peripheral nervous system manifestation [31]. These reports prompted more robust studies investigating the relationship between the COVID-19 vaccines and potential neurological side effects.

Studies then emerged calculating background incidence in order to determine whether a true change in BP incidence exists in relation to COVID-19 vaccinations. Researchers in Ontario, Canada, conducted a population-based retrospective observational study to estimate the background incidence of BP, finding the pre-pandemic mean annual rate of BP was 2.8 per 100,000 from the years 2015 to 2019 [32]. A multinational network cohort study including databases from Australia, France, Germany, Japan, Netherlands, Spain, United Kingdom, and United States, with a sample size of 126,661,070, notably found large variations between databases of different countries, suggesting rates of adverse events including BP should be compared to more localized background incidences [33].

Some studies claim an increased risk of BP in vaccinated patients. In a self-controlled case series in England, authors found a significantly increased rate of BP (17.9 cases per one million) following ChAdox1 vaccines; however, no association was found with the mRNA-1273 and BNT162b2 vaccine [15]. In another study comparing the inactivated CoronaVac vaccine and the mRNA-based vaccine, BNT162b2, authors conducted a retrospective study, based in Hong Kong, comparing the incidence of adverse events and all-cause mortality between the two. They analyzed a cohort of people who received at least one dose of either vaccine and found that among over 2 million people, there was a significantly higher rate of BP following the first dose of CoronaVac vs. BNT162b2 (67 versus 30 per 100,000 person-years; IRR = 1.95, 95% CI: 1.12–3.41, $p = 0.018$) [16]. In a study using a database of the largest healthcare system in Israel, there were 132 cases of BP out of 2,594,990 patients vaccinated with BNT162b2 after the first dose and 152 cases out of 2,434,674 s dose of the vaccine. This equated to standardized incidence ratios of 1.36 (95% CI: 1.14–1.61) and 1.16 (95% CI: 0.99–1.36), respectively, suggesting the possibility of an association between BP and the BNT162b2 mRNA vaccine [17]. However, other similarly designed studies failed to find an association between the two. A separate study taking place in Israel, for example, utilized a case-control design to evaluate patients recently vaccinated with BNT162b2. A proportion of patients with BP with exposure to the vaccine were compared to the overall number of patients with facial nerve palsy in prior years, and no association was found [18]. In addition, in a prospective study involving seven hospitals in Singapore, only 11 of 1,398,074 patients who were vaccinated with BNT162b2 and mRNA-1273 developed BP, and the authors were not able to establish any association [19]. In a self-controlled case series study assessing the risk of serious adverse events after BNT162b2, CoronaVac, and ChAdOx1 vaccines in Malaysia, authors were unable to find any increased risk of BP following either dose of all three vaccines 21 days after vaccination [20].

In two phase 3 COVID-19 vaccine trials, there were eight reported cases of BP amongst 73,868 total participants. Seven of these cases occurred in the vaccine group, which equates to an incidence of 19 per 100,000 [12,34,35]. The US Food and Drug Administration and the UK Medicine and Healthcare Products Regulatory Agency argue that these numbers are similar to the background rates of BP and in a disproportionality analysis by Renoud et al., there was no difference in reported adverse events of BP after COVID-19 vaccines compared to other viral vaccines [36]. It is important to note that facial paralysis is a known adverse event of vaccines, and that this phenomenon is not isolated to the COVID-19 vaccines; in a review of the vaccine adverse event reporting system (VAERS) database, the influenza vaccine had the greatest number of reported BP events, followed by varicella, and then human papilloma virus. The authors of this study note that the likelihood of BP remains very low overall at 0.26% over a 10-year span [37]. A different study using the VAERS database showed that reported levels of BP following COVID-19 mRNA vaccines are comparable to those of influenza before the COVID-19 pandemic [38].

Authors who found an association between the vaccine and BP conclude that despite this, the absolute or attributable risk is very low, and the benefits far outweigh the risks [17,39–41]. They highlight that the post-vaccine rates of adverse events, including BP, were similar to the expected background rates [11]. Furthermore, Tamaki et al. concluded that those with COVID-19 infection have a higher risk of BP than those who are vaccinated [12].

4. Mechanism of COVID-19 Infection and Vaccination and Bell's Palsy

Although there are a number of studies aiming to identify a connection between COVID-19 infection, vaccines, and BP, there is much to be discovered about the potential mechanism to explain such. The leading proposed etiology of BP is viral in nature, suggesting reactivation of HSV-1 at the geniculate ganglion as the possible cause [3,42]. Mouse models have shown the ability to induce facial nerve paralysis by infecting mice with HSV-1 [43]. In a mouse model of HSV-1-induced facial paralysis, Hato et al. found an increased level of nitric oxide, a free radical, and histologic evidence of demyelination in the mice experiencing facial paralysis. Their study suggested toxicity of nitric oxide on Schwann cells of the peripheral nervous system leading to nerve dysfunction. Their findings were supported by a significantly lower incidence of facial nerve dysfunction seen in mice treated with Edaravone, a free radical scavenger [44]. In the case of Ramsay Hunt Syndrome, facial paralysis is caused by the reactivation of varicella zoster virus, also at the geniculate ganglion [45]. The evidence of viral-induced facial paralysis suggests a possible route for COVID-19 infection to do the same. It has furthermore been proposed that coronaviruses are able to use olfactory nerves as the initial entrance into the central nervous system (CNS). Another hypothesis suggests "neuronal dissemination", a process of active transport that allows access to the CNS [46]. Another proposed mechanism of BP which could explain how COVID-19 causes neuropathy involves the principle of molecular mimicry, during which a foreign antigen, similar in structure to a self-antigen, causes immune-system sensitization. In the case of BP, this is thought to specifically affect the myelin sheath, impairing nerve conduction [47]. Coronaviruses use a glycoprotein that allows viral entry through the angiotensin-converting enzyme 2 receptor, which is often found on glial cells of the central and peripheral nervous system. It is suggested that this mechanism, also termed neurotropism, is one way the virus gains access to the nervous system [48].

It has been postulated that COVID-19 induces a hypercoagulable state, which may explain another way the virus affects our nervous system. In a systematic review by Parra-Medina et al., 60% of COVID-19 autopsies found microthrobi in the lung, heart, kidney, or liver. Furthermore, in a study by Karimi-Galougahi et al., positron emission tomography and computed tomography (PET/CT) obtained on a COVID-19-positive patient who presented with unilateral facial paralysis showed decreased metabolic activity within the affected facial nerve. This finding suggested a proposed mechanism of microthrombus-mediated pathology within the facial nerve or direct SARS-CoV-2 infection of the neurons or glial cells [49].

One mechanism proposing how BP may be caused by the COVID-19 vaccine is based on a theory that the pathogenesis of mRNA-vaccine-related BP is mediated by type I interferons. mRNA vaccines are known to cause a profound type I interferon response, and BP is a reported side effect seen in patients undergoing type I interferon therapy. Furthermore, type I interferon release is known to cause transient lymphopenia, which was the most common hematologic change seen during phase 1 trials of mRNA COVID-19 vaccines [47].

5. Conclusions

There is much to be discovered around the topic of COVID-19 as it relates to BP. Case reports of BP following both the COVID-19 vaccine and COVID-19 infection lack substantial evidence but opened the door for more robust studies.

Despite this, there has been no definitive evidence of an association between COVID-19 infection, COVID-19 vaccines, and BP.

Studies have mostly failed to identify incidences of BP that deviate significantly from pre-pandemic means.

The risk of BP following COVID-19 vaccines is no different from that seen with other viral vaccines.

Overall, the benefit of vaccination outweighs the risk of BP and there is insufficient evidence at this time to refute this.

Author Contributions: Conceptualization, E.N.T. and A.T.; methodology, E.N.T. and A.T.; formal analysis, E.N.T. and A.T.; investigation, E.N.T. and A.T.; resources, E.N.T. and A.T.; data curation, E.N.T., C.I.C. and A.T.; writing—original draft preparation, E.N.T. and A.T.; writing—review and editing, E.N.T., A.G., C.I.C., N.M.F., C.C.R., T.N.T., J.E.T., P.L., R.P.R., S.L. and A.T.; supervision, A.T. All authors have read and agreed to the published version of the manuscript.

Funding: This research received no external funding.

Conflicts of Interest: The authors declare no conflict of interest.

References

1. Zhang, W.; Xu, L.; Luo, T.; Wu, F.; Zhao, B.; Li, X. The etiology of Bell's palsy: A review. *J. Neurol.* **2020**, *267*, 1896–1905. [CrossRef]
2. Holland, N.J.; Bernstein, J.M. Bell's palsy. *BMJ Clin. Evid.* **2014**, *2014*, 1204. [PubMed]
3. Schirm, J.; Mulkens, P.S. Bell's palsy and herpes simplex virus. *APMIS* **1997**, *105*, 815–823. [CrossRef]
4. Nepal, G.; Rehrig, J.H.; Shrestha, G.S.; Shing, Y.K.; Yadav, J.K.; Ojha, R.; Pokhrel, G.; Tu, Z.L.; Huang, D.Y. Neurological manifestations of COVID-19: A systematic review. *Crit. Care* **2020**, *24*, 421. [CrossRef]
5. Iacono, A.; Pennisi, E.; Benincasa, C.; Marchetti, F. A case of facial nerve palsy in a pediatric patient associated with COVID-19. *Ital. J. Pediatr.* **2022**, *48*, 75. [CrossRef] [PubMed]
6. Afshar, Z.M.; Babazadeh, A.; Afsharian, M.; Vaziri, S.; Ebrahimpour, S. Bell's Palsy Associated with COVID-19 Infection: A Case Report. *Oman Med. J.* **2021**, *36*, e313. [CrossRef]
7. Lima, M.A.; Silva, M.T.T.; Soares, C.N.; Coutinho, R.; Oliveira, H.S.; Afonso, L.; Espíndola, O.; Leite, A.C.; Araujo, A. Peripheral facial nerve palsy associated with COVID-19. *J. Neurovirol.* **2020**, *26*, 941–944. [CrossRef]
8. Gupta, S.; Jawanda, M.K. Surge of Bell's Palsy in the era of COVID-19: Systematic review. *Eur. J. Neurol.* **2022**, *29*, 2526–2543. [CrossRef]
9. Islamoglu, Y.; Celik, B.; Kiris, M. Facial paralysis as the only symptom of COVID-19: A prospective study. *Am. J. Otolaryngol.* **2021**, *42*, 102956. [CrossRef]
10. Codeluppi, L.; Venturelli, F.; Rossi, J.; Fasano, A.; Toschi, G.; Pacillo, F.; Cavallieri, F.; Rossi, P.G.; Valzania, F. Facial palsy during the COVID-19 pandemic. *Brain Behav.* **2021**, *11*, e01939. [CrossRef]
11. Li, X.; Raventós, B.; Roel, E.; Pistillo, A.; Martinez-Hernandez, E.; Delmestri, A.; Reyes, C.; Strauss, V.; Prieto-Alhambra, D.; Burn, E.; et al. Association between COVID-19 vaccination, SARS-CoV-2 infection, and risk of immune mediated neurological events: Population based cohort and self-controlled case series analysis. *BMJ* **2022**, *376*, e068373. [CrossRef]
12. Tamaki, A.; Cabrera, C.I.; Li, S.; Rabbani, C.; Thuener, J.E.; Rezaee, R.P.; Fowler, N. Incidence of Bell Palsy in Patients With COVID-19. *JAMA Otolaryngol. Neck Surg.* **2021**, *147*, 767–768. [CrossRef]
13. Mutlu, A.; Kalcioglu, M.T.; Gunduz, A.Y.; Bakici, B.; Yilmaz, U.; Cag, Y. Does the SARS-CoV-2 pandemic really increase the frequency of peripheral facial palsy? *Am. J. Otolaryngol.* **2021**, *42*, 103032. [CrossRef]
14. Martin-Villares, C.; Alba, J.R.; Gonzalez-Gimeno, M.J. Data from 235 Cases of Bell's Palsy during COVID-19 Pandemic: Were There Clusters of Facial Palsy? *Neuroepidemiology* **2021**, *55*, 495–496. [CrossRef]
15. Walker, J.L.; Schultze, A.; Tazare, J.; Tamborska, A.; Singh, B.; Donegan, K.; Stowe, J.; Morton, C.E.; Hulme, W.J.; Curtis, H.J.; et al. Safety of COVID-19 vaccination and acute neurological events: A self-controlled case series in England using the OpenSAFELY platform. *Vaccine* **2022**, *40*, 4479–4487. [CrossRef]
16. Wong, C.K.H.; Lau, K.T.K.; Xiong, X.; Au, I.C.H.; Lai, F.T.T.; Wan, E.Y.F.; Chui, C.S.L.; Li, X.; Chan, E.W.Y.; Gao, L.; et al. Adverse events of special interest and mortality following vaccination with mRNA (BNT162b2) and inactivated (CoronaVac) SARS-CoV-2 vaccines in Hong Kong: A retrospective study. *PLoS Med.* **2022**, *19*, e1004018. [CrossRef]
17. Shibli, R.; Barnett, O.; Abu-Full, Z.; Gronich, N.; Najjar-Debbiny, R.; Doweck, I.; Rennert, G.; Saliba, W. Association between vaccination with the BNT162b2 mRNA COVID-19 vaccine and Bell's palsy: A population-based study. *Lancet Reg. Health-Eur.* **2021**, *11*, 100236. [CrossRef]
18. Shemer, A.; Pras, E.; Einan-Lifshitz, A.; Dubinsky-Pertzov, B.; Hecht, I. Association of COVID-19 Vaccination and Facial Nerve Palsy: A Case-Control Study. *JAMA Otolaryngol. Neck Surg.* **2021**, *147*, 739–743. [CrossRef]
19. Koh, J.S.; Hoe, R.H.M.; Yong, M.H.; Chiew, H.J.; Goh, Y.; Yong, K.P.; Tu, T.M.; Chan, D.W.S.; Tan, B.Y.-Q.; Yeo, L.L.L.; et al. Hospital-based observational study of neurological disorders in patients recently vaccinated with COVID-19 mRNA vaccines. *J. Neurol. Sci.* **2021**, *430*, 120030. [CrossRef]
20. Ab Rahman, N.; Lim, M.T.; Lee, F.Y.; Lee, S.C.; Ramli, A.; Saharudin, S.N.; King, T.L.; Jam, E.B.A.; Ayub, N.A.; Sevalingam, R.K.; et al. Risk of serious adverse events after the BNT162b2, CoronaVac, and ChAdOx1 vaccines in Malaysia: A self-controlled case series study. *Vaccine* **2022**, *40*, 4394–4402. [CrossRef]
21. Prado, M.B.; Adiao, K.J.B. Facial Diplegia as the Sole Manifestation of Post-Vaccination Guillain-Barre Syndrome: A Case Report and Literature Review. *Neurohospitalist* **2022**, *12*, 508–511. [CrossRef]
22. Poudel, S.; Nepali, P.; Baniya, S.; Shah, S.; Bogati, S.; Nepal, G.; Ojha, R.; Edaki, O.; Lazovic, G.; Kara, S. Bell's palsy as a possible complication of mRNA-1273 (Moderna) vaccine against COVID-19. *Ann. Med. Surg.* **2022**, *78*, 103897. [CrossRef]
23. Mirmosayyeb, O.; Barzegar, M.; Rezaei, M.; Baharlouie, N.; Shaygannejad, V. Bell's palsy after Sputnik V COVID-19 (Gam-COVID-Vac) vaccination. *Clin. Case Rep.* **2022**, *10*, e05468. [CrossRef]
24. Cellina, M.; D'Arrigo, A.; Floridi, C.; Oliva, G.; Carrafiello, G. Left Bell's palsy following the first dose of mRNA-1273 SARS-CoV-2 vaccine: A case report. *Clin. Imaging* **2022**, *82*, 1–4. [CrossRef]
25. Martin-Villares, C.; Vazquez-Feito, A.; Gonzalez-Gimeno, M.J.; de la Nogal-Fernandez, B. Bell's palsy following a single dose of mRNA SARS-CoV-2 vaccine: A case report. *J. Neurol.* **2022**, *269*, 47–48. [CrossRef]
26. Iftikhar, H.; Noor, S.M.U.; Masood, M.; Bashir, K. Bell's Palsy After 24 Hours of mRNA-1273 SARS-CoV-2 Vaccine. *Cureus* **2021**, *13*, e15935. [CrossRef]

27. Pothiawala, S. Bell's Palsy after Second Dose of Moderna COVID-19 Vaccine: Coincidence or Causation? *Acta Med. Litu.* **2021**, *28*, 298–301. [CrossRef]
28. Mussatto, C.C.; Sokol, J.; Alapati, N. Bell's palsy following COVID-19 vaccine administration in HIV+ patient. *Am. J. Ophthalmol. Case Rep.* **2022**, *25*, 101259. [CrossRef]
29. Repajic, M.; Lai, X.L.; Xu, P.; Liu, A. Bell's Palsy after second dose of Pfizer COVID-19 vaccination in a patient with history of recurrent Bell's palsy. *Brain Behav. Immun. Health* **2021**, *13*, 100217. [CrossRef]
30. Burrows, A.; Bartholomew, T.; Rudd, J.; Walker, D. Sequential contralateral facial nerve palsies following COVID-19 vaccination first and second doses. *BMJ Case Rep.* **2021**, *14*, e243829. [CrossRef]
31. Sriwastava, S.; Sharma, K.; Khalid, S.H.; Bhansali, S.; Shrestha, A.K.; Elkhooly, M.; Srivastava, S.; Khan, E.; Jaiswal, S.; Wen, S. COVID-19 Vaccination and Neurological Manifestations: A Review of Case Reports and Case Series. *Brain Sci.* **2022**, *12*, 407. [CrossRef]
32. Nasreen, S.; Calzavara, A.; Buchan, S.A.; Thampi, N.; Johnson, C.; Wilson, S.E.; Kwong, J.C. Background incidence rates of adverse events of special interest related to COVID-19 vaccines in Ontario, Canada, 2015 to 2020, to inform COVID-19 vaccine safety surveillance. *Vaccine* **2022**, *40*, 3305–3312. [CrossRef]
33. Li, X.; Ostropolets, A.; Makadia, R.; Shaoibi, A.; Rao, G.; Sena, A.G.; Martinez-Hernandez, E.; Delmestri, A.; Verhamme, K.; Rijnbeek, P.R.; et al. Characterizing the incidence of adverse events of special interest for COVID-19 vaccines across eight countries: A multinational network cohort study. *Medrxiv* **2021**, *373*, 1485. [CrossRef]
34. Polack, F.P.; Thomas, S.J.; Kitchin, N.; Absalon, J.; Gurtman, A.; Lockhart, S.; Perez, J.L.; Pérez Marc, G.; Moreira, E.D.; Zerbini, C.; et al. Safety and efficacy of the BNT162b2 mRNA COVID-19 vaccine. *N. Engl. J. Med.* **2020**, *383*, 2603–2615. [CrossRef]
35. Baden, L.R.; El Sahly, H.M.; Essink, B.; Kotloff, K.; Frey, S.; Novak, R.; Diemert, D.; Spector, S.A.; Rouphael, N.; Creech, C.B.; et al. Efficacy and Safety of the mRNA-1273 SARS-CoV-2 Vaccine. *N. Engl. J. Med.* **2021**, *384*, 403–416. [CrossRef]
36. Renoud, L.; Khouri, C.; Revol, B.; Lepelley, M.; Perez, J.; Roustit, M.; Cracowski, J.-L. Association of Facial Paralysis With mRNA COVID-19 Vaccines: A Disproportionality Analysis Using the World Health Organization Pharmacovigilance Database. *JAMA Intern. Med.* **2021**, *181*, 1243–1245. [CrossRef]
37. Ahsanuddin, S.; Nasser, W.; Roy, S.C.; Povolotskiy, R.; Paskhover, B. Facial paralysis and vaccinations: A vaccine adverse event reporting system review. *Fam. Pract.* **2021**, *39*, 80–84. [CrossRef]
38. Sato, K.; Mano, T.; Niimi, Y.; Toda, T.; Iwata, A.; Iwatsubo, T. Facial nerve palsy following the administration of COVID-19 mRNA vaccines: Analysis of a self-reporting database. *Int. J. Infect. Dis.* **2021**, *111*, 310–312. [CrossRef]
39. Wan, E.Y.F.; Chui, C.S.L.; Ng, V.W.S.; Wang, Y.; Yan, V.K.C.; Lam, I.C.H.; Fan, M.; Lai, F.T.T.; Chan, E.W.Y.; Li, X.; et al. Messenger RNA Coronavirus Disease 2019 (COVID-19) Vaccination with BNT162b2 Increased Risk of Bell's Palsy: A Nested Case-Control and Self-Controlled Case Series Study. *Clin. Infect. Dis.* **2022**, *published online*. [CrossRef]
40. Wan, E.Y.F.; Chui, C.S.L.; Lai, F.T.T.; Chan, E.W.Y.; Li, X.; Yan, V.K.C.; Gao, L.; Yu, Q.; Lam, I.C.H.; Chun, R.K.C.; et al. Bell's palsy following vaccination with mRNA (BNT162b2) and inactivated (CoronaVac) SARS-CoV-2 vaccines: A case series and nested case-control study. *Lancet Infect. Dis.* **2022**, *22*, 64–72. [CrossRef]
41. Cirillo, N.; Doan, R. The association between COVID-19 vaccination and Bell's palsy. *Lancet Infect. Dis.* **2022**, *22*, 5–6. [CrossRef] [PubMed]
42. Burgess, R.C.; Bale, J.F.; Michaels, L.; Smith, R. Polymerase Chain Reaction Amplification of Herpes Simplex Viral Dna from the Geniculate Ganglion of a Patient with Bell's Palsy. *Ann. Otol. Rhinol. Laryngol.* **1994**, *103*, 775–779. [CrossRef] [PubMed]
43. Takahashi, H.; Hitsumoto, Y.; Honda, N.; Hato, N.; Mizobuchi, M.; Murakami, S.; Kisaki, H.; Wakisaka, H.; Gyo, K. Mouse Model of Bell's palsy Induced by Reactivation of Herpes Simplex Virus Type 1. *J. Neuropathol. Exp. Neurol.* **2001**, *60*, 621–627. [CrossRef]
44. Hato, N.; Kohno, H.; Yamada, H.; Takahashi, H.; Gyo, K. Role of Nitric Oxide in the Onset of Facial Nerve Palsy by HSV-1 Infection. *JAMA Otolaryngol. Neck Surg.* **2013**, *139*, 1339–1342. [CrossRef]
45. Jeon, Y.; Lee, H. Ramsay Hunt syndrome. *J. Dent. Anesth. Pain Med.* **2018**, *18*, 333–337. [CrossRef]
46. Armocida, D.; Palmieri, M.; Frati, A.; Santoro, A.; Pesce, A. How SARS-CoV-2 can involve the central nervous system. A systematic analysis of literature of the department of human neurosciences of Sapienza University, Italy. *J. Clin. Neurosci.* **2020**, *79*, 231–236. [CrossRef]
47. Soeiro, T.; Salvo, F.; Pariente, A.; Grandvuillemin, A.; Jonville-Béra, A.-P.; Micallef, J. Type I interferons as the potential mechanism linking mRNA COVID-19 vaccines to Bell's palsy. *Therapies* **2021**, *76*, 365–367. [CrossRef]
48. Flores, G. SARS-CoV-2 (COVID-19) has neurotropic and neuroinvasive properties. *Int. J. Clin. Pract.* **2021**, *75*, e13708. [CrossRef]
49. Karimi-Galougahi, M.; Yousefi-Koma, A.; Raygani, N.; Bakhshayeshkaram, M.; Haseli, S. 18FDG-PET/CT Assessment of COVID-19-Induced Bell's Palsy. *Acad. Radiol.* **2021**, *28*, 144–145. [CrossRef]

encyclopedia

MDPI

Entry

The Post-Pandemic Transformation of Art and Architecture Libraries

Rose Orcutt [1,*], Lucy Campbell [2], Maya Gervits [3] and Barbara Opar [4]

1 University Libraries, University of Buffalo, Buffalo, NY 14214, USA
2 Richard P. Welsh Library, NewSchool of Architecture and Design, San Diego, CA 92101, USA
3 Barbara and Leonard Littman Architecture and Design Library, New Jersey Institute of Technology, Newark, NJ 07102, USA
4 King + King Architecture Library, Syracuse University, Syracuse, NY 13244, USA
* Correspondence: rmorcutt@buffalo.edu

Definition: This entry paper considers the impact of the COVID-19 pandemic on the processes and functions of art and architecture libraries in North America and distinguishes between temporary changes and those that will endure and are here to stay. COVID-19 impacted all aspects of human life, placing tremendous stress on institutions and individuals globally. Academic libraries responded to the crisis by bringing resources to communities remotely and keeping constituents engaged to maintain a sense of normalcy. While libraries in schools of architecture, art, and design, responded similarly to other academic libraries, they also had unique needs. This entry paper is informed by two surveys of art and architecture library staff and faculty, alongside a preliminary literature review. The results of the first survey were published in Art Documentation and the results and analysis of the second survey are forthcoming. Both temporary and long-standing changes were implemented to ensure uninterrupted service in academic institutions. Temporary solutions included extending loan periods, quarantining materials, enforcing social distancing, and expanding document delivery. Changes that will endure post-pandemic include the increased acquisition of digital materials, remote instruction and reference consultations, increased resource access, and the utilization of a vast array of technologies.

Keywords: COVID-19 pandemic; post-pandemic; libraries; online access; remote services; digitization; transformation; art and architecture; academic libraries

Citation: Orcutt, R.; Campbell, L.; Gervits, M.; Opar, B. The Post-Pandemic Transformation of Art and Architecture Libraries. *Encyclopedia* **2022**, 2, 1893–1901. https://doi.org/10.3390/encyclopedia2040131

Academic Editors: Fulvio Mazzocchi and Raffaele Barretta

Received: 25 October 2022
Accepted: 25 November 2022
Published: 30 November 2022

1. History

The recently published report *The Library of the Future* indicates that "the library profession, much like the library itself, is undergoing profound change" [1]. Indeed, following the COVID-19 pandemic, many library activities have moved online. Librarians have adapted and become "vital partners with scholars, instructors, students, and patrons in a way few had experienced before" [1].

December 2019 saw the first outbreak of the coronavirus disease in Wuhan, China. By mid-March 2020, all 50 of the United States had reported cases, leading to a rapid shutdown of businesses, cultural and religious institutions, and public and private educational facilities, including libraries. Few if any were prepared for the changes necessitated by the shutdown. Preparedness manuals offered little relevant content, and practices were rarely uniform even within institutions. We have now reached a point in the operation of libraries where predictions can be made about temporary workarounds versus changes that are here to stay.

Beginning in 2021, publications focused on library responses to COVID-19 were released, providing information on both public and academic libraries [2–5]. The majority address particular case studies, or specific library functions such as research productivity, management, copyright, or technological advancements. *The Handbook of Research on Library Response to the COVID-19 Pandemic* takes a scholarly approach to understanding how libraries transformed during the global health emergency. Chapters highlight a range of topics including crisis leadership, data management, and virtual programming. Library types from around the world are also represented. Chapters include *Opportunities and Challenges Offered by the Effects of the COVID-19 Pandemic on Academic Libraries* which proposes, "libraries cannot afford to close down their formal duties of providing information to the users ... The libraries should be in continuous coordination with the researchers conducting research in the field of the cure of the COVID-19" [6]. However, little attention has been paid to the specific response of architecture, art, and design libraries.

This entry applies to the information science field and information professions, more specifically to those in the art, architecture, and design disciplines. This content is informed by an exploratory review of current literature addressing responses and changes to academic library functions resulting from the COVID-19 pandemic, alongside two extensive surveys of library staff and faculty users. These surveys were circulated during the early and late stages of the pandemic. Detailed findings have been published [7].

2. Evaluation

2.1. *Customer Service and Reference*

2.1.1. Temporary Changes

Temporary measures allowed for the continuation of library services while addressing staff safety concerns. Collaboration between institutions was critical in formulating the format and extent of services and safety protocols. Organizations such as The Center for Disease Control and Prevention (CDC), and National Endowment for the Humanities (NEH), provided overall guidance, while, The International Federation of Library Associations and Institutions (IFLA), and American Library Association (ALA) shared library-specific best practices [8]. Many provided online discussion space and webinars, for example the Medical Library Association (MLA) published guidelines for appropriate COVID-19 preparation and practice [9]. Across architecture and design libraries, specific recommendations were shared via association and membership listservs. Measures included curbside pickup, social distancing signage, sanitizing spaces, alternative work schedules, restricting visitor numbers, the promotion of e-resources and e-services, and quarantining circulating materials (Table 1). In architecture, art, and design libraries, access to visual print materials remains integral to research practices. Quarantine and curbside pickup were dominant temporary responses. For example, 72% of architecture libraries reported offering curbside pickup services in Spring of 2021 [7]. However, these services have been terminated as patrons returned. After months of closures and restricted access, libraries reported 40–60% return of visitors in August 2022, compared to pre-pandemic levels, a number that is expected to increase [10].

Table 1. Circulation changes, temporary and/or permanent. These findings are informed by surveys and a review of the literature.

Circulation Changes	Temporary	Permanent	Notes
Building closures and/or limited access	X		
Reduced Operating Hours	X		A few institutions permanently adjusted hours of operation
Curbside Pickup	X		
Check out to lockers		X	

Table 1. *Cont.*

Circulation Changes	Temporary	Permanent	Notes
Extended loan periods	X		Some institutions may have studied and adjusted loan period structure post COVID-19
Fine forgiveness	X		
Glass/plexiglass desk partitions		X	
Staffing working from home full or part time			A few institutions have continued to allow staff to work off site some of the time. This service however does not lend itself well to off- site activities
Free mailing items to patrons	X		Mailing has continued but only for distance patrons- over 35 miles

2.1.2. Here to Stay

Following the COVID-19 pandemic, the concept of the art and architecture library being "open" no longer necessarily means the doors are unlocked. Instead, staff and materials are accessible and responsive to patrons digitally. As summarized by Dr. Todaro, "You can't see us, but we are here to help you" [11]. For libraries that established robust remote service models, service hours and access to physical spaces are now two different and distinct concepts. This change in both how libraries perceive their services and what users expect is likely to remain long term.

Guidelines changed over time as new information became available, for example studies on the effects of contact with different types of paper [12]. However, the guidelines provided by associations and professional organizations for quarantining were inconsistent and often contradictory. The recommendations varied between 2 and 8 days, and in September 2021, Northeast Document Conservation Center (NEDCC) suggested determining the length of the quarantine period by assessing the level of risk in each community [13]. Professional organizations have begun to develop standards and plans for managing communications, public health crisis, and access during lock down situations [14]. It is anticipated that with the benefit of hindsight some will publish informed and extensive guides that will serve as useful future-proofing tools.

Reference services have been permanently changed by COVID-19. When physical access to collections became impossible, reference librarians continued to assist patrons in creative ways. Patrons were referred to items available online, e-resources were ordered as surrogates, and staff with partial access to facilities scanned items for users (Table 2). These services have now become standard expectations where they were once exceptions.

Architecture literature continues to be heavily print reliant. The major periodical index, the *Avery Index to Architectural Periodicals*, is a bibliographic citation index, and the only reliable database to comprehensively search image saturated architecture periodicals. This continues to be a unique characteristic of libraries in the discipline. This discovery issue is specific to the field and this resource. While some older content has been made freely available online, the number of such titles is limited. The Avery also indexes many journals for which there is no online content. *The Architectural Review* has provided consistent online access for less than ten years, with very selective access to some older content. *Architectural Design* online is available only from 2005. Older content is important in architecture for historical and precedent research. Architectural research is image based and the quality and clarity of online images is paramount. With limited aggregator tools which in older cases are not sufficiently precise or uniform to direct patrons to online content. For example, a reference to the Seagram Building restaurant is cited as *Architectural Record.* 1959: 201–204. While there is freely available digital access to this journal through the *US Modernist Library*, the user needs more information to locate the source. Reference work is multifaceted, and in the case of architecture often involves in-depth content knowledge, for example detailed drawings of specific projects. It cannot be comprehensively conducted without access to materials, and older titles are often unavailable in e-formats. Architectural design is particularly challenging as few architectural monographs are digitized. While databases such as *DETAIL Inspiration* offer drawings, access is limited to newer projects. Similarly, architectural archives may be open access, but many offer low-resolution drawings. Others, such as *Le Corbusier Plans* are costly and extremely specialized.

Table 2. Reference Changes, temporary and/or permanent. These findings are informed by surveys and a review of the literature.

Reference Changes	Temporary	Permanent	Notes
Lack of access to physical content	X		
Greater reliance on purchased e-content		X	Many libraries are now selecting e-preferred for approval plans and some other content
Greater reliance on open access e-content		X	Archives such as *US Modernist* provide digitized content of core journals in the discipline
Lack of digital access to older content		X	While this is evolving, there is no consistent or intentional approach to digitizing older monographs or journal titles.
Concierge approach to reference work	X		Post COVID-19, many patrons have come to expect services like paging of books
Changes to how reference performed—reference interview curtailed or shortened	X		During COVID-19, many librarians shortened this process and simply supplied the patron with the desired content
Expansion of chat services		X	Patrons who had not previously used chat came to rely on this service
Zoom reference		X	Hybrid staffing has made this a desirable option for staff and some patrons
Hybrid work schedules		X	Most institutions have accepted hybridity as the new norm

2.2. *Outreach and Engagement*

2.2.1. Temporary Changes

Remote attendance changed outreach activities. Digital newsletters, emails, blogs, online exhibitions, and social media existed before the pandemic. However, reliance on these tools to promote resources, programming, and mental health checks increased as librarians sought to connect with isolated faculty and students. Online research guides became a prominent tool to present resources for class instruction. One analysis by Springshare found librarians created 26,000 new research guides in response to the pandemic [15]. Zoom sessions, Google Hangouts, and Microsoft Teams promoted scheduled public events such as book talks, lecture series, and presentations to patrons and sometimes increased attendance in comparison to in-person events, as people looked for ways to connect. Although these practices will continue to feature in library services, patrons and staff desire more in-person connections. Face-to-face activities are once again increasing.

2.2.2. Here to Stay

Despite the growing desire to meet in person, these events continue to incorporate online components. The hybrid environment is here to stay and is already impacting architectural education. A core practice in architecture and design education is the Lecture Series, in which prestigious guest speakers are invited to campus. Typically open to the public, these lectures are now being broadcast live online for free, opening them to a new audience of students and learners around the world. For libraries, the opportunity to support these efforts by providing resources and content has added value to their services. Libraries can promote lectures happening at universities in Hong Kong, Germany, or Brazil, while connecting users to relevant and unique content in their own collections.

2.3. *Collection Development*

2.3.1. Temporary Changes

Acquisition efforts shifted to electronic as opposed to analog materials, including books, journals, databases, and streaming videos. Some libraries implemented Controlled Digital Lending (CDL) to allow digital circulation of print materials including course reserve materials, and publishers bridged the gap by providing online access to critical resources for free or at reduced rates [16–18]. Initially the Internet Archive offered some 1.4 million titles through free CDL, although this initiative was quickly stymied by publisher concerns around intellectual property rights [19].

While collection development was pushed to a hybrid model, COVID-19 also led to budget concerns and policy changes. While academic libraries already preferenced e-formats in many disciplines, the arts retained greater flexibility and subject selectors made case-by-case judgments. To ensure 24/7 access, libraries mandated e-formats across disciplines, expanding access but drawing attention to the issues of e-format availability in the architecture and design disciplines.

2.3.2. Here to Stay

With decreased budgets, creative publishing methods, and where feasible the adoption of digital first strategies, librarians are cautiously participating in production processes for scholarly content. Open access publishing and Open Educational Resources (OER) are increasingly attractive alternatives as growing interest results in falling costs, expanded access, and most importantly, improved quality [20,21]. Although they have existed since the late nineties, OER have a reputation of low quality and inaccuracy. COVID-19 has changed those attitudes and signaled a willingness amongst educators to adopt and grow these free resources, making them available to remix, reuse, and adapt to course objectives.

While cost saving methods such as demand-driven acquisition, resource sharing, and consortiums are the new normal, print based collections in art and architecture will continue to struggle to maintain contemporary literature holdings. COVID-19 induced gaps in collections are unlikely to be filled because of because print budget has been reduced. Emphasis on lounge and study spaces and collaborative services with other departments has also led a trend towards reevaluating print holdings [1].

2.4. *Digital Resources*

2.4.1. Temporary Changes

Electronic books have existed since the digitization of the Declaration of Independence in 1971. However, widespread acceptance of the format really began just twenty years ago, and until recently the humanities have been particularly resistant [22–24]. Although they provide perpetual access, eBooks present issues such as managing logins, simultaneous use models, varying vendor platforms, and print quotas. eBook packages are rented and susceptible to continuous change. According to publisher agreements, content may disappear suddenly, creating uncertainty. Many libraries today employ evidence-based selection methods, so key titles are subject to removal if not consulted regularly. Despite these known issues architecture libraries were temporarily pushed to purchase eBooks exclusively.

According to a Motion Picture Association report, the number of subscribers to streaming services during the pandemic reached 1.1 billion [25]. The increased consumption of streaming media and vendor pricing models created a challenge for libraries to meet patrons' needs, especially in architecture libraries where film is an important visual learning resource. Some libraries developed policies and practices for converting DVDs to streaming content [26,27]. However, no standard controlled lending policies have been established to date. Institutions were slow to produce such copies, and a murky copyright environment meant most were only comfortable using this practice for required course materials or limited film snippets. With the return to in-person teaching, these efforts were largely abandoned.

2.4.2. Here to Stay

With the assumption that eBooks are favored by many patrons, some states such as Maryland and Rhode Island have introduced legislation mandating that eBook publishers must allow libraries to purchase eBooks at a "reasonable price" ensuring fair and balanced lending. These bills can be preempted by the federally mandated Copyright Act, as happened in New York. Nevertheless, this highlights the need for legislation and the possibility of bringing the issue to the state level to preserve the library's mission to make books available to the public at a reasonable cost [28].

Without a doubt, streaming media is both here to stay and has many advantages over outdated formats. Despite the TEACH Act, online teaching made it more problematic to use DVDs and resulted in increased use of platforms such as Kanopy, Swank, Artfilms Digital, Academic Video Online, OnArchitecture, and Pidgeon Digital. While these vendors provide robust collections, they are far from exhaustive. As a result, libraries must regularly negotiate streaming rights for specific titles which, although costly and available for a predetermined time, have become standard practice [29].

Libraries are continuing to struggle with providing online access to both new and older titles. While many vendors such as JSTOR provided expanded temporary or free access to certain collections during COVID-19, the industry has not responded satisfactorily to the ongoing needs of libraries [30]. Rather than provide unlimited or DRM free access to titles, many vendors have chosen to return to 1 or 3 simultaneous users. Multiple vendors provide access to popular titles, but few address the need for key older titles, especially in architecture. eBooks costs are rarely consistent, and while a few database vendors such as MADCAD are willing to expand access to certain resources for specific periods of time, this practice is rare. Surveying libraries and vendors for input on resource needs could be mutually beneficial.

2.5. *Technology*

2.5.1. Temporary Changes

Technology empowered libraries to maintain continuity and opened additional avenues for cooperation. Through collaborative efforts, they offered settings for new interactions and fostered engagement. Technology played a critical role in enabling online teaching, communications, and outreach. Popular communication software included Zoom, Jabber, Webex, and Google Meet. Mentimeter, Top Hat, and Canvas Tool Box helped increase interactivity, and smart video conferencing equipment such as Owl Pro facilitated both online teaching and group meetings. In architecture education, collaborative design software such as the Miro online whiteboard enabled studio culture to persist in a digital world. However, many of these solutions have since been discarded or neglected in favor of traditional studio practices.

2.5.2. Here to Stay

The high level of flexibility which technology facilitated will remain critical in a post-COVID-19 world. Some specialists predict that hybrid and HyFlex offerings will likely serve as a baseline for future operations [31,32]. Libraries and librarian roles are changing, and staffing patterns will follow suit. While many libraries are now permitting flexible scheduling and work from home, there are no uniform policies. Staffing patterns and roles and responsibilities vary from institution to institution. Guidelines and best practices could be established through a consensus of professional organizations. The move to hybrid delivery both in the classroom and for student services has increased expectations of technological expertise of staff. Remote communication techniques have been established and will continue.

Increased collaboration and aggressive adoption of new technologies became typical in education and research during the pandemic. Asynchronous learning provided opportunities for a more flexible educational process supporting students who were not always in the same time zones or unable to attend synchronous lectures. It allowed for increased participation and enhanced accessibility. At the same time, virtual meetings offered more dynamic and collaborative engagement, while requiring more nuanced scheduling, technical competence, and adequate infrastructure.

2.6. Remote Work Arrangements

2.6.1. Temporary Changes

The pandemic required almost everyone to work remotely. While this created flexibility in schedules, access to key resources were hard to obtain as the majority of architecture core texts remain print based. Remote work created blurred boundaries between work and home life. Librarians who cared for family, children, or the elderly had to balance work schedules with these responsibilities. The influx of virtual services such as Zoom, Google Meets, Slack, chat services, and similar platforms was a considerable positive aspect that facilitated interactions with students, staff, and faculty. These services allowed librarians to continue and even strengthen communication, teaching, and reference skills, proving the profession could function remotely [33].

2.6.2. Here to Stay

With the realization that work could be done at home, employees challenged the preceding notion of incapability to telecommute and pushed for more flex time. Librarians are re-assessing their work schedules; keeping the efficient productive responsibilities and obligations while focusing on efficient, uninterrupted operations. Working on-site may be necessitated by in-person meetings, class instruction, appointments, and faculty and student interactions. Virtual meetings, classes, appointments, and other activities could be accomplished remotely without the need to commute or be interrupted. Research has found that hybrid and flex schedules increase production and efficiency [34]. The ability to work remotely can reduce stress and help with individual mental health and wellbeing [35]. However, job related stresses such as inadequate pay, increased duties with no extra compensation, and unhealthy schedules has also led to the phenomenon of 'quiet quitting;' a push back on being undervalued [36]. Realistic goals should be set by supervisors who understand the employees' need for flexibility, thus creating a supportive workplace culture based on communication and mutual support [37]. The post-pandemic art and architecture library must seek new ways to think about information services and patron connections. Libraries must address change and acknowledge that the situation is different now and seek alternative ways of measuring the impact the library has on the campus community other than foot traffic and in-person interactions. In the aftermath of COVID19, additional assessment should be made to determine what has changed, what has improved and what issues still need resolution.

COVID-19's impact on academic art and architecture libraries has been transformative and clearly challenged librarians to creatively adapt. However, lessons learned have enabled libraries to be nimble, adapt quickly, learn new ways of doing things and expand services, practices, and goals.

Funding: This research received no external funding.

Institutional Review Board Statement: Not applicable.

Informed Consent Statement: Not applicable.

Conflicts of Interest: The authors declare no conflict of interest.

References

1. Carlson, S. *The Library of the Future: How the Heart of the Campus Is Transforming*; Chronicle of Higher Education, Inc.: Washington, DC, USA, 2022; pp. 39,50.
2. Ashiq, M.; Jabeen, F.; Mahmood, K. Transformation of Libraries During COVID-19 Pandemic: A Systematic Review. *J. Acad. Librariansh.* **2022**, *48*, 102534. Available online: https://www.ncbi.nlm.nih.gov/pmc/articles/PMC9046028/pdf/main.pdf (accessed on 25 October 2022). [CrossRef] [PubMed]
3. Dobreva, M.; Anghelescu, H. Libraries and COVID-19: Opportunities for Innovation. *IFLA J.* **2022**, *48*, 3–8. Available online: https://journals.sagepub.com/doi/10.1177/03400352221077748 (accessed on 25 October 2022). [CrossRef]
4. Louderback, P. During and Post COVID-19 Practices of a Regional Academic Library. *J. Libr. Adm.* **2021**, *61*, 726–734. [CrossRef]
5. Munip, L.; Tinik, L.; Borrelli, S.; Randone, G.R.; Paik, E.J. Lessons Learned: A Meta-Synthesis Examining Library Spaces, Services and Resources during COVID-19. *Libr. Manag.* **2022**, *43*, 80–92. [CrossRef]
6. Deol, N.K.; Brar, K.S. The Pandemic of COVID-19 and Role of Academic Libraries. *Libr. Philos. Pract.* 2021, p. 5099. Available online: https://digitalcommons.unl.edu/cgi/viewcontent.cgi?article=9434&context=libphilprac (accessed on 15 September 2022).
7. Orcutt, R.; Campbell, L.; Gervits, M.; Opar, B.; Edwards, K. COVID-19 Pandemic: Architecture Librarians Respond. *Art Doc.* **2021**, *40*, 123–140. [CrossRef]
8. American Library Association. Guidance Content & Protocols. Tools, Publications & Resources. 2022. Available online: https://www.ala.org/tools/covid/guidance-protocols (accessed on 14 September 2022).
9. Medical Library Association. COVID-19 Resources for Medical Librarians & Other Health Information Professionals. 2020. Available online: https://www.mlanet.org/page/covid-19-resources-for-medical-librarians (accessed on 16 August 2022).
10. Carlson, S.; Haricombe, L.J.; Ellis, E.; Schonfeld, R. The Future of Academic Libraries. 2022. Available online: https://occuspace.io/blog/future-of-academic-libraries (accessed on 20 September 2022).
11. Todaro, J. The Post-Pandemic Library: Managing Issues Now that They Are Our Daily Routine. 2022. Available online: https://www.nicheacademy.com/blog/the-post-pandemic-library (accessed on 25 October 2022).
12. OCLC. Realm Project. News. 28 October 2022. Available online: https://www.oclc.org/realm/news.html (accessed on 14 November 2022).
13. Northeast Document Conservation Center. 3.5 Disinfecting Books and Other Collections. 2021. Available online: https://www.nedcc.org/free-resources/preservation-leaflets/3.-emergency-management/3.5-disinfecting-books (accessed on 14 November 2022).
14. OCLC. Public Health Crisis Management Playbook for Archives, Libraries, and Museums. 2022. Available online: https://www.oclc.org/realm/public-health-crisis-playbook.html (accessed on 14 November 2022).
15. Talia. You've Switched to Remote Services … and the Numbers Show It, 2020. Springshare. Available online: https://blog.springshare.com/2020/04/28/youve-switched-to-remote-services-and-the-numbers-show-it/ (accessed on 5 May 2020).
16. Currier, C.; Centivany, A. Controlled Digital Lending. *Proc. Assoc. Inf. Sci. Technol.* **2021**, *58*, 80–91. Available online: https://asistdl.onlinelibrary.wiley.com/doi/pdfdirect/10.1002/pra2.438?download=true (accessed on 25 October 2022). [CrossRef]
17. Finlay, C.; Kopel, M.; Berney, T.; Nayyer, K.; Paolillo, M.; Walker, K. Controlled Digital Lending Environmental Scan Spring 2022. 2022. Available online: https://doi.org/1813/111412 (accessed on 25 October 2022).
18. Opar, B. They Stepped up: Vendors during the Coronavirus. Association of Collegiate Schools of Architecture, 2020. Association of Collegiate Schools of Architecture. Available online: https://www.acsa-arch.org/they-stepped-up-vendors-during-the-coronavirus/ (accessed on 17 June 2022).
19. Internet Archive. National Emergency Library, 2020. Internet Archive Blogs. Available online: http://blog.archive.org/national-emergency-library/ (accessed on 14 September 2022).
20. Wiley, D.; Green, C.; Soares, L. Dramatically Bringing down the Cost of Education with OER, 2012. The OER Knowledge Cloud. Available online: https://www.oerknowledgecloud.org/record1231 (accessed on 27 September 2022).
21. Ohler, L.A.; Pitts, J. From Peril to Promise: The Academic Library Post-COVID-19. *Coll. Res. Libr. News* **2021**, *82*, 41. [CrossRef]
22. Hawkins, D.T. Electronic Books: A Major Publishing Revolution. *Online* **2000**, *24*, 19.
23. Muthu, M. E-Books: An Overview. *Inf. Stud.* **2012**, *18*, 253.
24. Corlett-Rivera, K.; Hackman, T. E-Book Use and Attitudes in the Humanities, Social Sciences, and Education. *Portal Libr. Acad.* **2014**, *14*, 255–286. [CrossRef]
25. Motion Picture Association. Global Subscriptions to Online Video Services Exceeds One Billion for First Time Ever, New MPA Report Finds. 2021. Electronic Books: A Major Publishing Revolution. Available online: https://www.motionpictures.org/press/global-subscriptions-to-online-video-services-exceeds-one-billion-for-first-time-ever-new-mpa-report-finds/ (accessed on 9 August 2022).
26. Cooper, D.; Ruediger, D.; Skinner, M. Streaming Media Licensing and Purchasing Practices at Academic Libraries, 2022. Ithaka S+R. Available online: https://sr.ithaka.org/publications/streaming-media-licensing-and-purchasing-practices-at-academic-libraries/ (accessed on 3 September 2022).
27. Grove, T.M. Academic Library Video Services: Charting a Post-COVID Course. *PA Libr. Res. Pract.* **2021**, *9*, 101–110. [CrossRef]

28. Handler, S. Libraries, Publishers Battle over Terms for E-Books' Use. Bloomberg Law. 2022. Available online: https://news.bloomberglaw.com/ip-law/libraries-publishers-battle-over-terms-for-e-books-public-use (accessed on 5 September 2022).
29. Towery, S.; Price, A.N.; Cowen, K.E. Video Streaming Licenses: Using a Decision Tree and Workflow Chart. *J. Copyr. Educ. Librariansh.* **2019**, *3*, 7483. [CrossRef]
30. JSTOR. Expanded Access to Jstor during COVID-19 Crisis. 2020. Available online: https://about.jstor.org/news/expanded-access-to-jstor-during-covid-19-crisis/ (accessed on 14 September 2022).
31. Penrod, J. Staying Relevant: The Importance of Incorporating Hyflex Learning into Higher Education Strategy, 2022. EDUCAUSE Review. Available online: https://er.educause.edu/articles/2022/3/staying-relevant-the-importance-of-incorporating-hyflex-learning-into-higher-education-strategy (accessed on 14 September 2022).
32. Pang, A. 5 Emerging Technology Trends Higher Ed Is Watching for in 2022, 2022. EdTech: Focus on Higher Education. Available online: https://edtechmagazine.com/higher/article/2021/12/5-emerging-technology-trends-higher-ed-watching-2022 (accessed on 20 September 2022).
33. Radford, M.L.; Costello, L.; Montague, K. Surging Virtual Reference Services: COVID-19 a Game Changer. *Coll. Res. Libr. News* **2021**, *82*, 106. [CrossRef]
34. Hosoi, M.; Reiter, L.; Zabel, D. Reshaping Perspectives on Flexible Work: The Impact of COVID-19 on Academic Library Management. *Portal Libr. Acad.* **2021**, *21*, 695–713. [CrossRef]
35. Reynolds, B.W. The Mental Health Benefits of Remote and Flexible Work. Mental Health America. Available online: https://mhanational.org/blog/mental-health-benefits-remote-and-flexible-work (accessed on 11 October 2022).
36. Picchi, A. "Quiet Quitting": A Revolution in How We Work or the End of Working Hard? 2022. CBS News. Available online: https://www.cbsnews.com/news/what-is-quiet-quitting/ (accessed on 7 October 2022).
37. Bontrager, M.; Clinton, M.S.; Tyner, L. Flexible Work Arrangements: A Human Resource Development Tool to Reduce Turnover. *Adv. Dev. Hum. Resour.* **2021**, *23*, 124–141. [CrossRef]

encyclopedia MDPI

Entry

Gross Pathology in COVID-19

Bei Zhang

Department of Pathology and Laboratory Medicine, The Robert Larner, M.D. College of Medicine at University of Vermont, Burlington, VT 05405, USA; bei.zhang@med.uvm.edu

Definition: The global infectious disease COVID-19 is caused by SARS-CoV-2, a new member of the Coronaviridae family. Though presented as a novel disease that primarily affects the respiratory system, multi-organ involvement has been well-noticed and documented since the beginning of the pandemic. When performed properly with adequate safety measures, autopsy provides the most valuable information to decipher the pathogenesis of this novel disease, therefore providing a basis for clinical management. In addition to reviewing the macroscopic changes in organs and tissues involved in COVID-19, the relevant microscopic alterations and possible pathogenesis are also discussed.

Keywords: COVID-19; SARS-CoV-2; gross pathology; autopsy; post-mortem

Citation: Zhang, B. Gross Pathology in COVID-19. *Encyclopedia* **2022**, *2*, 1790–1802. https://doi.org/10.3390/encyclopedia2040123

Academic Editors: Stephen Bustin and Raffaele Barretta

Received: 12 August 2022
Accepted: 26 October 2022
Published: 28 October 2022

1. Introduction

Coronavirus disease (COVID-19), a novel seventh coronavirus disease, initially broke out in Wuhan, China, in December 2019 [1]. It quickly spread worldwide and became a pandemic, as declared by the World Health Organization in March 2020 [2]. As of Friday, 22 July 2022, more than 567 million have been affected, with more than 6.38 million deaths all over the world [3]. The unprecedented public health threat and the gravity of the situation have inevitably overwhelmed the healthcare system of many countries and created much turmoil and emerging challenges in many aspects of human life [4]. Social distancing has been used worldwide to limit the spread of the virus [5]. COVID-19 and its causative agent, severe acute respiratory syndrome coronavirus 2 (SARS-CoV-2), have been studied extensively.

The Coronaviridae family viruses are enveloped, positive-sense, single-stranded RNA viruses [6]. Previously, six coronaviruses have been identified to cause human diseases. Two of them, severe acute respiratory syndrome coronavirus (SARS-CoV) and Middle East respiratory syndrome coronavirus (MERS-CoV), can cause severe respiratory illness with fatality rates of 10% and 40%, respectively. In contrast, the other four usually cause mild upper respiratory diseases similar to the common flu [7,8].

SARS-CoV-2 is transmitted via inhalation or direct contact of the virus with the mucous membrane [9]. Like SARS-CoV, SARS-CoV-2 also binds to the angiotensin-converting enzyme 2 (ACE2) receptor primarily present on the surface of the alveolar epithelial cells in the lung, resulting in respiratory symptoms [7]. ACE2 is also found in the small intestinal epithelium, endothelial cells of blood vessels, alveolar macrophage and monocyte, and epithelial cells of trachea and bronchi, which may explain the multiple organ involvement in COVID-19 [7]. The virus contains four structural proteins: spike (S), envelope (E), membrane glycoprotein (M), and nucleocapsid phosphoprotein (N). The virus enters the cell via the interaction between the viral spike (S) protein and the host cell proteases, TMPRSS2 [10].

Like other coronaviruses, SARS-CoV-2 continuously develops mutations. Since the global outbreak, five major variants of concern (VOC) with increased transmissibility, varied virulence, evasion from therapeutic drugs, or decreased effectiveness of vaccines have been reported after the ancestral one. Those VOCs are alpha (B.1.1.7), beta (B.1.351), gamma (P.1), delta (B.1.617.2), and omicron (B.1.1.529) [11]. Selective pressures such as the use of monoclonal antibodies further drive the evolution of SARS-CoV-2, especially in immunocompromised patients [12].

Though often present as a mild disease with typical flu-like symptoms such as fever, cough, myalgia, or fatigue [13], about 19%, however, develop severe to critical disease that may result in progressive respiratory failure, presumably due to massive alveolar damage [5]. Deceased patients present with severe pneumonitis and advance to acute respiratory distress syndrome, often accompanied by multi-organ failure [14], which may be contributed by severe endothelial damage, disseminated intravascular coagulation, and a cytokine storm [15,16]. The severity and prognosis of the disease seem to be associated with age; gender; blood group A; cigarette smoking; obesity; and a variety of comorbidities, including coronary artery disease, diabetes mellitus, chronic kidney disease, hypertension, congestive heart failure, and chronic obstructive pulmonary disease [14,17]. Most fatal cases have significant underlying diseases, with systemic hypertension and diabetes mellitus being the most common [18]. Besides the comorbidities listed above, HIV infection and tuberculosis are common among COVID-19 decedents in Africa [19].

The complexity of COVID-19 has been made well aware of since its outbreak. It is a multiorgan disease that presents with a broad spectrum of clinical manifestations and a wide range of degrees of severity [13,14,20]. For example, autopsies have revealed the systemic multiorgan involvement of vessels in the lungs, heart, kidney, liver, GI tract, kidney, brain, and skin [21]. Gross examination of involved organs obtained from autopsy provides valuable information, which is imperative for elucidating the pathogenesis of COVID-19 and laying out the basis for clinical management.

2. COVID-19 Autopsy

The importance of autopsy in deciphering the pathogenesis of a novel disease such as COVID-19 is undisputable [22]. It is one of the primary ways to access organs to perform gross examinations.

Initially, autopsies on deceased COVID-19 patients were scarce due to significant concerns, such as the risk of contagiousness, lack of healthcare specialists, and the abrupt outbreak of the disease [23]. The autopsy of COVID-19 patients is limited mainly due to strict biosafety measures and infection control over specimen collection and handling. Because of this, there was a minimal number of publications on postmortem findings in COVID-19 [24,25].

SARS-CoV-2 presents particular hazards to the professionals working in the lab or clinical settings [26,27]. Exposure risk levels of autopsies and specimen handling from deceased COVID-19 patients are considered "very high" [28]. Therefore, implementing strict security measures to manage the diseased from COVID-19 is essential in protecting healthcare professionals and family members, decreasing the risk of exposure, and preventing infection expansion [29]. Based on previous guidelines for working with SARS-CoV and MERS-CoV, the WHO and the CDC released postmortem guidance regarding COVID-19 [30]. The College of American Pathologists (CAP) endorsed the postmortem guidance from the CDC about specimen collection and handling involving confirmed or suspected COVID-19 [31]. Such administrative support and biosafety guidelines have promoted autopsy in COVID-19, which helps tremendously in gaining better knowledge about this new and complex infectious disease. It is essential that each lab access the risk, follow the protocol, and abide by the rules for biosafety practice.

After obtaining informed consent from the patient's next of kin, an autopsy of COVID-19 should be performed in an autopsy suite that is adequately equipped. The essentials include an appropriately functioning ventilation system capable of six complete air exchanges in an hour with negative pressure and HEPA filters [8,32]. Airborne Infection Isolation Rooms (AIIRs) are recommended by the CDC when conducting autopsies of COVID-19 patients [30]. The number of personnel in the autopsy room should be minimized, and aerosol formation should be avoided as much as possible. Essential personal protective equipment

(PPE) includes a fluid-resistant gown and apron, double gloves with cut-proofing, a surgical cap, face shields or goggles, boots or overshoes, and an N95 respirator face mask or equivalent [29,33]. Whole-body suits with individual respirators are not necessary [27].

Before the autopsy investigation and during the external examination, nasopharyngeal and oropharyngeal swabs are collected for diagnostic or virological research [34]. Each involved organ system is explored by following standard operating procedures. For example, the "en bloc" extraction technique can be used to obtain the respiratory block, including the tongue, hypopharynx, larynx, trachea, bronchi, and lungs [34]. Intro-autopsy swabs can then be collected from the removed and opened respiratory block [34]. A thorough examination of the brain is performed by adopting the protocol for Creutzfeldt-Jakob Disease brain autopsies [35]. Representative tissue samples obtained from the involved organs are first fixed in formalin for 24–48 h or even 72 h to inactivate the virus and then processed for histology examination sectioning and examination [33,35,36]. A new set of tools are used for each organ to avoid cross-contamination. Diagnostic testing for COVID-19 is performed by real-time reverse transcriptase PCR using swabs taken from the trachea, lung parenchyma, pericardium, pleural cavity, etc. [33].

Though creating critical challenges in the autopsy as a novel infectious disease for many institutions and clinics, autopsies for COVID-19 can be performed routinely by adequately trained personnel who carefully adhere to the most updated safety guidelines. As the pandemic evolves, more and more postmortem examinations have been performed to elaborately study the macroscopic changes in the multiple organs affected by the virus, aiming to elucidate the pathogenesis of the disease and the exact cause of death.

Multiple autopsy clinics have established a new biobanking model with shared and centralized biomaterial and data management. Such established autopsy networks provide high-quality biosample collection, data analysis and reports to support disease-related research, health policymaking, and public discussion [37]. By promoting communication and collaboration across different institutions, autopsy and an accompanied centralized model of biobanking have significantly increased the systemic understanding of COVID-19, which set up a successful model for studying other infectious diseases as well [37].

When safety regulations are too stringent to meet or the fear of contraction is too big to overcome, postmortem biopsies can be an acceptable and reasonable alternative, providing significant histopathological findings [38].

3. Pulmonary Findings in COVID-19

The respiratory tract is the primary target of SARS-CoV-2, with acute respiratory distress syndrome (ARDS) being the most common cause of death [18].

In general and grossly, the lungs are heavier due to edema, congestion is notable, and consolidation or hemorrhage may or may not be present (Figure 1). Microscopically, it is featured as diffuse alveolar damage (DAD) of the acute or organizing phases or a mixture of both [18]. ARDS/DAD has been the number one immediate cause of death in COVID-19, followed by multi-organ failure and bacterial pulmonary superinfection [39]. The pathological changes in the lung are varied depending on the stages and duration of the disease and the severity of the pulmonary damage.

Significant generalized pulmonary edema can be present at the early stage. The lungs weigh heavier than usual. Consistency of the lower lobes is slightly increased, with capillary endotheliitis infiltrated by neutrophils. Microthrombi formation in alveolar capillaries and small pulmonary vessels are seen microscopically. Inflammatory exudates with neutrophils, multinucleated giant cells, and scanty hyaline membranes are observed as well, but no focal changes are macroscopically visible, except the cutting surface is slightly sticky [36].

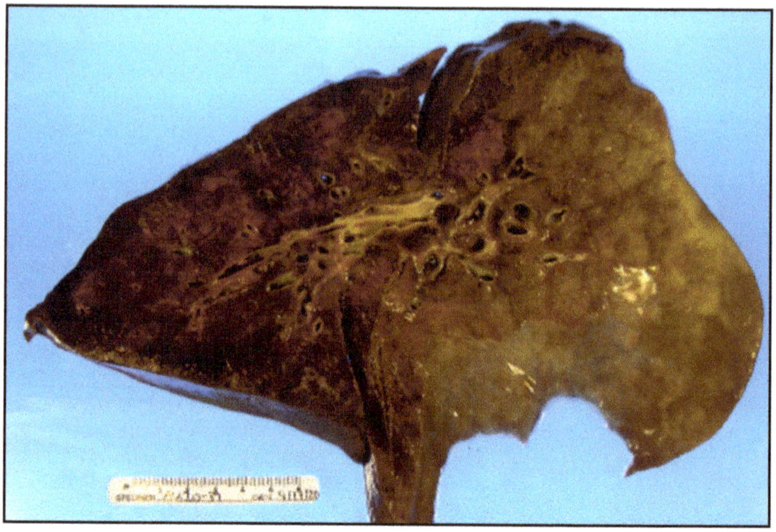

Figure 1. A heavy lung from a deceased COVID-19 patient with patchy consolidation and hemorrhage. Figure courtesy of Dr. Sharon Mount from the University of Vermont Medical Center.

As the disease progresses, pulmonary edema becomes more remarkable, and consolidation occurs at both lower lobes. Thrombi are visible in small to medium-sized pulmonary arteries and veins at the cutting surface. The affected part changes color to dark red and is consolidated without air, suggesting lobar pneumonia [33]. Focal changes around thrombi include hemorrhage (petechial), consolidation, and fresh infarction indicated by discoloration. Accompanied histological changes demonstrate diffuse alveolar damage with fibrin deposition, fibromyxoid exudates, hyaline membrane, and an increased number of macrophages within the alveoli [33,36].

Consolidation expands to the upper and lower lobes of the lungs as the disease progresses. Both the size and the weight of the lungs increase significantly. The accompanied histological changes are consistent with prolonged ARDS featured by extensive epithelium hyperplasia and focal squamous metaplasia. Concentrically arranged fibroblasts and central accumulation of inflammatory cells inside the alveoli are seen at the organizing stage [36]. Hyperplasia and shedding of type II pneumocytes are quite notable [33].

Without medical treatment, the onset of severe acute lung injury can be very rapid, with all lobes affected equally. The cross-section reveals edema, diffused firm, and rubbery parenchyma without any mass. The parenchyma is colored from pale pink to dark with scattered hemorrhagic areas that are not well-defined. The bronchi are filled with frothy proteinaceous exudates. The corresponding microscopic findings are consistent with the early exudative phase of acute lung injury featured by hyaline membrane formation and hyperplasia of type II pneumocytes with atypical changes [40]. Lymphocytic infiltration is consistent with viral pneumonia [33].

The pleural is slightly thickened with decreased effusion [41]. Purulent sputum and pleural effusion with turbid fluid can be seen in the pleural cavity. Fibrinous exudate can be found over the visceral pleura in some cases [33].

Neither redness nor erosion is seen at the trachea and bronchi, but reactive and atypical epithelium changes are observed microscopically [40]. Frothy secretions of gray-white colored viscous fluid are prevalent in the airways, including the larynx, with or without mucous plugging [40,42]. Superimposed bronchopneumonia can present due to bacterial or fungal infection and has been found in a significant number of cases that are most likely bacterial-related [43,44]. It can be focal or diffused. Tracheitis has been reported [45]. Such findings are not surprising considering the expression of ACE-2 receptors at the upper respiratory tract [46].

Hilar lymph nodes are enlarged, with the gross section surface varying from white to black [40]. Mediastinal lymph nodes can be enlarged, too [47].

4. Cardiovascular Findings in COVID-19

Cardiovascular co-morbidities are common in COVID-19 [48]. The multiple cardiovascular complications worsened or induced by SARS-CoV-2 include myocardial infarction (MI), myocarditis, acute coronary syndromes, arrhythmias, heart failure, cardiogenic shock, and sudden cardiac death [49]. Myocardial injury indicated by an increased level of troponin I is a common finding in COVID-19 patients [50,51]. A significant number of deaths are attributed to heart failure induced by COVID-19 without previous cardiovascular disease history [52]. The diversified cardiovascular consequences are caused by infiltration of inflammatory cells due to viral attack, the release of a large variety of pro-inflammatory cytokines, and micro-thrombosis due to endothelial damage [50]. Hypoxia caused by ARDS also contributes significantly to heart failure [14].

The gross weight of the infected heart can be normal but is mostly increased due to hypertrophy, edema, and chamber dilation [53,54]. The thickness of the myocardial wall is usually normal or slightly below normal [53]. The myocardium can have a firm texture and shows a red-brown color [47,55]. Intracardiac and coronary thrombosis is the most petrifying finding, with thrombin rich in platelets, fibrin, and neutrophil extracellular traps found in the chambers, coronary arteries, or veins [53,56]. In general, the three primary gross pathological findings are myocardial ischemia, thrombosis, and cardiac dilation, especially at the right heart [53]. Myocardial fibrosis, the end stage of cardiac injury, is found in about 25% of cases [53]. Senile amyloidosis is found in some cases [45]. The virus has been detected in the myocardium in about half of the cases without necessarily all resulting in myocarditis [51]. Myocarditis is much less frequently reported than expected, which turns out to be a rare sequela of certain cohort studies [18]. Pericardial effusion has been found in some COVID-19 patients who died from cardiogenic shock. Pericarditis has also been reported [57]. It is important to note that many postmortem findings in the hearts of COVID-19 patients are consequences of pre-existing chronic conditions. In the absence of ARDS/DAD or COVID-19 pneumonia, SARS-CoV-2 is most likely a contributing rather than a direct cause of death [18].

Vascular injury has been consistently reported in deceased COVID-19 patients [58]. Endotheliitis has been reported in multiple organs, including the heart, kidney, small bowel, and lungs, which could be caused by either the host's inflammatory response or direct infection by the virus [59]. COVID-19 patients are prone to develop arterial, venous, and microvascular thrombosis, with pulmonary arterial thrombosis being the most common pattern in post-mortem studies [60,61]. The combination of diffused alveolar damage and thrombosis contributes to the rapid deterioration of severe COVID-19 cases. Thrombosis has been observed in small and medium-sized pulmonary arteries, even with prophylactic anticoagulant therapy, indicating profound coagulopathy [36] (Figure 2). Deep venous thrombosis (DVT) is found in a significant number of COVID-19 patients [62,63]. Cerebral DVT leads to encephalopathy [64]. Other systemic thromboses reported include thrombosis at the ophthalmic artery, femoral artery, portal vein, and superior mesenteric artery [61,65]. The COVID-19 thrombi are more likely to occur at the small peripheral blood vessels such as capillaries or arterioles and to consist of fibrin and platelets [66]. Damage or damage-associated molecular patterns caused by invasion of the endothelial cell of the virus, including the release of cytokines, activation of leukocytes, platelets, and completement, are thought to be contributors to the hyper coagulated state of COVID-19 [61].

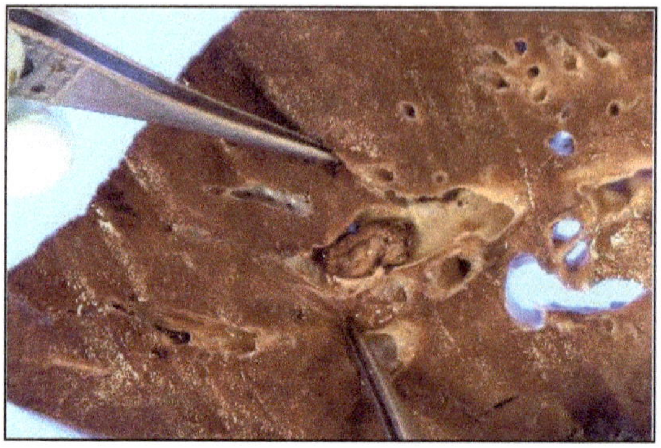

Figure 2. A thromboembolus at the right lower lobe of the lung of a deceased COVID-19 patient. Figure courtesy of Dr. Sharon Mount from the University of Vermont Medical Center.

5. Other Gross Pathological Findings in COVID-19

As the leading mortality cause of severe COVID-19, ARDS/CAD is not specific but seen in various direct or indirect lung injuries, including other respiratory viral infections. However, the disproportional hypoxia to radiographic abnormalities and multi-organ failure distinguish severe COVID-19 from other respiratory infectious diseases that end with ARDS/CAD [66]. Such a hallmark of COVID-19 is attributed to systemic endothelitis that disturbs the anti-coagulatory property of endothelium. This also explains why patients with certain pre-existing conditions are more likely to progress to severe COVID-19. All those conditions, including old age, hypertension, diabetes, and obesity, share one thing in common: altered endothelial metabolism [67]. A cytokine release syndrome induced by severe inflammation contributes to the adverse course of COVID-19 and multiple organ damage. The severity of the disease can be directly linked to the dramatic rise of a specific subset of cytokines, including IL-6, associated with mortality [68]. It is important to note that increased levels of specific cytokines are also predictable for mild COVID-19, for example, CCL17 [69]. The released pro-inflammatory cytokines trigger the capillary leaking syndrome, leading to disseminated intravascular coagulation (DIC) [70]. Local overactivation of completement is another important factor to consider in regarding organ damage, especially the lungs and kidneys [71]. RT-PCR has demonstrated invasion of SARS-CoV-2 at multiple organ systems besides the respiratory and cardiovascular systems [66,72–74]. The virus makes its way into those organs by binding the ACE2 receptors or through the blood circulation [7,13]. NRP-1 receptor has been reported to potentiate SARS-CoV-2 entry into the cell [75].

Renal complications are common and associated with a high mortality rate of COVID-19 [76]. Renal signs of shock are seen grossly in most autopsies [45]. Clinical manifestations range from mild proteinuria to acute kidney injury (AKI), most subclinical and AKI seen in severe cases [77]. Besides the mechanisms mentioned earlier of organ damage caused by SAR-CoV-2, disturbance of the renin-angiotensin-aldosterone (RAAS) regulation system is another critical detrimental factor. The binding of the virus to its receptor ACE2 downregulates the enzymatic activity of ACE2, which catalyzes the production of angiotensins that are cardio/renal protective [78]. Acute infarction and cortical necrosis have been reported [59,79]. The pitting and coarseness of the renal capsule, representing the arterionephrosclerosis observed microscopically, is typically seen in comorbidities such as hypertension and diabetes. Intrinsic acute kidney injury (AKI) is thought to be the most common form of AKI in COVID-19 patients, as evidenced by histopathological findings including acute tubular necrosis, loss of luminal brush border, eosinophilic hyaline casts, detached tubular epithelial cells, microthrombi, and fibrosis at the interstitium without glomerular injury and lymphocyte infiltration [74]. Small fibrin thrombi of the glomeruli indicate early signs of DIC [41]. Other reported genitourinary system pathological findings include prostate vein thrombosis, testicular atrophy, or testicular parenchyma damage [66].

The neurological and psychiatric symptoms presented by the COVID-19 patients suggest the involvement of both the central and peripheral nervous systems. The invasion of the central nervous system occurs via the route of the blood or nerves, with the aid of the deteriorated blood–brain barrier by the cytokine storm, whereas the infection at the peripheral nervous system is most likely immune-mediated [80]. The spectrum of neurological manifestations includes the more specific ones, such as anosmia and hypogeusia, and the nonspecific ones such as fatigue, headache, dizziness, and nausea [73,81]. The most frequently reported gross anomalies in the brain are ischemia, hemorrhage, and edema [73]. The neurons that execute cognitive functions seem more likely to be affected [82]. Microglial activation has been observed in many studies [80]; other abnormal histological findings such as microthrombi [83], brain stem encephalitis [72], and myelin loss are also reported [84]. Neurosensory skin system involvement has been evidenced by more and more reported cutaneous neurosensory symptoms. Burning pain or itching sensations start proximally in a diffused pattern irrespective of dermatomes. The affected skin area is erythematous with red-purple color. Histological examinations demonstrate hypertrophic nerve fibers without inflammation [85].

Gastrointestinal symptoms are common and can be the only manifestation, leading to delayed diagnosis of COVID-19. The symptoms are nonspecific, with loss of appetite and diarrhea being the most common [86]. Multiple punctate hemorrhages in the mucosa of the stomach and duodenum have been reported [41]. Acute mesenteric ischemia (AMI) is a rare but life-threatening emergent thrombotic complication of COVID-19 caused by arterial or venous thrombosis [87,88]. Exploratory laparotomy reveals the superior mesenteric artery without pulse and the gangrenous small intestine [89]. Thrombosis can occur at the portal or mesenteric veins as well [90].

Abnormal liver function is common in COVID-19 patients, especially in older and/or severe cases. The factors causing liver damage include direct attack by the virus, cytokine storm, hypoxia, and hepatotoxic drugs [91]. The compromised liver function indicated by elevated levels of liver enzymes can be persistent and chronic, with males being more susceptible to it [92]. Steatosis is the most common hepatic finding in COVID-19 autopsy. The liver is larger with fatty changes consistent with the common comorbidities of COVID-19, such as hypertension, obesity, and diabetes [54]. Ischemic and necrotic changes in the liver have been reported. Acute portal thrombosis secondary to COVID-19 has turned out not to be a rare case [65]. The hepatic sinus may become congested and dark red due to micro thrombosis [92]. The damaged liver can profoundly affect other organ systems and interfere with anti-viral treatment. For example, the skin color becomes darker in rare cases of COVID-19 due to adrenocortical insufficiency caused by decreased inactivation of estrogen by the liver [92].

Significantly increased incidence of type I diabetes mellitus during the pandemic calls for attention to the involvement of the pancreas in COVID-19 [93]. The rapid postmortem autolysis of the pancreas makes it quite a challenge to study it in much detail from autopsy, and gross examinations have not reported any severe injuries [80], but decreased insulin production and glucose-stimulated secretion after SARS-CoV-2 infection have been discovered [94].

Dysregulated immune responses and the typical peripheral lymphopenia in severe COVID-19 indicates the involvement of lymphoid organs [80]. The spleen can be impaired in COVID-19 by direct viral assault, cytokine storm, thrombosis, or lymphocyte apoptosis [95]. The spleen may serve as the reservoir of SARS-CoV-2, which may account for the recurrence of COVID-19 [96]. Grossly, the spleen is contracted by the shrinking capsule. Infarction, thrombi, and hemorrhage are common findings [97]. Several cases of spontaneous splenic rupture related to COVID-19 have been reported. The lacerations can be multiple, accompanied by hemorrhage or hematoma, necrosis, and blood clots [98]. Microscopically, neutrophil infiltration in the red pulp, necrosis, reduction in lymphoid follicles, and white pulp atrophy have been observed. Arterial thrombosis and fibrous tissue proliferation at the sinus are the common causes of spleen infarction. Persistent depletion of IgM memory B cells is associated with a higher mortality rate and increased risk of superimposed bacterial infections [38,95]. Mediastinal lymphadenopathy has been detected in hospitalized patients and, more often, in severe COVID-19 [99]. Enlarged intrathoracic lymph nodes were found in autopsy [97]. Characteristic lymph node changes include edema, capillary congestion, and hemorrhage. Histopathological alterations are manifested by disrupted boundaries between follicles and paracortical zones, focal necrosis and apoptosis, and reduction in or atrophy of lymphoid follicles and white pulp [97,99]. Blockage of lymphatic vessels by fibrin blots has been reported, indicating the coagulopathies associated with COVID-19 are not limited to blood vasculature [100].

In severe cases, cardiomegaly, liver damage, intestinal mucositis, and hemorrhage can be present altogether, besides respiratory symptoms [36]. Multiple organ failures are observed in many patients and may be contributed by the pro-inflammatory cytokine storm involving a variety of ILs, interferon-gamma, and activated macrophages [15,36].

6. Conclusions

- COVID-19 can be a multi-organ systemic disease. COVID-19 has often been considered a respiratory viral disease, yet it is clear that SARS-CoV-2 affects multiple extrapulmonary organs besides the lungs. It can spread systemically, which may explain the lingering symptoms of long-COVID. The complexity of COVID-19 has been made aware of as the pandemic evolved. The virus has been found in macrophages, monocytes, and endothelial cells at multiple blood–physiology barriers [101]. The mechanism of organ injury includes direct viral attack, hypoxia, and inflammatory response secondary to viral infection.
- The sequelae of COVID-19 can be highly individualized. Pathological studies have revealed that pre-existing conditions play critical roles in the clinical course of COVID-19. The most common comorbidities include systemic hypertension, diabetes, obesity, and coronary artery disease [18].
- The pathogenesis of long-COVID is still under investigation. It takes a varied length of time to recover from COVID-19 infection. A significant number of patients reported lasting symptoms over twelve weeks after acute infection, known as long-COVID, "long haulers", or long-COVID syndrome [102]. The occurrence of long-COVID is not necessarily directly related to the severity of the initial disease [103]. The constellation of the symptoms such as fatigue, muscle weakness, dyspnea, pain, discomfort, etc. indicates the involvement of multiple organ systems and can significantly affect the quality of the patient's life. The evolution of long-COVID can be attributed to either direct viral attacks or the outcomes of viral attacks, including inflammation and oxidative stress [104].
- Testing for a broader group of potential causative agents is necessary for acute diagnosis and appropriate patient management. The respiratory distress and the gross pathological changes observed in COVID-19 are not specific. Complete pathological examination using ancillary tools such as cytology, electron microscopy, and other tissue techniques are beneficial for making an accurate diagnosis, differentiation from other coronavirus infections, and deepening our understanding of the pathogenesis of COVID-19 as a newly emerging disorder.

Funding: This research received no external funding.

Data Availability Statement: All references used in this review can be found at PubMed.

Acknowledgments: I greatly appreciate Sharon Mount's advice in preparing the paper and providing two autopsy photos.

Conflicts of Interest: The authors declare no conflict of interest.

References

1. Zavascki, A.P.; Falci, D.R. Clinical Characteristics of COVID-19 in China. *N. Engl. J. Med.* **2020**, *382*, 1859. [CrossRef] [PubMed]
2. Mahase, E. COVID-19: WHO declares pandemic because of "alarming levels" of spread, severity, and inaction. *BMJ* **2020**, *368*, m1036. [CrossRef] [PubMed]
3. JHU. COVID-19 Dashboard. Available online: https://coronavirus.jhu.edu/map.html (accessed on 31 May 2021).
4. Beneke, R.; Leithäuser, R.M. COVID-19: Impact of a "Global Player"-A Reflection 1 Year On. *Int. J. Sports Physiol. Perform* **2021**, *16*, 323–324. [CrossRef] [PubMed]
5. Hassan, S.A.; Sheikh, F.N.; Jamal, S.; Ezeh, J.K.; Akhtar, A. Coronavirus (COVID-19): A Review of Clinical Features, Diagnosis, and Treatment. *Cureus* **2020**, *12*, e7355. [CrossRef] [PubMed]
6. Lu, G.; Liu, D. SARS-like virus in the Middle East: A truly bat-related coronavirus causing human diseases. *Protein Cell* **2012**, *3*, 803–805. [CrossRef] [PubMed]
7. Lin, P.; Wang, M.; Wei, Y.; Kim, T.; Wei, X. Coronavirus in human diseases: Mechanisms and advances in clinical treatment. *MedComm* **2020**, *1*, 270–301. [CrossRef]
8. Calabrese, F.; Pezzuto, F.; Fortarezza, F.; Hofman, P.; Kern, I.; Panizo, A.; von der Thüsen, J.; Timofeev, S.; Gorkiewicz, G.; Lunardi, F. Pulmonary pathology and COVID-19: Lessons from autopsy. The experience of European Pulmonary Pathologists. *Virchows Arch.* **2020**, *477*, 359–372. [CrossRef]
9. (CDC). Centers for Disease Control and Prevent. Scientific Brief: SARS-CoV-2 Transmission. Available online: https://www.cdc.gov/coronavirus/2019-ncov/science/science-briefs/sars-cov-2-transmission.html?CDC_AA_refVal=https%3A%2F%2Fwww.cdc.gov%2Fcoronavirus%2F2019-ncov%2Fscience%2Fscience-briefs%2Fscientific-brief-sars-cov-2.html#anchor_1619805167515 (accessed on 22 May 2021).
10. Marsh, M.; Helenius, A. Virus entry: Open sesame. *Cell* **2006**, *124*, 729–740. [CrossRef]
11. WHO. Tracking SARS-CoV-2 variants. Available online: https://www.who.int/en/activities/tracking-SARS-CoV-2-variants (accessed on 26 July 2022).
12. Scherer, E.M.; Babiker, A.; Adelman, M.W.; Allman, B.; Key, A.; Kleinhenz, J.M.; Langsjoen, R.M.; Nguyen, P.V.; Onyechi, I.; Sherman, J.D.; et al. SARS-CoV-2 Evolution and Immune Escape in Immunocompromised Patients. *N. Engl. J. Med.* **2022**, *386*, 2436–2438. [CrossRef]
13. Huang, C.; Wang, Y.; Li, X.; Ren, L.; Zhao, J.; Hu, Y.; Zhang, L.; Fan, G.; Xu, J.; Gu, X.; et al. Clinical features of patients infected with 2019 novel coronavirus in Wuhan, China. *Lancet* **2020**, *395*, 497–506. [CrossRef]
14. Zhou, F.; Yu, T.; Du, R.; Fan, G.; Liu, Y.; Liu, Z.; Xiang, J.; Wang, Y.; Song, B.; Gu, X.; et al. Clinical course and risk factors for mortality of adult inpatients with COVID-19 in Wuhan, China: A retrospective cohort study. *Lancet* **2020**, *395*, 1054–1062. [CrossRef]
15. Li, H.; Liu, L.; Zhang, D.; Xu, J.; Dai, H.; Tang, N.; Su, X.; Cao, B. SARS-CoV-2 and viral sepsis: Observations and hypotheses. *Lancet* **2020**, *395*, 1517–1520. [CrossRef]
16. Stasi, A.; Castellano, G.; Ranieri, E.; Infante, B.; Stallone, G.; Gesualdo, L.; Netti, G.S. SARS-CoV-2 and Viral Sepsis: Immune Dysfunction and Implications in Kidney Failure. *J. Clin. Med.* **2020**, *9*, 4057. [CrossRef] [PubMed]
17. Al-Ansari, R.Y.; Alshaer, A.; Al-Anazi, A.; Al-Otaibi, N.; Abdalla, L.; Al-Tarrah, S.; Shilash, A.; Al-Zahrani, N. ABO in Correlation to the Requirement of Mechanical Ventilation and Mortality in Critically Ill Patients With COVID-19. *J. Hematol.* **2021**, *10*, 64–70. [CrossRef]
18. Hooper, J.E.; Padera, R.F.; Dolhnikoff, M.; da Silva, L.F.F.; Duarte-Neto, A.N.; Kapp, M.E.; Lacy, J.M.; Mauad, T.; Saldiva, P.H.N.; Rapkiewicz, A.V.; et al. A Postmortem Portrait of the Coronavirus Disease 2019 (COVID-19) Pandemic: A Large Multi-institutional Autopsy Survey Study. *Arch. Pathol. Lab. Med.* **2021**, *145*, 529–535. [CrossRef]
19. Himwaze, C.M.; Telendiy, V.; Maate, F.; Songwe, M.; Chanda, C.; Chanda, D.; Julius, P.; Mumba, C.; Marimo, C.; Hamukale, A.; et al. Post Mortem examination of Hospital Inpatient COVID-19 Deaths in Lusaka, Zambia—A Descriptive Whole Body Autopsy Series. *Int. J. Infect. Dis.* **2021**, *108*, 363–369. [CrossRef]
20. Weiss, P.; Murdoch, D.R. Clinical course and mortality risk of severe COVID-19. *Lancet* **2020**, *395*, 1014–1015. [CrossRef]
21. Xu, Z.; Shi, L.; Wang, Y.; Zhang, J.; Huang, L.; Zhang, C.; Liu, S.; Zhao, P.; Liu, H.; Zhu, L.; et al. Pathological findings of COVID-19 associated with acute respiratory distress syndrome. *Lancet Respir. Med.* **2020**, *8*, 420–422. [CrossRef]
22. Sperhake, J.P. Autopsies of COVID-19 deceased? Absolutely! *Leg. Med.* **2020**, *47*, 101769. [CrossRef]
23. Sapino, A.; Facchetti, F.; Bonoldi, E.; Gianatti, A.; Barbareschi, M.; SIAPEC. The autopsy debate during the COVID-19 emergency: The Italian experience. *Virchows Arch.* **2020**, *476*, 821–823. [CrossRef]
24. Barton, L.M.; Duval, E.J.; Stroberg, E.; Ghosh, S.; Mukhopadhyay, S. COVID-19 Autopsies, Oklahoma, USA. *Am. J. Clin. Pathol.* **2020**, *153*, 725–733. [CrossRef]
25. Wichmann, D.; Sperhake, J.P.; Lütgehetmann, M.; Steurer, S.; Edler, C.; Heinemann, A.; Heinrich, F.; Mushumba, H.; Kniep, I.; Schröder, A.S.; et al. Autopsy Findings and Venous Thromboembolism in Patients With COVID-19: A Prospective Cohort Study. *Ann. Intern. Med.* **2020**, *173*, 268–277. [CrossRef] [PubMed]
26. Kaufer, A.M.; Theis, T.; Lau, K.A.; Gray, J.L.; Rawlinson, W.D. Laboratory biosafety measures involving SARS-CoV-2 and the classification as a Risk Group 3 biological agent. *Pathology* **2020**, *52*, 790–795. [CrossRef] [PubMed]
27. Hanley, B.; Lucas, S.B.; Youd, E.; Swift, B.; Osborn, M. Autopsy in suspected COVID-19 cases. *J. Clin. Pathol.* **2020**, *73*, 239–242. [CrossRef] [PubMed]

28. OSHA. Postmortem Care Workers and Employers. Available online: https://www.osha.gov/coronavirus/control-prevention/postmortem-care (accessed on 20 May 2021).
29. Baj, J.; Ciesielka, M.; Buszewicz, G.; Maciejewski, R.; Budzyńska, B.; Listos, P.; Teresiński, G. COVID-19 in the autopsy room-requirements, safety, recommendations and pathological findings. *Forensic Sci. Med. Pathol.* **2021**, *17*, 101–113. [CrossRef]
30. CDC. Collection and Submission of Postmortem Specimens from Deceased Persons with Confirmed or Suspected COVID-19. Available online: https://www.cdc.gov/coronavirus/2019-ncov/hcp/guidance-postmortem-specimens.html (accessed on 20 May 2021).
31. CAP. Amended COVID-19 Autopsy Guideline Statement from the CAP Autopsy Committee. Available online: https://documents.cap.org/documents/COVID-Autopsy-Statement.pdf (accessed on 20 May 2021).
32. Basso, C.; Calabrese, F.; Sbaraglia, M.; Del Vecchio, C.; Carretta, G.; Saieva, A.; Donato, D.; Flor, L.; Crisanti, A.; Dei Tos, A.P. Feasibility of postmortem examination in the era of COVID-19 pandemic: The experience of a Northeast Italy University Hospital. *Virchows Arch.* **2020**, *477*, 341–347. [CrossRef]
33. Youd, E.; Moore, L. COVID-19 autopsy in people who died in community settings: The first series. *J. Clin. Pathol.* **2020**, *73*, 840–844. [CrossRef]
34. Santurro, A.; Scopetti, M.; D'Errico, S.; Fineschi, V. A technical report from the Italian SARS-CoV-2 outbreak. Postmortem sampling and autopsy investigation in cases of suspected or probable COVID-19. *Forensic Sci. Med. Pathol.* **2020**, *16*, 471–476. [CrossRef]
35. Fu, L.; Zak, T.; Shanes, E. A Framework for Maintaining a Fully Operational Autopsy Service at a Large Academic Teaching Institution During a Global Pandemic. *Acad. Pathol.* **2021**, *8*, 23742895211006821. [CrossRef]
36. Bösmüller, H.; Traxler, S.; Bitzer, M.; Häberle, H.; Raiser, W.; Nann, D.; Frauenfeld, L.; Vogelsberg, A.; Klingel, K.; Fend, F. The evolution of pulmonary pathology in fatal COVID-19 disease: An autopsy study with clinical correlation. *Virchows Arch.* **2020**, *477*, 349–357. [CrossRef]
37. Domke, L.M.; Klein, I.M.; Hartmann, L.; Schwab, C.; Marx, A.; Werner, M.; Möller, P.; Fend, F.; Bösmüller, H.; Schirmacher, P. Biobanking in times of crisis—The COVID-19 Autopsy and Biosample Registry Baden-Wuerttemberg. *Pathol. Res. Pract.* **2022**, *237*, 154011. [CrossRef] [PubMed]
38. Yurdaisik, I.; Demiroz, A.S.; Oz, A.B.; Akker, M.; Agirman, A.; Aksoy, S.H.; Nurili, F. Postmortem Biopsies of the Lung, Heart, Liver, and Spleen of COVID-19 Patients. *Cureus* **2021**, *13*, e20734. [CrossRef] [PubMed]
39. von Stillfried, S.; Bülow, R.D.; Röhrig, R.; Boor, P.; German Registry of COVID-19 Autopsies (DeRegCOVID), D.R.C. First report from the German COVID-19 autopsy registry. *Lancet. Reg. Health Eur.* **2022**, *15*, 100330. [CrossRef] [PubMed]
40. Suess, C.; Hausmann, R. Gross and histopathological pulmonary findings in a COVID-19 associated death during self-isolation. *Int. J. Legal. Med.* **2020**, *134*, 1285–1290. [CrossRef]
41. Adachi, T.; Chong, J.M.; Nakajima, N.; Sano, M.; Yamazaki, J.; Miyamoto, I.; Nishioka, H.; Akita, H.; Sato, Y.; Kataoka, M.; et al. Clinicopathologic and Immunohistochemical Findings from Autopsy of Patient with COVID-19, Japan. *Emerg. Infect. Dis.* **2020**, *26*, 2157–2161. [CrossRef]
42. Attoh, S.; Segborwotso, R.P.; Akoriyea, S.K.; Teddy, G.; Edusei, L.; Hobenu, F.; Agyemang-Bediako, K.; Toppar, A.; Fatchu, R.D.; Akakpo, P.K. COVID-19 autopsy reports from the Ga-East Municipal and the 37 Military Hospitals in Accra, Ghana. *Ghana Med. J.* **2020**, *54*, 52–61. [CrossRef]
43. Grosse, C.; Grosse, A.; Salzer, H.J.F.; Dünser, M.W.; Motz, R.; Langer, R. Analysis of cardiopulmonary findings in COVID-19 fatalities: High incidence of pulmonary artery thrombi and acute suppurative bronchopneumonia. *Cardiovasc. Pathol.* **2020**, *49*, 107263. [CrossRef]
44. Tian, S.; Xiong, Y.; Liu, H.; Niu, L.; Guo, J.; Liao, M.; Xiao, S.Y. Pathological study of the 2019 novel coronavirus disease (COVID-19) through postmortem core biopsies. *Mod. Pathol.* **2020**, *33*, 1007–1014. [CrossRef]
45. Menter, T.; Haslbauer, J.D.; Nienhold, R.; Savic, S.; Hopfer, H.; Deigendesch, N.; Frank, S.; Turek, D.; Willi, N.; Pargger, H.; et al. Postmortem examination of COVID-19 patients reveals diffuse alveolar damage with severe capillary congestion and variegated findings in lungs and other organs suggesting vascular dysfunction. *Histopathology* **2020**, *77*, 198–209. [CrossRef]
46. Verger, A.; Rousseau, P.F.; Malbos, E.; Chawki, M.B.; Nicolas, F.; Lançon, C.; Khalfa, S.; Guedj, E. Involvement of the cerebellum in EMDR efficiency: A metabolic connectivity PET study in PTSD. *Eur. J. Psychotraumatol.* **2020**, *11*, 1767986. [CrossRef]
47. Lacy, J.M.; Brooks, E.G.; Akers, J.; Armstrong, D.; Decker, L.; Gonzalez, A.; Humphrey, W.; Mayer, R.; Miller, M.; Perez, C.; et al. COVID-19: Postmortem Diagnostic and Biosafety Considerations. *Am. J. Forensic Med. Pathol.* **2020**, *41*, 143–151. [CrossRef] [PubMed]
48. Halushka, M.K.; Vander Heide, R.S. Myocarditis is rare in COVID-19 autopsies: Cardiovascular findings across 277 postmortem examinations. *Cardiovasc. Pathol.* **2021**, *50*, 107300. [CrossRef] [PubMed]
49. Boukhris, M.; Hillani, A.; Moroni, F.; Annabi, M.S.; Addad, F.; Ribeiro, M.H.; Mansour, S.; Zhao, X.; Ybarra, L.F.; Abbate, A.; et al. Cardiovascular Implications of the COVID-19 Pandemic: A Global Perspective. *Can. J. Cardiol.* **2020**, *36*, 1068–1080. [CrossRef] [PubMed]
50. Adeghate, E.A.; Eid, N.; Singh, J. Mechanisms of COVID-19-induced heart failure: A short review. *Heart Fail. Rev.* **2021**, *26*, 363–369. [CrossRef] [PubMed]

51. Escher, F.; Pietsch, H.; Aleshcheva, G.; Bock, T.; Baumeier, C.; Elsaesser, A.; Wenzel, P.; Hamm, C.; Westenfeld, R.; Schultheiss, M.; et al. Detection of viral SARS-CoV-2 genomes and histopathological changes in endomyocardial biopsies. *ESC Heart Fail.* **2020**, *7*, 2440–2447. [CrossRef]
52. Chen, T.; Wu, D.; Chen, H.; Yan, W.; Yang, D.; Chen, G.; Ma, K.; Xu, D.; Yu, H.; Wang, H.; et al. Clinical characteristics of 113 deceased patients with coronavirus disease 2019: Retrospective study. *BMJ* **2020**, *368*, m1091. [CrossRef]
53. Roshdy, A.; Zaher, S.; Fayed, H.; Coghlan, J.G. COVID-19 and the Heart: A Systematic Review of Cardiac Autopsies. *Front. Cardiovasc. Med.* **2020**, *7*, 626975. [CrossRef]
54. Elsoukkary, S.S.; Mostyka, M.; Dillard, A.; Berman, D.R.; Ma, L.X.; Chadburn, A.; Yantiss, R.K.; Jessurun, J.; Seshan, S.V.; Borczuk, A.C.; et al. Autopsy Findings in 32 Patients with COVID-19: A Single-Institution Experience. *Pathobiology* **2021**, *88*, 56–68. [CrossRef]
55. Fox, S.E.; Akmatbekov, A.; Harbert, J.L.; Li, G.; Quincy Brown, J.; Vander Heide, R.S. Pulmonary and cardiac pathology in African American patients with COVID-19: An autopsy series from New Orleans. *Lancet Respir. Med.* **2020**, *8*, 681–686. [CrossRef]
56. Nicolai, L.; Leunig, A.; Brambs, S.; Kaiser, R.; Weinberger, T.; Weigand, M.; Muenchhoff, M.; Hellmuth, J.C.; Ledderose, S.; Schulz, H.; et al. Immunothrombotic Dysregulation in COVID-19 Pneumonia Is Associated With Respiratory Failure and Coagulopathy. *Circulation* **2020**, *142*, 1176–1189. [CrossRef]
57. Hanley, B.; Jensen, M.; Osborn, M. Emerging spectrum of COVID-19-related cardiopulmonary pathology in adults. *Diagn. Histopathol.* **2021**, *27*, 317–324. [CrossRef] [PubMed]
58. Sadeghzadeh-Bazargan, A.; Rezai, M.; Nobari, N.N.; Mozafarpoor, S.; Goodarzi, A. Skin manifestations as potential symptoms of diffuse vascular injury in critical COVID-19 patients. *J. Cutan. Pathol.* **2021**, *48*, 1266–1276. [CrossRef] [PubMed]
59. Varga, Z. Endotheliitis in COVID-19. *Pathologe* **2020**, *41*, 99–102. [CrossRef]
60. Romanova, E.S.; Vasilyev, V.V.; Startseva, G.; Karev, V.; Rybakova, M.G.; Platonov, P.G. Cause of death based on systematic post-mortem studies in patients with positive SARS-CoV-2 tissue PCR during the COVID-19 pandemic. *J. Intern. Med.* **2021**, *290*, 655–665. [CrossRef]
61. Manolis, A.S.; Manolis, T.A.; Manolis, A.A.; Papatheou, D.; Melita, H. COVID-19 Infection: Viral Macro- and Micro-Vascular Coagulopathy and Thromboembolism/Prophylactic and Therapeutic Management. *J. Cardiovasc. Pharmacol. Ther.* **2021**, *26*, 12–24. [CrossRef]
62. Rouyer, O.; Pierre-Paul, I.N.; Balde, A.T.; Jupiter, D.; Bindila, D.; Geny, B.; Wolff, V. High Prevalence of Deep Venous Thrombosis in Non-Severe COVID-19 Patients Hospitalized for a Neurovascular Disease. *Cerebrovasc. Dis. Extra* **2020**, *10*, 174–180. [CrossRef] [PubMed]
63. Cai, C.; Guo, Y.; You, Y.; Hu, K.; Cai, F.; Xie, M.; Yang, L.; Ling, K.; Ye, D.; Misra, S.; et al. Deep Venous Thrombosis in COVID-19 Patients: A Cohort Analysis. *Clin. Appl. Thromb. Hemost.* **2020**, *26*, 1076029620982669. [CrossRef]
64. Hoelscher, C.; Sweid, A.; Ghosh, R.; Al Saiegh, F.; Keppetipola, K.M.; Farrell, C.J.; Jallo, J.; Jabbour, P.; Tjoumakaris, S.; Gooch, M.R.; et al. Cerebral deep venous thrombosis and COVID-19: Case report. *J. Neurosurg.* **2020**, *135*, 17–20. [CrossRef]
65. Hassan, W.; Ramadan, H.K. COVID-19 as a novel etiology of portal vein thrombosis: Change in the current management concepts. *Infect. Dis.* **2021**, *53*, 148–150. [CrossRef]
66. Satturwar, S.; Fowkes, M.; Farver, C.; Wilson, A.M.; Eccher, A.; Girolami, I.; Pujadas, E.; Bryce, C.; Salem, F.; El Jamal, S.M.; et al. Postmortem Findings Associated With SARS-CoV-2: Systematic Review and Meta-analysis. *Am. J. Surg. Pathol.* **2021**, *45*, 587–603. [CrossRef]
67. Maccio, U.; Zinkernagel, A.S.; Shambat, S.M.; Zeng, X.; Cathomas, G.; Ruschitzka, F.; Schuepbach, R.A.; Moch, H.; Varga, Z. SARS-CoV-2 leads to a small vessel endotheliitis in the heart. *EBioMedicine* **2021**, *63*, 103182. [CrossRef] [PubMed]
68. McGonagle, D.; Sharif, K.; O'Regan, A.; Bridgewood, C. The Role of Cytokines including Interleukin-6 in COVID-19 induced Pneumonia and Macrophage Activation Syndrome-Like Disease. *Autoimmun. Rev.* **2020**, *19*, 102537. [CrossRef]
69. Sugiyama, M.; Kinoshita, N.; Ide, S.; Nomoto, H.; Nakamoto, T.; Saito, S.; Ishikane, M.; Kutsuna, S.; Hayakawa, K.; Hashimoto, M.; et al. Serum CCL17 level becomes a predictive marker to distinguish between mild/moderate and severe/critical disease in patients with COVID-19. *Gene* **2021**, *766*, 145145. [CrossRef] [PubMed]
70. Henderson, L.A.; Canna, S.W.; Schulert, G.S.; Volpi, S.; Lee, P.Y.; Kernan, K.F.; Caricchio, R.; Mahmud, S.; Hazen, M.M.; Halyabar, O.; et al. On the Alert for Cytokine Storm: Immunopathology in COVID-19. *Arthritis Rheumatol.* **2020**, *72*, 1059–1063. [CrossRef]
71. Niederreiter, J.; Eck, C.; Ries, T.; Hartmann, A.; Märkl, B.; Büttner-Herold, M.; Amann, K.; Daniel, C. Complement Activation. *Front. Immunol.* **2022**, *13*, 835156. [CrossRef] [PubMed]
72. Delavari, F.; Varzaneh, F.N.; Rezaei, N. Neurologic Manifestations of COVID-19. *Adv. Exp. Med. Biol.* **2021**, *1318*, 343–353. [CrossRef]
73. Al-Sarraj, S.; Troakes, C.; Hanley, B.; Osborn, M.; Richardson, M.P.; Hotopf, M.; Bullmore, E.; Everall, I.P. Invited Review: The spectrum of neuropathology in COVID-19. *Neuropathol. Appl. Neurobiol.* **2021**, *47*, 3–16. [CrossRef]
74. Diao, B.; Wang, C.; Wang, R.; Feng, Z.; Zhang, J.; Yang, H.; Tan, Y.; Wang, H.; Liu, L.; Liu, Y.; et al. Human kidney is a target for novel severe acute respiratory syndrome coronavirus 2 infection. *Nat. Commun.* **2021**, *12*, 2506. [CrossRef]
75. Cantuti-Castelvetri, L.; Ojha, R.; Pedro, L.D.; Djannatian, M.; Franz, J.; Kuivanen, S.; van der Meer, F.; Kallio, K.; Kaya, T.; Anastasina, M.; et al. Neuropilin-1 facilitates SARS-CoV-2 cell entry and infectivity. *Science* **2020**, *370*, 856–860. [CrossRef]

76. Pei, G.; Zhang, Z.; Peng, J.; Liu, L.; Zhang, C.; Yu, C.; Ma, Z.; Huang, Y.; Liu, W.; Yao, Y.; et al. Renal Involvement and Early Prognosis in Patients with COVID-19 Pneumonia. *J. Am. Soc. Nephrol.* **2020**, *31*, 1157–1165. [CrossRef]
77. Martinez-Rojas, M.A.; Vega-Vega, O.; Bobadilla, N.A. Is the kidney a target of SARS-CoV-2? *Am. J. Physiol. Renal. Physiol.* **2020**, *318*, F1454–F1462. [CrossRef] [PubMed]
78. Apetrii, M.; Enache, S.; Siriopol, D.; Burlacu, A.; Kanbay, A.; Kanbay, M.; Scripcariu, D.; Covic, A. A brand-new cardiorenal syndrome in the COVID-19 setting. *Clin. Kidney J.* **2020**, *13*, 291–296. [CrossRef] [PubMed]
79. Project, C.; Autopsias, P. The first COVID-19 autopsy in Spain performed during the early stages of the pandemic. *Rev. Esp. Patol.* **2020**, *53*, 182–187. [CrossRef]
80. Jonigk, D.; Werlein, C.; Acker, T.; Aepfelbacher, M.; Amann, K.U.; Baretton, G.; Barth, P.; Bohle, R.M.; Büttner, A.; Büttner, R.; et al. Organ manifestations of COVID-19: What have we learned so far (not only) from autopsies? *Virchows Arch.* **2022**, *481*, 139–159. [CrossRef] [PubMed]
81. Vakili, K.; Fathi, M.; Hajiesmaeili, M.; Salari, M.; Saluja, D.; Tafakhori, A.; Sayehmiri, F.; Rezaei-Tavirani, M. Neurological Symptoms, Comorbidities, and Complications of COVID-19: A Literature Review and Meta-Analysis of Observational Studies. *Eur. Neurol.* **2021**, *84*, 307–324. [CrossRef] [PubMed]
82. Yang, A.C.; Kern, F.; Losada, P.M.; Agam, M.R.; Maat, C.A.; Schmartz, G.P.; Fehlmann, T.; Stein, J.A.; Schaum, N.; Lee, D.P.; et al. Dysregulation of brain and choroid plexus cell types in severe COVID-19. *Nature* **2021**, *595*, 565–571. [CrossRef]
83. Bryce, C.; Grimes, Z.; Pujadas, E.; Ahuja, S.; Beasley, M.B.; Albrecht, R.; Hernandez, T.; Stock, A.; Zhao, Z.; AlRasheed, M.R.; et al. Pathophysiology of SARS-CoV-2: The Mount Sinai COVID-19 autopsy experience. *Mod. Pathol.* **2021**, *34*, 1456–1467. [CrossRef]
84. Reichard, R.R.; Kashani, K.B.; Boire, N.A.; Constantopoulos, E.; Guo, Y.; Lucchinetti, C.F. Neuropathology of COVID-19: A spectrum of vascular and acute disseminated encephalomyelitis (ADEM)-like pathology. *Acta Neuropathol.* **2020**, *140*, 1–6. [CrossRef]
85. Grieco, T.; Gomes, V.; Rossi, A.; Cantisani, C.; Greco, M.E.; Rossi, G.; Sernicola, A.; Pellacani, G. The Pathological Culprit of Neuropathic Skin Pain in Long COVID-19 Patients: A Case Series. *J. Clin. Med.* **2022**, *11*, 4474. [CrossRef]
86. Mao, R.; Qiu, Y.; He, J.S.; Tan, J.Y.; Li, X.H.; Liang, J.; Shen, J.; Zhu, L.R.; Chen, Y.; Iacucci, M.; et al. Manifestations and prognosis of gastrointestinal and liver involvement in patients with COVID-19: A systematic review and meta-analysis. *Lancet Gastroenterol. Hepatol.* **2020**, *5*, 667–678. [CrossRef]
87. Calcagno, E.; Sogunro, O.; Nepal, P.; Assaker, R.; Sapire, J. COVID-19 induced mesenteric venous infarction. *Radiol. Case Rep.* **2021**, *16*, 1999–2002. [CrossRef] [PubMed]
88. Segovia, F.D.; Ream, S.; Dang, T.; Chaganti, B.T.; Ortega, A.J.; Rhee, S.; Borges, J.C. COVID-19-Associated Superior Mesenteric Artery Thrombosis and Acute Intestinal Ischemia. *Cureus* **2022**, *14*, e27722. [CrossRef] [PubMed]
89. Ammar, A.S.; Naqi, S.A.; Ashraf, M.; Saleem, M.; Raza, H.A.; Haider, U. A rare case report of short bowel anastomosis after acute mesenteric ischaemia in COVID-19 postive patient. *J. Pak. Med. Assoc.* **2022**, *72*, 1222–1224. [CrossRef] [PubMed]
90. Batra, S.; Nair, A.G.; Syal, K. An Unusual Presentation of Superior Mesenteric Venous Occlusion in Mild COVID-19. *Indian J. Clin. Biochem.* **2022**, 1–4. [CrossRef]
91. Bertolini, A.; van de Peppel, I.P.; Bodewes, F.A.J.A.; Moshage, H.; Fantin, A.; Farinati, F.; Fiorotto, R.; Jonker, J.W.; Strazzabosco, M.; Verkade, H.J.; et al. Abnormal Liver Function Tests in Patients With COVID-19: Relevance and Potential Pathogenesis. *Hepatology* **2020**, *72*, 1864–1872. [CrossRef]
92. Li, P.; Liu, Y.; Cheng, Z.; Yu, X.; Li, Y. COVID-19-associated liver injury: Clinical characteristics, pathophysiological mechanisms and treatment management. *Biomed. Pharmacother.* **2022**, *154*, 113568. [CrossRef]
93. Kayhan, S.; Hepsen, S.; Kalkisim, H.K.; Sendur, I.N.; Altay, F.A.; Yalcindag, A. The evaluation of pancreas β-cell autoantibodies in non-diabetic COVID-19 patients. *Arch. Endocrinol. Metab.* **2022**, *66*, 459–465. [CrossRef]
94. Szarpak, L.; Pruc, M.; Najeeb, F.; Jaguszewski, M.J. POST-COVID-19 and the pancreas. *Am. J. Emerg. Med.* **2022**, *59*, 174–175. [CrossRef]
95. Cococcia, S.; Lenti, M.V.; Santacroce, G.; Achilli, G.; Borrelli de Andreis, F.; Di Sabatino, A. Liver-spleen axis dysfunction in COVID-19. *World J. Gastroenterol.* **2021**, *27*, 5919–5931. [CrossRef]
96. Petroianu, A. COVID-19 recurrence associated with the virus storage in the Spleen. *Rev. Assoc. Med. Bras.* **2022**, *68*, 751–753. [CrossRef]
97. Liu, Q.; Shi, Y.; Cai, J.; Duan, Y.; Wang, R.; Zhang, H.; Ruan, Q.; Li, J.; Zhao, L.; Ping, Y.; et al. Pathological changes in the lungs and lymphatic organs of 12 COVID-19 autopsy cases. *Natl. Sci. Rev.* **2020**, *7*, 1868–1878. [CrossRef] [PubMed]
98. Trabulsi, N.H.; Alshammakh, S.S.; Shabkah, A.A.; Aladawi, M.; Farsi, A.H. Spontaneous rupture of spleen in a patient with COVID-19 disease: Case report and review of the literature. *J. Surg. Case Rep.* **2022**, *2022*, rjac124. [CrossRef] [PubMed]
99. Abdullaev, A.; Odilov, A.; Ershler, M.; Volkov, A.; Lipina, T.; Gasanova, T.; Lebedin, Y.; Babichenko, I.; Sudarikov, A. Viral Load and Patterns of SARS-CoV-2 Dissemination to the Lungs, Mediastinal Lymph Nodes, and Spleen of Patients with COVID-19 Associated Lymphopenia. *Viruses* **2021**, *13*, 1410. [CrossRef]
100. MacDonald, M.E.; Weathered, R.K.; Stewart, E.C.; Magold, A.I.; Mukherjee, A.; Gurbuxani, S.; Smith, H.; McMullen, P.; Mueller, J.; Husain, A.N.; et al. Lymphatic coagulation and neutrophil extracellular traps in lung-draining lymph nodes of COVID-19 decedents. *Blood Adv.* 2022; *in press*. [CrossRef] [PubMed]
101. Yao, X.H.; Luo, T.; Shi, Y.; He, Z.C.; Tang, R.; Zhang, P.P.; Cai, J.; Zhou, X.D.; Jiang, D.P.; Fei, X.C.; et al. A cohort autopsy study defines COVID-19 systemic pathogenesis. *Cell Res.* **2021**, *31*, 836–846. [CrossRef]

102. Baig, A.M. Chronic COVID syndrome: Need for an appropriate medical terminology for long-COVID and COVID long-haulers. *J. Med. Virol.* **2021**, *93*, 2555–2556. [CrossRef]
103. Radtke, T.; Ulyte, A.; Puhan, M.A.; Kriemler, S. Long-term Symptoms After SARS-CoV-2 Infection in Children and Adolescents. *JAMA* **2021**, *326*, 869–871. [CrossRef]
104. DePace, N.L.; Colombo, J. Long-COVID Syndrome and the Cardiovascular System: A Review of Neurocardiologic Effects on Multiple Systems. *Curr. Cardiol. Rep.* **2022**. [CrossRef]

encyclopedia

MDPI

Entry

COVID-19-Associated Encephalopathy (COVEP): Basic Aspects of Neuropathology

George S. Stoyanov [1,*], Dimo Stoyanov [2], Martin Ivanov [2], Anton B. Tonchev [2], Hristo Popov [1] and Lilyana Petkova [1]

1 Department of General and Clinical Pathology, Forensic Medicine and Deontology, Faculty of Medicine, Medical University—Varna "Prof. Dr. Paraskev Stoyanov", 9002 Varna, Bulgaria
2 Department of Anatomy and Cell Biology, Faculty of Medicine, Medical University—Varna "Prof. Dr. Paraskev Stoyanov", 9002 Varna, Bulgaria
* Correspondence: georgi.stoyanov@mu-varna.bg

Definition: SARS-CoV-2, a member of the betacoronavirus group and causative agent of COVID-19, is a virus affecting multiple systems, not only the respiratory. One of the systems affected by the virus is the central nervous system, with neuropathological studies reporting a wide set of morphological phenomena—neuroinflammation, vascular and blood-brain barrier alterations, neurodegeneration, and accelerated aging, while contradicting data is present on the direct neuroinvasive potential of the virus and active viral replication within neurons. The depicted changes, other than an acute effect (which may contribute to the death of the patient) also have chronic sequelae in the context of post-COVID syndrome cognitive impediments, sleep, and mood disorders. The following chapter describe the basic neuropathological aspects of SARS-CoV-2 as based on the present evidence in scientific literature and propose the term COVEP—COVID-associated encephalopathy—to unite the undisputed effects of the infection on nervous system morphology and function.

Keywords: SARS-CoV-2; COVID-19; central nervous system; anosmia; neuropathology; encephalopathy

Citation: Stoyanov, G.S.; Stoyanov, D.; Ivanov, M.; Tonchev, A.B.; Popov, H.; Petkova, L. COVID-19-Associated Encephalopathy (COVEP): Basic Aspects of Neuropathology. *Encyclopedia* **2022**, 2, 1773–1789. https://doi.org/10.3390/encyclopedia2040122

Academic Editors: Stephen Bustin and Raffaele Barretta

Received: 29 August 2022
Accepted: 14 October 2022
Published: 27 October 2022

1. Introduction

The novel coronavirus disease, which began its outbreak in 2019 (COVID-19) caused by severe acute respiratory syndrome coronavirus 2 (SARS-CoV-2), has emerged as a multisystem disease [1–3]. While initially regarded as a respiratory system disease, one of the earliest peculiarities of the disease was the development of anosmia (loss of smell sensation) and ageusia (loss of taste perception) by those infected, which pointed toward nervous system involvement as well [4–9]. Since then, many other aspects of the disease have emerged, such as renal involvement (COVAN), myopericarditis and endotheliitis, gastrointestinal system disorders, and many more [10–17]. With the emergence of new variants of SARS-CoV-2 that cause severe disease in significantly fewer people while also being severely more infective, the scientific focus has gradually shifted toward the chronic sequelae of infection: post-COVID syndromes where once more the nervous system takes center stage [18–23].

2. Applications and Influences

As a multisystem infection, it is essential not to underestimate or focus the chronic or acute sequelae of COVID-19 purely to the respiratory system [21,23–25]. A myriad of symptoms in the acute and chronic phases of the disease show signs of its effect on the central nervous system—anosmia, ageusia, migraine headaches, confusion, clouding of consciousness, memory problems, etc., [8,22,26–28].

3. COVID-19 and the Brain

Coronaviruses, as a diffuse group of viruses, have shown many properties and organ targets in their biology [3,6,29–31]. The previous two coronaviruses of concern—severe acute respiratory syndrome coronavirus (SARS) and middle eastern respiratory syndrome coronavirus (MERS)—also had signs pointing toward central nervous system involvement, including morphological ones [26,29,32–34]. Furthermore, close relatives to SARS-CoV-2 have been known to cause encephalitis in other animals, such as the mouse hepatitis virus, which is known to have significant neurotropic properties [35–37].

The mechanisms of neuroinvasion to this point are still not well known, but there are several candidates, including direct invasion through the cribriform plate, neuronal pathway invasion, and hematogenous dissemination through COVID-19-induced endotheliitis [38–40]. Direct invasion through the cribriform plate and nasal to meningeal dissemination is a well-known mechanism utilized by viruses, including some other members of the coronavirus family and bacteria [22,38,40–42]. Direct neuronal invasion is a mechanism typical for neurotropic viruses, in which once the viral particles enter the neuronal body they travel antero- and retrograde through it, with the mechanism being suggested not only for the nasal cavity nerve endings and bodies but also for pulmonary and gastrointestinal ones as well; after this, the newly produced viral particles infect neighboring neurons and repeat the chain [22,43–46]. The third and most important mechanism, as it plays a role not only in the direct neuronal involvement of SARS-CoV-2 but also in its myriad of vascular complications, is that of endothelialitis, in which the endothelial cells of the blood vessels are infected and undergo subsequent desquamation and necrosis [22,29,38,39,47–49]. Neuroinvasion through this mechanism would induce direct viral damage to the central nervous system neurons and toxic harm as well, as the endothelial cell damage would disrupt the blood–brain barrier [50–54]. Limited data on the choroid plexus further suggests that there may be choroid tropism of the virus, with secondary blood-cerebrospinal fluid disruption [55].

Another suggested mechanism by which SARS-CoV-2 can affect the central nervous system is that of inflammatory cell mediation. Direct immune cell invasion, although primarily affecting the immune response and cytokine storm onset, is also an important mechanism by which unaffected organs can be directly infected by viral shedding from circulating infected immune cells, especially if they migrate to the parenchyma [56,57].

Further unknowns are raised by the exact mechanism by which SARS-CoV-2 can affect the functioning of the central nervous system. While neuroinvasion refers to the ability of the viral particles to enter the CNS, that by itself does not directly indicate a pathological sequence [58]. Neurotropism on the other hand reflects on the ability of the virus to successfully enter the CNS cells, while neurovirulence reflects on the pathogenic capabilities of the virus in the nervous system—direct or indirect—without neurotropism [58]. While undoubtably SARS CoV-2 has neuroinvasive potential through multiple mechanisms, the neuroinvasive aspects have been confirmed only in vitro, with most postmortem studies disputing this mechanism [43,59,60]. On the other hand, multiple postmortem studies indicate a myriad of pathological changes, ranging from necrotic and degenerative to inflammatory and reactive, indicating that even in the absence of neurotropism, there are signs of neurovirulence [38,58,61,62].

3.1. Meninges

Reports on meningitis and meningeal involvement in COVID-19 are relatively scarce. Most scientific literature reports signs of meningism—severe headaches, disorientation, and neck stiffness, with some also noting seizures [26,38,63]. In most of these cases, aseptic meningitis is diagnosed in a predominantly severe clinical course setting, although in some patients, meningism may be the initial presentation of the disease [26,63]. Only a handful of reports were able to isolate SARS-CoV-2 from the cerebrospinal fluid of such patients [64,65]. On the other hand, there are multiple reports of co-infection meningitis occurring in sepsis and in secondary bacterial infections during COVID-19 [66]. Most morphological studies reporting cases without morphological evidence of a superimposed infection report meningeal histopathological changes consisting of severe edema, focal microhemorrhages, and lymphocytic infiltration [9]. Involvement of the meninges based on the endotheliitis mechanism is most likely to explain the clinical symptoms as based on the morphology—vascular damage would cause the edema and lymphocytic infiltration, with only those having sufficient hemorrhages, i.e., viral particles entering from the blood—giving a positive result upon laboratory test for SARS-CoV-2 from the cerebrospinal fluid [8,13,16,39,47]. Of course, the direct invasion through the cribriform plate is also a viable and highly likely mechanism, although it is ill-supported by the morphological findings [8].

3.2. Cerebrum

As in nearly all aspects of neuropathology, the gross changes in the brain are mostly minimal and predominantly nonspecific, manifested by cerebral edema resulting in cerebellar tonsillar herniation into the foramen magnum, edema of the meninges, and focal vascular changes, predominantly petechial hemorrhages in severe cases [67].

The focal point of COVID-19-induced neuropathological damage is, of course, the direct effects of the virus on the central nervous system, predominantly the cerebrum. These can be viewed in several different mechanisms; the first and most profound clinically is that of hypoxia-induced hypoperfusion due to the pulmonary changes induced by the virus; due to decreased oxygen saturation, neurons start undergoing hypoxic and hence degenerative change, with this mechanism being most prominent in patients with a severe clinical course—hypoxic brain injury [50–53]. The second mechanism corresponding well to the clinical manifestation is that of endothelialitis, where the desquamated endothelial cells cause a predisposition for thrombosis and vascular ruptures, resulting in the clinically well-documented higher incidence of cerebrovascular disease in COVID-19 [68–70]. This mechanism would also lead to blood–brain barrier disruption and the onset of neuronal degeneration through toxin-induced damage [22,53,71]. The third and final mechanism is the direct neuronal invasion of SARS-CoV-2 and viral-induced damage to neurons—viral encephalitis [22,29,38].

3.2.1. Cerebral Hypoxic Brain Injury and Hypoperfusion

Hypoxic brain injury, also referred to as anoxic and hypoxic-ischemic brain injury, is a complex neuropathological process in which neurons undergo first degenerative and, subsequently, necrotic change due to insufficient oxygen supplementation [72]. The causative agents for the decreased oxygen saturation or vascular perfusion are multiple and vary from direct reduction of plasma oxygen, as in COVID-19, temporary vascular obstruction or flow reduction, as in trauma, to cardiac arrest, carbon monoxide poisoning, etc., [50,71–73]. This mechanism would directly correlate with the morphology observed in fatal cases of COVID-19, as those patients typically have a significant decrease in oxygen saturation [74,75]. Interestingly, the long-term consequences of hypoxic brain injury correlate highly to the so-called "brain fog" in the context of post-COVID syndrome—transient clouding of consciousness, cognitive disabilities, attention deficit, sleep disorders, executive dysfunction, etc., [62,76]. These mechanisms of brain injury are well-supported by neuropathological data depicting foci of micronecrosis and hemorrhages, axonal degeneration and microgliopathy [54,62,77–79]. However, they would not apply to people experiencing the same symptoms in the context of post-COVID syndrome without suffering from a severe form of the disease in the acute phase, with significant pulmonary involvement and hypoxia [22,24,80].

3.2.2. Vascular Incidents

As mentioned several times, endotheliitis is a focal point of SARS-CoV-2-induced organ pathology, and the central nervous system is no exception here [13,16,39,47–49,70,81,82]. Other than disruption of the structure of the blood–brain barrier, direct viral replication within the vascular endothelial cells and their following desquamation and necrosis results in exposing the endothelial cell basal lamina collagen, which acts as a tissue factor in the activation of the coagulation cascade and hence enacts Virchow's triad, leading to vascular thrombosis formation [83–87]. As a result, the autochthonous thrombi in predominantly small and medium-sized blood vessels lead to focal ischemia and neuronal necrosis—cerebral infarction (clinically referred to as stroke), a well-reported sequence of SARS-CoV-2 infection [22,29,68–71]. Besides autochthonous thrombi, the multiple systems involved by endotheliitis and further cardiovascular sequelae also allow for more significant ischemic incidents due to thromboembolism to the brain [68,78,88]. Other than ischemic incidents, these patients also have a higher likelihood of developing cerebral hemorrhages (clinically referred to as hemorrhagic stroke), as well as thrombosis of the dural sinuses (cerebral venous sinus thrombosis) [68,71].

The extent of microvascular damage to the central nervous system should also not be underestimated, even when there is a lack of microvascular thrombi, as some capillaries in the context of endotheliitis completely lose their endothelium and collapse, resulting in a string-like transformation [89]. These may play a key role in COVID-induced neuropathological damage, as these inactive and disappearing capillaries induce hypoxia in the peripheral tissues [90].

3.2.3. Encephalitis and Encephalopathy

As already mentioned, a focal point of research is the direct neurotropic effect of SARS-CoV-2 and its potential to lead to encephalitis, as in some of its close relatives [29,35,36,91–93]. In the initial phases of the pandemic, multiple studies reported encephalitis in COVID-19 patients ranging from panencephalitis to acute hemorrhagic, acute necrotizing, limbic, and autoimmune encephalitis [82,91–102]. In the case of confirmed limbic and autoimmune encephalitis, SARS-CoV-2 can be both a triggering and a concomitant factor, as has been reported with other viruses [103,104]. For necrotizing and hemorrhagic-necrotic encephalitis cases, the relationship has since become more dubious in the absence of histology, as most of these reports are based on neuroradiology and can be mimicked by the systemic and vascular effects of the virus [82,97–99]. The relationships and capabilities of SARS-CoV-2 to lead to the development of true encephalitis are further disputed by most morphological studies, as despite histology the morphological changes may be highly similar to those of encephalitis, and while there are data on micro- and astroglyopathy, as well as cytotoxic T lymphocyte infiltration, immunologically only a few studies have isolated viral presence in the central nervous system [9,62,67,78,105,106]. Worthy of note is the heterogeneity of reported locations of encephalitis by some studies; while most depict the brainstem as the most severely affected location, others point toward the limbic systems or isolated cortical and subcortical areas of the frontal lobe [9,89,94,98,104,107]. Here it is essential to mention that while neuroinflammation and encephalitis are often used as synonyms and have similar mechanisms and morphology, encephalitis refers to active infection-induced inflammation of the brain parenchyma, while neuroinflammation (clinically referred to as encephalopathy in some cases, i.e., hepatic encephalopathy) refers purely to the presence of an inflammatory reaction in the brain, predominantly due to neuronal loss leading to the release of inflammatory cytokines, as seen in a myriad of conditions—neurovirulence [108–110]. Based on the presence of inflammatory reaction, lack of undisputable evidence of the viral presence, and the evident neuronophagia overpowering the inflammatory response, these data point more towards encephalopathy than encephalitis [111–116].

3.2.4. Neurodegeneration

Given the mechanisms described so far and their inevitable neuronal degeneration and necrosis spectrum of sequelae, they are predominantly the ones occurring in severe and fatal cases [26,68,89]. Accumulating evidence suggests additional mechanisms associated with SARS-CoV-2 infection that could trigger or accelerate already-developed neurodegenerative disorders [117,118].

Some studies suggest that the viral surface structure acts as a binding site for heparin and accelerates the aggregation and displacement of heparin-binding proteins such as Aβ, α-synuclein, tau, prion, and TDP-43 RRM, resulting in initiation or acceleration of the associated neurodegenerative pathways [119,120]. Other studies have also suggested that within the host cells, the SARS-CoV-2 viral protein interacts with multiple intracellular pathways associated with aging, taking part in vesicle trafficking, lipid modifications, RNA processing and regulation, ubiquitin ligases, and mitochondrial activity, while at the same time depleting intracellular iron and further hindering mitochondrial function [59,60,117]. Furthermore, as the virus enters the host cell through the ACE-2 receptor, viral interaction may lead to decreased functionality, reducing the neuroprotective effects of ACE-2 [121,122]. These mechanisms would have implications for the central nervous system and multiple other organ sites, where resident cellular mitotic activity is low. However, based on the dispute over viral presence within neurons, this intracellular pathway of accelerated aging is dubious at this point and heralds significant future research [78,123].

One group of patients with neurodegenerative diseases severely affected by SARS-CoV-2 infection are those with Parkinson's disease. Multiple case reports and cohort studies have reported a significant functional and cognitive decline in these patients, with these patients also being more likely to expire from COVID-19 [124,125]. The exact mechanism of accelerated degeneration in these patients is also highly disputed, with some studies supporting the direct neuroinvasive potential of SARS-CoV-2 and pointing toward the brainstem as the most affected area in the encephalitis spectrum; others propose an ACE-2 suppression-associated mechanism, as the receptor is significantly expressed in dopaminergic neurons, while others point to the fact that infection-associated acceleration in Parkinson's disease is a typical hallmark of the disease and that progressive decline in these patients is predominantly due to physical and other therapies being discontinued during lockdowns [117,124–128]. One further fact supporting these claims is the isolation of coronavirus antibodies against other members of the viral family from the cerebrospinal fluid of patients with Parkinson's disease in the past decades [128,129].

Furthermore, discontinuation of non-medication treatment and social isolation during lockdowns has been shown to have adverse functional effects, not only on patients with chronic diseases, including neurodegenerative ones such as Alzheimer's disease, but significantly on neuropsychiatric diseases such as depression, anxiety, and post-traumatic stress disorder [117].

3.2.5. Hippocampal Damage

The hippocampus is a small and fragile structure within the brain with vast implications for neurodegenerative and other conditions, as it is a crucial area for adult neurogenesis [130]. As the hippocampus has been identified to play a role in a myriad of conditions, some studies have also tried to elaborate on its possible damage in the context of SARS-CoV-2 infection, as some of the long-term sequelae of the infection, such as brain fog, are indicative of hippocampal damage [62,130,131]. Clinical studies have established hippocampal hyperintensity and atrophy on brain MRI scans, suggesting a de novo process during COVID-19 [132]. Morphological studies have shown aberrant permeability of the blood–brain barrier due to endotheliitis, perivascular and pericellular microcalcifications, and neuronal loss in the dentate gyrus resulting in "skip" lesions and loss of doublecortin-positive immature neurons [133,134]. Although no viral RNA was isolated, the hippocampus in these studies showed microglial activation, T lymphocyte infiltration, and increases in the levels of interleukins 1 and 6, suggestive of a neuroinflammation cascade, with the result also being recreated in an animal model of SARS-CoV-2 infection—neurovirulence [133]. Furthermore, spatial and architectural changes were noted not only in the neuronal and microglial but also in the astrocytic cellular populations, as well as changes in the cellular morphology [135,136].

3.3. Olfactory Epithelium and Olfactory Bulbs

One of the most striking early features that first suggested nervous system involvement in COVID-19 was the onset of anosmia and ageusia, features rarely reported in the previous two coronaviruses of concern—SARS-CoV and MERS-CoV [7,8,27–29,137,138].

SARS-CoV-2, as a virus with undisputed epitheliotropic features like most members of the coronavirus family, was quickly established to infect respiratory epithelial cells, with the nasal cavity and pharynx epithelia being no exception; hence the nasal swab tests for diagnosis proved highly efficient [139–141].

While initially regarded as due to nasal obstruction, it soon became apparent that anosmia develops due to complex mechanisms [8,131]. Initial reports on olfactory epithelia showed olfactory mucosa involvement, with active viral replication in sustentacular cells (sensory neuron supporting cells), but not esthesiocytes (olfactory sensory neurons), with sustentacular cell involvement also allowing for probable leptomeningeal spread as well (Figure 1) [8,141]. As the sustentacular cells have many functions, among which are odorant endocytosis, local homeostasis regulation, and esthesiocyte cilia structural support, a functional aberration in them inhibits the proper function of the receptor neurons [8]. Further clinical-based neuroradiology reports described olfactory bulb edema and subsequent atrophy during and after infection [9,142–144]. Initial histopathology suggested changes associated with direct viral-induced damage to the bulbs with edema, inflammatory cell infiltration, microglial nodules and severe neuronal degeneration, and neuronal necrosis with areas of colliquation, suggestive of necrotizing olfactory bulbitis (Figure 1) [9]. Further reports supported the presence of neuroinflammation and degenerative changes within the olfactory bulbs and additional endotheliitis-associated blood–brain barrier injury and suggested the presence of viral RNA (Figure 1) [61,78,105,145–148]. A promising sign for the reversible nature of SARS-CoV-2 induced nervous system pathology is the recovery of smell sensation, albeit delayed in most patients after COVID-19, probably linked to adult neurogenesis in the bulb [7,149,150]. This mechanism would also be in play in the regeneration of the esthesiocytes and their sustentacular cell in the respiratory part of the nasal mucosa [151]. However, one of the most detailed studies to date indicated that there are no pathological sequelae in the olfactory nerves and bulb, but rather that all of these changes are attributed to the nasal mucosa infection [141].

Unlike anosmia, the mechanisms for ageusia remain widely unelaborated upon (Figure 1) [152–154].

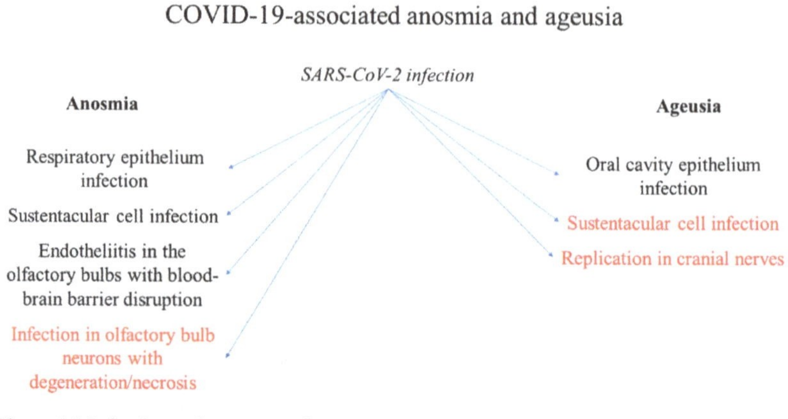

Figure 1. Mechanisms of anosmia and ageusia onset in COVID-19; red denotes disputed mechanisms.

3.4. *Cerebellum, Spinal Cord and Peripheral Nervous System*

Few studies have focused on the cerebellum, presenting predominantly neuroinflammatory change [67,105,155]. Interestingly enough, there have been clinical reports on the onset of cerebellar dysfunction leading to ataxia, with some reports also focusing on accelerated aging and neurodegeneration [101,156–158].

At this stage, severe morphological lesions induced in the spinal cord by SARS-CoV-2 infection have not been proven, with the most frequently reported vascular and ischemic incidents being meningeal and minor neuroinflammation with accompanying degenerative changes [77,89,107,159]. Individual cases of transverse myelitis have also been reported associated with the infection [160,161].

Peripheral neuropathy is a relatively common complication, especially in critically ill patients, and tends to correspond with the extent of time spent in intensive care units [161]. Direct damage to the peripheral nerves is also discussed, with some studies isolating viral particles and RNA from peripheral nerves, including cranial ones [159,161–163]. The resulting neuritis has been reported to affect the musculoskeletal system with the onset of type two muscle atrophy [163]. Further supporting the presence of peripheral nervous system involvement, direct or indirect, is the increased likelihood of COVID-19 patients developing Guillain-Barré syndrome [22,38,106,131].

3.5. *Post-COVID Syndrome and Brain Fog*

Post-COVID syndrome, also referred to as long COVID and persistent COVID, represents a wide group of symptoms and complaints reported by patients after acute SARS-CoV-2 infection [21,24,147,160,164]. While initially focusing on persistent respiratory system symptoms such as post-infectious asthma and pulmonary fibrosis, symptoms soon expanded to the cardiovascular, endocrine, and nervous systems [165–169]. Persistent anosmia and dysosmia were among the first reported long symptoms of the nervous system, with fatigue and tiredness, insomnia, mood changes, and difficulties in concentrating soon after that [170–175]. According to some studies, the long-lasting nervous system sequelae of COVID-19 are highly selective, with individuals reporting cognitive deficit and depression while alertness and orientation remained intact [174]. These symptoms are more likely to develop in patients with severe clinical disease but have also been described as the only symptom of the infection [24,99,170,175]. While the mechanisms for this remain widely unknown, functional studies report that most patients experiencing these symptoms show biomarkers of protracted inflammation, while cortical areas of the brain are hypometabolic, especially in the frontal and parietal lobes [173]. Thankfully these memory-related areas of the brain show a gradual improvement in their metabolic function, with most patients slowly regaining baseline cognition functions [173].

3.6. COVEP

Based on the accumulated body of evidence, despite some facts being disputable, SARS-CoV-2 infection is a true multisystem disease that affects the central nervous system [10,17,24,39,69,77–79,106,111,115,131,135,162,176,177]. Despite some evidence pointing toward active viral replication within neurons and others disputing it, the neuropathological consensus, for the most part, is that during active COVID-19 infection, there is a presence of neuroinflammation, neuronal degeneration, and an admixture of vascular phenomena such as endotheliitis, blood–brain barrier disruption, and vascular incidents, as well as hypoxic changes (Figure 2) [22,71,79,101,131,176]. Despite some of the presented evidence being contradictory to the others, the protracted central nervous system complaints reported from patients surviving SARS-CoV-2 infection show disruption of brain metabolism and function, with a steady improvement in overall cognitive functioning [173]. Hence, a proposed nomenclature change would be to implement the terminological use of COVID-associated encephalopathy (COVEP). The proposed nomenclature can unite the neuroinflammatory nature with vascular and degenerative phenomena observed in the brains of the deceased as well as the neurocognitive function of survivors, further underlining the truly multifaceted nature of COVID-19 and the multiple systems it can affect with varying clinical severity other than the respiratory system, as with similar nomenclature changes that have already been implemented, e.g., COVAN [10].

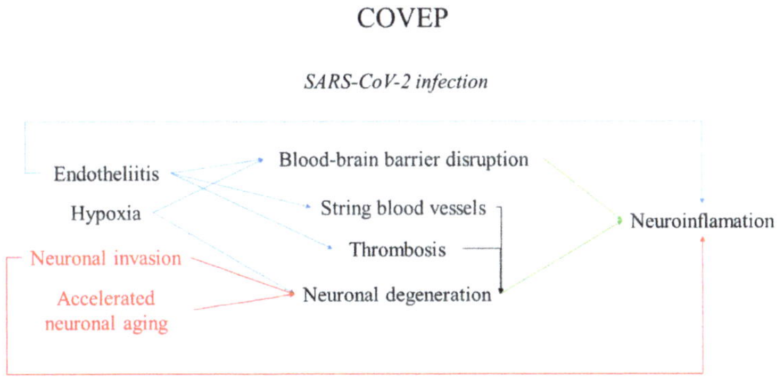

Figure 2. Mechanisms of neurological damage associated with COVID-19—COVEP; red denotes disputed mechanisms.

3.7. Lessons from the Past—Previous Pandemics and von Economo Encephalitis

COVID-19 is not the first coronavirus disease to cause a severe health concern, nor is it likely to be the last [30]. In the previous two decades, closely related members of the betacoronavirus subfamily—SARS and MERS—have also caused outbreaks of worrying diseases [1,6,29,30,178]. SARS-CoV and MERS-CoV are also highly unlikely to be the first coronaviruses to cause severe illness in humans, as coronaviruses are known to cause severe disease in various animals and have accompanied humanity for most of its recent existence [36,129,179–183]. Despite serological evidence lacking, based on the clinical picture and symptoms reported by the patients, some of which are highly similar to those induced by SARS-CoV-2 (mainly loss of taste and smell, clouding of consciousness, and encephalitis symptoms, all rarely seen in influenza), it is highly likely that the last great pandemic of the nineteenth century (1889–1891), the so-called Russian or Asian influenza, was also caused by a member of the coronavirus family [184,185].

Furthermore, another alarm bell rung based on the clinical manifestations of COVEP and a previous epidemic central nervous system disease was that of the probability of COVEP developing into a von Economo or von Economo-like lethargic encephalitis [100]. While von Economo disease is frequently misinterpreted as post-infectious parkinsonism developing in patients after the 1918–1920 Spanish influenza pandemic, it is essential to note that the first cases were described in 1917, well over a year before the onset of Spanish influenza [100,186–188]. Furthermore, since then serological data from sporadic cases do not confirm influenza viral particles, while being more indicative of an enterovirus causative agent [189]. Multiple reports have since tried to bridge the gap between COVID-19 and von Economo encephalitis, however, the main presenting symptoms of von Economo's of somnolent-ophthalmoplegic, hyperkinetic, and amyostatic-akinetic forms with the development of post-encephalic parkinsonism do not fit the spectrum of clinical sequelae of COVEP [187].

4. Conclusions

- COVID-associated encephalopathy—COVEP—is a common clinical manifestation in severe cases of SARS-CoV-2 infection.
- The basis of COVEP is the presence of neuroinflammatory changes, predominantly located in the brainstem and temporal lobe; vascular, degenerative, and hypoxic phenomena also play a significant role in its development.
- These combined changes result in altered sensation, e.g., smell and taste; mood swings; cognitive impediments; insomnia; and severe complications—infarctions, hemorrhages, and neurodegeneration, with these symptoms persisting some time after the infection has been eradicated.
- The neurotropism, neurovirulence, and neuroinvasion of SARS-CoV-2 are still disputable in their mechanisms and direct and indirect effects on the central nervous system.

Author Contributions: G.S.S. and A.B.T. conceptualized the manuscript; G.S.S., H.P. and L.P. performed detailed review on clinical and pathological phenomena; M.I. and L.P. performed detailed review on neuroanatomy and processes; G.S.S., H.P. and L.P. wrote the initial draft; M.I. conceptualized the figures; H.P., L.P., M.I. and D.S. performed major text edits; A.B.T. critically reviewer the manuscript and approved its version submitted for publication. All authors have read and agreed to the published version of the manuscript.

Funding: This research received no external funding.

Institutional Review Board Statement: Not applicable.

Data Availability Statement: Not applicable.

Conflicts of Interest: The authors declare no conflict of interest.

References

1. Guarner, J. Three Emerging Coronaviruses in Two DecadesThe Story of SARS, MERS, and Now COVID-19. *Am. J. Clin. Pathol.* **2020**, *153*, 420–421. [CrossRef]
2. Gorbalenya, A.E.; Baker, S.C.; Baric, R.S.; de Groot, R.J.; Drosten, C.; Gulyaeva, A.A.; Haagmans, B.L.; Lauber, C.; Leontovich, A.M.; Neuman, B.W.; et al. The species Severe acute respiratory syndrome-related coronavirus: Classifying 2019-nCoV and naming it SARS-CoV-2. *Nat. Microbiol.* **2020**, *5*, 536–544. [CrossRef]
3. Li, X.; Zai, J.; Zhao, Q.; Nie, Q.; Li, Y.; Foley, B.T.; Chaillon, A. Evolutionary history, potential intermediate animal host, and cross-species analyses of SARS-CoV-2. *J. Med. Virol.* **2020**, *92*, 602–611. [CrossRef]
4. Borczuk, A.C.; Salvatore, S.P.; Seshan, S.V.; Patel, S.S.; Bussel, J.B.; Mostyka, M.; Elsoukkary, S.; He, B.; Del Vecchio, C.; Fortarezza, F.; et al. COVID-19 pulmonary pathology: A multi-institutional autopsy cohort from Italy and New York City. *Mod. Pathol.* **2020**, *33*, 2156–2168. [CrossRef] [PubMed]
5. Stoyanov, G.S.; Yanulova, N.; Stoev, L.; Zgurova, N.; Mihaylova, V.; Dzhenkov, D.L.; Stoeva, M.; Stefanova, N.; Kalchev, K.; Petkova, L. Temporal Patterns of COVID-19-Associated Pulmonary Pathology: An Autopsy Study. *Cureus* **2021**, *13*, e20522. [CrossRef] [PubMed]

6. Rockx, B.; Kuiken, T.; Herfst, S.; Bestebroer, T.; Lamers, M.M.; Munnink, B.B.O.; De Meulder, D.; Van Amerongen, G.; Van Den Brand, J.; Okba, N.M.A.; et al. Comparative pathogenesis of COVID-19, MERS, and SARS in a nonhuman primate model. *Science* **2020**, *368*, 1012–1015. [CrossRef] [PubMed]
7. Paolo, G. Does COVID-19 cause permanent damage to olfactory and gustatory function? *Med. Hypotheses* **2020**, *143*, 110086. [CrossRef] [PubMed]
8. Butowt, R.; von Bartheld, C.S. Anosmia in COVID-19: Underlying Mechanisms and Assessment of an Olfactory Route to Brain Infection. *Neuroscientist* **2020**, *27*, 582–603. [CrossRef]
9. Stoyanov, G.S.; Petkova, L.; Dzhenkov, D.L.; Sapundzhiev, N.R.; Todorov, I. Gross and Histopathology of COVID-19 with First Histology Report of Olfactory Bulb Changes. *Cureus* **2020**, *12*, e11912. [CrossRef] [PubMed]
10. Velez, J.C.Q.; Caza, T.; Larsen, C.P. COVAN is the new HIVAN: The re-emergence of collapsing glomerulopathy with COVID-19. *Nat. Rev. Nephrol.* **2020**, *16*, 565–567. [CrossRef]
11. Ng, J.H.; Zaidan, M.; Jhaveri, K.D.; Izzedine, H. Acute tubulointerstitial nephritis and COVID-19. *Clin. Kidney J.* **2021**, *14*, 2151–2157. [CrossRef] [PubMed]
12. Siripanthong, B.; Nazarian, S.; Muser, D.; Deo, R.; Santangeli, P.; Khanji, M.Y.; Cooper, L.T.; Chahal, C.A.A. Recognizing COVID-19–related myocarditis: The possible pathophysiology and proposed guideline for diagnosis and management. *Heart Rhythm* **2020**, *17*, 1463–1471. [CrossRef] [PubMed]
13. Varga, Z.; Flammer, A.J.; Steiger, P.; Haberecker, M.; Andermatt, R.; Zinkernagel, A.S.; Mehra, M.R.; Schuepbach, R.A.; Ruschitzka, F.; Moch, H. Endothelial cell infection and endotheliitis in COVID-19. *Lancet* **2020**, *6736*, 19–20. [CrossRef]
14. Aloysius, M.M., Thatti, A.; Gupta, A.; Sharma, N.; Bansal, P.; Goyal, H. COVID-19 presenting as acute pancreatitis. *Pancreatology* **2020**, *20*, 1026–1027. [CrossRef]
15. Kainth, M.K.; Goenka, P.K.; Williamson, K.A.; Fishbein, J.S.; Subramony, A.; Barone, S.; Belfer, J.A.; Feld, L.M.; Krief, W.I.; Palumbo, N.; et al. Early Experience of COVID-19 in a US Children's Hospital. *Pediatrics* **2020**, *146*, 2020003186. [CrossRef] [PubMed]
16. Bradley, B.T.; Maioli, H.; Johnston, R.; Chaudhry, I.; Fink, S.L.; Xu, H.; Najafian, B.; Deutsch, G.; Lacy, J.M.; Williams, T.; et al. Histopathology and ultrastructural findings of fatal COVID-19 infections in Washington State: A case series. *Lancet* **2020**, *396*, 320–332. [CrossRef]
17. Buja, L.M.; Wolf, D.; Zhao, B.; Akkanti, B.; McDonald, M.; Lelenwa, L.; Reilly, N.; Ottaviani, G.; Elghetany, M.T.; Trujillo, D.O.; et al. The emerging spectrum of cardiopulmonary pathology of the coronavirus disease 2019 (COVID-19): Report of 3 autopsies from Houston, Texas, and review of autopsy findings from other United States cities. *Cardiovasc. Pathol.* **2020**, *48*, 107233. [CrossRef]
18. Hoffmann, M.; Krüger, N.; Schulz, S.; Cossmann, A.; Rocha, C.; Kempf, A.; Nehlmeier, I.; Graichen, L.; Moldenhauer, A.S.; Winkler, M.S.; et al. The Omicron variant is highly resistant against antibody-mediated neutralization: Implications for control of the COVID-19 pandemic. *Cell* **2022**, *185*, 447–456.e11. [CrossRef]
19. Karim, S.S.A.; Karim, Q.A. Omicron SARS-CoV-2 variant: A new chapter in the COVID-19 pandemic. *Lancet* **2021**, *398*, 2126. [CrossRef]
20. Del Rio, C.; Omer, S.B.; Malani, P.N. Winter of Omicron—The Evolving COVID-19 Pandemic. *JAMA* **2022**, *327*, 319–320. [CrossRef]
21. Shaw, B.; Daskareh, M.; Gholamrezanezhad, A. The lingering manifestations of COVID-19 during and after convalescence: Update on long-term pulmonary consequences of coronavirus disease 2019 (COVID-19). *Radiol. Med.* **2021**, *126*, 40–46. [CrossRef] [PubMed]
22. Ellul, M.A.; Benjamin, L.; Singh, B.; Lant, S.; Michael, B.D.; Easton, A.; Kneen, R.; Defres, S.; Sejvar, J.; Solomon, T. Neurological associations of COVID-19. *Lancet Neurol.* **2020**, *19*, 767–783. [CrossRef]
23. Torres-Castro, R.; Vasconcello-Castillo, L.; Alsina-Restoy, X.; Solis-Navarro, L.; Burgos, F.; Puppo, H.; Vilaró, J. Respiratory function in patients post-infection by COVID-19: A systematic review and meta-analysis. *Pulmonology* **2021**, *27*, 328. [CrossRef] [PubMed]
24. Oronsky, B.; Larson, C.; Hammond, T.C.; Oronsky, A.; Kesari, S.; Lybeck, M.; Reid, T.R. A Review of Persistent Post-COVID Syndrome (PPCS). *Clin. Rev. Allergy Immunol.* **2021**, *1*, 1–9. [CrossRef] [PubMed]
25. Wu, Y.C.; Chen, C.S.; Chan, Y.J. The outbreak of COVID-19: An overview. *J. Chin. Med. Assoc.* **2020**, *83*, 217. [CrossRef] [PubMed]
26. Prakash, A.; Singh, H.; Sarma, P.; Bhattacharyya, A.; Dhibar, D.P.; Balaini, N.; Shree, R.; Goyal, M.; Modi, M.; Medhi, B. nCoV-2019 infection induced neurological outcome and manifestation, linking its historical ancestor SARS-CoV and MERS-CoV: A systematic review and meta analysis. *Sci. Rep.* **2021**, *11*, 12888. [CrossRef]
27. Vargas-Gandica, J.; Winter, D.; Schnippe, R.; Rodriguez-Morales, A.G.; Mondragon, J.; Escalera Antezana, J.P.; del Pilar Trelles-Thorne, M.; Bonilla-Aldana, D.K.; Rodriguez-Morales, A.J.; Paniz-Mondolfi, A. Ageusia and anosmia, a common sign of COVID-19? A case series from four countries. *J. Neurovirol.* **2020**, *26*, 785–789. [CrossRef]
28. Walker, A.; Pottinger, G.; Scott, A.; Hopkins, C. Anosmia and loss of smell in the era of covid-19. *BMJ* **2020**, *370*, m2808. [CrossRef]
29. Alshebri, M.S.; Alshouimi, R.A.; Alhumidi, H.A.; Alshaya, A.I. Neurological Complications of SARS-CoV, MERS-CoV, and COVID-19. *SN Compr. Clin. Med.* **2020**, *2*, 2037–2047. [CrossRef]

30. Peeri, N.C.; Shrestha, N.; Siddikur Rahman, M.; Zaki, R.; Tan, Z.; Bibi, S.; Baghbanzadeh, M.; Aghamohammadi, N.; Zhang, W.; Haque, U. The SARS, MERS and novel coronavirus (COVID-19) epidemics, the newest and biggest global health threats: What lessons have we learned? *Int. J. Epidemiol.* **2020**, *49*, 717–726. [CrossRef]
31. McIntosh, K. Coronaviruses: A Comparative Review. In *Current Topics in Microbiology and Immunology*; Springer: Berlin/Heidelberg, Germany, 1974; pp. 85–129. [CrossRef]
32. Ng, D.L.; Al Hosani, F.; Keating, M.K.; Gerber, S.I.; Jones, T.L.; Metcalfe, M.G.; Tong, S.; Tao, Y.; Alami, N.N.; Haynes, L.M.; et al. Clinicopathologic, Immunohistochemical, and Ultrastructural Findings of a Fatal Case of Middle East Respiratory Syndrome Coronavirus Infection in the United Arab Emirates, April 2014. *Am. J. Pathol.* **2016**, *186*, 652–658. [CrossRef] [PubMed]
33. Alsaad, K.O.; Hajeer, A.H.; Al Balwi, M.; Al Moaiqel, M.; Al Oudah, N.; Al Ajlan, A.; AlJohani, S.; Alsolamy, S.; Gmati, G.E.; Balkhy, H.; et al. Histopathology of Middle East respiratory syndrome coronovirus (MERS-CoV) infection—Clinicopathological and ultrastructural study. *Histopathology* **2018**, *72*, 516–524. [CrossRef] [PubMed]
34. Ding, Y.; Wang, H.; Shen, H.; Li, Z.; Geng, J.; Han, H.; Cai, J.; Li, X.; Kang, W.; Weng, D.; et al. The clinical pathology of severe acute respiratory syndrome (SARS): A report from China. *J. Pathol.* **2003**, *200*, 282–289. [CrossRef] [PubMed]
35. McIntosh, K.; Becker, W.B.; Chanock, R.M. Growth in suckling-mouse brain of 'IBV-like' viruses from patients with upper respiratory tract disease. *Proc. Natl. Acad. Sci. USA* **1967**, *58*, 2268–2273. [CrossRef] [PubMed]
36. Lavi, E.; Fishman, P.S.; Highkin, M.K.; Weiss, S.R. Limbic encephalitis after inhalation of a murine coronavirus. *Lab. Investig.* **1988**, *58*, 31–36.
37. Pereira Oliveira, G.; Kroon, E.G. Mouse hepatitis virus: A betacoronavirus model to study the virucidal activity of air disinfection equipment on surface contamination. *J. Virol. Methods* **2021**, *297*, 114274. [CrossRef]
38. Ahmed, M.U.; Hanif, M.; Ali, M.J.; Haider, M.A.; Kherani, D.; Memon, G.M.; Karim, A.H.; Sattar, A. Neurological Manifestations of COVID-19 (SARS-CoV-2): A Review. *Front. Neurol.* **2020**, *11*, 518. [CrossRef]
39. Vrints, C.J.M.; Krychtiuk, K.A.; Van Craenenbroeck, E.M.; Segers, V.F.; Price, S.; Heidbuchel, H. Endothelialitis plays a central role in the pathophysiology of severe COVID-19 and its cardiovascular complications. *Acta Cardiol.* **2020**, *76*, 109–124. [CrossRef]
40. Van Riel, D.; Verdijk, R.; Kuiken, T. The olfactory nerve: A shortcut for influenza and other viral diseases into the central nervous system. *J. Pathol.* **2015**, *235*, 277–287. [CrossRef]
41. Cooper, K.W.; Brann, D.H.; Farruggia, M.C.; Bhutani, S.; Pellegrino, R.; Tsukahara, T.; Weinreb, C.; Joseph, P.V.; Larson, E.D.; Parma, V.; et al. COVID-19 and the Chemical Senses: Supporting Players Take Center Stage. *Neuron* **2020**, *107*, 219–233. [CrossRef]
42. Zhu, N.; Wang, W.; Liu, Z.; Liang, C.; Wang, W.; Ye, F.; Huang, B.; Zhao, L.; Wang, H.; Zhou, W.; et al. Morphogenesis and cytopathic effect of SARS-CoV-2 infection in human airway epithelial cells. *Nat. Commun.* **2020**, *11*, 3910. [CrossRef] [PubMed]
43. Li, Y.C.; Bai, W.Z.; Hashikawa, T. The neuroinvasive potential of SARS-CoV-2 may play a role in the respiratory failure of COVID-19 patients. *J. Med. Virol.* **2020**, *92*, 552–555. [CrossRef] [PubMed]
44. Alenquer, M.; Amorim, M.J.; Graham, S.; Modis, Y. Exosome Biogenesis, Regulation, and Function in Viral Infection. *Viruses* **2015**, *7*, 5066–5083. [CrossRef]
45. Wong, S.H.; Lui, R.N.S.; Sung, J.J.Y. Covid-19 and the digestive system. *J. Gastroenterol. Hepatol.* **2020**, *35*, 744–748. [CrossRef]
46. Swanson, P.A.; McGavern, D.B. Viral diseases of the central nervous system. *Curr. Opin. Virol.* **2015**, *11*, 44–54. [CrossRef] [PubMed]
47. Ackermann, M.; Verleden, S.E.; Kuehnel, M.; Haverich, A.; Welte, T.; Laenger, F.; Vanstapel, A.; Werlein, C.; Stark, H.; Tzankov, A.; et al. Pulmonary Vascular Endothelialitis, Thrombosis, and Angiogenesis in COVID-19. *N. Engl. J. Med.* **2020**, *383*, 120–128. [CrossRef] [PubMed]
48. Angeles Montero-Fernandez, M.; Pardo-Garcia, R. Histopathology features of the lung in COVID-19 patients. *Diagn. Histopathol.* **2021**, *27*, 123–127. [CrossRef] [PubMed]
49. Bösmüller, H.; Matter, M.; Fend, F.; Tzankov, A. The pulmonary pathology of COVID-19. *Virchows Arch.* **2021**, *478*, 137–150. [CrossRef]
50. Kumar, A.; Mittal, R.; Khanna, H.D.; Basu, S. Free Radical Injury and Blood-Brain Barrier Permeability in Hypoxic-Ischemic Encephalopathy. *Pediatrics* **2008**, *122*, e722–e727. [CrossRef]
51. Lee, W.L.A.; Michael-Titus, A.T.; Shah, D.K. Hypoxic-Ischaemic Encephalopathy and the Blood-Brain Barrier in Neonates. *Dev. Neurosci.* **2017**, *39*, 49–58. [CrossRef]
52. Kuperberg, S.J.; Wadgaonkar, R. Sepsis-associated encephalopathy: The blood-brain barrier and the sphingolipid rheostat. *Front. Immunol.* **2017**, *8*, 597. [CrossRef] [PubMed]
53. Daneman, R.; Prat, A. The Blood–Brain Barrier. *Cold Spring Harb. Perspect. Biol.* **2015**, *7*, a020412. [CrossRef] [PubMed]
54. Glatzel, M. Neuropathology of COVID-19: Where are the neuropathologists? *Brain Pathol.* **2020**, *30*, 729. [CrossRef] [PubMed]

55. Pellegrini, L.; Albecka, A.; Mallery, D.L.; Kellner, M.J.; Paul, D.; Carter, A.P.; James, L.C.; Lancaster, M.A. SARS-CoV-2 Infects the Brain Choroid Plexus and Disrupts the Blood-CSF Barrier in Human Brain Organoids. *Cell Stem Cell* **2020**, *27*, 951–961.e5. [CrossRef]
56. Boumaza, A.; Gay, L.; Mezouar, S.; Diallo, A.B.; Michel, M.; Desnues, B.; Raoult, D.; La Scola, B.; Halfon, P.; Vitte, J.; et al. Monocytes and macrophages, targets of SARS-CoV-2: The clue for COVID-19 immunoparalysis. *bioRxiv* **2020**. [CrossRef]
57. Ferreira, A.C.; Soares, V.C.; de Azevedo-Quintanilha, I.G.; Dias, S.d.S.G.; Fintelman-Rodrigues, N.; Sacramento, C.Q.; Mattos, M.; de Freitas, C.S.; Temerozo, J.R.; Teixeira, L.; et al. SARS-CoV-2 engages inflammasome and pyroptosis in human primary monocytes. *Cell Death Discov.* **2021**, *7*, 43. [CrossRef]
58. Bauer, L.; Laksono, B.M.; de Vrij, F.M.S.; Kushner, S.A.; Harschnitz, O.; van Riel, D. The neuroinvasiveness, neurotropism, and neurovirulence of SARS-CoV-2. *Trends Neurosci.* **2022**, *45*, 358. [CrossRef]
59. Sfera, A.; Osorio, C.; Maguire, G.; Rahman, L.; Afzaal, J.; Cummings, M.; Maldonado, J.C. COVID-19, ferrosenescence and neurodegeneration, a mini-review. *Prog. Neuro-Psychopharmacol. Biol. Psychiatry* **2021**, *109*, 110230. [CrossRef]
60. Lippi, A.; Domingues, R.; Setz, C.; Outeiro, T.F.; Krisko, A. SARS-CoV-2: At the Crossroad between Aging and Neurodegeneration. *Mov. Disord.* **2020**, *35*, 716–720. [CrossRef]
61. Serrano, G.E.; Walker, J.E.; Arce, R.; Glass, M.J.; Vargas, D.; Sue, L.I.; Intorcia, A.J.; Nelson, C.M.; Oliver, J.; Papa, J.; et al. Mapping of SARS-CoV-2 Brain Invasion and Histopathology in COVID-19 Disease. *medRxiv* **2021**. [CrossRef]
62. Al-Sarraj, S.; Troakes, C.; Hanley, B.; Osborn, M.; Richardson, M.P.; Hotopf, M.; Bullmore, E.; Everall, I.P. Invited Review: The spectrum of neuropathology in COVID-19. *Neuropathol. Appl. Neurobiol.* **2021**, *47*, 3–16. [CrossRef] [PubMed]
63. Naz, S.; Hanif, M.; Haider, M.A.; Ali, M.J.; Ahmed, M.U.; Saleem, S. Meningitis as an Initial Presentation of COVID-19: A Case Report. *Front. Public Health* **2020**, *8*, 474. [CrossRef] [PubMed]
64. Yousefi, K.; Poorbarat, S.; Abasi, Z.; Rahimi, S.; Khakshour, A. Viral Meningitis Associated with COVID-19 in a 9-year-old Child: A Case Report. *Pediatr. Infect. Dis. J.* **2021**, *40*, E87–E98. [CrossRef]
65. Khodamoradi, Z.; Hosseini, S.A.; Gholampoor Saadi, M.H.; Mehrabi, Z.; Sasani, M.R.; Yaghoubi, S. COVID-19 meningitis without pulmonary involvement with positive cerebrospinal fluid PCR. *Eur. J. Neurol.* **2020**, *27*, 2668–2669. [CrossRef]
66. Gallacher, S.D.; Seaton, A. Meningococcal meningitis and COVID-19 co-infection. *BMJ Case Rep. CP* **2020**, *13*, e237366. [CrossRef]
67. Colombo, D.; Falasca, L.; Marchioni, L.; Tammaro, A.; Adebanjo, G.A.R.; Ippolito, G.; Zumla, A.; Piacentini, M.; Nardacci, R.; Del Nonno, F. Neuropathology and Inflammatory Cell Characterization in 10 Autoptic COVID-19 Brains. *Cells* **2021**, *10*, 2262. [CrossRef] [PubMed]
68. Tsivgoulis, G.; Palaiodimou, L.; Zand, R.; Lioutas, V.A.; Krogias, C.; Katsanos, A.H.; Shoamanesh, A.; Sharma, V.K.; Shahjouei, S.; Baracchini, C.; et al. COVID-19 and cerebrovascular diseases: A comprehensive overview. *Ther. Adv. Neurol. Disord.* **2020**, *13*, 1756286420978004. [CrossRef]
69. Reddy, S.T.; Garg, T.; Shah, C.; Nascimento, F.A.; Imran, R.; Kan, P.; Bowry, R.; Gonzales, N.; Barreto, A.; Kumar, A.; et al. Cerebrovascular Disease in Patients with COVID-19: A Review of the Literature and Case Series. *Case Rep. Neurol.* **2020**, *12*, 199–209. [CrossRef]
70. Qi, X.; Keith, K.A.; Huang, J.H. COVID-19 and stroke: A review. *Brain Hemorrhages* **2021**, *2*, 76–83. [CrossRef]
71. Zirpe, K.G.; Dixit, S.; Kulkarni, A.P.; Sapra, H.; Kakkar, G.; Gupta, R.; Bansal, A.R.; Garg, A.; Dash, S.K.; Gurnani, A.; et al. Pathophysiological Mechanisms and Neurological Manifestations in COVID-19. *Indian J. Crit. Care Med.* **2020**, *24*, 975. [CrossRef]
72. Busl, K.M.; Greer, D.M. Hypoxic-ischemic brain injury: Pathophysiology, neuropathology and mechanisms. *NeuroRehabilitation* **2010**, *26*, 5–13. [CrossRef] [PubMed]
73. Dougherty, J.H.; Rawlinson, D.G.; Levy, D.E.; Plum, F. Hypoxic-ischemic brain injury and the vegetative state. *Neurology* **1981**, *31*, 991. [CrossRef] [PubMed]
74. Dzieciatkowski, T.; Szarpak, L.; Filipiak, K.J.; Jaguszewski, M.; Ladny, J.R.; Smereka, J. COVID-19 challenge for modern medicine. *Cardiol. J.* **2020**, *27*, 175–183. [CrossRef]
75. Hu, B.; Guo, H.; Zhou, P.; Shi, Z.L. Characteristics of SARS-CoV-2 and COVID-19. *Nat. Rev. Microbiol.* **2021**, *19*, 141–154. [CrossRef]
76. Anderson, C.A.; Arciniegas, D.B. Cognitive sequelae of hypoxic-ischemic brain injury: A review. *NeuroRehabilitation* **2010**, *26*, 47–63. [CrossRef] [PubMed]
77. Reichard, R.R.; Kashani, K.B.; Boire, N.A.; Constantopoulos, E.; Guo, Y.; Lucchinetti, C.F. Neuropathology of COVID-19: A spectrum of vascular and acute disseminated encephalomyelitis (ADEM)-like pathology. *Acta Neuropathol.* **2020**, *140*, 1–6. [CrossRef] [PubMed]
78. Thakur, K.T.; Miller, E.H.; Glendinning, M.D.; Al-Dalahmah, O.; Banu, M.A.; Boehme, A.K.; Boubour, A.L.; Bruce, S.S.; Chong, A.M.; Claassen, J.; et al. COVID-19 neuropathology at Columbia University Irving Medical Center/New York Presbyterian Hospital. *Brain* **2021**, *144*, 2696–2708. [CrossRef]
79. Deigendesch, N.; Sironi, L.; Kutza, M.; Wischnewski, S.; Fuchs, V.; Hench, J.; Frank, A.; Nienhold, R.; Mertz, K.D.; Cathomas, G.; et al. Correlates of critical illness-related encephalopathy predominate postmortem COVID-19 neuropathology. *Acta Neuropathol.* **2020**, *140*, 583–586. [CrossRef]

80. Fabbri, V.P.; Foschini, M.P.; Lazzarotto, T.; Gabrielli, L.; Cenacchi, G.; Gallo, C.; Aspide, R.; Frascaroli, G.; Cortelli, P.; Riefolo, M.; et al. Brain ischemic injury in COVID-19-infected patients: A series of 10 post-mortem cases. *Brain Pathol.* **2021**, *31*, 205. [CrossRef]
81. Arrossi, A.V.; Farver, C. The pulmonary pathology of COVID-19. *Clevel. Clin. J. Med.* 2020, *in press*. [CrossRef]
82. Mullaguri, N.; Sivakumar, S.; Battineni, A.; Anand, S.; Vanderwerf, J. COVID-19 Related Acute Hemorrhagic Necrotizing Encephalitis: A Report of Two Cases and Literature Review. *Cureus* **2021**, *13*, e14236. [CrossRef] [PubMed]
83. Kumar, D.R.; Hanlin, E.R.; Glurich, I.; Mazza, J.J.; Yale, S.H. Virchow's Contribution to the Understanding of Thrombosis and Cellular Biology. *Clin. Med. Res.* **2010**, *8*, 168. [CrossRef] [PubMed]
84. Kushner, A.; West, W.P.; Pillarisetty, L.S. Virchow Triad. *Radiopaedia* **2021**. [CrossRef]
85. Van Der Meijden, P.E.J.; Munnix, I.C.A.; Auger, J.M.; Govers-Riemslag, J.W.P.; Cosemans, J.M.E.M.; Kuijpers, M.J.E.; Spronk, H.M.; Watson, S.P.; Renné, T.; Heemskerk, J.W.M. Dual role of collagen in factor XII–dependent thrombus formation. *Blood* **2009**, *114*, 881–890. [CrossRef]
86. Chaudhry, R.; Usama, S.M.; Babiker, H.M. *Physiology, Coagulation Pathways*; StatPearls: Tampa, FL, USA, 2021.
87. Farndale, R.W.; Sixma, J.J.; Barnes, M.J.; De Groot, P.G. The role of collagen in thrombosis and hemostasis. *J. Thromb. Haemost.* **2004**, *2*, 561–573. [CrossRef]
88. Nishiga, M.; Wang, D.W.; Han, Y.; Lewis, D.B.; Wu, J.C. COVID-19 and cardiovascular disease: From basic mechanisms to clinical perspectives. *Nat. Rev. Cardiol.* **2020**, *17*, 543–558. [CrossRef]
89. Metodiev, D.; Toshev, Y.; Anachkov, K.; Minkin, K.; Nachev, S. Two Cases of Encephalitis with Brainstem Involvement and Microglial Activation in SARS-CoV-2 Infection. *J. Neurol. Neurobiol.* **2021**, *7*, 1–5. [CrossRef]
90. Brown, W.R. A review of string vessels or collapsed, empty basement membrane tubes. *J. Alzheimer's Dis.* **2010**, *21*, 725–739. [CrossRef]
91. Ye, M.; Ren, Y.; Lv, T. Encephalitis as a clinical manifestation of COVID-19. *Brain Behav. Immun.* **2020**, *88*, 945. [CrossRef]
92. Jebril, N. Viral Encephalitis Associated with COVID-19: A Review of the Literature and Two Cases. *SSRN Electron. J.* **2020**, *12*, 1–6. [CrossRef]
93. Haider, A.; Siddiqa, A.; Ali, N.; Dhallu, M. COVID-19 and the Brain: Acute Encephalitis as a Clinical Manifestation. *Cureus* **2020**, *12*, e10784. [CrossRef] [PubMed]
94. Zambreanu, L.; Lightbody, S.; Bhandari, M.; Hoskote, C.; Kandil, H.; Houlihan, C.F.; Lunn, M.P. A case of limbic encephalitis associated with asymptomatic COVID-19 infection. *J. Neurol. Neurosurg. Psychiatry* **2020**, *91*, 1229–1230. [CrossRef] [PubMed]
95. Bhagat, R.; Kwiecinska, B.; Smith, N.; Peters, M.; Shafer, C.; Palade, A.; Sagi, V. New-Onset Seizure with Possible Limbic Encephalitis in a Patient with COVID-19 Infection: A Case Report and Review. *J. Investig. Med. High Impact Case Rep.* **2021**, *9*, 1–7. [CrossRef]
96. Burr, T.; Barton, C.; Doll, E.; Lakhotia, A.; Sweeney, M. N-Methyl-d-Aspartate Receptor Encephalitis Associated with COVID-19 Infection in a Toddler. *Pediatr. Neurol.* **2021**, *114*, 75. [CrossRef] [PubMed]
97. Gadani, S.; Cohen, A. Acute Necrotizing Encephalitis as an Early Manifestation of COVID-19. *Cureus* **2022**, *14*, e.27928. [CrossRef] [PubMed]
98. Ghosh, R.; Dubey, S.; Finsterer, J.; Chatterjee, S.; Ray, B.K. SARS-CoV-2-Associated Acute Hemorrhagic, Necrotizing Encephalitis (AHNE) Presenting with Cognitive Impairment in a 44-Year-Old Woman without Comorbidities: A Case Report. *Am. J. Case Rep.* **2020**, *21*, e925641-1. [CrossRef]
99. Zamani, R.; Pouremamali, R.; Rezaei, N. Central neuroinflammation in COVID-19: A systematic review of 182 cases with encephalitis, acute disseminated encephalomyelitis, and necrotizing encephalopathies. *Rev. Neurosci.* **2022**, *33*, 397–412. [CrossRef]
100. Badrfam, R.; Zandifar, A. From encephalitis lethargica to COVID-19: Is there another epidemic ahead? *Clin. Neurol. Neurosurg.* **2020**, *196*, 106065. [CrossRef]
101. Hayashi, M.; Sahashi, Y.; Baba, Y.; Okura, H.; Shimohata, T. COVID-19-associated mild encephalitis/encephalopathy with a reversible splenial lesion. *J. Neurol. Sci.* **2020**, *415*, 116941. [CrossRef]
102. Chalil, A.; Baker, C.S.; Johnston, R.B.; Just, C.; Debicki, D.B.; Mayich, M.S.; Bosma, K.J.; Steven, D.A. Acute Hemorrhagic Encephalitis Related to COVID-19. *Neurol. Clin. Pract.* **2021**, *11*, e147–e151. [CrossRef]
103. Venkatesan, A.; Benavides, D.R. Autoimmune Encephalitis and Its Relation to Infection. *Curr. Neurol. Neurosci. Rep.* **2015**, *15*, 3. [CrossRef] [PubMed]
104. Bustin, S.; Shnayder, N.A.; Sirbiladze, T.K.; Demko, I.V.; Petrova, M.M.; Nasyrova, R.F. Limbic Encephalitis Associated with COVID-19. *Encyclopedia* **2021**, *2*, 26–35. [CrossRef]
105. Matschke, J.; Lütgehetmann, M.; Hagel, C.; Sperhake, J.P.; Schröder, A.S.; Edler, C.; Mushumba, H.; Fitzek, A.; Allweiss, L.; Dandri, M.; et al. Neuropathology of patients with COVID-19 in Germany: A post-mortem case series. *Lancet Neurol.* **2020**, *19*, 919–929. [CrossRef]
106. Younger, D.S. Postmortem neuropathology in COVID-19. *Brain Pathol.* **2021**, *31*, 385. [CrossRef] [PubMed]
107. Metodiev, D.; Toshev, Y.; Anachkov, K.; Sarbyanova, N.; Nachev, S. Three Cases of Encephalopathy/Disseminated Encephalomyelitis in SARS-CoV-2 Infection. *Acta Med. Bulg.* **2022**, *49*, 51–56. [CrossRef]
108. Lyman, M.; Lloyd, D.G.; Ji, X.; Vizcaychipi, M.P.; Ma, D. Neuroinflammation: The role and consequences. *Neurosci. Res.* **2014**, *79*, 1–12. [CrossRef]
109. DiSabato, D.J.; Quan, N.; Godbout, J.P. Neuroinflammation: The devil is in the details. *J. Neurochem.* **2016**, *139*, 136–153. [CrossRef]

110. Jayakumar, A.R.; Rama Rao, K.V.; Norenberg, M.D. Neuroinflammation in Hepatic Encephalopathy: Mechanistic Aspects. *J. Clin. Exp. Hepatol.* **2015**, *5*, S21–S28. [CrossRef]
111. Cosentino, G.; Todisco, M.; Hota, N.; Della Porta, G.; Morbini, P.; Tassorelli, C.; Pisani, A. Neuropathological findings from COVID-19 patients with neurological symptoms argue against a direct brain invasion of SARS-CoV-2: A critical systematic review. *Eur. J. Neurol.* **2021**, *28*, 3856–3865. [CrossRef]
112. Maiese, A.; Manetti, A.C.; Bosetti, C.; Del Duca, F.; La Russa, R.; Frati, P.; Di Paolo, M.; Turillazzi, E.; Fineschi, V. SARS-CoV-2 and the brain: A review of the current knowledge on neuropathology in COVID-19. *Brain Pathol.* **2021**, *31*, e13013. [CrossRef]
113. Babkina, A.S.; Golubev, A.M.; Ostrova, I.V.; Volkov, A.V.; Kuzovlev, A.N. Brain morphological changes in covid-19. *Obs. Reanimatol.* **2021**, *17*, 4–15. [CrossRef]
114. Lee, M.H.; Perl, D.P.; Steiner, J.; Pasternack, N.; Li, W.; Maric, D.; Safavi, F.; Horkayne-Szakaly, I.; Jones, R.; Stram, M.N.; et al. Neurovascular injury with complement activation and inflammation in COVID-19. *Brain* **2022**, *145*, 2555–2568. [CrossRef] [PubMed]
115. Al-Dalahmah, O.; Thakur, K.T.; Nordvig, A.S.; Prust, M.L.; Roth, W.; Lignelli, A.; Uhlemann, A.C.; Miller, E.H.; Kunnath-Velayudhan, S.; Del Portillo, A.; et al. Neuronophagia and microglial nodules in a SARS-CoV-2 patient with cerebellar hemorrhage. *Acta Neuropathol. Commun.* **2020**, *8*, 147. [CrossRef] [PubMed]
116. Boldrini, M.; Canoll, P.D.; Klein, R.S. How COVID-19 Affects the Brain. *JAMA Psychiatry* **2021**, *78*, 682–683. [CrossRef]
117. Chandra, A.; Johri, A. A Peek into Pandora's Box: COVID-19 and Neurodegeneration. *Brain Sci.* **2022**, *12*, 190. [CrossRef]
118. Tavassoly, O.; Safavi, F.; Tavassoly, I. Seeding Brain Protein Aggregation by SARS-CoV-2 as a Possible Long-Term Complication of COVID-19 Infection. *ACS Chem. Neurosci.* **2020**, *11*, 3704–3706. [CrossRef]
119. Idrees, D.; Kumar, V. SARS-CoV-2 spike protein interactions with amyloidogenic proteins: Potential clues to neurodegeneration. *Biochem. Biophys. Res. Commun.* **2021**, *554*, 94–98. [CrossRef]
120. Ramani, A.; Müller, L.; Ostermann, P.N.; Gabriel, E.; Abida-Islam, P.; Müller-Schiffmann, A.; Mariappan, A.; Goureau, O.; Gruell, H.; Walker, A.; et al. SARS-CoV-2 targets neurons of 3D human brain organoids. *EMBO J.* **2020**, *39*, e106230. [CrossRef]
121. Dolatshahi, M.; Sabahi, M.; Aarabi, M.H. Pathophysiological Clues to How the Emergent SARS-CoV-2 Can Potentially Increase the Susceptibility to Neurodegeneration. *Mol. Neurobiol.* **2021**, *58*, 2379–2394. [CrossRef]
122. Bennion, D.M.; Haltigan, E.; Regenhardt, R.W.; Steckelings, U.M.; Sumners, C. Neuroprotective mechanisms of the ACE2-angiotensin-(1-7)-Mas axis in stroke. *Curr. Hypertens. Rep.* **2015**, *17*, 3. [CrossRef]
123. Solomon, I.H.; Normandin, E.; Bhattacharyya, S.; Mukerji, S.S.; Keller, K.; Ali, A.S.; Adams, G.; Hornick, J.L.; Padera, R.F.; Sabeti, P. Neuropathological Features of COVID-19. *N. Engl. J. Med.* **2020**, *383*, 989–992. [CrossRef] [PubMed]
124. Fearon, C.; Fasano, A.; Safra Program in Parkinson's Disease; Shulman, G. Parkinson's Disease and the COVID-19 Pandemic. *J. Parkinson's Dis.* **2021**, *11*, 431–444. [CrossRef] [PubMed]
125. Cartella, S.M.; Terranova, C.; Rizzo, V.; Quartarone, A.; Girlanda, P. COVID-19 and Parkinson's disease: An overview. *J. Neurol.* **2021**, *268*, 4415–4421. [CrossRef] [PubMed]
126. Cavallieri, F.; Fioravanti, V.; Toschi, G.; Grisanti, S.; Napoli, M.; Moratti, C.; Pascarella, R.; Versari, A.; Fraternali, A.; Casali, M.; et al. COVID-19 and Parkinson's disease: A casual association or a possible second hit in neurodegeneration? *J. Neurol.* **2022**, *269*, 59–61. [CrossRef] [PubMed]
127. Pavel, A.; Murray, D.K.; Stoessl, A.J. COVID-19 and selective vulnerability to Parkinson's disease. *Lancet Neurol.* **2020**, *19*, 719. [CrossRef]
128. Antonini, A.; Leta, V.; Teo, J.; Chaudhuri, K.R. Outcome of Parkinson's Disease Patients Affected by COVID-19. *Mov. Disord.* **2020**, *35*, 905. [CrossRef]
129. Fazzini, E.; Fleming, J.; Fahn, S. Cerebrospinal fluid antibodies to coronavirus in patients with Parkinson's disease. *Mov. Disord.* **1992**, *7*, 153. [CrossRef]
130. Anand, K.; Dhikav, V. Hippocampus in health and disease: An overview. *Ann. Indian Acad. Neurol.* **2012**, *15*, 239. [CrossRef]
131. Lou, J.J.; Movassaghi, M.; Gordy, D.; Olson, M.G.; Zhang, T.; Khurana, M.S.; Chen, Z.; Perez-Rosendahl, M.; Thammachantha, S.; Singer, E.J.; et al. Neuropathology of COVID-19 (neuro-COVID): Clinicopathological update. *Free Neuropathol.* **2021**, *2*, 2. [CrossRef]
132. Moriguchi, T.; Harii, N.; Goto, J.; Harada, D.; Sugawara, H.; Takamino, J.; Ueno, M.; Sakata, H.; Kondo, K.; Myose, N.; et al. A first case of meningitis/encephalitis associated with SARS-Coronavirus-2. *Int. J. Infect. Dis.* **2020**, *94*, 55. [CrossRef]
133. Klein, R.; Soung, A.; Sissoko, C.; Nordvig, A.; Canoll, P.; Mariani, M.; Jiang, X.; Bricker, T.; Goldman, J.; Rosoklija, G.; et al. COVID-19 induces neuroinflammation and loss of hippocampal neurogenesis. *Res. Sq.* 2021, *preprint*. [CrossRef]
134. Stoyanov, G.; Stoyanov, D.; Ivanov, M.; Ionchev, A.; Petkova, L.; Dzhenkov, D. Histopathological aspects of SARS-CoV-2-induced hippocampal damage. In Proceedings of the Black Sea Neurogenesis, Varna, Bulgaria, 26–28 May 2022; p. 31.
135. Poloni, T.E.; Medici, V.; Moretti, M.; Visonà, S.D.; Cirrincione, A.; Carlos, A.F.; Davin, A.; Gagliardi, S.; Pansarasa, O.; Cereda, C.; et al. COVID-19-related neuropathology and microglial activation in elderly with and without dementia. *Brain Pathol.* **2021**, *31*, e12997. [CrossRef] [PubMed]
136. Bayat, A.-H.; Azimi, H.; Hassani Moghaddam, M.; Ebrahimi, V.; Fathi, M.; Vakili, K.; Mahmoudiasl, G.-R.; Forouzesh, M.; Boroujeni, M.E.; Nariman, Z.; et al. COVID-19 causes neuronal degeneration and reduces neurogenesis in human hippocampus. *Apoptosis* 2022, *preprint*. [CrossRef] [PubMed]

137. Equilis, O.; Lekaj, K.; Fattani, S.; Wu, A.; Liu, G. Proposed mechanism for anosmia during COVID-19: The role of local zinc distribution. *J. Transl. Sci.* **2020**, *7*, 66–78. [CrossRef]
138. Al-Ani, R.M.; Acharya, D. Prevalence of Anosmia and Ageusia in Patients with COVID-19 at a Primary Health Center, Doha, Qatar. *Indian J. Otolaryngol. Head Neck Surg.* 2020, *preprint*. [CrossRef]
139. Vinh, D.B.; Zhao, X.; Kiong, K.L.; Guo, T.; Jozaghi, Y.; Yao, C.; Kelley, J.M.; Hanna, E.Y. Overview of COVID-19 testing and implications for otolaryngologists. *Head Neck* **2020**, *42*, 1629–1633. [CrossRef]
140. Zitek, T. The Appropriate Use of Testing for COVID-19. *West J. Emerg. Med.* **2020**, *21*, 470. [CrossRef]
141. Khan, M.; Yoo, S.J.; Clijsters, M.; Backaert, W.; Vanstapel, A.; Speleman, K.; Lietaer, C.; Choi, S.; Hether, T.D.; Marcelis, L.; et al. Visualizing in deceased COVID-19 patients how SARS-CoV-2 attacks the respiratory and olfactory mucosae but spares the olfactory bulb. *Cell* **2021**, *184*, 5932–5949.e15. [CrossRef]
142. Chiu, A.; Fischbein, N.; Wintermark, M.; Zaharchuk, G.; Yun, P.T.; Zeineh, M. COVID-19-induced anosmia associated with olfactory bulb atrophy. *Neuroradiology* **2020**, *63*, 147–148. [CrossRef]
143. Laurendon, T.; Radulesco, T.; Mugnier, J.; Gérault, M.; Chagnaud, C.; El Ahmadi, A.A.; Varoquaux, A. Bilateral transient olfactory bulb edema during COVID-19-related anosmia. *Neurology* **2020**, *95*, 224–225. [CrossRef]
144. Aragão, M.F.V.V.; Leal, M.C.; Cartaxo Filho, O.Q.; Fonseca, T.M.; Valença, M.M. Anosmia in COVID-19 Associated with Injury to the Olfactory Bulbs Evident on MRI. *Am. J. Neuroradiol.* **2020**, *41*, 1703–1706. [CrossRef] [PubMed]
145. Schurink, B.; Roos, E.; Radonic, T.; Barbe, E.; Bouman, C.S.C.; de Boer, H.H.; de Bree, G.J.; Bulle, E.B.; Aronica, E.M.; Florquin, S.; et al. Viral presence and immunopathology in patients with lethal COVID-19: A prospective autopsy cohort study. *Lancet Microbe* **2020**, *1*, e290–e299. [CrossRef]
146. Meinhardt, J.; Radke, J.; Dittmayer, C.; Franz, J.; Thomas, C.; Mothes, R.; Laue, M.; Schneider, J.; Brünink, S.; Greuel, S.; et al. Olfactory transmucosal SARS-CoV-2 invasion as a port of central nervous system entry in individuals with COVID-19. *Nat. Neurosci.* **2020**, *24*, 168–175. [CrossRef] [PubMed]
147. Xydakis, M.S.; Albers, M.W.; Holbrook, E.H.; Lyon, D.M.; Shih, R.Y.; Frasnelli, J.A.; Pagenstecher, A.; Kupke, A.; Enquist, L.W.; Perlman, S. Post-viral effects of COVID-19 in the olfactory system and their implications. *Lancet Neurol.* **2021**, *20*, 753–761. [CrossRef]
148. Lopez, G.; Tonello, C.; Osipova, G.; Carsana, L.; Biasin, M.; Cappelletti, G.; Pellegrinelli, A.; Lauri, E.; Zerbi, P.; Rossi, R.S.; et al. Olfactory bulb SARS-CoV-2 infection is not paralleled by the presence of virus in other central nervous system areas. *Neuropathol. Appl. Neurobiol.* **2022**, *48*, e12752. [CrossRef]
149. Lledo, P.M.; Valley, M. Adult olfactory bulb neurogenesis. *Cold Spring Harb. Perspect. Biol.* **2016**, *8*, 1–14. [CrossRef]
150. Doeppner, T.R.; Herz, J.; Bähr, M.; Tonchev, A.B.; Stoykova, A. Zbtb20 Regulates Developmental Neurogenesis in the Olfactory Bulb and Gliogenesis after Adult Brain Injury. *Mol. Neurobiol.* **2019**, *56*, 567–582. [CrossRef]
151. Baig, A.M. Loss of smell in COVID-19: Reasons for variable recovery patterns from anosmia. *Neural Regen. Res.* **2022**, *17*, 1623. [CrossRef]
152. Shanyoor, S.J.; Ali Naji, Z.M. Association of Leptin and Ghrelin Serum Levels with Anosmia and Ageusia in Iraqi COVID-19 Infected Patients. *Pak. J. Med. Health. Sci.* **2022**, *16*, 832. [CrossRef]
153. Xu, W.; Sunavala-Dossabhoy, G.; Spielman, A.I. Chemosensory loss in COVID-19. *Oral Dis.* 2022, *preprint*. [CrossRef]
154. Sampaio Rocha-Filho, P.A.; Albuquerque, P.M.; Carvalho, L.C.L.S.; Dandara Pereira Gama, M.; Magalhães, J.E. Headache, anosmia, ageusia and other neurological symptoms in COVID-19: A cross-sectional study. *J. Headache Pain* **2022**, *23*, 2. [CrossRef] [PubMed]
155. Ciolac, D.; Crivorucica, I.; Zota, E.; Gorincioi, N.; Efremova, D.; Manea, D.; Crivorucica, V.; Ciocanu, M.; Groppa, S.A. Extensive cerebellar involvement and cognitive impairment in COVID-19-associated acute necrotizing encephalopathy. *Ther. Adv. Neurol. Disord.* **2021**, *14*, 1756286420985175. [CrossRef]
156. Fadakar, N.; Ghaemmaghami, S.; Masoompour, S.M.; Shirazi Yeganeh, B.; Akbari, A.; Hooshmandi, S.; Ostovan, V.R. A First Case of Acute Cerebellitis Associated with Coronavirus Disease (COVID-19): A Case Report and Literature Review. *Cerebellum* **2020**, *19*, 911–914. [CrossRef] [PubMed]
157. Povlow, A.; Auerbach, A.J. Acute Cerebellar Ataxia in COVID-19 Infection: A Case Report. *J. Emerg. Med.* **2021**, *60*, 73–76. [CrossRef] [PubMed]
158. Reiken, S.; Sittenfeld, L.; Dridi, H.; Liu, Y.; Liu, X.; Marks, A.R. Alzheimer's-like signaling in brains of COVID-19 patients. *Alzheimer's Dement.* **2022**, *18*, 955–965. [CrossRef]
159. Kahan, J.; Gibson, C.J.; Strauss, S.B.; Bronstein, M.; Winchell, R.J.; Barie, P.S.; Segal, A.Z. Cervical spinal cord infarction associated with coronavirus infectious disease (COVID)-19. *J. Clin. Neurosci.* **2021**, *87*, 89–91. [CrossRef]
160. Kara, S.; Candelore, T.; Youssef, P.; Nedd, K. Evidence of Post-COVID-19 Transverse Myelitis Demyelination. *Cureus* **2021**, *13*, e19087. [CrossRef]
161. Nersesjan, V.; Amiri, M.; Lebech, A.M.; Roed, C.; Mens, H.; Russell, L.; Fonsmark, L.; Berntsen, M.; Sigurdsson, S.T.; Carlsen, J.; et al. Central and peripheral nervous system complications of COVID-19: A prospective tertiary center cohort with 3-month follow-up. *J. Neurol.* **2021**, *268*, 3086–3104. [CrossRef]

162. Bulfamante, G.; Bocci, T.; Falleni, M.; Campiglio, L.; Coppola, S.; Tosi, D.; Chiumello, D.; Priori, A. Brainstem neuropathology in two cases of COVID-19: SARS-CoV-2 trafficking between brain and lung. *J. Neurol.* **2021**, *268*, 4486–4491. [CrossRef]
163. Suh, J.; Mukerji, S.S.; Collens, S.I.; Padera, R.F.; Pinkus, G.S.; Amato, A.A.; Solomon, I.H. Skeletal Muscle and Peripheral Nerve Histopathology in COVID-19. *Neurology* **2021**, *97*, e849.58. [CrossRef]
164. Zhao, Y.M.; Shang, Y.M.; Song, W.B.; Li, Q.Q.; Xie, H.; Xu, Q.F.; Jia, J.L.; Li, L.M.; Mao, H.L.; Zhou, X.M.; et al. Follow-up study of the pulmonary function and related physiological characteristics of COVID-19 survivors three months after recovery. *eClinicalMedicine* **2020**, *25*, 100463. [CrossRef] [PubMed]
165. Busse, W.W.; Lemanske, R.F.; Gern, J.E. Role of viral respiratory infections in asthma and asthma exacerbations. *Lancet* **2010**, *376*, 826–834. [CrossRef]
166. Ayoubkhani, D.; Khunti, K.; Nafilyan, V.; Maddox, T.; Humberstone, B.; Diamond, I.; Banerjee, A. Post-covid syndrome in individuals admitted to hospital with COVID-19: Retrospective cohort study. *BMJ* **2021**, *372*, n693. [CrossRef] [PubMed]
167. Anaya, J.M.; Rojas, M.; Salinas, M.L.; Rodríguez, Y.; Roa, G.; Lozano, M.; Rodríguez-Jiménez, M.; Montoya, N.; Zapata, E.; Monsalve, D.M.; et al. Post-COVID syndrome. A case series and comprehensive review. *Autoimmun. Rev.* **2021**, *20*, 102947. [CrossRef]
168. Vasarmidi, E.; Tsitoura, E.; Spandidos, D.; Tzanakis, N.; Antoniou, K. Pulmonary fibrosis in the aftermath of the COVID-19 era (Review). *Exp. Ther. Med.* **2020**, *20*, 2557–2560. [CrossRef]
169. Naik, P.K.; Moore, B.B. Viral infection and aging as cofactors for the development of pulmonary fibrosis. *Expert Rev. Respir. Med.* **2010**, *4*, 759. [CrossRef]
170. Becker, J.H.; Lin, J.J.; Doernberg, M.; Stone, K.; Navis, A.; Festa, J.R.; Wisnivesky, J.P. Assessment of Cognitive Function in Patients after COVID-19 Infection. *JAMA Netw. Open* **2021**, *4*, e2130645. [CrossRef]
171. Bertuccelli, M.; Ciringione, L.; Rubega, M.; Bisiacchi, P.; Masiero, S.; Del Felice, A. Cognitive impairment in people with previous COVID-19 infection: A scoping review. *Cortex* **2022**, *154*, 212–230. [CrossRef]
172. Penninx, B.W.J.H. Psychiatric symptoms and cognitive impairment in "Long COVID": The relevance of immunopsychiatry. *World Psychiatry* **2021**, *20*, 357. [CrossRef]
173. Blazhenets, G.; Schroeter, N.; Bormann, T.; Thurow, J.; Wagner, D.; Frings, L.; Weiller, C.; Meyer, P.T.; Dressing, A.; Hosp, J.A. Slow but Evident Recovery from Neocortical Dysfunction and Cognitive Impairment in a Series of Chronic COVID-19 Patients. *J. Nucl. Med.* **2021**, *62*, 910–915. [CrossRef]
174. Lamontagne, S.J.; Winters, M.F.; Pizzagalli, D.A.; Olmstead, M.C. Post-acute sequelae of COVID-19: Evidence of mood & cognitive impairment. *Brain Behav. Immun. Health* **2021**, *17*, 100347. [CrossRef] [PubMed]
175. Ceban, F.; Ling, S.; Lui, L.M.W.; Lee, Y.; Gill, H.; Teopiz, K.M.; Rodrigues, N.B.; Subramaniapillai, M.; Di Vincenzo, J.D.; Cao, B.; et al. Fatigue and cognitive impairment in Post-COVID-19 Syndrome: A systematic review and meta-analysis. *Brain Behav Immun.* **2022**, *101*, 93–135. [CrossRef] [PubMed]
176. Abdel-Mannan, O.; Eyre, M.; Löbel, U.; Bamford, A.; Eltze, C.; Hameed, B.; Hemingway, C.; Hacohen, Y. Neurologic and Radiographic Findings Associated with COVID-19 Infection in Children. *JAMA Neurol.* **2020**, *77*, 1440–1445. [CrossRef] [PubMed]
177. Singh, A.K.; Gillies, C.L.; Singh, R.; Singh, A.; Chudasama, Y.; Coles, B.; Seidu, S.; Zaccardi, F.; Davies, M.J.; Khunti, K. Prevalence of co-morbidities and their association with mortality in patients with COVID-19: A systematic review and meta-analysis. *Diabetes Obes. Metab.* **2020**, *22*, 1915–1924. [CrossRef]
178. Andersen, K.G.; Rambaut, A.; Lipkin, W.I.; Holmes, E.C.; Garry, R.F. The proximal origin of SARS-CoV-2. *Nat. Med.* **2020**, *26*, 450–452. [CrossRef]
179. Wertheim, J.O.; Chu, D.K.W.; Peiris, J.S.M.; Kosakovsky Pond, S.L.; Poon, L.L.M. A case for the ancient origin of coronaviruses. *J. Virol.* **2013**, *87*, 7039–7045. [CrossRef]
180. Corman, V.M.; Muth, D.; Niemeyer, D.; Drosten, C. Hosts and Sources of Endemic Human Coronaviruses. *Adv. Virus Res.* **2018**, *100*, 163. [CrossRef]
181. Lalchhandama, K. The chronicles of coronaviruses: The electron microscope, the doughnut, and the spike. *Sci. Vis.* **2020**, *20*, 78–92. [CrossRef]
182. Fehr, A.R.; Perlman, S. Coronaviruses: An overview of their replication and pathogenesis. *Methods Mol. Biol.* **2015**, *1282*, 1–23. [CrossRef]
183. Woo, P.C.Y.; Lau, S.K.P.; Lam, C.S.F.; Lau, C.C.Y.; Tsang, A.K.L.; Lau, J.H.N.; Bai, R.; Teng, J.L.L.; Tsang, C.C.C.; Wang, M.; et al. Discovery of Seven Novel Mammalian and Avian Coronaviruses in the Genus Deltacoronavirus Supports Bat Coronaviruses as the Gene Source of Alphacoronavirus and Betacoronavirus and Avian Coronaviruses as the Gene Source of Gammacoronavirus and Deltacoronavirus. *J. Virol.* **2012**, *86*, 3995. [CrossRef]
184. Vijgen, L.; Keyaerts, E.; Moës, E.; Thoelen, I.; Wollants, E.; Lemey, P.; Vandamme, A.-M.; Van Ranst, M. Complete Genomic Sequence of Human Coronavirus OC43: Molecular Clock Analysis Suggests a Relatively Recent Zoonotic Coronavirus Transmission Event. *J. Virol.* **2005**, *79*, 1595. [CrossRef] [PubMed]
185. Brüssow, H.; Brüssow, L. Clinical evidence that the pandemic from 1889 to 1891 commonly called the Russian flu might have been an earlier coronavirus pandemic. *Microb. Biotechnol.* **2021**, *14*, 1860. [CrossRef] [PubMed]
186. Reid, A.H.; Mccall, S.; Henry, J.M.; Taubenberger, J.K. Experimenting on the Past: The Enigma of von Economo's Encephalitis Lethargica. *J. Neuropathol. Exp. Neurol.* **2001**, *60*, 663–670. [CrossRef] [PubMed]

187. Von Dickman, M.S. Economo Encephalitis. *Arch. Neurol.* **2001**, *58*, 1696–1698. [CrossRef] [PubMed]
188. Hoffman, L.A.; Vilensky, J.A. Encephalitis lethargica: 100 years after the epidemic. *Brain* **2017**, *140*, 2246–2251. [CrossRef] [PubMed]
189. Herishanu, Y.; Noah, Z. On Acute Encephalitic Parkinsonian Syndrome. *Eur. Neurol.* **1973**, *10*, 117–124. [CrossRef]

encyclopedia

Entry

Implementation of Blended Learning during COVID-19

Santiago Batista-Toledo * and Diana Gavilan

Department of Marketing, Complutense University of Madrid, 28040 Madrid, Spain
* Correspondence: sabatist@ucm.es

Definition: Blended learning (BL) is a teaching model that combines face-to-face activities in the classroom with activities outside the classroom through the introduction of technology that is computer-based, distance, or mobile learning, among others. There are several BL models to adopt, depending on the importance and extent to which the technology is used. It brings great benefits to the learner and involves teachers in the design of new teaching methods.

Keywords: blended learning; synchronous learning; asynchronous learning experience; COVID-19; higher education

Citation: Batista-Toledo, S.; Gavilan, D. Implementation of Blended Learning during COVID-19. *Encyclopedia* **2022**, *2*, 1763–1772. https://doi.org/10.3390/encyclopedia2040121

Academic Editors: Stephen Bustin and Raffaele Barretta

Received: 14 September 2022
Accepted: 24 October 2022
Published: 26 October 2022

1. Introduction

The COVID-19 pandemic precipitated a profound change in the global educational system, transforming the way in which education was delivered. According to UNESCO [1], 81.8% of students globally, at different academic levels, were affected by the total or partial closure of education centres. Initially, due to the lockdown, the education centers were forced to shut down, thereby shifting teaching to online platforms and resulting in an increase of up to 200% in the use of educational applications [2]. As the health situation improved, students gradually moved back to face-to-face classrooms, giving rise, in many cases, to the teaching model known as blended learning (BL), which combines face-to-face and online learning strategies.

BL allowed a partial return to the desired 'normality,' respecting the current sanitary measures of social distancing and seating capacity. However, BL also posed a challenge to the actors involved in the learning process—teachers, students, and institutions—given the infrastructure and organization required to successfully carry it out.

In universities, the implementation of BL has been prolonged more than in other levels of education, such as primary and secondary since higher education seemed to be less vulnerable to the need to return to the face-to-face teaching model. Information technology has changed the role of faculty members and the teaching–learning process itself [3]; therefore, in higher education institutions, students were prone to combine face-to-face instruction with on-line instructional resources, understanding the physical presence of the professor as a complementary form of communication [4]. This has had a more visible impact, affecting the characteristics linked to the essence of universities, such as student mobility, research, and knowledge transfer [5].

In addition, BL has had an impact on several aspects of university life, such as teaching, learning, social relations, costs, and the use of technology, all of which have turned the educational community into a true laboratory of innovation. This new educational context and the existence of new health crises resulting in situations like the one we have experienced make it necessary to study and understand how the COVID-19 pandemic has affected the educational framework, as well as its academic implications (performance, costs, quality of teaching, etc.). This will make it possible, firstly, to determine the real viability of this teaching model in educational and organizational terms and, consequently, to develop measures and policies that will favor its correct functioning in the future.

In fact, as can be seen in Figure 1, in a survey conducted in 2020 in 29 countries around the world about the future of higher education, a majority of the participants stated that they considered teaching in universities would be carried out under the BL modality five years from now [6]. The survey showed that the respondents considered blended and online teaching as normal and key, which emphasizes the importance of understanding this type of modality.

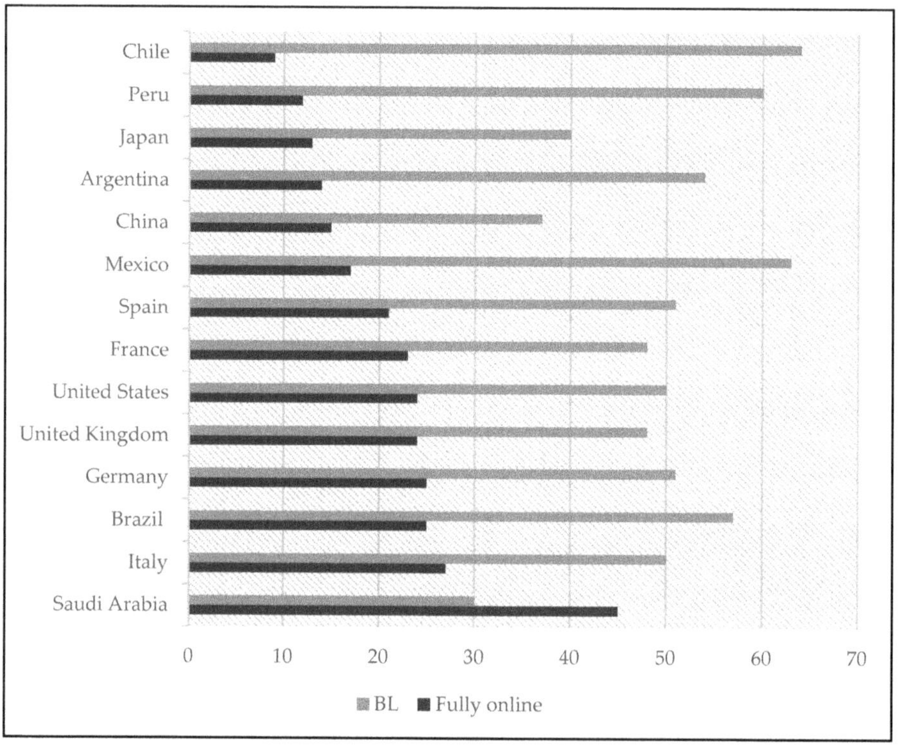

Figure 1. Sample of responses from the survey about the teaching modalities that will be used in the future for higher education.

It is also worth mentioning the different measures that were adopted by the countries considered. In general terms, universities extended deadlines for assignments or exams and modified evaluation methods. For instance, in Argentina, an online portal was developed with content for teachers and students, and in Spain, computer resources were purchased for vulnerable families. In the field of research, United Kingdom and United States created platforms to promote collaboration and inter-university research on COVID-19 [5].

The objective of this study is to show the impact of BL implementation in higher education during the pandemic. Although BL has had a gradual implementation, the pandemic forced universities to implement this type of teaching immediately to the whole community of higher education. Therefore, it is of interest to analyze the impact of BL in the experience of students and professors during COVID-19. To this end, the results of numerous academic studies are collected from the perspective of the experience of students, professors, and universities. It concludes with the challenges posed by BL during the pandemic and in the post-pandemic future. In this regard, this chapter conceptualizes the BL model, its dimensions, and the way it may be implemented. Moreover, it describes the consequences of BL experienced by both teachers and students during the COVID-19 pandemic. Finally, the technical and infrastructural implications that universities have faced while implementing BL are presented, as well as the challenges institutions will face in managing an adequate BL approach that meets their needs. To this end, the research carried out during the pandemic between 2020 and 2022 is analyzed. Understanding what the experience of BL has been like until now is crucial for the development of measures and policies favoring its correct functioning in the future.

2. Description of Blended Learning

The beginnings of BL date back to the mid-19th century when Sir Issac Pitman introduced distance learning by sending materials to his students through the mail. However, it was not until the 1960s and 1970s that the first incorporation of technology as a means of distance learning occurred. In particular, Stanford University, which was one of the first organizations to adopt distance learning, used a video network model that allowed its students to learn without the physical presence of a professor. As early as the 1990s, specific learning systems—such as CD-ROMs and web resources—were actually deve-loped, allowing teaching and training outside the classroom, thereby enhancing this type of teaching. Several continuous technological advances, from the early 2000s to the present, have been shaping what we know today as BL [7].

The definition of the phenomenon of BL itself is reflected in its evolution over the years. One of the first academic definitions of BL was from Garrison and Kanuka [8], who defined BL as 'the thoughtful integration of classroom face-to-face learning experiences with online learning experiences' (page 96). Likewise, the authors stated that for BL to take place, there must be a balance between face-to-face and online teaching methods so that neither dominates the other. However, this definition—as well as BL itself—has evolved into broader concepts closer to the definitions given by Goncharov et al. [9] or Siripongdee et al. [10]. Therefore, BL is a process of assimilating knowledge, skills, and methods through a combination of face-to-face, computer-based, distance, and mobile learning, creating an environment that allows for the incorporation and combination of any technology in or outside the classroom. Consequently, a wide variety of BL models have emerged [9]:

- Station rotation: Face-to-face and technology-based activities are alternated while students work in small groups. The teacher decides the content of the activity and gives the students a suitable tool.
- Lab rotation: Students are first taught by a teacher in a classroom and then work individually in a computer class to consolidate and build upon what they have already learned in class.
- Flipped: The student learns the theoretical material independently outside the classroom, deciding on how and when to learn. The classroom focuses on active learning, where the teacher encourages the students to clear their doubts and challenge their understanding.
- Individual rotation: Each student has a specific learning program, rotating through different activities based on their interests and abilities.
- Flexible: Students learn independently outside the classroom using online resources. Once in the classroom, they discuss what they have learned.
- Self-mix: Students choose the type of online learning they want to supplement the face-to-face classes with.
- Enriched virtual: Students mainly complete their learning online but spend several hours face-to-face with a teacher solving doubts and deepening their understanding of the concepts.

These models show the evolution of BL to satisfy the emerging needs of students and teachers. The mixture of technology-based resources with the presence of a teacher varies within each model. Eventually, technology outweighs the teacher, who becomes a guide and support for the student. This gives the student greater autonomy and decision-making ability in the learning process. This evolution also showcases the main features of BL, which are face-to-face and self-paced, as well as distant and ubiquitous [10].

In this regard, the BL case studies during COVID-19 included the use of digital applications to replace blackboards and the classroom and the encouragement of group work or the leadership assumed by the different members of the university community in carrying out their activities [11]. Other case studies pointed to the improvement in performance compared to the face-to-face modality [12].

3. The Impact of Blended Learning in Higher Education

The impact of BL has been a topic of continuous research interest in recent years around the world due to its importance in higher education. In this sense, and for the purpose of this paper, in addition to the research carried out during the pandemic, the research completed prior to the pandemic will be described in order to understand and compare the results of this phenomenon over time. Likewise, it is specified that the COVID-19 period frames the studies carried out from February 2020 to September 2021, corresponding to the phases of implementation of sanitary measures, whereas the pre-COVID-19 period refers to those studies prior to the indicated dates.

3.1. Pre-COVID-19 Period

Academically, student autonomy is one of the main benefits of BL as it allows the students to decide their own learning pace [7]. This increases the student's individual work and extends their learning outside the classroom, thus generating a continuous learning process instead of limiting learning process to the classroom [13]. Moreover, this dissociation of learning within the classroom and the addition of technological resources have made it possible for teachers to communicate with students outside of the classroom [7]. It involves a learner-centered learning style, which enhances student performance and skill achievement [14]. Specifically, compared to conventional lectures, the learner's abilities to process and acquire knowledge and solve problems are emphasized.

However, Ma and Lee [15], in a comparison between the three teaching models—face-to-face, online, and BL—stated that even though BL increases student satisfaction with respect to the other teaching models, students engagement and performance in BL model do not show a significant improvement, contradicting what is mentioned above.

One of the main characteristics of BL is the incorporation of technology. This fact favors the development of students and teachers with greater technological skills [7]. This was demonstrated by Hadiyanto et al. [14] in their research that indicated significant differences in the acquisition of digital skills in BL with respect to face-to-face classes.

For universities, it generated greater flexibility and the capacity for greater reach as it enabled them to offer more courses and programs to a larger volume of students [13]. This, in turn, led to more efficient use of the available resources [9].

From a social point of view, BL occasionally means that students are not physically present in the same place but do more individualized work. However, communication between students and teachers, as well as among students themselves, is increased. This is because BL provides the opportunity, through online activities, for social interactions to take place outside of the classroom, which has a positive impact on the students' social and communicative skills [14]. These interactions, either synchronous or asynchronous, result in the creation of a community between students and teachers [9].

Negatively, BL presents problems in terms of accessibility and equality. The need for computer equipment and internet access is a problem for students with fewer resources. It is for this reason that universities, especially public universities that guarantee equal access to the educational system for all, must support this group of students in order to maintain quality education [16].

3.2. COVID-19 Period

Students were satisfied with BL because they found it to be an environment conducive to learning, as this modality allowed for the incorporation of interesting content in face-to-face classes and effective interaction with the faculty [17]. However, students did not see this incorporation of interesting content in virtual classes [18]. This modality, in comparison with the fully online teaching modality, gave them the opportunity to have at any time and place the materials explained in class [19], in addition to having the possibility to avail the teacher's support outside of the classroom [20].

Individually, the students highlighted the flexibility they had with BL to organize their time and follow the pace of study that best suited them [17,18,21]. In particular, the fact that they did not have to travel to the university for classes saved them time that they invested in studying or in other activities. This allowed the students to be more liberated and more engaged in their learning, thus improving their academic performance [18,19]. However, they found it difficult to combine online and face-to-face activities as, in many cases, both of these overlapped [17,22].

Despite all of this, in their study, Gazica et al. [23] concluded that students reported higher levels of motivation, commitment, and fulfillment of expectations created in the face-to-face modality and preferred it over BL.

In the case of teachers, there is less research. Even so, teachers consider BL as a desirable future option due to the richness that the combination of face-to-face and online classes would bring to the learning experience [24]. As for students, introducing new content to the classes was one of the main features highlighted by teachers. Performing online activities on what was explained in the class, such as discussion forums or quizzes, allowed teachers to carry out teaching methods that were adapted to the needs of all students [25].

The web resources and online lecture recordings were highlighted by the teachers as a positive of BL, as those allowed the students to view the lecture materials as many times as they wanted. This, according to the teachers, improved the students' understanding of the subject matter [25].

The entry of technology and its importance in the development of the different activities have had implications on students. Many students perceived that BL made it difficult for them to adequately demonstrate their knowledge. This was because the students did not have the necessary training to handle and solve the problems using the different tools, generating in them the assumption that they did not show an adequate performance [21].

The teachers also found it difficult to use the online tools due to their lack of technological knowledge. One of the main problems was caused by having to request the students to keep their cameras active during online lectures, given the implications in terms of the privacy that this entailed [26]. Finally, some researchers have reported teachers' concerns about the threatening role that the entry of technology poses to their status. Specifically, they argue that modalities such as BL, which give students greater autonomy in their learning, may reduce their importance and need as actors in training. Consequently, these teachers question the capacity of online materials as substitutes for face-to-face classes [27].

In terms of socialization, the advent of BL has reduced in-person interactions among students, leading, in some cases, to a sense of social isolation among the students [21]. However, online communications in the realization of lecture activities, together with the use of social networks, have mitigated the feeling of isolation expressed by students [28]. This has strengthened relationships among the students and between the students and the teachers, creating a community that encouraged collaboration [17]. An example of this was the creation of online forums where students shared ideas and which brought teachers closer to students [27], resulting in classroom dynamics favorable for greater interactions [25].

BL has also allowed students to experience a comfortable transition from fully online to face-to-face teaching, making them feel confident about the existing health situation [22]. It was also favorable for students with mobility problems or disabilities as they were no longer obliged to travel to the university to receive the teaching, and this did not affect their learning process [18].

4. The Challenges and Opportunities of BL Implementation in Higher Education during the COVID-19 Period and Post-Pandemic

Table 1 presents the main results of both periods, showing the overlap in academic-related results and the differences in the technological and social aspects.

Table 1. Summary of the main results for each period analyzed.

	Pre COVID-19 Period	COVID-19 Period	
Academic experience	Student autonomy	Student autonomy	[7,17,19]
	Greater performance	Greater performance	[14,18,19]
	New teaching methods	New teaching methods	[7,25]
Technological experience	Lack of technological knowledge	Lack of technological knowledge	[14,21]
	Acquisition of digital skills	Loss of privacy	[14,26]
Social experience	Greater communication	Greater communication	[7,9,28]
	Problems of accessibility and equality	Favorable for students with mobility problems	[16,18]

Nevertheless, COVID-19 and the arrival of BL compelled universities to face a series of challenges for which they were not prepared. Since the beginning of the health crisis, universities had to ensure continuity in teaching, necessitating training programs for teachers on the different online tools, as well as the new pedagogical ways of teaching [29,30]. Simultaneously, universities had to invest in infrastructure and equipment to provide their centers, students, and teachers with the necessary resources to ensure that the learning process was effectively carried out in the new environment [31,32].

The universities had to develop strategies to ensure that everyone could access and attend their classes while safeguarding the students' safety from possible contagion [33]. Additionally, they had to address the potential digital divide that could affect some of the students through the provision of computer aids and equipment, as well as by developing legal frameworks to regulate issues related to the introduction of technology, such as privacy concerns (due to the obligation to activate cameras) and student assessments [34].

However, the implementation of BL has brought several opportunities for universities and educational institutions. The pandemic emphasized the development of contingency plans to be better prepared for future situations similar to this one and in enacting a rapid response. Blended learning highlighted the need to create continuous training plans for teachers and students using online tools. Likewise, in the same way the methods of teaching are changing, the students' ways of choosing the university where they will develop their studies are also changing, taking into consideration the capacity of the universities to face adverse situations in a manner that does not affect their learning. Therefore, having pre-established plans can become a determining factor in students' future university choices [32].

In this regard, the experience with BL during COVID-19 sheds light on the future of universities. Blended learning could be a potential way of attracting students [31], regardless of their location [33]. This would make it possible for universities to expand around the world while also achieving higher revenues. In addition, with students' regular use of university-managed online systems, universities could obtain a greater amount of data on their behavior that would enable them to improve their decision making and strategy development.

In summary, and according to the results of the previous research, to implement BL, it is necessary to take into account several challenges, aligned with those mentioned by Khan [35] but, specifically, with what is shown in Figure 2.

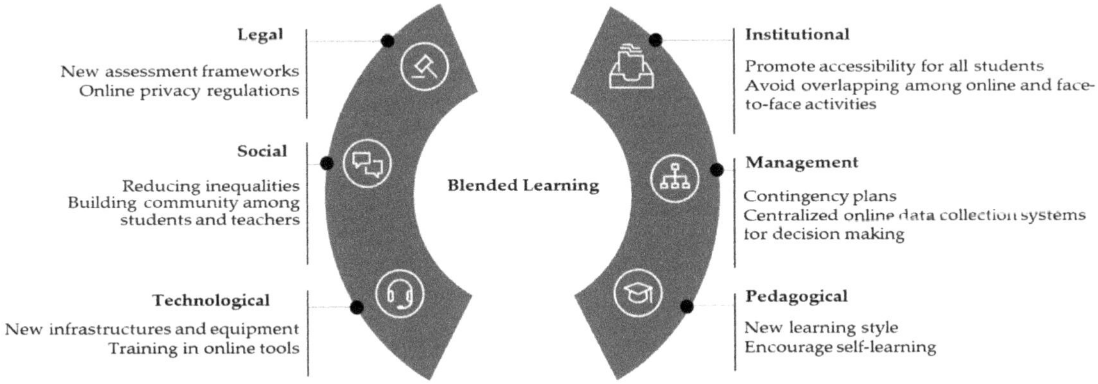

Figure 2. The challenges in and the course of action for implementing blended learning based on the COVID-19 experience.

Universities must facilitate the correct development of teaching and, in doing so, recognize the need to develop timetables and equipment in accordance with those teaching needs. A new and specific legal framework that guarantees privacy and ensures a suitable context for assessment is essential. Other challenges involve the teachers, who must be open to learning new tools and teaching methods based on greater communication with their students.

However, the major challenge with the most implications for the future is the ability to turn BL into a scalable teaching model. The high number of students in public universities, as well as the limited means available, leads to prioritizing those dimensions that best meet the needs of the university and the students. Therefore, a strong institutional leadership commitment to the implementation of such a model will be essential. This commitment must be long-lasting due to the complexity of the project and must seek the financial and personnel support necessary for success.

Other studies already agree with the challenges raised. The continuation of BL, or specific plans for its implementation, are necessary to be prepared for future situations, in addition to promoting the digital transformation of universities [36]. The problems of accessibility and inequality, especially in developing countries, require political intervention. However, solutions that involve the development of personalized educational tools and more effective pedagogies that do not prejudice the opportunity for learning are also being considered [37]. Other studies support the scalability of implementation, which should be accompanied by clear and precise measures to avoid overloading teachers [38], and we give special mention to one of the main problems discussed by Baloran [39] in relation to mental health during the pandemic. The issues of accessibility and socialization that BL can generate and exert on students' situations of anxiety are problems for which HEIs must have plans and tools to accompany and help students.

5. Conclusions

The study conducted shows BL as a teaching model that has been growing steadily to promote the development of knowledge and skills in higher education institutions [14], and that the pandemic has boosted its value. From the analysis and comparison of the results obtained from the literature, a series of conclusions about BL and its implementation can be drawn:

- The existing health situation does not seem to have altered the results obtained for BL from before the pandemic.
- The pandemic has accelerated the implementation of BL and has made it emerge as the future of universities for the globalization of teaching [40].

- Although the sudden implementation of BL has revealed the challenges that may ensue (infrastructure, lack of training, and digital divide), its positive contributions have been put into evidence (both in academic terms and resource management efficiency).
- BL can improve the quality of teaching and promote a more rational use of the technological and economic resources of universities [9] without jeopardizing academic work [41].
- BL is postulated as the first option to enrich the experience and effectiveness of student learning in new educational environments [10].
- The need to reach more students in the future while maintaining social experiences along the learning process makes BL the most viable option [16].
- The training of university faculty in the use of technology and in new teaching methodologies is the basis for the successful implementation of BL.
- Since BL is a broad concept, it is important to adopt a combination of technologies in or outside the classroom that best fits the needs of students and teachers.
- Prior research shows that the style of the teacher, the backgrounds of the students, and the subject in which the academic experience is measured can condition the results obtained [10].
- The efforts and the institutional will to implement this teaching model are necessary conditions for its correct development. BL is not about doing the same old things through a new medium [8].

In short, BL during COVID-19 developed in a complex situation, but in spite of this, BL has been able to extract the advantages of face-to-face and online teaching, demonstrating it to be a suitable teaching model and one that enhances the experience of students and teachers.

Author Contributions: Conceptualization, D.G. and S.B.-T.; resources, S.B.-T.; data curation, S.B.-T.; writing—original draft preparation, S.B.-T.; writing—review and editing, D.G.; visualization, D.G.; supervision, D.G.; project administration, D.G. All authors have read and agreed to the published version of the manuscript.

Funding: This research received no external funding.

Institutional Review Board Statement: Not applicable.

Informed Consent Statement: Not applicable.

Acknowledgments: This research has received the support of the Student Observatory of the Complutense University of Madrid, through Project POE 17-212.

Conflicts of Interest: The authors declare no conflict of interest.

References

1. UNESCO. Seguimiento Global de los Cierres de Escuelas. 2022. Available online: https://es.unesco.org/covid19/educationresponse (accessed on 7 July 2022).
2. World Economic Forum. La pandemia COVID-19 ha Cambiado la Educación Para Siempre. Así es Como. 2020. Available online: https://es.weforum.org/agenda/2020/05/la-pandemia-covid-19-ha-cambiado-la-educacion-para-siempre-asi-es-como/ (accessed on 7 July 2022).
3. Connick, G.P. Issues and Trends to Take Us into the Twenty-First Century. *New Dir. Teach. Learn.* **1997**, *1997*, 5–12. [CrossRef]
4. Jusoff, K.; Khodabandelou, R. Preliminary Study on the Role of Social Presence in Blended Learning Environment in Higher Education. *Int. Educ. Stud.* **2009**, *2*, 79–83. [CrossRef]
5. Conferencia de Rectores de las Universidades Españolas. La Universidad Frente a la Pandemia. 2020. Available online: https://www.crue.org/wp-content/uploads/2020/12/La-Universidad-frente-a-la-Pandemia.pdf (accessed on 10 July 2022).
6. La Educación del Futuro Será Online? Available online: https://es.statista.com/grafico/23692/encuesta-educacion-superior-online-o-presencial/ (accessed on 8 September 2022).
7. Singh, J.; Steele, K.; Singh, L. Combining the Best of Online and Face-to-Face Learning: Hybrid and Blended Learning Approach for COVID-19, Post Vaccine, & Post-Pandemic World. *J. Educ. Technol. Syst.* **2021**, *50*, 140–171. [CrossRef]
8. Garrison, D.R.; Kanuka, H. Blended learning: Uncovering its transformative potential in higher education. *Internet High. Educ.* **2004**, *7*, 95–105. [CrossRef]

9. Goncharov, V.V.; Stepanova, D.I.; Kovalev, D.V.; Kovaleva, T.A.; Batyrshina, A.R. Blended learning perspectives for students (university experience under constraints due to COVID-19 pandemic). *Rev. Incl.* **2020**, *7*, 288–300. Available online: https://revistainclusiones.org/index.php/inclu/article/view/1370 (accessed on 7 July 2022).
10. Siripongdee, K.; Pimdee, P.; Tuntiwongwanich, S. A blended learning model with IoT-based technology: Effectively used when the COVID-19 pandemic? *J. Educ. Gift. Young Sci.* **2020**, *8*, 905–917. [CrossRef]
11. Baumber, A.; Allen, L.; Key, T.; Kligyte, G.; Melvold, J.; Pratt, S. Teaching resilience: Enabling factors for effective responses to covid-19. *Stud. Success* **2021**, *12*, 1–12. [CrossRef]
12. Alsalhi, N.R.; Eltahir, M.; Dawi, E.; Abdelkader, A.; Zyoud, S. The Effect of Blended Learning on the Achievement in a Physics Course of Students of a Dentistry College: A Case Study at Ajman University. *Electron. J. E-Learn.* **2021**, *19*, 1–17. [CrossRef]
13. Singh, H. Building Effective Blended Learning Programs. *Educ. Technol.* **2003**, *43*, 51–54.
14. Hadiyanto, H.; Failasofah, F.; Armiwati, A.; Abrar, M.; Thabran, Y. Students' Practices of 21st Century Skills between Conventional learning and Blended Learning. *J. Univ. Teach. Learn. Pract.* **2021**, *18*, 7. [CrossRef]
15. Ma, L.; Lee, C.S. Evaluating the effectiveness of blended learning using the ARCS model. *J. Comput. Assist. Learn.* **2021**, *37*, 1397–1408. [CrossRef]
16. Carius, A.C. Network Education and Blended Learning: Cyber University concept and Higher Education post COVID-19 Pandemic. *Res. Soc. Dev.* **2020**, *9*, e8209109340. [CrossRef]
17. Lin, S.L.; Wen, T.H.; Ching, G.S.; Huang, Y.C. Experiences and challenges of an english as a medium of instruction course in taiwan during COVID-19. *Int. J. Environ. Res. Public Health* **2021**, *18*, 12920. [CrossRef]
18. Buck, E.; Tyrrell, K. Block and blend: A mixed method investigation into the impact of a pilot block teaching and blended learning approach upon student outcomes and experience. *J. Furth. High. Educ.* **2022**, 1–14. [CrossRef]
19. Peimani, N.; Kamalipour, H. The Future of Design Studio Education: Student Experience and Perception of Blended Learning and Teaching during the Global Pandemic. *Educ. Sci.* **2022**, *12*, 140. [CrossRef]
20. Finlay, M.J.; Tinnion, D.J.; Simpson, T. A virtual versus blended learning approach to higher education during the COVID-19 pandemic: The experiences of a sport and exercise science student cohort. *J. Hosp. Leis. Sport Tour. Educ.* **2022**, *30*, 100363. [CrossRef]
21. Bezliudna, V.; Shcherban, I.; Kolomiyets, O.; Mykolaiko, V.; Bezliudnyi, R. Master Students' Perceptions of Blended Learning in the Process of Studying English during COVID 19 Pandemic in Ukraine. *Rupkatha J. Interdiscip. Stud. Humanit.* **2021**, *13*, 1–14. [CrossRef]
22. Potra, S.; Pugna, A.; Pop, M.-D.; Negrea, R.; Dungan, L.; González-Zamar, M.-D.; Vázquez-Cano, E.; López Meneses, E. Facing COVID-19 Challenges: 1st-Year Students' Experience with the Romanian Hybrid Higher Educational System. *Int. J. Environ. Res. Public Health* **2021**, *18*, 3058. [CrossRef]
23. Gazica, M.W.; Leto, G.D.; Irish, A.L. The effects of unexpected changes to content delivery on student learning outcomes: A psychological contract perspective during the COVID-19 era. *Psychol. Sch.* **2022**, *59*. [CrossRef]
24. Müller, A.M.; Goh, C.; Lim, L.Z.; Gao, X. COVID-19 Emergency eLearning and Beyond: Experiences and Perspectives of University Educators. *Educ. Sci.* **2021**, *11*, 19. [CrossRef]
25. Robson, L.; Gardner, B.; Dommett, E.J. The Post-Pandemic Lecture: Views from Academic Staff across the UK. *Educ. Sci.* **2022**, *12*, 123. [CrossRef]
26. Green, J.K. Designing Hybrid Spaces for Learning in Higher Education Health Contexts. *Postdigital Sci. Educ.* **2022**, *4*, 93–115. [CrossRef]
27. Calderón, A.; Scanlon, D.; MacPhail, A.; Moody, B. An integrated blended learning approach for physical education teacher education programmes: Teacher educators' and pre-service teachers' experiences. *Phys. Educ. Sport Pedagog.* **2021**, *26*, 562–577. [CrossRef]
28. Asghar, M.Z.; Iqbal, A.; Seitamaa-Hakkarainen, P.; Barbera, E. Breaching learners' social distancing through social media during the covid-19 pandemic. *Int. J. Environ. Res. Public Health* **2021**, *18*, 11012. [CrossRef]
29. Simón, Y.V.; Melian, I.G.G.; da Silva, C. Blended learning for doctoral training in the context of the COVID-19 pandemic. *Rev. Tempos E Espaços Em Educ.* **2022**, *15*, 2. [CrossRef]
30. Verde, A.; Valero, J.M. Teaching and Learning Modalities in Higher Education During the Pandemic: Responses to Coronavirus Disease 2019 From Spain. *Front. Psychol.* **2021**, *12*, 3376. [CrossRef]
31. Roatta, S.; Tedini, D. La pandemia del COVID-19 y el aprendizaje semipresencial en la educación superior. *Rev. Iberoam. De Tecnol. En Educ. Y Educ. En Tecnol.* **2021**, *28*, 318–323. [CrossRef]
32. Al-Sholi, H.Y.; Shadid, O.R.; Alshare, K.A.; Lane, M. An agile educational framework: A response for the COVID 19 pandemic. *Cogent Educ.* **2021**, *8*, 1980939. [CrossRef]
33. Yang, B.; Huang, C. Turn crisis into opportunity in response to COVID-19: Experience from a Chinese University and future prospects. *Stud. High. Educ.* **2021**, *46*, 121–132. [CrossRef]
34. Area-Moreira, M.; Bethencourt-Aguilar, A.; Martín-Gómez, S.; Nicolás-Santos, M.A.B.S. Analysis of Higher Education Policies in Spain for Covid-19: Adapted Presence. *Rev. De Educ. A Distancia* **2021**, *21*, 19. [CrossRef]
35. Khan, B.H. The Global E-Learning Framework. In *Challenges and Opportunities for the Global Implementation of E-Learning Frameworks*, 1st ed.; Khan, B.H., Affouneh, S., Salha, S.H., Khlaif, Z.N., Eds.; IGI Global: Hershey, PA, USA, 2021; pp. 1–14.

36. Ngoatle, C.; Mothiba, T.M.; Ngoepe, M.A. Navigating through COVID-19 Pandemic Period in Implementing Quality Teaching and Learning for Higher Education Programmes: A Document Analysis Study. *Int. J. Environ. Res. Public Health* **2022**, *19*, 11146. [CrossRef] [PubMed]
37. Pokhrel, S.; Chhetri, R. A literature review on impact of COVID-19 pandemic on teaching and learning. *High. Educ. Future* **2021**, *8*, 133–141. [CrossRef]
38. Zhang, C.; Wen, M.; Tong, K.; Chen, Z.; Wen, Q.; Yang, T.; Liu, Q. Institutional Adoption and Implementation of Blended Learning in the Era of Intelligent Education. *Appl. Sci.* **2022**, *12*, 8846. [CrossRef]
39. Baloran, E.T. Knowledge, Attitudes, Anxiety, and Coping Strategies of Students during COVID-19 Pandemic. *J. Loss Trauma* **2020**, *25*, 635–642. [CrossRef]
40. Pham, H.H.; Ho, T.T.H. Toward a 'new normal' with e-learning in Vietnamese higher education during the post COVID-19 pandemic. *High. Educ. Res. Dev.* **2020**, *39*, 1327–1331. [CrossRef]
41. Ożadowicz, A. Modified blended learning in engineering higher education during the COVID-19 lockdown-building automation courses case study. *Educ. Sci.* **2020**, *10*, 292. [CrossRef]

encyclopedia

Entry

SARS, MERS and COVID-19-Associated Renal Pathology

Hristo Popov [1,*], George S. Stoyanov [1], Lilyana Petkova [1], Dimo Stoyanov [2], Martin Ivanov [2] and Anton B. Tonchev [2]

1 Department of General and Clinical Pathology, Forensic Medicine and Deontology, Faculty of Medicine, Medical University—Varna "Prof. Dr. Paraskev Stoyanov", 9002 Varna, Bulgaria
2 Department of Anatomy and Cell Biology, Faculty of Medicine, Medical University—Varna "Prof. Dr. Paraskev Stoyanov", 9002 Varna, Bulgaria
* Correspondence: popov12@abv.bg

Definition: Coronaviruses are a large group of RNA viruses, the most notable representatives of which are SARS-CoV, MERS-CoV and SARS-CoV-2. Human coronavirus infections were first documented in the 1960s, when members causing seasonal common colds were successfully replicated in human embryonal trachea and kidney cell cultures and classified based on electron microscopy. The history of coronaviruses stretched far back to that point, however, with some representatives causing disease in animals identified several decades prior and evolutionary data pointing towards the origin of this viral group more than 55 million years ago. In the short time period of research since they were discovered, coronaviruses have shown significant diversity, genetic peculiarities and varying tropism, resulting in the three identified causative agents of severe disease in humans—SARS, MERS and the most recent one, COVID-19, which has surpassed the previous two due to causing a pandemic resulting in significant healthcare, social and political consequences. Coronaviruses are likely to have caused pandemics long before, such as the so-called Asian or Russian influenza. Despite being epitheliotropic viruses and predominantly affecting the respiratory system, these entities affect multiple systems and organs, including the kidneys. In the kidneys, they actively replicate in glomerular podocytes and epithelial cells of the tubules, resulting in acute kidney injury, seen in a significant percentage of severe and fatal cases. Furthermore, the endothelial affinity of the viruses, resulting in endotheliitis, increases the likelihood of thrombotic microangiopathy, damaging the kidneys in a two-hit mechanism. As such, recently, COVAN has been a suggested nomenclature change indicating renal involvement in coronavirus infections and its long-lasting consequences.

Keywords: SARS (CoV); MERS (CoV); SARS-CoV-2; COVID-19; COVAN; nephropathology; coronavirus-associated nephritis; multisystem infection

Citation: Popov, H.; Stoyanov, G.S.; Petkova, L.; Stoyanov, D.; Ivanov, M.; Tonchev, A.B. SARS, MERS and COVID-19-Associated Renal Pathology. *Encyclopedia* **2022**, *2*, 1710–1721. https://doi.org/10.3390/encyclopedia2040117

Academic Editors: Stephen Bustin and Raffaele Barretta

Received: 29 August 2022
Accepted: 28 September 2022
Published: 9 October 2022

1. Introduction

Coronaviruses are representatives of a large group of RNA viruses [1]. According to their structure, these viruses have relatively large sizes, varying between 80 and 120 μm, but some members are characterized by smaller and significantly larger sizes—from 50 to 400 μm, with a molecular mass of about 40,000 kilodaltons [1–4]. The viral single-stranded RNA is enveloped by a double lipid membrane in which transmembrane and structural proteins are integrated, including the so-called spike proteins [5]. Formed in this way, the virion has a characteristic rayed surface, visible in electron microscopy and computer modeled reconstructions [1]. From this characteristic surface structure of the virions, they derive their name—*corona* viruses [1,6]. It is through these membrane-associated proteins that the virions bind to cell receptors, during which the viral endocytosis in the host cell takes place. Immediately after virion endocytosis, viral "undressing" occurs in the host cell's cytoplasm and viral RNA is released [7]. The structure of this RNA, with a 5′ methylated cap and a 3′ polyadenylated tail, allows it to be recognized by the granulated endoplasmic reticulum as an mRNA and thus initiate direct replication of new structural proteins for the assembly of new virions, by synthesizing a replication–transcription complex [6].

The replication–transcription complex allows the viral RNA to be replicated in multiple steps, the viral structures to be transcribed and, in the presence of at least two viral RNAs, even from another virus family, in the host cell, to recombine the sources [6]. Errors in the first two described stages and the third stage of the process give the characteristics of high mutagenicity and emergence of new virus variants; a critical clarification is that such mutant and/or recombined forms are not always vital [8]. Furthermore, the hijacking of the host cell not only disrupts its metabolism and homeostasis, leading to induced apoptosis or necrosis, but can also lead to structural, functional, or mutation alterations occurring in it [9].

After the synthesis of the necessary genetic and structural material, the process of virion assembly begins, taking place predominantly in the Golgi complex, after which new virions are released from the cell by mediated exocytosis and/or cell destruction (necrosis) and can directly infect other cells [6].

Coronaviruses exhibit epithelial tropism, with individual members having specific tissue, organ and even species tropism, as well as different modes of transmission [10]. The most common infection transmission mechanism is airborne, while there are also data on fecal–oral transmission (alimentary)—coronavirus gastroenteritis in pigs [6,10–12]. Given the diversity of structural proteins, the cellular receptors used for endocytosis vary between different entities, with the most commonly used ones being the ACE-2 and alanine aminopeptidase receptors [6,13].

As a group of viruses, they cause diseases in a large proportion of mammals, including humans, as well as in birds, i.e., are a typical example of anthropozoonosis [6,14,15]. Characteristic of the course of these infections is the involvement of the respiratory system, with the majority of representatives involving the upper respiratory tract and causing seasonal common colds with acute, predominantly serous rhinosinusitis, conjunctivitis, otitis, pharyngitis and laryngitis [14,16]. Classically, these infections are not severe; they are transient, no specific treatment is available, and if necessary, the treatment is symptomatic—nasal decongestants, antipyretics and vitamins [16].

The earliest documented data on coronavirus infections date back to the 1920s, when they were described as causing severe bronchitis in newly hatched chicks, with extremely high mortality ranging from 40% to 90% [15,17]. Newly hatched chicks had severe respiratory symptoms, and the isolated virus was named infectious bronchitis virus in 1933 and cultivated in 1937 [18,19]. In the 1940s, viral infections in mice causing encephalitis and hepatitis were also described, and at a later stage, it was understood that the three viruses described so far belong to the same group [4,20]. Human coronaviruses were described in the 1960s as the causes of common seasonal colds, in which it was impossible to cultivate the causative agent using conventional methods used for adenoviruses and rhinoviruses [21,22]. Cultivation was achieved only a few years later using tissue cultures from human embryonal trachea [23]. Descriptions of similar viruses followed in the same decade, some of which were replicated successfully in human embryonal kidney cell cultures [23–25]. Utilizing electron microscopy, it was established that all the viral pathogens described so far have a characteristic shape and membrane protrusions, which is why they were united in a joint group called coronaviruses, which later included many more representatives, based on genetic analysis, with varying organ tropism and severity of symptoms [25,26].

Evolutionarily, the earliest established ancestor of modern coronaviruses is thought to have existed about 10,000 years ago, with some evidence suggesting the presence of similar viruses about 55 million years ago in bats and birds [27]. This evolutionary theory of the origin of modern coronaviruses is well supported by the fact that the natural reservoir and source of new variants are most often bats and birds [28].

The modern classification of viruses defines these viruses in the family *coronaviridae*, with two subfamilies, *letovirinae* and *orthocoronavirinae*, of which the characteristics and entities described so far are representatives [10,29]. The *orthocoronavirinae* subfamily, in turn, consists of four *genera*—alpha, beta, gamma and delta coronavirus [27]. Alpha- and betacoronaviruses have the greatest infectious affinity for the human population, while gamma and delta are primarily zoonotic infections [10,29–31]. Betacoronaviruses are of fundamental importance to the human population, whose representations include the three most severe infections with such viruses—SARS, MERS and COVID-19 [12,32,33]. It is important to note that while the betacoronavirus family is a close relative, SARS-CoV and SARS-CoV-2 are members of the *subgenus sarbecovirus*, while MERS is a more distant relative—a member of the *subgenus* of *merbecovirus*.

Although the clinical picture in humans is relatively mild, except for some virus types, coronaviruses are thought to have caused epidemic outbreaks of severe disease long before they were identified, most often interpreted as influenza infections [6,14,16,34,35]. For example, the last major pandemic of the 19th century—the so-called Asian or Russian influenza, which caused a pandemic outbreak in 1889–1890, long considered to be influenza type 1—had similar symptoms to COVID-19, including neurological symptoms—loss of taste and smell, clouding of consciousness and encephalitis-like symptoms, all rarely seen in influenza [14,36,37]. Of course, serological data from the period do not exist, and proving a phylogenetic relationship is practically impossible.

Since emerging in late 2019, the most recent representative of severe coronaviruses, SARS-CoV-2 has led to multiple consequences, from medical and social to political and philosophical [38–41]. The clinical disease the virus causes, coronavirus disease, identified in 2019 (COVID-19), while initially regarded as a respiratory infection, has shown its multisystem nature [42,43]. While most cases present with and have the most severe clinical symptoms from the respiratory system, case reports, small cohort studies and systemic research have genuinely shown the systemic nature of the virus due to its epitheliotropism and rapid dissemination (Figure 1) [40,44–49]. The characteristics of the virus and the disease it causes are broadly representative of coronaviruses, and its pathological effects are highly similar to those of the previous two significant outbreaks—SARS and MERS.

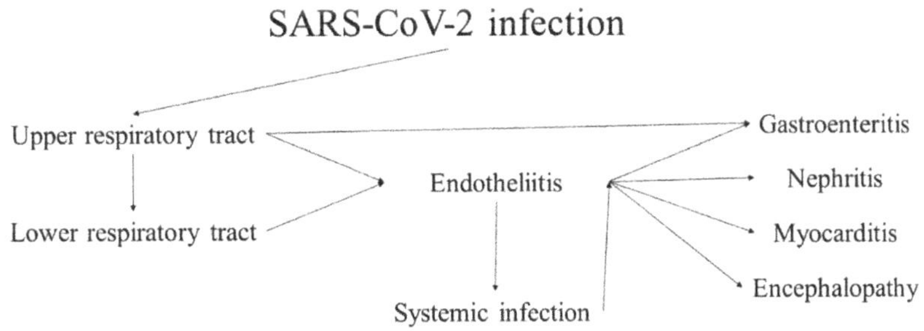

Figure 1. Progression and sequelae of SARS-CoV-2 infection (COVID-19).

2. Applications and Influences

Knowledge of the viral mechanism established in close relatives and the systemic effects of the infection are essential in caring for and treating ill patients, especially those in critical condition. Focus purely on the most severely affected system, i.e., the respiratory system, even with optimal care, while negating the effects of the virus on other systems may lead to rapid deterioration due to multisystem infection and the death of the patients, even in the absence of severe pathological effects to the respiratory system.

3. Coronaviruses and the Kidney

As already mentioned, SARS-CoV-2 is not the first entry of coronaviruses to cause an outbreak with severe health concerns in the last two decades. However, SARS-CoV-2 follows the same structural organization and similarities for tropism not only with other humans but also with animal coronaviruses that have yet to jump to human hosts. Severe acute respiratory syndrome coronavirus (SARS-CoV) and Middle Eastern respiratory syndrome coronavirus (MERS-CoV), although much less studied, are close relatives of SARS-CoV-2, and looking back at the limited reports of those infections gave some of the first hints and the possible multisystem involvement caused by these viruses and the potential health complications [33,50,51]. Furthermore, these historical data also underline the systemic effects of coronaviruses, not only the respiratory ones, but also their renal tropism, as one of the earliest ways of cultivating them was using human embryonal kidney cell cultures.

3.1. SARS-CoV

The first identified coronavirus entry of concern, SARS-CoV, began its spread in 2002 as an infection in southern China [13]. The clinical course of the disease was severe, with predominantly respiratory symptoms and a mortality rate of 11% [34,52]. A total of just over 8000 cases have been identified, of which almost 800 are fatal, with the highest mortality rate noted in the age groups over 65 years old, where it is closer to 55%, and in all age groups, the prognosis is worse in men [52,53].

Thankfully, no new disease cases have been reported worldwide since 2004, with the last reported cases linked to intra-laboratory transmission in the virus study [54].

Explainable given the small number of infected patients and deaths worldwide, data on morphological changes caused by SARS-CoV are limited, and most of them focus on the lung parenchyma changes. In a report of eight autopsy cases, Franks et al. showed morphologic changes of diffuse alveolar damage clinically correlated with patients' main clinical features of acute respiratory distress syndrome, namely pulmonary hyaline membranes, hyperplasia of type 2 pneumocytes with multinucleation, macrophage infiltration with multinucleation, squamous metaplasia, and in patients surviving more than ten days after onset of the symptomatology and organization with interstitial fibroblastic proliferation, morphological changes virtually identical to those caused by SARS-CoV-2 [55].

Lang et al., for their part, reported three autopsy cases with gross hemorrhagic areas in the subpleural aspects of the lungs, as well as a histological finding represented by intestinal lymphoplasmacytic infiltration, capillary microthrombi, fibrin thrombi in larger vessels and diffuse alveolar damage with hyaline membranes, which the authors interpret as hemorrhagic inflammation, due to erythrocytic effusion in the alveolar spaces [56]. Other, albeit non-specific, changes have been described in the spleen with follicular atrophy and acute hemorrhage [56]. Again in a report of three autopsy cases, Ding et al. reported gross consolidation of the lung parenchyma, with acute focal hemorrhages and necrotic areas [57]. The histological finding is comparable to that described so far, except for intracytoplasmic inclusions in the alveolar epithelium, which are positive for Macchiavello staining [57]. A fundamental contribution of Ding's report is the description of the extrapulmonary manifestations of the infection, which confirm follicular atrophy and acute hemorrhages in the splenic parenchyma. On the side of changes in the organs not described in the previous two reports, the authors focus on the endothelial cells in the venous vessels of the heart, which are swollen, and the vessel walls are edematous with lymphocytic infiltration, a finding that we can interpret as endotheliitis–vasculitis, without a significant morphological finding in cardiomyocytes themselves [57]. In the liver, steatosis was described, and centroacinar necrosis was extensive in two cases, as well as perivascular lymphocytic infiltration around venous vessels [57]. In the brain parenchyma, in two of the cases, in addition to advanced cerebral edema with neuronal degeneration, the authors also described perivenous vasculitis–encephalitis with focal demyelination; in the muscles, myositis of the lower limbs was established with degenerative changes and lymphocytic inflammatory infiltration in and around the small arteries and veins [57]. In the bone marrow, changes with reduction in parenchyma were described, mainly due to the decrease in granulocyte–megakaryocytic lineages and background proliferation of polychromatophilic erythroblasts [57]. Areas of necrosis and a mononuclear inflammatory infiltrate—lymphocytes and macrophages, associated with venous blood vessels as well as independently scattered in the interstitium of the kidney—with similar changes noted in the adrenal glands as well [57].

Although obtained from a small number of autopsy cases, the three independent reports show similarities in the type of lung and splenic damage, with Ding's report also showing the potential for extrapulmonary multiorgan involvement in the endotheliitis-venous vasculitis type and interstitial nephritis with necrosis [57]. Further research underlined the viral tropism to three main sites—the respiratory, gastrointestinal and urinary system—with the virus successfully replicating in the epithelial cells of the proximal tubules in the kidney, with the results being replicated ex vivo, leading to acute kidney injury with acute tubular necrosis in around 10% of cases [58–62]. However, those who developed acute kidney injury had an almost always lethal outcome [60,61].

Despite the limited literature data, the histopathology of SARS is virtually identical to that induced by SARS-CoV-2 [55–57,63–66].

3.2. MERS-CoV

The next known representative of coronaviruses causing severe clinical disease, MERS, began its spread in 2012 in Saudi Arabia [67,68]. The symptoms are similar to the previous representative with a severe clinical course. Unlike the interrupted epidemic chain of SARS, cases of MERS continue to be diagnosed to this day, and the main reason for this is the substantial spread in the natural reservoir of the infection—camels [69–71]. The main reported cases of infection transmission are primarily associated with the medical care of critically ill patients, indicating a low anthropogenic transmission potential of the virus [72–74].

The continuation of the epidemic chain also leads to new variations of the initially described virus, such as the initially described variant called Clades A (EMC/2012 and Jordan-N3/2012), while in recent years, a new variant called Clades B has emerged which, although genotypically different, leads to a similar course of the disease [75,76].

To date, nearly 3000 cases have been reported, of which nearly 900 have been fatal [77].

Again, due to the small number of cases, there are extremely few morphological reports of organ changes in cases with fatal MERS. In a report of a deceased 33-year-old male patient with T-cell lymphoma, Alsaad used an innovative technique for postmortem tissue examination by means of through-cut necropsy of lung, kidney, liver, heart, brain, and peripheral muscles taken 45 min after death [78]. Here, it is worth noting that the used methodology, although not perfect in terms of the completeness of the morphological examination, is innovative and simultaneously applicable and significantly safer in the necropsy examination of deceased patients from infectious diseases with unclear pathogenesis, organ damage, high contagiousness index and/or mortality—hazard groups three and four [79,80]. The morphological findings in the lungs show relative similarity to the lesions in SARS—diffuse alveolar damage, fibrin effusion in the alveolar spaces, interstitial infiltration by B lymphocytes and macrophages, parenchymal necrosis and subendothelial infiltration by T lymphocytes in medium-sized vessels [78]. In terms of liver changes, in addition to chronic portal hepatitis, centroacinar necrosis with polymorphonuclear infiltration was also found [78]. Degenerative-inflammatory changes with lymphocytic infiltration in the endo- and perimysium were found in the skeletal muscles [78]. No morphological changes were detected in the heart and brain [78]. In the renal parenchyma, the changes clinically correlate with acute renal failure (acute tubular injury)—dilatation of the proximal tubules with advanced cellular edema [78]. By means of electron microscopy, Alsaad also established the presence of virions in the cytoplasm and close to the nuclear membrane in pneumocytes, macrophages in the lung and muscle, as well as in the epithelial cells of the proximal segment of the renal tubules, showing a tropism of infection, not only to the lung but also to the kidney [78].

In another autopsy case report published by Ng, performed on a 45-year-old obese male, a different technique for decreasing the infectious risk of postmortem examination was applied [81]. To minimize the risk of transmission to the medical staff, the autopsy was performed ten days postmortem, during which the deceased's body was stored at 4 degrees Celsius [81]. The report also describes the gross organ findings, including 5 L of pleural effusion, 150 mL of pericardial effusion and an unspecified amount of ascites fluid, without describing the characteristics of the effusion itself (serous, fibrinous, purulent, hemorrhagic, etc.) [81]. The lungs were grossly enlarged and heavy, diffusely consolidated [81]. The morphology of lung injury is comparable to that described in Alsaad's report, with an acute phase of diffuse alveolar damage—interalveolar edema, fibrin effusion with the formation of pulmonary hyaline membranes, thickened alveolar septa, hyperplasia of type 2 pneumocytes, multinuclear syncytial cells and mixed interstitial and peribronchial infiltrate [81]. Viral particles were detected via immunohistochemistry, mainly in epithelial cells of bronchial glands and pneumocytes and macrophages [81]. Severe hypertensive changes with focal interstitial inflammation were described in the kidney [81]. No specific changes were described in the lymph nodes (reactive changes), spleen (reactive changes), bone marrow (preserved hematopoiesis with increased granulopoiesis), heart (hypertensive heart) and central nervous system [81]. In the liver, steatosis, focal calcifications and portal hepatitis were described [81]. Except for the lung parenchyma, no viral particles were detected via immunohistochemistry [81].

From a clinical perspective, more than 50% of critically ill cases develop acute kidney injury, requiring renal replacement therapy [82]. Other than direct tubular cell infection and necrosis, it has also been suggested that the effects of MERS-CoV on the kidney are also due to the induction of apoptosis in these cells [83–85].

There are also data on the morphology of chronic renal consequences of MERS in a patient who underwent a kidney biopsy eight weeks after infection due to newly appearing symptoms [85]. Morphologically, the changes were represented by acute tubular necrosis and sclerosis with protein casts and tubulointerstitial nephritis without glomerulosclerosis present [85]. However, no viral particles were detected in the biopsy [85].

Once again, as with SARS, MERS-induced histopathological changes are virtually identical to those induced by SARS-CoV-2 [55,56,63,78,81].

3.3. SARS-CoV-2

The literature is increasingly enriched with data on morphological changes in the kidney during and after SARS-CoV-2 infection, given the high frequency of clinically reported renal complications, including acute kidney injury and chronic kidney failure developing after infection [48,86,87].

At the beginning of the pandemic, initial reports on kidney morphology, predominantly case reports and small cohort studies, reported changes akin to tubulointerstitial nephritis—lymphocytic infiltration and tubular degeneration [66,87].

Evidence suggests that acute kidney injury is clinically and morphologically observed in about 50% of severe and fatal cases [88]. Most often, morphological changes are associated with acute tubular injury with epithelial swelling and necrosis, interstitial lymphocyte and macrophage infiltration and an admixture of cast nephropathy phenomena, with electron microscopy, also suggesting that there is active viral replication within the tubular epithelial cells leading to their degeneration and necrosis and inducing nephritis [87–89]. Interstitial changes reported in around 10% of fatal cases are also thrombosis, endotheliitis, cortical necrosis and infarctions, as well as myoglobin casts due to rhabdomyolysis [88]. From the glomerular aspects of the kidney injury, fatal cases often show predisposing injury such as hypertensive and diabetic nephropathy; however, it is interesting that these cases also show a significant percentage, varying around 10% as based on most studies, with thrombotic microangiopathy—glomerular capillary loop fibrin thrombi [88,90]. Interestingly, thrombotic microangiopathy in these patients develops in the context of active anticoagulant treatment, and it is suggested that without the administration of anticoagulants, a significantly higher percentage of patients with COVID-19 would develop this morphological phenomenon of glomerular injury [86,87,90]. Electron microscopy of renal tissue samples also suggests direct podocyte injury and direct viral replication in them, leading to podocyte feet shortening, desquamation and subsequent hyperplasia—a collapsing glomerulopathy form of focal segmental glomerulosclerosis, which to a large extent, in addition to the vascular changes, contributes significantly to the decreased renal function and kidney injury onset [89,91–96]. Other than the collapsing glomerulopathy form of focal segmental glomerulosclerosis, cases of pauci-immune crescentic glomerulonephritis have also been described [97].Thankfully, most patients who survive show at least moderate improvement in kidney function after COVID-19 [90]. In our practice, we have encountered patients that have previously had no kidney-related health concerns but several weeks after a mild clinical form of COVID-19 saw a rapid decrease in kidney function and required dialysis, with several other reports also depicting similar disease courses [90].

Other reported types of non-specific injury to the parenchyma, even in the context of no previous clinical signs or symptoms, have broadly been accepted as a previously unrecognized co-morbidity and include varying types of glomerulonephritis and amyloidosis [87,88,90,91].

In addition to the native kidney, data are also available for acute injury in transplanted kidneys with antibody-mediated rejection developing several weeks after COVID-19 [90,98]. In a small sample, despite most of the patients not having a severe form of COVID-19, allograft biopsy showed rejection phenomena—acute and chronic, as well as acute tubular injury and collapsing, perihilar, tip-lesion and focal segmental glomerulosclerosis, with some patients requiring dialysis due to the allograft injury [98].

3.4. COVAN

The accumulated data on COVID-19 patients, combined with the limited data available on patients with SARS and MERS, underline not only the presence of an epitheliotropism in this viral family but also the ability of severe clinical variants to manifest not as an organ-specific and limited disease, but as an actual multisystem disease. As renal involvement is relatively common in the course of COVID-19 and has a significant morphological substrate COVID-19-associated nephropathy, COVAN has been a suggested nomenclature addition to signify not only the possible acute but also chronic sequelae in these patients, especially in preexisting renal diseases (Figure 2) [48,99–102]. However, renal involvement is not universal and varies in severity; a genetic predisposition has also been suggested in people with African ancestry and APOL1 genotype [99].

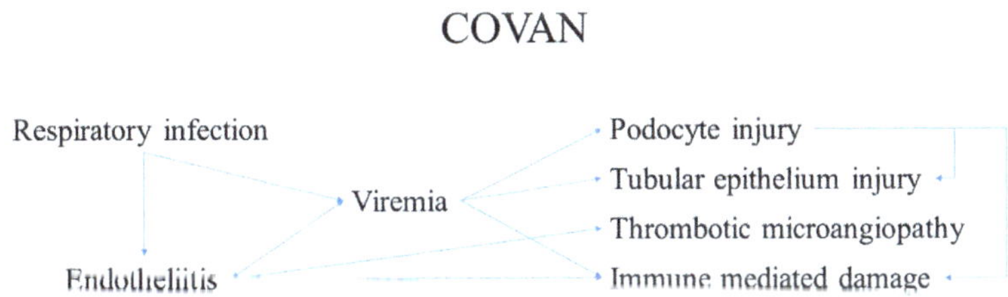

Figure 2. Development and components of COVAN.

In retrospect, COVAN, despite being discussed only in narrow fields and poorly presented to the general public, is a logical component of the disease. The presence of direct viral replication in renal epithelial cells explains the presence and a concentration correlated with the epidemiological process of SARS-CoV-2 RNA in municipal wastewater, while solid fracture wastewater concentration, while also probably correlated with COVAN, is more indicative of gastrointestinal involvement as well [103,104].

4. Conclusions and Prospects

- Coronaviruses are epitheliotropic viruses, with three variants of concern emerging over the last two decades;
- While respiratory symptoms dominate these diseases' clinical course, many other systems and organs are also a direct viral target;

- One of these is the kidney. The renal involvement, designated as COVAN, is due to:
    - direct viral replication and damage to the podocytes;
    - Direct viral replication and damage to tubule epithelial cells, resulting in:
        - glomerulopathy and tubule-interstitial nephritis with acute kidney injury, latent kidney injury and chronic kidney injury, requiring dialysis in such patients;
- One of the main non-direct components of COVAN is the development of thrombotic microangiopathy, even in the context of active anticoagulant treatments, indicating a two-hit mechanism;
- Awareness of these complications, active monitoring and preventive as well as systemic treatment will inevitably decrease mortality and improve life quality in the context of post-COVID-19 syndrome.

Author Contributions: H.P. and G.S.S. conceptualized the study; H.P. and G.S.S. performed initial literature review; H.P. performed detailed review on historical data; H.P., A.B.T., M.I., D.S. and L.P. performed review on morphology and mechanisms; G.S.S., M.I., D.S. and L.P. conceptualized and produced the figures; H.P., G.S.S. and L.P. wrote the initial manuscript; A.B.T., D.S. and M.I. performed critical revisions; A.B.T. revised and approved the final version of the manuscript for submitting; H.P., G.S.S. and A.B.T. performed revisions after review. All authors have read and approve the final version of the published manuscript.

Funding: This research received no external funding.

Institutional Review Board Statement: Not applicable.

Data Availability Statement: Not applicable.

Conflicts of Interest: The authors declare no conflict of interest.

References

1. Goldsmith, C.S.; Tatti, K.M.; Ksiazek, T.G.; Rollin, P.E.; Comer, J.A.; Lee, W.W.; Rota, P.A.; Bankamp, B.; Bellini, W.J.; Zaki, S.R. Ultrastructural characterization of SARS coronavirus. *Emerg. Infect. Dis.* **2004**, *10*, 320–326. [CrossRef] [PubMed]
2. Masters, P.S. The molecular biology of coronaviruses. *Adv. Virus Res.* **2006**, *66*, 193–292. [CrossRef] [PubMed]
3. Neuman, B.W.; Kiss, G.; Kunding, A.H.; Bhella, D.; Baksh, M.F.; Connelly, S.; Droese, B.; Klaus, J.P.; Makino, S.; Sawicki, S.G. A structural analysis of M protein in coronavirus assembly and morphology. *J. Struct. Biol.* **2011**, *174*, 11–22. [CrossRef]
4. Lalchhandama, K. The chronicles of coronaviruses: The electron microscope, the doughnut, and the spike. *Sci. Vis.* **2020**, *20*, 78–92. [CrossRef]
5. Godet, M.; L'Haridon, R.; Vautherot, J.F.; Laude, H. TGEV corona virus ORF4 encodes a membrane protein that is incorporated into virions. *Virology* **1992**, *188*, 666. [CrossRef]
6. Fehr, A.R.; Perlman, S. Coronaviruses: An overview of their replication and pathogenesis. *Methods Mol. Biol.* **2015**, *1282*, 1–23. [CrossRef]
7. Simmons, G.; Zmora, P.; Gierer, S.; Heurich, A.; Pöhlmann, S. Proteolytic activation of the SARS-coronavirus spike protein: Cutting enzymes at the cutting edge of antiviral research. *Antivir. Res.* **2013**, *100*, 605–614. [CrossRef] [PubMed]
8. Su, S.; Wong, G.; Shi, W.; Liu, J.; Lai, A.C.K.; Zhou, J.; Liu, W.; Bi, Y.; Gao, G.F. Epidemiology, Genetic Recombination, and Pathogenesis of Coronaviruses. *Trends Microbiol.* **2016**, *24*, 490–502. [CrossRef] [PubMed]
9. Zhu, N.; Wang, W.; Liu, Z.; Liang, C.; Wang, W.; Ye, F.; Huang, B.; Zhao, L.; Wang, H.; Zhou, W. Morphogenesis and cytopathic effect of SARS-CoV-2 infection in human airway epithelial cells. *Nat. Commun.* **2020**, *11*, 1–8. [CrossRef]
10. Family—Coronaviridae. *Virus Taxon.* **2012**, 806–828. [CrossRef]
11. Decaro, N. Alphacoronavirus. *Springer Index Viruses* **2011**, 371–383. [CrossRef]
12. Decaro, N. Betacoronavirus. *Springer Index Viruses* **2011**, 385–401. [CrossRef]
13. Li, F.; Li, W.; Farzan, M.; Harrison, S.C. Structure of SARS coronavirus spike receptor-binding domain complexed with receptor. *Science* **2005**, *309*, 1864–1868. [CrossRef]
14. King, A. An uncommon cold. *New Sci.* **2020**, *246*, 32. [CrossRef]
15. Estola, T. Coronaviruses, a new group of animal RNA viruses. *Avian Dis.* **1970**, *14*, 330–336. [CrossRef]
16. Liu, P.; Shi, L.; Zhang, W.; He, J.; Liu, C.; Zhao, C.; Kong, S.K.; Loo, J.F.C.; Gu, D.; Hu, L. Prevalence and genetic diversity analysis of human coronaviruses among cross-border children. *Virol. J.* **2017**, *14*, 1–8. [CrossRef]
17. Fabricant, J. The early history of infectious bronchitis. *Avian Dis.* **1998**, *42*, 648–650. [CrossRef] [PubMed]
18. Bushnell, L.D.; Brandly, C.A. Laryngotracheitis in Chicks. *Poult Sci.* **1933**, *12*, 55–60. [CrossRef]
19. Decaro, N. Gammacoronavirus‡: Coronaviridae. *Springer Index Viruses* **2011**, 403. [CrossRef]

20. McIntosh, K. Coronaviruses: A Comparative Review. *Curr. Top. Microbiol. Immunol./Ergeb. Mikrobiol. Immun.* **1974**, 85–129. [CrossRef]
21. Kahn, J.S.; McIntosh, K. History and recent advances in coronavirus discovery. *Pediatr. Infect. Dis. J.* **2005**, *24*, S223–S227. [CrossRef]
22. Mahase, E. Covid-19: First Coronavirus was described in The BMJ in 1965. *BMJ* **2020**, *369*, m1547. [CrossRef] [PubMed]
23. Tyrrell, D.A.J.; Bynoe, M.L. Cultivation of a Novel Type of Common-Cold Virus in Organ Cultures. *Br. Med. J.* **1965**, *1*, 1467–1470. [CrossRef] [PubMed]
24. Hamre, D.; Procknow, J.J. A new virus isolated from the human respiratory tract. *Proc. Soc. Exp. Biol. Med.* **1966**, *121*, 190–193. [CrossRef] [PubMed]
25. Almeida, J.D.; Tyrrell, D.A. The morphology of three previously uncharacterized human respiratory viruses that grow in organ culture. *J. Gen. Virol.* **1967**, *1*, 175–178. [CrossRef] [PubMed]
26. McIntosh, K.; Becker, W.B.; Chanock, R.M. Growth in suckling-mouse brain of 'IBV-like' viruses from patients with upper respiratory tract disease. *Proc. Natl. Acad. Sci. USA* **1967**, *58*, 2268–2273. [CrossRef] [PubMed]
27. Wertheim, J.O.; Chu, D.K.W.; Peiris, J.S.M.; Kosakovsky Pond, S.L.; Poon, L.L.M. A case for the ancient origin of coronaviruses. *J. Virol.* **2013**, *87*, 7039–7045. [CrossRef] [PubMed]
28. Woo, P.C.Y.; Lau, S.K.P.; Lam, C.S.F.; Lau, C.C.; Tsang, A.K.; Lau, J.H.; Bai, R.; Teng, J.L.; Tsang, C.C.; Wang, M. Discovery of Seven Novel Mammalian and Avian Coronaviruses in the Genus Deltacoronavirus Supports Bat Coronaviruses as the Gene Source of Alphacoronavirus and Betacoronavirus and Avian Coronaviruses as the Gene Source of Gammacoronavirus and Deltacoronavirus. *J. Virol.* **2012**, *86*, 3995–4008. [CrossRef] [PubMed]
29. Fan, Y.; Zhao, K.; Shi, Z.L.; Zhou, P. Bat Coronaviruses in China. *Viruses* **2019**, *11*, 210. [CrossRef] [PubMed]
30. Alfarouk, K.O.; AlHoufie, S.T.S.; Ahmed, S.B.M.; Shabana, M.; Ahmed, A.; Alqahtani, S.S.; Alqahtani, A.S.; Alqahtani, A.M.; Ramadan, A.M.; Ahmed, M.E. Pathogenesis and Management of COVID-19. *J. Xenobiot.* **2021**, *11*, 6. [CrossRef] [PubMed]
31. Coronaviridae Study Group of the International Committee on Taxonomy of Viruses. The species Severe acute respiratory syndrome-related coronavirus: Classifying 2019-nCoV and naming it SARS-CoV-2. *Nat. Microbiol.* **2020**, *5*, 536–544. [CrossRef] [PubMed]
32. Rockx, B.; Kuiken, T.; Herfst, S.; Bestebroer, T.; Lamers, M.M.; Oude Munnink, B.B.; de Meulder, D.; van Amerongen, G.; van den Brand, J.; Okba, N.M.A. Comparative pathogenesis of COVID-19, MERS, and SARS in a nonhuman primate model. *Science* **2020**, *368*, 1012–1015. [CrossRef] [PubMed]
33. Guarner, J. Three Emerging Coronaviruses in Two DecadesThe Story of SARS, MERS, and Now COVID-19. *Am. J. Clin. Pathol.* **2020**, *153*, 420–421. [CrossRef] [PubMed]
34. Forgie, S.; Marrie, T.J. Healthcare-associated atypical pneumonia. *Semin. Respir. Crit. Care Med.* **2009**, *30*, 67–85. [CrossRef]
35. Corman, V.M.; Muth, D.; Niemeyer, D.; Drosten, C. Hosts and Sources of Endemic Human Coronaviruses. *Adv. Virus Res.* **2018**, *100*, 163. [CrossRef] [PubMed]
36. Brüssow, H.; Brüssow, L. Clinical evidence that the pandemic from 1889 to 1891 commonly called the Russian flu might have been an earlier coronavirus pandemic. *Microb. Biotechnol.* **2021**, *14*, 1860. [CrossRef]
37. Vijgen, L.; Keyaerts, E.; Moës, E.; Thoelen, I.; Wollants, E.; Lemey, P.; Vandamme, A.M.; Van Ranst, M. Complete Genomic Sequence of Human Coronavirus OC43: Molecular Clock Analysis Suggests a Relatively Recent Zoonotic Coronavirus Transmission Event. *J. Virol.* **2005**, *79*, 1595. [CrossRef]
38. Phillips, N. The coronavirus is here to stay - here's what that means. *Nature* **2021**, *590*, 382–384. [CrossRef]
39. Andersen, K.G.; Rambaut, A.; Lipkin, W.I.; Holmes, E.C.; Garry, R.F. The proximal origin of SARS-CoV-2. *Nat. Med.* **2020**, *26*, 450–452. [CrossRef]
40. Dzieciatkowski, T.; Szarpak, L.; Filipiak, K.J.; Jaguszewski, M.; Ladny, J.R.; Smereka, J. COVID-19 challenge for modern medicine. *Cardiol. J.* **2020**, *27*, 175–183. [CrossRef]
41. Lai, J.W.; Cheong, K.H. Superposition of COVID-19 waves, anticipating a sustained wave, and lessons for the future. *BioEssays* **2020**, *42*, 2000178. [CrossRef]
42. Hu, B.; Guo, H.; Zhou, P.; Shi, Z.L. Characteristics of SARS-CoV-2 and COVID-19. *Nat. Rev. Microbiol.* **2021**, *19*, 141–154. [CrossRef]
43. Popov, G.T.; Baymakova, M.; Vaseva, V.; Kundurzhiev, T.; Mutafchiyski, V. Clinical Characteristics of Hospitalized Patients with COVID-19 in Sofia, Bulgaria. *Vector Borne Zoonotic Dis.* **2020**, *20*, 910–915. [CrossRef] [PubMed]
44. Nishiga, M.; Wang, D.W.; Han, Y.; Lewis, D.B.; Wu, J.C. COVID-19 and cardiovascular disease: From basic mechanisms to clinical perspectives. *Nat. Rev. Cardiol.* **2020**, *17*, 543–558. [CrossRef]
45. Khanna, R.C.; Cicinelli, M.V.; Gilbert, S.S.; Honavar, S.G.; Murthy, G.V.S. COVID-19 pandemic: Lessons learned and future directions. *Indian J. Ophthalmol.* **2020**, *68*, 703. [CrossRef]
46. Buja, L.M.; Wolf, D.; Zhao, B.; Akkanti, B.; McDonald, M.; Lelenwa, L.; Reilly, N.; Ottaviani, G.; Elghetany, M.T.; Trujillo, D.O.; et al. The emerging spectrum of cardiopulmonary pathology of the coronavirus disease 2019 (COVID-19): Report of 3 autopsies from Houston, Texas, and review of autopsy findings from other United States cities. *Cardiovasc. Pathol.* **2020**, *48*, 107233. [CrossRef] [PubMed]

47. Siripanthong, B.; Nazarian, S.; Muser, D.; Deo, R.; Santangeli, P.; Khanji, M.Y.; Cooper, L.T., Jr.; Chahal, C.A.A. Recognizing COVID-19–related myocarditis: The possible pathophysiology and proposed guideline for diagnosis and management. *Heart Rhythm* **2020**, *17*, 1463–1471. [CrossRef]
48. Legrand, M.; Bell, S.; Forni, L.; Joannidis, M.; Koyner, J.L.; Liu, K.; Cantaluppi, V. Pathophysiology of COVID-19-associated acute kidney injury. *Nat. Rev. Nephrol.* **2021**, *17*, 751–764. [CrossRef] [PubMed]
49. Abdel-Mannan, O.; Eyre, M.; Löbel, U.; Bamford, A.; Eltze, C.; Hameed, B.; Hemingway, C.; Hacohen, Y. Neurologic and Radiographic Findings Associated With COVID-19 Infection in Children. *JAMA Neurol.* **2020**, *77*, 1440–1445. [CrossRef] [PubMed]
50. Bradley, B.T.; Bryan, A. Emerging respiratory infections: The infectious disease pathology of SARS, MERS, pandemic influenza, and Legionella. *Semin. Diagn. Pathol.* **2019**, *36*, 152–159. [CrossRef] [PubMed]
51. Peeri, N.C.; Shrestha, N.; Siddikur Rahman, M.; Zaki, R.; Tan, Z.; Bibi, S.; Baghbanzadeh, M.; Aghamohammadi, N.; Zhang, W.; Haque, U. The SARS, MERS and novel coronavirus (COVID-19) epidemics, the newest and biggest global health threats: What lessons have we learned? *Int. J. Epidemiol.* **2020**, *49*, 717–726. [CrossRef] [PubMed]
52. Chan-Yeung, M.; Xu, R.H. SARS: Epidemiology. *Respirology* **2003**, *8*, S9. [CrossRef]
53. Consensus Document on the Epidemiology of Severe Acute Respiratory Syndrome. (SARS). Available online: http://apps.who.int/iris/handle/10665/70863 (accessed on 17 August 2022).
54. Stephenson, J. SARS in China. *JAMA* **2004**, *291*, 2534. [CrossRef]
55. Franks, T.J.; Chong, P.Y.; Chui, P.; Galvin, J.R.; Lourens, R.M.; Reid, A.H.; Selbs, E.; McEvoy, C.P.; Hayden, C.D.; Fukuoka, J.; et al. Lung pathology of severe acute respiratory syndrome (SARS): A study of 8 autopsy cases from Singapore. *Hum. Pathol.* **2003**, *34*, 743–748. [CrossRef]
56. Lang, Z.W.; Zhang, L.J.; Zhang, S.J.; Meng, X.; Li, J.Q.; Song, C.Z.; Sun, L.; Zhou, Y.S.; Dwyer, D.E. A clinicopathological study of three cases of severe acute respiratory syndrome (SARS). *Pathology* **2003**, *35*, 526–531. [CrossRef] [PubMed]
57. Ding, Y.; Wang, H.; Shen, H.; Li, Z.; Geng, J.; Han, H.; Cai, J.; Li, X.; Kang, W.; Weng, D.; et al. The clinical pathology of severe acute respiratory syndrome (SARS): A report from China. *J. Pathol.* **2003**, *200*, 282–289. [CrossRef] [PubMed]
58. Ding, Y.; He, L.; Zhang, Q.; Li, Z.; Geng, J.; Han, H.; Cai, J.; Li, X.; Kang, W.; Weng, D.; et al. Organ distribution of severe acute respiratory syndrome (SARS) associated coronavirus (SARS-CoV) in SARS patients: Implications for pathogenesis and virus transmission pathways. *J. Pathol.* **2004**, *203*, 622–630. [CrossRef]
59. Zhang, Q.L.; Ding, Y.Q.; Hou, J.L.; He, L.; Huang, Z.X.; Wang, H.J.; Cai, J.J.; Zhang, J.H.; Zhang, W.L.; Geng, J.; et al. [Detection of severe acute respiratory syndrome (SARS)-associated coronavirus RNA in autopsy tissues with in situ hybridization]. *Di Yi Jun Yi Da Xue Xue Bao* **2003**, *23*, 1125–1127. [PubMed]
60. Chu, K.H.; Tsang, W.K.; Tang, C.S.; Lam, M.F.; Lai, F.M.; To, K.F.; Fung, K.S.; Tang, H.L.; Yan, W.W.; Chan, H.W.; et al. Acute renal impairment in coronavirus-associated severe acute respiratory syndrome. *Kidney Int.* **2005**, *67*, 698–705. [CrossRef]
61. Pacciarini, F.; Ghezzi, S.; Canducci, F.; Sims, A.; Sampaolo, M.; Ferioli, E.; Clementi, M.; Poli, G.; Conaldi, P.G.; Baric, R.; et al. Persistent Replication of Severe Acute Respiratory Syndrome Coronavirus in Human Tubular Kidney Cells Selects for Adaptive Mutations in the Membrane Protein. *J. Virol.* **2008**, *82*, 5137–5144. [CrossRef] [PubMed]
62. Satija, N.; Lal, S.K. The Molecular Biology of SARS Coronavirus. *Ann. N. Y. Acad. Sci.* **2007**, *1102*, 26–38. [CrossRef] [PubMed]
63. Stoyanov, G.S.; Yanulova, N.; Stoev, L.; Zgurova, N.; Mihaylova, V.; Dzhenkov, D.L.; Stoeva, M.; Stefanova, N.; Kalchev, K.; Petkova, L. Temporal Patterns of COVID-19-Associated Pulmonary Pathology: An Autopsy Study. *Cureus* **2021**, *13*. [CrossRef] [PubMed]
64. Bradley, B.T.; Maioli, H.; Johnston, R.; Chaudhry, I.; Fink, S.L.; Xu, H.; Najafian, B.; Deutsch, G.; Lacy, J.M.; Williams, T.; et al. Histopathology and ultrastructural findings of fatal COVID-19 infections in Washington State: A case series. *Lancet* **2020**, *396*, 320–332. [CrossRef]
65. Hariri, L.P.; North, C.M.; Shih, A.R.; Israel, R.A.; Maley, J.H.; Villalba, J.A.; Vinarsky, V.; Rubin, J.; Okin, D.A.; Sclafani, A.; et al. Lung Histopathology in Coronavirus Disease 2019 as Compared With Severe Acute Respiratory Sydrome and H1N1 Influenza: A Systematic Review. *Chest* **2021**, *159*, 73–84. [CrossRef]
66. Stoyanov, G.S.; Petkova, L.; Dzhenkov, D.L.; Sapundzhiev, N.R.; Todorov, I. Gross and Histopathology of COVID-19 With First Histology Report of Olfactory Bulb Changes. *Cureus* **2020**, *12*. [CrossRef]
67. Zaki, A.M.; van Boheemen, S.; Bestebroer, T.M.; Osterhaus, A.D.M.E.; Fouchier, R.A.M. Isolation of a novel coronavirus from a man with pneumonia in Saudi Arabia. *N. Engl. J. Med.* **2012**, *367*, 1814–1820. [CrossRef]
68. Assiri, A.; Al-Tawfiq, J.A.; Al-Rabeeah, A.A.; Al-Rabiah, F.A.; Al-Hajjar, S.; Al-Barrak, A.; Flemban, H.; Al-Nassir, W.N.; Balkhy, H.H.; Al-Hakeem, R.F.; et al. Epidemiological, demographic, and clinical characteristics of 47 cases of Middle East respiratory syndrome coronavirus disease from Saudi Arabia: A descriptive study. *Lancet Infect. Dis.* **2013**, *13*, 752–761. [CrossRef]
69. Hemida, M.G.; Perera, R.A.; Wang, P.; Alhammadi, M.A.; Siu, L.Y.; Li, M.; Poon, L.L.; Saif, L.; Alnaeem, A.; Peiris, M. Middle East Respiratory Syndrome (MERS) coronavirus seroprevalence in domestic livestock in Saudi Arabia, 2010 to 2013. *Euro Surveill* **2013**, *18*, 659. [CrossRef]
70. Azhar, E.I.; El-Kafrawy, S.A.; Farraj, S.A.; Hassan, A.M.; Al-Saeed, M.S.; Hashem, A.M.; Madani, T.A. Evidence for camel-to-human transmission of MERS coronavirus. *N. Engl. J. Med.* **2014**, *370*, 2499–2505. [CrossRef]
71. Briese, T.; Mishra, N.; Jain, K.; Zalmout, I.S.; Jabado, O.J.; Karesh, W.B.; Daszak, P.; Mohammed, O.B.; Alagaili, A.N.; Lipkin, W.I. Middle East respiratory syndrome coronavirus quasispecies that include homologues of human isolates revealed through whole-genome analysis and virus cultured from dromedary camels in Saudi Arabia. *mBio* **2014**, *5*, 14. [CrossRef] [PubMed]

72. Assiri, A.; McGeer, A.; Perl, T.M.; Price, C.S.; Al Rabeeah, A.A.; Cummings, D.A.; Alabdullatif, Z.N.; Assad, M.; Almulhim, A.; Makhdoom, H.; et al. Hospital outbreak of Middle East respiratory syndrome coronavirus. *N. Engl. J. Med.* **2013**, *369*, 407–416. [CrossRef]
73. Who Mers-Cov Research Group. State of Knowledge and Data Gaps of Middle East Respiratory Syndrome Coronavirus (MERS-CoV) in Humans. *PLoS Curr.* **2013**, *5*. [CrossRef]
74. Cauchemez, S.; Fraser, C.; Van Kerkhove, M.D.; Donnelly, C.A.; Riley, S.; Rambaut, A.; Enouf, V.; van der Werf, S.; Ferguson, N.M. Middle East respiratory syndrome coronavirus: Quantification of the extent of the epidemic, surveillance biases, and transmissibility. *Lancet Infect. Dis.* **2014**, *14*, 50–56. [CrossRef]
75. Chu, D.K.W.; Poon, L.L.M.; Gomaa, M.M.; Shehata, M.M.; Perera, R.A.; Abu Zeid, D.; El Rifay, A.S.; Siu, L.Y.; Guan, Y.; Webby, R.J.; et al. MERS coronaviruses in dromedary camels, Egypt. *Emerg. Infect. Dis.* **2014**, *20*, 1049–1053. [CrossRef]
76. Saey, T.H. Story one: Scientists race to understand deadly new virus: SARS-like infection causes severe illness, but may not spread quickly among people. *Sci. News* **2013**, *183*, 5–6. [CrossRef]
77. WHO EMRO. Middle East Respiratory Syndrome. Available online: http://www.emro.who.int/health-topics/mers-cov/mers-outbreaks.html (accessed on 17 August 2022).
78. Alsaad, K.O.; Hajeer, A.H.; Al Balwi, M.; Al Moaiqel, M.; Al Oudah, N.; Al Ajlan, A.; AlJohani, S.; Alsolamy, S.; Gmati, G.E.; Balkhy, H.; et al. Histopathology of Middle East respiratory syndrome coronovirus (MERS-CoV) infection—Clinicopathological and ultrastructural study. *Histopathology* **2018**, *72*, 516–524. [CrossRef]
79. Lacy, J.M.; Brooks, E.G.; Akers, J.; Armstrong, D.; Decker, L.; Gonzalez, A.; Humphrey, W.; Mayer, R.; Miller, M.; Perez, C.; et al. COVID-19: Postmortem Diagnostic and Biosafety Considerations. *Am. J. Forensic Med. Pathol.* **2020**, *41*, 143. [CrossRef]
80. Kim, M.-Y.; Cheong, H.; Kim, H.-S. Medicine TWG for SAG for C-19 from TKS for L: Proposal of the Autopsy Guideline for Infectious Diseases: Preparation for the Post-COVID-19 Era (abridged translation). *J. Korean Med. Sci.* **2020**, *35*, 3. [CrossRef]
81. Ng, D.L.; Al Hosani, F.; Keating, M.K.; Gerber, S.I.; Jones, T.L.; Metcalfe, M.G.; Tong, S.; Tao, Y.; Alami, N.N.; Haynes, L.M.; et al. Clinicopathologic, Immunohistochemical, and Ultrastructural Findings of a Fatal Case of Middle East Respiratory Syndrome Coronavirus Infection in the United Arab Emirates, April 2014. *Am. J. Pathol.* **2016**, *186*, 652–658. [CrossRef]
82. Arabi, Y.M.; Arifi, A.A.; Balkhy, H.H.; Najm, H.; Aldawood, A.S.; Ghabashi, A.; Hawa, H.; Alothman, A.; Khaldi, A.; Al Raiy, B. Clinical course and outcomes of critically ill patients with middle east respiratory syndrome coronavirus infection. *Ann. Intern. Med.* **2014**, *160*, 389–397. [CrossRef] [PubMed]
83. Eckerle, I.; Müller, M.A.; Kallies, S.; Gotthardt, D.N.; Drosten, C. In-vitro renal epithelial cell infection reveals a viral kidney tropism as a potential mechanism for acute renal failure during Middle East Respiratory Syndrome (MERS) Coronavirus infection. *Virol. J.* **2013**, *10*, 1–5. [CrossRef] [PubMed]
84. Yeung, M.L.; Yao, Y.; Jia, L.; Chan, J.F.; Chan, K.H.; Cheung, K.F.; Chen, H.; Poon, V.K.; Tsang, A.K.; To, K.K.; et al. MERS coronavirus induces apoptosis in kidney and lung by upregulating Smad7 and FGF2. *Nat. Microbiol.* **2016**, *1*, 1–8. [CrossRef] [PubMed]
85. Cha, R.H.; Yang, S.H.; Moon, K.C.; Joh, J.S.; Lee, J.Y.; Shin, H.S.; Kim, D.K.; Kim, Y.S. A Case Report of a Middle East Respiratory Syndrome Survivor with Kidney Biopsy Results. *J. Korean Med. Sci.* **2016**, *31*, 635–640. [CrossRef]
86. Silver, S.A.; Beaubien-Souligny, W.; Shah, P.S.; Harel, S.; Blum, D.; Kishibe, T.; Meraz-Munoz, A.; Wald, R.; Harel, Z. The Prevalence of Acute Kidney Injury in Patients Hospitalized With COVID-19 Infection: A Systematic Review and Meta-analysis. *Kidney Med.* **2021**, *3*, 83–98. [CrossRef]
87. Ng, J.H.; Zaidan, M.; Jhaveri, K.D.; Izzedine, H. Acute tubulointerstitial nephritis and COVID-19. *Clin. Kidney J.* **2021**, *14*, 2151–2157. [CrossRef]
88. Rivero, J.; Merino-López, M.; Olmedo, R.; Garrido-Roldan, R.; Moguel, B.; Rojas, G.; Chavez-Morales, A.; Alvarez-Maldonado, P.; Duarte-Molina, P.; Castaño-Guerra, R.; et al. Association between Postmortem Kidney Biopsy Findings and Acute Kidney Injury from Patients with SARS-CoV-2 (COVID-19). *Clin. J. Am. Soc. Nephrol.* **2021**, *16*, 685–693. [CrossRef]
89. Diao, B.; Wang, C.C.; Wang, R.; Journet, J.; Lariotte, A.C.; Aubignat, D.; Rebibou, J.M.; De La Vega, M.F.; Legendre, M.; Belliot, G.; et al. Human kidney is a target for novel severe acute respiratory syndrome coronavirus 2 infection. *Nat. Commun.* **2021**, *12*, 1–9. [CrossRef]
90. Akilesh, S.; Nast, C.C.; Yamashita, M.; Henriksen, K.; Charu, V.; Troxell, M.L.; Kambham, N.; Bracamonte, E.; Houghton, D.; Ahmed, N.I.; et al. Multicenter Clinicopathologic Correlation of Kidney Biopsies Performed in COVID-19 Patients Presenting With Acute Kidney Injury or Proteinuria. *Am. J. Kidney Dis.* **2021**, *77*, 82–93. [CrossRef]
91. Caramaschi, S.; Kapp, M.E.; Miller, S.E.; Eisenberg, R.; Johnson, J.; Epperly, G.; Maiorana, A.; Silvestri, G.; Giannico, G.A. Histopathological findings and clinicopathologic correlation in COVID-19: A systematic review. *Mod. Pathol.* **2021**, *34*, 1614–1633. [CrossRef]
92. Gupta, R.K.; Bhargava, R.; Shaukat, A.A.; Albert, E.; Leggat, J. Spectrum of podocytopathies in new-onset nephrotic syndrome following COVID-19 disease: A report of 2 cases. *BMC Nephrol.* **2020**, *21*, 1–7. [CrossRef]
93. Deshmukh, S.; Zhou, X.J.; Hiser, W. Collapsing glomerulopathy in a patient of Indian descent in the setting of COVID-19. *Ren. Fail.* **2020**, *42*, 877. [CrossRef] [PubMed]
94. Pasupulati, A.K. Is Podocyte Injury During COVID-19 Infection Contributes To Proteinuria and A Threat To Renal Failure ? *J. Clin. Nephrol. Res.* **2020**, *7*, 7–1096.

95. Sharma, Y.; Nasr, S.H.; Larsen, C.P.; Kemper, A.; Ormsby, A.H.; Williamson, S.R. COVID-19–Associated Collapsing Focal Segmental Glomerulosclerosis: A Report of 2 Cases. *Kidney Med.* **2020**, *2*, 493–497. [CrossRef]
96. Magoon, S.; Bichu, P.; Malhotra, V.; Alhashimi, F.; Hu, Y.; Khanna, S.; Berhanu, K. COVID-19–Related Glomerulopathy: A Report of 2 Cases of Collapsing Focal Segmental Glomerulosclerosis. *Kidney Med.* **2020**, *2*, 488–492. [CrossRef] [PubMed]
97. Sharma, P.; Uppal, N.N.; Wanchoo, R.; Shah, H.H.; Yang, Y.; Parikh, R.; Khanin, Y.; Madireddy, V.; Larsen, C.P.; Jhaveri, K.D.; et al. COVID-19–Associated Kidney Injury: A Case Series of Kidney Biopsy Findings. *J. Am. Soc. Nephrol.* **2020**, *31*, 1948–1958. [CrossRef] [PubMed]
98. Basic-Jukic, N.; Coric, M.; Bulimbasic, S.; Dika, Z.; Juric, I.; Furic-Cunko, V.; Katalinic, L.; Kos, J.; Fistrek, M.; Kastelan, Z.; et al. Histopathologic findings on indication renal allograft biopsies after recovery from acute COVID-19. *Clin. Transplant.* **2021**, *35*, e14486. [CrossRef]
99. Velez, J.C.Q.; Caza, T.; Larsen, C.P. COVAN is the new HIVAN: The re-emergence of collapsing glomerulopathy with COVID-19. *Nat. Rev. Nephrol.* **2020**, *16*, 565–567. [CrossRef]
100. Bouquegneau, A.; Erpicum, P.; Grosch, S.; Habran, L.; Hougrand, O.; Huart, J.; Krzesinski, J.M.; Misset, B.; Hayette, M.P.; Delvenne, P.; et al. COVID-19–associated Nephropathy Includes Tubular Necrosis and Capillary Congestion, with Evidence of SARS-CoV-2 in the Nephron. *Kidney360* **2021**, *2*, 639. [CrossRef]
101. Meijers, B.; Hilbrands, L.B. The clinical characteristics of coronavirus-associated nephropathy. *Nephrol. Dial. Transplant.* **2020**, *35*, 1279–1281. [CrossRef]
102. Shetty, A.A.; Tawhari, I.; Safar-Boueri, L.; Seif, N.; Alahmadi, A.; Gargiulo, R.; Aggarwal, V.; Usman, I.; Kisselev, S.; Gharavi, A.G.; et al. COVID-19-associated glomerular disease. *J. Am. Soc. Nephrol.* **2021**, *32*, 33–40. [CrossRef]
103. Nemudryi, A.; Nemudraia, A.; Wiegand, T.; Surya, K.; Buyukyoruk, M.; Cicha, C.; Vanderwood, K.K.; Wilkinson, R.; Wiedenheft, B. Temporal Detection and Phylogenetic Assessment of SARS-CoV-2 in Municipal Wastewater. *Cell Rep. Med.* **2020**, *1*, 100098. [CrossRef] [PubMed]
104. Kitamura, K.; Sadamasu, K.; Muramatsu, M.; Yoshida, H. Efficient detection of SARS-CoV-2 RNA in the solid fraction of wastewater. *Sci. Total Environ.* **2021**, *763*, 144587. [CrossRef] [PubMed]

encyclopedia MDPI

Entry

SARS-CoV-2 Associated Pulmonary Pathology

George S. Stoyanov [1,*], Hristo Popov [1], Lilyana Petkova [1], Dimo Stoyanov [2], Martin Ivanov [2] and Anton B. Tonchev [2]

1 Department of General and Clinical Pathology, Forensic Medicine and Deontology, Faculty of Medicine, Medical University—Varna "Prof. Dr. Paraskev Stoyanov", 9002 Varna, Bulgaria
2 Department of Anatomy and Cell Biology, Faculty of Medicine, Medical University—Varna "Prof. Dr. Paraskev Stoyanov", 9002 Varna, Bulgaria
* Correspondence: georgi.geesh@gmail.com

Definition: Severe acute respiratory syndrome coronavirus 2 (SARS-CoV-2) is a novel entry in the betacoronaviridae group of coronaviruses. This is the second member of this group, and the third of the family overall to emerge in the last 20 years, which has caused significant health concerns due to the clinical severity and spread of the disease it causes—coronavirus disease identified in 2019 (COVID-19). While initially emerging as a respiratory disease, and while most cases experience symptoms predominantly from this system, SARS-CoV-2 has emerged as a multisystem pathogen. From a pathomorphological point of view, the severity of changes in the respiratory system can be summed up as diffuse alveolar damage—desquamation of the alveolar epithelium with exudative and proliferative changes—pulmonary hyaline membranes, Clara cell hyperplasia, squamous cell metaplasia, and fibrosis. The second most prominent way the disease affects the lung is through endotheliitis—damage to the endothelial cells of the pulmonary vasculature, predominantly affecting the medium and large caliber blood vessels that cause the well-established clinical phenomenon of thrombosis/thromboembolism of the pulmonary vasculature. As the spread of the disease continues with the emergence of new variants and the number of cases continues to grow, including a large percentage of recurrent cases, it is essential to remember that the viral effects are not only acute but, due to the proliferative phenomena, can produce chronic sequelae. Therefore, in the background of dwindling publication interest, it is critical to focus on the histopathological aspects of the pulmonary disease, with the goal of better understanding the effects of the virus on the organism and identifying probable future complications after infection.

Keywords: SARS-CoV-2; COVID-19; pathology; autopsy; diffuse alveolar damage; pulmonary pathology; virus-induced lung damage; long COVID

Citation: Stoyanov, G.S.; Popov, H.; Petkova, L.; Stoyanov, D.; Ivanov, M.; Tonchev, A.B. SARS-CoV-2 Associated Pulmonary Pathology. *Encyclopedia* **2022**, 2, 1698–1709. https://doi.org/10.3390/encyclopedia2040116

Academic Editor: Stephen Bustin and Raffaele Barretta

Received: 30 July 2022
Accepted: 22 September 2022
Published: 30 September 2022

1. Introduction

The novel representative of coronaviruses (SARS-CoV-2) and the clinical disease it causes (COVID-19), which emerged at the end of 2019, have led to healthcare and social consequences not seen in the last 100 years [1–6]. The rapid spread of the infection, the severe organ damage to multiple systems, and the lack of effective prevention forced the World Health Organization (WHO) to officially declare a pandemic of the disease [7–9]. Given the new nature of the infectious agent and the many unknowns surrounding it, the WHO implemented protocols developed during the most closely related infectious agents—MERS and SARS-CoV, namely, social distance, personal protective equipment, quarantine of healthy disease carriers and contacts of the sick, and strict monitoring of the epidemiological process [10–12]. The severe health challenges including the unknowns surrounding the course of the disease and the epidemiological process, the large number of healthy infection spreaders, the severe clinical course with high and sometimes sudden mortality in some patients, the lack of healthcare personnel, and effective prevention and misinformation (at the beginning of the pandemic due to lack of scientifically proven facts, and, in the later stages, for non-medical reasons) led to the mobilization of medical science in the study of SARS-CoV-2 not only towards the origin of the virus and the study of its clinical consequences and morphology, but also to the rapid development of effective vaccine prophylaxis, largely possible based on the experience gained in the previous two severe coronavirus diseases [9,13–16].

With the abatement of the pandemic in 2022 and given the mutational variants of the disease leading to a significantly milder clinical course and a decrease in overall mortality, as well as due to the availability of widespread effective vaccine prevention, not only the public but also the publication interest in the subject has gradually subsided [17–19]. The question remains open not only about the origin of the virus and, to a large extent, the characteristics regarding organ involvement, but above all about the chronic consequences of the illness, which the medical community has yet to face [20–27].

Historically, this is not the first time that medicine has encountered a similar situation; numerous pandemics, not only of viral origin but also of bacterial origin, have led to the permanent disability of those who have suffered, and subsequently to the development of new and, at first glance, unexpected long-term consequences [28]. A relatively recent example is the HIV-AIDS infection, which, in addition to immune deficiency, has been proven to lead to many severe consequences, including neoplasia and dementia [29–32]. In the history of medicine, there are many more such examples, such as von Economo's disease (lethargic encephalitis), often confused as a consequence of the Spanish flu; although, the epidemic process began several years before it and led to postencephalitic parkinsonism [33–35].

It is for these reasons that it is necessary to retain the interest of medical science in the matter of the detailed study of the acute and chronic effects of the virus that are yet to be encountered and that can be used in combating future pandemic variants of coronavirus infections [36–39].

Autopsies of patients with COVID-19 have revealed a myriad of gross and especially histological changes in multiple internal organs, namely, the lungs, where the changes lead to the dominating clinical symptom of hypoxia, but also the liver, heart, and other organs [40–44]. It is important, however, that autopsies reveal only the most severe effects of the disease in patients who had either a severe protracted clinical course or those who expired suddenly. It is highly likely that in cases with a moderate clinical course, either a significantly less diffuse and developed set of complications is present or it did not manifest at all.

Furthermore, it is likely that in patients with mild clinical disease, a whole new spectrum of changes can be present, with all of these further developing and evolving into chronic changes in the spectrum of post-COVID syndrome. Post-COVID syndrome, or long COVID or persistent COVID, are a direct result of the persistent damage caused by the viral infection. While mainly focusing on the diverse pulmonary pathology, which leads to chronic complications, this spectrum also includes sequelae from other systems and organs, such as the kidneys, cardiovascular, gastrointestinal, and especially the central nervous system [21,45–48].

Safety Precautions during Autopsy—Determining the Hazard Group

As the causative agent of the disease has been identified by the WHO as a pandemic entity, special precautions must be taken during the autopsy of suspected, probable, and identified cases [49]. Furthermore, as a general precautionary rule in the presence of diffusely spreading infectious pandemic entities, safety precautions should be taken in all cases, even if the autopsy case is not suspected or even has been ruled out to be a carrier of the disease.

For autopsy practice, especially for infectious disease entries, cases are separated into hazard groups (HG) based on the ability of the pathogens to infect new hosts, the severity of the disease it causes, and the presence of effective prevention, treatment, or the lack thereof [50]. HG1 refers to pathogens that are unlikely to cause human disease, cause minimal illness, or there is effective prevention and treatment; HG2 refers to pathogens that can lead to infection in the personnel but are unlikely to spread to the general population, and there is effective prevention and treatment; HG3 refers to pathogens that cause severe disease to the personnel and can spread to the community, but there is effective prevention and treatment; and HG4 refers to pathogens that cause severe diseases, can spread in the general population, and there is no effective prevention and treatment. It is essential to know that in many regions, based on their legislation, HG4 autopsies are counter-indicated, while in others, HG4 is mandated as it is viewed as a threat to national and regional security [49,51–54].

During the initial phases of the pandemic, there was a broad discussion regarding which HG COVID-19 should be placed in, with initial decisions putting it in HG4, and, hence, the number of autopsy cases was very low [49,51,55]. As data started to accumulate and there was a relatively low incidence of periautopsy infection, it was gradually moved down to HG3 and, in some areas after the introduction of vaccinations, even to HG2. Based, however, on the significant mutation frequency of the virus and the evasion of acquired immunity by the new variants, in the future, it would be sound to keep SARS-CoV-2 in HG3 to prevent the spreading of potentially deadly variants of the virus to healthcare personnel and the population in general [56].

2. Gross Findings

The respiratory system in patients who have died from COVID-19 shows a myriad of gross changes. The mucous membranes of the trachea and bronchi are moderate to severely erythematous, most prominently in the interchondral areas, and often have scattered mucosal hemorrhages and ulcerations (Figure 1) [57]. In the thoracic cavity, a large subset of patients had pleural effusions, varying from serous to hemorrhagic [41]. The characteristics of the pleural surface correspond to the presence and nature of pleural effusions, ranging from preserved pleural surfaces to edematous ones, diffusely scattered fibrin deposits, or hemorrhagic areas [58]. However, the lungs have the most striking changes to them. They are significantly enlarged, weighing more than a kilogram (i.e., more than twice their average weight), and can reach nearly two kilograms in the most severe cases. The parenchyma is firm to the touch, red-violet, and often deformed (Figure 1) [55,59–61]. On sectioning, the cut surface is diffusely consolidated, with a scant amount of mucohemmorhagic fluid flowing from it spontaneously when the parenchyma is compressed [60,61]. In cases with extremely severe parenchymal involvement, hepatization results in the bulging of the large and medium-sized blood vessels, giving the parenchyma a beef meat appearance (Figure 1). A large subset of patients also have a positive gross probe for pulmonary thromboembolism, and the vessel section reveals thrombi in smaller branches of the vessels, some in different stages of organization and/or areas of hemorrhagic infarction [44,62,63].

Normal lung		SARS-CoV-2 associated gross pulmonary changes	
Weight		Weight	
Left	Right	First 10 days	After the 10th day
~400g	~450g	Up to more than 1kg each	~800g each
Soft, pinkish parenchyma, on section aerated		Firm and deformed, red-purple parenchyma, consolidated and airless, with beef meat appearance	Firm and deformed, violet-gray parenchyma, consolidated, few aerated zones may be noted peripherally

Figure 1. Comparison between gross features of normal lung and SARS-CoV-2 infected lung.

In patients with a more protracted clinical course (survival more than ten days from the onset of symptoms), the lungs are relatively lighter, regularly around 800–900 g, and grossly have a more grayish-red-violet color; they are firmer to palpation, deformed, and some peripheral areas may have reaeration resembling emphysematous deformation (Figure 1) [60]. When a secondary bacterial infection is superimposed, areas of suppuration and/or abscessation are visible in the parenchyma, and the bronchi are filled with purulent-hemorrhagic exudate [44,59,63]. In some patients, a fungal superinfection may be present, with aspergillus and mucormycosis being the most commonly isolated causative agents [64,65].

In chronically and severely ill patients and the elderly, the lungs may have significantly fewer changes, varying from focal and mild consolidation to nearly normal-looking lungs, with some cases showing only histological changes [58–60].

Histology largely depends on the innate resilience of the organism and the virulence and pathogenicity of the viral variant. In most cases, however, there are at least minimal signs of diffuse alveolar damage correlating to the clinical constellation of acute respiratory distress syndrome [44,55,59].

Practical Tips for Obtaining Respiratory System Specimens

In our practice, the authors have implemented a harvesting protocol for respiratory system specimens, intending to identify, even if minimally present, the changes induced by the virus on histology. When obtaining samples from the respiratory system, the authors open the ribcage with bone cutters, which is an important safety tip, as if opened with an electrical saw, as in some institutions, the vibrations produced can mobilize vital viral particles and spread them in the air, increasing the risk for the personnel present. Secondly, the respiratory system is sectioned only after in situ probing of the pulmonary artery for the presence of large thrombi/emboli. Once the respiratory system is eviscerated, the authors take at least three tissue specimens from every pulmonary lobe—one hilar, one central, and one peripheral, with other areas harvested as desired by the obductor. Furthermore, the authors take specimens from the trachea, bronchial bifurcation, and principal bronchi.

3. Histological Findings

The histological findings are largely non-specific, as similar changes can be observed in MERS, SARS-CoV-2, respiratory syncytial virus, pandemic variants of influenza and others, and some opportunistic viral infections to the lung and respiratory system [66–71].

3.1. Trachea and Large Bronchi

The trachea and large bronchi in patients with COVID-19 generally have histologic findings of extensive desquamation of the respiratory epithelium, basal cell hyperplasia, scant interstitial infiltration by lymphocytes, and goblet cell hyperplasia in the submucosal glands (Figure 2) [57].

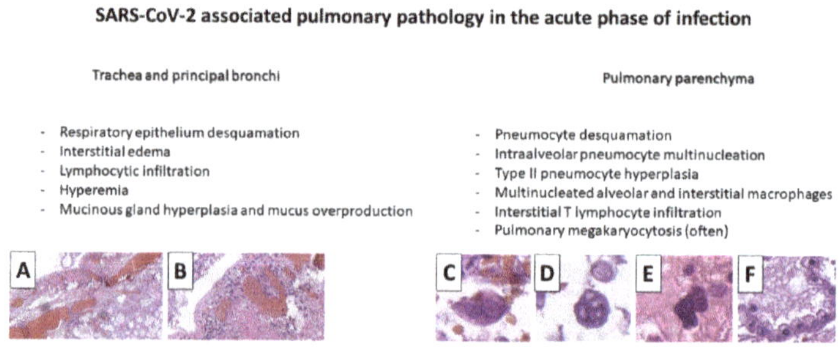

Figure 2. Histological features of SARS-CoV-2-induced damage in the trachea, principal bronchi, and the acute phase of pulmonary involvement: (**A**) respiratory epithelium desquamation, edema, lymphocytic infiltration, and mucinous gland hyperplasia in the trachea; (**B**) lymphocytic infiltrate in the tracheal submucosa around hyperemic blood vessels; (**C**) alveolar multinucleated cell of pneumocyte origin; (**D**) alveolar multinucleated cell of macrophage origin; (**E**) pulmonary megakaryocyte; (**F**) type II pneumocyte hyperplasia. Note: Histology sections adapted from ref. [60].

3.2. Pulmonary Histopathology

As already mentioned, pulmonary histopathology is non-specific and follows the pattern of diffuse alveolar damage and vascular endothelial damage—its two coexisting forms.

Diffuse alveolar damage consists of severe damage to the respiratory and alveolar epithelium, occurring in two primary forms—an exudative phase (acute), which is observed in patients who die within the first week of the onset of symptoms, and a proliferative (initial and advanced) phase, which is observed in patients with survival of more than ten days from the onset of symptoms [44,59,72]. The initial phase of proliferative diffuse alveolar damage combines the findings of the exudative and advanced proliferative phases [44,60,69].

3.2.1. Acute Phase of the Infection—Diffuse Alveolar Damage

The first histological changes observed in the exudative phase of diffuse alveolar damage (patients who died by the seventh day from the onset of symptoms) are the desquamation of the epithelium of the terminal bronchioles and alveoli, as well as the hyperplasia of type II pneumocytes, the formation of alveolar and interstitial multinucleated cells, scarce interstitial infiltration comprised by predominantly T lymphocytes, intra-alveolar and interstitial macrophage infiltration with multinucleation, and occasionally pulmonary megakaryocytes (Figure 2) [58,60,63]. The alveolar multinucleated cells originating from pneumocytes have characteristically ground glass opacity cytoplasm, peripheral inclusions, up to six nuclei (predominantly, these cells have two or three nuclei) with a central, sometimes ruby-red nucleoli, and a diameter varying between 20 and 40 μm (Figure 2) [60,61]. The second type of multinucleated cells, with macrophage origin, also presents intra-alveolarly, but the cells are mostly interstitially located, smaller (about 20 μm in diameter), primarily trinucleated, but may have up to seven nuclei, and their cytoplasm is more basophilic and positive for CD68 (Figure 2) [59–61,73].

3.2.2. Organization Phase of Diffuse Alveolar Damage

In patients with a survival of about ten days from the onset of symptoms, a transformation of changes with an initial phase of organization is observed. Alveolar macrophages decrease in number, and in the terminal and respiratory bronchioles, there is hyperplasia of Clara-type cells—non-ciliated cells of the bronchioles—with a secretory function (Figure 3) [60]. Other than their secretory function, which plays a significant role in local homeostasis regulation and stress response, these cells also play a role in tissue repair as they serve as a regeneratory "reservoir" but are also susceptible to metaplastic change [74]. Fibrous changes also begin with the thickening of the alveolar walls and focal interstitial fibrosis (Figure 3) [41,44,58,63].

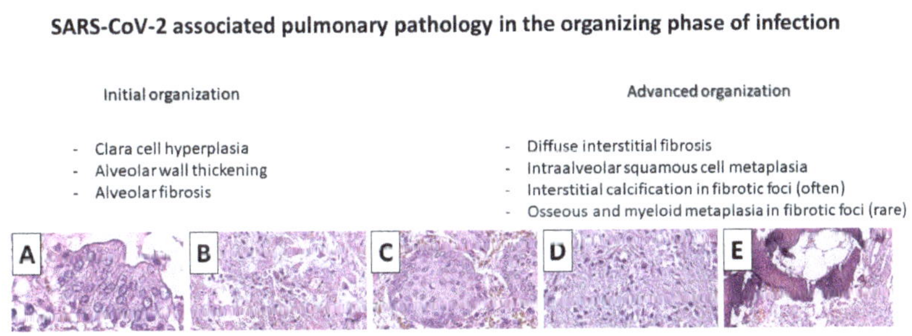

Figure 3. Organizational changes in COVID-19: (**A**) Clara cell hyperplasia in alveolar tracts and alveoli; (**B**) fibrosis with thickening of the alveolar septa; (**C**) intra-alveolar squamous cell metaplasia; (**D**) diffuse fibrosis; (**E**) osteoid and myeloid metaplasia in fibrotic foci. Note: Histology sections adapted from ref. [60].

In patients who died 15 days after the onset of symptoms, advanced organization of the lung parenchyma can be noted, with pronounced fibrosis—diffuse interstitial, thickening of the alveolar septa to a bronchiolitis obliterans organizing pneumonia pattern with intra-alveolar fibroblastic proliferation and alveolar obliteration [47,60,75].

In this phase, several interesting phenomena can also be observed, the most striking of which is the transformation (metaplasia) of Clara-type cells into squamous epithelium that diffusely fills the alveoli and respiratory tracts without the involvement of the larger bronchi (Figure 3) [60,63]. Secondary to fibrosis, diffuse calcium deposition can also be observed in some cases with further osteoid and myeloid metaplasia (Figure 3) [43,60].

3.3. *Vascular Changes*

The second most prominent group of changes—those of the pulmonary blood vessels—is more monomorphic and does not undergo such great dynamics. These changes manifest with endotheliitis (endothelialitis)—swelling, palisading, and desquamation of the endothelium of the larger vessels with focal intravascular endothelial proliferation in the regeneration phase (Figure 4) [57,60,62,76,77]. CD34-labeled vessels show extensive areas of endothelial desquamation, with sometimes interconnected endothelial cells freely "hanging" in the lumens of large vessels like a curtain (Figure 4). Interestingly smaller blood vessels, especially capillaries, do not constitute such an endothelial change [60].

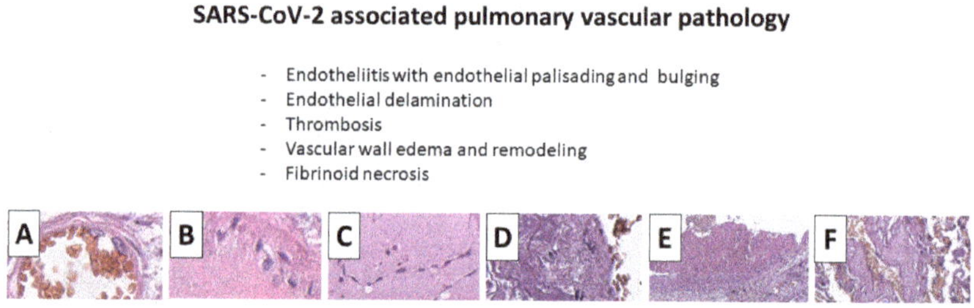

Figure 4. SARS-CoV-2 associated pulmonary vasculature pathology: (**A**) endothelial cell edema; (**B**) endothelial cell palisading; (**C**) endothelial cell desquamation in groups; (**D**) fibrinoid necrosis; (**E**) fibrin thrombus with organization partially attached to the wall of a large vessel; (**F**) homogenization and thickening of the vascular wall. Note: Histology sections adapted from ref. [60].

These described endothelial changes have two immediate effects—thrombosis, a well clinically manifested phenomenon, and degenerative changes in the vascular wall due to increased permeability [60,62,77,78].

Although pulmonary thrombosis is clinically comparable to thromboembolic disease, given the severe single-vessel involvement and advanced organization in some cases, it is more likely an autochthonous thrombosis of the pulmonary circulation (Figure 4) [44,62,77–79].

The changes in the vessel wall as a result of the increased permeability are represented by distortion of the cellular arrangement in the structure of the vascular wall and degeneration of the extracellular matrix—the walls of the vessels are eccentrically thickened, acellular and amorphic, akin to hyalinized, with focal fibrinoid necrosis, lymphocytic infiltrate in the vascular wall, and subintimal foamy macrophages may be observed in some cases (Figure 4) [60].

Special histochemical stains show that these changes develop due to simple extracellular matrix edema, with only focally positive proteinaceous deposits (PAS-positive), while Congo red, Phosphotungstic acid hematoxylin (PTAH) and Van Gieson stains, Masson trichrome, and Alcian blue are negative (Figure 4) [60]. Immunohistochemically, the larger vessels show a distortion of the smooth muscle cell arrangement and focal loss of fibroblasts (Figure 4). It is important to note that the changes described up to this point involve the vessels of mostly medium and small caliber, with the larger vessels having less pronounced changes, while in the microcirculation, these changes are hardly noticeable.

Precisely because of this, as already mentioned, fibrin thrombi are present in these branches in most of the cases, while thrombi in the microcirculation are present in a significantly smaller proportion of patients.

3.4. Non-Time Associated Changes

Changes observed in the lung parenchyma, which are not associated with the time since the onset of infection, are again non-specific and associated with diffuse alveolar damage (pulmonary hyaline membranes) and secondary infections [41,58,59,63,72,73,80].

3.4.1. Pulmonary Hyaline Membranes

Pulmonary hyaline membranes (alveolar fibrinous exudate) present with classic morphology; however, the intra-alveolar edema in these areas has a more vacuolated appearance due to increased albumin (Figure 5) [58,60,63]. It is important to note that hyaline membranes are only seen in half of the patients who have expired from COVID-19 [43,57,59,60,63]. These reflect the severe direct alveolar epithelium damage and the dysregulation of alveolar homeostasis. The spectrum of vascular phenomena also plays a big part in it, as the alveolar walls are comprised of capillaries. At the onset of hyaline membranes, the alveoli are no longer able to carry out their gas exchanging function. As such, the condition of these patients deteriorates rapidly with a sudden drop in peripheral oxygen saturation [81–83]. Furthermore, as already stated, these changes do not appear in a time-related manner and can be seen in the exudative, early, and late organizational phases of diffuse alveolar damage [59,60]. In patients with more prolonged survival, mainly those on invasive lung ventilation, the hyaline membranes are thick and layered, in some areas resembling intra-alveolar globules.

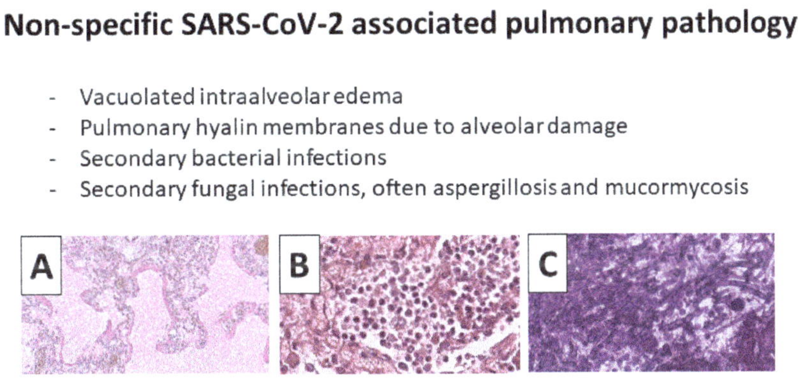

Figure 5. Non-specific pulmonary changes associated with SARS-CoV-2 infection, Hyaline membranes, and edema in COVID-19: (**A**) pulmonary hyaline membranes and vacuolated intra-alveolar edema; (**B**) secondary bacterial infection (purulent bronchopneumonia); (**C**) secondary fungal infection.

3.4.2. Secondary Infections

Secondary infections, in the form of suppuration and abscessation in the lung parenchyma, as a time-independent complication, can develop in around one-third of patients, regardless of antibiotic prophylaxis, and can be not only bacterial but also fungal, with aspergillus and mucormycosis being the most prevalently isolated pathogens from this group (Figure 5) [64,65].

3.5. Practical Tips for Reporting Histopathology in Autopsy Protocols

If the patient tests positive antemortem, then COVID-19, as a socially significant disease, should be noted as the main/principal disease that unlocked the mechanisms of tanatogenesis [50]. In cases where the patient has multiple severe conditions, such as malignancy, other infectious diseases (e.g., tuberculosis), or immune suppression, all of these should be mentioned together as primary diseases, while COPD, CVDs, etc., should be specified as background diseases [50].

In cases where the patient was not tested antemortem or tested negative, but the clinical symptoms and morphology are compatible with COVID-19, then instead of COVID-19 being recognized as the primary disease, the main illness should be specified as an acute viral infection and its components listed, such as diffuse alveolar damage in organization phase with alveolar and interstitial multinucleated cells, scant lymphocytic interstitial infiltration, Clara cell hyperplasia, squamous cell metaplasia, fibrosis, and medium caliber pulmonary vessel degeneration and thrombosis. While many institutions allow for postmortem PCR tests and recognize them as valid, hence, for postmortem COVID-19 diagnosis, it is important to note that all commercially available tests have been validated for use only on the living, and none for postmortem evaluation. Immunohistochemistry on neutral formaldehyde-fixated tissue specimens, although a validated method for postmortem evaluation, should also be noted as not always being reliable depending on the antibody used, i.e., if the antibody targets a frequently mutated part of the antigenic structure of the virus, it may not detect a positive case. At the same time, cross-reactivity with other members of the coronaviridae family should not be underestimated, such as SARS-CoV, and MERS, which present with virtually identical morphology, as well as different non-pandemic variants of coronaviruses such as those causing seasonal common cold [44,51,68,73,84].

4. Conclusions

- The pulmonary pathology induced by SARS-CoV-2 follows a relatively strict pattern of evolution with:
    - ➢ Diffuse alveolar damage—desquamation of the alveolar epithelium with exudative and proliferative changes—pulmonary hyaline membranes, Clara cell hyperplasia, squamous cell metaplasia, and fibrosis;
    - ➢ Endotheliitis—endothelial cell infection, edema, bulging, desquamation, and vascular thrombosis with vascular wall remodeling;
    - ➢ Opportunity for secondary infections—bacterial and fungal.
- These changes are not pathognomonic COVID-19, as multiple other viruses, including some other coronaviruses (SARS-CoV-2 and MERS), present with similar morphology.
- The described acute changes have further implications to chronic sequele in the respiratory and cardiovascular systems.

Author Contributions: G.S.S. and L.P. conceptualized the study; G.S.S. and H.P. performed the initial literature review; G.S.S. and D.S. performed detailed review on available data of acute effects; L.P. and M.I. performed detailed review on chronic effects; D.S., M.I. and A.B.T. reviewed the mechanisms of viral biology and functional changes; G.S.S. and H.P. wrote the initial draft; G.S.S., D.S., M.I. and H.P. devised the figures; A.B.T., M.I., H.P. and L.P. revised the initial draft critically; A.B.T. performed the final revision and approved the manuscript for submission. All authors have read and agreed to the published version of the manuscript.

Funding: This research received no external funding.

Institutional Review Board Statement: Not applicable.

Informed Consent Statement: Not applicable.

Data Availability Statement: Not applicable.

Conflicts of Interest: The authors declare no conflict of interest.

References

1. Li, X.; Zai, J.; Zhao, Q.; Nie, Q.; Li, Y.; Foley, B.T.; Chaillon, A. Evolutionary history, potential intermediate animal host, and cross-species analyses of SARS-CoV-2. *J. Med. Virol.* **2020**, *92*, 602–611. [CrossRef] [PubMed]
2. Andersen, K.G.; Rambaut, A.; Lipkin, W.I.; Holmes, E.C.; Garry, R.F. The proximal origin of SARS-CoV-2. *Nat. Med.* **2020**, *26*, 450–452. [CrossRef] [PubMed]

3. Wu, Y.-C.; Chen, C.-S.; Chan, Y.-J. The outbreak of COVID-19: An overview. *J. Chin. Med. Assoc.* **2020**, *83*, 217–220. [CrossRef] [PubMed]
4. Liu, Q.; Luo, D.; Haase, J.E.; Guo, Q.; Wang, X.Q.; Liu, S.; Xia, L.; Liu, Z.; Yang, J.; Yang, B.X. The experiences of health-care providers during the COVID-19 crisis in China: A qualitative study. *Lancet Glob. Health* **2020**, *8*, e790–e798. [CrossRef]
5. Sun, N.; Wei, L.; Shi, S.; Jiao, D.; Song, R.; Ma, L.; Wang, H.; Wang, C.; Wang, Z.; You, Y.; et al. A qualitative study on the psychological experience of caregivers of COVID-19 patients. *Am. J. Infect. Control* **2020**, *48*, 592–598. [CrossRef]
6. De Brier, N.; Stroobants, S.; Vandekerckhove, P.; De Buck, E. Factors affecting mental health of health care workers during coronavirus disease outbreaks (SARS, MERS & COVID-19): A rapid systematic review. *PLoS ONE* **2020**, *15*, e0244052. [CrossRef]
7. Wang, C.; Horby, P.W.; Hayden, F.G.; Gao, G.F. A novel coronavirus outbreak of global health concern. *Lancet* **2020**, *395*, 470–473. [CrossRef]
8. Hu, B.; Guo, H.; Zhou, P.; Shi, Z.-L. Characteristics of SARS-CoV-2 and COVID-19. *Nat. Rev. Microbiol.* **2021**, *19*, 141–154. [CrossRef] [PubMed]
9. Baloch, S.; Baloch, M.A.; Zheng, T.; Pei, X. The Coronavirus Disease 2019 (COVID-19) Pandemic. *Tohoku J. Exp. Med.* **2020**, *250*, 271–278. [CrossRef]
10. Guarner, J. Three Emerging Coronaviruses in Two Decades the Story of SARS, MERS, and Now COVID-19. *Am. J. Clin. Pathol.* **2020**, *153*, 420–421. [CrossRef]
11. Peeri, N.C.; Shrestha, N.; Rahman, M.S.; Zaki, R.; Tan, Z.; Bibi, S.; Baghbanzadeh, M.; Aghamohammadi, N.; Zhang, W.; Haque, U. The SARS, MERS and novel coronavirus (COVID-19) epidemics, the newest and biggest global health threats: What lessons have we learned? *Int. J. Epidemiol.* **2020**, *49*, 717–726. [CrossRef] [PubMed]
12. Dagens, A.; Sigfrid, L.; Cai, E.; Lipworth, S.; Cheung, V.; Harris, E.; Bannister, P.; Rigby, I.; Horby, P. Scope, quality, and inclusivity of clinical guidelines produced early in the COVID-19 pandemic: Rapid review. *BMJ* **2020**, *369*, m1936. [CrossRef] [PubMed]
13. Dzieciatkowski, T.; Szarpak, L.; Filipiak, K.J.; Jaguszewski, M.; Ladny, J.R.; Smereka, J. COVID-19 challenge for modern medicine. *Cardiol. J.* **2020**, *27*, 175–183. [CrossRef] [PubMed]
14. Harris, C.; Carson, G.; Baillie, J.K.; Horby, P.; Nair, H. An evidence-based framework for priority clinical research questions for COVID-19. *J. Glob. Health* **2020**, *10*, 11001. [CrossRef] [PubMed]
15. Khalifa, S.A.M.; Mohamed, B.S.; Elashal, M.H.; Du, M.; Guo, Z.; Zhao, C.; Musharraf, S.G.; Boskabady, M.H.; El-Seedi, H.H.R.; Efferth, T.; et al. Comprehensive Overview on Multiple Strategies Fighting COVID-19. *Int. J. Environ. Res. Public Health* **2020**, *17*, 5813. [CrossRef]
16. Kuhn, S.A.K.; Lieb, R.; Freeman, D.; Andreou, C.; Zander-Schellenberg, T. Coronavirus conspiracy beliefs in the German-speaking general population: Endorsement rates and links to reasoning biases and paranoia. In *Psychological Medicine*; Cambridge University Press: Cambridge, UK, 2021; pp. 1–15. [CrossRef]
17. Karim, S.S.A.; Karim, Q.A. Omicron SARS-CoV-2 variant: A new chapter in the COVID-19 pandemic. *Lancet* **2021**, *398*, 2126–2128. [CrossRef]
18. Del Rio, C.; Omer, S.B.; Malani, P.N. Winter of Omicron—The Evolving COVID-19 Pandemic. *JAMA* **2022**, *327*, 319. [CrossRef]
19. Hoffmann, M.; Krüger, N.; Schulz, S.; Cossmann, A.; Rocha, C.; Kempf, A.; Nehlmeier, I.; Graichen, L.; Moldenhauer, A.-S.; Winkler, M.S.; et al. The Omicron variant is highly resistant against antibody-mediated neutralization: Implications for control of the COVID-19 pandemic. *Cell* **2022**, *185*, 447–456.e11. [CrossRef]
20. Phillips, N. The coronavirus is here to stay—here's what that means. *Nature* **2021**, *590*, 382–384. [CrossRef]
21. Torres-Castro, R.; Vasconcello-Castillo, L.; Alsina-Restoy, X.; Solis-Navarro, L.; Burgos, F.; Puppo, H.; Vilaró, J. Respiratory function in patients post-infection by COVID-19: A systematic review and meta-analysis. *Pulmonology* **2021**, *27*, 328. [CrossRef]
22. Shaw, B.; Daskareh, M.; Gholamrezanezhad, A. The lingering manifestations of COVID-19 during and after convalescence: Update on long-term pulmonary consequences of coronavirus disease 2019 (COVID-19). *Radiol. Med.* **2021**, *126*, 40–46. [CrossRef] [PubMed]
23. Zhao, Y.-M.; Shang, Y.-M.; Song, W.-B.; Li, Q.-Q.; Xie, H.; Xu, Q.-F.; Jia, J.-L.; Li, L.-M.; Mao, H.-L.; Zhou, X.-M.; et al. Follow-up study of the pulmonary function and related physiological characteristics of COVID-19 survivors three months after recovery. *eClinicalMedicine* **2020**, *25*, 100463. [CrossRef] [PubMed]
24. Castagnoli, R.; Votto, M.; Licari, A.; Brambilla, I.; Bruno, R.; Perlini, S.; Rovida, F.; Baldanti, F.; Marseglia, G.L. Severe Acute Respiratory Syndrome Coronavirus 2 (SARS-CoV-2) Infection in Children and Adolescents: A Systematic Review. *JAMA Pediatr.* **2020**, *174*, 882–889. [CrossRef] [PubMed]
25. Dehingia, N.; Raj, A. Sex differences in COVID-19 case fatality: Do we know enough? *Lancet Glob. Heal.* **2021**, *9*, e14–e15. [CrossRef]
26. Lazzerini, M.; Putoto, G. COVID-19 in Italy: Momentous decisions and many uncertainties. *Lancet Glob. Health* **2020**, *8*, e641–e642. [CrossRef]
27. Levin, A.T.; Hanage, W.P.; Owusu-Boaitey, N.; Cochran, K.B.; Walsh, S.P.; Meyerowitz-Katz, G. Assessing the age specificity of infection fatality rates for COVID-19: Systematic review, meta-analysis, and public policy implications. *Eur. J. Epidemiol.* **2020**, *35*, 1123–1138. [CrossRef]
28. Huremović, D. Brief History of Pandemics (Pandemics Throughout History). In *Psychiatry of Pandemics*; Springer: Cham, Switzerland, 2019; pp. 7–35. [CrossRef]
29. Quinn, T.C. HIV epidemiology and the effects of antiviral therapy on long-term consequences. *AIDS* **2008**, *22*, S7–S12. [CrossRef]

30. Clutton, G.; Xu, Y.; Baldoni, P.L.; Mollan, K.R.; Kirchherr, J.; Newhard, W.; Cox, K.; Kuruc, J.D.; Kashuba, A.; Barnard, R.; et al. The differential short- and long-term effects of HIV-1 latency-reversing agents on T cell function. *Sci. Rep.* **2016**, *6*, 30749. [CrossRef]
31. Lake, J.E.; Currier, J.S. Metabolic disease in HIV infection. *Lancet Infect. Dis.* **2013**, *13*, 964–975. [CrossRef]
32. Degano, B.; Yaïci, A.; Le Pavec, J.; Savale, L.; Jaïs, X.; Camara, B.; Humbert, M.; Simonneau, G.; Sitbon, O. Long-term effects of bosentan in patients with HIV-associated pulmonary arterial hypertension. *Eur. Respir. J.* **2009**, *33*, 92–98. [CrossRef]
33. Dickman, M.S. von Economo Encephalitis. *Arch. Neurol.* **2001**, *58*, 1696–1698. [CrossRef] [PubMed]
34. Reid, A.; McCall, S.; Henry, J.M.; Taubenberger, J.K. Experimenting on the Past: The Enigma of von Economo's Encephalitis Lethargica. *J. Neuropathol. Exp. Neurol.* **2001**, *60*, 663–670. [CrossRef] [PubMed]
35. Hoffman, L.A.; Vilensky, J.A. Encephalitis lethargica: 100 years after the epidemic. *Brain* **2017**, *140*, 2246–2251. [CrossRef] [PubMed]
36. Assaad, R.; El-Adaway, I.H. Guidelines for Responding to COVID-19 Pandemic: Best Practices, Impacts, and Future Research Directions. *J. Manag. Eng.* **2021**, *37*, 6021001. [CrossRef]
37. Khanna, R.C.; Cicinelli, M.V.; Gilbert, S.S.; Honavar, S.G.; Murthy, G.S.V. COVID-19 pandemic: Lessons learned and future directions. *Indian J. Ophthalmol.* **2020**, *68*, 703–710. [CrossRef]
38. Saqr, M.; Wasson, B. COVID-19: Lost opportunities and lessons for the future. *Int. J. Health Sci.* **2020**, *14*, 4.
39. Lai, J.W.; Cheong, K.H. Superposition of COVID-19 waves, anticipating a sustained wave, and lessons for the future. *BioEssays* **2020**, *42*, e2000178. [CrossRef]
40. Siripanthong, B.; Nazarian, S.; Muser, D.; Deo, R.; Santangeli, P.; Khanji, M.Y.; Cooper, L.T.; Chahal, C.A.A. Recognizing COVID-19–related myocarditis: The possible pathophysiology and proposed guideline for diagnosis and management. *Hear. Rhythm* **2020**, *17*, 1463–1471. [CrossRef]
41. Buja, L.M.; Wolf, D.A.; Zhao, B.; Akkanti, B.; McDonald, M.; Lelenwa, L.; Reilly, N.; Ottaviani, G.; Elghetany, M.T.; Trujillo, D.O.; et al. The emerging spectrum of cardiopulmonary pathology of the coronavirus disease 2019 (COVID-19): Report of 3 autopsies from Houston, Texas, and review of autopsy findings from other United States cities. *Cardiovasc. Pathol.* **2020**, *48*, 107233. [CrossRef]
42. Haider, A.; Siddiqa, A.; Ali, N.; Dhallu, M. COVID-19 and the Brain: Acute Encephalitis as a Clinical Manifestation. *Cureus* **2020**, *12*, e10784. [CrossRef]
43. Menezes, R.G.; Rizwan, T.; Ali, S.S.; Hasan, W.; Khetpal, A.; Aqil, M.; Madadin, M.; Siddiqi, T.J.; Usman, M.S. Postmortem findings in COVID-19 fatalities: A systematic review of current evidence. *Leg. Med.* **2022**, *54*, 102001. [CrossRef]
44. Montero-Fernandez, M.A.; Pardo-Garcia, R. Histopathology features of the lung in COVID-19 patients. *Diagn. Histopathol.* **2021**, *27*, 123–127. [CrossRef] [PubMed]
45. Anaya, J.-M.; Rojas, M.; Salinas, M.L.; Rodríguez, Y.; Roa, G.; Lozano, M.; Rodríguez-Jiménez, M.; Montoya, N.; Zapata, E.; Monsalve, D.M.; et al. Post-COVID syndrome. A case series and comprehensive review. *Autoimmun. Rev.* **2021**, *20*, 102947. [CrossRef] [PubMed]
46. Ceban, F.; Ling, S.; Lui, L.M.; Lee, Y.; Gill, H.; Teopiz, K.M.; Rodrigues, N.B.; Subramaniapillai, M.; Di Vincenzo, J.D.; Cao, B.; et al. Fatigue and cognitive impairment in Post-COVID-19 Syndrome: A systematic review and meta-analysis. *Brain Behav. Immun.* **2022**, *101*, 93–135. [CrossRef]
47. Oronsky, B.; Larson, C.; Hammond, T.C.; Oronsky, A.; Kesari, S.; Lybeck, M.; Reid, T.R. A Review of Persistent Post-COVID Syndrome (PPCS). *Clin. Rev. Allergy Immunol.* **2021**, *1*, 1–9. [CrossRef]
48. Ayoubkhani, D.; Khunti, K.; Nafilyan, V.; Maddox, T.; Humberstone, B.; Diamond, I.; Banerjee, A. Post-covid syndrome in individuals admitted to hospital with COVID-19: Retrospective cohort study. *BMJ* **2021**, *372*, n693. [CrossRef]
49. Kim, M.-Y.; Cheong, H.; Kim, H.-S. Medicine TWG for SAG for C-19 from TKS for L: Proposal of the Autopsy Guideline for Infectious Diseases: Preparation for the Post-COVID-19 Era (abridged translation). *J. Korean Med. Sci.* **2020**, *35*, e310. [CrossRef]
50. Lee, J.A. Guidelines on autopsy practice. In *The Royal College of Pathologists*; The Royal College of Pathologists: London, UK, 2002.
51. Hanley, B.; Lucas, S.B.; Youd, E.; Swift, B.; Osborn, M. Autopsy in suspected COVID-19 cases. *J. Clin. Pathol.* **2020**, *73*, 239–242. [CrossRef]
52. Schwartz, D.A.; Herman, C.J. Editorial Response: The Importance of the Autopsy in Emerging and Reemerging Infectious Dis-eases. *Clin. Infect. Dis.* **1996**, *23*, 248–254. [CrossRef]
53. Buja, L.M.; Barth, R.F.; Krueger, G.R.; Brodsky, S.V.; Hunter, R.L. The Importance of the Autopsy in Medicine: Perspectives of Pathology Colleagues. *Acad. Pathol.* **2019**, *6*. [CrossRef]
54. Nolte, K.B.; Muller, T.B.; Denmark, A.M.; Burstein, R.; Villalobos, Y.A. Design and Construction of a Biosafety Level 3 Autopsy Laboratory. *Arch. Pathol. Lab. Med.* **2021**, *145*, 407–414. [CrossRef] [PubMed]
55. Barton, L.M.; Duval, E.J.; Stroberg, E.; Ghosh, S.; Mukhopadhyay, S. COVID-19 Autopsies, Oklahoma, USA. *Am. J. Clin. Pathol.* **2020**, *153*, 725–733. [CrossRef] [PubMed]
56. Lacy, J.M.; Brooks, E.G.; Akers, J.; Armstrong, D.; Decker, L.; Gonzalez, A.; Humphrey, W.; Mayer, R.; Miller, M.; Perez, C.; et al. COVID-19: Postmortem Diagnostic and Biosafety Considerations. *Am. J. Forensic Med. Pathol.* **2020**, *41*, 143–151. [CrossRef]
57. Bradley, B.T.; Maioli, H.; Johnston, R.; Chaudhry, I.; Fink, S.L.; Xu, H.; Najafian, B.; Deutsch, G.; Lacy, J.M.; Williams, T.; et al. Histopathology and ultrastructural findings of fatal COVID-19 infections in Washington State: A case series. *Lancet* **2020**, *396*, 320–332. [CrossRef]

58. Arrossi, A.V.; Farver, C. The pulmonary pathology of COVID-19. *Clevel. Clin. J. Med.* **2020**, *89*. [CrossRef]
59. Borczuk, A.C.; Salvatore, S.P.; Seshan, S.V.; Patel, S.S.; Bussel, J.B.; Mostyka, M.; Elsoukkary, S.; He, B.; DEL Vecchio, C.; Fortarezza, F.; et al. COVID-19 pulmonary pathology: A multi-institutional autopsy cohort from Italy and New York City. *Mod. Pathol.* **2020**, *33*, 1–13. [CrossRef] [PubMed]
60. Stoyanov, G.S.; Yanulova, N.; Stoev, L.; Zgurova, N.; Mihaylova, V.; Dzhenkov, D.L.; Stoeva, M.; Stefanova, N.; Kalchev, K.; Petkova, L. Temporal Patterns of COVID-19-Associated Pulmonary Pathology: An Autopsy Study. *Cureus* **2021**, *13*, e20522. [CrossRef]
61. Stoyanov, G.S.; Petkova, L.; Dzhenkov, D.L.; Sapundzhiev, N.R.; Todorov, I. Gross and Histopathology of COVID-19 With First Histology Report of Olfactory Bulb Changes. *Cureus* **2020**, *12*, e11912. [CrossRef]
62. Ackermann, M.; Verleden, S.E.; Kuehnel, M.; Haverich, A.; Welte, T.; Laenger, F.; Vanstapel, A.; Werlein, C.; Stark, H.; Tzankov, A.; et al. Pulmonary Vascular Endothelialitis, Thrombosis, and Angiogenesis in Covid-19. *N. Engl. J. Med.* **2020**, *383*, 120–128. [CrossRef]
63. Bösmüller, H.; Matter, M.; Fend, F.; Tzankov, A. The pulmonary pathology of COVID-19. *Virchows Arch.* **2021**, *478*, 137–150. [CrossRef]
64. Bhatt, K.; Agolli, A.; Patel, M.H.; Garimella, R.; Devi, M.; Garcia, E.; Amin, H.; Domingue, C.; Del Castillo, R.G.; Sanchez-Gonzalez, M. High mortality co-infections of COVID-19 patients: Mucormycosis and other fungal infections. *Discoveries* **2021**, *9*, e126. [CrossRef] [PubMed]
65. Zurl, C.; Hoenigl, M.; Schulz, E.; Hatzl, S.; Gorkiewicz, G.; Krause, R.; Eller, P.; Prattes, J. Autopsy Proven Pulmonary Mucormycosis Due to *Rhizopus microsporus* in a Critically Ill COVID 19 Patient with Underlying Hematological Malignancy. *J. Fungi* **2021**, *7*, 88. [CrossRef] [PubMed]
66. Alsaad, K.O.; Hajeer, A.H.; Balwi, M.A.; Moaiqel, M.A.; Oudah, N.A.; Ajlan, A.A.; Aljohani, S.; Alsolamy, S.; Gmati, G.E.; Balkhy, H.; et al. Histopathology of Middle East respiratory syndrome coronovirus (MERS-CoV) infection—clinicopathological and ultrastructural study. *Histopathology* **2018**, *72*, 516–524. [CrossRef] [PubMed]
67. Ng, D.L.; Hosani, F.A.; Keating, M.K.; Gerber, S.I.; Jones, T.L.; Metcalfe, M.G.; Tong, S.; Tao, Y.; Alami, N.N.; Haynes, L.M.; et al. Clinicopathologic, Immunohistochemical, and Ultrastructural Findings of a Fatal Case of Middle East Respiratory Syndrome Coronavirus Infection in the United Arab Emirates, April 2014. *Am. J. Pathol.* **2016**, *186*, 652–658. [CrossRef] [PubMed]
68. Bradley, B.T.; Bryan, A. Emerging respiratory infections: The infectious disease pathology of SARS, MERS, pandemic influenza, and Legionella. *Semin. Diagn. Pathol.* **2019**, *36*, 152–159. [CrossRef]
69. Ding, Y.; Wang, H.; Shen, H.; Li, Z.; Geng, J.; Han, H.; Cai, J.; Li, X.; Kang, W.; Weng, D.; et al. The clinical pathology of severe acute respiratory syndrome (SARS): A report from China. *J. Pathol.* **2003**, *200*, 282–289. [CrossRef]
70. Nicholls, J.M.; Poon, L.L.; Lee, K.C.; Ng, W.F.; Lai, S.T.; Leung, C.Y.; Chu, C.M.; Hui, P.K.; Mak, K.L.; Lim, W.; et al. Lung pathology of fatal severe acute respiratory syndrome. *Lancet* **2003**, *361*, 1773–1778. [CrossRef]
71. Lang, Z.-W.; Zhang, L.-J.; Zhang, S.-J.; Meng, X.; Li, J.-Q.; Song, C.-Z.; Sun, L.; Zhou, Y.-S.; Dwyer, D.E. A clinicopathological study of three cases of severe acute respiratory syndrome (SARS). *Pathology* **2003**, *35*, 526–531. [CrossRef]
72. Calabrese, F.; Pezzuto, F.; Fortarezza, F.; Hofman, P.; Kern, I.; Panizo, A.; von der Thüsen, J.; Timofeev, S.; Gorkiewicz, G.; Lunardi, F. Pulmonary pathology and COVID-19: Lessons from autopsy. The experience of European Pulmonary Pathologists. *Virchows Arch.* **2020**, *477*, 359–372. [CrossRef]
73. Hariri, L.P.; North, C.M.; Shih, A.R.; Israel, R.A.; Maley, J.H.; Villalba, J.A.; Vinarsky, V.; Rubin, J.; Okin, D.A.; Sclafani, A.; et al. Lung Histopathology in Coronavirus Disease 2019 as Compared with Severe Acute Respiratory Sydrome and H1N1 Influenza: A Systematic Review. *Chest* **2021**, *159*, 73–84. [CrossRef]
74. Stripp, B.; Reynolds, S. CLARA CELLS. In *Encyclopedia of Respiratory Medicine*; Elsevier: Amsterdam, The Netherlands, 2006; pp. 471–478. [CrossRef]
75. Vasarmidi, E.; Tsitoura, E.; Spandidos, D.; Tzanakis, N.; Antoniou, K. Pulmonary fibrosis in the aftermath of the Covid-19 era (Review). *Exp. Ther. Med.* **2020**, *20*, 2557–2560. [CrossRef] [PubMed]
76. Varga, Z.; Flammer, A.J.; Steiger, P.; Haberecker, M.; Andermatt, R.; Zinkernagel, A.S.; Mehra, M.R.; Schuepbach, R.A.; Ruschitzka, F.; Moch, H. Endothelial Cell Infection and Endotheliitis in COVID-19. *Lancet* **2020**, *395*, 1417–1418. [CrossRef]
77. Vrints, C.J.M.; Krychtiuk, K.A.; Van Craenenbroeck, E.M.; Segers, V.F.; Price, S.; Heidbuchel, H. Endothelialitis plays a central role in the pathophysiology of severe COVID-19 and its cardiovascular complications. *Acta Cardiol.* **2020**, *76*, 109–124. [CrossRef] [PubMed]
78. Becker, R.C. COVID-19-associated vasculitis and vasculopathy. *J. Thromb. Thrombolysis* **2020**, *50*, 499–511. [CrossRef]
79. Nishiga, M.; Wang, D.W.; Han, Y.; Lewis, D.B.; Wu, J.C. COVID-19 and cardiovascular disease: From basic mechanisms to clinical perspectives. *Nat. Rev. Cardiol.* **2020**, *17*, 543–558. [CrossRef] [PubMed]
80. Suess, C.; Hausmann, R. Gross and histopathological pulmonary findings in a COVID 19 associated death during self-isolation. *Int. J. Legal Med.* **2020**, *134*, 1285–1290. [CrossRef] [PubMed]
81. Jefferies, A.L.; Coates, G.; O'Brodovich, H. Pulmonary Epithelial Permeability in Hyaline-Membrane Disease. *N. Engl. J. Med.* **1984**, *311*, 1075–1080. [CrossRef]

82. Capers, T.H.; Minden, B. Pulmonary fibrinolysins in hyaline membrane formation in adults. *Am. J. Med.* **1964**, *36*, 377–381. [CrossRef]
83. Capers, T.H. Pulmonary hyaline membrane formation in the adult: A clinicopathologic study. *Am. J. Med.* **1961**, *31*, 701–710. [CrossRef]
84. Rockx, B.; Kuiken, T.; Herfst, S.; Bestebroer, T.; Lamers, M.M.; Munnink, B.B.O.; de Meulder, D.; van Amerongen, G.; van den Brand, J.; Okba, N.M.A.; et al. Comparative pathogenesis of COVID-19, MERS, and SARS in a nonhuman primate model. *Science* **2020**, *368*, 1012–1015. [CrossRef]

encyclopedia MDPI

Entry

COVID-19 and Peace in Conflict-Affected Areas

Emmanuel Chiwetalu Ossai [1,2]

1 Department of Religion and Cultural Studies, First Floor, Russwurm Building, Faculty of the Social Sciences, University of Nigeria, Nsukka 410001, Nigeria; chiwetalu.ossai@unn.edu.ng
2 School of Divinity, University of Edinburgh, New College, Mound Place, Edinburgh EH1 2LX, UK

Definition: The relationship between COVID-19 and peace has been considered from a variety of perspectives. In addition, different empirical studies on the link between the pandemic and peace in conflict-affected areas exist. However, little work has been performed on examining these studies to highlight key findings on the theme of COVID-19 and peace in conflict-affected areas. A conflict-affected area is a country, or part of a country, where widespread violence or armed conflict was present when COVID-19 emerged in December 2019, or that was transitioning from recent armed conflict to peace by the time the disease arose. What do we know, so far, about how peace has been affected by the COVID-19 pandemic in conflict-affected areas? To address this question, this paper begins by recognizing the multidimensionality of peace and clarifying that the main aspects of peace in conflict-affected areas being considered in the article are relations between conflict parties, peace efforts, and peace processes. Afterwards, the paper discusses existing evidence regarding the impact of COVID-19 and state responses to it on these components of peace in conflict-affected areas. The conflict-affected areas considered include Afghanistan, Colombia, Iraq, Israel-Palestine, Libya, Myanmar, Nigeria, South Sudan, Syria, the Philippines, Yemen, and other zones. The central finding of the article is that the existing studies on COVID-19 and peace in conflict-affected areas present mixed findings. On the one hand, the virus generated opportunities for cooperation between conflict parties in some cases, such as in the West Bank and Gaza Strip of Israel-Palestine. However, on the other hand, it created conditions that enabled conflict and impeded peace efforts and processes in many or most conflict-affected areas. The paper explains that two factors that determined how the disease affected peace in conflict-affected and non-conflict-affected areas are the pre-COVID-19 political and socio-economic conditions in an area, and how state and non-state actors responded to the pandemic. The article closes with a summary of the discussion and identification of its major limitations.

Keywords: COVID-19; peace; COVID-19 and peace; COVID-19 in conflict-affected areas; impact of COVID-19

Citation: Ossai, E.C. COVID-19 and Peace in Conflict-Affected Areas. *Encyclopedia* **2022**, *2*, 1678–1687. https://doi.org/10.3390/encyclopedia2040114

Academic Editors: Stephen Bustin and Raffaele Barretta

Received: 10 August 2022
Accepted: 26 September 2022
Published: 28 September 2022

1. Introduction

COVID-19 arose in late December 2019 in Wuhan, China. By early April 2020, close to 2 million cases and over 100 thousand deaths had been reported worldwide in more than 200 "countries, areas or territories" [1]. These numbers increased in subsequent months, while different governments and peoples adopted a variety of responses to the disease. The current paper draws on the existing literature about the disease and its impact to provide an overview of its relationship with peace in conflict-affected areas. A "conflict-affected area" is a country, or part of a country, where widespread violence or armed conflict was present when COVID-19 emerged in December 2019, or that was transitioning from recent armed conflict to peace by the time the disease arose [2–6]. This introductory section is followed by a segment where attention is given to the importance of clarifying what is meant by "peace" in the discussion on COVID-19 and peace. The clarification is useful mainly because peace is a multidimensional concept, which has been used in multiple ways in different contexts. After the section, the paper explains that to fully understand the impact of COVID-19 on peace, at least three stages of its influence should be considered. These are short-term, medium-term, and long-term stages and effects. After discussing these, the article draws on the existing academic literature on COVID-19 and peace to describe the different ways the virus and responses to it have affected peace in conflict-affected areas.

2. The Concept of Peace

"COVID-19 and Peace" is a broad topic under which one could place or discuss various themes. Peace-related issues whose link with COVID-19 have been discussed include peacekeeping, peacebuilding, the military, food security, civil society, democratic processes, governance, human rights, humanitarian actions, terrorism, international relations, the international system, political stability, state-society relations, socio-economic inequalities, gender-based violence, conflict, fragile states, the economy, refugees, Internally Displaced Persons (IDPs), violent crime, discrimination, peace processes, security, cooperation, diplomacy, regional tension, politics, elections, justice, interpersonal and intergroup relations, and cybercrime. It is useful to clarify how the term peace is applied in the discussion. Peace is often used to refer to the absence of war or physical violence. Additionally, it has been understood as being of two major kinds, which are negative (absence of direct violence) and positive (absence of direct, structural, and cultural violence) [7–9]. However, peace research has shown the complexity and multidimensionality of the term. Peace has different meanings and applications in different contexts [10]. In addition to positive and negative peace, various other kinds of peace have been identified by researchers [8,10–14].

The two concepts of "relational peace" and "situational peace" [10] are useful in the study of the relationship between COVID-19 and peace. With the understanding that peace has situational and relational dimensions, the inquirer would be interested in how COVID-19 has affected relations between individuals and groups, and the situation or condition in a given area—for example, in terms of the absence of direct violence. Regarding human relations, the researcher may also be more specific about the kind being explored. For example, in a study [14] about the impact of COVID-19 on peace in Nigeria, the author gave major attention to relations between Christians and Muslims in the country and concluded that the pandemic had a positive effect on Christian-Muslim relations, given that it drew the different believers together in COVID-19 response. This is similar to the effect that the 2013/2015 Ebola Virus Epidemic in Upper West Africa had on the peoples of Guinea, Liberia and Sierra Leone, who are said to have "stood together" to fight a disease that was rightly perceived as "a common threat" [15]. Given the multidimensionality of peace, specificity about what is meant by "peace" is useful in the discussion on COVID-19 and peace. Due to space constraints, the current paper will focus mainly on the impact of COVID-19 on relations between conflict parties, peace efforts, and peace processes in conflict-affected areas. Before this is discussed in Section 4, it is useful to reflect briefly on the issue of "impact" in the following segment.

3. How Do We Understand the Impact of COVID-19 on Peace?

Many peace researchers would agree that its impact on global peace or on peace in any given area can be understood in terms of short-term, medium-term, and long-term effects [16–19]. The short-term impact is the effect it had in the period that commenced when the emergence of the disease was announced in December 2019 and ended in the weeks or months of 2021 following different countries' adoption of various "urgent" strategies to curb the spread of the disease. This could be called "the emergency period" [16]. To understand the long-term impact of the disease on peace, one may consider what takes place in the period of recovery from the pandemic, which could be referred to as "the recovery period" [16]. An intermediate period could be examined for the medium-term effects of the disease. This is the time between the emergency and recovery period. It is not clear when the emergency period of the COVID-19 pandemic ended or when one should regard as the beginning of the recovery period. Different countries have had different experiences. Most of the existing studies on COVID-19 and different dimensions of peace, some of which were consulted while writing this paper, are based on data collected in the years 2020 and 2021, which include the emergency period and months that could be regarded as the medium-term. The following section of the paper mainly discusses the effects of the pandemic and responses to the pandemic in this 2020-2021 timeframe, especially in 2020.

4. Survey of COVID-19 and Peace in Conflict-Affected Areas

Apart from adverse effects on peace, the outbreak of infectious diseases may produce positive peace-related outcomes in society. For example, it could reveal the weaknesses of a given peace strategy, which might then trigger the need or will to improve it, before or after the crisis has been controlled. In some conflict zones, infectious disease outbreaks create opportunities for cooperation between conflict parties, which could be grasped [14,16]. This cooperation caused by diseases is part of what is at times referred to as "disaster diplomacy" or "disaster-related cooperation", which also includes cooperation resulting from the emergence of other kinds of crises, such as natural disasters [16,17,20,21]. Additionally, the outbreak of infectious diseases is said to create conditions that discourage war. For example, it causes economic challenges, which might reduce a state's, or an actor's, capability to start or sustain a war [14]. Most of the existing studies on COVID-19 suggest that its effects have been largely negative, but it seems the pandemic and state responses to it have had mixed effects on peace in conflict-affected areas [14]. While they seemed to reduce conflict or cause cooperation between conflict parties in some cases, they created conditions that enabled conflict in other areas.

The emergence of the disease and subsequent global efforts to curb its spread led to a reduction in the intensity of some conflicts in different zones [14,22]. For example, Ide [23] finds that in the first half of 2020, the pandemic led to a temporary decline in armed conflict events in some conflict-affected areas, including Afghanistan, Colombia, Thailand, and Yemen. He recognizes, however, that there might have been other factors not related to COVID-19 that contributed to the decline in conflict. For example, he notes that the February 2020 peace deal between the United States of America (USA) and the Taliban did influence the Afghanistan case. On the other hand, a report published by the Armed Conflict Location and Event Data Project (ACLED) in 2021 shows that "most wars continued to rage" one year after the COVID-19 situation emerged [24]. Ide [23] observes that although Afghanistan, Colombia, Thailand, and Yemen experienced a temporary decline in armed conflict in early 2020 partly due to the pandemic, armed conflict events seem not to have decreased in the same period in some other areas, such as India, Iraq, Libya, Pakistan, and the Philippines. In fact, according to Ide [23] and Polo [25], it appears that there was rather an increase in armed conflict events in some countries, such as Iraq, Libya, Pakistan, and the Philippines after March 2020, in part due to issues not related to COVID-19. Mehrl and Thurner [26] also found that armed conflicts increased in some parts of the Middle East during the shutdowns in early 2020, but they reduced in Europe, South Asia, and the Caucasus. The pandemic had mixed effects on the Israeli-Palestinian conflict, as shown in Lehrs' [16] analysis of its influence on relations between some key parties in the conflict from March 2020 to September 2020. These parties include Israel and the Palestinian Authority in the West Bank, Israel and the Palestinian community in East Jerusalem, and Israel and the Hamas government in the Gaza strip [16].

In the West Bank, Israel and the Palestinian Authority cooperated at the initial stage when they understood that joint efforts were required to control the virus. In a period when the leaderships of the two parties did not have much communication, the pandemic led to a phone call between the Israeli President, Reuven Rivlin, and the Palestinian President, Mahmoud Abbas, on 18 March 2020, some days after the first case of the virus was declared in Israel on 27 February 2020 [16]. In addition, Israel delivered COVID-19 testing materials to the Palestinian Authority, medical personnel from both parties took part in joint training sessions, discussions between finance ministers of both parties regarding the economic dimensions of the pandemic took place, and financial aid was provided for the Palestinians by Israel [16]. However, Lehrs [16] observes that the interest in cooperation declined as the emergency period passed. The initial cooperation was limited, and it did not prevent violent incidents from occurring in the West Bank. In fact, by the end of May 2020, the situation had changed "from one of cooperation to one of conflict", partly because of some political changes in Israel and because of a perception in Israel that the virus was largely under control [16]. Although the second wave of the infection in Israel, which began in late June, seemed to re-focus the Israeli leadership and public interest on the virus, the conflict between Israel and the Palestinian Authority in the West Bank persisted. The first wave of the virus triggered cooperation between the parties, but the second wave did not [16].

Contradictory effects were also recorded in East Jerusalem. The spread of the virus from March 2020 caused tension between Israeli authorities and the Palestinians, but the situation also led to cooperation between Israeli actors and the Palestinians in the region, and among the Palestinians, who set up committees to provide COVID-19-related assistance to residents of the area [16]. In the Gaza strip, the crisis led to cooperation between the Hamas government, the Palestinian Authority, and Israel, for example, in terms of the coordination of humanitarian efforts [16]. However, the virus later became an issue of conflict between the parties. For example, Hamas demanded ventilators from Israel and even threatened to "take them by force from Israel" if they were not provided, and Israel seemed to require Hamas' release of the bodies of Israeli soldiers in exchange for COVID-19 assistance [16]. By August 2020, the conflict between the Israelis and the Palestinians had escalated despite the initial cooperation, to the point that at least two rockets were launched from Gaza into Israel in August, leading to Israeli military responses [16]. In general, it seems the pandemic has not caused any lasting positive change in the Israeli-Palestinian conflict. As Lehrs [16] explains, it neither produced "a new peacemaking process" nor "a dramatic improvement in relations" between the conflict parties. What is clear, however, is that although pre-disaster conditions in the region shaped the COVID-19 experiences in these three parts of Israel-Palestine, the pandemic promoted cooperation and equally created conditions that enabled conflict.

On 23 March 2020, UN Secretary-General, Antonio Guterres. called for a global humanitarian ceasefire in conflict zones to enable COVID-19 efforts. In response to this, the Saudi-backed coalition in Yemen announced on 8 April 2020 that it would cease all military operations in the country from 9 April 2020 to support coronavirus response, even though no cases had been reported in Yemen. Although many hoped that the declaration would create opportunities for cooperation between the conflict parties, it did not stop the escalation of violence days after the declaration, as Houthi forces are said to have taken advantage of the COVID-19 situation to recruit members and advance their operations [19]. As Montevecchio [19] puts it, this led to the arrest of the "progress towards peace" in Yemen. The UN appeal for a ceasefire initially generated "often unilateral ceasefire agreements" [27] in some conflict zones, including Yemen, Colombia, Cameroon, and the Philippines [19,27,28]. However, the declarations hardly received general acceptance and support from the conflict parties in the areas and therefore, rarely had major lasting effects on hostilities [19,27,28].

As of 11 March 2020, when the World Health Organization (WHO) declared the COVID-19 outbreak a pandemic, at least six United Nations (UN) peacekeeping missions were active in Africa [29]. These include the UN Multidimensional Integrated Stabilization Mission in the Central African Republic (MINUSCA), the UN Multidimensional Integrated Stabilization Mission in Mali (MINUSMA), the UN Interim Security Force for Abyei (UNISFA), The UN Mission in South Sudan (UNMISS), the UN Organization Stabilization Mission in the Democratic Republic of the Congo (MONUSCO), and the African Union-United Nations Mission in Darfur (UNAMID) [29]. In these conflict-affected areas, the pandemic led to cooperation between the UN peacekeepers and the governments of the countries in the coordination of COVID-19 efforts [29]. However, it is not clear whether there has been any lasting positive effect that this cooperation or the pandemic had on the armed conflicts in these African countries. Instead, it is reported that the restrictive measures imposed by the states to mitigate the spread of the virus hampered peace efforts in the countries [29]. For example, Peter [30] and Montevecchio [19] have observed that the pandemic and restrictive measures put in place to control it hindered the implementation of the Revitalized peace Agreement on the Resolution of the Conflict in the Republic of South Sudan (R-ARCSS), which the parties in the South Sudanese conflict signed in Addis Ababa, Ethiopia, on 12 September 2018. In some other conflict zones outside Africa, the pandemic mainly worsened the conflict situation and impeded, rather than aided, peace processes. For instance, in Myanmar, the COVID-19 situation is believed to have deepened the political, economic, and humanitarian crisis that was existing before the first case of the infection in the country was reported on 23 March 2020 [31]. In addition, peace processes in Colombia, the Philippines and Ukraine were slowed down [32], and different studies have shown how UN and non-UN peace work in Africa and other regions were hampered [14,33–38]. The pandemic and the restrictive measures taken by governments also created conditions that led to an increase in local violence in the Democratic Republic of the Congo (DRC), Kenya, Libya, Nigeria, and South Sudan, among other countries within and outside Africa [28].

Global and regional cooperation emerged in response to the pandemic, as in the case of the member states of the South African Development Community (SADC) [39]. Yet, the pandemic raised tensions between countries as in the case of China and the USA. It created security gaps, which terror groups and other violent non-state actors took advantage of. For example, in July 2020, the UN warned that ISIS was exploiting the COVID-19 situation to relaunch operations in Iraq and Syria-in a period when the control of the disease's spread was a priority of most or all governments [40]. In some parts of northern Nigeria where armed bandits attacked communities before the COVID-19 period, communal attacks are said to have increased during the lockdown [14]. Terror groups in the northeast region of the country, including Boko Haram, also took advantage of the disease outbreak to intensify their operations and recruit more members [41].

5. What Determined COVID-19's Impact on Peace?

Although this paper does not do a comprehensive assessment of the different variables that have determined the effect of the pandemic on peace in conflict-affected and non-conflict-affected areas, it will highlight the important role played by two broad factors. These are the pre-COVID-19 political and socio-economic conditions in an area, and how state and non-state actors responded to the pandemic. These factors are discussed below.

5.1. Pre-Existing Conditions

One factor that helped to determine how the pandemic affected peace in different countries is the political and socio-economic situation in the areas before the emergence of COVID-19. This, in turn, helped to shape how different governments responded to the disease. In other words, pre-COVID-19 country-specific conditions and government response were influential determinants of the impact of the pandemic on peace [14,15,42–46]. Different societies experienced the COVID-19 pandemic in different ways. Truly, there were experiences which could be found in more than one area. For example, in some countries where the state ordered a shutdown to curtail the disease's spread, economic difficulties were experienced by large numbers of people. Furthermore, similar religious interpretations and conspiracy theories regarding the disease existed in various societies. In addition, there were fears about COVID-19 vaccination in the West and other countries in the Global South. These similarities notwithstanding, every country where COVID-19 cases were reported had its own unique pre-COVID-19 political and socio-economic conditions, which helped to shape how it responded to the disease, and the impact the disease and the responses had on the society. For example, before the emergence of the disease, some states had a relatively high degree of economic capability and stability, which in turn enabled their governments to ease the economic problems that a COVID-19 shutdown might cause. Other countries where this economic feature was lacking were unable to sustain a system that alleviated the problems resulting from the shutdown. It appears that social unrest was more likely to emerge in areas where COVID-19 restrictive measures were ordered with little or no implementation of economic support policies [43].

In addition, some states had major security problems before the emergence of the disease. COVID-19 seemed to compound the previously existing poor security situation in some of these areas. Armed conflict weakens medical institutions in the area where the conflict takes place, thereby impairing the societies' ability to properly manage an infectious disease outbreak. On the other hand, the spread of an infectious disease might also produce conditions that enable or motivate violence. Hence, the relationship between infectious diseases and conflict is "symbiotic" [22]. The absence of armed conflict and the presence of other peaceful conditions in a society are part of what affects its ability to "anticipate, detect, and coordinate response and recovery" from a disease outbreak situation such as that of COVID-19 [47]. Additionally, it is believed that by worsening conditions that contribute to conflict in conflict-affected areas, COVID-19 might have delayed the realization of peace in the societies. For example, through reduced economic activity and job losses, it increased youth unemployment and youth poverty, which in turn might have aided armed groups' recruitment of new members amid the pandemic [25]. For these reasons, peace actors have been largely concerned about the situation in conflict-affected zones in the COVID-19 period.

Existing studies on COVID-19 and peace in conflict-affected areas show that mostly short-lived cooperation between conflict parties has emerged from the pandemic. This article suggests that one way to understand this limited impact of COVID diplomacy is to think about the complex nature of peace and conflict and the pre-COVID-19 conflict situations in conflict-affected areas. As Ide [23] rightly observes, "armed conflicts are complex, dynamic and multi-faceted phenomena". Similarly, peace in any given conflict-affected or non-conflict-affected area is generally shaped by multiple factors, including political, economic, ethnoreligious, and other kinds of variables, depending on the context [14,48–50]. The prevention of armed conflicts and the causation of sustainable peace in conflict-affected areas require more than the health diplomacy that the need to control COVID-19 generates [14]. It seems that the status of different intrastate conflicts before the emergence of COVID-19 helped to determine the extent to which the conflict parties were committed to advancing any peace talks during the COVID-19 period.

For COVID diplomacy to generate continued cooperation or peace talks between conflict parties, it appears that one necessary condition is that the parties should be willing to extend cooperation beyond the immediate COVID-19 context or be committed to doing so. Such acceptance or commitment might be partially or fully based on a conflict party's understanding that the continued communication or cooperation would or could lead to the partial or total resolution of its central concerns, for which it is involved in the conflict. If the state of the conflict before the emergence of COVID-19 and COVID diplomacy was that of significant distance from resolution, it would be unsurprising if no further peace talks emerge from COVID-19 response. However, that is not to say that there are not other factors apart from pre-COVID-19 conditions which could affect conflict parties' commitment to post-COVID-19 peace talks. This paper recognizes the potency of COVID-19 efforts to facilitate communication and cooperation between conflict parties. In addition, COVID-19 has obstructed peace work that was going on before its emergence and worsened conditions that drive conflict in different areas. Therefore, the point in the current section is not that there is a straightforward link between pre-COVID-19 conflict situation, COVID-19-related cooperation, and post-COVID-19 communication and cooperation between conflict parties in conflict-affected areas. Instead, the point is that pre-existing conflict situations in conflict-affected areas might have helped to determine conflict parties' willingness to promote post-COVID-19 communication, cooperation or peace talks in conflict zones.

5.2. Responses to the Pandemic

To explain how the responses of state and non-state actors to the spread of the virus affected peace, this section pays attention to governments' local COVID-19 efforts and the instrumentalization of the COVID-19 situation by armed groups. As the virus spread across the globe in early 2020, different governments felt the urgent need to curb its spread. Two kinds of responses to the virus produced by this sense of urgency are the introduction of restrictive measures, and cooperation between state and non-state actors in the coordination of COVID-19 efforts. For example, cooperation between different governmental and non-governmental actors in conflict-affected areas emerged in Israel-Palestine and Nigeria [14,16]. A strategy that was widely adopted to curtail the spread of the virus is the use of shutdowns, which many governments in the Global North and Global South introduced in early 2020. Although shutdowns were common, they played out in different societies in different ways. For example, some governments provided financial support for residents during the shutdown, but others provided little or no support. This influenced the behavior of the masses and levels of social unrest during the shutdown [43]. For example, in some areas in Africa where the financial intervention of the state was poor or non-existent, shutdowns led to criminal activity. In parts of Nigeria, residents were less likely to follow the government's shutdown directives, and some people resorted to robbery to get the resources they needed to survive in a period when there was minimal economic activity [14].

Shutdowns generally had a link with protest events. At the beginning of the implementation of shutdowns in many countries in early 2020, there was a significant reduction in demonstrations globally. Understandably, this was because restrictions on people's movement meant that people spent more time away from the public space. However, protest events reemerged later as the shutdown continued [44,51]. It has been reported that there were more demonstrations in 2020 than there were before the emergence of COVID-19 in 2019 [24]. Hence, the relationship between the pandemic or shutdown policies and demonstrations has been understood as being "U-shaped" [44]. Some of the protests condemned government responses to the pandemic, but there were protests related to other pre-COVID-19 matters [24]. It is estimated that about 33,247 of the protests that occurred in 2020 were "directly related to COVID-19" [22].

In early 2020, the need to control the spread of the virus drew the attention of governments in conflict-affected and non-conflict-affected zones. In areas where governments were fighting armed groups before the emergence of the virus, such as Iraq, Libya, Nigeria, and Syria, the governments' attention to COVID-19 and the adverse impact of the pandemic on state economic and military strength created opportunities for armed groups to extend their political and territorial control [14,23,25,52]. In addition, as governments were preoccupied with managing the COVID-19 situation among their local populations, international and UN-led peace efforts declined, and this contributed to the escalation of violence in some areas, such as Libya in early 2020 [23,25,42]. Even though it seems there was a temporary decline in armed conflict events in Afghanistan in early 2020 [23], the Taliban seized the pandemic as an opportunity to intensify their attacks against the Afghan government in that period [25].

6. Conclusions

- The relationship between COVID-19 and peace has been explored from a variety of perspectives. Different studies on the link between COVID 19 and peace in conflict-affected areas exist, but little work has been done on assessing them to understand their key points.
- This article has discussed the major research findings on the impact of COVID-19 and state responses to it on some aspects of peace in conflict-affected areas, including relations between conflict parties, peace efforts and peace processes. The conflict-affected areas considered include Afghanistan, Colombia, Iraq, Israel-Palestine, Libya, Myanmar, Nigeria, South Sudan, Syria, the Philippines, Yemen, and other zones.

- The central finding of the paper is that the existing studies on COVID-19 and peace in conflict-affected areas present mixed findings. On the one hand, the virus generated opportunities for cooperation between conflict parties in some cases, such as in the West Bank and Gaza Strip of Israel-Palestine. However, on the other hand, it created conditions that enabled conflict and impeded peace efforts and processes in many or most conflict-affected areas.
- Given that peace in conflict-affected areas is broader than the issues that have been the primary foci of this paper, a more comprehensive review of existing evidence is required to get a wider understanding of the impact of the virus on peace in the areas.
- In addition, since the global COVID-19 situation is still evolving, its full impact on peace in conflict-affected areas will be understood when its long-term effects are examined in future.
- This paper will be useful in future analyses. It has considered existing evidence on how COVID-19 affected relations between conflict parties, peace efforts, and peace processes in conflict-affected areas.

Funding: This research received no external funding.

Institutional Review Board Statement: Not applicable.

Informed Consent Statement: Not applicable.

Data Availability Statement: Data sharing is not applicable.

Acknowledgments: I am grateful for the help of the editorial team of *Encyclopedia*. I sincerely thank Niall Martin and Jenny Martin for proofreading the manuscript.

Conflicts of Interest: The author declares no conflict of interest.

References

1. Anyanwu, M.U.; Festus, I.J.; Nwobi, O.C.; Jaja, C.-J.I.; Oguttu, J.W. A Perspective on Nigeria's Preparedness, Response and Challenges to Mitigating the Spread of COVID-19. *Challenges* **2020**, *11*, 22. Available online: https://www.mdpi.com/2078-1547/11/2/22# (accessed on 10 August 2021). [CrossRef]
2. Strand, H.; Dahl, M. *Defining Conflict-Affected Countries*; UNESCO: Paris, France, 2010; pp. 1–18. Available online: https://www.prio.org/publications/4817 (accessed on 27 June 2022).
3. OECD. *OECD Due Diligence Guidance for Responsible Supply Chains of Minerals from Conflict-Affected and High-Risk Areas*, 2nd ed.; OECD Publishing: Paris, France, 2013. Available online: https://www.oecd.org/corporate/mne/mining.htm (accessed on 18 May 2022).
4. Malmstrom, C. *Commission Recommendation (EU) 2018/1149—Of 10 August 2018—On Non-Binding Guidelines for the Identification of Conflict-Affected and High-Risk Areas and Other Supply Chain Risks under Regulation (EU) 2017/821 of the European Parliament and of the Council*; European Parliament and of the Council: Brussels, Belgium, 2018.
5. World Bank Classification of Fragile and Conflict-Affected Situations. Available online: https://www.worldbank.org/en/topic/fragilityconflictviolence/brief/harmonized-list-of-fragile-situations (accessed on 8 August 2022).
6. Responsible Minerals Initiative (RMI), Conflict-Affected and High-Risk Areas (CAHRAs). Available online: https://www.responsiblemineralsinitiative.org/minerals-due-diligence/risk-management/conflict-affected-and-high-risk-areas/ (accessed on 8 August 2022).
7. Galtung, J. Positive and Negative Peace. In *Peace and Conflict Studies: A Reader*; Webel, C., Johansen, J., Eds.; Routledge: Abingdon, UK, 2012; pp. 75–80.
8. Hognuld, K.; Soderberg, M. Beyond the Absence of War: The Diversity of Peace in Post-Settlement Societies. *Rev. Int. Stud.* **2010**, *36*, 367–390. [CrossRef]
9. Wagner, R.V. Distinguishing between Positive and Negative Approaches to Peace. *J. Soc. Issues* **1988**, *44*, 1–15. [CrossRef]
10. Jarstad, A.; Eklund, N.; Johansson, P.; Olivius, E.; Saati, A.; Sahovic, D.; Strandh, V.; Soderstrom, J.; Wimelius, M.; Akebo, M. Three Approaches to Peace: A Framework for Describing and Exploring Varieties of Peace. *Umea Work. Pap. Peace Confl. Stud.* **2019**, *12*, 124. Available online: http://www.diva-portal.org/smash/get/diva2:1375816/FULLTEXT02.pdf (accessed on 3 May 2021).
11. Hawksley, T.; Mitchell, J. Introduction. In *Peacebuilding and the Arts*; Mitchell, J., Vincett, G., Hawksley, T., Culbertson, H., Eds.; Palgrave Macmillan: Cham, Switzerland, 2020; pp. 1–31.
12. Little, D. Peace, Justice, and Religion. In *What is a Just Peace?* Allan, P., Keller, A., Eds.; Oxford University Press: New York, NY, USA, 2006; pp. 149–175.
13. Philpott, D. *Just and Unjust Peace*; Oxford University Press: New York, NY, USA, 2012.

14. Ossai, E. Crises, Conflict and Cooperation: The Two-Sided Impact of COVID-19 on Peace in Nigeria. *Afr. Secur.* **2021**, *14*, 410–438. [CrossRef]
15. Richards, P. *Ebola: How a People's Science Helped End an Epidemic*; Zed Books: London, UK, 2016.
16. Lehrs, L. Conflict and Cooperation in the Age of COVID-19: The Israeli-Palestinian Case. *Int. Aff.* **2021**, *97*, 1843–1862. [CrossRef]
17. Ganapati, N.; Kelman, I.; Koukis, T. Analysing Greek-Turkish Disaster-Related Cooperation: A Disaster Diplomacy Perspective. *Coop. Confl.* **2010**, *45*, 162–185. [CrossRef]
18. Onuma, H.; Shin, K.; Managi, S. Short-, Medium-, and Long-Term Growth Impacts of Catastrophic and Non-Catastrophic Natural Disasters. *Econ. Disaster Clim. Chang.* **2021**, *5*, 53–70. [CrossRef]
19. Montevecchio, C. The Peace Dimension of the COVID-19 Pandemic. *J. Soc. Encount.* **2021**, *5*, 37–50.
20. Kelman, I. Acting on Disaster Diplomacy. *J. Int. Aff.* **2006**, *59*, 215–240. Available online: https://www.jstor.org/stable/24358434 (accessed on 20 July 2022).
21. Ker-Lindsay, J. Greek-Turkish Rapprochement: The Impact of Disaster Diplomacy? *Camb. Rev. Int. Aff.* **2000**, *14*, 215–232. [CrossRef]
22. Gugushvili, A.; McKee, M. The COVID-19 Pandemic and War. *Scand. J. Public Health* **2021**, *50*, 16–18. [CrossRef] [PubMed]
23. Ide, T. COVID-19 and Armed Conflict. *World Dev.* **2021**, *140*, 105355. [CrossRef] [PubMed]
24. Kishi, R. A Year of COVID-19: The Pandemic's Impact on Global Conflict and Demonstration Trends. Armed Conflict Location and & Event Data Project (ACLED). April 2021. Available online: https://reliefweb.int/report/world/year-covid-19-pandemic-s-impact-global-conflict-and-demonstration-trends (accessed on 3 August 2021).
25. Polo, S.M.T. A Pandemic of Violence? The Impact of COVID-19 on Conflict. *Peace Econ. Peace Sci. Public Policy* **2020**, *26*. [CrossRef]
26. Mehrl, M.; Thurner, P.W. The Effect of the COVID-19 Pandemic on Global Armed Conflict: Early Evidence. *Political Stud. Rev.* **2020**, *19*, 286–293. [CrossRef]
27. Mustasilta, K. *The Effects of the COVID-19 Pandemic on Peace and Conflict*; IPI Global Observatory: New York, NY, USA, 2020.
28. Bell, C.; Epple, T.; Pospisil, J. *The Impact of COVID-19 on Peace and Transition Processes: Tracking the Trends*; Political Settlements Research Programme (PSRP); University of Edinburgh: Edinburgh, UK, 2020. Available online: https://www.politicalsettlements.org/wp-content/uploads/2020/06/Nexus-Report-Digital.pdf (accessed on 7 June 2022).
29. Makosso, A. United Nations Peacekeeping Operations in the Era of COVID-19. *J. Intell. Confl. Warf.* **2020**, *3*, 26–39. [CrossRef]
30. Peter, M. *COVID-19 and Fragile Peace Process in South Sudan*; Institute of Social Policy and Research: Juba, South Sudan, 2020. [CrossRef]
31. Transnational Institute. *No One Left Behind? COVID-19 and the Struggle for Peace and Justice in Myanmar*; Transnational Institute: Amsterdam, The Netherlands, 2021.
32. Santos, A.; Salamat, N.; Bolukoglu, S.; Baron, B.; Choi, C.; Gasperetti, H. Lockdown on Peace? COVID-19's Impact on Women Peacebuilders. *Soc Polit* **2022**, jxab050. [CrossRef]
33. De Coning, C. COVID-19 and the Resilience of Africa's Peace and Security Networks. *Afr. Secur.* **2021**, *14*, 341–369. [CrossRef]
34. De Coning, C. The Impact of COVID-19 on Peace Operations. *IPI Global Observatory*. 2 April 2020. Available online: https://theglobalobservatory.org/2020/04/impact-covid-19-peace-operations/ (accessed on 2 June 2022).
35. Obi, C.; Kabandula, A. Special Issue on "COVID-19, Peace and Security in Africa: Challenges and Opportunities". *Afr. Secur.* **2021**, *14*, 307–317. [CrossRef]
36. Van der Lijn, J. *The Impact of the COVID-19 Pandemic on Multilateral Peace Operations*; Stockholm International Peace Research Institute: Stockholm, Sweden, 2022.
37. International Alert. *Can We Build Peace from a Distance? The Impact of COVID-19 on the Peacebuilding Sector*; International Alert: London, UK, 2020.
38. Herbert, S.; Marquette, H. *COVID-19, Governance, and Conflict: Emerging Impacts and Future Evidence Needs*; Institute of Development Studies: Brighton, UK, 2021.
39. Joseph, J. The South African Development Community (SADC) and COVID-19: Revisiting Security Community in SADC. *EUREKA Soc. Humanit.* **2021**, *5*, 69–81. [CrossRef]
40. Cruickshank, P. ISIS Exploiting Coronavirus Security Gaps to Relaunch Insurgency, UN Report Warns. *CNN News*. 23 July 2020. Available online: https://edition.cnn.com/2020/07/23/politics/isis-coronavirus-un-terrorism-report/index.html (accessed on 20 August 2021).
41. Iweze, D. COVID-19 and Nigeria's Counterinsurgency Operations in the Northeast. *Kujenga Amani (Social Science Research Council)*. 4 June 2020. Available online: https://kujenga-amani.ssrc.org/2020/06/04/covid-19-and-nigerias-counterinsurgency-operations-in-the-northeast/ (accessed on 20 August 2021).
42. Hilhorst, D.; Mena, R. When COVID-19 Meets Conflict: Politics of the Pandemic Response in Fragile and Conflict-Affected States. *Disasters* **2021**, *45*, S174–S194. [CrossRef] [PubMed]
43. Wood, R.; Reinhardt, G.Y.; Rezaeedaryakenari, B.; Windsor, L.C. Resisting Lockdown: The Influence of COVID-19 Restrictions on Social Unrest. *Int. Stud. Q.* **2022**, *66*, sqac015. [CrossRef]
44. Berman, N.; Couttenier, M.; Monnet, N.; Ticku, R. Shutdown Policies and Conflict Worldwide. *AMSE Work. Papers* **2022**, *50*, 240–255. [CrossRef] [PubMed]
45. Menzel, C. *The Impact of Outbreaks of Infectious Diseases on Political Stability: Examining the Examples of Ebola, Tuberculosis and Influenza*; Fundacion Konrad Adenauer A.C.: Ciudad de México, Mexico, 2017.

46. Long, W. *Pandemics and Peace: Public Health Cooperation in Zones of Conflict*; United States Institute of Peace: Washington, DC, USA, 2011.
47. Syropoulos, S.; Puschett, E.; Leidner, B. Positive and Negative Peace as Predictors of Pandemic Preparedness: Evidence from a Micro- and Macro-Level Investigation during the Onset of the COVID-19 Pandemic. *Polit Psychol.* **2021**, *42*, 729–745. [CrossRef] [PubMed]
48. Ossai, E.C. I Respect My Imam, But I Can't Fight Even If He Tells Me to Fight. I Am Peaceful for Myself and My Family': Are We Overestimating Religion in Peace Dynamics? *Islam Christ. Muslim Relat.* **2021**, *32*, 181–202. [CrossRef]
49. Ossai, E.C. We Aren't Killing Each Other, but We Bear Grudges That Could Be Sparked': How Interreligious 'Peace' and Non-Peace Coexist in a West African City. *Islam Christ. Muslim Relat.* **2020**, *31*, 307–323. [CrossRef]
50. Ossai, E.C. Impact of Religion on Interreligious Peace: Evidence from Zones of Peace in Abuja, Nigeria. Ph.D. Thesis, University of Edinburgh, Edinburgh, UK, 2021. [CrossRef]
51. Bloem, J.R.; Salemi, C. COVID-19 and Conflict. *World Dev.* **2021**, *140*, 105294. [CrossRef]
52. Blanc, J.; Brown, F. Conflict Zones in the Time of Coronavirus: War and War by Other Means. Available online: https://carnegieendowment.org/2020/12/17/conflict-zones-in-time-of-coronavirus-war-and-war-by-other-means-pub-83462 (accessed on 10 September 2022).

encyclopedia MDPI

Entry

COVID-19 Pandemic as a Transitional Event: From the Perspective of the Transition Theory

Eamin Z. Heanoy [1,*], Tugba Uzer [2] and Norman R. Brown [1]

1 Department of Psychology, University of Alberta, Edmonton, AB T6G 2E9, Canada
2 Department of Psychology, TED University, Ankara 06420, Turkey
* Correspondence: heanoy@ualberta.ca

Definition: The COVID-19 pandemic has affected every aspect of people's lives across the globe. It is also unique in the way it changed their lives. In this entry, a framework, the Transition Theory, is outlined, which is used to interpret the transitional properties of this pandemic, the ways it differs from other transitional events, and how it impacts the lives and well-being of the individuals. The prediction is that people might consider the pandemic as an important life transition event only if there is a little similarity between their pre-pandemic and post pandemic lives. Individual differences also need to be considered as those whose lives have been directly affected by the pandemic experience a greater COVID-related change (e.g., job loss vs. no job loss). Lastly, the transitional impact of the pandemic might have a strong link with people's mental outcomes. These notions call for a longitudinal approach to get an accurate understanding of the pandemic experience while this world-changing event unfolds rather than in retrospect.

Keywords: COVID-19; pandemic; transition theory; life elements; transitional impact; well-being

Citation: Heanoy, E.Z.; Uzer, T.; Brown, N.R. COVID-19 Pandemic as a Transitional Event: From the Perspective of the Transition Theory. *Encyclopedia* **2022**, 2, 1602–1610. https://doi.org/10.3390/encyclopedia2030109

Academic Editors: Harry H. X. Wang and Raffaele Barretta

Received: 25 July 2022
Accepted: 9 September 2022
Published: 15 September 2022

1. Introduction

In December 2019, the world saw the emergence of a novel coronavirus disease (COVID-19) which the World Health Organization (WHO) officially labeled a pandemic on 11 March 2020 [1]. As of May 2022, over 500 million positive cases and over 6 million deaths were recorded [2]. To curb the spread of the virus, isolation, social distancing, and other restrictions were put in place [3,4]. As a result, people had to reconfigure aspects of their environments and their routines to adapt to the pandemic-related changes they were experiencing (e.g., online classes, work from home). Furthermore, people's economic stability had a hard hit as financial markets fell and unemployment rates rose. Thus, the pandemic affected life across the globe to some extent in terms of their financial, social, and day-to-day activities. In addition, the pandemic came to dominate the news cycle and social interaction [5,6].

Given the breadth and scope of the pandemic, it is intuitively clear that the pandemic has created a "new normal", or a pandemic period [7]. Considering life events that require an adjustment in a person's accustomed way of life, the COVID-19 pandemic could undoubtedly be counted as one of the most important life events or, in other words, an event of transition that has significantly impacted the lives of people from around the world. How the pandemic has changed people's lives, the nature and extent of these changes, and the effect these changes have had on people's well-being are less clear. It is relatively early to provide a complete empirical explanation of these issues, but given what we know about life transitions, their aspects of it, and their impact on the well-being status [8–18], it is possible to speculate about them in an informed manner. This entry, speaking in broader terms, aims to explain whether the COVID-19 pandemic could be considered a distinctive (life) transition, and its qualitative impact. This is discussed in a few different steps: first, a theoretical framework, the Transition Theory, is outlined, which provides means for understanding the onset of the COVID-19 pandemic as a transitional event; second, discussed how the pandemic appears to be different from other transitional life events; finally, to take into account how the pandemic has been likely to affect people's lives, memories, and well-being.

2. Overview of the Transition Theory—Definition of Transition and Its Properties

According to the Transition Theory [7,17,19,20], a transition is an event or series of events that causes fundamental changes in the "fabric of daily life"—what people do, where they do it, and with whom. During regular periods, when life is relatively stable, we spend most of our time engaging in mundane activities (e.g., commuting, and socializing) [21,22]. During a transition, this stability is interrupted. As a result, the familiar elements (e.g., people, location, objects) of our lives are removed, partially or fully. At the same time, we are introduced to a new set of life elements, marking the beginning of a new period in our lives and the end of the old one. Over time and with repeated exposure, some of these new elements might become familiar and eventually come to represent life, hence, defining the post-transitional period [7,20].

To explain this notion, two separate examples are provided. First, a person who has immigrated to another country has to go through a significant transition, as they have left their stable life behind (e.g., a graduate in the USA) and ended up in a different country with a different role (e.g., a lecturer in the UK). This introduces a new set of life elements (e.g., new neighbors, new stores) which, due to recurrent exposure, leads them towards a new stable post-transitional life period. Second, an individual went on a trip to Japan which introduced another set of novel life elements, but unlike the first example, these new elements had no lasting effect. This was because, at one point, the vacation was over, the individual came back home, and life returned to its normal course. Thus, rather than a stable post-transition period, a "brief interlude" was created. It is important to keep in mind that some of the life elements at any given point are always familiar (e.g., the spouse, the children, the exercise) while others are novel (e.g., a new colleague, a new cafe). That being said, some familiar elements from the pre-transitional period are retained across the transition while others are not (abandoned). Eventually, the post-transitional period should give rise to a new set of familiar life elements.

Hence, the transition could be understood from two aspects. One, where the post-transitional period is very much similar to the pre-transitional period, i.e., the retained life elements are many and the abandoned and/or new elements are few. Two, when pre- and post-transitional periods are very different, i.e., the retained elements are few and the abandoned and/or new elements are many. Thus, numerically speaking, transitions could affect lives through the process of addition (i.e., yielding larger new elements), subtraction (yielding smaller retained elements and larger abandoned elements), or both [7].

Assessment of the Impact of a Transition—Transitional Impact Scale

Since its development, the Transitional Impact Scale (TIS-12) has been used by researchers to assess how candidate transitional events impact the lives of people [15,16,18,23–25]. This 12-item TIS separately evaluates the material and psychological impacts of a transitional event, together explaining the overall changes brought to a person's life. Material impacts indicate the adjustment people have to make to their way of living, including changes in their residence, possessions, day-to-day activities, and people with whom they socialize. Psychological changes concern changes in people's beliefs, life viewpoints, attitudes, self-perception, ethics, and morality. For each TIS item, such as "This event has changed the activities I engage in," the participants had to rate their agreement on a five-point Likert scale ranging from 1 (completely disagree) to 5 (completely agree). In theory, if an event scores higher than three (neutral), that indicates a moderate impact on life at the minimum. In general, major transitions that define important life chapters, e.g., immigration, tend to elicit TIS scores of 4.0 or higher [16,18,23,25,26].

The overall impact of a transitional event on an individual's life is determined by material and psychological changes brought by that event. These two types of changes are to some degree independent, such that psychological change can occur in the absence of material change. For instance, a religious conversion after experiencing trauma would be an example of a dramatic psychological change but a weak material change [15,24]. In contrast, high degrees of material change tend to correspond to high degrees of psychological change, e.g., immigration [27].

While measuring the transitional impact of an event, individual differences also need to be considered. For example, "starting university" might be considered a more impactful transition for the students who left their homes and live in a university dormitory ("dormies") compared to the students who continue living with their parents ("homies"). Likewise, for those immigrating from one country to another, relocation might be a more influential transition in contrast to those relocating within the same state, i.e., from one city to another.

3. COVID-19 Pandemic as an Event of Transition—Features, Assessment, and Scope

The pandemic has caused a substantial change in people's personal, social, and economic life as people have been facing isolation, concern about being infected, life activities, and work-related disruption [28–32]. Some of the changes, especially during the early days of the pandemic, have entailed the move of learning and office work online, closure of retail establishments, cancellation of all recreational activities and social gatherings, people being forced to stay in and as a result, spending more time on social media, and so on. Thus, considering its near-universal scope, this pandemic could be seen as a potentially important, and possibly the largest collective transition of all time [6,7].

Broadly speaking, this pandemic is unique in the way it has affected people's lives. On the one hand, given its pervasive nature, the pandemic should have brought marked changes to everyone's regular lives. On the other hand, the pandemic is likely to affect the lives of some people more than those of others. For example, the widespread job loss during the pandemic or at least in its early phase; people who have lost their jobs should, on average, experience greater COVID-related changes than those who have not [6,28]. These points are further elaborated below.

3.1. Difference between the COVID-19 Transition and Other Life Transitions

Usually, a transition involves the accumulation of changes in a person's life, that is, replacement of old life elements with new ones, e.g., house, shops, neighbors (Figure 1, Panel 1), but one of the atypical features of the COVID-19 pandemic is that it appears to have altered our lives by narrowing them. Simply put, at least during the lockdown, the new normal differed from the old one by largely limiting what we could do and where we could do it. This led us to experience a unique type of transition—"transition-by-omission"—where the set of abandoned familiar elements was much greater than the new set of life elements (Figure 1, Panel 2).

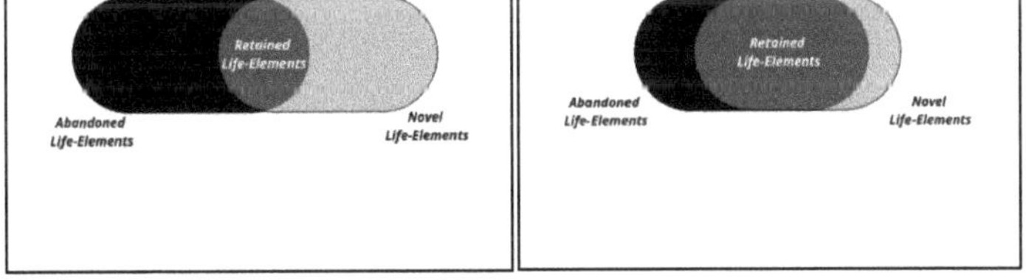

Figure 1. Transition—life elements are replaced, e.g., immigration (**Panel 1**). Transition—life elements are omitted/excluded, e.g., the COVID-19 pandemic (**Panel 2**).

The notion that the COVID-19 pandemic onset was experienced as transition-by-omission as supported by a recent study where 1215 North Americans responded to an online survey [6]. A couple of findings were particularly interesting. First, Cronbach's Alpha of this TIS scale usually ranges from 0.80 to 0.90 [15,24], indicating that major life transitions, such as relocation, typically bring about a synchronized change in many aspects of a person's life. On the other hand, the pandemic produced a Cronbach's Alpha of 0.60, implying that some elements of a person's life were changing but others were not. This point was explained in the second finding. Two of the five items of the material TIS which concerned the activities people engaged in (mean = 3.95) and the places where they spent their time (mean = 3.33) received moderately high scores. The other items, which concerned people (mean = 2.87), belongings (mean = 1.98), and general material circumstances (mean = 2.76), produced ratings at or below the midpoint of the scale. One way to interpret these findings is that, at the outset of the pandemic, many areas went into lockdown. As a result, people could not go where they had been going previously and could not do what they had been doing previously. However, people were, for the most part, still living in the same place they had been living before the pandemic and were spending time with a subset of people with whom they had already been familiar (e.g., family members). Thus, these data indicate that the fabric of daily life has changed for many people, but it was not changed in a wholesome manner [6,7].

In terms of psychological change, people provided moderately high ratings for three out of five items. These concerned attitudes (mean = 3.47), emotional response (mean = 3.43), and thoughts about different things in their lives (mean = 3.71). The other two items, which addressed the sense of self (mean = 2.99) and an understanding of right and wrong (mean = 2.13), received ratings at or below the midpoint of the scale. One explanation could be that the unprecedented nature of the pandemic has caused people to be distressed and have negative affective thoughts. Thus, people have reacted to this atypical period by reevaluating their feelings, thoughts, and perspective towards life, which has brought about a considerable amount of psychological change [6,33].

Therefore, from the Transition Theory perspective, many people have gone through a relatively brief and shallow adjustment period, such as those who have retained their employment, their house, and/or continued their studies during the pandemic. More specifically, these people have faced a decline of familiar elements in their stable daily life to some level, but a moderate increase after some time. This decline was the result of introducing a fair number of new elements (e.g., online classes, video meetings, masks) and a notable decrease in the number of familiar elements (e.g., in-person classes, social gatherings). The stability in life was expected to return rather quickly because life under lockdown tends to be largely repetitive. As a result, the newly introduced life elements should lose their novelty fast. It is true that the pandemic has been disruptive, but compared to other life-changing events (e.g., relocation to a foreign country), life during the pandemic was quite similar to the pre-pandemic one, at least from a materialistic viewpoint (e.g., family dinner, living place, etc.).

3.2. *COVID-19 Transition—Period of Enduring or an Interlude?*

Public events sometimes define the lifetime periods of individuals [18,20,34–37]. This would only happen when a population undergoes a major "collective transition", a transition that brings rapid, fundamental, and enduring changes in the lives of all affected people [7,17,18]. Typically, after this transition, there is a sharp decrease in the stability of people's lives, and this instability sometimes lasts for an extended period. This, in turn, would lead to the gradual establishment of the post-transitional life period which is often different from the earlier (pre-transitional) life period.

During the pandemic or at least at the outset, several billion people have been under lockdown, isolation, or quarantine. The lives these people were living (or are still living) have been different to some extent from the lives they lived before the pandemic. Therefore, the novel coronavirus produced the largest collective transition of all time, at least in the numerical sense. A couple of questions come forward– in the future, will people frequently mention the pandemic while talking about different events from their lives (e.g., "this happened before COVID")? Will people consider the pandemic as an important period and, therefore, think of it as of one of their major life events? [17,38–42]. The answers lie in the prediction of how people might remember the impact of the COVID-19 pandemic on their lives. Prior studies demonstrated that even very important public events (e.g., the 9/11 attacks and the collapse of the Soviet Union) were not regarded as major life events as they did not bring "fundamental and enduring changes" in the lives of all the people who were affected [23,35,36].

Therefore, to speculate whether this COVID-19 transition would be long-standing or just a period of exceptional experience, it is necessary to consider the level of fundamental and enduring changes it brings to people's lives. It is apparent that we are living in a period of new normal that is at least moderately stable and somewhat different from the pre-COVID-19 period. It is also evident that regardless of its near-universal scope, the immediate effect of the pandemic was largely different from one place to another (e.g., in Mexico with a 5.6% case–fatality ratio vs. Japan with a 0.4% case–fatality ratio) [43], from one person to another (e.g., a laid-off restaurant worker vs. a faculty member working from home), and from one timepoint to another (before lockdown vs. after lockdown). The degree to which the life after the pandemic, which may also be called as the next new normal, would be different from the pre-pandemic period. This is a crucial point, as not all transitional events are counted as important; rather, only some distinct, identifiable periods should become a significant part of a person's life. Generally speaking, from the viewpoint of the Transition Theory, a transition is considered important and life-altering when it produces a long-lasting effect and shapes the course of an individual's life [18,40,41,44–46]. Thus, in other words, if a person's post-pandemic life is quite similar to his or her pre-pandemic life, they might well remember the pandemic as a notable period, but retrospectively, should not consider it to be a major life-changing event. Rather, they should regard the Pandemic period more as an extended interlude (e.g., an exchange semester in a foreign country) [7]. The intuition here is that if the pandemic could not produce fundamental and enduring changes in the fabric of daily life of an individual, in a general sense, it should not be marked as one of the most important life-changing events or transitional events of this individual.

Lastly, as mentioned earlier, the COVID-19 pandemic could be seen as an extensive collective transition from a historical viewpoint. It should be mentioned that the Transition Theory treats the personal and collective transition similarly. Thus, as the theory predicts, like any other transition, the COVID-19 pandemic will be considered a major life event only if it brings about a fundamental change in a person's life. This should be true regardless of the pandemic's scope, its cultural and historical importance [18–20]. If those aforementioned social aspects of the pandemic play a significant role in deciding whether the COVID-19 period will be regarded as a major event in an individual's life, then keeping the effect of the transition fixed, this COVID-19 period should be common in the regions where the pandemic had a hard hit and less common in relatively unaffected areas. In another scenario, given the pandemic's breadth and scope, there is a possibility that the 'life at the time of the pandemic' might be a lasting conversational topic for everyone, even for those who were less affected or unaffected, marking it as an important life event [47,48].

3.3. Functionality of the TIS—Measuring the Transitional Impact of the Pandemic

People experiencing transitions after major events (e.g., wars, disasters) have to leave their old routines, take part in many one-off events, and have many first time experiences [49,50]. Likewise, in this pandemic, everyone has had several COVID-19-related first-time experiences, such as online learning, cleaning routine, remote working, sanitization, etc. As discussed earlier, in its near-universal scope, the pandemic, at least at the outset, changed our lives in terms of the activities we do, the people we spend time with, the places we visit, our thoughts, emotions, etc. Hence, the abovementioned

Transitional Impact Scale is a useful measurement tool to identify and assess the material and psychological aspects of an individual's life that has changed due to the pandemic, simultaneously indicating its transitional properties. In line with the Transition Theory, it is reasonable to expect that those who have experienced a greater COVID-19-related change should produce a higher TIS rating than those who have not. This notion was supported by a recent web-based study [6] where those who lost their job as a direct result of the pandemic provided a higher material and psychological TIS rating than those who did not (Table S1). In the research setting, the transitional impact of the pandemic could also be measured by asking participants to provide an open-ended narrative about their pandemic-related experience in combination with TIS [7,33,41,51]. This mixed approach has a merit of overcoming the limitation posed by rating-based instruments alone as responses are collected in an unsolicited manner [32]. People might describe in detail how the pandemic has disrupted their lives by restricting where and what they could do, whom they could meet, changing goals and plans, and experiencing poor emotions [33], increasing the external validity of TIS.

Association with Well-Being Consequences

Prior studies have demonstrated that major life transitions also affect people's overall well-being [8,11,13,14]. To elaborate on that, life transitions or public transitional events could be very stressful, and that links transitional events to mental health issues [52]. Considering the COVID-19 pandemic, as per the Transition Theory, an event of a transition, it brought about a sudden end to routine life and led to a different one, at least during its onset. This adjustment with sudden/new changes (aka transition) is related to a poor well-being outcome [28–30]. Given that the pandemic has generated a great deal of uncertainty and uneasiness [53,54], many have indicated that life during the pandemic is depressing, anxiety-provoking, and stressful [31,55,56]. Especially those whose lives have been directly affected by the pandemic (e.g., residence-displaced, study-disrupted, business-folded) have experienced amplified negative well-being [57–59]. Thus, it could be understood that there is potentially a strong link between the transitional impact of the pandemic and the psychological distress it caused. In numeric terms, the TIS rating, particularly, the material TIS should be a robust predictor of well-being measures, indicating that people have an adverse reaction to the negative consequences of their changing life circumstances [6]. This implies that the TIS instrument could not only identify the quantity and quality of changes brought by the pandemic experience, but also their relation to mental outcomes such as anxiety, depression, and PTSD evoked by the pandemic [24].

3.4. Future Scope of Research

The unusual feature of this pandemic has the potential to attribute to extending the Transition Theory [7,20]. One possible way to do this is by comparing the TIS ratings between two groups—one who have lost their job and the other who have lost their close ones, both as a direct consequence of the pandemic. The aim is to see which group will be more likely to consider the COVID-19 pandemic as a major event in their life period. The expectation is that the job loss group should provide a significantly higher rating in the material and psychological subscale of TIS than the loss of close others group. This is because the job loss group should experience both higher material and psychological change compared to those who have lost their significant ones (high psychological but relatively low material change). More concretely, if the material impact of the COVID-19 pandemic is stronger than its psychological impact, then this should demonstrate that the COVID-19 pandemic satisfies the definition of major life transitions provided by the Transition Theory [15,16,24].

4. Conclusions

Undoubtedly, the COVID-19 pandemic is distinctive in many ways in its near-universal scope and the way it has affected our lives to various degrees—permanently altering for some while temporarily changing for others. The Transition Theory provides an explanation to understand at least some of its uniqueness. From this perspective of the Transition Theory, the beginning of the COVID-19 pandemic can be denoted as a transition by omission, one that has engendered a relatively shallow decline and then a sharp increase in the steadiness of a person's life, leading to a somewhat stable pandemic period. The speculation here is that people will consider the pandemic to be an important transition period only if their pre-pandemic and post-pandemic lives are less similar; or else, this pandemic period will be regarded as an extended interlude [7]. Nevertheless, the COVID-19 pandemic will be viewed as a significant event leaving an impression on people's lives. What is less clear is how this pandemic-specific transition will continue to impact the lives of individuals. The authors believe that there will be a long-term impact of the pandemic as sometimes people's immediate and later reaction to a crisis varies in degrees, especially when that crisis keeps affecting their lives. In other words, the pandemic could pose a nonlinear trajectory as at one-point people might start returning to their normal life. Short-term approaches like cross-sectional studies have shortcomings in their capacity of measuring this "change over time" trend or the cumulative effect of the pandemic. This is because they are carried out at a one-time point or over a short period which makes it difficult to determine the temporal link between the pandemic and its associated changes [60]. This notion calls for a longitudinal approach to assess the pandemic's transitional impact because over time, some people get accustomed to a relatively small adjustment to their routines while others scramble with radical life changes. Understanding this particular differential impact could provide a guiding framework of developing a tailored distress-specific intervention which would not only have the value of dealing with the ongoing pandemic, but also of addressing future ones.

Supplementary Materials: The following supporting information can be downloaded at: https://www.mdpi.com/article/10.3390/encyclopedia2030109/s1, Table S1: Average ratings on COVID-TIS from 1 (strongly disagree) to 5 (strongly agree).

Author Contributions: Conceptualization, E.Z.H. and N.R.B.; methodology, E.Z.H. and T.U.; writing—original draft preparation, E.Z.H.; writing—review and editing, T.U. and N.R.B.; visualization, E.Z.H.; supervision, N.R.B. and T.U.; funding acquisition, N.R.B. All authors have read and agreed to the published version of the manuscript.

Funding: This research was funded by the third author's Natural Sciences and Engineering Research Council of Canada (NSERC) Discovery Grant, RES0038944.

Institutional Review Board Statement: Not applicable.

Informed Consent Statement: Not applicable.

Data Availability Statement: Not applicable.

Conflicts of Interest: The authors declare no conflict of interest.

References

1. World Health Organization. Director-General's Opening Remarks at the Media Briefing on COVID-19 [Speech Transcription]. 2020. Available online: https://www.who.int/dg/speeches/detail/who-director-general-s-openingremarks-at-the-mediabriefing-on-covid-19---11-march-2020 (accessed on 3 May 2020).
2. WHO Coronavirus (COVID-19) Dashboard. Available online: https://covid19.who.int/ (accessed on 30 May 2022).
3. Wang, C.; Pan, R.; Wan, X.; Tan, Y.; Xu, L.; Ho, C.S.; Ho, R.C. Immediate psychological responses and associated factors during the initial stage of the 2019 coronavirus disease (COVID-19) epidemic among the general population in China. *Public Health* **2020**, *17*, 1729. [CrossRef] [PubMed]
4. Ren, S.Y.; Gao, R.D.; Chen, Y.L. Fear can be more harmful than the severe acute respiratory syndrome coronavirus 2 in controlling the corona virus disease 2019 epidemic. *World J. Clin. Cases* **2020**, *8*, 652–657. [CrossRef] [PubMed]
5. Oh, S.H.; Lee, S.Y.; Han, C. The Effects of Social Media Use on Preventive Behaviors during Infectious Disease Outbreaks: The Mediating Role of Self-relevant Emotions and Public Risk Perception. *Health Commun.* **2021**, *36*, 972–981. [CrossRef]
6. Heanoy, E.Z.; Shi, L.; Brown, N.R. Assessing the Transitional Impact and Mental Health Consequences of the COVID-19 Pandemic Onset. *Front. Psychol.* **2020**, *11*, 3715. [CrossRef]

7. Brown, N.R. The possible effects of the COVID-19 pandemic on the contents and organization of autobiographical memory: A Transition-Theory perspective. *Cognition* **2021**, *212*, 104694. [CrossRef]
8. Holmes, T.H.; Rahe, R.H. The social readjustment rating scale. *J. Psychosom. Res.* **1967**, *11*, 213–222. [CrossRef]
9. Wyler, A.R.; Masuda, M.; Holmes, T.H. Magnitude of life events and seriousness of illness. *Psychosom. Med.* **1971**, *33*, 115–122. [CrossRef]
10. Sarason, I.G.; Johnson, J.H.; Siegel, J.M. Assessing the impact of life changes: Development of the life experiences survey. *J. Consult. Clin. Psychol.* **1978**, *46*, 932–946. [CrossRef]
11. Wheaton, B. Life transitions, role histories, and mental health. *Am. Sociol. Rev.* **1990**, *55*, 209–223. [CrossRef]
12. Turner, R.J.; Wheaton, B. The assessment of stress using life events scale. In *Measuring Stress: A Guide for Health and Social Scientists*; Cohen, S., Kessler, R.C., Gordon, L.U., Eds.; Oxford University Press: New York, NY, USA, 1995; pp. 29–53.
13. Rutter, M. Transitions and turning points in developmental psychopathology: As applied to the age span between childhood and mid-adulthood. *Int. J. Behav. Dev.* **1996**, *19*, 603–626. [CrossRef]
14. Tennant, C. Life events, stress and depression: A review of recent findings. *Aust. N. Z. J. Psychiatry* **2002**, *36*, 173–182. [CrossRef]
15. Svob, C.; Brown, N.R.; Reddon, J.R.; Uzer, T.; Lee, P.J. The transitional impact scale: Assessing the material and psychological impact of life transitions. *Behav. Res. Methods* **2014**, *46*, 448–455. [CrossRef] [PubMed]
16. Shi, L.; Brown, N.R. The effect of immigration on the contents and organization of autobiographical memory: A transition-theory perspective. *J. Appl. Res. Mem. Cogn.* **2016**, *5*, 135–142. [CrossRef]
17. Brown, N.R.; Schweickart, O.; Svob, C. The effect of collective transitions on the organization and contents of autobiographical memory: A transition theory perspective. *Am. J. Psychol.* **2016**, *129*, 259–282. [CrossRef] [PubMed]
18. Gu, X.; Tse, C.S.; Brown, N.R. The effects of collective and personal transitions on the organization and contents of autobiographical memory in older Chinese adults. *Mem. Cogn.* **2017**, *45*, 1335–1349. [CrossRef]
19. Brown, N.R.; Hansen, T.G.B.; Lee, P.J.; Vanderveen, S.A.; Conrad, F.G. Historically defined autobiographical periods: Their origins and implications. In *Under-Standing Autobiographical Memory: Theories and Approaches*; Berntsen, D., Rubin, D., Eds.; Cambridge University Press: Cambridge, UK, 2012; pp. 160–180.
20. Brown, N.R. Transition theory: A minimalist perspective on the organization of autobiographical memory. *J. Appl. Res. Mem. Cogn.* **2016**, *5*, 128–134. [CrossRef]
21. Kahneman, D.; Krueger, A.B.; Schkade, D.A.; Schwarz, N.; Stone, A.A. A survey method for characterizing daily life experience: The day reconstruction method. *Science* **2004**, *306*, 1776–1780. [CrossRef]
22. White, M.P.; Dolan, P. Accounting for the richness of daily activities. *Psychol. Sci.* **2009**, *20*, 1000–1008. [CrossRef]
23. Nourkova, V.V.; Brown, N.R. Assessing the impact of "The Collapse" on the organization and content of autobiographical memory in the former Soviet Union. *J. Soc.* **2015**, *71*, 324–337. [CrossRef]
24. Uzer, T. Validity and reliability testing of the transitional impact scale. *Stress. Health* **2020**, *36*, 478–486. [CrossRef]
25. Uzer, T.; Beşiroğlu, L.; Karakılıç, M. Event centrality, transitional impact and symptoms of posttraumatic stress in a clinical sample. *Anxiety Stress Coping* **2020**, *33*, 75–88. [CrossRef] [PubMed]
26. Uzer, T.; Brown, N.R. Disruptive individual experiences create lifetime periods: A study of autobiographical memory in persons with spinal cord injury. *Appl. Cogn. Psychol.* **2015**, *29*, 768–774. [CrossRef]
27. Svob, C.; Brown, N.R. Intergenerational transmission of the reminiscence bump and biographical conflict knowledge. *Psychol. Sci.* **2012**, *23*, 1404–1409. [CrossRef] [PubMed]
28. Fitzpatrick, K.M.; Harris, C.; Drawve, G. Fear of COVID-19 and the mental health consequences in America. *Psychol. Trauma Theory Res. Pract. Policy* **2020**, *12*, S17–S21. [CrossRef] [PubMed]
29. Tull, M.T.; Edmonds, K.A.; Scamaldo, K.M.; Richmond, J.R.; Rose, J.P.; Gratz, K.L. Psychological outcomes associated with stay-at-home orders and the perceived impact of COVID-19 on daily life. *Psychiatry Res.* **2020**, *289*, 113098. [CrossRef]
30. Shigemura, J.; Ursano, R.J.; Morganstein, J.C.; Kurosawa, M.; Benedek, D.M. Public responses to the novel 2019 coronavirus (2019-nCoV) in Japan: Mental health consequences and target populations. *Psychiatry Clin. Neurosci.* **2020**, *74*, 281. [CrossRef]
31. Choi, E.P.H.; Hui, B.P.H.; Wan, E.Y.F. Depression and anxiety in Hong Kong during COVID-19. *Int. J. Environ. Res. Public Health* **2020**, *17*, 3740. [CrossRef]
32. Whitehead, B.R.; Torossian, E. Older adults' experience of the COVID-19 pandemic: A mixed-methods analysis of stresses and joys. *Gerontologist* **2021**, *61*, 36–47. [CrossRef]
33. Heanoy, E.Z.; Nadler, E.H.; Lorrain, D.; Brown, N.R. Exploring People's Reaction and Perceived Issues of the COVID-19 Pandemic at Its Onset. *Int. J. Environ. Res. Public Health* **2021**, *18*, 10796. [CrossRef]
34. Bohn, A.; Habermas, T. Living in history and living by the cultural life script: How older Germans date their autobiographical memories. *Memory* **2016**, *24*, 482–495. [CrossRef]
35. Brown, N.R.; Lee, P.J. Public events and the organization of autobiographical memory: An overview of the Living-in-History Project. *Behav. Sci. Terror. Political Aggress.* **2010**, *2*, 133–149. [CrossRef]
36. Brown, N.R.; Lee, P.J.; Krslak, M.; Conrad, F.G.; Hansen, T.; Havelka, J.; Reddon, J.R. Living in history: How war, terrorism, and natural disaster affect the organization of autobiographical memory. *Psychol. Sci.* **2009**, *20*, 399–405. [CrossRef] [PubMed]
37. Zebian, S.; Brown, N.R. Living in history in Lebanon: The influence of chronic social upheaval on the organization of autobiographical memory. *Memory* **2014**, *22*, 194–211. [CrossRef]
38. Friedman, W.J. Memory for the time of past events. *Psychol. Bull.* **1993**, *113*, 44–66. [CrossRef]

39. Shum, M.S. The role of temporal landmarks in autobiographical memory processes. *Psychol. Bull.* **1998**, *124*, 423–442. [CrossRef]
40. Habermas, T.; Bluck, S. Getting a life: The emergence of the life story in adolescence. *Psychol. Bull.* **2000**, *126*, 748–769. [CrossRef]
41. McAdams, D.P. The psychology of life stories. *Rev. Gen. Psychol.* **2001**, *5*, 100–122. [CrossRef]
42. Thomsen, D.K. Autobiographical periods: A review and central components of a theory. *Rev. Gen. Psychol.* **2015**, *19*, 294–310. [CrossRef]
43. Johns Hopkins Coronavirus Resource Center. Mortality Analysis. Available online: https://coronavirus.jhu.edu/data/mortality (accessed on 19 May 2022).
44. Gu, X.; Tse, C.; Brown, N.R. Factors that modulate the intergenerational transmission of autobiographical memory from older to younger generations. *Memory* **2020**, *28*, 204–215. [CrossRef]
45. Thomsen, D.K.; Jensen, T.; Holm, T.; Olesen, M.H.; Schnieber, A.; Tønnesvang, J. A 3.5 year diary study: Remembering and life story importance are predicted by different event characteristics. *Conscious. Cogn.* **2015**, *36*, 180–195. [CrossRef]
46. Thomsen, D.K.; Berntsen, D. The cultural life script and life story chapters contribute to the reminiscence bump. *Memory* **2008**, *16*, 420–436. [CrossRef] [PubMed]
47. Cohn, M.A.; Mehl, M.R.; Pennebaker, J.W. Linguistic markers of psychological change surrounding September 11, 2001. *Psychol. Sci.* **2004**, *15*, 687–693. [CrossRef] [PubMed]
48. Hirst, W.; Echterhoff, G. Remembering in conversations: The social sharing and reshaping of memories. *Annu. Rev. Psychol.* **2012**, *63*, 55–79. [CrossRef]
49. Robinson, J.A. First Experience Memories: Contexts and Functions in Personal Histories. In *Theoretical Perspectives on Autobiographical Memory*; Conway, M.A., Rubin, D.C., Spinnler, H., Wagenaar, W.A., Eds.; Springer: Dordrecht, The Netherlands, 1992; pp. 223–239.
50. Rubin, D.C.; Rahhal, T.A.; Poon, L.W. Things learned in early adulthood are remembered best. *Mem. Cognit.* **1998**, *26*, 3–19. [CrossRef] [PubMed]
51. Thomsen, D.K. There is more to life stories than memories. *Memory* **2009**, *17*, 445–457. [CrossRef]
52. Lundberg, U.; Theorell, T.; Lind, E. Life changes and myocardial infarction: Individual differences in life change scaling. *J. Psychosom. Res.* **1975**, *19*, 27–32. [CrossRef]
53. McGinty, E.E.; Presskreischer, R.; Han, H.; Barry, C.L. Psychological distress and loneliness reported by US adults in 2018 and April 2020. *JAMA* **2020**, *324*, 93–94. [CrossRef]
54. Zandifar, A.; Badrfam, R. Iranian mental health during the COVID-19 epidemic. *Asian J. Psychiatry* **2020**, *51*, 101990. [CrossRef]
55. Xiang, Y.T.; Yang, Y.; Li, W.; Zhang, L.; Zhang, Q.; Cheung, T.; Ng, C.H. Timely mental health care for the 2019 novel coronavirus outbreak is urgently needed. *Lancet Psychiatry* **2020**, *7*, 228–229. [CrossRef]
56. Torales, J.; O'Higgins, M.; Castaldelli-Maia, J.M.; Ventriglio, A. The outbreak of COVID-19 coronavirus and its impact on global mental health. *Int. J. Soc. Psychiatry* **2020**, *66*, 317–320. [CrossRef]
57. Crayne, M.P. The traumatic impact of job loss and job search in the aftermath of COVID-19. *Psychol. Trauma.* **2020**, *12*, S180. [CrossRef] [PubMed]
58. Purtle, J. COVID-19 and mental health equity in the United States. *Soc. Psychiatry Psychiatr. Epidemiol.* **2020**, *55*, 969–971. [CrossRef] [PubMed]
59. Killgore, W.D.; Cloonan, S.A.; Taylor, E.C.; Dailey, N.S. Mental health during the first weeks of the COVID-19 pandemic in the United States. *Front. Psychiatry* **2021**, *12*, 561898. [CrossRef] [PubMed]
60. Levin, K. Study design III: Cross-sectional studies. *Evid. Based Dent.* **2006**, *7*, 24–25. [CrossRef] [PubMed]

encyclopedia

MDPI

Entry

Telework: Before and after COVID-19

Mirela Cătălina Türkeș [1,*] and Daniela Roxana Vuță [2]

1 Faculty of Economics and Business Administration, Dimitrie Cantemir Christian University, 040051 Bucharest, Romania
2 Faculty of Economic Sciences and Business Administration, Transilvania University of Brasov, 1 Colina Universitatii Street, Building A, 500068 Brasov, Romania; daniela.vuta@unitbv.ro
* Correspondence: mirela.turkes@ucdc.ro; Tel.: +40-728-176-475

Definition: Telework is, today, a voluntary form of work organization in which the employee is located outside the employer's premises, at home or elsewhere, under a telework contract, uses information and communication technologies (ICT) and works according to a predetermined schedule on the basis of an agreed supervisory mechanism and an online reporting system on the work undertaken.

Keywords: teleworking evolution; COVID-19; work legislation; work–life balance

1. History

During the COVID-19 pandemic, teleworking became the "new normal," changing people's lives and affecting working relationships. More than ever, it has inspired researchers from different fields of activity: economic, sociology, medical, ethical, etc. Reviewing the literature, this entry rediscovered the concept of "teleworking" and how it evolved in the context of socio-economic development from 2000 to 2019. In the context of the crisis generated by the COVID-19 pandemic, this entry looked for answers regarding the changes produced by teleworking, one of the main forms of adapting employment to social distancing. What changes have been made to the legal and contractual regulations? How was the work schedule organized and the working time recorded? How was the training provided and performance management carried out? What measures have been taken regarding the socio-fiscal protection, occupational safety, and work health of employees? What were the effects of digitalization? How has the work–life balance changed? In terms of results, there is clear evidence that telework leads to increased professional satisfaction, higher productivity, and reduced administrative costs, representing a viable future option.

Telework is a compound term originated by joining two components, "telou" (distance) from the Greek language and the word "tripalliare" (work) of Latin origin [1]. The term can also be found in the specialized literature under the appellation of remote work [2], working at a distance [3], teleworking [4], telecommuting [5], working from home (WFH) [6], mobile work [7], remote e-working [8], and work from anywhere [9]. It is worth noting that the term "telecommuting" appears almost exclusively in articles published in the North American media, while in European publications, the preferred term seems to be "telework."

The premises for the emergence of telework were created during the Industrial Revolution in telecommunications in the early nineteenth century. Once the federal postal service, telegraphs, photographs, and telephones were introduced, it generated the transition from a society based on voice communication, art, and writings (letters, newspapers, and books) to an industrialized one, marked by the development of the social division of labor, emergence of new branches of production, new industrial, commercial and transport centers, and expansion of economic, commercial, and communication relations.

Over time, researchers have tried to provide a unitary and well-accepted definition for telework, but with little success. A definition that covers the essence of telework and

Citation: Türkeș, M.C.; Vuță, D.R. Telework: Before and after COVID-19. *Encyclopedia* **2022**, 2, 1370–1383. https://doi.org/10.3390/encyclopedia2030092

Academic Editors: Stephen Bustin, Milva Pepi and Raffaele Barretta

Received: 30 March 2022
Accepted: 14 July 2022
Published: 18 July 2022

differentiates it from other forms of work in the context of changes over time seems an impossible endeavor.

In the 1980s, Grant et al. (1985) [10] characterized teleworking as "one kind of remote working, or doing normal work activities while away from one's normal workplace." Other researchers have issued narrow definitions, such as: "working away from the central office" [11], "for employees to work out of their homes" [12], and "working at home" [13]. If computer and communications technology are considered [14], the definition of remote work is expanded to include aspects of the processes required to organize work outside the normal organizational boundaries of space and time.

In the second half of the twentieth century, the digital revolution, through the integration of digital computers and communication technologies, gradually allowed the transition from mechanical and analog electronic technology to digital electronics. The advent of the Internet, the introduction of the home computer, the invention of the World Wide Web, the provision of the first online services by its members, the transition to digital television, the use of mobile phones, online social networks, and the increase in the number of users have marked the beginning of an era of information and communication technologies in the production process, machines gradually diminishing the need for human intervention. In this context of the digital economy, the interest in teleworking has increased and international institutions, and contemporary researchers have developed new modern approaches to this concept.

In 1996, the International Labor Organization (ILO) saw work from home as a form of work organization in which the employee is located at a distance from the organization's headquarters or production units and cannot have personal contact with co-workers [15]. In 2020, the same organization expands the definition of telework, saying that it represents work performed outside the employer's headquarters, at the employee's home, or elsewhere by using information and communication technologies (ICT), such as smartphones, tablets, laptops, and desktop computers, etc., and carried out based on a voluntary agreement between the employer and the employee, based on some previously established hours/ schedule, agreed on surveillance mechanism, and some arrangements for reporting the work undertaken [16].

In addition to the above, in 2008, the European Commission proposed several recommendations on teleworking, such as voluntary choice of teleworking, the right to return to work at the organization's headquarters, the guarantee of maintaining the status of the employee, providing equal treatment, the employer's obligation to inform, train and evaluate the teleworker, coverage of the costs of teleworking arrangements by the employer, ensuring the protection of all teleworkers in the field of occupational safety and health (OSH), concluding insurance and confidentiality contracts with teleworkers, respecting the rights and obligations of teleworkers, and facilitating access to telework [17].

In the context of the European Employment Strategy, negotiated agreements between the European Council and several social partners for the modernization of the labor organization led to the issuance of Directives 91/533/EEC [18] and 2019/1152 [19], which regulated new teleworking-specific information, such as a telework employment agreement, telework voluntariness and reversibility, telework working instruments, equal treatment and non-discrimination of teleworkers, the privacy of teleworkers, and vulnerable groups of workers.

Some older studies present teleworking as a flexible way of working that involves the accomplishment of a wide range of remote work activities, electronic information processing, and using telecommunications to maintain the employer–employee relationship while performing full-time or part-time work [20,21]. Authors use terms such as "telework," "telecommuting," or "remote work," which generally refer to lucrative activities or work tasks carried out outside the office, either at home or elsewhere, and relying on new technologies [22–25]

The aim of the entry is to analyze the evolution of telework as a flexible and modern way of working before and after the COVID-19 pandemic, but also the psycho-socio-economic implications generated on the activity of European enterprises.

The first objective of the entry is to identify several specific aspects of telework, also highlighting its evolutionary change and socio-economic implications until 2019. Following the change in the way we connect, communicate, and work, the second objective examines the changes in telework regarding legal and contractual regulations, work arrangements, working time, measures regarding socio-fiscal protection, work safety, the health of employees, digitalization, and work-life balance, all as a form of adapting to the sensitive socio-economic context generated by the COVID-19 pandemic. The third objective involves making a forecast of the evolution of the number of teleworkers between 2022 and 2025 in the EU (27 countries), which was made by using the Time Series Modeler procedure.

In the context of increasingly competitive and intensely digitized economies, this entry contributes to the literature by presenting the deepest transformations suffered by this voluntary form of work organization, from its appearance to the present.

2. The Evolution of Telework between 1990–2019

Current trends and future evolutions of telework have been the subject of numerous international studies. Specialists grouped the statistics related to telework, considering the degree of penetration in different countries, the potential for adaptation, and future growth. Thus, Huws (1991) [26] explored the meanings attributed to homeworkers and the present and future extent of teleworking. According to Gareis and Kordey (2000) [27], at the end of 1999, nine million EU residents were teleworking, and their number was to increase between 5–22.8% by 2005 in the most developed countries, such as France, Italy, Germany, Spain, and the United Kingdom.

From 2011 to 2019, the share of employed persons working from home in the total employment has experienced a different evolution from country to country. In Belgium, the share of employed persons working from home decreased from 9.9% in 2011 to 6.6% in 2018. In Figure 1, a similar evolution is observed in Denmark, where the share of employed persons working from home decreased from 12.0% (2011) to 7.9% (2019). At the opposite pole are Malta and Finland, where the share of employees working at home increased by 4.2 and, respectively, 3.6 in the same period [28].

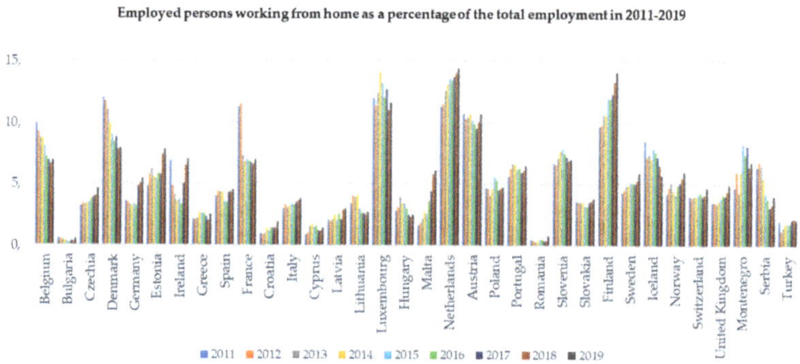

Figure 1. Employed persons working from home as a percentage of the total employment in 2011–2019.

In the European Union (EU), the share of people aged between 15 and 64 working from home out of the total employment increased from 5.4% in 2019 to 12.0% in 2020 and 13.2% in 2021 [28]. The highest shares of females working from home were recorded in Finland (13.3%), the Netherlands (12.5%), and Luxembourg (12.4%). A special situation is observed in the Netherlands (15.4%) and Finland (14.7%), where the share of males who worked from home during the pandemic was higher than that of females (see Figure 2).

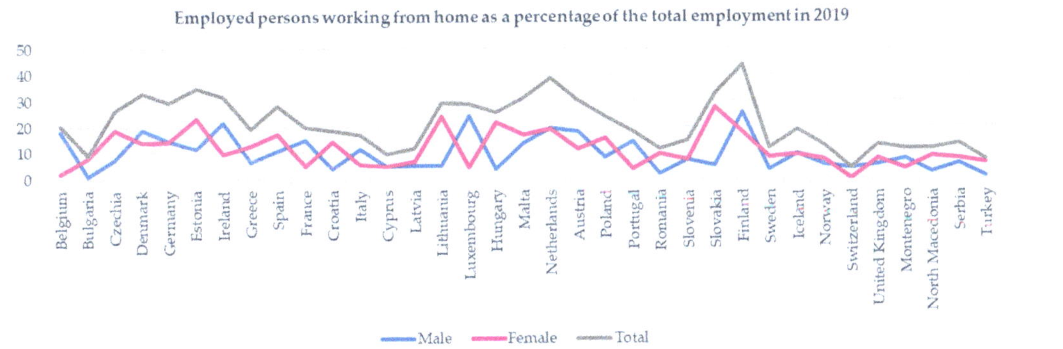

Figure 2. Employed persons working from home as a percentage of the total employment in 2019.

Dangelmaier et al., in 1999 [29], estimated that the penetration of teleworking in the U.S. would have increased to 25% by 2001. At the same time, other surveys indicated high rates of telework in Scandinavian countries and the Netherlands [30]. Grimes (2000) [31], analyzing the development perspectives of rural areas, considered that the social dimension must be connected with the technological dimension, focused on the installation of the necessary infrastructure and equipment, and that teleworking is the ideal form to be promoted in these areas. The results of a 1993 study showed that in New Zealand, the number of teleworkers had increased, especially among low-skilled technical workers, professionals, or innovative small businesses at home [32]. Another study from Latvia shows that, in the context of globalization, the integration of information and communication technologies, as well as the change of professional responsibilities, the demand for telework increases regardless of criteria, such as gender, age, and place of residence of the respondents. Moreover, the inhabitants of less populated areas are interested in socializing, and professional networking activities and are looking for a job in smart centers specially created for remote work [33]. Hesse (1995) [34] shows that the potential for teleworking will increase over time, presenting the example of the U.S. Department of Defense, which has expanded telecommuting arrangements for its employees with disabilities and designed the technologies needed for this form of work in the short and long term.

In recent years, more and more studies have shown that the use of teleworking brings many benefits to individuals, organizations, and society. These are presented in Table 1.

Table 1. The multiple benefits brought by telework.

<table>
<tr><th colspan="3">The Benefits Brought by Telework</th></tr>
<tr><td>1.</td><td colspan="2">Individuals</td></tr>
<tr><td></td><td>→ contribute to achieving a better work–life balance;
→ obtaining a flexible schedule, working in a coworking space or on vacation;
→ decreasing the expenses regarding transport, clothes, and food;
→ reducing stress and burnout syndrome (professional burnout);
→ developing telework-specific skills.</td><td>[35–39]</td></tr>
<tr><td>2.</td><td colspan="2">Organizations</td></tr>
<tr><td></td><td>→ reducing administrative costs;
→ growing labour productivity;
→ increasing employee engagement;
→ finding new ways of employee recruitment.</td><td>[39–41]</td></tr>
</table>

Table 1. *Cont.*

	The Benefits Brought by Telework	
3.	**Society**	
	→ new job opportunities for rural residents and small communities; → more time for parents to spend with their children while balancing their professional and personal interests; → reduced commuting to and from work; → facilitates its replacement with voluntary actions directed at people without food or shelter or with abandoned pets; → reducing environmental pollution, consumption of non-renewable resources, and lowering waste levels; → leads to reduced discrimination; → increases the opportunity to find a job for people with health problems and veterans; → improves public health; → creates the opportunity to extend one's career beyond retirement.	[42]

The existing literature highlights a series of studies that analyze the attitudes and perceptions of managers and employees related to telework. Some managers, although reporting positive attitudes towards telework, still show high resistance, although this could become a significant form of work [43]. Silva-C (2019) [44] noted that specific managerial practices, employee productivity, and the improvement of information security tools in organizations are the main factors affecting managers' attitudes towards adopting teleworking practices. For young workers who use information and communication technologies (ICT) easily, telework has become a natural part of work, while for older workers, it has become a form of postponing or staying active after retirement.

For enterprises, teleworking can also be seen as an opportunity to hire young and older people, ensure working patterns' diversification, and experience exchange [45].

3. Telework and COVID-19 Pandemic

With the outbreak of the COVID-19 pandemic, telework represented, on the one hand, a form of workforce adaptation to new social distancing conditions and, on the other hand, a method of organizing the activity of enterprises and employment. Telework rapidly extended, and many employees were forced to work from home, which, for a significant part of them, was a novelty. Moreover, the implementation of telework was one of the measures highly recommended or imposed by government institutions, which had to be accepted by employees and employers through agreements as a measure of maintaining an important part of the human capital and an opportunity to implement new informational communication technologies. In addition to the legal and contractual implications, both EU and national regulations on teleworking during the COVID-19 pandemic have undergone a series of changes related to work organization, tasks, working time, training, and performance management, and socio-fiscal protection, occupational safety and health measures, digitalization, and work–life balance.

3.1. Legal and Contractual Implications

In most EU countries, teleworking has been regulated by one of the following three methods: statutory legislation, social dialogue, and collective bargaining. If in some countries, there were statutory definitions and specific legislation included in the labor code and related rules (Belgium, Bulgaria, Czech Republic, Spain, Germany, Estonia, France, Greece, Hungary, Croatia, Italy, Lithuania, Luxembourg, Malta, the Netherlands, Poland, Portugal, Romania, Slovenia, and Slovakia), in others (Austria, Cyprus, Denmark, Finland, Ireland, Latvia, and Sweden), statutory legislation on teleworking has been regulated by laws on data protection, working time, and the safety and health of employees [46].

Individual and collective labor contracts were updated with new conditions in countries such as Romania, Bulgaria, Hungary, Luxembourg, and Slovenia, while in others (France, Estonia, Spain, Malta, Croatia, Italy, Portugal, and Greece) it was enough only to conclude written agreements. According to Hendrickx et al. (2020) [47], the Belgian government adopted a series of labor market-related measures, amending the legal regulations on teleworking and social distancing while implementing the Belgian temporary unemployment system. To reduce the effects of the pandemic, the French government introduced partial unemployment measures, thus distributing the efforts between the state, employers, and employees and limiting the loss of jobs [48].

3.2. Work Organization and Working Time

As the COVID-19 pandemic spread rapidly, more and more European enterprises were forced to introduce temporary leave, reduce wages, reduce working hours, temporarily or permanently suspend their activities, operate redundancies, or reduce the number of jobs. A significant part of the active European population was forced to choose between teleworking or part-time work, where the activities of the enterprises allowed it. In the case of teleworking, most of the changes included: work schedule modifications agreed upon by both parties or a pre-set schedule introduced by the employer, workload management, recording (monitoring) of the hours worked (limited, normal, and overtime), defining job autonomy with consequences on the priority and content of professional tasks, and others. Recent studies have shown that most teleworkers have experienced extended work schedules as a result of prolonged working hours during the evening and on weekends or due to the extension of meetings with clients or work teams to meet the demands of work [49–51]. Other theorists studying the effects of team member diversity on work dynamics and performance in the Global Virtual Team (GVT) showed that it generally has a substantial effect on effectiveness, while contextual diversity has a positive influence on task outcomes, and personal diversity has a negative impact on psychological outcomes [52–54]. Andrade and Petiz Lousã (2021) [55] showed that teleworking has brought about major changes in employees' work routines, such as increased overtime, overloaded roles, training on the use of technology after working hours, low work autonomy, and a blurred line between paid work and personal life.

3.3. Training and Performance Management

During the COVID-19 pandemic, enterprises identified new opportunities and faced new challenges related to staff training and professional improvement. On the one hand, telework required a different way of managing remote work teams and a distinct way of recruiting staff, while, on the other hand, it led to developing new skills needed to cope with a crisis, protecting the well-being of employees, and maintaining organizational performance.

Through the available devices and platforms, the enterprises had the opportunity to implement multiple initiatives, such as communication and collaboration with their employees, training programs to acquire the skills and knowledge necessary for successful teleworking, and motivation to support labor productivity and business performance. To foster performance, enterprises had to provide their employees with high-effective work equipment, adequate security conditions, training for leadership and communication skills in times of crisis, instructions for efficient time management, indications for minimizing health risks, options for maintaining the balance between work and personal life, and recommendations for adopting healthy eating habits and sufficient time for rest, etc. Buomprisco et al. (2021) [56] analyzed the effects of teleworking on workers' health and safety and highlighted the need to raise awareness among managers and teleworkers on the importance and right of having rest breaks during the working day, as well as the positive impact on health. Organizations had to teach their employees about the inherent risks in using data display screens [57], the use of e-learning platforms [58], or telementoring platforms for practical training [59].

One important challenge managers had to face was to maintain a high standard of performance, from the team level to the overall organizational performance, while fulfilling their commitments to employees, customers, stakeholders, and other beneficiaries. Kim et al. (2021) [60], assessing the role of supervisors in managing/ motivating teleworkers, showed that supervision, which includes results-based management and confidence-building efforts, has contributed substantially to improving organizational performance where teleworking has been applied. Bușu and György (2021) [61] demonstrated the influence of professional teleworking activities on employee performance in the context of adapting the new work system. Moreover, they claimed that the impact of teleworking on business performance was conditioned by several determining factors, such as the adequate management of human resources, capitalization of the positive aspects of teleworking, the ability to actively involve all staff, and the ability to reward teleworkers for the work performed and to prevent their resistance to change. The study conducted by Jamal et al. (2021) [62] showed that the presence of autonomy, the flexibility of working hours, and the existence of technological resources have contributed to improving the work–life balance, raising work productivity and performance, and increasing employees' satisfaction in full-time telework.

3.4. Socio-Fiscal Protection, Occupational Safety, and Health

With the transition to telework, employees have been exposed to various physical and psychological risks to their health and safety when working. For this reason, the organizations responsible for the health and safety of their teleworkers had to identify and effectively manage these occupational risks. During the COVID-19 pandemic, teleworking for most employees meant longer time spent in front of the computer.

Therefore, the physical health threats category includes the risks generated by prolonged office work in front of laptops. Ergonomic problems often lead to many diseases, such as scoliosis, myopia, diabetes, cardiovascular diseases, obesity, and/or can cause negative effects on the health of employees, such as back pain, neck pain, shoulder pain, tired eyes, etc. The psychological risks faced by teleworkers refer to isolation, overwork, stress, anxiety, depression, anger, insomnia, etc. [63].

Analyzing the significant impact of the intrusive type of management on employees during telework, Magnavita et al. (2021) [64] showed that performing tasks outside the working hours generated occupational stress, less happiness, anxiety, and depression. According to Brooks et al., 2021 [65], multi-week quarantine and social distancing had a strong impact on the entire population, leading to "emotional disorders, depression, stress, low mood, irritability, insomnia, post-traumatic stress symptoms, anger, and emotional exhaustion." Carillo et al., 2021 [49], highlighted how the crisis generated by the COVID-19 pandemic had profound implications on teleworkers, leading to professional isolation, a difficult work environment, and increased work and stress. Overall, the coronavirus pandemic has led to changes in occupational safety and health rules. Regarding how to promote employee health while working from home, several studies revealed the significant influence of teleworking on the mental and physical health of employees and proposed new recommendations for employers and employees to optimize their health (Oakman et al., 2020 and Turkes et al., 2021) [66,67]. Belzunegui-Eraso and Erro-Garcés (2020) [68] analyzed how to implement telework as a security practice to cope with the first wave of the COVID-19 disease crisis. Baert et al. (2020) [69] examined the perceptions of Flemish employees about teleworking and observed that some consider telework and digital conferencing as actions needed to retain employment during the COVID-19 crisis, while others admit that it diminishes their opportunities and weakens ties with their colleagues and their employer (43%).

Authorities have adopted socio-fiscal measures to help employees overcome the problems generated by the COVID-19 pandemic and to support those who carry out telework activities. For example, the Italian government targeted multiple measures, such as income support, parental leave, rest and/or leave, dismissal, and specific legislation to maintain the health and safety of employees in telework but also to prevent the spread of the coronavirus at the workplace (Biasi*, 2020) [70].

According to Budacia (2021) [71], one of the social protection measures implemented in Romania during the pandemic was a non-taxable income within the limit of 400 lei per month, granted to employees who carried out teleworking activities to cover the expenses of utilities and purchases of office equipment. Cuerdo-Vilches (2021) [72] conducted an online survey to study the perception of Spanish employees about the workspace and its adequacy. The adequacy of teleworking spaces was insufficient for one-third of households, the number of people working or studying at home was extremely high, employees had to quickly improvise exclusive teleworking spaces, and the availability of digital resources was limited.

3.5. Digitalization

Digitalization, a socio-technical process that continuously evolves at the individual, organizational, societal, and global levels [73], is considered the key to innovation, competitiveness, and the growth of society [74]. Through its specific tools (cloud computing, software, platforms for teaching and learning, etc.) and complex technologies, digitalization creates the opportunity to increase organizational performance and work productivity, improve management practices, and create higher remuneration for new jobs created. In the context of teleworking and extensive usage of the Internet, the adoption of digital technologies by enterprises has led to new opportunities for teleworkers, a different way of organizing work, additional safety and health norms, new requirements for digital skills, labor standards, and a high interest towards the well-being of teleworkers. According to Stoica et al. (2021) [75], the spectacular development of information and communication technology corroborated with modern management (anthropocentric, systemic, product-oriented, etc.) led, in particular, to the creation of a new infrastructure for telework and, in general, to the creation of a global Internet network, in which digital technologies (cloud computing, Big Data, artificial intelligence, Internet of Things (IoT), Internet of Everything (IoE), etc.) are an integral part of the ecosystem of today's telemarketing paradigm. Sapfirova et al. 2021 [76], studying the impact of digitalization on legal regulations, labor relations, and the protection of labor rights, noticed the need to redefine the rights and obligations of employees and employers who have adopted this modern form of teleworking. It reiterated the employee's obligation to inform the employer about the equipment used during teleworking, as well as the employer's obligation to provide the teleworker with the equipment, technical support, and digital training necessary for carrying out the work activity.

3.6. Work–Life Balance

During the COVID-19 pandemic, telework was implemented in different circumstances than usual, more involuntary than voluntarily. For a significant part of the employees, work was carried out either remotely or working in the employer's location, full-time or part-time.

Few studies highlight the positive experiences employees had while working from home during the pandemic. Several employees admitted that telework has also produced positive effects, such as increased efficiency, a flexible work schedule [77], less commuting time, lower stress of travel to the employer's location, reduced risk of exhaustion [69], and new technology-related skills [78].

However, the biggest challenge for teleworkers during the pandemic remains the conflict between work and personal life. Recent studies show that maintaining a work–life balance has been an impossible task. Most employees said that teleworking generated a series of negative effects, such as an increased number of overtime hours, lack of hours reserved for rest and personal life, inefficient management of their workload [79], expansion availability of work-related functions, reduced well-being, higher risk of stress, etc. [56]. In part, these have created an inability to effectively disconnect from work due to a combination of daily stressors, which eventually leads to anxiety, burnout syndrome, or other associated illnesses [80].

Investigating the impact of telework on employee life and its contribution to the prospect of work–life conflict, Zhang et al. (2020) [81] demonstrated that children play a vital role in telework behavior as an important feature of the stage of family life that is complexly associated with telework behavior. Consequently, telework increases the conflict between "work–family" or "family–work," triggering the redistribution of domestic tasks in couples and aggravating gender differences. Before the pandemic, telework was associated with large gender differences, especially with housework and work interruptions for women. During the pandemic, more than a third of the employees worked from home, with the share of the female being higher than that of men. A recent UK study shows an illustrative case law relevant to the Equality Act, demonstrating that the challenges faced by employees, regardless of gender, are similar when teleworking is applied in the longer term [82].

The COVID-19 pandemic has profoundly affected the sphere of human life but also the protective behavior adopted by each country. Beyond the negative effects on mental health (anxiety, depression, stress, post-traumatic stress disorder, etc.), the crisis has affected the cultural dimension, creating more individualism, distance from power, uncertainty, and lack of transparency from public institutions [83–85].

An opinion poll among Austrian employees revealed that men have a more favorable attitude towards teleworking than females, and gender and age stereotypes have no effect on the 41% of Austrian employees who worked remotely during the pandemic [86–88]. At the end of 2020, the share of males (employees) working from home in the total employment in the EU reached 11.2%, while that of females reached 13%. (See Figure 3). In Romania, the share of employed persons working from home registered an upward trend, increasing from 0.8% in 2019 to 2.5% in 2020. The highest shares among the "male population" were recorded in Luxembourg (22.5%) and Ireland (21.3%), followed by the Netherlands (18.8%), Austria (17.5%), and Belgium (16.2%). On the opposite spectrum were situated countries such as Bulgaria (0.6%) and Turkey (0.9%). In terms of the "female population" who worked from home, the first places are occupied by Finland (25.5%) and Luxembourg (23.9%), and the last places are attributed to North Macedonia (3.8%), Romania (3.7%), and Bulgaria (1.9%) (See Figure 4) The share of men who worked from home continues to exceed that of the "females" in several countries, as follows: Netherlands (18.8% male; 16.7% female), Germany (13.8% male, 13.0% female), Iceland (9.1% male; 8.3% female) and Norway (5.1% male; 4.1% female).

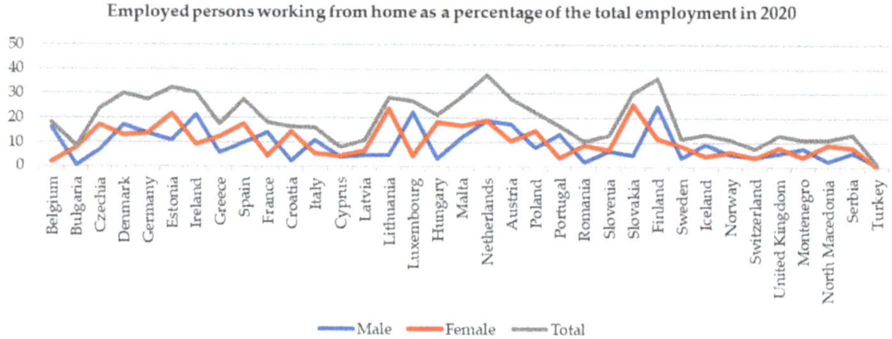

Figure 3. Employed persons working from home as a percentage of the total employment in 2020.

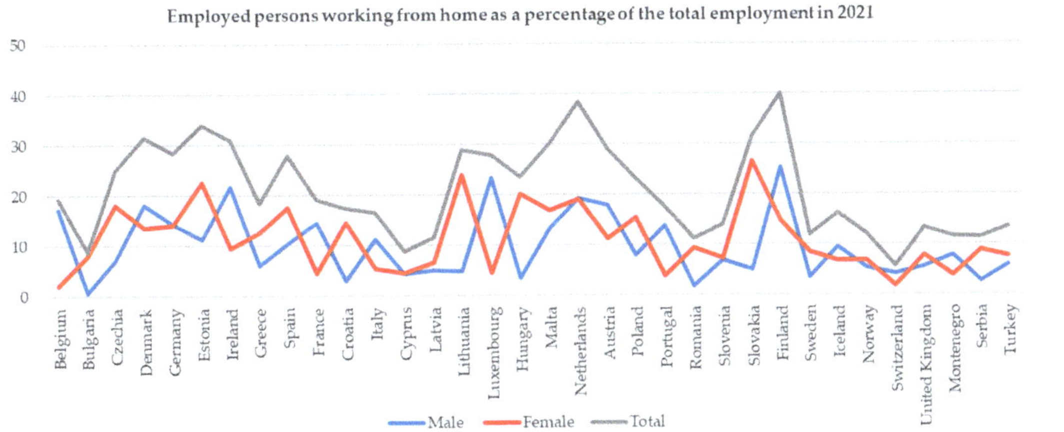

Figure 4. Employed persons working from home as a percentage of the total employment in 2021.

In 2021, the share of employees working from home in the total employment slowly continued its upward trend (see Figure 4), reaching maximum levels for men in Finland (25.8%), Luxembourg (24.3%), and Ireland (21.9%), while for women in the Netherlands (19.6%), Germany (14.7%), Iceland (11.2%) [28].

Given both the above-mentioned aspects and the database provided by Eurostat, a forecast has been made to highlight the future trends in the number of people who will work remotely (teleworkers) until 2025 in the EU (27 countries), using the Time Series Modeler procedure from the SPSS program. Figure 5 shows the clear, strong upward trend of the number of teleworkers in the EU from 2011 to 2021 compared to the previous period.

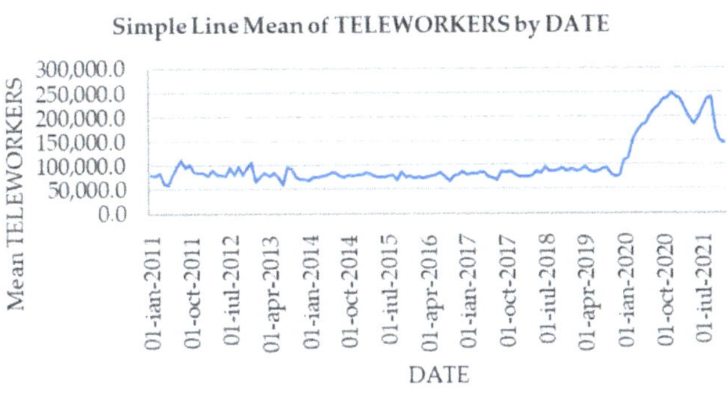

Figure 5. A simple line means of teleworkers in the UE during 2011–2021 by date.

In Table 2, the value of the stationary R-square (0.530 < 1) indicates a good, correct fit of the model and explains the variation observed in the Ljung–Box statistical series.

Table 2. Model fit statistics—teleworkers between 2022–2025.

Model	Number of Predictors	Model Fit Statistics	Ljung–Box Q (18)			Number of Outliers
		Stationary R-Squared	Statistics	DF	Sig.	
Teleworkers-Model_1	0	0.530	0.934	20.843	15	0.142

The significance value (0.142), greater than 0.05, is not significant; therefore, the model is specified correctly.

Figure 6 indicates the observed values of the dependent series, the values for the forecast period, the values for the estimation period, and the confidence intervals for the forecast period. In conclusion, the model predicted an upward evolution of the number of teleworkers in the EU for the forecasted period from 2022–2025.

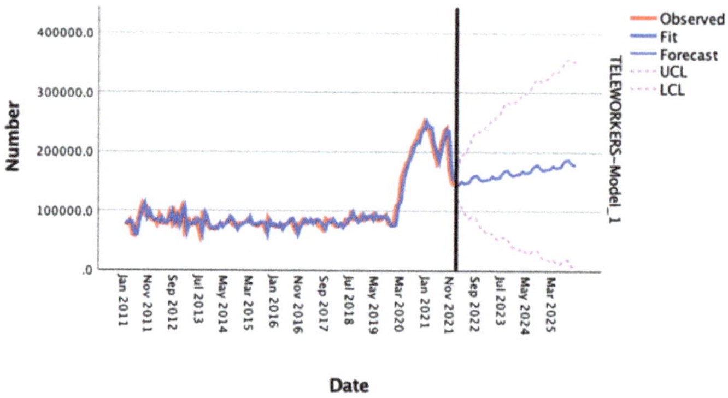

Figure 6. Predicted and observed values—teleworkers between 2011–2025.

4. Future Direction

While before the COVID-19 pandemic, telework seemed an unrealizable dream for some employees, today it represents the future of work. Rejected in the past, due to the lack of certainties regarding the implementation of labor relations and due to a low degree of technology, and temporarily recommended by governments during the state of alert and imposed unilaterally on employees, telework required a complete, modern design for the professional activity to be carried out at optimal parameters. Moreover, it came as a vital alternative for enterprises to ensure business continuity and performance standards.

By 2020, many enterprises have implemented telework in full or temporarily or have introduced mixed working solutions, in which a physical presence at the office alternates with telework, and most likely, they intend to use this viable model in the future. Regardless of the official recommendations for physical distance or the limitation of social interactions, implementing telework within enterprises was mainly possible due to five recognizable advantages of teleworking, namely: tested productivity, employee motivation, reduced employee fluctuation, reduction of administrative costs, and environmental protection.

Given that more and more employees are working from home, teleworking is no longer a Millennial trend but a way of life, where employees are happier and more productive, and organizations operate more efficiently and profitably.

Further research should focus, during and after the COVID-19 crisis, both on the evaluation of the situation of remote work within organizations and on the knowledge of the perceptions of Romanian employees regarding the use of telework.

Author Contributions: Conceptualization, M.C.T.; methodology, M.C.T.; software, M.C.T. and D.R.V.; validation, M.C.T.; formal analysis, M.C.T.; investigation, M.C.T. and D.R.V.; resources, M.C.T. and D.R.V.; data curation, M.C.T.; writing—original draft preparation, M.C.T. and D.R.V.; writing—review and editing. All authors have read and agreed to the published version of the manuscript.

Funding: This research received no external funding.

Institutional Review Board Statement: Not applicable.

Informed Consent Statement: Not applicable.

Data Availability Statement: Not applicable.

Conflicts of Interest: The author declares no conflict of interest.

Entry Link on the Encyclopedia Platform: https://encyclopedia.pub/entry/25214.

References

1. Padilla-Meléndez, A.; Del Aguila-Obra, A.R.; Analysis of Telework in the Context of E-Collaboration. Enciclopedia de la e-Colaboración. Grupo De la Idea. En Prensa, 2007. Available online: http://www.ieev.uma.es/ebusiness/papers/Mis%20publicaciones/Analysis%20of%20Telework%20in%20the%20context%20of%20Ecollaboration_chap_2006.pdf (accessed on 28 January 2022).
2. Barsness, Z.I.; Diekmann, K.A.; Seidel, M.D.L. Motivation and opportunity: The role of remote work, demographic dissimilarity, and social network centrality in impression management. *Acad. Manag. J.* **2005**, *48*, 401–419. [CrossRef]
3. Hamblin, H. Employees' perspectives on one dimension of labour flexibility: Working at a distance. *Work Employ. Soc.* **1995**, *9*, 473–498. [CrossRef]
4. Haddon, L.; Lewis, A. The experience of teleworking: An annotated review. *Int. J. Hum. Resour. Manag.* **1994**, *5*, 193–223. [CrossRef]
5. Butler, E.S.; Aasheim, C.; Williams, S. Does telecommuting improve productivity? *Commun. ACM* **2007**, *50*, 101–103. [CrossRef]
6. Rupietta, K.; Beckmann, M. Working from home: What is the effect on employees' effort? *WWZ Work. Pap.* **2016**, *7*, 1–40. [CrossRef]
7. Chatterjee, S.; Chakraborty, S.; Sarker, S.; Sarker, S.; Lau, F.Y. Examining the success factors for mobile work in healthcare: A deductive study. *Decis. Support Syst.* **2009**, *46*, 620–633. [CrossRef]
8. Grant, C.A.; Wallace, L.M.; Spurgeon, P.C. An exploration of the psychological factors affecting remote e-worker's job effectiveness, well-being and work-life balance. *Empl. Relat.* **2013**, *35*, 527–546. [CrossRef]
9. Choudhury, P.; Foroughi, C.; Larson, B. Work-from-anywhere: The productivity effects of geographic flexibility. *Strateg. Manag. J.* **2021**, *42*, 655–683. [CrossRef]
10. Grant, K.A. How Practical Is Teleworking? *Can. Datasyst.* **1985**, *17*, 1–25.
11. Kelly, M.M. The Next Workplace Revolution: Telecommuting. *Superv. Manag.* **1985**, *30*, 2–7.
12. Regenye, S. Telecommuting. *J. Inf. Manag.* **1985**, *6*, 15–23.
13. Shamir, B.; Salomon, I. Work-at-home and the quality of working life. *Acad. Manag. Rev.* **1985**, *10*, 455–464. [CrossRef]
14. Olsen, M.H. Work at home for computer professionals: Current attitudes and future prospects. *ACM* **1989**, *7*, 317–338. [CrossRef]
15. ILO. Recommendation No. 184, Concerning Home Work. 1996. Available online: https://www.ilo.org/dyn/normlex/en/f?p=NORMLEXPUB:12100:0::NO::P12100_ILO_CODE:R184 (accessed on 28 February 2022).
16. ILO. *Practical Guide on Teleworking during the COVID-19 Pandemic and Beyond. A Practical Guide*; International Labour Office: Geneva, Switzerland, 2020; Available online: https://www.ilo.org/wcmsp5/groups/public/---ed_protect/---protrav/---travail/documents/instructionalmaterial/wcms_751232.pdf (accessed on 1 May 2022).
17. European Commission. Report on the Implementation of the European Social Partners' Framework Agreement on Telework, Commission Staff Working Paper. 2008. Available online: https://eur-lex.europa.eu/legal-content/EN/TXT/PDF/?uri=CELEX:52008SC2178&from=EN (accessed on 28 February 2022).
18. European Council. Directive No. 91/533/EEC, of 14 October 1991, on an Employer's Obligation to Inform Employees of the Conditions Applicable to the Contract or Employment Relationship. *Off. J. Eur. Communities* **1991**, *288*, 32–35. Available online: http://eur-lex.europa.eu/legal-content/EN/TXT/PDF/?uri=CELEX:31991L0533&from=EN (accessed on 28 February 2022).
19. European Parliament and European Council. *Directive (EU) 2019/1152, of 20 June 2019, on Transparent and Predictable Working Conditions in the European Union*; European Parliament and European Council: Brussels, Belgium, 2019; Volume L186, pp. 105–121. Available online: https://eur-lex.europa.eu/legal-content/EN/TXT/PDF/?uri=CELEX:32019L1152&from=EN (accessed on 28 February 2022).
20. Gray, M.; Hudson, N.; Gordon, G. Teleworking explained. *Long Range Plan.* **1996**, *29*, 910.
21. Fritz, M.E.W.; Higa, K.; Narasimhan, S. Toward a telework taxonomy and test for suitability: A synthesis of the literature. *Group Decis. Negot.* **1995**, *4*, 311–334. [CrossRef]
22. Rodríguez, M. El teletrabajo en el mundo y Colombia. *Redalyc Gac. Labor.* **2007**, *13*, 29–42.
23. Gallardo, R.; Whitacre, B. 21st century economic development: Telework and its impact on local income. *Reg. Sci. Policy Pract.* **2018**, *10*, 103–123. [CrossRef]
24. Lachapelle, U.; Tanguay, G.A.; Neumark-Gaudet, L. Telecommuting and sustainable travel: Reduction of overall travel time, increases in non-motorised travel and congestion relief? *Urban Stud.* **2018**, *55*, 2226–2244. [CrossRef]
25. Toscano, F.; Zappalà, S. Social Isolation and Stress as Predictors of Productivity Perception and Remote Work Satisfaction during the COVID-19 Pandemic: The Role of Concern about the Virus in a Moderated Double Mediation. *Sustainability* **2020**, *12*, 9804. [CrossRef]
26. Huws, U. Telework: Projections. *Futures* **1991**, *23*, 19–31. [CrossRef]
27. Gareis, K.; Kordey, N. The spread of telework in 2005. E-business: Key Issues. In *Applications and Technologies*; IOS Press: Amsterdam, The Netherlands, 2000; pp. 83–90.
28. Eurostat. Data Base. 2021. Available online: https://ec.europa.eu/eurostat/data/database?node_code=lfsa_ehomp (accessed on 23 February 2022).

29. Dangelmaier, W.; Forster, D.; Horsthemke, V.; Kress, S. Penetration and outlook of telework in Europe—An Internet snapshot. In Proceedings of the 32nd Annual Hawaii International Conference on Systems Sciences, Maui, HI, USA, 5–7 January; 1999; p. 16. [CrossRef]
30. Van Klaveren, M.; Tijdens, K. Telework: Regulated or deregulated? In Proceedings of the 22nd International Labour Process Conference, Amsterdam, The Netherlands, 5–7 April 2004; pp. 256–257.
31. Grimes, S. Rural areas in the information society: Diminishing distance or increasing learning capacity? *J. Rural Stud.* **2000**, *16*, 13–21. [CrossRef]
32. Schoeffel, P.; Loveridge, A.; Davidson, C. Telework: Issues for New Zealand. *Prometheus* **1993**, *11*, 45–60. [CrossRef]
33. Vitola, A.; Baltina, I. An evaluation of the demand for telework and smart work centres in rural areas: A case study from Latvia. *Eur. Countrys.* **2013**, *5*, 251–264. [CrossRef]
34. Hesse, B.W. Curb cuts in the virtual community: Telework and persons with disabilities. In Proceedings of the Twenty-Eighth Annual Hawaii International Conference on System Sciences, Wailea, HI, USA, 3–6 January 1995; Volume 4, pp. 418–425. [CrossRef]
35. Greer, T.W.; Payne, S.C. Overcoming telework challenges: Outcomes of successful telework strategies. *Psychol.-Manag. J.* **2014**, *17*, 87–111. [CrossRef]
36. Algrari, A.Y. The influences of telecommuting on teleworkers skills. *IOSR J. Comput. Eng.* **2017**, *19*, 45–48. [CrossRef]
37. Tavares, A.I. Telework and health effects review. *Int. J. Healthc.* **2017**, *3*, 30–36. [CrossRef]
38. Beauregard, T.A.; Basile, K.A.; Canónico, E. Telework: Outcomes and facilitators for employees. In *The Cambridge Handbook of Technology and Employee Behavior*; Landers, R.N., Ed.; Cambridge University Press: Cambridge, UK, 2019; pp. 511–543. ISBN 9781108649636.
39. Dima, A.-M.; Ţuclea, C.-E.; Vrânceanu, D.-M.; Ţigu, G. Sustainable Social and Individual Implications of Telework: A New Insight into the Romanian Labor Market. *Sustainability* **2019**, *11*, 3506. [CrossRef]
40. Mahler, J. The telework divide: Managerial and personnel challenges of telework. *Rev. Public Pers. Adm.* **2012**, *32*, 407–418. [CrossRef]
41. Lister, K.; Harnish, T. Telework and its effects in the United States. In *Telework in the 21st Century 29 November 2019*; Edward Elgar Publishing: Cheltenham, UK, 2019; pp. 128–170. [CrossRef]
42. Frumkin, H. COVID-19, the built environment, and health. *Environ. Health Perspect.* **2021**, *129*, 075001. [CrossRef]
43. Scholefield, G.; Peel, S. Managers' attitudes to teleworking. *N. Z. J. Employ. Relat.* **2009**, *34*, 1–13.
44. Silva-C, A. The attitude of managers toward telework, why is it so difficult to adopt it in organizations? *Technol. Soc.* **2019**, *59*, 101133. [CrossRef]
45. Arvola, R.; Tint, P.; Kristjuhan, Ü.; Siirak, V. Impact of telework on the perceived work environment of older workers. *Sci. Ann. Econ. Bus.* **2017**, *64*, 199–214. [CrossRef]
46. Euroagenda. Regulating Telework in a Post-COVID_19 Europe, 2021. Available online: https://euagenda.eu/upload/publications/telework--20post-covid.pdf (accessed on 28 February 2022).
47. Hendrickx, F.; Taes, S.; Wouters, M. COVID-19 and labour law in Belgium. *Eur. Labour Law J.* **2020**, *11*, 276–285. [CrossRef]
48. Sachs, T. COVID-19 and labour law in France. *Eur. Labour Law J.* **2020**, *11*, 286–291. [CrossRef]
49. Carillo, K.; Cachat-Rosset, G.; Marsan, J.; Saba, T.; Klarsfeld, A. Adjusting to epidemic-induced telework: Empirical insights from teleworkers in France. *Eur. J. Inf. Syst.* **2021**, *30*, 69–88. [CrossRef]
50. Forte, T.; Santinha, G.; Carvalho, S.A. The COVID-19 Pandemic Strain: Teleworking and Health Behavior Changes in the Portuguese Context. *Healthcare* **2021**, *9*, 1151. [CrossRef]
51. Mar, S.; Buzeti, J. Working in Public Administration during Nonwork Time during the COVID-19 Pandemic. *Cent. Eur. Pub. Admin. Rev.* **2021**, *19*, 223. [CrossRef]
52. Jimenez, A.; Boehe, D.M.; Taras, V.; Caprar, D.V. Working across boundaries: Current and future perspectives on global virtual teams. *J. Int. Manag.* **2007**, *23*, 341–349. [CrossRef]
53. Taras, V.; Caprar, D.V.; Rottig, D.; Sarala, R.M.; Zakaria, N.; Zhao, F.; Jiménez, A.; Wankel, C.; Lei, W.S.; Minor, M.S.; et al. A global classroom? Evaluating the effectiveness of global virtual collaboration as a teaching tool in management education. *Acad. Manag. Learn. Educ.* **2013**, *12*, 414–435. [CrossRef]
54. Taras, V.; Baack, D.; Caprar, D.; Dow, D.; Froese, F.; Jimenez, A.; Magnusson, P. Diverse effects of diversity: Disaggregating effects of diversity in global virtual teams. *J. Int. Manag.* **2019**, *25*, 100689. [CrossRef]
55. Andrade, C.; Petiz Lousã, E. Telework and Work–Family Conflict during COVID-19 Lockdown in Portugal: The Influence of Job-Related Factors. *Adm. Sci.* **2021**, *11*, 103. [CrossRef]
56. Buomprisco, G.; Ricci, S.; Perri, R.; De Sio, S. Health and telework: New challenges after COVID-19 pandemic. *Eur. J. Environ. Public Health* **2021**, *5*, 0073. [CrossRef]
57. Diallo, A.F.; Alabi, O.; Groves, A.; Johnson, A.E.; Okoro, F.; Ramos, S.R.; Nelson, R.K.; Boutjdir, M. Training Underrepresented Early-Career Faculty in Cardiovascular Health Research during COVID-19: Structural Inequities and Health Disparity. *Ethn. Dis.* **2021**, *31*, 411. [CrossRef]
58. Malureanu, A.; Panisoara, G.; Lazar, I. The Relationship between Self-Confidence, Self-Efficacy, Grit, Usefulness, and Ease of Use of eLearning Platforms in Corporate Training during the COVID-19 Pandemic. *Sustainability* **2021**, *13*, 6633. [CrossRef]
59. Greenberg, J.A.; Schwarz, E.; Paige, J.; Dort, J.; Bachman, S. At-home hands-on surgical training during COVID19: Proof of concept using a virtual telementoring plat-form. *Surg. Endosc.* **2021**, *35*, 1963–1969. [CrossRef]

60. Kim, T.; Mullins, L.B.; Yoon, T. Supervision of telework: A key to organizational performance. *Am. Rev. Public Adm.* **2021**, *51*, 263–277. [CrossRef]
61. Busu, M.; Gyorgy, A. The Mediating Role of the Ability to Adapt to Teleworking to Increase the Organizational Performance. *Amfiteatru Econ. J.* **2021**, *23*, 654. [CrossRef]
62. Jamal, M.T.; Anwar, I.; Khan, N.A.; Saleem, I. Work during COVID-19: Assessing the influence of job demands and resources on practical and psychological outcomes for employees. *Asia-Pac. J. Bus. Adm.* **2021**, *13*, 293–319. [CrossRef]
63. de Macêdo, T.A.M.; Cabral, E.L.D.S.; Silva Castro, W.R.; de Souza Junior, C.C.; da Costa Junior, J.F.; Pedrosa, F.M.; da Silva, A.B.; de Medeiros, V.R.F.; de Souza, R.P.; Cabral, M.A.L.; et al. Ergonomics and telework: A systematic review. *Work* **2020**, *66*, 777–788. [CrossRef]
64. Magnavita, N.; Tripepi, G.; Chiorri, C. Telecommuting, Off-Time Work, and Intrusive Leadership in Workers' Well-Being. *Int. J. Environ. Res. Public Health* **2021**, *18*, 3330. [CrossRef] [PubMed]
65. Brooks, S.K.; Webster, R.K.; Smith, L.E.; Woodland, L.; Wessely, S.; Greenberg, N.; Rubin, G.J. The psychological impact of quarantine and how to reduce it: Rapid review of the evidence. *Lancet* **2020**, *395*, 912–920. [CrossRef]
66. Oakman, J.; Kinsman, N.; Stuckey, R.; Graham, M.; Weale, V. A rapid review of mental and physical health effects of working at home: How do we optimise health? *BMC Public Health* **2020**, *20*, 1–13. [CrossRef] [PubMed]
67. Turkeș, M.C.; Stăncioiu, A.F.; Băltescu, C.A. Telework during the COVID-19 Pandemic—An Approach from the Perspective of Romanian. *Amfiteatru Economic.* **2021**, *23*, 525–542. [CrossRef]
68. Belzunegui-Eraso, A.; Erro-Garcés, A. Teleworking in the Context of the COVID-19 Crisis. *Sustainability* **2020**, *12*, 3662. [CrossRef]
69. Baert, S.; Lippens, L.; Moens, E.; Weytjens, J.; Sterkens, P. The COVID-19 Crisis and Telework: A Research Survey on Experiences, Expectations and Hopes. IZA Discussion, Paper No. 13229. 2020. Available online: https://ssrn.com/abstract=3596696 (accessed on 1 May 2022).
70. Biasi, M. COVID-19 and labour law in Italy. *Eur. Labour Law J.* **2020**, *11*, 306–313. [CrossRef]
71. Budacia, L.C.G. Fiscal, legal and accounting aspects regarding telework in Romania. *J. Inf. Syst. Oper. Manag.* **2021**, *15*, 51–57.
72. Cuerdo-Vilches, T.; Navas-Martín, M.Á.; March, S.; Oteiza, I. Adequacy of telework spaces in homes during the lockdown in Madrid, according to socioeconomic factors and home features. *Sustain. Cities Soc.* **2021**, *75*, 103262. [CrossRef]
73. Legner, C.; Eymann, T.; Hess, T.; Matt, C.; Böhmann, T.; Drews, P.; Mädche, A.; Urbach, N.; Ahlemann, F. Digitalization: Opportunity and challenge for the business and information systems engineering community. *Bus. Inf. Syst. Eng.* **2017**, *59*, 301–308. [CrossRef]
74. Bălăcescu, A.; Pătraşcu, A.; Păunescu, L.M. Adaptability to Teleworking in European Countries. *Amfiteatru Econ.* **2021**, *23*, 683–699. [CrossRef]
75. Stoica, M.; Ghilic-Micu, B.; Mircea, M. The Telework Paradigm in the IoE Ecosystem—A Model for the Teleworker Residence Choice in Context of Digital Economy and Society. *Econ. Comput. Econ. Cybern. Stud. Res.* **2021**, *55*, 263–278. [CrossRef]
76. Sapfirova, A.A.; Volkova, V.V.; Petrushkina, A.V. Impact of the Digital Economy on the Legal Regulation of Labor Relations and Protection of Labor Rights. In *Current Problems and Ways of Industry Development: Equipment and Technologies*; Lecture Notes in Networks and, Systems; Shakirova, O.G., Bashkov, O.V., Khusainov, A.A., Eds.; Springer: Cham, Switzerland, 2021; Volume 200, pp. 719–725. [CrossRef]
77. Putra, K.C.; Pratama, T.A.; Linggautama, R.A.; Prasetyaningtyas, S.W. The Impact of Flexible Working Hours, Remote Working, and Work Life Balance to Employee Satisfaction in Banking Industry during COVID-19 Pandemic Period. *J. Bus. Manag. Rev.* **2020**, *1*, 341–353. [CrossRef]
78. Hughes, C. The Changing Learning Technological Landscape for Trainers in the Wake of COVID-19. *Adv. Dev. Hum. Resour.* **2021**, *23*, 66–74. [CrossRef]
79. Rodríguez-Modroño, P.; López-Igual, P. Job Quality and Work—Life Balance of Teleworkers. *Int. J. Environ. Res. Public Health* **2021**, *18*, 3239. [CrossRef]
80. Lizana, P.A.; Vega-Fernadez, G.; Gomez-Bruton, A.; Leyton, B.; Lera, L. Impact of the COVID-19 Pandemic on Teacher Quality of Life: A Longitudinal Study from before and during the health crisis. *Int. J. Environ. Res. Public Health* **2021**, *18*, 3764. [CrossRef] [PubMed]
81. Zhang, S.; Moeckel, R.; Moreno, A.T.; Shuai, B.; Gao, J. A work-life conflict perspective on telework. *Transp. Res. Part A Policy Pract.* **2020**, *141*, 51–68. [CrossRef] [PubMed]
82. Nath, V.; Lockwood, G. Implications of the UK Equality Law for tele-homeworking: COVID-19 and beyond. *Int. J. Law Manag.* **2022**, *64*, 253–272. [CrossRef]
83. Balcombe, L.; De Leo, D. Digital Mental Health Amid COVID-19. *Encyclopedia* **2021**, *1*, 1047–1057. [CrossRef]
84. Bueno-Guerra, N. COVID-19 and Psychological Impact. *Encyclopedia* **2022**, *2*, 400–408. [CrossRef]
85. Nair, N.; Selvaraj, P.; Nambudiri, R. Culture and COVID-19: Impact of Cross Cultural Dimensions on Behavioral Responses. *Encyclopedia* **2022**, *2*, 1210–1224. [CrossRef]
86. Beno, M. Home-based Telework and the Role of Gender Results of a Study in Austria. In *CONF-IRM*; Association for Information Systems: Atlanta, GA, USA, 2019; pp. 1–12.
87. Yang, W.; Gao, H.; Yang, Y.; Liao, J. Embodied Carbon in China's Export Trade: A Multi Region Input-Output Analysis. *Int. J. Environ. Res. Public Health* **2022**, *19*, 3894. [CrossRef] [PubMed]
88. Yang, W.; Gao, H.; Yang, Y. Analysis of Influencing Factors of Embodied Carbon in China's Export Trade in the Background of "Carbon Peak" and "Carbon Neutrality". *Sustainability* **2022**, *14*, 3308. [CrossRef]

encyclopedia

MDPI

Entry

Culture and COVID-19: Impact of Cross-Cultural Dimensions on Behavioral Responses

Nisha Nair [1,*,†], Patturaja Selvaraj [2,†] and Ranjeet Nambudiri [2,3,†]

1 Katz Graduate School of Business, University of Pittsburgh, Pittsburgh, PA 15260, USA
2 Management Department, Gettysburg College, Gettysburg, PA 17325, USA; pselvara@gettysburg.edu (P.S.); ranjeet@iimidr.ac.in (R.N.)
3 Indian Institute of Management, Indore 453556, India
* Correspondence: nnair@pitt.edu
† All authors are joint first authors.

Definition: The global pandemic of COVID-19 has impacted every sphere of human life across all nations of the world. Countries adapted and responded to the crisis in different ways with varied outcomes and different degrees of success in mitigation efforts. Studies have examined institutional and policy-based responses to the pandemic. However, to gain a holistic understanding of the pandemic response strategy and its effectiveness, it is also important to understand the cultural foundations of a society driving its response behavior. Towards that end, this entry focuses on a few key cultural dimensions of difference across countries and proposes that national culture is related to the protective behavior adopted by societies during COVID-19. The cultural dimensions examined in relation to COVID-19 include the dimensions of individualism vs. collectivism, power distance, uncertainty avoidance, masculinity and femininity, and future orientation. Inferences are drawn from academic research, published data, and discernible indicators of social behavior. The entry provides pointers for each dimension of culture and proposes that cultural awareness be made an important element of policy making while responding to crises such as COVID-19.

Keywords: culture; COVID-19; pandemic; cultural dimensions; individualism vs. collectivism; power distance; uncertainty avoidance; masculinity and femininity; future orientation

Citation: Nair, N.; Selvaraj, P.; Nambudiri, R. Culture and COVID-19: Impact of Cross-Cultural Dimensions on Behavioral Responses. *Encyclopedia* **2022**, 2, 1210–1224. https://doi.org/10.3390/encyclopedia2030081

Academic Editors: Stephen Bustin and Raffaele Barretta

Received: 30 May 2022
Accepted: 27 June 2022
Published: 1 July 2022

1. Introduction

For many, the unprecedented COVID-19 pandemic, which began spreading across the globe in January 2020, has been the first and only pandemic people have witnessed in their lifetime [1]. The pandemic has been a crisis of unprecedented proportion which brought with it conditions never encountered by the current generations. Governments and people across the world have been left scrambling to contain the spread of the virus and to adopt effective risk mitigation strategies, even after pharmaceutical interventions such as vaccines have come on the horizon [2]. The scale of damage that the SARS-CoV-2 virus has unleashed in terms of the lives lost, harmful mental and physical health consequences [3], and constraints on public health systems [4] has been unprecedented. As of May 2022, more than 520 million cases of COVID-19 and 6.2 million fatalities have been reported worldwide, with the United States, India, Brazil, France, Germany, the United Kingdom, and Russia having reported the largest number of cases [5]. On the other hand, countries such as New Zealand, Egypt, Sri Lanka, and Norway reportedly had fewer than 1.2 million cases [5]. Governments have exhibited wide variations in their responses to the pandemic. Some countries experienced nation-wide lockdowns such as India and China, while others adopted softer approaches such as that of Sweden [6–9]. Similarly, the societal response to the pandemic has also varied significantly. It can be argued that to understand a COVID-19 response strategy it is important to understand the interaction of both the formal (institutional mechanisms) and the informal (cultural underpinnings) elements guiding decision making [10].

There is increasing recognition today that one cannot understand pandemic responses without adopting a behavioral science approach [11–13]. Consequently, there is a mounting body of work in this direction with several published works focusing on understanding responses to the COVID-19 pandemic through a behavioral lens [13,14]. Early in the pandemic, when pharmaceutical interventions were limited, some researchers called for recognizing and changing behavior to control the transmission of the virus [12]. Several studies have emerged pointing to differences in country-level responses. For example, one such study [9] points to differences in cross-country perceptions of risk influencing social distancing amidst the pandemic.

Different cultures react and behave differently to threat perceptions based on shared belief systems [15]. Differences is how people behave in a social context are often grounded in varying expectations and learned behavior acquired through socialization [16]. National cultures shape people's behaviors [15,17,18] and have been shown to predict people's wellbeing amidst the pandemic [19]. This is particularly relevant in times of crisis such as the pandemic when people tend to adhere more strongly to prevailing social norms [20]. Indicative of the powerful effect of culture in shaping behavior amidst the pandemic, in a recent study using econometric data, culture has in fact been shown to act as a substitute for state action in ensuring compliance with COVID-19 policies [21]. Thus, if culture has the potency to supplement or replace policy, it merits attention to understand the cultural dimensions shaping and guiding behavior, which can augment policy-level interventions to manage the ongoing pandemic.

Culture has been widely studied for many decades. Geert Hofstede's cultural diversity model is considered one of the major frameworks for understanding culture [15–17]. Since human behavior is a reflection of the underlying values that people subscribe to [22], it is worthwhile to reflect on the values that shape this behavior at the cross-cultural level. One of the earliest ways of understanding cross-cultural values or dimensions of difference was offered by Hofstede based on data from across 64 countries [17]. Hofstede conceptualized cultural differences emerging from differences in values categorized along certain dimensions [16,23]. The original four dimensions of difference across cultures were identified as individualism versus collectivism, power distance, uncertainty avoidance, and masculinity versus femininity [16,23]. Other dimensions such as long-term versus short-term were later included in the conceptualization. Individualism versus collectivism captures the dichotomy of independence versus interdependence, or loyalty to oneself compared to that towards the group [24,25]. It refers to the extent to which people affiliate with loosely or tightly knit social groups [25]. Power distance refers to the acceptance of power differentials in a society, while uncertainty avoidance refers to the extent of perceived discomfort with ambiguities or uncertainties in a society [16,18,26]. Masculinity versus femininity refers to the extent to which cultures prefer equality or egalitarianism between the sexes in a society. It captures the degree to which cultures are prone towards competition and assertiveness, or caring and nurturance [16,26]. The long-term versus short-term dimension refers to a cultural orientation that is rooted in either the present or the future [27].

This entry explores some of the above dimensions of cross-cultural difference as it relates to understanding or shaping behavior amidst the pandemic. In the following sections, the entry examines the relevant cultural dimensions and attempt to synthesize emerging literature linking cultural dimensions to the pandemic. The effect of cultural dimensions on variations in behavior will also be illustrated through some country-level differences, where available. In offering this overview of culture and COVID-19, we aim to understand the relevant cultural variables influencing and guiding human behavior at the collective level amidst a crisis such as the current pandemic.

2. COVID-19 and Cultural Differences between Individualism and Collectivism

A wealth of cross-cultural research has established the individualism versus collectivism dimension as one of the most vital dimensions capable of explaining differences between countries [28]. Being the most used dimension in cross-cultural research, individualism/collectivism is also thought to have the greatest predictive power [29].

The measure of individualism/collectivism is an indication of whether people tend to value individual goals, interests, and needs, or emphasize collective concerns and goals [24,25]. In other words, individualistic cultures focus on prioritizing personal needs above that of the group [16] while collectivist cultures tend to put more emphasis on group harmony over personal needs and interests [30]. As a cultural value, collectivism relates to ties between people. People who subscribe to a collectivist social value tend to interact cooperatively, embodying interdependence and recognizing mutual duties and obligations to one another [25]. Thus, collectivism is characterized by a strong sense of community, loyalty, trust, and respect towards one another and willingness to forgo individual needs in the interest of collective needs and goals. Individualistic societies on the other hand tend to value personal freedom and do not feel a compulsion to adhere to collective norms or goals.

Prior research has shown that collectivists are more likely to display adaptive responses in times of crisis [31]. Research has also established that in collectivist cultures people tend to adhere to social norms and demonstrate greater compliance as opposed to individualistic cultures [32]. A collectivist belief orientation would urge the protection of collective interests over efforts to maintain independent selves [33]. Further, given the perceived threat of community-based sanctions [34] for violating social norms in collectivist societies, people are more likely to participate in mitigation efforts during the pandemic to limit the growth of COVID-19.

Emerging studies are supporting the view that a collectivistic mindset drives willingness to engage in behaviors that can curtail the spread of the virus. Cultural factors were found to account for a large portion of the explanatory power for variation in COVID-19 containment efforts across nations [14]. Research has shown that individualists and collectivists tend to behave differently as far as virus containment measures such as social distancing is concerned [20]. Empirical studies are emerging showing behaviors such as mask wearing, social distancing, and intention to vaccinate are connected to collectivist mindsets or collectivistic cultures [20,35,36]. Using data from 67 countries varying on individualism and collectivism, Lu and colleagues [36] have been able to show that mask wearing was more common in countries high in collectivism and less so where individualism was high. Whether variations in individualism–collectivism led to different outcomes in terms of case rate and mortality rate was investigated in another research [14] across 54 countries, indicating that collectivism had a significant impact on containing the pandemic and on flattening the curve.

Individualism, on the other hand, has been linked to negative outcomes in relation to the COVID-19 pandemic. Examining intentions to reduce the spread of the virus, a study [20] found that individualism negatively predicted intention to engage in social distancing, mediated through belief in conspiracy theories and powerlessness. Early in the pandemic, cultures that were high on individualism were found to experience higher infected cases and death than collectivist cultures [14]. Other studies have shown that individualist cultures have contributed to worsening fatality rates, compared to nations with a collectivist culture [37]. The cultural norm of individualism has also been shown to have a positive effect on the growth rate of COVID-19 cases based on a time series analysis of data from 107 countries [8]. More recently, individualism has been linked to higher disease prevalence [21] and a higher mortality rate in a study across 110 countries considering climate risk and the COVID-19 mortality rate [38]. Another study [6] using data from 111 countries examined variations in behavior in relation to lockdown measures instituted by governments to curb the spread of the virus, finding support for the view that individualism has made government interventions harder, as opposed to a collectivist dynamic which is more geared towards promoting compliance with COVID-19 policies.

Even at the level of individual experience of the pandemic's effects, individualism has been linked to higher experienced stress and isolation [19]. Some emerging research on the experience of social isolation amidst an ongoing pandemic suggests that collectivist societies are better equipped to deal with social isolation beget by pandemic conditions, with worry, fear, and anxiety being kept in check through networks of social connections [3]. Recent research has in fact shown that an individualist mindset led to a reduced intention to vaccinate compared with collectivism [35].

Looking at country-level data, the United States has recorded the largest number of infected cases and suffered a disproportionately higher number of lost lives to COVID-19 compared to all other countries in the first year of the pandemic [39]. Americans typically tend to be high on individualism [17,25,40], with American society marked by a preference for independence and a prioritization of individual freedom over collective welfare. In fact, as some note, there is even a resistance against the collective [41]. It can be argued that the fatalities suffered in the United States owing to the COVID-19 pandemic are partly attributable to the premium placed on individual freedom, independence, and autonomy, all captured through the cultural orientation of individualism [39]. This focus on individualism may have prompted a lack of adherence to public health measures in pursuit of individual freedom and liberty. People in individualistic societies tend to prioritize their own selves and wellbeing over those of others. There were even news reports [42] in the early days of the pandemic of beaches in Florida being crammed with people enjoying their spring break, with little thought to health advisories such as social distancing to mitigate the virus spread. In the US, even well-established practices such as mask wearing for containing the pandemic [43] have been met with resistance and have been portrayed as an affront to people's freedoms [39]. Thus, with the prevalent individualist ethos, what we may have seen in the US is the prioritization of individual choice and personal freedom at the cost of collective consequences.

On the other hand, collectivist countries such as South Korea and Singapore emphasized civic efforts such as persistent mask wearing [44], while individualistic nations such as the US and Italy found it challenging to encourage the adoption of mitigation efforts from early on in the pandemic [45]. For another collectivist country, Slovakia, some research [46] has shown a link between collectivism among Slovaks and containing the pandemic through engagement in prosocial behavior. Similarly, in collectivist China, there appeared to be greater adherence to lockdown rules [6] compared to the United States with its high individualism and lesser willingness to abide by COVID-19 policy recommendations. Considering a month-long period of government intervention on the case rate and pandemic-induced mortality rate, researchers [14] found that collectivist countries such as China, Japan, South Korea, and Singapore witnessed fewer cases compared to the more individualistic Western European and North American cultures. Based on emerging research, it can therefore be inferred:

Key Takeaway: The cultural dimension of collectivism is positively related to higher engagement in COVID-19 protective behaviors such as mask wearing and social contact avoidance, compared to more individualistic cultures.

Behaviors aligned with individualism are more likely to be harmful during times of crises with intensifying cases in individualistic countries emerging from an unwillingness to sacrifice individual needs or give up personal freedoms in the interest of collective welfare. By contrast, in collectivist societies, people tend to act as a group, with group success and objectives taking precedence over individual liberties or autonomy. There appears to be higher altruism and more effective rule observation in a collectivistic dynamic, which makes the implementation of COVID-19 policies such as lockdowns or mask wearing easier and more uniform in their adoption across a society. Highlighting collectivism and concern for others by focusing on the individual's role in benefiting the larger good can thus be a powerful narrative in shaping people's sensibilities to contribute towards efforts in limiting the spread of the virus. It can encourage mitigation efforts and the willingness of a society to collectively curb the growth of the pandemic.

3. COVID-19 and the Cultural Norm of Power Distance

One of the dimensions of cross-cultural difference is power distance, which is an indication of people's attitude to power. Hofstede [26] argues that some countries are more unequal than others, with a high power distance culture characterized by higher deference shown to authority and authority figures, compared with those in low power distance cultures. It is indicative of the extent to which individuals with less power in society accept and expect that power is distributed unequally [47] and how much they endorse authority and power differences in a society [48]. Thus, power distance refers to how people react and behave in relation to power and power differentials in a society.

Power distance has been positively linked to conformity [49]. Individuals in high power distance countries are more willing to accept and observe rules from authority figures [48] and tend to be more willing to follow guidelines [50]. People in low power distance countries tend to be more willing to challenge authority and are generally perceived as being less submissive than individuals in high power distance cultures [51]. Countries higher in power distance are thus able to exercise greater authoritarian behavior and elicit desired compliance, compared to countries lower in power distance.

There is some emerging evidence [52] that in societies with high power distance, people's responses to mobility restrictions instituted by governments amidst the COVID-19 pandemic have generally been more favorable, compared with countries having a lower power distance. Subscribing to the values of power distance means that individuals are willing to acknowledge the role of the government and willingly comply with many tough measures instituted amidst the pandemic such as protracted lockdowns [7]. In another recent study [53], the moderating role of power distance was studied among consumers in relation to compliance with expected behaviors during the pandemic such as mask wearing. Results indicate that when countries have high power distance, along with other intervening factors, it can lead to greater compliance with expected behaviors. Since high power distance countries are more likely to evidence obedience and willingness to be led by others [54], there will likely be more effective participation in risk mitigation efforts, while countries low in power distance, being characterized by an emphasis on free will and with a greater predilection to challenge experts [55], are less likely to be effective in mitigation efforts.

In high power distant and collectivist countries such as South Korea, China, India, Singapore, Taiwan, the Philippines, and Vietnam, the high power distance coupled with high collectivism can create conditions for better enforceability of government-run initiatives to control the spread of the virus, as some researchers have proposed [7,56]. In both Vietnam and South Korea, surveillance apps were used by the government amidst the pandemic [44,57] and has been met with little resistance. In countries such as South Korea, China, India, Singapore, Taiwan, and Vietnam, people have been willing to comply with government-led measures such as downloading apps on their mobile phones, granting health authorities access to detail call records for contact tracing, and other such surveillance of the populace, geared towards curbing the spread of the virus [7]. It is likely to be the high power distance which has allowed countries such as Taiwan to institute something like an 'electronic fence' to track an individual's location via GPS and mobile phones, inviting police intervention whenever there is non-compliance to government measures put in place to curb the spread of COVID-19 [7]. There also appears to be high approval among the public for such practices in Taiwan even with hefty fines as high as $33,000 for non-compliance, given the high power distance and cultural beliefs that such sacrifices are necessary to keep the country safe [58].

In contrast, countries low in power distance such as the US, Italy, Norway, and Germany, where governments are viewed less deferentially, have had limited success in using governmental measures to curb the virus spread. Even with a technologically advanced app for contact tracing such as the one developed in Germany, the app could not be mandated but only voluntarily used [59]. With its low power distance, both the US and Germany saw people protesting mitigation efforts [56]. In Norway too such an app for contact tracing had to be discontinued after its initial launch in the face of public disapproval and criticism [60]. Given the extremely low power distance in the US and strong data protection and privacy laws preventing government use of individual data [61], no such app even took shape in the US. In a separate study [52], it was demonstrated that government-induced social contact restrictions were higher in India and Namibia (high power distant countries) compared to the US or Germany (countries with low power distance). Another study of several European countries showed that power distance had a significant negative effect on the rate of increase in COVID-19 [62]. In separate research [8], it was observed that government intervention weakened the growth rate of virus transmission, and this effect was most significant in collectivist and high power distant countries, therefore suggesting that high power distance can have a moderating effect on the efficacy of other emergency response measures adopted by governments in times of crises, such as the COVID-19 pandemic. Thus, we can conclude:

Key Takeaway: Adherence to health policy guidelines and government mandates and restrictions to curb the spread of COVID-19 is higher in high power distance countries than in low power distance countries.

As discussed above, differences in behavioral responses in terms of abiding by preventive measures during the pandemic can be attributed to power distance norms prevalent in a country. High power distance ensures better enforceability of government diktats such as lockdowns, mask wearing, or quarantine rules put in place to control the spread of the virus. When this is combined with high collectivism, there tends to be high support for government mandates and less overall resistance to tough measures such as surveillance or extended lockdowns, as the welfare of the group takes precedence over individual rights and autonomy. In high power distance countries, even seemingly harsh measures invoked during the pandemic such as surveillance of the citizenry are rationalized by the populace as a necessary tradeoffs of relinquishing individual liberties to ensure the safety and wellbeing of the collective. Even with the availability of pharmaceutical interventions such as vaccination, in low power distant countries where there is a greater tendency to question or challenge authority [51], adoption rates can suffer as has been evidenced in countries such as the United States [2]. High power distance in effect allows governments to be more authoritative and pursue more stringent measures. Nations high in power distance have an advantage in containing the pandemic, as they face lesser resistance from the public to policy measures that might infringe on people's freedoms, and people are generally more willing to comply with necessary restrictions and interventions required to contain the spread of the outbreak.

4. COVID-19 and the Cultural Dimension of Uncertainty Avoidance

Uncertainty avoidance deals with the tolerance that a society has for ambiguous conditions. It has been noted [17,26] that members of certain societies are more comfortable in predictable and structured situations (high uncertainty avoidance) while other societies seem to thrive in conditions of ambiguity and unpredictability (low uncertainty avoidance).

Several studies have examined the outcomes and correlates of uncertainty avoidance, indicating that high uncertainty avoidance is associated with a lower propensity for risk and a greater desire for expectedness. In a study with 303 participants from Spain, Germany, and Sweden [63], it was noted that customers who came from high uncertainty avoidance cultures were less satisfied with service defect situations than those from low uncertainty avoidance cultures. This points towards a greater tolerance for ambiguity in low uncertainty avoidance cultures. Societies that are high on uncertainty avoidance are characterized by higher stress and lower scores on subjective wellbeing [26]. In such societies, individuals have shown a lower propensity to switch jobs since new and different roles are often considered threats, with people attempting to bring a sense of stability and predictability in their lives [64]. It has been posited [65] that uncertainty avoidance is an antecedent of risk perception, with decision makers in such cultures preferring the conservative choice in order to increase predictability and control [66]. Uncertainty avoidance has also been studied as a moderator of the relationship between leadership behavior and innovative work, suggesting a stronger correlation in high uncertainty avoidance cultures [67]. With samples drawn from India, the United States, Brazil and the United Kingdom, a separate study [68] found that uncertainty avoidance moderated the relationship between intention to use mobile banking and its actual use, with a stronger relationship found in higher uncertainty avoidance cultures. Another study [69] conducted with participants from a high uncertainty avoidance culture (Turkey) and a low uncertainty avoidance culture (Malaysia) found that the cultural dimension had an influence on customer loyalty. A study conducted in Norway (known to be moderate in uncertainty avoidance) showed that uncertainty avoidance was a strong predictor of interest in valid and established genetic testing methods for highly penetrative diseases [70]. This finding assumes significance for the current essay which attempts to understand the relationship between dimensions of national culture and the COVID response behavior of societies.

Unexpected events with a global impact (such as the pandemic, a financial market meltdown, an oil crisis, etc.) create conditions of ambiguity and carry a high risk of decision failures. Given that uncertainty avoidance cultures are prone to risk aversion and conservatism in decision making [64,65], it seems reasonable to argue that the uncertainty avoidance dimension of a national culture is related to the COVID-19 protective behaviors adopted by nations and societies. Erman and Medeiros [71] gathered COVID-19-related data from over 73 countries and adopted meta-analytic methods to show that uncertainty avoidance and other cultural dimensions were independent predictors of test positivity, case infection, and mortality risk. Separately, a linkage between uncertainty avoidance and higher rates of COVID-19 infection has been suggested [64] with the argument that countries high in uncertainty avoidance are more likely to resist changes in social structure. This would render strategies such as mandatory mask wearing and social contact avoidance less efficient, thus increasing infection rates from the virus. Uncertainty avoidance has also been linked to the risk perception of tourists in the COVID-19 context [72,73]. Another study posited uncertainty avoidance to moderate the relationship between the stringency of lockdown processes and country-level innovation, albeit with limited support for the relationship [74].

Considering uncertainty avoidance scores for a few countries [75], it appears that uncertainty avoidance may have a correlation with the COVID-19 protective behaviors of societies. A recent study by the University of Michigan [76] classified Vietnam, a culture low in uncertainty avoidance, as among the few nations which exhibited a rapid public health response by successfully imposing social and behavioral changes such as social contact avoidance and mandatory mask wearing. Similarly, Singapore, considered low in uncertainty avoidance [75], saw the government imposing high monitoring and control measures [77]. For instance, students who reported back to the colleges were asked to record and report their temperature several times in a day and entry into public places such as the libraries and cafeterias were strictly regulated for a longer duration [77]. Aggressive contact tracing measures such as scanning the identification documents of people at supermarkets and other public locations were part of a centralized control approach [77]. This seems in line with the view that low uncertainty avoidance cultures are more likely to be open to stricter control measures. On the other hand, Germany, a high uncertainty avoidance society [77], witnessed many anti-lockdown protests during the pandemic, indicating that high uncertainty avoidance cultures are less likely to impose stringent measures such as lockdowns or mandatory mask wearing. The following takeaway therefore emerges:

Key Takeaway: Cultures low in uncertainty avoidance are more likely to have a tolerance for varied risk mitigation strategies requiring behavioral changes than cultures high in uncertainty avoidance.

In the initial stages of the pandemic when vaccines were still under development, the only method of preventing the spread of the virus was through behavioral changes in society. This included measures such as social contact avoidance, mandatory mask wearing, repeated washing of the hands, and avoiding public areas. Government interventions included lockdowns of varying intensity and duration as well as strict regulation of the above-mentioned measures. It can be argued that acceptance or resistance of social and behavioral changes induced by the pandemic are likely to be affected by the uncertainty avoidance propensities of societies. Thus, nations low on uncertainty avoidance found it simpler to implement stringent social and behavioral changes during the pandemic. People in low uncertainty avoidance cultures tend to tolerate uncertainty and ambiguities better than those in high uncertainty avoidance cultures. Hence, it becomes easier to introduce varied policy interventions without backlash or resistance from people.

5. COVID-19 and Cultural Orientations of Masculinity and Femininity

Masculinity and femininity denote differences in cultures based on perceived masculine and feminine values. According to Hofstede [47], masculinity and femininity are in relation to differences in emotional roles between the sexes. The values of assertiveness and competition are categorized as masculine, and the values of care, compassion, and modesty as feminine in this conceptualization [26,47]. "Cultural masculinity stands for a focus on ego, money, things, and work; cultural femininity for a focus on relationships, people, and quality of life." [47] (p. 72). It is argued that "women in feminine countries have the same modest, caring values as the men; in masculine countries, they are somewhat assertive and competitive, but not as much as the men, so that these countries show a gap between men's values and women's values." [47] (p. 63). Thus, a culture high in masculinity is interpreted as one where there are differences in values and work roles along gendered lines, while cultures high in femininity can be considered as more egalitarian and less polarized in values between the genders. Countries high on masculinity tend to focus on material, career, and business success, with cooperative behavior not much appreciated in such societies, while countries high on femininity tend to focus on modesty and give importance to quality of life, kindness, and empathy [78]. Feminine societies are thus thought to stress the importance of a work–life balance, have minimal emotional and social role differentiation between the genders, express sympathy and support for the weaker in society, and have the values of caring and being modest subscribed to by both genders [26], whereas masculine societies support explicit emotional and social differentiation amongst the genders, have an admiration for stronger people, and have work deemed as central, to an extent where it often takes precedence over the family [26].

Research has shown masculinity to be high in Japan, Germany, Austria, and Switzerland, and as moderately high in English-speaking Western countries such as the United Kingdom and the United States [26]. For example, South Koreans are considered to be less assertive and competitive than Americans, thus scoring lesser in masculinity than the United States [79]. Femininity is deemed high in the Netherlands and Nordic countries such as Norway, Sweden, and Denmark, and moderately high in countries such as France, Chile, and Thailand [26,47].

The United States (high on masculinity) and Norway and Denmark (high on femininity) handled COVID-19 very differently. Norway acted fast and went into lockdown in mid-March of 2020. It closed schools, restaurants, gyms, and other public places and banned cultural and sports activities and the entry of people from other countries [80]. It resulted in a lower number of people being infected and in a lower death rate per capita in comparison to the United States [80]. In the US, the federal government did not mandate the closure of schools unilaterally but left it to the individual schools to assess the situation and decide about the closure [81]. When some states in the US started introducing masking requirements, there was resistance to follow the mask mandates at the individual level [82]. Additionally, in the US, the federal government and state governments were sending conflicting and mixed messages [83]. Overall, resistance to the pandemic-induced restriction was high in the US. In contrast, the robust social security system in Norway with free-cost education, a public financed health care system, paid maternity and parental leave, and low-cost childcare (making it a more egalitarian society and high on feminine cultural norms) helped Norway tide over the pandemic with much more ease than many other countries [83,84]. In the United States, the then President faced major criticisms for his failure to protect the people of the U.S. from the COVID-19 pandemic [85], while the prime minister of Norway was lauded for handling the crisis with kindness and compassion [83,85,86]. Another Scandinavian country, Denmark, a feminine society with a smaller gap between rich and poor, was less hit by the pandemic [87]. Denmark registered fewer infected cases and deaths compared to the United States [87,88]. Being one of the first countries in Europe to take swift action to ban large gatherings and impose restrictions on travel, Denmark saw the closure of daycares, schools, and universities early on in the pandemic [87]. Given the preference for work–life balance, a feminine cultural norm [17], people in Denmark took to the new normal fairly quickly and smoothly, making the adoption of the pandemic-induced restrictions easier [87]. In contrast, in the United States, with the fear of job loss, expensive college education and health care systems, and rising fears of economic insecurity [89], there was greater resistance to pandemic-imposed restrictions [89]. This entry can therefore surmise the following:

Key Takeaway: Feminine cultural norms enable higher receptivity and societal tolerance for pandemic-induced shocks compared to masculine cultural norms.

Feminine dominant societies prioritize concern for the weaker community members and also elevate women to top managerial and political positions [86]. For countries like Norway and Denmark, with a dominant feminine culture, there also tends to be wider societal support for policies geared towards the larger public good [86]. Pandemic-induced restrictions such as forced work from home also allowed for a better work–family integration, a value cherished in societies that follow feminine cultural norms.

6. COVID-19 and the Cultural Dimension of Long-Term versus Short-Term Focus

One of the ways in which cultures differ is grounded in how people perceive time. Differences in time orientation has thus emerged as another dimension of cross-cultural difference [90]. One set of this difference refers to the distinction between monochronic and polychronic cultures, and another captures a differing focus on the past, present, and future [90,91]. A past orientation emphasizes a view towards the past and focuses on the maintenance or restoration of traditions, while a future orientation stresses a mindful awareness of the future and actions and behaviors grounded in things such as planning and delayed gratification, with a view towards ensuring a better future [92]. A future orientation is akin to Hofstede's conceptualization of the cultural dimension of long-term versus short-term focus [27].

Cultures high on short-term orientation show a preference for immediate rewards and individualism, while those with a longer-term orientation tend to focus on long-term goals and are more likely to be collectivist in orientation [27]. Having a future orientation has also been tied to protective behaviors such as engaging in social contact avoidance [52]. There is some evidence that a future orientation is linked to people's abilities to set goals for their future health [93]; thus, it should follow that even with regard to the pandemic, a future orientation should be instrumental in setting goals that move the needle towards a pandemic-free world. A case in point is China, which is high on long-term orientation [18,24]. The country was among the first to use technology aids such as facial recognition for identifying and isolating affected individuals [7] as well as implementing rapid nucleic acid testing, which seems to indicate a futuristic orientation towards prevention rather than containment. There is also some emerging research that suggests countries higher in long-term orientation have been better able to avoid higher fatality rates compared with those having a preference for a short-term orientation [37].

Lu and colleagues [36] examined the masking behavior of people from 29 countries. These included countries high on future orientation such as South Korea and Singapore as well as countries with a short-term orientation such as Canada and the United States. The results indicated that people in Singapore and South Korea showed a greater propensity to wear masks during the pandemic. Research indicated that countries with a high long-term orientation were able to successfully implement COVID-19 protocols such as social contact avoidance and mask wearing [7]. For instance, in South Korea and Singapore, the governments found it easier to implement social contact avoidance and persistent masking [44] while mandatory mask wearing was met with significant resistance in the United States [43]. As mentioned earlier, Taiwan, a nation with a high long-term orientation, was able to implement an "electronic fence" for surveillance and contact tracing [7]. Therefore, it can be surmised:

Key Takeaway: A future or long-term orientation will be positively associated with increased protective behaviors amidst the pandemic.

Considering a pandemic-free world as the aspired future state, cultures with a dominant future orientation are more likely to engage in practices and behaviors that help drive towards this desired future, even if it discomfits the present. The degree to which cultures have a long-term or future orientation could therefore suggest whether people are willing to sacrifice personal liberties and autonomy in the present, such as refraining from socializing, in order to move towards the desirable future of a pandemic-free existence.

7. Conclusions

Much has happened since the COVID-19 pandemic was first detected. In the early stages, prior to the development of vaccines, most countries deployed social and behavioral strategies of varying nature, including nation-wide or localized lockdowns, social contact avoidance, and mask wearing, among others. Different nations implemented travel restrictions of varying intensity and duration [94]. Access to vaccines also varied across nations, with the US and the UK making vaccines available much earlier than many other nations [95]. The pandemic itself has witnessed multiple waves across 2020–2022, with new mutations appearing [96]. Amidst this evolving situation, attention to cultural factors can go a long way in both understanding what is fueling behavior responses and designing effective interventions and policy recommendations.

Examining the role of cross-cultural factors in driving pandemic responses, our analysis revealed that cultural dispositions can either aid or thwart effective responses during times of crisis, such as that of the pandemic. Hofstede's [15–17] model has also been previously applied to understand behavior during other crisis contexts such as the global financial crisis [97]. Cultural characteristics such as individualism can be a drawback in times of emergencies such as the pandemic, where in the absence of effective checks for furthering individual interests, it can create conditions that can potentially accelerate the spread of the pandemic. There is emerging evidence that a cultural preference for individualism makes it challenging to promote risk mitigation behaviors such as vaccination and mask wearing [36]. During a global crisis, when concern for others drives pandemic containment behaviors such as social contact avoidance, mask wearing, vaccination, and adherence to risk mitigation strategies, an overt emphasis on seeking and fulfilling one's individual needs for autonomy and disregard for how one's actions could contribute towards the spread of the virus can be catastrophic. On the other hand, a collectivistic orientation has been a useful cultural trait in limiting the spread of the virus. Promoting collectivism, where possible, may be a way to strengthen policy measures to contain the pandemic and increase people's engagement with efforts in this direction [20].

Similarly, having high power distance as a cultural norm can be useful to ensure compliance with and the adoption of government mandates and policy recommendations in times of crises. Whatever be the drawbacks of having high power distance, in times of crises when expert guidelines and adherence to government mandates are crucial for crisis resolution, high power distance can come in handy to ensure high compliance and less resistance to authority.

Another cultural norm that seems to be advantageous in a time of crisis is a feminine cultural norm, with values of compassion and egalitarianism fueling adequate responses supported by the larger community. Feminine cultural norms potentially indicate a higher tolerance for absorbing shocks during a crisis situation compared with masculine cultures.

It also appears that nations with high uncertainty avoidance faced challenges while implementing control measures for managing the pandemic such as lockdown, curfews, social contact avoidance, and mandatory mask wearing. Owing to the preference for order and stability, any initiatives or attempts to manage the crisis that is shrouded in further uncertainty is likely to be met with some degree of resistance in high uncertainty avoidance cultures. Thus, policy makers are advised to recognize that having a sound rationalization for instituting measures for risk mitigation may not be sufficient in itself if it does not address peoples' misgivings or concerns with ambiguity.

Finally, the cultural value of future orientation or long-term focus can also come in handy to make the many inconveniences necessitated for the management of the pandemic, such as restrictions on personal mobility, tolerable. Mobilizing individual action to engage in such sacrifices are also made easy when there is a long-term cultural orientation. A long-term cultural orientation can thus help build resilience in the face of an ongoing crisis, making tough decisions more palatable.

Thus, what can be inferred from exploring the cultural underpinnings of behavior is that certain cultural norms tend to be more conducive to the facilitation of risk mitigation strategies versus others, such as collectivist orientations, high power distance, low uncertainty avoidance, feminine cultural norms, and a long-term or future cultural orientation.

In arguing for considering the role of cultural differences in shaping pandemic behavior, while looking at the cultural differences driving divergent behavioral responses, the entry has illustrated with a few country-level responses wherever information is available and the linkage to behavior can be inferred. The country-level illustrations are only indicative and are in no way meant to be exhaustive or to be interpreted as a suggestion that all countries with similar cultural norms will behave in analogous ways. Thus, this entry does not purport to explain behavioral responses for all countries using the cultural model of Hofstede or make the claim that all countries subscribing to the same cultural norm will behave the same way. There will surely be instances when a particular country meets with less or more success in tackling the pandemic than other countries with similar cultural dispositions. Clearly, there are numerous other factors that influence effectiveness of pandemic responses such as economic factors, population density and size of a country, vaccination availability, governmental action/non action, and effective public health systems, among others. The larger point is that culture is one of the factors that appears to have some bearing on how groups of people behave amidst the pandemic and should be considered as another useful tool in a country's arsenal to fight the pandemic.

The continually evolving nature of the pandemic must also be acknowledged and borne in mind. What is true of a country's response today may change in the future as the pandemic changes, the political will and resources available to fight the pandemic changes, and newer interventions continue to be developed. Therefore, while thinking of a country's pandemic response, it is useful to keep in mind that this is also susceptible to variation and influence by a number of other intervening factors, given the ongoing nature of the pandemic. Thus, the current entry is limited to understanding pandemic behavior at specific moments in time, but this literature is continually being added to and country-level responses and the management of the pandemic is also ever morphing even as this entry is being written.

While the entry is a commentary on the possible relationship between the cultural dimensions proposed by Hofstede [16,17] and the pandemic response behaviors of societies, it does not claim to be a propositional inventory but instead arguments are based on an integration of the extant literature and demonstrable information on the actual responses of societies. Given that pandemic response strategies have evolved with growing information about the virus [96], the entry recommends a longitudinal time lagged analysis of data to draw firm conclusions about the nature of the relationship between cultural dimensions and COVID response behavior.

An understanding of how cultural norms influence people's behavior can be a useful tool in shaping and implementing policy interventions to manage the ongoing pandemic or the future of such crises. Our cultural analysis of behavior linked to COVID-19 offers one lens for thinking about what can enable or disrupt even the best thought out mitigation efforts amidst an ongoing crisis. Given differences in cultural orientations and ensuing the behavioral tendencies of people, a one-size-fits-all approach to navigating and managing the pandemic may not always be effective. Governments thus need to incorporate cultural awareness into their policy decisions for emergency preparedness and instituting containment measures and interventions, as the COVID-19 pandemic has shown us. Even with regard to any future global crisis, our analysis reveals that cultural norms can play a powerful role in disposing people to react and behave in particular ways. Effective risk mitigation strategies are therefore ones which factor in cultural norms to either use to their advantage or to actively design policy interventions to counter cultural tendencies that can subvert effective crisis resolution.

Author Contributions: Conceptualization, N.N., P.S. and R.N.; methodology, N.N., P.S. and R.N.; formal analysis, N.N., P.S. and R.N.; writing—original draft preparation, N.N., P.S. and R.N.; writing—review and editing, N.N., P.S. and R.N. All authors have read and agreed to the published version of the manuscript.

Funding: This research received no external funding.

Institutional Review Board Statement: Not applicable.

Informed Consent Statement: Not applicable.

Conflicts of Interest: The authors declare no conflict of interest.

References

1. Honigsbaum, M. *The Pandemic Century: A History of Global Contagion from the Spanish Flu to COVID-19*; WH Allen: London, UK, 2020.
2. Saif, K.; Zou, B.; Adler-Milstein, J. Factors and reasons associated with low COVID-19 vaccine uptake among highly hesitant communities in the US. *Am. J. Infect. Control* **2022**, *50*, 262–267.
3. Hussein, N.H. COVID-19 in a collectivist culture: Social isolation and maintenance of social relations. *Int. J. Sociol. Soc. Policy* **2022**, *42*, 276–288. [CrossRef]
4. McGee, A.; Carter, D. The equivalence thesis and the last ventilator. *J. Appl. Philos.* **2022**, *39*, 297–312. [CrossRef]
5. World Health Organization. Available online: https://covid19.who.int/ (accessed on 9 May 2022).
6. Chen, C.; Frey, C.B.; Presidente, G. Culture and contagion: Individualism and compliance with COVID-19 policy. *J. Econ. Behav. Organ.* **2021**, *19*, 191–200. [CrossRef]
7. Gupta, M.; Shoja, A.; Mikalef, P. Toward the understanding of national culture in the success of non-pharmaceutical technological interventions in mitigating COVID-19 pandemic. *Ann. Oper. Res.* **2021**, *3*, 1–18. [CrossRef]
8. Dheer, R.J.S.; Egri, C.P.; Treviño, L.J. A cross-cultural exploratory analysis of pandemic growth: The case of COVID-19. *J. Int. Bus. Stud.* **2021**, *52*, 1871–1892. [CrossRef]
9. Milani, F. COVID-19 outbreak, social response, and early economic effects: A global VAR analysis of cross-country interdependencies. *J. Popul. Econ.* **2021**, *34*, 223–252. [CrossRef]
10. Geva-May, I.; Hoffman, D.C.; Muhleisen, J. Twenty years of comparative policy analysis: A survey of the field and a discussion of topics and methods. *J. Comp. Policy Anal. Res. Pract.* **2018**, *20*, 18–35. [CrossRef]
11. Bavel, J.J.V.; Baicker, K.; Boggio, P.S.; Capraro, V.; Cichocka, A.; Cikara, M.; Crockett, M.J.; Crum, A.J.; Douglas, K.M.; Druckman, J.N.; et al. Using social and behavioural science to support COVID-19 pandemic response. *Nat. Hum. Behav.* **2020**, *4*, 460–471. [CrossRef]
12. West, R.; Michie, S.; Rubin, G.J.; Amlôt, R. Applying principles of behaviour change to reduce SARS-CoV-2 transmission. *Nat. Hum. Behav.* **2020**, *4*, 451–459. [CrossRef]
13. Nair, N.; Selvaraj, P. Using a cultural and social identity lens to understand pandemic responses in the US and India. *Int. J. Cross Cult. Manag.* **2021**, *21*, 545–568. [CrossRef]
14. Cao, C.; Li, N.; Liu, L. Do national cultures matter in the containment of COVID-19? *Int. J. Sociol. Soc. Policy* **2020**, *40*, 939–961. [CrossRef]
15. Triandis, H.C. The self and social behavior in differing cultural contexts. *Psychol. Rev.* **1989**, *96*, 506–520. [CrossRef]

16. Hofstede, G.; Hofstede, G.J.; Minkov, M. *Cultures and Organizations: Software of the Mind: Intercultural Cooperation and Its Importance for Survival*, 3rd ed.; McGraw-Hill: New York, NY, USA, 2010.
17. Hofstede, G. *Culture's Consequences: International Differences in Work-Related Values*; Sage: Beverly Hills, CA, USA, 1980.
18. Hofstede, G. *Culture's Consequences: Comparing Values, Behaviors, Institutions, and Organizations across Nations*, 2nd ed.; Sage: Thousand Oaks, CA, USA, 2001.
19. Kowal, M.; Coll-Martín, T.; Ikizer, G.; Rasmussen, J.; Eichel, K.; Studzińska, A.; Koszałkowska, K.; Karwowski, M.; Najmussaqib, A.; Pankowski, D.; et al. Who is the most stressed during the COVID-19 pandemic? Data from 26 countries and areas. *Appl. Psychol. Health Well-Being* **2020**, *12*, 946–966. [CrossRef]
20. Biddlestone, M.; Green, R.; Douglas, K.M. Cultural orientation, power, belief in conspiracy theories, and intentions to reduce the spread of COVID-19. *Br. J. Soc. Psychol.* **2020**, *59*, 663–673. [CrossRef]
21. He, Z.; Jiang, Y.; Chakraborti, R.; Berry, T.D. The impact of national culture on COVID-19 pandemic outcomes. *Int. J. Soc. Econ.* **2022**, *49*, 313–335. [CrossRef]
22. Han, S. Understanding cultural differences in human behavior: A cultural neuroscience approach. *Curr. Opin. Behav. Sci.* **2015**, *3*, 68–72. [CrossRef]
23. Hofstede, G.; Bond, M.H. The Confucius connection: From cultural roots to economic growth. *Organ. Dyn.* **1988**, *16*, 5–21. [CrossRef]
24. Hofstede, G. Culture and organizations. *Int. Stud. Manag. Organ.* **1980**, *10*, 15–41. [CrossRef]
25. Triandis, H.C. *Individualism & Collectivism*; Westview Press: Boulder, CO, USA, 1995; p. 259.
26. Hofstede, G. Dimensionalizing cultures: The Hofstede model in context. Online Read. *Psychol. Cult.* **2011**, *2*, 8. Available online: http://scholarworks.gvsu.edu/orpc/vol2/iss1/8 (accessed on 8 May 2022).
27. Hofstede, G.; Minkov, M. Long-versus short-term orientation: New perspectives. *Asia Pac. Bus. Rev.* **2010**, *16*, 493–504. [CrossRef]
28. Triandis, H.C. Individualism-collectivism and personality. *J. Personal.* **2001**, *69*, 907–924. [CrossRef]
29. Taras, V.; Steel, P.; Kirkman, B.L. Improving national cultural indices using a longitudinal meta-analysis of Hofstede's dimensions. *J. World Bus.* **2012**, *47*, 329–341. [CrossRef]
30. Triandis, H.C.; McCusker, C.; Hui, C.H. Multimethod probes of individualism and collectivism. *J. Personal. Soc. Psychol.* **1990**, *59*, 1006–1020. [CrossRef]
31. Murray, D.R.; Trudeau, R.; Schaller, M. On the origins of cultural differences in conformity: Four tests of the pathogen prevalence hypothesis. *Personal. Soc. Psychol. Bull.* **2011**, *37*, 318–329. [CrossRef]
32. Kim, M.S. Cross-cultural comparisons of the perceived importance of conversational constraints. *Hum. Commun. Res.* **1994**, *21*, 128–151. [CrossRef]
33. Kitayama, S.; Park, J.; Miyamoto, Y.; Date, H.; Boylan, J.M.; Markus, H.R.; Karasawa, M.; Kawakami, N.; Coe, C.L.; Love, G.D.; et al. Behavioral adjustment moderates the link between neuroticism and biological health risk: A US–Japan comparison study. *Personal. Soc. Psychol. Bull.* **2018**, *44*, 809–822. [CrossRef]
34. Heinrichs, N.; Rapee, R.M.; Alden, L.A.; Bögels, S.; Hofmann, S.G.; Oh, K.J.; Sakano, Y. Cultural differences in perceived social norms and social anxiety. *Behav. Res. Ther.* **2006**, *44*, 1187–1197. [CrossRef]
35. Courtney, E.P.; Felig, R.N.; Goldenberg, J.L. Together we can slow the spread of COVID-19: The interactive effects of priming collectivism and mortality salience on virus-related health behavior intentions. *Br. J. Soc. Psychol.* **2022**, *61*, 410–431. [CrossRef]
36. Lu, J.G.; Jin, P.; English, A.S. Collectivism predicts mask use during COVID-19. *Proc. Natl. Acad. Sci. USA* **2021**, *118*, e2021793118. [CrossRef]
37. Oey, E.; Rahardjo, B.S. Does culture influence our ways in handing COVID-19? *Int. J. Sociol. Soc. Policy* **2021**, *41*, 1149–1169. [CrossRef]
38. Ozkan, A.; Ozkan, G.; Yalaman, A.; Yildiz, Y. Climate risk, culture and the COVID-19 mortality: A cross-country analysis. *World Dev.* **2021**, *141*, 105412. [CrossRef] [PubMed]
39. Kitayama, S.; Camp, N.P.; Salvador, C.E. Culture and the COVID-19 pandemic: Multiple mechanisms and policy implications. *Soc. Issues Policy Rev.* **2022**, *16*, 164–211. [CrossRef]
40. Schwartz, S.H. Universals in the content and structure of values: Theoretical advances and empirical tests in 20 countries. *Adv. Exp. Soc. Psychol.* **1992**, *25*, 1–65. [CrossRef]
41. Markus, H.R.; Kitayama, S. A collective fear of the collective: Implications for selves and theories of selves. *Personal. Soc. Psychol. Bull.* **1994**, *20*, 568–579. [CrossRef]
42. Kesslen, B. As Florida Coronavirus Cases Surge, Spring Breakers Express Regret. NBC News. Available online: https://www.nbcnews.com/news/us-news/floridacoronavirus-cases-surge-spring-breakers-express-regret-n1168686 (accessed on 10 May 2022).
43. Lyu, W.; Wehby, G.L. Community use of face masks and COVID-19: Evidence from a natural experiment of state mandates in the US: Study examines impact on COVID-19 growth rates associated with state government mandates requiring face mask use in public. *Health Aff.* **2020**, *39*, 1419–1425. [CrossRef]
44. Fisher, M.; Sang-Hun, C. How South Korea Llattened the Curve. *The New York Times*. Available online: https://www.nytimes.com/2020/03/23/world/asia/coronavirus-south-korea-flatten-curve.html (accessed on 11 May 2022).
45. Pisano, G.P.; Sadun, R.; Zanini, M. Lessons from Italy's Response to Coronavirus. *Harvard Business Review*. 2020. Available online: https://vwww.hbs.edu/faculty/Pages/item.aspx?num=57971 (accessed on 8 May 2022).

46. Čavojová, V.; Adamus, M.; Ballová Mikušková, E. You before me: How vertical collectivism and feelings of threat predicted more socially desirable behaviour during COVID-19 pandemic. *Curr. Psychol.* **2022**, 1–12, (advance online publication). [CrossRef]
47. Hofstede, G.; McCrae, R.R. Personality and culture revisited: Linking traits and dimensions of culture. *Cross-Cult. Res.* **2004**, *38*, 52–88. [CrossRef]
48. Taras, V.; Kirkman, B.L.; Steel, P. Examining the impact of culture's consequences: A three-decade, multilevel, meta-analytic review of Hofstede's cultural value dimensions. *J. Appl. Psychol.* **2010**, *95*, 405–439. [CrossRef] [PubMed]
49. Carl, D.; Gupta, V.; Javidan, M. Power distance. In *Culture, Leadership, and Organizations the GLOBE Study of 62 Societies*; House, R.J., Hanges, P.J., Javidan, M., Dorfman, P.W., Gupta, V., Eds.; Sage: Thousand Oaks, CA, USA, 2004; pp. 513–563.
50. Smith, P.B.; Peterson, M.F.; Schwartz, S.H. Cultural values, sources of guidance, and their relevance to managerial behavior: A 47-nation study. *J. Cross-Cult. Psychol.* **2002**, *33*, 188–208. [CrossRef]
51. Daniels, M.A.; Greguras, G.J. Exploring the nature of power distance: Implications for micro-and macro-level theories, processes, and outcomes. *J. Manag.* **2014**, *40*, 1202–1229. [CrossRef]
52. Messner, W. The association of cultural and contextual factors with social contact avoidance during the COVID-19 pandemic. *PLoS ONE* **2021**, *16*, e0261858. [CrossRef]
53. Matta, S.; Rogova, N.; Luna-Cortés, G. Investigating tolerance of uncertainty, COVID-19 concern, and compliance with recommended behavior in four countries: The moderating role of mindfulness, trust in scientists, and power distance. *Personal. Individ. Differ.* **2022**, *186*, 111352. [CrossRef]
54. Ji, Y.; Zhou, E.; Li, C.; Yan, Y. Power distance orientation and employee help seeking: Trust in supervisor as a mediator. *Soc. Behav. Personal.* **2015**, *43*, 1043–1054. [CrossRef]
55. De Meulenaer, S.; De Pelsmacker, P.; Dens, N. Power distance, uncertainty avoidance, and the effects of source credibility on health risk message compliance. *Health Commun.* **2018**, *33*, 291–298. [CrossRef]
56. Nienaber, M.; Chambers, M. Germans Stage Protests Against Lockdown Measures, Social Distancing Rules. *Reuters*. Available online: https://www.reuters.com/news/picture/germans-stageprotests-against-lockdown-idUSKBN22S0MS (accessed on 12 May 2022).
57. Pollack, T.; Thwaites, G.; Rabaa, M.; Choisy, M.; van Doorn, R.; Luong, D.H.; Tan, D.Q.; Quang, T.D.; Dinh, P.C.; Nghia, N.D.; et al. Emerging COVID-19 Success Story: Vietnam's Commitment to Containment. 2020. Available online: https://ourworldindata.org/covid-exemplar-vietnam (accessed on 12 May 2022).
58. Lee, W.-Y.; McCauley, E.; Abadi, M. Taiwan Used Police Surveillance, Government Tracking, and $33,000 Fines to Contain Its Coronavirus Outbreak. 2020. Available online: https://www.businessinsider.com/taiwan-coronavirus-surveillance-masks-china-2020-6 (accessed on 12 May 2022).
59. Busvine, D. Explainer: Europe Steps Up Tech Battle vs. Coronavirus with German App. 2020. Available online: https://www.reuters.com/article/us-health-coronavirus-germany-app-explai/explainer-europe-steps-uptech-battle-vs-coronavirus-with-german-app-idUSKBN23M1HM (accessed on 12 May 2022).
60. Reuters. Norway to Halt COVID-19 Track and Trace App on Data Protection Concerns. 2020. Available online: https://www.reuters.com/article/us-health-coronavirus-norway-apps/norway-to-halt-covid-19-track-andtrace-app-on-data-protection-concerns-idUSKBN23M18T (accessed on 13 May 2022).
61. Kluth, A. If We Must Build a Surveillance State, Let's Do It Properly. 2020. Available online: https://www.bloomberg.com/opinion/articles/2020-04-22/taiwan-offers-the-best-model-for-coronavirus-data-tracking (accessed on 13 May 2022).
62. Gokmen, Y.; Baskici, C.; Ercil, Y. The impact of national culture on the increase of COVID-19: A cross-country analysis of European countries. *Int. J. Intercult. Relat.* **2021**, *81*, 1–8. [CrossRef]
63. Reimann, M.; Lünemann, U.F.; Chase, R.B. Uncertainty avoidance as a moderator of the relationship between perceived service quality and customer satisfaction. *J. Serv. Res.* **2008**, *11*, 63–73. [CrossRef]
64. Voegel, J.; Wachsman, Y. The effect of culture in containing a pandemic: The case of COVID-19. *J. Risk Res.* **2021**, 1–9. [CrossRef]
65. Kozak, M.; Crotts, J.C.; Law, R. The impact of the perception of risk on international travelers. *Int. J. Tour. Res.* **2007**, *9*, 233–242. [CrossRef]
66. Parnell, J.A. Crisis management and strategic orientation in Small and Medium-sized Enterprises (SMEs) in Peru, Mexico and the United States. *J. Contingencies Crisis Manag.* **2015**, *23*, 221–233. [CrossRef]
67. Afsar, B.; Masood, M. Transformational leadership, creative self-efficacy, trust in supervisor, uncertainty avoidance, and innovative work behavior of nurses. *J. Appl. Behav. Sci.* **2018**, *54*, 36–61. [CrossRef]
68. Picoto, W.N.; Pinto, I. Cultural impact on mobile banking use–A multi-method approach. *J. Bus. Res.* **2021**, *124*, 620–628. [CrossRef]
69. Ndubisi, N.O.; Malhotra, N.K.; Ulas, D.; Ndubisi, G.C. Examining uncertainty avoidance, relationship quality, and customer loyalty in two cultures. *J. Int. Consum. Mark.* **2012**, *24*, 320–337. [CrossRef]
70. Wolff, K.; Nordin, K.; Brun, W.; Berglund, G.; Kvale, G. Affective and cognitive attitudes, uncertainty avoidance and intention to obtain genetic testing: An extension of the theory of planned behavior. *Psychol. Health* **2011**, *26*, 1143–1155. [CrossRef]
71. Erman, A.; Medeiros, M. Exploring the effect of collective cultural attributes on COVID-19-related public health outcomes. *Front. Psychol.* **2021**, *12*, 884. [CrossRef]
72. Godovykh, M.; Pizam, A.; Bahja, F. Antecedents and outcomes of health risk perceptions in tourism, following the COVID-19 pandemic. *Tour. Rev.* **2021**, *76*, 737–748. [CrossRef]

73. Chua, B.L.; Al-Ansi, A.; Lee, M.J.; Han, H. Impact of health risk perception on avoidance of international travel in the wake of a pandemic. *Curr. Issues Tour.* **2021**, *24*, 985–1002. [CrossRef]
74. Kapoor, H.; Ticku, A.; Tagat, A.; Karandikar, S. Innovation in isolation? *COVID-19 lockdown stringency and culture-innovation relationships. Front. Psychol.* **2021**, *12*, 83.
75. Hofstede. Available online: https://www.hofstede-insights.com/country-comparison (accessed on 8 May 2022).
76. Pires, F. How Countries on Five Continents Responded to the Pandemic, Helping Shape Future of Health Policy. 2021. Available online: https://news.umich.edu/how-countries-on-five-continents-responded-to-the-pandemic-helping-shape-future-of-health-policy/ (accessed on 18 May 2022).
77. Bremmer, I. The Best Global Responses to the COVID-19 Pandemic: One Year Later. *Time*. 2021. Available online: https://time.com/5851633/best-global-responses-covid-19/ (accessed on 8 May 2022).
78. Gallego-Álvarez, I.; Pucheta-Martínez, M.C. Hofstede's cultural dimensions and R&D intensity as an innovation strategy: A view from different institutional contexts. *Eurasian Bus. Rev.* **2021**, *11*, 191–220.
79. Cheong, H.J.; Mohammed-Baksh, S. US and Korean consumers: A cross-cultural examination of product information-seeking and-giving. *J. Promot. Manag.* **2020**, *26*, 893–910. [CrossRef]
80. McLaughlin, K. Sweden Has Nearly 10 Times the Number of COVID-19 Related Deaths than Its Nordic Neighbors. Here's Where It Went Wrong. *Insider*. Available online: https://www.businessinsider.com/how-sweden-and-norway-handled-coronavirus-differently-2020-4 (accessed on 19 May 2022).
81. Sawchuk, S. To Close or Not? *How Superintendents Decide to Shut Down Schools*. Available online: https://www.edweek.org/leadership/to-close-or-not-how-superintendents-decide-to-shut-down-schools/2020/03 (accessed on 18 May 2022).
82. Vargas, E.D.; Sanchez, G.R. American Individualism Is an Obstacle to Wider Mask Wearing in the US. Available online: https://www.brookings.edu/blog/up-front/2020/08/31/american-individualism-is-an-obstacle-to-wider-mask-wearing-in-the-us/ (accessed on 18 May 2022).
83. Bennett, J. Norway Handles COVID-19 Better than the US—Opinion. *Newsweek*. Available online: https://www.newsweek.com/norway-handles-covid-19-better-us-opinion-1574902 (accessed on 18 May 2022).
84. Ursin, G.; Skjesol, I.; Tritter, J. The COVID-19 pandemic in Norway: The dominance of social implications in framing the policy response. *Health Policy Technol.* **2020**, *9*, 663–672. [CrossRef]
85. Johnson, C.; Williams, B. Gender and political leadership in a time of COVID. *Politics Gend.* **2020**, *16*, 943–950. [CrossRef]
86. Windsor, L.C.; Yannitell Reinhardt, G.; Windsor, A.J.; Ostergard, R.; Allen, S.; Burns, C.; Giger, J.; Wood, R. Gender in the time of COVID-19: Evaluating national leadership and COVID-19 fatalities. *PLoS ONE* **2020**, *15*, e0244531. [CrossRef] [PubMed]
87. Olagnier, D.; Mogensen, T.H. The Covid-19 pandemic in Denmark: Big lessons from a small country. *Cytokine Growth Factor Rev.* **2020**, *53*, 10–12. [CrossRef] [PubMed]
88. Petersen, M.B.; Bor, A. Denmark Appears to Have Beaten COVID-19—for Now. Here's How It Did it. *The Washington Post*. Available online: https://www.washingtonpost.com/politics/2021/09/20/denmark-appears-have-beaten-covid-19-now-here-is-how-it-did-it/ (accessed on 20 May 2022).
89. Konish, L. 71% of Americans Are Worried Social Security Will Run out of Money in Their Lifetimes. Why Experts Say that Won't Happen. *NBC News*. 2021. Available online: https://www.cnbc.com/2021/07/06/many-fear-social-security-will-run-out-of-money-why-that-wont-happen.html (accessed on 20 May 2022).
90. Mayfield, M.; Mayfield, J.; Martin, D.; Herbig, P. Time perspectives of the cross-cultural negotiations process. *Am. Bus. Rev.* **1997**, *15*, 78–85.
91. Hall, E.T. *Beyond Culture*; Anchor Books: New York, NY, USA, 1976.
92. Kluckhohn, F.R.; Strodtbeck, F.L. *Variations in Value Orientation*; Harper & Row: New York, NY, USA, 1961.
93. Laditka, S.B.; Laditka, J.N. Moxie matters: Associations of future orientation with active life expectancy, Aging Ment. *Health* **2017**, *21*, 1040–1046. [CrossRef]
94. Chinazzi, M.; Davis, J.T.; Ajelli, M.; Gioannini, C.; Litvinova, M.; Merler, S.; Piontti, A.P.Y.; Mu, K.; Rossi, L.; Sun, K.; et al. The effect of travel restrictions on the spread of the 2019 novel coronavirus (COVID-19) outbreak. *Science* **2020**, *368*, 395–400. [CrossRef]
95. Mullard, A. How COVID vaccines are being divvied up around the world. *Nature* **2020**, *30*, 10.1038. [CrossRef]
96. Maragakis, L. Corona Virus Second Wave, Third Wave and Beyond: What Causes a COVID Surge. 2021. Available online: https://www.hopkinsmedicine.org/health/conditions-and-diseases/coronavirus/first-and-second-waves-of-coronavirus (accessed on 17 May 2022).
97. Baltacı, A.; Cergibozan, R.; Ari, A. Cultural values and the global financial crisis: A missing link? *Eurasian Econ. Rev.* **2022**, 1–23. [CrossRef]

encyclopedia

Entry

Otovestibular Symptoms of COVID-19 and Its Vaccines/Treatments

Marcello Cherchi [1,2]

1 Ken and Ruth Davee Department of Neurology, Northwestern University Feinberg School of Medicine, Chicago, IL 60611, USA; m-cherchi2@northwestern.edu; Tel.: +1-312-274-0197
2 Chicago Dizziness and Hearing, Chicago, IL 60611, USA

Definition: The rapidly developing literature regarding COVID-19 and its treatments has documented an impressive breadth of pathology across multiple organ systems. In this entry, researchers highlight the audiologic and vestibular manifestations that have been reported in association with COVID-19, its vaccines, and some of its treatments.

Keywords: COVID-19; vestibular; vertigo; auditory; hearing loss; tinnitus; otovestibular; vaccines

1. Introduction

The coronavirus disease pandemic that began in 2019 (COVID-19) poses a range of challenges for patients, physicians, and health care delivery systems. The pandemic's rapidly changing consequences have necessitated commensurately rapid evolution in our understanding of this disease; thus, it is no exaggeration to say that manuscripts on this topic are already out of date even before going to press. The most common presentations (fever, respiratory symptoms, and fatigue) have understandably commanded the most attention, but experience has shown that most organ systems can suffer involvement. Auditory abnormalities and disorders of balance are not among the most common, but accumulating evidence suggests that they are not rare either. In this entry, the author reviews what is known and acknowledge what is not known about the audiologic and vestibular symptoms that have been associated with the disease itself. The author then closes with some comments regarding audiologic and vestibular symptoms reported in association with the vaccines and some of the antiviral treatments for the disease.

2. Pathobiology of COVID-19

Transmission of SARS-CoV-2 and entry through the respiratory tract is fairly well understood. Our understanding of how SARS-CoV-2 enters the nervous system is evolving.

2.1. How SARS-CoV-2 Infects the Body

The severe acute respiratory syndrome coronavirus type 2 ("SARS-CoV-2") is a member of a family of coronaviruses. This family comprises single-stranded RNA viruses. From their lipid bilayer envelope protrude spike glycoproteins that function as "hooks" that facilitate entry into host cells, where they replicate, and from where they propagate. The spoke glycoproteins bind to angiotensin-converting enzyme receptors [1,2] that are densely expressed in cells in the pulmonary system, which is believed to be the mechanism by which the most common initial symptoms of this infection involve the respiratory tract. However, the infection does not remain confined to the respiratory tract. A more detailed discussion of the molecular aspects underlying this mechanism can be found elsewhere in this Encyclopedia [3].

Citation: Cherchi, M. Otovestibular Symptoms of COVID-19 and Its Vaccines/Treatments. *Encyclopedia* **2022**, 2, 1200–1209. https://doi.org/10.3390/encyclopedia2030080

Academic Editors: Stephen Bustin and Raffaele Barretta

Received: 23 May 2022
Accepted: 25 June 2022
Published: 30 June 2022

2.2. How SARS-CoV-2 Infects the Nervous System

Investigators have a limited understanding of the factors that make an individual vulnerable to the coronavirus and the mechanisms by which these viruses invade the central nervous system (CNS) [4,5], though there is evidence [6] of cells within the CNS that express angiotensin converting enzyme receptors—even if at a lower density than found in the lower respiratory tract. It appears that after these viruses have invaded the CNS, they are capable of advancing via axonal transport [5].

It has long been known that other coronaviruses can invade the central nervous system, as they have been isolated in the brain and spinal cord tissue or the cerebrospinal fluid of patients suffering from a variety of neurological diseases such as encephalitis [7–11], acute disseminated encephalomyelitis [12], optic neuritis [13], Parkinson's disease [14], and multiple sclerosis [15–17]. For some of these diseases (e.g., multiple sclerosis, Parkinson's disease) it seems somewhat unlikely that coronaviruses play a causative role, whereas in others (e.g., optic neuritis, encephalitis, and encephalomyelitis), it is reasonable to entertain the possibility that the viruses themselves are the etiopathogenetic factor.

Early in the pandemic, clinicians began reporting neurologic symptoms in individuals infected with SARS-CoV-2 [18,19] who had been hospitalized [20], especially among those in intensive care units [21]. Data regarding SARS-CoV-2 [22–24] suggest that its capacity to invade the central nervous system is similar to that of other members of the coronavirus family [25], though there also appear to be clear differences [2], such as the predilection of SARS-CoV-2 to cause anosmia and ageusia [26–30], which in turn suggests involvement of cranial nerves. Therefore it is logical to consider whether cranial nerve involvement by SARS-CoV-2 is the mechanism underlying other focal neurological manifestations, such as the vestibular and auditory symptoms observed in patients presenting to primary care offices, emergency rooms, and otoneurology/neuro-otology clinics.

Early in the pandemic, the author began evaluating patients with laboratory confirmation of SARS-CoV-2 infection who complained of auditory symptoms (such as hearing loss or tinnitus) and/or dizziness. This matches the evolving clinical literature, which reports dizziness [31], auditory symptoms (such as hearing loss or tinnitus), or both [32].

3. Auditory and Vestibular Symptoms Associated with COVID-19

The author will briefly review the representative literature regarding COVID-19 and auditory and vestibular symptoms; the author discusses that it is difficult to prove a causal relationship between the infection and these symptoms; and researchers outline several pathogenetic hypotheses regarding the mechanisms that have been proposed in support of the idea that the relationship might be causal.

3.1. COVID-19 Associated with Auditory Disorders

The literature is accumulating regarding an association between COVID-19 infection and hearing loss. While a few papers failed to find any relationship between COVID-19 and hearing loss [33,34], a growing number of case reports [35–41] and case series [42–46] have documented clear instances of hearing loss in the context of SARS-CoV-2 infection. The summary article by De Luca et al. [47] reviewed numerous case reports and a case series of COVID-19 patients, including both sexes, with a broad range of ages (18–84 years), with unilateral or bilateral typically sudden onset sensorineural hearing loss. The summary article by Fancello et al. [48] reviewed numerous case reports and two case series of COVID-19 patients, including both sexes, with a similarly broad range of ages, with unilateral (more common) or bilateral (less common) sudden sensorineural hearing loss. The prospective single-institution study by Dusan et al. [42] reported a similar variety.

A smaller but growing literature is also beginning to document an association between COVID-19 and tinnitus [36,37,39,44,45,48–53]. In many cases, the tinnitus accompanies hearing loss [36,37,39]. Some of the literature describes tinnitus occurring with or without concomitant hearing loss [52] or without any reported hearing loss [53].

3.2. COVID-19 Associated with Disequilibrium

A case series from Wuhan of 799 patients described dizziness as a symptom in 8% of confirmed COVID-19 patients [54]. Another study, also from Wuhan, of 214 confirmed cases of COVID-19 that specifically asked patients about neurological symptoms reported dizziness in 16.8% of patients [28]. A study of 509 patients from several hospitals in Chicago reported dizziness in 29.7% of cases [20]. The variability reflected in this broad range (8–29.7%) among individual studies has been noted in reviews [31], though it is clear that there is increasing recognition of an association between COVID-19 and vestibular disorders [48]. The ability of COVID-19 to cause auditory and vestibular symptoms appears to be distinct from the other SARS coronaviruses [55].

3.3. Potential Mechanisms for Auditory and Vestibular Symptoms from SARS-CoV-2

In view of the emerging evidence of cochlear symptoms (hearing loss, tinnitus) and vestibular symptoms (dizziness) occurring in the context of COVID-19 infection, most reviews of this subject are concluding that the relationship between COVID-19 and audiovestibular dysfunction may be causal rather than simply associative [48,55–65].

In COVID-19 patients with auditory and vestibular symptoms, otovestibular testing is sometimes abnormal [63], though the mechanism by which SARS-CoV-2 causes such dysfunction is unclear. The author discusses several candidate mechanisms here.

First, as mentioned earlier, SARS-CoV-2 seems capable of affecting individual cranial nerves, manifesting with ophthalmoparesis [66], optic neuritis [13], and anosmia [26–30]. It is therefore logical to consider the possibility of SARS-CoV-2 involving the vestibulocochlear nerve, manifesting as vestibular neuritis [67–70] and/or cochlear neuritis or labyrinthitis. It should be noted, however, that some publications [71] describing "COVID-19 vestibular neuritis" appear to base the diagnosis on clinical criteria rather than on objective otovestibular testing; so, this remains a conjecture requiring further study.

Second, there is emerging evidence that the SARS-CoV-2 virus can directly infect inner ear hair cells [72], which may underlie reported cases of labyrinthitis [73]. Whether such involvement by SARS-CoV-2 in turn increases the risk for other specific otologic diseases, such as Ménière's disease [74] and benign paroxysmal positional vertigo [75,76], remains unclear.

A third potential mechanism for inner ear dysfunction due to COVID-19 infection is labyrinthine ischemia secondary to hypoxia [32]. COVID-19 infection increases the risk of thrombosis and can deoxygenate erythrocytes; since the inner ear's circulation is entirely dependent on the small and tenuous labyrinthine artery, this mechanism is plausible.

A fourth potential mechanism is hematologic, via intralabyrinthine hemorrhage, though so far this appears rare [35,77].

A fifth potential mechanism, at least for vestibular (not auditory) symptoms, is that SARS-CoV-2 appears to induce autonomic dysfunction in some patients [78–82]; so, orthostatic intolerance (generally postural orthostatic tachycardia) may be another mechanism by which SARS-CoV-2 provokes dizziness [83–89].

4. Auditory and Vestibular Symptoms Associated with Vaccination for SARS-CoV-2 and Treatment for COVID-19

Concerted research and pharmaceutical efforts have been directed at developing vaccines for SARS-CoV-2 and treatments for COVID-19. As these interventions have come to market, new questions have been raised regarding potential adverse effects, including auditory and vestibular symptoms. Here, the author briefly reviews several studies and reports regarding the vaccines and antiviral agents. Other interventions, such as interleukin modulators (anakinra, tocilizumab, and sarilumab) and other immunomodulators being used on an experimental basis in patients who are in (or who are at risk of entering) intensive care units, are covered elsewhere [90].

4.1. *Vaccines for COVID-19*

As of this writing, several vaccines have received FDA approval for use [91–93]. A broader review of possible adverse effects associated with the vaccines can be found elsewhere in this volume [94]. Researchers have received questions from patients regarding whether the vaccines themselves can cause otovestibular symptoms or exacerbate pre-existing otovestibular diseases. There are still insufficient data to answer these questions confidently. Our general experience so far has been that (1) apparent adverse effects from the vaccines have been transient, lasting days to weeks; (2) although symptoms from COVID-19 infection itself can be very mild, they can also be devastating (if a patient survives) or lethal. On the whole, the potential protection conferred by receiving the vaccines appears greatly to outweigh the risk of the vaccines.

4.1.1. Vaccines for COVID-19 and Dizziness

The literature regarding potential adverse effects from the Pfizer vaccine (BNT162b2 mRNA) is somewhat difficult to interpret as it pertains to vestibular symptoms. The original trial [92] included 43,548 participants (of whom 21,720 received the intervention and 21,828 received a placebo). The report, and its supplementary material, do not list dizziness/vertigo as an adverse event. However, a much smaller study (Kadali, Janagama et al. 2021) of 1245 recipients of the vaccine (no placebo arm), documented that out of 803 patients with "generalized" or "neurological" symptoms, 67 (8.34%) reported "dizziness," and 20 (2.49%) reported "vertigo." There has additionally been a case report of postural orthostatic tachycardia occurring following receipt of this vaccine [95]. There is a case report [70] of a patient who received the Pfizer vaccine and subsequently developed vestibular neuritis (supposedly corroborated on video head impulse testing), but whether this relationship was causal or associative is not known.

It is also difficult to interpret the literature about the Moderna vaccine's (mRNA-1273) association with vestibular symptoms. The original trial [91] studied 30,420 participants (of whom 15,210 received the vaccine and 15,210 received a placebo). Symptoms of "dizziness and "vertigo" were reported as adverse effects of zero patients in the trial's supplementary material. In contrast, a much smaller study of 432 vaccine recipients [96] reported "vertigo like symptoms" in 15 (3.47%) patients and "dizziness" in 63 (14.58%) patients.

It is similarly difficult to interpret the literature about the Johnson & Johnson's Janssen vaccine (Ad26.COV2.S). The original trial [93] included 39,260 participants (of whom 19,630 received the vaccine and 19,630 received placebo). The supplementary material from the trial reported that no vaccine recipients endorsed symptoms of "dizziness" or "vertigo." Yet, the product monograph (https://covid-vaccine.canada.ca/info/pdf/janssen-covid-19-vaccine-pm-en.pdf, accessed 26 June 2022) that reviewed data from 43,783 participants (of whom 21,895 received the vaccine and 21,888 received placebo) stated 13 patients in the treatment group and 7 patients in the placebo group endorsed the symptom of "vertigo."

4.1.2. Vaccines for COVID-19 and Hearing Loss

The Centers for Disease Control's Vaccine Adverse Effects Reporting System (CDC VAERS) provides publicly available data regarding the two mRNA vaccines (Pfizer and Moderna). Analysis of these data revealed 40 cases of unilateral sensorineural hearing loss (confirmed on audiometric testing) thought "most likely" to be attributable to the vaccines themselves [97]. The report indicated that the unilateral hearing loss occurred within 3 weeks (mean 4 days) of having received the vaccines. The calculated incidence was 0.3 cases per 100,000 individuals (i.e., 3 per million).

4.1.3. Vaccines for COVID-19 and Tinnitus

Tinnitus has been less studied as a potential adverse effect of COVID-19 vaccines, but emerging literature is beginning to discuss this [98,99].

4.2. Anti-Viral Therapies for COVID-19

For an individual already infected with COVID-19 the vaccines play no role in acute management, but treatments aiming at the virus itself are being investigated. These have recently been reviewed elsewhere [100]. Some of these agents are already known to be ototoxic, such as chloroquine, hydroxychloroquine, and ivermectin.

As of this writing there was considerable interest in the combination antiviral agent Paxlovid, which contains ritonavir (an agent already used in the treatment of HIV) and nirmatrelvir (an investigational agent); unfortunately, there is almost no literature about the potential ototoxicity of these agents; ritonavir is also one component of the combination antiviral drug, Kaletra (which also contains lopinavir), which has been reported to cause reversible bilateral hearing loss [101], but whether that property is due to ritonavir or lopinavir remains unclear.

Bamlanivimab (LY-CoV555 by Lilly) is a neutralizing IgG1 antibody for SARS-CoV-2 [102]. In a randomized phase 3 trial of 1035 patients [103], of whom 518 individuals received bamlanivimab in combination with another antiviral agent (etesevimab), and 517 individuals received a placebo, the symptom of "dizziness" was reported in four patients (0.8%) from the treatment group and three patients (0.6%) from the control group. The comparable rate of this symptom in both groups and the fact that the intervention group received a combination agent (bamlanivimab + etesevimab) makes it unclear what risk of vestibular symptoms bamlanivimab actually incurs.

Molnupiravir (MK-4882/EIDD-2801 by Merck) is a nucleotide analogue that inhibits SARS-CoV-2 replication. In a randomized phase 3 trial completed by 1411 patients [104], of whom 710 individuals received molnupiravir and 701 individuals received placebo, the symptom of "dizziness" was reported in 1% of the treatment group and 0.7% of the placebo group. The comparable rate of this symptom in both groups makes it unclear what risk of vestibular symptoms molnupiravir actually incurs.

5. Summary

The accumulating literature suggests that audiologic and vestibular systems can occur in association with COVID-19 infection; such symptoms are not among the most common, nor are they rare. Whether the relationship is causal is difficult to establish, even though some data (such as evidence of viral infection of inner ear hair cells) are quite suggestive of causality. The mechanism through which auditory and vestibular symptoms could be provoked by COVID-19 remains unclear; proposed mechanisms include vestibular (or vestibulocochlear) neuritis; direct infection of cochlear and/or vestibular hair cells; labyrinthine ischemia; intralabyrinthine hemorrhage; and autonomic dysfunction. The pandemic has lasted long enough for investigators to begin to recognize "long-haul" COVID-19 symptoms, often defined as symptoms persisting >6 months beyond initial infection; a recent study of such patients reported that symptoms such as dizziness and tinnitus, if present at the initial evaluation, were either still present or had actually increased by the time of the followup evaluation at 6–9 months [49].

While it is sensible to include COVID-19 on a differential diagnosis during a pandemic, it behooves the clinician to bear in mind that other diseases still merit consideration, and reasonable alternative explanations for a given symptom should be entertained.

As an example, there are emerging reports of patients with diagnosed COVID-19 infection who also appear to have vestibular neuritis. While it may be impossible at this time to ascertain whether the vestibular neuritis is due to COVID-19 itself or has occurred independently, it is still important to identify vestibular hypofunction in this circumstance, because such a deficit is potentially treatable with appropriately targeted vestibular rehabilitation therapy. Thus, in our patients diagnosed with COVID-19 who appear to have an acute vestibular syndrome, researchers recommend undertaking at least a screening otovestibular workup for vestibular weakness, including video head impulse testing, videonystagmography, and ocular and cervical vestibular evoked myogenic potentials; if these results are compatible with vestibular weakness (whether unilateral or bilateral), then referral for vestibular rehabilitation therapy is logical.

Auditory and vestibular symptoms are also being reported in association with the vaccines and treatments for COVID-19. While causality has not yet been proven, this relationship warrants further scrutiny. However, in view of the evidence of "long-haul" COVID-19 symptoms (mentioned earlier), and the absence (so far) of evidence for similarly lasting symptoms from vaccines and treatments for COVID-19, our current impression is that the overall the risk of harm from the vaccines and treatments seems significantly lower than the risks of SARS-CoV-2 infection itself.

6. Conclusions

- The acute, potentially life-threatening manifestations of COVID-19 certainly merit the greatest scrutiny of public health officials, researchers and clinicians. However, once such threats are treated or excluded, the longer-term consequences of COVID-19 are becoming more apparent.
- Among those consequences are auditory and vestibular symptoms associated with COVID-19 itself and with its vaccines and treatments. While these consequences may not be lethal, they still impose significant morbidity which, in turn, can incur non-trivial economic consequences at the individual level and at the broader population-based level.
- Greater understanding of these auditory and vestibular symptoms associated with COVID-19, its vaccines, and its treatments will be achieved partly through continued epidemiologic monitoring.
- Greater understanding of the pathobiological mechanisms underlying these symptoms will require more systematic evaluation of these patients, beginning with more regularly applied audiologic and vestibular testing. Facilitating such evaluations may require changes at the health-care-systems level, perhaps through promulgating practice guidelines.

Accumulating and analyzing such data will improve the likelihood of correctly diagnosing, and perhaps eventually treating, these aspects of the disease.

Funding: This research received no external funding.

Institutional Review Board Statement: This review article did not require ethical approval from the author's institutional review board.

Informed Consent Statement: This study did not involve any patients.

Data Availability Statement: This study reviewed literature, and did not collect any new data.

Conflicts of Interest: The author declares no conflict of interest.

References

1. Yan, R.; Zhang, Y.; Li, Y.; Xia, L.; Guo, Y.; Zhou, Q. Structural basis for the recognition of SARS-CoV-2 by full-length human ACE2. *Science* **2020**, *367*, 1444–1448. [CrossRef]
2. Ceccarelli, M.; Berretta, M.; Rullo, E.V.; Nunnari, G.; Cacopardo, B. Differences and similarities between Severe Acute Respiratory Syndrome (SARS)-CoronaVirus (CoV) and SARS-CoV-2. Would a rose by another name smell as sweet? *Eur. Rev. Med. Pharmacol. Sci.* **2020**, *24*, 2781–2783.
3. De Masi, L.; Argenio, M.A.; Giordano, D.; Facchiano, A. Molecular Aspects of Spike—ACE2 Interaction. *Encyclopedia* **2022**, *2*, 96–108. [CrossRef]
4. Dales, S. Factors controlling coronavirus infections and disease of the central nervous system. A review. *Adv. Exp. Med. Biol.* **1995**, *380*, 13–22. [PubMed]
5. Dube, M.; Le Coupanec, A.; Wong, A.H.M.; Rini, J.M.; Desforges, M.; Talbot, P.J. Axonal Transport Enables Neuron-to-Neuron Propagation of Human Coronavirus OC43. *J. Virol.* **2018**, *92*, e00404–e00418. [CrossRef]
6. Baig, A.M.; Khaleeq, A.; Ali, U.; Syeda, H. Evidence of the COVID-19 Virus Targeting the CNS: Tissue Distribution, Host-Virus Interaction, and Proposed Neurotropic Mechanisms. *ACS Chem. Neurosci.* **2020**, *11*, 995–998. [CrossRef]
7. Morfopoulou, S.; Brown, J.R.; Davies, E.G.; Anderson, G.; Virasami, A.; Qasim, W.; Chong, W.K.; Hubank, M.; Plagnol, V.; Desforges, M.; et al. Human Coronavirus OC43 Associated with Fatal Encephalitis. *N. Engl. J. Med.* **2016**, *375*, 497–498. [CrossRef]

8. Arabi, Y.M.; Harthi, A.; Hussein, J.; Bouchama, A.; Johani, S.; Hajeer, A.H.; Saeed, B.T.; Wahbi, A.; Saedy, A.; AlDabbagh, T.; et al. Severe neurologic syndrome associated with Middle East respiratory syndrome corona virus (MERS-CoV). *Infection* **2015**, *43*, 495–501. [CrossRef]
9. Li, Y.; Li, H.; Fan, R.; Wen, B.; Zhang, J.; Cao, X.; Wang, C.; Song, Z.; Li, S.; Li, X.; et al. Coronavirus Infections in the Central Nervous System and Respiratory Tract Show Distinct Features in Hospitalized Children. *Intervirology* **2016**, *59*, 163–169. [CrossRef]
10. Nilsson, A.; Edner, N.; Albert, J.; Ternhag, A. Fatal encephalitis associated with coronavirus OC43 in an immunocompromised child. *Infect. Dis.* **2020**, *52*, 419–422. [CrossRef]
11. Shnayder, N.A.; Sirbiladze, T.K.; Demko, I.V.; Petrova, M.M.; Nasyrova, R.F. Limbic Encephalitis Associated with COVID-19. *Encyclopedia* **2022**, *2*, 26–35. [CrossRef]
12. Yeh, E.A.; Collins, A.; Cohen, M.E.; Duffner, P.K.; Faden, H. Detection of coronavirus in the central nervous system of a child with acute disseminated encephalomyelitis. *Pediatrics* **2004**, *113*, e73–e76. [PubMed]
13. Dessau, R.B.; Lisby, G.; Frederiksen, J.L. Coronaviruses in spinal fluid of patients with acute monosymptomatic optic neuritis. *Acta Neurol. Scand.* **1999**, *100*, 88–91. [CrossRef] [PubMed]
14. Fazzini, E.; Fleming, J.; Fahn, S. Cerebrospinal fluid antibodies to coronavirus in patients with Parkinson's disease. *Mov. Disord.* **1992**, *7*, 153–158. [CrossRef]
15. Burks, J.S.; DeVald, B.L.; Jankovsky, L.D.; Gerdes, J.C. Two coronaviruses isolated from central nervous system tissue of two multiple sclerosis patients. *Science* **1980**, *209*, 933–934. [CrossRef]
16. Salmi, A.; Ziola, B.; Hovi, T.; Reunanen, M. Antibodies to coronaviruses OC43 and 229E in multiple sclerosis patients. *Neurology* **1982**, *32*, 292–295. [CrossRef]
17. Hovanec, D.L.; Flanagan, T.D. Detection of antibodies to human coronaviruses 229E and OC43 in the sera of multiple sclerosis patients and normal subjects. *Infect. Immun.* **1983**, *41*, 426–429. [CrossRef]
18. Koralnik, I.J.; Tyler, K.L. COVID-19: A Global Threat to the Nervous System. *Ann. Neurol.* **2020**, *88*, 1–11. [CrossRef]
19. Pinzon, R.T.; Wijaya, V.O.; Buana, R.B.; Al Jody, A.; Nunsio, P.N. Neurologic Characteristics in Coronavirus Disease 2019 (COVID-19): A Systematic Review and Meta-Analysis. *Front. Neurol.* **2020**, *11*, 565. [CrossRef]
20. LLiotta, E.M.; Batra, A.; Clark, J.R.; Shlobin, N.A.; Hoffman, S.C.; Orban, Z.S.; Koralnik, I.J. Frequent neurologic manifestations and encephalopathy-associated morbidity in Covid-19 patients. *Ann. Clin. Transl. Neurol.* **2020**, *7*, 2221–2230. [CrossRef]
21. Pinna, P.; Grewal, P.; Hall, J.P.; Tavarez, T.; Dafer, R.M.; Garg, R.; Osteraas, N.D.; Pellack, D.R.; Asthana, A.; Fegan, K.; et al. Neurological manifestations and COVID-19: Experiences from a tertiary care center at the Frontline. *J. Neurol. Sci.* **2020**, *415*, 116969. [CrossRef] [PubMed]
22. Nath, A. Neurologic complications of coronavirus infections. *Neurology* **2020**. [CrossRef] [PubMed]
23. Poyiadji, N.; Shahin, G.; Noujaim, D.; Stone, M.; Patel, S.; Griffith, B. COVID-19-associated Acute Hemorrhagic Necrotizing Encephalopathy: CT and MRI Features. *Radiology* **2020**, *296*, E119–E120. [CrossRef] [PubMed]
24. Filatov, A.; Sharma, P.; Hindi, F.; Espinosa, P.S. Neurological complications of coronavirus disease (COVID-19): Encephalopathy. *Cureus* **2020**, *12*, e7352. [CrossRef]
25. Zubair, A.S.; McAlpine, L.S.; Gardin, T.; Farhadian, S.; Kuruvilla, D.E.; Spudich, S. Neuropathogenesis and Neurologic Manifestations of the Coronaviruses in the Age of Coronavirus Disease 2019: A Review. *JAMA Neurol.* **2020**, *77*, 1018–1027. [CrossRef]
26. Giacomelli, A.; Pezzati, L.; Conti, F.; Bernacchia, D.; Siano, M.; Oreni, L.; Rusconi, S.; Gervasoni, C.; Ridolfo, A.L.; Rizzardini, G.; et al. Self-reported olfactory and taste disorders in SARS-CoV-2 patients: A cross-sectional study. *Clin. Infect. Dis.* **2020**. [CrossRef]
27. Gautier, J.F.; Ravussin, Y. A New Symptom of COVID-19: Loss of Taste and Smell. *Obesity* **2020**, *28*, 848. [CrossRef]
28. Mao, L.; Jin, H.; Wang, M.; Hu, Y.; Chen, S.; He, Q.; Chang, J.; Hong, C.; Zhou, Y.; Wang, D.; et al. Neurologic Manifestations of Hospitalized Patients With Coronavirus Disease 2019 in Wuhan, China. *JAMA Neurol* **2020**, *77*, 683–690. [CrossRef]
29. Mermelstein, S. Acute anosmia from COVID-19 infection. *Pract. Neurol.* **2020**, *20*, 343–344. [CrossRef]
30. Vavougios, G.D. Potentially irreversible olfactory and gustatory impairments in COVID-19: Indolent vs. fulminant SARS-CoV-2 neuroinfection. *Brain. Behav. Immun.* **2020**, *87*, 107–108. [CrossRef]
31. Saniasiaya, J.; Kulasegarah, J. Dizziness and COVID-19. *Ear Nose Throat J.* **2021**, *100*, 29–30. [CrossRef] [PubMed]
32. Kaliyappan, K.; Chen, Y.C.; Krishnan Muthaiah, V.P. Vestibular Cochlear Manifestations in COVID-19 Cases. *Front. Neurol.* **2022**, *13*, 850337. [CrossRef] [PubMed]
33. Bhatta, S.; Sharma, S.; Sharma, D.; Maharjan, L.; Bhattachan, S.; Sah, M.K.; Singhal, A.; Ghanpur, A.D.; Ganesuni, D. Study of Hearing Status in COVID 19 Patients: A Multicentered Review. *Indian J. Otolaryngol. Head Neck Surg.* **2021**, 1–7. [CrossRef] [PubMed]
34. Chari, D.A.; Parikh, A.; Kozin, E.D.; Reed, M.; Jung, D.H. Impact of COVID-19 on Presentation of Sudden Sensorineural Hearing Loss at a Single Institution. *Otolaryngol. Head Neck Surg.* **2021**, *165*, 163–165. [CrossRef]
35. Chern, A.; Famuyide, A.O.; Moonis, G.; Lalwani, A.K. Bilateral Sudden Sensorineural Hearing Loss and Intralabyrinthine Hemorrhage in a Patient With COVID-19. *Otol. Neurotol.* **2021**, *42*, e10–e14. [CrossRef]
36. Chirakkal, P.; Al Hail, A.N.; Zada, N.; Vijayakumar, D.S. COVID-19 and Tinnitus. *Ear Nose Throat J.* **2021**, *100*, 160S–162S. [CrossRef]
37. Degen, C.; Lenarz, T.; Willenborg, K. Acute Profound Sensorineural Hearing Loss After COVID-19 Pneumonia. *Mayo Clin. Proc.* **2020**, *95*, 1801–1803. [CrossRef]

38. Edwards, M.; Muzaffar, J.; Naik, P.; Coulson, C. Catastrophic bilateral sudden sensorineural hearing loss following COVID-19. *BMJ Case Rep.* **2021**, *14*, e243157. [CrossRef]
39. Gerstacker, K.; Speck, I.; Riemann, S.; Aschendorff, A.; Knopf, A.; Arndt, S. Deafness after COVID-19? *HNO* **2021**, *69*, 92–95. [CrossRef]
40. Koumpa, F.S.; Forde, C.T.; Manjaly, J.G. Sudden irreversible hearing loss post COVID-19. *BMJ Case Rep.* **2020**, *13*, e238419. [CrossRef]
41. Lamounier, P.; Franco Goncalves, V.; Ramos, H.V.L.; Gobbo, D.A.; Teixeira, R.P.; Dos Reis, P.C.; Bahmad, F., Jr.; Candido Costa, C. A 67-Year-Old Woman with Sudden Hearing Loss Associated with SARS-CoV-2 Infection. *Am. J. Case Rep.* **2020**, *21*, e927519. [CrossRef] [PubMed]
42. Dusan, M.; Milan, S.; Nikola, D. COVID-19 caused hearing loss. *Eur. Arch. Otorhinolaryngol.* **2021**, *279*, 2363–2372. [CrossRef] [PubMed]
43. Fidan, V.; Akin, O.; Koyuncu, H. Rised sudden sensorineural hearing loss during COVID-19 widespread. *Am. J. Otolaryngol.* **2021**, *42*, 102996. [CrossRef] [PubMed]
44. Gosavi, S.; Nagarajan, S.; Shah, N.J.; Thomas, N.A.T.; Kumar, K.R.; Sangole, V. ENT Symptomology in Active COVID-19 Patients in our Tertiary Care Centre. *Indian J. Otolaryngol. Head Neck Surg.* **2021**, 1–6. [CrossRef]
45. Munro, K.J.; Uus, K.; Almufarrij, I.; Chaudhuri, N.; Yioe, V. Persistent self-reported changes in hearing and tinnitus in post-hospitalisation COVID-19 cases. *Int. J. Audiol.* **2020**, *59*, 889–890. [CrossRef]
46. Ricciardiello, F.; Pisani, D.; Viola, P.; Cristiano, E.; Scarpa, A.; Giannone, A.; Longo, G.; Russo, G.; Bocchetti, M.; Coppola, C.; et al. Sudden Sensorineural Hearing Loss in Mild COVID-19: Case Series and Analysis of the Literature. *Audiol. Res.* **2021**, *11*, 313–326. [CrossRef]
47. De Luca, P.; Scarpa, A.; Ralli, M.; Tassone, D.; Simone, M.; De Campora, L.; Cassandro, C.; Di Stadio, A. Auditory Disturbances and SARS-CoV-2 Infection: Brain Inflammation or Cochlear Affection? Systematic Review and Discussion of Potential Pathogenesis. *Front. Neurol.* **2021**, *12*, 707207. [CrossRef]
48. Fancello, V.; Hatzopoulos, S.; Corazzi, V.; Bianchini, C.; Skarzynska, M.B.; Pelucchi, S.; Skarzynski, P.H.; Ciorba, A. SARS-CoV-2 (COVID-19) and audio-vestibular disorders. *Int. J. Immunopathol. Pharmacol.* **2021**, *35*, 20587384211027373. [CrossRef]
49. Ali, S.T.; Kang, A.K.; Patel, T.R.; Clark, J.R.; Perez-Giraldo, G.S.; Orban, Z.S.; Lim, P.H.; Jimenez, M.; Graham, E.L.; Batra, A.; et al. Evolution of neurologic symptoms in non-hospitalized COVID-19 "long haulers". *Ann. Clin. Transl. Neurol.* **2022**, *35*, 20587384211027373. [CrossRef]
50. Beukes, E.; Ulep, A.J.; Eubank, T.; Manchaiah, V. The Impact of COVID-19 and the Pandemic on Tinnitus: A Systematic Review. *J. Clin. Med.* **2021**, *10*, 2763. [CrossRef]
51. Beukes, E.W.; Baguley, D.M.; Jacquemin, L.; Lourenco, M.; Allen, P.M.; Onozuka, J.; Stockdale, D.; Kaldo, V.; Andersson, G.; Manchaiah, V. Changes in Tinnitus Experiences During the COVID-19 Pandemic. *Front. Public Health* **2020**, *8*, 592878. [CrossRef] [PubMed]
52. Elibol, E. Otolaryngological symptoms in COVID-19. *Eur. Arch. Otorhinolaryngol.* **2021**, *278*, 1233–1236. [CrossRef] [PubMed]
53. LLiang, Y.; Xu, J.; Chu, M.; Mai, J.; Lai, N.; Tang, W.; Yang, T.; Zhang, S.; Guan, C.; Zhong, F.; et al. Neurosensory dysfunction: A diagnostic marker of early COVID-19. *Int J Infect Dis* **2020**, *98*, 347–352. [CrossRef] [PubMed]
54. Chen, T.; Wu, D.; Chen, H.; Yan, W.; Yang, D.; Chen, G.; Ma, K.; Xu, D.; Yu, H.; Wang, H.; et al. Clinical characteristics of 113 deceased patients with coronavirus disease 2019: Retrospective study. *BMJ* **2020**, *368*, m1091. [CrossRef] [PubMed]
55. Almufarrij, I.; Uus, K.; Munro, K.J. Does coronavirus affect the audio-vestibular system? A rapid systematic review. *Int. J. Audiol.* **2020**, *59*, 487–491. [CrossRef]
56. Karimi-Galougahi, M.; Naeini, A.S.; Raad, N.; Mikaniki, N.; Ghorbani, J. Vertigo and hearing loss during the COVID-19 pandemic—Is there an association? *Acta Otorhinolaryngol. Ital.* **2020**, *4*, 463–465. [CrossRef]
57. Maharaj, S.; Bello Alvarez, M.; Mungul, S.; Hari, K. Otologic dysfunction in patients with COVID-19: A systematic review. *Laryngoscope Investig. Otolaryngol.* **2020**, *5*, 1192–1196. [CrossRef]
58. AlJasser, A.; Alkeridy, W.; Munro, K.J.; Plack, C.J. Is COVID-19 associated with self-reported audio-vestibular symptoms? *Int. J. Audiol.* **2021**, 1–9. [CrossRef]
59. Almufarrij, I.; Munro, K.J. One year on: An updated systematic review of SARS-CoV-2, COVID-19 and audio-vestibular symptoms. *Int. J. Audiol.* **2021**, *60*, 935–945. [CrossRef]
60. Chao, C.H.; Young, Y.H. Evolution of incidence of audiovestibular disorders during the pandemic COVID-19 period. *Eur. Arch. Otorhinolaryngol.* **2021**, *279*, 3341–3345. [CrossRef]
61. Gallus, R.; Melis, A.; Rizzo, D.; Piras, A.; De Luca, L.M.; Tramaloni, P.; Serra, A.; Longoni, E.; Soro, G.M.; Bussu, F. Audiovestibular symptoms and sequelae in COVID-19 patients. *J. Vestib. Res. Equilib. Orientat.* **2021**, *31*, 381–387. [CrossRef] [PubMed]
62. Jafari, Z.; Kolb, B.E.; Mohajerani, M.H. Hearing Loss, Tinnitus, and Dizziness in COVID-19: A Systematic Review and Meta-Analysis. *Can. J. Neurol. Sci.* **2021**, 1–12. [CrossRef] [PubMed]
63. Tan, M.; Cengiz, D.U.; Demir, I.; Demirel, S.; Colak, S.C.; Karakas, O.; Bayindir, T. Effects of Covid-19 on the audio-vestibular system. *Am. J. Otolaryngol.* **2021**, *43*, 103173. [CrossRef]
64. Viola, P.; Ralli, M.; Pisani, D.; Malanga, D.; Sculco, D.; Messina, L.; Laria, C.; Aragona, T.; Leopardi, G.; Ursini, F.; et al. Tinnitus and equilibrium disorders in COVID-19 patients: Preliminary results. *Eur. Arch. Otorhinolaryngol.* **2021**, *278*, 3725–3730. [CrossRef] [PubMed]

65. Wichova, H.; Miller, M.E.; Derebery, M.J. Otologic Manifestations After COVID-19 Vaccination: The House Ear Clinic Experience. *Otol. Neurotol.* **2021**, *42*, e1213–e1218. [CrossRef]
66. Dinkin, M.; Gao, V.; Kahan, J.; Bobker, S.; Simonetto, M.; Wechsler, P.; Harpe, J.; Greer, C.; Mints, G.; Salama, G.; et al. COVID-19 presenting with ophthalmoparesis from cranial nerve palsy. *Neurology* **2020**, *95*, 221–223. [CrossRef]
67. Malayala, S.V.; Raza, A. A Case of COVID-19-Induced Vestibular Neuritis. *Cureus* **2020**, *12*, e8918. [CrossRef]
68. Vanaparthy, R.; Malayala, S.V.; Balla, M. COVID-19-Induced Vestibular Neuritis, Hemi-Facial Spasms and Raynaud's Phenomenon: A Case Report. *Cureus* **2020**, *12*, e11752. [CrossRef]
69. Mat, Q.; Noel, A.; Loiselet, L.; Tainmont, S.; Chiesa-Estomba, C.M.; Lechien, J.R.; Duterme, J.P. Vestibular Neuritis as Clinical Presentation of COVID-19. *Ear. Nose. Throat. J.* **2021**, 145561321995021. [CrossRef]
70. Jeong, J. Vestibular neuritis after COVID-19 vaccination. *Hum. Vaccin Immunother.* **2021**, *17*, 5126–5128. [CrossRef]
71. Malayala, S.V.; Mohan, G.; Vasireddy, D.; Atluri, P. A case series of vestibular symptoms in positive or suspected COVID-19 patients. *Infez. Med.* **2021**, *29*, 117–122. [PubMed]
72. Jeong, M.; Ocwieja, K.E.; Han, D.; Wackym, P.A.; Zhang, Y.; Brown, A.; Moncada, C.; Vambutas, A.; Kanne, T.; Crain, R.; et al. Direct SARS-CoV-2 infection of the human inner ear may underlie COVID-19-associated audiovestibular dysfunction. *Commun. Med.* **2021**, *1*, 44. [CrossRef]
73. Perret, M.; Bernard, A.; Rahmani, A.; Manckoundia, P.; Putot, A. Acute Labyrinthitis Revealing COVID-19. *Diagnostics* **2021**, *11*, 482. [CrossRef] [PubMed]
74. Lovato, A.; Frosolini, A.; Marioni, G.; de Filippis, C. Higher incidence of Meniere's disease during COVID-19 pandemic: A preliminary report. *Acta Otolaryngol.* **2021**, *141*, 921–924. [CrossRef] [PubMed]
75. Picciotti, P.M.; Passali, G.C.; Sergi, B.; De Corso, E. Benign Paroxysmal Positional Vertigo (BPPV) in COVID-19. *Audiol Res* **2021**, *11*, 418–422. [CrossRef]
76. Maslovara, S.; Kosec, A. Post-COVID-19 Benign Paroxysmal Positional Vertigo. *Case Rep. Med.* **2021**, *2021*, 9967555. [CrossRef]
77. Narozny, W.; Tretiakow, D.; Skorek, A. Intralabyrinthine Hemorrhage in a Patient with Covid-19—A Challenge for an Otologist. *Otol. Neurotol.* **2021**, *42*, e967. [CrossRef]
78. Shouman, K.; Vanichkachorn, G.; Cheshire, W.P.; Suarez, M.D.; Shelly, S.; Lamotte, G.J.; Sandroni, P.; Benarroch, E.E.; Berini, S.E.; Cutsforth Gregory, J.K.; et al. Autonomic dysfunction following COVID-19 infection: An early experience. *Clin. Auton. Res.* **2021**, *31*, 385–394. [CrossRef]
79. Dani, M.; Dirksen, A.; Taraborrelli, P.; Torocastro, M.; Panagopoulos, D.; Sutton, R.; Lim, P.B. Autonomic dysfunction in 'long COVID': Rationale, physiology and management strategies. *Clin. Med.* **2021**, *21*, e63–e67. [CrossRef]
80. Goodman, B.P.; Khoury, J.A.; Blair, J.E.; Grill, M.F. COVID-19 Dysautonomia. *Front. Neurol.* **2021**, *12*, 624968. [CrossRef]
81. Lo, Y.L. COVID-19, fatigue, and dysautonomia. *J. Med. Virol.* **2021**, *93*, 1213. [CrossRef] [PubMed]
82. Eshak, N.; Abdelnabi, M.; Ball, S.; Elgwairi, E.; Creed, K.; Test, V.; Nugent, K. Dysautonomia: An Overlooked Neurological Manifestation in a Critically ill COVID-19 Patient. *Am. J. Med. Sci.* **2020**, *360*, 427–429. [CrossRef] [PubMed]
83. Miglis, M.G.; Prieto, T.; Shaik, R.; Muppidi, S.; Sinn, D.-I.; Jaradeh, S. A case report of postural tachycardia syndrome after COVID-19. *Clin. Auton. Res.* **2020**, *30*, 449–451. [CrossRef]
84. Johansson, M.; Ståhlberg, M.; Runold, M.; Nygren-Bonnier, M.; Nilsson, J.; Olshansky, B.; Bruchfeld, J.; Fedorowski, A. Long-Haul Post-COVID-19 Symptoms Presenting as a Variant of Postural Orthostatic Tachycardia Syndrome: The Swedish Experience. *JACC Case Rep.* **2021**, *3*, 573–580. [CrossRef] [PubMed]
85. Kanjwal, K.; Jamal, S.; Kichloo, A.; Grubb, B.P. New-onset Postural Orthostatic Tachycardia Syndrome Following Coronavirus Disease 2019 Infection. *J. Innov. Card Rhythm. Manag.* **2020**, *11*, 4302–4304. [CrossRef]
86. Schofield, J.R. Persistent Antiphospholipid Antibodies, Mast Cell Activation Syndrome, Postural Orthostatic Tachycardia Syndrome and Post-COVID Syndrome: 1 Year On. *Eur. J. Case Rep. Intern. Med.* **2021**, *8*, 002378. [CrossRef]
87. Goldstein, D.S. The possible association between COVID-19 and postural tachycardia syndrome. *Heart Rhythm.* **2021**, *18*, 508–509. [CrossRef]
88. Novak, P. Post COVID-19 syndrome associated with orthostatic cerebral hypoperfusion syndrome, small fiber neuropathy and benefit of immunotherapy: A case report. *eNeurologicalSci* **2020**, *21*, 100276. [CrossRef]
89. Blitshteyn, S.; Whitelaw, S. Postural orthostatic tachycardia syndrome (POTS) and other autonomic disorders after COVID-19 infection: A case series of 20 patients. *Immunol. Res.* **2021**, *69*, 205–211. [CrossRef]
90. Skarzynska, M.B.; Matusiak, M.; Skarzynski, P.H. Adverse Audio-Vestibular Effects of Drugs and Vaccines Used in the Treatment and Prevention of COVID-19: A Review. *Audiol. Res.* **2022**, *12*, 224–248. [CrossRef]
91. Baden, L.R.; El Sahly, H.M.; Essink, B.; Kotloff, K.; Frey, S.; Novak, R.; Diemert, D.; Spector, S.A.; Rouphael, N.; Creech, C.B.; et al. Efficacy and Safety of the mRNA-1273 SARS-CoV-2 Vaccine. *N. Engl. J. Med.* **2021**, *384*, 403–416. [CrossRef] [PubMed]
92. Polack, F.P.; Thomas, S.J.; Kitchin, N.; Absalon, J., Gurtman, A.; Lockhart, S.; Perez, J.L.; Perez Marc, G.; Moreira, E.D.; Zerbini, C.; et al. Safety and Efficacy of the BNT162b2 mRNA Covid-19 Vaccine. *N. Engl. J. Med.* **2020**, *383*, 2603–2615. [CrossRef] [PubMed]
93. Sadoff, J.; Gray, G.; Vandebosch, A.; Cardenas, V.; Shukarev, G.; Grinsztejn, B.; Goepfert, P.A.; Truyers, C.; Fennema, H.; Spiessens, B.; et al. Safety and Efficacy of Single-Dose Ad26.COV2.S Vaccine against COVID-19. *N. Engl. J. Med.* **2021**, *384*, 2187–2201. [CrossRef] [PubMed]
94. Ajmera, K.M. Adverse Events Profile of COVID-19 Preventative Strategies. *Encyclopedia* **2022**, *2*, 457–465. [CrossRef]

95. Reddy, S.; Reddy, S.; Arora, M. A Case of Postural Orthostatic Tachycardia Syndrome Secondary to the Messenger RNA COVID-19 Vaccine. *Cureus* **2021**, *13*, e14837. [CrossRef] [PubMed]
96. Kadali, R.A.K.; Janagama, R.; Peruru, S.; Gajula, V.; Madathala, R.R.; Chennaiahgari, N.; Malayala, S.V. Non-life-threatening adverse effects with COVID-19 mRNA-1273 vaccine: A randomized, cross-sectional study on healthcare workers with detailed self-reported symptoms. *J. Med. Virol.* **2021**, *93*, 4420–4429. [CrossRef] [PubMed]
97. Formeister, E.J.; Chien, W.; Agrawal, Y.; Carey, J.P.; Stewart, C.M.; Sun, D.Q. Preliminary Analysis of Association Between COVID-19 Vaccination and Sudden Hearing Loss Using US Centers for Disease Control and Prevention Vaccine Adverse Events Reporting System Data. *JAMAOtolaryngol. Head Neck Surg.* **2021**, *147*, 674–676. [CrossRef] [PubMed]
98. Ahmed, S.H.; Waseem, S.; Shaikh, T.G.; Qadir, N.A.; Siddiqui, S.A.; Ullah, I.; Waris, A.; Yousaf, Z. SARS-CoV-2 vaccine-associated-tinnitus: A review. *Ann. Med. Surg.* **2022**, *75*, 103293. [CrossRef]
99. Parrino, D.; Frosolini, A.; Gallo, C.; De Siati, R.D.; Spinato, G.; de Filippis, C. Tinnitus following COVID-19 vaccination: Report of three cases. *Int. J. Audiol.* **2021**, *61*, 526–529. [CrossRef]
100. Coffin, A.B.; Boney, R.; Hill, J.; Tian, C.; Steyger, P.S. Detecting Novel Ototoxins and Potentiation of Ototoxicity by Disease Settings. *Front. Neurol.* **2021**, *12*, 725566. [CrossRef]
101. Williams, B. Ototoxicity may be associated with protease inhibitor therapy. *Clin. Infect. Dis.* **2001**, *33*, 2100–2102. [CrossRef] [PubMed]
102. Orders, M. An EUA for Bamlanivimab-A Monoclonal Antibody for COVID-19. *JAMA* **2021**, *325*, 880–881.
103. Dougan, M.; Nirula, A.; Azizad, M.; Mocherla, B.; Gottlieb, R.L.; Chen, P.; Hebert, C.; Perry, R.; Boscia, J.; Heller, B.; et al. Bamlanivimab plus Etesevimab in Mild or Moderate COVID-19. *N. Engl. J. Med.* **2021**, *385*, 1382–1392. [CrossRef] [PubMed]
104. Jayk Bernal, A.; Gomes da Silva, M.M.; Musungaie, D.B.; Kovalchuk, E.; Gonzalez, A.; Delos Reyes, V.; Martín-Quirós, A.; Caraco, Y.; Williams-Diaz, A.; Brown, M.L.; et al. Molnupiravir for Oral Treatment of Covid-19 in Nonhospitalized Patients. *N. Engl. J. Med.* **2022**, *386*, 509–520. [CrossRef] [PubMed]

encyclopedia

Entry

COVID-19: Gender and Outcomes

Alfonso Ilardi

Department of Internal Medicine, Inmates Ward, "Antonio Cardarelli" Hospital, Via A. Cardarelli, 9, 80131 Naples, Italy; alfonso.ilardi@aocardarelli.it

Definition: The existence of differences in susceptibility to SARS-CoV-2 infection between males and females in both incidence and outcomes is well documented in the scientific literature. These differences, which are still underestimated, may have important implications in terms of prevention, diagnosis, and treatment of COVID-19, with significant prognostic consequences. The greater severity of the infection observed in males, even more so if they are elderly, would seem, according to current knowledge, to be due to multiple influences: immunological and endocrinological, but also genetic and behavioral.

Keywords: immunosenescence; coronavirus; Angiotensin Converting Enzyme 2 (ACE2); dendritic cells; estradiol

1. Introduction

Since the outbreak of the current pandemic, it has been clear that the severity of infection was greater in older people, depending on the burden of comorbidities [1], and most likely related to the decay of immune functions, referred to as immunosenescence, which occurs as the physiological aging process advances. The latter is characterized by a progressive failure of innate and especially acquired immunity, secondary to the decreased availability of naïve peripheral T and B cells, which tend to be gradually depleted by repeated microbiological exposure throughout life [2].This depletion is accompanied by the expansion of some memory cell subsets, which leads to a significant imbalance in the relationship with naïve cells. The result is a reduced availability of cells oriented towards immune responses to new pathogens and an increased susceptibility to infection [3,4].

Another widely recognized aspect of the aging process is theprofound structural changes that occur to the rib cage (stiffening from calcification and kyphosis from osteoporosis), reducing its compliance and impairing the complete emptying of the lungs at expiration with an increase in residual volume. There is also an increase in the size of the distal airspaces due to the loss of supporting tissue and a progressive reduction in the strength of the respiratory muscles. These effects reduce the reserve capacity of the whole system, increasing the vulnerability to functional failure in situations of increased ventilatory demand [5].

The aforementioned issues do not discount the weight of comorbidities on the severity of the infection. In the cohort of patients evaluated by Grasselli and co-workers, about 1550 subjects were admitted to the Intensive Care Unit (ICU), and at least one comorbidity was recorded in 68% of cases [6].

A lower percentage (23.7%) was reported in Guan's study of 1099 patients. However, in this cohort, the infection was classified as severe in only 173 patients [7].

The data on the type of preexisting disorder is also of significance. Case fatality is highest in patients with defined comorbidities, such as cardiovascular disease, diabetes mellitus, hypertension, chronic respiratory disease, and cancer [8]. Of these, hypertension is the most common in patients with COVID-19 and hypertensive patients have a higher disease severity and admission rate to the ICU than those with normal blood pressure [6,9].

Citation: Ilardi, A. COVID-19: Gender and Outcomes. *Encyclopedia* **2022**, *2*, 864–872. https://doi.org/10.3390/encyclopedia2020056

Academic Editors: Stephen Bustin and Raffaele Barretta

Received: 6 March 2022
Accepted: 16 April 2022
Published: 22 April 2022

Therefore, since hypertension has a higher prevalence in males than in females, at least until the onset of menopause [10], the possible link between hypertension and the severity of COVID-19 should also be investigated. According to some authors, it should be attributable to endothelial dysfunction, which preexists with the infection but promotes its progression through a state of hypercoagulability, and to dysregulation of the Renin-Angiotensin System (RAS). The latter would be favored by downregulation of the ACE2 enzyme, on the surface of pneumocytes, with reduced production of Ang 1-7 and an increase of the pro-oxidative and pro-inflammatory actions of Ang II [11].

However, even irrespective of age and comorbidities, the greater severity of infection observed in males, makes this subset at higher risk for admission to the ICU [6,12], as well as having a higher mortality rate [13,14].

This was also supported by Peckam's meta-analysis, which selected 107 studies from all over the world with a total of 3,111,714 patients. The analysis shows that males and females are at equivalent risk of infection, with males being associated with the development of severe disease as measured by admission to the ICU [15].

Although the current epidemiological situation is in constant evolution, the trend does not seem to have changed substantially.

In England, the majority of deaths in COVID-19 patients (99%), from March 2020 to April 2021, occurred in adults aged 45 years and older, and from this threshold age, most deaths were in males [16].

In Italy, the most recent data provided by the National Institute of Health document that the number of positive swabs is higher in females between the ages of 20 and 55. Conversely, the incidence curves of hospital admissions, including those in the ICU, begin to differ after the age of 40, with a greater slope in males than in females [17].

The aim of this entry is to explore the above gender-correlated differences, with particular focus on risk factors that are thought to have the greatest impact on important clinical outcomes.

2. Risk Factors

The observed differences between the sexes may have different assumptions: behavioral, endocrinological, immunological, as well as genetic. These factors have come more strongly to the attention of the scientific community since the pandemic SARS, which originated in China in 2002. Over the years it has become clear that their knowledge and management can provide useful contributions both in terms of preventive strategies and the identification of potential therapeutic targets. This last aspect is even more important if framed within the context of gender-orientedpharmacology, which highlights and defines the differences in the efficacy and safety of drugs according to gender.

2.1. *Behavioural Factors*

The adoption of healthy lifestyles by females is considered to be one of the contributing factors. For example, in this subgroup, there is lower consumption of cigarettes and alcohol [18].

However, it should be emphasized, especially with regard to smoking status, that its impact on the two sexes varies between countries. Developed countries have a higher prevalence of female smokers than developing countries, while the prevalence of male smokers tends to be more or less similar [19].However, among non-daily smokers, women have lower cigarette consumption and nicotine dependence [20].

At the same time, significant differences were observed among females and males in the perception of illness in terms of both severity and compliance. As reported in a survey involving 21,649 subjects from eight different countries (Australia, Austria, France, Germany, Italy, New Zealand, UK and USA), this perception, which appears less relevant in young people, tends to increase with age, although males with symptoms of illness are more likely to adhere to containment measures (interpersonal distance, hand washing, and correct use of personal protective equipment) [21].

Significant differences also emerged between the two sexes in their responses to stress triggered by lockdown and prolonged restriction actions. The study by Salfi and coworkers demonstrates, within the Italian population, a different temporal pattern of sleep disturbances and mental health status during the pandemic. Although the scores recorded in females were higher than males over time, especially at the beginning of the lockdown, the gender gap progressively narrowed. In the long term, women seemed to be more resilient than men, showing a tendency to improve in terms of anxiety, depression, and insomnia [22].

The different responses would be due to the emergence of two different reactive patterns: a fight-or-flight pattern in males and a tend-and-befriend pattern in females [23]. The latter can further explain the greater acceptance by females of the rules and restrictions imposed by the health emergency.

On the other hand, increased levels of perceived stress in males may also have significant effects on immune-mediated responses. In fact, it is known that under conditions of chronic stress, the cytotoxic action of Natural Killer cells is reduced, with suppression of the lymphocyte proliferative response and attenuation of humoral responses [24].

A further observationofthe gap between the two sexes, disadvantaging the females in this case, can be observed in the under-60 age group and is related to the characteristics of the working pattern. The direct care of the sick members of the family, who are often elderly, as well as the care of children, especially those of school age, could represent a source of increased exposure to infection in females, a relationship, moreover, already suggested by Monto about twenty years ago [25].

Moreover, in this age group, women are highly represented in the health professions, especially among nurses and the risk of respiratory infections among health care workers is also well described [26].

Indeed, it is estimated that women currently represent more than 70% of the global health workforce, and this representation rises to 90% in the nursing professions [27].

2.2. Endocrine and Immunological Factors

The interfering effect of immunological and hormonal factors on susceptibility to infection and its progression is a complex study area.

First of all, we must consider the potential role of androgens as a restraining factor in the cytokine response, with higher levels of TNF-α and IL1-β seen in androgen-deficient males [28].

In this regard, it has been demonstrated that androgens suppress the activity of transcription factors (NF-kB) by increasing the expression of peroxisome proliferator-activated receptor (PPAR) in T cells [29].

However, suppressing the cytokine response should make younger males more vulnerable. This hypothesis is disproved by available epidemiological data [17].

Alternatively, overexpression of the integral membrane glycoprotein Angiotensin Converting Enzyme 2 (ACE2), which acts as a gateway for coronavirus, might be considered [30].

This function is related to its binding with the viral Spike protein, which protrudes from the surface, causing the virus to take on a crown-like appearance. The key role of ACE2 has been widely confirmed by several studies, which have also shown that the affinity of the Spike-protein of the new coronavirus is higher than that of the Spike-protein of SARS-CoV [31].

The enzyme, like its counterpart, the Angiotensin Converting Enzyme (ACE), plays an essential role in modulating sodium balance and vasoconstriction and is highly expressed not only in the lungs but also in other organs [32]. Particularly in the lungs, more than 80% of the cells expressing this metalloproteinase on the surface are type II pneumocytes, explaining the increased vulnerability of the lower respiratory tract to infection [33].

The key action of ACE2 is the conversion of the octapeptide Ang II to its metabolite Angiotensin-(1–7), which performs opposite actions to those of Angiotensin II, a molecule with vasopressive, profibrotic, and proliferative properties [34].

However, the interaction of the virus with ACE2 may favor its downregulation with a loss of enzyme function. The higher concentration of the enzyme at the alveolar cell surface, observed in males, suggests that the downregulation phenomenon mentioned above is more extensive and potentially unbalancing; i.e., the increased production of Ang II and subsequent over-stimulation of the AT1 receptor (AT1R) could contribute to additional or worsening lung damage in this subgroup of patients. Indeed, it has been suggested that the loss of ACE2 activity may result, via the AT1R, in an increase in vascular permeability with the destruction of the alveolar barrier and the extravasal collection of inflammatory cells [35].

Conversely, high concentrations of estradiol reduce ACE2 expression in the lungs, with opposite effects in the presence of decreased levels [36,37].

Additional to these observations is the finding that estrogens affect the expression of the AT1R and ACE, promoting the concurrent decrease in plasma renin activity [38]. The reduced concentration of AT1R could, therefore, exert a dampening effect on lung damage in women.

A further issue for discussion is the possible imbalance between the enzyme bound to the plasma membrane and the soluble form (sACE2), which is released into the circulation through the action of tumor necrosis factor-alpha convertase (ADAM17). It could be assumed that an increased circulating fraction reduces the compensatory power of ACE2. Since males exhibit higher plasma concentrations of sACE2 relative to children and women [39], the greater severity of the disease in males should be secondary to an accentuation of the pathogenic sequences triggered by the infection [40].

However, Yang and coworkers' study reported that, in patients with higher circulating levels of the enzyme ectodomain, the outcome improved, suggesting a protective effect of sACE2 against acute lung injury [41].

From this perspective, it could be assumed that sACE2, acting as a decoy for the coronavirus, prevents the downregulation of the cell surface enzyme and subsequent over-stimulation of the AT1R [42].

The different immunological reactivity detectable in the two sexes is more accurately defined. Indeed, females are more likely to develop a vigorous immunological response following an infection, in both innate and acquired immunity [43]. From an evolutionary viewpoint, this high level of responsiveness increases their survival and hence the reproductive capacity of the species [33]. This is supported by the observation in animal studies that infections tend to occur more severely in the middle-aged than in the young and old [43].

The above differences should be related to the estrogenic effects mediated by specific receptors (e.g., ERα), which promote gene transcription after interaction with an appropriate ligand [44]. It has been established that signals triggered by ERα activation are involved in the differentiation of various subsets of dendritic cells (DCs), which are essential for the activation of specific naïve T cells and their subsequent differentiation into effector T cells [45].

In addition to the classical DCs (cDCs), which specialize in antigen processing and presentation, there are monocyte-derived CD11b+ inflammatory/migratory DCs, which display many of the characteristics of cDCs, Langerhans cells, and plasmacytoid DCs (pDCs). CDCs, with their distinctive dendritic appearance, are specialized in antigen processing and presentation. In contrast, pDCs have a spherical shape, have no phagocytic functions, and are unable to present exogenous antigens to CD4+ T cells [45].

They are activated by specific pattern recognition receptors (PRRs).Among these receptors is Toll-Like-Receptor 7 (TLR-7), an endosomal innate immune sensor, which recognizes single-stranded RNA sequences, including the coronavirus genome [33].

These cells are also able to produce large amounts of type I Interferons (IFN) in response to viral infections [45,46], although all nucleated cells can in fact produce type I IFN. The signals triggered by these mediators induce transient lymphopenia, which is due to the rapid migration of lymphocytes into secondary lymphoid organs [47].

However, the production and release time of these compounds can be critical for protection, because a possible slowdown can have negative inflammatory effects. In this regard, the reaction can be regarded as more timely and quantitatively more intense in females [43].

2.3. Genetic Factors

A genetic hypothesis has been advanced to overcome the traditional estrogen/androgen hormone dichotomy and to support the differences in immunological reactivity. Such an assumption makes possible an extension of the differences between the sexes to a broader age range [48].

In mammals, females carry a pair of X chromosomes in their somatic cells, each of which consists of 154 Mb, about three times the 59 Mb of the Y chromosome. To balance the dosage of genes carried by the X chromosome between males and females, one of the two X chromosomes is randomly inactivated in female embryos, and DNA methylation is one of the factors contributing to gene silencing on the inactivated X chromosome [49].

Due to the randomness of this inactivation, some cells will have an active X chromosome of maternal origin and others a paternal chromosome [50].

However, about 15% of X-linked genes escape X-inactivation in women [49]. TLR7, encoded on the X chromosome, is one of the molecules able to escape the inactivation process, and this allows females to carry higher amounts of this receptor [51].

Consequently, its level of activity in pDCs results in higher IFNα production in females than in males after stimulation [33].

Such an observation is particularly attractive when one considers that coronavirus (SARS-CoV-1) is a weak IFN inducer due to its ability to inhibit TLR7-mediated signals. This would suggest that inhibition of antiviral responses in females is reduced [52].

In addition, early activation of IFN release may improve the protection of the host against the cytokine storm that in males is associated with later secretion of these mediators [43].

As a link between innate and adaptive immunity, it is interesting to highlight that IFNα release results in up-regulation of TLR7 receptors onendosomal compartmentsof naïve B lymphocytes. This up-regulation allows immediate expansion and differentiation of B cells, with the production of IgM and inflammatory cytokines. Therefore, in females, which produce more TLR7, antibody production will be more pronounced [33].

On the male side, androgens are reported to inhibit B-cell lymphopoiesis; indeed, gonadectomy in male mice activates B-cell lymphopoiesis in the bone marrow, an effect that can be reversed by the administration of testosterone [53]. This effect would be achieved both directly, through androgen receptors, and indirectly, through the upregulation of TGFβ production by marrow stromal cells, which suppresses B-lymphopoietic activity [54].

A recent study reported the presence of neutralizing autoantibodies (immunoglobulin G) against at least one type I IFN in patients with life-threatening COVID-19 (101/987, 10.2%): against IFN-α (36 patients), against interferon-ω (13 patients), or against both (52 patients). Instead, neutralizing autoantibodies were absent in asymptomatic individuals and in patients with mild SARS CoV-2 infection [55]. Among patients with severe SARS-CoV-2 related pneumonia and anti-IFNs antibodies, males were highly predominant (95/101, 94%).

Additionallysignificant is the observation that the prevalence of these Abs tends to increase with age, although they were detected from 25 to 87 years old [55].This may account for the increased vulnerability to infection described in the elderly, regardless of comorbidities.

Post-Transcriptional Gene Regulation

In post-transcriptional gene regulation, a pivotal position is currently assigned to small non-coding RNA molecules of about 22 nucleotides in length, called microRNAs (miRNAs, miRs) [56].

It is estimated that up to 4% of the entire genome encodes about 400 miRs, which in turn are involved in the regulation of about 1/3 of the whole genome [57].This regulation is achieved by binding to complementary sequences within the 3′untranslated region (UTR) of the target mRNA, with a blockade of translation or rapid mRNA degradation [58].

These small molecules are involved in a number of biological processes, from apoptosis to tumorigenesis and, as reported, in the regulation of immune responses [59].

One of the first studies to highlight this relationship showed that miR-146 is a negative regulator of signals mediated by Toll-like Receptors [60]—signals that are known to be activated by the recognition of specific molecular patterns, associated with pathogenic microorganisms (PAMPs: pathogen-associated molecular patterns), or released from damaged tissues (DAMPs: damage-associated molecular patterns) [61].

It was subsequently established that IFNβ inhibits replication of the hepatitis C virus in the human hepatoma cell line Huh7 by inducing miRNAs that target the viral genome [62].

Since about a hundred miRs are encoded by the X chromosome but only four are encoded by the Y chromosome [63], it is easily predictable that these molecules are differentially expressed in both sexes, promoting different susceptibilities to infectious and autoimmune diseases.

This difference in expression could be further enhanced by estrogen receptors as transcription factors that regulate the genesis of miRs [64].

3. Conclusions

The availability of sex-disaggregated data during the current pandemic has opened a wide window on the existing gaps between males and females in both incidence and fatality rates. These differences can be ascribed to several factors.

- First, it is well-documented that there are differences in lifestyle between sexes, with lower alcohol and tobacco consumption in women. Moreover, significant differences have been also reported in response to the stress imposed by the pandemic and lockdown. Females demonstrated greater adherence to non-pharmacological prevention measures (interpersonal distance, hand washing, correct use of personal protective equipment) than males but they also showed greater resilience, lower levels of anxiety, depression and insomnia triggered by lockdown.
- Second, differences have been observed in terms of immunological reactivity. The latter could be influenced by the patient's hormonal profile, which favors – in the male sex – an increased expression of ACE2 on the surface of the alveolar cells. This molecule, acting as receptor for the viral spike-protein, is internalized following interaction with its ligand. Internalization would lead to an imbalance in ACE-controlled activities, i.e., increased Ang II production with overstimulation of AT1R. This results in an increased vascular permeability and overflow of inflammatory cells.
- Finally, in addition to the above-mentioned differences, specific genetic interferences have a significant modulating role. Due to the different gene load carried by the X and Y chromosomes, in order to ensure balancing, one of the two X chromosomes is randomly inactivated in female embryos. However, about 15% of X-linked genes escape this random inactivation process (e.g., the gene encoding for TLR7). Therefore, in females there is a greater production of INFs with positive effects both on the production of inflammatory cytokines and on B-cells expansion. It has been recently reported that patients with life-threatening COVID-19 have neutralized antibodies against at least one type I IFN; among patients with IFNs antibodies, males are largely predominant. Genetic interference may be further accentuated by the post-transcriptional control exerted by the so-called miRNAs, which are encoded in large numbers by the X chromosome but in very low amounts by the Y chromosome.

Adequate knowledge of these multiple differences may allow a more comprehensive investigation of their origins, identifying possible therapeutic targets and selecting the most effective preventive strategies.

Funding: This research received no external funding.

Acknowledgments: Many thanks to Ciro Rosario Ilardi for helpful suggestions.

Conflicts of Interest: The author declare no conflict of interest.

References

1. Ya'Qoub, L.; Elgendy, I.Y.; Pepine, C.J. Sex and Gender Differences in COVID-19: More to be learned! *Am. Heart J. Plus Cardiol. Res. Pract.* **2021**, *3*, 100011. [CrossRef]
2. Aiello, A.; Farzaneh, F.; Candore, G.; Caruso, C.; Davinelli, S.; Gambino, C.M.; Ligotti, M.E.; Zareian, N.; Accardi, G. Immunosenescence and Its Hallmarks: How to Oppose Aging Strategically? A Review of Potential Options for Therapeutic Intervention. *Front. Immunol.* **2019**, *10*, 2247. [CrossRef]
3. Farber, D.; Yudanin, N.; Restifo, N. Human memory T cells: Generation, compartmentalization and homeostasis. *Nat. Rev. Immunol.* **2014**, *14*, 24–35. [CrossRef]
4. Nikolich-Zugich, J.; Rudd, B.D. Immune memory and aging: An infinite or finite resource? *Curr. Opin. Immunol.* **2010**, *22*, 535–540. [CrossRef]
5. Sharma, G.; Goodwin, J. Effect of aging on respiratory system physiology and immunology. *Clin. Interv. Aging* **2006**, *1*, 253–260. [CrossRef]
6. Grasselli, G.; Zangrillo, A.; Zanella, A. Baseline Characteristics and Outcomes of 1591 Patients Infected With SARS-CoV-2 Admitted to ICUs of the Lombardy Region, Italy. *JAMA* **2020**, *323*, 1574–1581. [CrossRef]
7. Guan, W.J.; Ni, Z.Y.; Hu, Y.; Liang, W.H.; Qu, C.Q.; He, J.X.; Liu, L.; Shan, H.; Lei, C.L.; Hui, D.S.C.; et al. Clinical Characteristics of Coronavirus Disease 2019 in China. *N. Engl. J. Med.* **2020**, *382*, 1708–1720. [CrossRef]
8. Onder, G.; Rezza, G.; Brusaferro, S. Case-fatality rate and characteristics of patients dying in relation to COVID-19 in Italy. *JAMA* **2020**, *323*, 1775–1776. [CrossRef]
9. Wang, D.; Hu, B.; Hu, C.; Zhu, F.; Liu, X.; Zhang, J.; Wang, B.; Xiang, H.; Cheng, Z.; Xiong, Y.; et al. Clinical characteristics of 138 hospitalized patients with 2019 novel coronavirus–infected pneumonia in Wuhan, China. *JAMA* **2020**, *323*, 1061–1069. [CrossRef]
10. Ramirez, L.A.; Sullivan, J.C. Sex Differences in Hypertension: Where We Have Been and Where We Are Going. *Am. J. Hypertens.* **2018**, *31*, 1247–1254. [CrossRef]
11. Muhamad, S.-A.; Ugusman, A.; Kumar, J.; Skiba, D.; Hamid, A.A.; Aminuddin, A. COVID-19 and Hypertension: The What, the Why, and the How. *Front. Physiol.* **2021**, *12*, 665064. [CrossRef]
12. Alkhouli, M.; Nanjundappa, A.; Annie, F.; Bates, M.C.; Bhatt, D.L. Sex differences in case fatality rate of COVID-19: Insights from a multinational registry. *Mayo Clin. Proc.* **2020**, *95*, 1613–1620. [CrossRef]
13. Iaccarino, G.; Grassi, G.; Borghi, C.; Carugo, S.; Fallo, F.; Ferri, C.; Giannattasio, C.; Grassi, D.; Letizia, C.; Mancusi, C.; et al. Gender differences in predictors of intensive care units admission among COVID-19 patients: The results of the SARS-RAS study of the Italian Society of Hypertension. *PLoS ONE* **2020**, *15*, e0237297. [CrossRef]
14. Su, W.; Qiu, Z.; Zhou, L.; Hou, J.; Wang, Y.; Huang, F.; Zhang, Y.; Jia, Y.; Zhou, J.; Liu, D.; et al. Sex differences in clinical characteristics and risk factors for mortality among severe patients with COVID-19: A retrospective study. *Aging* **2020**, *12*, 18833–18843. [CrossRef]
15. Peckham, H.; de Gruijter, N.M.; Raine, C.; Radziszewska, A.; Ciurtin, C.; Wedderburn, L.R.; Rosser, E.C.; Webb, K.; Deakin, C.T. Male sex identified by global COVID-19 meta-analysis as a risk factor for death and ITU admission. *Nat. Commun.* **2020**, *11*, 6317. [CrossRef]
16. Scientific Advisory Group for Emergencies and Department of Health and Social Care. Direct and Indirect Health Impacts of COVID-19 in England. 2021; Published 17 September 2021. Available online: https://assets.publishing.service.gov.uk/government/uploads/system/uploads/attachment_data/file/1018698/S1373_Direct_and_Indirect_Health_Impacts_of_C19_Detailed_Paper_.pdf. (accessed on 25 January 2022).
17. CovidStat INFN—Datidell'ISS. Available online: https://covid19.infn.it/iss/ (accessed on 25 January 2022).
18. Bwire, G.M. Coronavirus: Why Men are More Vulnerable to COVID-19 Than Women? *SNCompr. Clin. Med.* **2020**, *2*, 874–876. [CrossRef]
19. Ng, M.; Freeman, M.K.; Fleming, T.D.; Robinson, M.; Dwyer-Lindgren, L.; Thomson, B.; Wollum, A.; Sanman, E.; Wulf, S.; Lopez, A.D.; et al. Smoking prevalence and cigarette consumption in 187 countries, 1980–2012. *JAMA* **2014**, *311*, 183–192. [CrossRef]
20. Allen, A.M.; Scheuermann, T.S.; Nollen, N.; Hatsukami, D.; Ahluwalia, J.S. Gender Differences in Smoking Behavior and Dependence Motives Among Daily and Nondaily Smokers. *Nicotine Tob. Res.* **2016**, *18*, 1408–1413.
21. Galasso, V.; Pons, V.; Profeta, P.; Becher, M.; Brouard, S.; Foucault, M. Gender differences in COVID-19 attitudes and behavior: Panel evidence from eight countries. *Proc. Natl. Acad. Sci. USA* **2020**, *117*, 27285–27291. [CrossRef]
22. Salfi, F.; Lauriola, M.; Amicucci, G.; Corigliano, D.; Viselli, L.; Tempesta, D.; Ferrara, M. Gender-related time course of sleep disturbances and psychological symptoms during the COVID-19 lockdown: A longitudinal study on the Italian population. *Neurobiol. Stress* **2020**, *13*, 100259.
23. Taylor, S.E.; Klein, L.C.; Lewis, B.P.; Gruenewald, T.L.; Gurung, R.A.; Updegraff, J.A. Biobehavioral responses to stress in females: Tend-and-befriend, not fight-or-flight. *Psychol. Rev.* **2000**, *107*, 411. [CrossRef] [PubMed]

24. Dhabhar, F.S. Effects of stress on immune function: The good, the bad, and the beautiful. *Immunol. Res.* **2014**, *58*, 193–210. [CrossRef] [PubMed]
25. Monto, A.S. Epidemiology of viral respiratory infections. *Am. J. Med.* **2002**, *112*, 4S–12S. [CrossRef]
26. Menzies, D.; Joshi, R.; Pai, M. Risk of tuberculosis infection and disease associated with work in health care settings. *Int. J. Tuberc. Lung Dis.* **2007**, *11*, 593–605.
27. Shannon, G.; Minckas, N.; Tan, D.; Haghparast-Bidgoli, H.; Batura, N.; Mannell, J. Feminisation of the health workforce and wage conditions of health professions: An exploratory analysis. *Hum. Resour. Health* **2019**, *17*, 72. [CrossRef]
28. Ilardi, A.; Politi, C.; Ciarambino, T. COVID-19: Could sex and age be a risk factor? *Minerva Med.* **2020**. [CrossRef]
29. Klein, S.; Flanagan, K. Sex differences in immune responses. *Nat. Rev. Immunol.* **2016**, *16*, 626–638. [CrossRef]
30. Zhang, H.; Penninger, J.M.; Li, Y.; Zhong, N.; Slutsky, A.S. Angiotensin-converting enzyme 2 (ACE2) as a SARS-CoV-2 receptor: Molecular mechanisms and potential therapeutic target. *Intensive Care Med.* **2020**, *46*, 586–590. [CrossRef]
31. Mercurio, I.; Tragni, V.; Busto, F.; De Grassi, A.; Pierri, C.L. Protein structure analysis of the interactions between SARS-CoV-2 spike protein and the human ACE2 receptor: From conformational changes to novel neutralizing antibodies. *Cell. Mol. Life Sci.* **2021**, *78*, 1501–1522. [CrossRef]
32. Hamming, I.; Timens, W.; Bulthuis, M.L.C.; Lely, A.T.; Navis, G.J.; van Goor, H. Tissue distribution of ACE2 protein, the functional receptor for SARS coronavirus. A first step in understanding SARS pathogenesis. *J. Pathol.* **2004**, *203*, 631–637. [CrossRef]
33. Gadi, N.; Wu, S.C.; Spihlman, A.P.; Moulton, V.R. What's Sex Got to Do With COVID-19? Gender-Based Differences in the Host Immune Response to Coronaviruses. *Front. Immunol.* **2020**, *11*, 2147. [CrossRef] [PubMed]
34. Turner, A.J.; Julian, A.; Hiscox, J.A.; Hooper, N.M. ACE2: From vasopeptidase to SARS virus receptor. *Trends Pharmacol. Sci.* **2004**, *25*, 291–294. [CrossRef] [PubMed]
35. Lambert, D.W.; Yarski, M.; Warner, F.J.; Thornhill, P.; Parkin, E.T.; Smith, A.I.; Hooper, N.M.; Turner, A.J. Tumor necrosis factor-alpha convertase (ADAM17) mediates regulated ectodomain shedding of the severe-acute respiratory syndrome coronavirus (SARS-CoV) receptor, angiotensin-converting enzyme-2 (ACE2). *J. Biol. Chem.* **2005**, *280*, 30113–30119. [CrossRef]
36. Pinna, G. Sex and COVID-19: A Protective Role for Reproductive Steroids. *Trends Endocrinol. Metab.* **2021**, *32*, 3–6. [CrossRef]
37. Baristaite, G.; Gurwitz, D. Estradiol reduces ACE2 and TMPRSS2 mRNA levels in A549 human lung epithelial cells. *Drug Dev. Res.* **2022**, 1–6. [CrossRef]
38. McGuire, B.B.; Watson, R.W.G.; Pérez-Barriocanal, F.; Fitzpatrick, J.M.; Docherty, N. Gender differences in the renin-angiotensin and nitric oxide systems: Relevance in the normal and diseased kidney. *Kidney Blood Press. Res.* **2007**, *30*, 67–80. [CrossRef]
39. Swärd, P.; Edsfeldt, A.; Reepalu, A.; Jehpsson, L.; Rosengren, B.E.; Karlsson, M.K. Age and sex differences in soluble ACE2 may give insights for COVID-19. *Crit. Care* **2020**, *24*, 221. [CrossRef]
40. Larouche-Lebel, É.; Loughran, K.A.; Oyama, M.A.; Solter, P.F.; Laughlin, D.S.; Sánchez, M.D.; Assenmacher, C.A.; Fox, P.R.; Fries, R.C. Plasma and tissue angiotensin converting enzyme 2 activity and plasma equilibrium concentrations of angiotensin peptides in dogs with heart disease. *J. Vet. Intern. Med.* **2019**, *33*, 1571–1584. [CrossRef]
41. Yang, P.; Gu, H.; Zhao, Z.; Wang, W.; Cao, B.; Lai, C.; Yang, X.; Zhang, L.; Duan, Y.; Zhang, S.; et al. Angiotensin-converting enzyme 2 (ACE2) mediates influenza H7N9 virus-induced acute lung injury. *Sci. Rep.* **2014**, *4*, 7027. [CrossRef]
42. Medina-Enríquez, M.M.; Lopez-León, S.; Carlos-Escalante, J.A.; Aponte-Torres, Z.; Cuapio, A.; Wegman-Ostrosky, T. ACE2: The molecular doorway to SARS-CoV-2. *Cell Biosci.* **2020**, *10*, 148. [CrossRef]
43. Channappanavar, R.; Fett, C.; Mack, M.; Ten Eyck, P.P.; Meyerholz, D.K.; Perlman, S. Sex-Based Differences in Susceptibility to Severe Acute Respiratory Syndrome Coronavirus Infection. *J. Immunol.* **2017**, *198*, 4046–4053. [CrossRef]
44. Heldring, N.; Pike, A.; Andersson, S.; Matthews, J.; Cheng, G.; Hartman, J.; Tujague, M.; Strom, A.; Treuter, E.; Warner, M.; et al. Estrogen receptors: How do they signal and what are their targets. *Physiol. Rev.* **2007**, *87*, 905–931. [CrossRef] [PubMed]
45. Satpathy, A.; Wu, X.; Albring, J.; Murphy, K.M. Re(de)fining the dendritic cell lineage. *Nat. Immunol.* **2012**, *13*, 1145–1154. [CrossRef] [PubMed]
46. Gilliet, M.; Cao, W.; Liu, Y.J. Plasmacytoid dendritic cells: Sensing nucleic acids in viral infection and autoimmune diseases. *Nat. Rev. Immunol.* **2008**, *8*, 594–606. [CrossRef]
47. Kamphuis, E. Type I interferons directly regulate lymphocyte recirculation and cause transient blood lymphopenia. *Blood* **2006**, *108*, 3253–3261. [CrossRef]
48. Laffont, S.; Guéry, J.C. Deconstructing the sex bias in allergy and autoimmunity: From sex hormones and beyond. *Adv. Immunol.* **2019**, *142*, 35–64.
49. Hewagama, A. Role of X-Chromosome encoded miRNAs in Autoimmunity: Suppressing the suppressor and female predisposition. *Rheumatol. Curr. Res.* **2013**, *3*, 118. [CrossRef]
50. Fang, H.; Disteche, C.M.; Berletch, J.B. X Inactivation and Escape: Epigenetic and Structural Features. *Front. Cell Dev. Biol.* **2019**, *7*, 219. [CrossRef]
51. Souyris, M.; Mejía, J.E.; Chaumeil, J.; Guéry, J.-C. Female predisposition to TLR7-driven autoimmunity: Gene dosage and the escape from X chromosome inactivation. *Semin. Immunopathol.* **2019**, *41*, 153–164. [CrossRef]
52. Li, S.-W.; Wang, C.-Y.; Jou, Y.-J.; Huang, S.-H.; Hsiao, L.-H.; Wan, L.; Lin, Y.-J.; Kung, S.-H.; Lin, C.-W. SARS Coronavirus papain-like protease Inhibits the TLR7 signaling pathway through removing Lys63-linked polyubiquitination of TRAF3 and TRAF6. *Int. J. Mol. Sci.* **2016**, *17*, 678. [CrossRef]
53. GubbelsBupp, M.R.; Jorgensen, T.N. Androgen-Induced Immunosuppression. *Front. Immunol.* **2018**, *9*, 794. [CrossRef] [PubMed]

54. Olsen, N.J.; Gu, X.; Kovacs, W.J. Bone marrow stromal cells mediate androgenic suppression of B lymphocyte development. *J. Clin. Investig.* **2001**, *108*, 1697–1704. [CrossRef] [PubMed]
55. Bastard, P.; Rosen, L.B.; Zhang, Q.; Michailidis, E.; Hoffmann, H.H.; Zhang, Y.; Dorgham, K.; Philippot, Q.; Rosain, J.; Béziat, V.; et al. Autoantibodies against type I IFNs in patients with life-threatening COVID-19. *Science* **2020**, *370*, eabd4585. [CrossRef] [PubMed]
56. Lewis, B.P.; Burge, C.B.; Bartel, D.P. Conserved seed pairing, often flanked by adenosines, indicates that thousands of human genes are microRNA targets. *Cell* **2005**, *120*, 15–20. [CrossRef]
57. Gu, S.; Jin, L.; Zhang, F.; Sarnow, P.; Kay, M.A. Biological basis for restriction of microRNA targets to the 3′ untranslated region in mammalian mRNAs. *Nat. Struct. Mol. Biol.* **2009**, *16*, 144–150. [CrossRef]
58. Moulton, V.R. Sex Hormones in Acquired Immunity and Autoimmune Disease. *Front. Immunol.* **2018**, *9*, 2279. [CrossRef]
59. Dai, R.; Phillips, R.A.; Zhang, Y.; Khan, D.; Crasta, O.; Ahmed, S.A. Suppression of LPS-induced Interferon-γ and nitric oxide in splenic lymphocytes by select estrogen-regulated microRNAs: A novel mechanism of immune modulation. *Blood* **2008**, *112*, 4591–4597. [CrossRef]
60. Taganov, K.D.; Boldin, M.P.; Chang, K.-J.; Baltimore, D. NF-kappaB-dependent induction of microRNA miR-146, an inhibitor targeted to signaling proteins of innate immune responses. *Proc. Natl. Acad. Sci. USA* **2006**, *103*, 12481–12486. [CrossRef]
61. Chen, G.Y.; Nuñez, G. Sterile inflammation: Sensing and reacting to damage. *Nat. Rev. Immunol.* **2010**, *10*, 826–837. [CrossRef]
62. Pedersen, I.M.; Cheng, G.; Wieland, S.; Volinia, S.; Croce, C.M.; Chisari, F.V.; David, M. Interferon modulation of cellular microRNAs as an antiviral mechanism. *Nature* **2007**, *449*, 919–922. [CrossRef]
63. Pérez-Cremades, D.; Mompeón, A.; Vidal-Gómez, X.; Hermenegildo, C.; Novella, S. Role of miRNA in the Regulatory Mechanisms of Estrogens in Cardiovascular Ageing. *Oxid. Med. Cell. Longev.* **2018**, *2018*. [CrossRef] [PubMed]
64. Castellano, L.; Giamas, G.; Jacob, J.; Coombes, R.C.; Lucchesi, W.; Thiruchelvam, P.; Barton, G.; Jiao, L.R.; Wait, R.; Waxman, J.; et al. The estrogen receptor-alpha-induced microRNA signature regulates itself and its transcriptional response. *Proc. Natl. Acad. Sci. USA* **2009**, *106*, 15732–15737. [CrossRef] [PubMed]

encyclopedia

Entry

COVID-19 in the Construction Sector

Ruben Rodríguez Elizalde

Faculty of Economics and Business, Universitat Oberta de Catalunya (UOC), Rambla del Poblenou, 156, 08018 Barcelona, Spain; ruben.rodriguezelizalde@gmail.com

Definition: This section analyzes the influence of COVID-19 in the construction sector. Construction workers' high vulnerability to the spread of the virus motivated this entry. The construction sector's peculiarities and some work procedure characteristics in this sector make telecommuting impossible in most activities. In addition, most of the states and national governments declared the construction sector essential activity due to its high economic impact. The working conditions in this sector are very special: constant trips to work in groups, work group execution with little interpersonal distance, group travel, stays and accommodations away from home, meals in restaurants or work canteens, lunch in restaurants or work canteens, etc. Due to all of this, the contagion rate was very high during the pandemic months. Even today, it is still considered one of the most dangerous sectors for these purposes. With all this in mind, here we discuss why it is difficult to minimize the spread of the virus for construction workers, summarize how to assess exposure risk grades for construction job tasks, and provide possible protection requirements for the different exposure risk grades.

Keywords: COVID-19; construction sector; building work; civil work

Citation: Elizalde, R.R. COVID-19 in the Construction Sector. *Encyclopedia* **2022**, 2, 717–728. https://doi.org/10.3390/encyclopedia2020050

Academic Editors: Stephen Bustin and Raffaele Barretta

Received: 6 March 2022
Accepted: 6 April 2022
Published: 13 April 2022

1. Introduction

The year 2020 changed humanity. In March 2020, a global pandemic was declared due to the new coronavirus SARS-CoV-2. This virus produces the disease known as COVID-19 [1]. Since the pandemic's declaration, the virus has kept the entire world on edge, with borders closed for many months and millions of citizens confined at home.

COVID-19 infections have proliferated very quickly around the world. During the first few months, governments made extraordinary decisions to limit the virus spread and prevent health systems collapsing.

Two years later, scientists still have some confusion about the virus's mechanism operation and its effect on the human body. However, everybody knows this virus is highly contagious and its effects can be very harmful and even deadly.

The construction sector's activity includes all types of building (residential and non-residential) construction, rehabilitation, maintenance, and demolition. It includes civil engineering works also, such as roads, railways, or pipeline transport execution, all their complementary works (such as bridges or tunnels), and the rest of public service system execution [2].

Several market groups are involved in the construction sector, such as architectural and engineering design, materials and equipment production, transportation, or energy and waste management, to name just a few. Construction creates value thanks to the transformation of basic raw materials into capital goods, which are essential for economic activity and the provision of infrastructure services [2]. Its labor and economic importance is unquestionable.

Therefore, the Occupational Safety and Health Administration (an agency from the United States Department of Labor) includes within the sector, in addition to employers and construction workers, those engaged in carpentry, ironworking, plumbing, electrical, heating, ventilation, air conditioning, masonry and concrete work, utility construction work, and earthmoving activities [3].

Construction sector activity can have a great impact on generating economic income and reducing poverty. Its potential to create employment is considerable due to its labor-intensive nature and its links with many other economic sectors as well.

Before the pandemic, the construction sector represented about 7.7% of global employment [4]. Forecasts for 2020 were that construction would contribute 13.4% of the global GDP, but the COVID-19 crisis changed everything [5].

2. Industrial Hygiene and Construction

Industrial hygiene is a preventive technique. There are very varied definitions for industrial hygiene. Almost all of them have essentially the same orientation and meaning: it tries to prevent occupational diseases [6]. To achieve this, industrial hygiene acts on the risk factors of a physical, chemical, or biological nature, measuring and assessing the contaminants present in the work to eliminate them or, if this is not possible, to reduce them [7].

Therefore, industrial hygiene is the occupational risk prevention technique responsible for identifying, evaluating, and controlling hygienic risks originating in the workplace which can endanger the workers' health through the work environment. It can also be considered a non-medical technique for occupational diseases prevention by controlling the contaminants that cause these diseases in work environment.

Therefore, there is a clear and primary objective: to protect and promote workers' health and well-being and the environment in general through the preventive measures in workplace series adoption.

An important part of labor production processes is producing changes in the work environment. These modifications provoke a series of aggressive agents for the health of the workers. These harmful agents are pollutants or contaminants.

A pollutant or contaminant is a substance, a form of energy, or a living being (or a part of a living being) present in the work environment which, at a sufficient concentration, can get into the environment. It can pass from the environment to the human body, causing negative or harmful effects to the health of a worker. Thus, it gives rise to hygienic risk: the probability of suffering alterations to one's health due to the action of contaminants present in the environment during the performance of a certain job.

According to current legislation, environmental condition exposure in the workplace cannot put workers' safety and health at risk. Therefore, a company must adopt adequate preventive and control measures in the presence of every contaminant.

Safety at work is the most attended preventive technique in the construction sector. However, industrial hygiene is also very important. Construction sector workers are exposed to risks associated with contaminating agents in their workplaces daily, including noise, mechanical vibrations, solar radiation (workers outdoors), or dangerous substances such as chemicals, crystalline silica dust, or even asbestos, one of the most dangerous substances still present in old buildings.

The SARS-CoV-2 coronavirus is a virus. Consequently, it is a biological contaminant. Biological contaminants are organisms with a certain life cycle which cause, when entering the human body, a negative effect on one's health, which is different in each case (always depending on the causal agent). This life cycle includes the reproduction and growth processes [8]. Therefore, biological contaminants can be, in addition to viruses, bacteria, fungi, or parasites, for example.

In general, the construction sector does not include activities where biological risk is an occupational risk [9]. Under normal conditions (before the pandemic), contagions among construction workers could only occur exceptionally.

It differentiates construction from other activities, such as social and health activities [10]. In them, COVID-19 contagion is considered an occupational health issue. However, the virus's incidence in the construction sector has been considered a public health issue [11] from the beginning. Contagion risk is not related to the work execution processes.

3. COVID-19 Risk Assessment Construction

The intervention of the company in all occupational risk management is crucial. The company must support its occupational risk prevention service because it is key to this.

Although it is not an occupational hazard, but it is a matter of public health, the risk of contagion from coronavirus is not an exception. Despite the vaccines, companies' actions against exposure to SARS-COV-2 were crucial, are crucial, and will continue being crucial. Companies have had to adapt their activities with recommendations and updated prevention measures to avoid possible contagion. These measures were (ranked in order):

1. Organizational measures;
2. Collective protection measures;
3. Individual or personal protection measures;
4. Special measures for especially vulnerable workers.

All the above measures must always be in accordance with the level of risk. In addition, the company has to study all cases of contagion and contact that have occurred in the company. The company also has to collaborate to manage temporary disabilities.

Legislation and states have required the cooperation of companies with health authorities in every way to detect all cases compatible with COVID-19 and their contacts as soon as possible. Only then is transmission controlled.

Companies have to assess the risk of exposure to which workers may be exposed in each of the differentiated tasks they perform. Companies must follow the recommendations issued by the prevention service regarding the risk of exposure and protection against it. Prevention services have to recommend following the guidelines and recommendations given by health authorities.

Construction companies have not been an exception. Construction companies have had to comply with the regulations and recommendations and try to protect their workers just like the rest of the companies, despite the difficulties imposed by the sector.

Any decision making on the preventive measures to be adopted in each company must be based on information collected through the specific exposure risk assessment, which will always be carried out in accordance with the information provided by the health authorities.

Depending on the nature of the activities and the transmission mechanisms of the SARS-CoV-2 coronavirus, we can establish the different exposure scenarios in which workers can be found, which are presented in the following table, in order to establish the required preventive measures.

Below are the classification criteria followed by the Spanish Ministry of Health [12], which distinguishes the following types of exposure:

1. Risk exposure: A work situation where close contact with a case of coronavirus infection (or suspected infection) may occur;
2. Low exposure risk: A work situation where the worker may be related to a suspected or confirmed case without being in close contact;
3. Low exposure probability: Workers without direct attention to the public or workers who, if they attend directly to the public, do it at more than 2 meters of distance or have collective protection elements that serve as a barrier which prevent possible contacts (such as, for example, a glass partition).

To break down these categories, the Ministry prepared Table 1.

According to Table 1, construction site personnel belong to the risk exposure category. A construction site, whether civil work or building work, is a situation in which close contact with a possible case of a worker infected with COVID-19 cannot be avoided.

Table 1. Exposure risk degrees to SARS-CoV-2 coronavirus in the work environment [12].

Exposure Risk	Low Exposure Risk	Low Exposure Probability
Health care personnel and non-care personnel who care for COVID-19 suspected cases or COVID-19 confirmed cases. Medical transport technicians, who can transfer and contact directly COVID-19 suspected cases or COVID-19 confirmed cases. It is impossible to avoid close contact with a COVID-19 suspected case or a COVID-19 confirmed case at work.	Health professionals without close contact with a suspected case of COVID-19 or a confirmed case of COVID-19 in their work activity. This is the case of, for example, transfer companions, guards, stretcher bearers, or hospital cleaning staff. Laboratory personnel responsible for virological diagnostic tests. Non-health professionals who come into contact with possibly contaminated medical material, fomites, or waste. Home help for asymptomatic contacts.	Workers without direct attention to the public, from more than 2 m away, or with collective protection measures to avoid contact.

Another example more applied to the case was given by the Occupational Safety and Health Administration [3] agency from the United States Department of Labor. To evaluate the exposure risk, OSHA developed Table 2, which describes construction work tasks associated with the exposure risk levels.

Table 2. Construction work tasks associated with exposure risk levels [3].

Lower (Caution)	Medium	High	Very High
Tasks that allow employees to remain at least 1.85 m apart and involve little contact with the public, visitors, or customers.	Tasks that require workers to be within 1.85 m of one another. Tasks that require workers to be in close contact (within 1.85 m) with customers, visitors, or members of the public.	Entering an in-door work site occupied by people such as other workers, customers, or residents suspected of having or known to have COVID-19, including when an occupant of the site reports signs and symptoms consistent with COVID-19. Note: Employers may consider delaying this work by following the guidance below.	Category not applicable for most anticipated work tasks.

In civil works, it is usual to work outdoors, supposing a ventilated environment and synonymous security. The same happens in the initial phases of construction work for buildings (e.g., soil movements and excavations or execution of foundations and structures) It is important that before the coronavirus pandemic, studies already showed that 52% of indoor air pollution is due to inadequate ventilation. In contrast, 5% is due to microbial contamination, and 3% is due to building constituent materials [13].

Apart from this, in each work environment, it is necessary to analyze the existing risk for each trade present and for each task to be carried out, always depending on the environment where the work is carried out. Despite this, it is very difficult to control exposure risk, as it depends on every worker's attitude. In construction sites, getting workers to wear a mask permanently and adopt distancing measures is a daily battle, especially in hot areas or in summertime. The following photographs (Figures 1–5) show examples of construction activities, in civil work and building work, where the safety distance was not respected and workers did not always wear mask protection.

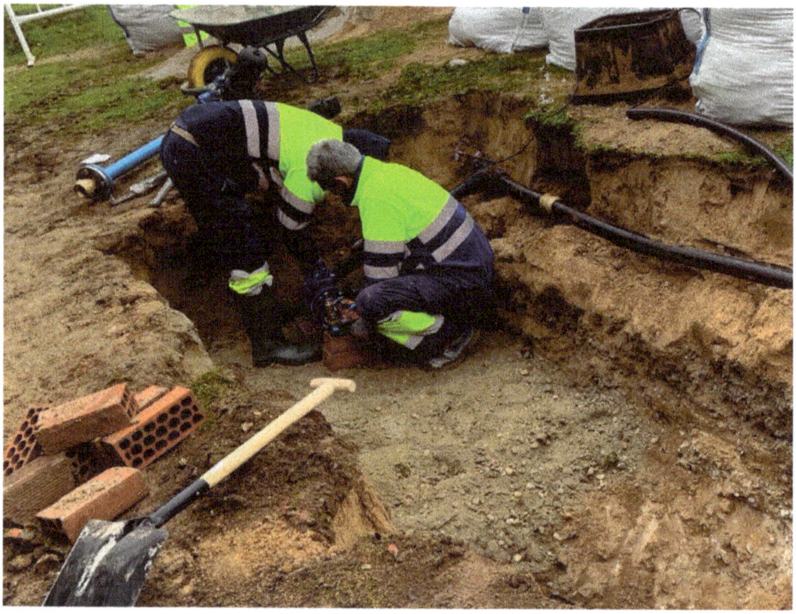

Figure 1. Workers finishing hydraulic pump placement in civil work for water conduction. The work had to be performed in pairs without a safe distance (author's photograph).

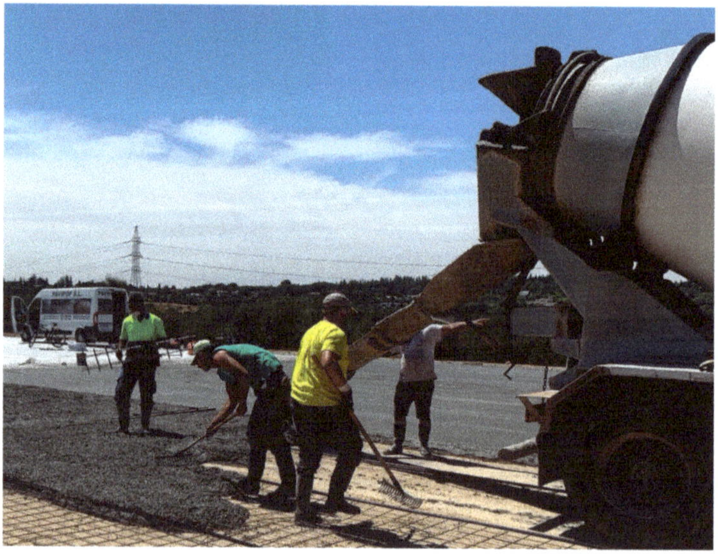

Figure 2. Workers spreading concrete on an open-air screed without keeping safety distance (author's photograph).

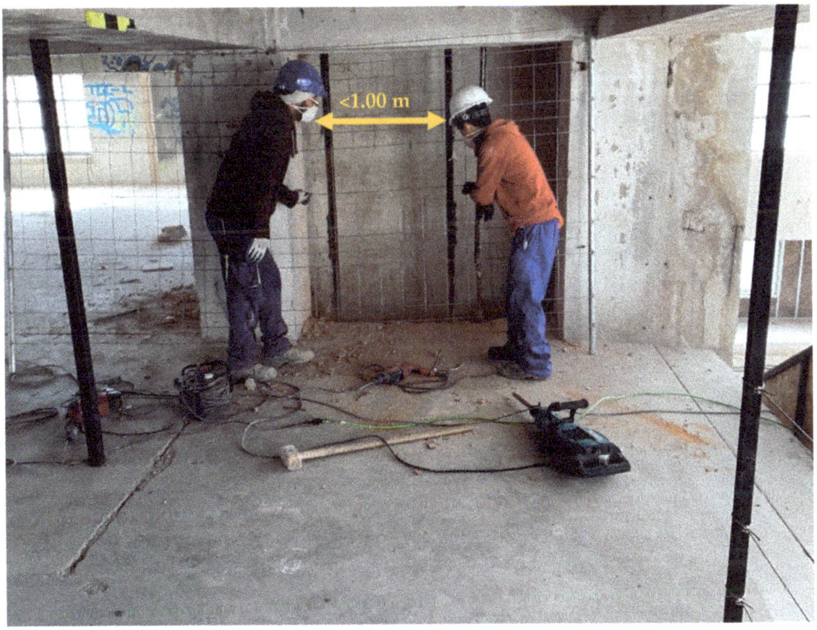

Figure 3. Workers exchanging a protection element in an elevator shaft in a building's interior rehabilitation work. The photograph indicates the separation distance between workers (author's photograph).

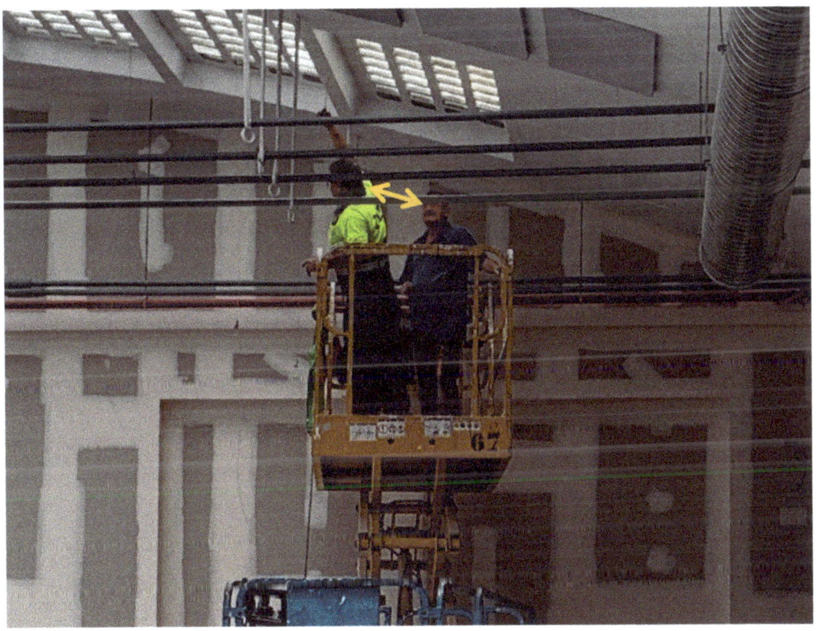

Figure 4. Workers installing false ceiling supports on a lifting platform. The photograph marks the distance between the workers, which is lower than 1.00 m (author's photograph).

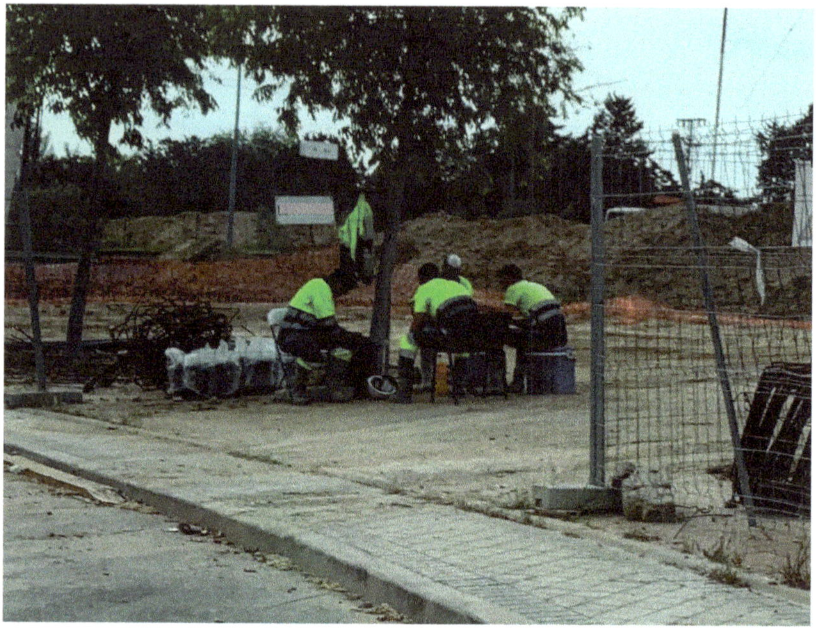

Figure 5. Workers having lunch outside the dining booth and not keeping a safe distance (author's photograph).

In this sector, many activities cannot be carried out alone; many activities need work teams, where there is a lot of proximity between workers.

This is aggravated by the usual practices of many workers in the sector. A lot of workers have lunch and dinner together in bars and restaurants or in work canteens (closed environments). A lot of workers go to a bar at the end of the day to drink in a group. A lot of workers stay in rooms or shared housing on weekdays. A lot of workers go to work on public transport or travel as a group in a common vehicle. All of this is common in the sector. Companies cannot control this, as doing so is impossible [14].

Indeed, most infections have not occurred on construction sites but on public transport or in shared vehicles, as well as in the case of posted workers in shared flats and, above all, in the personal environment of the worker [15].

Although most infections have not occurred on construction sites [16], an infected worker at a site is a potential risk, especially for building construction work. It is very difficult to control this, and it was even more difficult even in previous months when there was a testing deficit.

Added to this is the importance of the figure of the asymptomatic patient, one of the greatest difficulties of this pandemic [17].

4. COVID-19 Protection and Prevention in Construction

As we said before, companies have to assess the risk of exposure for all their workers. Thus, they will be able to fulfill their obligation to guarantee effective protection for the safety and health of their workers.

In the particular case of the coronavirus, companies must follow health authorities' guidelines and recommendations [1,3,12,14].

Common recommendations include the following:

- Hand hygiene: This is the main measure for COVID-19 infection prevention and control. From the beginning, the importance of personal hygiene measures was highlighted. It was essential to reinforce personal hygiene measures in all areas of work and in any exposure scenario. For this, companies had to provide all the means necessary for workers to clean themselves properly.

- Respiratory protection. This includes the following:
    a. Respiratory protection mask use.
    b. Covering the nose and mouth when coughing or sneezing. During 2020, masks were in short supply. People had to look for alternative solutions, and one of them was covering with a handkerchief, which was disposed of afterward in the garbage (always with a lid and pedal). When handkerchiefs were not available, people used the insides of their elbows for this, and thus their hands were not contaminated.
    c. Not touching the eyes, nose, or mouth.
- Respiratory hygiene habits: Society has become aware of the importance of ventilation in recent months. In this sense, building work is more dangerous than civil work generally. For this reason, construction works carried out in a closed area require regular ventilation.
- Maintenance physical separation distance: Various studies have given rise to the distance fluctuating in its value. Right here, we have seen how the Spanish authorities established 1.50 m and the American authorities raised it to 1.85 m (6 feet).

According to the different types of exposure, the Spanish Ministry of Health established the protection requirements [12] listed in Table 3.

Table 3. Requirements for exposure risk degrees to SARS-CoV-2 in the work environment [12].

Exposure Risk	Low Exposure Risk	Low Exposure Probability
Personal protective equipment components for biological protection and for aerosol and splash protection under certain circumstances. It depends on the specific exposure risk evaluation in each case.	Personal protective equipment components for biological protection. It depends on the specific exposure risk evaluation in each case.	Personal protective equipment use is not necessary. In special circumstances, respiratory protection or protective gloves may be necessary. Do not forget that collective protection reduces risk, and personal protection only reduces damage.

As we have seen in previous subsections, it is advisable to use mobility options that best guarantee an interpersonal distance of at least 1.50 m whenever possible.

One of the characteristics of construction work is the intervention of numerous figures in the management of people's occupational health and safety. Coordination and cooperation between all figures is relevant, with each one from the role that corresponds to playing, promoting, assessing, agreeing, planning, implementing, and controlling the extraordinary measures that are necessary to avoid contagion by SARS-CoV-2 [14].

These measures probably affect the technical and organizational conditions of the work and the execution times and costs of the work. However, it is essential to accept these extraordinary changes as well as integrate the recommendations and instructions issued by the health authorities at all times in order to stop the pandemic and reduce the number of those affected.

When de-escalation started, to return to work after the worst months of the pandemic, all these measures had to be taken into account [18].

5. Impact of COVID-19 on the Construction Sector

The construction sector reaches beyond construction sites. There are many sectors and areas that directly or indirectly depend on it. Everything covered by the construction sector has already been mentioned in Section 1 [2].

The risk of contagion on a construction site is really high, as we saw in Section 3. A worker's illness and, above all, a worker's death are preventable misfortunes, and these are occupational health and safety failures.

Protection of the health of workers (and non-workers as well) has been a maxim throughout the pandemic. This meant paralyzing a very important part of world's economic activity. Despite being declared an essential activity, this stoppage affected the construction sector in a lot of countries [19]. There are many trades involved in a construction site from the project phase to the completion of execution of the work. All of them have been affected by the pandemic in one way or another [20]. This is explained by the economic importance of the construction sector. For example, 11.2 million people work in the construction sector in the USA [21]. Latin American countries invest an average of 28% of their total average spending in public transport infrastructure, which includes land transport, rail transport, and air transport, among others. These same countries invest an average of 19.7% of spending in housing construction and the construction of community services, such as public water supply networks and public electricity supply networks [22].

On an economic level, the problem has gone beyond the construction site; it has affected supply chains and transport, caused labor shortages and unemployment, caused problems of contractual implication, and of course, it has brought financial problems [18]. Investment in construction has a multiplying effect on the economy, generating indirect employment and boosting other industries that are part of the production chain. Likewise, this sector employs a high proportion of the unskilled and socioeconomically vulnerable population that depends on daily income, affecting populations that do not have an "economic cushion" that allows them to support themselves for a long time [2].

For the protection and prevention measures of COVID-19 at construction sites analyzed in Section 4, which include compliance with the guidelines of the WHO and the corresponding government, maintenance of social distance, and the use of protective equipment [18], it was necessary to add other structural measures. These measures could be grouped into two groups able, at this point, to assess the effectiveness of several of them, which have been adopted:

1. Technical, logistical, and organizational measures to be adopted by companies with public administration help: Here would be the increase in remote work (something difficult in a sector where few workers can telecommute), the use of 3D printing, and modular or prefabricated construction [19], in which certain elements of construction are manufactured in an industrial plant, where procedures are more controlled and hygiene and social distance measures can be better applied. It has already been pointed out that construction activities were considered essential activities in a lot of countries, so they continued operating throughout the pandemic months. In fact, the construction sector is essential for the economy. Therefore, this sector is key to the economic recovery of a lot of countries. The security measures and protocols to reduce the spread of COVID-19, which began at every construction site, are very important to ensure that reactivation [18].
2. Fiscal and financial measures encouraged by public administrations: Some countries have adopted fiscal and financial measures for the construction sector. With them, the states tried to reduce the negative impact on employment and avoid the bankruptcy of more companies in the sector. There are several interesting experiences in this regard. The experiences of some countries serve as an example:
    a. Belgium, where companies in the sector came to temporarily close in the hardest months of the pandemic. Due to this situation, the National Unemployment Office paid up to 70% of the workers' salaries [23,24].
    b. Canada, which offered a colossal amount of money (CAD 65 billion) for business credit financing in certain sectors, notably construction [25].
    c. Argentina, which subsidized loans from companies related to construction [26].
    d. Israel, which increased by 2% the percentage of the credit portfolios of banks that financed companies in the construction sector [27,28].

6. Conclusions

- The coronavirus pandemic has caused illness, death, and economic hardship around the world. In addition to the threat to public health, social and economic shocks endanger the livelihoods and well-being of millions of workers, including those in the construction industry.
- In general, the construction sector does not include activities where biological risk is an occupational hazard because contagion from construction workers could only occur exceptionally. However, the virus affects everyone, both workers and non-workers, and every worker can carry it to work. Minimizing the spread of the virus was and remains a top priority. It can be particularly difficult for construction workers, as most of them are unable to telecommute and often work in close proximity to each other in an ever-changing work environment.
- This paper sections described that, depending on the nature of the activities and SARS-CoV-2 coronavirus transmission mechanisms, the different risk scenarios in which the workers can be found can be established. The stated criteria define three scenarios: risk, low risk, and low exposure probability, with a table that provides examples of working personnel or situations that meet the definitions to be located in each risk scenario. Afterward, a new table established the requirements to determine the measures to be adopted in each specific situation. These are, as the document clearly indicates, examples of activities or work situations and not an exhaustive list of them. Workers cannot be placed in any of the three defined scenarios permanently and generally but always depending on the nature of the activities and the exposure risk assessment. The preventive measures to be adopted in each case will be determined based on the specific evaluation of the risk of exposure. This evaluation is the only technical activity that can serve as a basis for making preventive technical decisions adapted to each case.
- The evaluation criteria have shown that full construction worker protection is very difficult (if not impossible). Within the risk scenarios for exposure to coronavirus, construction workers and the nature of the work they carry out (in the absence of collective protection) are in a situation of risk exposure. This risk is higher or lower depending on the type of work and the type of construction work. Open-air civil work is not the same as an interior reform in a building. For this reason, within the tasks associated with the levels of exposure risk, a distinction is made between a low level, medium level, high level, or very high level of risk. However, none of these contemplate null risk or nonexistent risk. Furthermore, the low level included the caution in parentheses. In addition, these evaluations have also served to demonstrate cleaning measures' importance and work organization and distribution measures' importance, especially with regard to travel, access to the work site for staff, and the operator's location in the workplace to maintain s safe distance.
- The measures of social distancing, cleaning, and disinfection within the workplace require pedagogy, where easy-to-understand guides and training courses for workers are necessary.
- The measures within the work must be complemented with measures that promote safety in transport, with the performance of risk analysis at the construction sites and consensus on the measures among the intervening agents (companies, clients or public administration, and workers).
- Fiscal and financial measures were and are necessary to reactivate the construction sector. All public measures must be adapted to the context of each country. Many of these measures are proving to be effective in the short term and may help companies and projects that were underway before the pandemic to survive. However, after 2 years of the pandemic, it is necessary to think about reforms in the construction sector in the long term. It should not be forgotten that only a few workers in the sector can telecommute. For that, and also thanks to that, the pandemic showed that the

digitization of many services was possible. There was a notable deficit in this area, and there is still much to be done.

Funding: This research received no external funding.

Conflicts of Interest: The author declares no conflict of interest.

References

1. World Health Organization. Coronavirus Disease (COVID-19). Available online: https://www.who.int/health-topics/coronavirus#tab=tab_1 (accessed on 2 February 2022).
2. International Labour Organization. Good Practices and Challenges in Promoting Decent Work in Construction and Infrastructure Projects. 2015. Available online: https://www.ilo.org/wcmsp5/groups/public/---ed_dialogue/---sector/documents/publication/wcms_416378.pdf (accessed on 22 January 2022).
3. Occupational Safety and Health Administration. COVID-19 Control and Prevention. Construction Work. Available online: https://www.osha.gov/coronavirus/control-prevention/construction (accessed on 29 December 2021).
4. International Labour Organization. ILO Monitor: COVID-19 and the World of Work. 2020. Available online: https://www.ilo.org/wcmsp5/groups/public/---dgreports/---dcomm/documents/briefingnote/wcms_740877.pdf (accessed on 21 January 2022).
5. Global Construction Perspectives y Oxford Economics. *Global Construction 2030: A Global Forecast for the Construction Industry to 2030*; Global Construction Perspectives and Oxford Economics: London, UK, 2015.
6. International Labour Organization. Occupational Safety and Health Management System. 2016. Available online: https://www.ilo.org/wcmsp5/groups/public/---africa/---ro-abidjan/---sro-cairo/documents/publication/wcms_622420.pdf (accessed on 29 December 2021).
7. Occupational Safety and Health Administration. Industrial Hygiene. Available online: https://www.osha.gov/sites/default/files/training-library_industrial_hygiene.pdf (accessed on 29 December 2021).
8. Rice, P. Industrial Hygiene for the Construction Industry. In Proceedings of the ASSE Professional Development Conference and Exposition, Las Vegas, NV, USA, 24 June 2013. Available online: https://aeasseincludes.assp.org/proceedings/2013/docs/702.pdf (accessed on 31 January 2022).
9. Lippy, B.; West, G.H.; Gillen, M.; Betit, E.; Goldenhar, L.M.; Memarian, B.; Rinehart, B.; Barlet, G.; Fletcher, M.K.; Brooks, S.; et al. Industrial Hygiene Issues in Construction. In *Patty's Industrial Hygiene*, 7th ed.; Cohersen, B., Ed.; Wiley: Hoboken, NJ, USA, 2021; Volume 4.
10. World Health Organization. COVID-19: Occupational Health and Safety for Health Workers. 2021. Available online: https://apps.who.int/iris/rest/bitstreams/1329986/retrieve (accessed on 2 February 2022).
11. World Health Organization. Considerations for Implementing and Adjusting Public Health and Social Measures in the Context of COVID-19. 2021. Available online: https://apps.who.int/iris/rest/bitstreams/1351572/retrieve (accessed on 2 February 2022).
12. Ministerio de Sanidad. Procedimiento de Actuación para los Servicios de Prevención de Riesgos Laborales frente a la Exposición al SARS-CoV-2. 2020. Available online: https://www.sanidad.gob.es/profesionales/saludPublica/ccayes/alertasActual/nCov/documentos/PrevencionRRLL_COVID-19.pdf (accessed on 2 February 2022).
13. Todd, L.A. Evaluación del Medio Ambiente de Trabajo. In *Enciclopedia de Salud y Seguridad en el Trabajo*; Stellman, J.M., Ed.; Ministerio de Trabajo y Asuntos Sociales: Madrid, España, 1998; Capítulo 30. Higiene Industrial; Available online: https://www.insst.es/documents/94886/161958/Cap%C3%ADtulo+30.+Higiene+industrial (accessed on 2 February 2022).
14. Ministerio de Sanidad. Directrices de Buenas Prácticas en las Obras de Construcción. Medidas para la Prevención de Contagios del SARS-CoV-2. 2020. Available online: https://www.insst.es/documents/94886/717230/Directrices%20de%20buenas%20pr%C3%A1cticas%20en%20obras%20de%20construcci%C3%B3n%2026.04.20.pdf/4adee5b0-2177-4cbb-bfc2-9a5736672ca0 (accessed on 2 February 2022).
15. Hatoum, M.B.; Faisal, A.; Nassereddine, H.; Sarvari, H. Analysis of COVID-19 Concerns Raised by the Construction Workforce and Development of Mitigation Practices. 2021. Available online: https://www.frontiersin.org/articles/10.3389/fbuil.2021.688495/full (accessed on 31 January 2022).
16. Bushman, D.; Sekaran, J.; Jeffery, N.; Rath, C.; Ackelsberg, J.; Weiss, D.; Wu, W.; Van Oss, K.; Johnston, K.; Huang, J.; et al. Coronavirus Disease 2019 (COVID-19) Outbreaks at 2 Construction Sites—New York City, October–November 2020. *Clin. Infect. Dis.* **2021**, *73*, S81–S83. [CrossRef] [PubMed]
17. Bousquin, J. Study: Construction Has the Highest COVID-19 Rate of Nearly Any Industry. 2020. Available online: https://www.constructiondive.com/news/study-construction-has-the-highest-covid-19-rate-of-nearly-any-industry/592171/ (accessed on 2 February 2022).
18. Gan, W.H.; Koh, D. COVID-19 and return-to-work for the construction sector: Lessons from Singapore. *Saf. Health Work* **2021**, *12*, 277–281. [CrossRef] [PubMed]
19. Biswas, A.; Ghosh, A.; Kar, A.; Mondal, T.; Ghosh, B.; Bardhan, P.K. The impact of COVID-19 in the construction sector and its remedial measures. *J. Phys. Conf. Ser.* **2021**, *1797*, 012054. Available online: https://iopscience.iop.org/article/10.1088/1742-6596/1797/1/012054/pdf (accessed on 4 March 2022). [CrossRef]

20. Ogunnusi, M.; Hamma-Adama, M.; Salman, H.; Kouider, T. COVID-19 pandemic: The effects and prospects in the construction industry. *Int. J. Real Estate Stud.* **2020**, *14*, 120–128. Available online: https://www.utm.my/intrest/files/2020/11/2_Final_MS_CRES-Covid-025.pdf (accessed on 4 March 2022).
21. Alsharef, A.; Banerjee, S.; Jamil Uddin, S.M.; Albert, A.; Jaselskis, E. Early impacts of the COVID-19 pandemic on the United States construction industry. *Int. J. Environ. Res. Public Health* **2021**, *18*, 1559. [CrossRef] [PubMed]
22. Armendáriz, E.; Carrasco, H. El gasto en inversión pública de América Latina: Cuánto, quién y en qué. In *Inter—American Development Bank IDB-DP-697*; Banco Interamericano de Desarrollo: Washington, DC, USA, 2019. [CrossRef]
23. Caprioni, M. COVID-19—Belgian government takes measures for those who can and can't work. In *The National Law Review*; National Law Forum LLC: Chicago, IL, USA, 2020; Volume X. Available online: https://www.natlawreview.com/article/covid-19-belgian-government-takes-measures-those-who-can-and-can-t-work#google_vignette (accessed on 2 March 2022).
24. International Monetary Fund. Policy Responses to COVID-19. 2021. Available online: https://www.imf.org/en/Topics/imf-and-covid19/Policy-Responses-to-COVID-19#B (accessed on 31 January 2022).
25. International Monetary Fund. Policy Responses to COVID-19. 2021. Available online: https://www.imf.org/en/Topics/imf-and-covid19/Policy-Responses-to-COVID-19#C (accessed on 31 January 2022).
26. International Monetary Fund. Policy Responses to COVID-19. 2021. Available online: https://www.imf.org/en/Topics/imf-and-covid19/Policy-Responses-to-COVID-19#A (accessed on 31 January 2022).
27. Bank of Israel. The Banking system and the construction and real estate activity segment: Extent of exposure and credit—Risk levels. In *Information Published by the Bank of Israel Due to the Corona Epidemic*; Bank of Israel: Jerusalem, Israel, 2021. Available online: https://www.boi.org.il/en/BankingSupervision/Survey/Documents/202129en.pdf (accessed on 3 March 2022).
28. International Monetary Fund. Policy Responses to COVID-19. 2021. Available online: https://www.imf.org/en/Topics/imf-and-covid19/Policy-Responses-to-COVID-19#I (accessed on 31 January 2022).

encyclopedia

MDPI

Review

Simple Formulae, Deep Learning and Elaborate Modelling for the COVID-19 Pandemic

Athanassios S. Fokas [1,2,3,*], Nikolaos Dikaios [3], Sotirios Tsiodras [4] and George A. Kastis [3]

1 Department of Applied Mathematics and Theoretical Physics, University of Cambridge, Cambridge CB3 0WA, UK
2 Viterbi School of Engineering, University of Southern California, Los Angeles, CA 90089, USA
3 Mathematics Research Center, Academy of Athens, 11527 Athens, Greece; ndikaios@academyofathens.gr (N.D.); gkastis@academyofathens.gr (G.A.K.)
4 Fourth Department of Internal Medicine, Attikon University Hospital, National and Kapodistrian University of Athens, 12462 Athens, Greece; tsiodras@med.uoa.gr
* Correspondence: tf227@cam.ac.uk

Abstract: Predictive modelling of infectious diseases is very important in planning public health policies, particularly during outbreaks. This work reviews the forecasting and mechanistic models published earlier. It is emphasized that researchers' forecasting models exhibit, for large t, algebraic behavior, as opposed to the exponential behavior of the classical logistic-type models used usually in epidemics. Remarkably, a newly introduced mechanistic model also exhibits, for large t, algebraic behavior in contrast to the usual Susceptible-Exposed-Infectious-Removed (SEIR) models, which exhibit exponential behavior. The unexpected success of researchers' simple forecasting models provides a strong support for the validity of this novel mechanistic model. It is also shown that the mathematical tools used for the analysis of the first wave may also be useful for the analysis of subsequent waves of the COVID-19 pandemic.

Keywords: COVID-19; forecasting model; SARS-CoV-2; variant of concern; VOC

Citation: Fokas, A.S.; Dikaios, N.; Tsiodras, S.; Kastis, G.A. Simple Formulae, Deep Learning and Elaborate Modelling for the COVID-19 Pandemic. *Encyclopedia* **2022**, 2, 679–689. https://doi.org/10.3390/encyclopedia2020047

Academic Editors: Stephen Bustin and Raffaele Barretta

Received: 16 January 2022
Accepted: 31 March 2022
Published: 6 April 2022

Publisher's Note: MDPI stays neutral with regard to jurisdictional claims in published maps and institutional affiliations.

1. Introduction

The first period of the COVID-19 pandemic in Europe, often referred to as 'the first wave', provides an ideal situation for the retrospective study of the various mathematical formulations used for modelling the dynamics of this viral epidemic. Indeed, during this phase, many European countries employed similar measures for combating the spread of the epidemic, and moreover, the pandemic was dominated by a single viral strain. Such a study is not only useful for academic purposes, but also, importantly, could identify an accurate mathematical formalism that could be used in a variety of epidemiological phenomena.

In the framework introduced by Holmdahl and Buckee [1], epidemiological models are broadly divided into two categories: *forecasting* and *mechanistic*. The former models fit a specific formula to the data, and then attempt to predict the dynamics of the quantity under consideration. The main limitation of these models is that they usually remain valid for a short period of time, and specifically only if the epidemiological situation remains unchanged. For example, they can be used during a lockdown period, but will not make accurate predictions after the lockdown is lifted. In contrast to forecasting models, mechanistic models can make predictions even when the relevant circumstances change. The main limitation of the forecasting models is the difficulty of determining the parameters specifying them.

In what follows, the researchers first discuss specific forecasting and mechanistic models introduced by the collaborative efforts published in [2–8]. In particular, the researchers provide an explanation for the remarkable success of researchers' simple forecasting models for predicting the dynamics of the first wave. The researchers then emphasize that the tools introduced for the analysis of the first wave can also be useful for analyzing subsequent waves of the COVID-19 pandemic. This is illustrated with a brief discussion of the second wave.

2. The Success of the Novel Formulae as Opposed to the Logistic Formula

A novel class of forecasting models was presented in [2,3]. Although, as correctly noted in [9], the forecasting models are 'not well suited for long-term predictions,' the researchers' class of forecasting models provided highly accurate long-term predictions both for the number of deaths caused by COVID-19 and the number of reported infected cases. Specifically, by training researchers' novel formulae (i.e., by fixing the constant parameters appearing in theses formulae) using data for the accumulative number of deaths in a given country until 1 May 2020, it was possible to make predictions for a period of more than 3.5 months. A typical example is shown in in Figure 1: for the COVID-19 epidemic in Italy, it is seen that there was no deviation between the curve depicting the number of deaths and the curve constructed via the model formula. Incidentally, although this formula was trained using dates during the lockdown period, its predictions remained accurate even after the easing of the lockdown conditions; possible explanations for this unexpected fact are discussed in [4].

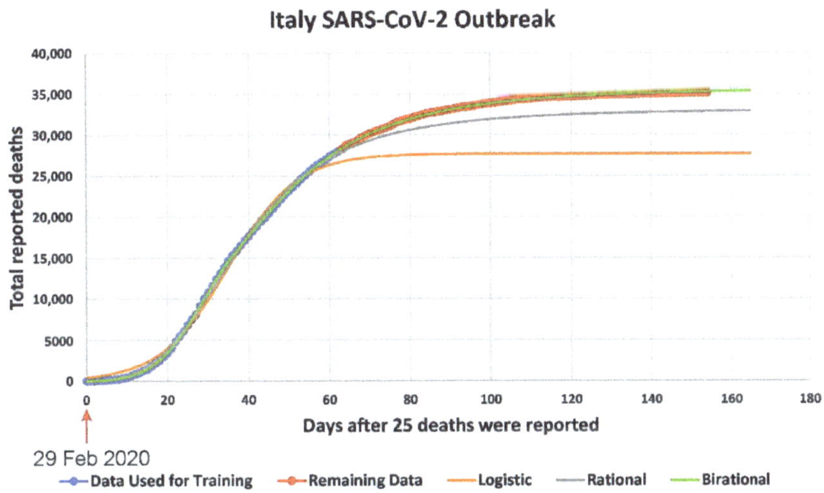

Figure 1. Predictions for the number of deaths in Italy. Comparison of the predictions of researchers' formulae for the number of reported deaths using data only until 1 May 2020, versus the actual data until 1 August 2020 (predictions for 92 days). The thick blue data-points depict the data used for calibrating the formulae and the red data-points depict the data used for checking the predictions of the 3 formulae.

In researchers' previous work [2,3], the usual logistic formula used in epidemiology is replaced by a different formula, called the *rational formula*. The logistic and rational formulae are given, respectively, by

$$N(t) = \frac{N_f}{1 + \beta e^{-kt}} \tag{1}$$

and

$$N(t) = \frac{N_f}{1 + \beta (1 + dt)^{-k}}. \tag{2}$$

In these formulae $N(t)$ denotes the cumulative number of deaths (or reported infected cases) at time t; the parameters N_f, k, β, and d are constants that can be determined by 'training' the model using the given data.

In addition to the rational formula, researchers also used a simple variant of this formula, called *birational* [2,3]. The birational formula is similar to the rational formula, but the associated parameters are different before and after a fixed time point. Both the rational and birational formulae are based on a particular nonlinear ordinary differential equation, called the Riccati equation. This equation is specified by the constant parameter, N_f, denoting the final total number of deceased (or infected individuals), and by a time-dependent function, a(t). Remarkably, although this Riccati equation is a nonlinear equation that involves time-dependent coefficients, it can be solved in closed form. Its solution depends on N_f, a(t), and on a parameter related to the constant that arises in integrating this equation. In the particular case that a(t) is a constant, the explicit solution of the above Riccati equation becomes the classical logistic Formula (1). If a(t) = kd/(1 + dt), then it becomes Formula (2).

3. Deep Learning

In previous work [2], researchers also investigated deep learning algorithms, and in particular, the bidirectional long short-term memory (BiLSTM) network, which is a powerful generalization of recurrent neural networks (RNN) that can capture long-term dependencies while at the same time avoiding the problem of vanishing/exploding gradients. RNN can capture sequential information but cannot learn from long term dependencies. A common problem with RNN, particularly when many hidden layers are used, is the vanishing or the exploding of the gradient in the backpropagation algorithm occurring during the process of updating the weights. Hochreiter and Schmidhuber introduced in [10] the Long Short-Term Memory (LSTM) networks that can capture long term dependencies and at the same time avoid the problem of vanishing/exploding gradients. LSTM networks are a type of RNN, where a memory cell maintains its state over time; they use gates to decide whether to flow information in (keep) or out (forget) of the memory cell.

Graves and Schmidhuber introduced in [11] the BiLSTM networks; this development was motivated by the Bidirectional RNN networks, introduced earlier by Schuster and Paliwal in [12], where the training runs forwards and backwards using two separate RNN. Consequently, the main difference is the training sequence: in the LSTM, the sequence runs backwards, preserving information from the future, whereas in the BiLSTM training, the sequence runs backward and forward, preserving information from both the past and the future. The BiLSTM networks are well suited for time series prediction and can potentially completely capture the contextual information of the time series.

The rational and birational formulae are, in a sense, optimal, since such elaborate deep learning algorithms investigated in [2] could not improve the predictions obtained by using these simple analytic formulae.

What is the critical difference between the logistic and the rational formulae? Although, for large time, t, both the logistic and the rational formulae tend to a constant, N_f, namely, the plateau reached by the epidemic, this constant is approached with exponential and algebraic rates, respectively. Indeed, for large t, Equations (1) and (2) yield the following asymptotic expressions:

$$N(t) \sim N_f\left(1-\beta e^{-kt}\right), \qquad t \to \infty \tag{3}$$

and

$$N(t) \sim N_f\left(1-\frac{\beta}{d^k}t^{-k}\right), \qquad t \to \infty \tag{4}$$

It is interesting to note that given a set of data, it is always possible to choose the constant parameters that specify these two formulae, so that they can match the given data extremely well. However, when these formulae are used to predict the dynamics of the epidemic, it becomes clear that the curve obtained via the logistic formula immediately begins to deviate from the curve of the real data, whereas the rational formula yields excellent predictions.

Regarding the algebraic decay, it is worth noting the following observation: whereas physical phenomena are often accurately modelled by exponential processes, social phenomena usually require an algebraic formalism.

4. A Typical Susceptible-Exposed-Infected-Recovered (SEIR) Type Model

In summary, the analysis of the real data from several European countries during the first wave of the COVID-19 epidemic suggests that the long-time behavior of the dynamics of the underlying processes is characterized by an algebraic as opposed to an exponential decay. This raises the following important question: do the mechanistic equations used to model these dynamics exhibit large t algebraic decay? This important question is discussed below.

It is well known that the most widely used mechanistic models are the so-called susceptible-exposed-infected-recovered (SEIR) type models. A typical such model was analyzed in [5,6]. This model consists of six ordinary differential equations modelling the number of infected, asymptomatic, sick, recovered, hospitalized, and deceased. Numerous other investigators have analyzed similar models, which include the well know works of [13]. Different SEIR models use different number of 'compartments,' but the essential physiological hypothesis used for deriving these models is the same.

The large time asymptotics of the model of [5] are analyzed in [7], where it is shown that this SEIR model exhibits exponential decay. It is natural to expect that all other SEIR type models will exhibit a similar behavior, which is inconsistent with the summary at the beginning of this section.

By modelling in [7] a physiologically important mechanism, which was until recently ignored, an additional nonlinear effect was introduced in the six ordinary differential equations presented in [5]. Remarkably, for large t, the novel model introduced in [7] exhibits algebraic decay, consistent with the decay exhibited by the real data. It is noted that the new physiological mechanism used in [7] was first introduced in [8,14] in connection with a simpler model.

5. From the First to the Second Wave

RNA viruses, as exemplified by influenza, may acquire mutations that can have a significant effect on their biological behavior [15,16]. Viruses' mutation rates are affected by various factors inherent to their replication such as the polymerase action, or external to the virus itself such as environmental effects. The precise contribution of these effects and how natural selection acts to optimize these rates remains unknown. The novel coronavirus, even before harboring genetic changes like the D614G polymorphism, was already fit enough to cause a pandemic.

The novel pandemic coronavirus SARS-CoV-2 acquired mutations early on [17], which altered some of its essential characteristics, affecting diagnosis [18], disease phenotype and severity [19,20], therapeutic interventions [21], and vaccine efficacy [22].

The exact public health impact of the early mutations remains debatable. By April 2020, strains carrying the D614G mutation [23,24] became prevalent in Europe, the USA, and Canada [23]. In particular, in a study in Houston, Texas, USA, the D614G variant strain gradually fully dominated the local epidemic [25]. The high prevalence of this strain was also confirmed in a UK study involving the analysis of 25,000 genomes [26]. In human infections, this strain was reported to be associated with a fitness advantage, as well as with greater transmissibility [23] and higher viral loads.

A difference in the growth rates between the higher levels of recorded infections and lower levels of respective number of deaths during the evolution of the pandemic, and especially during the second surge of the infection, is evident in the examination of the epidemic curves available from the European Centre for Disease Control [27,28]. A number of different factors may be associated with this 'paradox,' including increased testing, better health system capacity, earlier treatment, and increased levels of immunity in local populations. The possibility that the virus—due to structural differences—has evolved to be associated with less virulence, has been reported at the experimental level [29]. In this context, studies investigating the effect of earlier mutations including the D614G polymorphism showed that infections with D614G carrying strains were associated with higher viral loads in the upper respiratory tracts and a fitness advantage, leading to increased transmissibility [23,30–34]. Two large genomic analysis studies suggested otherwise [26,35]; they did not find convincing evidence with regards to infectivity or virulence [26,35]. The question of establishing whether this strain is indeed more infectious or less virulent remains crucial with regards to virus evolution to less virulent forms [36]. In the meantime, the world is faced with the emergence of new variants [37–50].

5.1. Predictions for the Number of Reported Infected Cases and the Number of the Deceased for the Second Wave in Portugal

In order to show that the techniques developed for the first wave can also be used for the analysis of subsequent waves, researchers applied the rational and logistic formulae to the cumulative number of deaths and reported infected cases for the second wave of Portugal. These formulae provided accurate predictions for the relevant dynamics (Figure 2). The data were fitted up to 27 December 2020, the last day before the first appearance of the UK lineage. Therefore, the researchers' curves determine what the plateau for reported cases and deaths would have been without the emergence of the UK lineage. For the number of deaths, the logistic formula predicted a plateau on 21 February 2021 with 6002 deaths for the second wave and 7798 total deaths overall; the rational formula predicted a plateau on 2 March 2021 with 6432 deaths for the second wave and 8228 total deaths overall. The plateau is defined *as the point when the rate of deaths for the given wave is 5% of the maximum rate.* It should be noted that in order to get accurate predictions, the model should employ data at least up to a short period after the time when the rate of deaths reached a *maximum*. In Portugal, for the deaths of the second wave, this occurred on 6 December 2020.

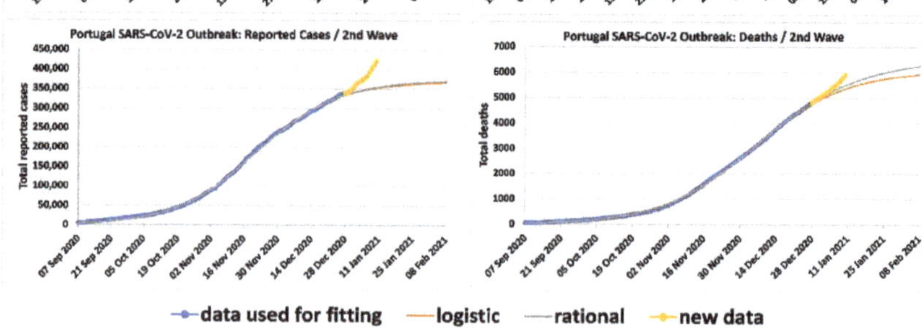

Figure 2. Comparisons between the actual reported cases and actual deaths for the first and second waves in Portugal vs. the fitted logistic and rational formulae. The data were fitted up to 27 December 2020, the last day before the first appearance of the UK lineage. The third wave in Portugal began on 28 December 2020.

For the number of reported infected cases for Portugal, the logistic formula predicted a plateau on 2 February 2021 with 364,526 cases for the second wave and 420,123 total cases overall; the rational formula predicted a plateau on 5 February 2021 with 369,040 cases for the second wave and 424,637 total cases overall. In Portugal, the rate of infections of the third wave reached a maximum on 21 November 2020.

5.2. Higher Infectivity and Lower Virulence

In order to compare the infectivity and virulence of the first two waves, additional techniques are needed. In this regard, first, researchers computed the rates dN/dt directly from the data, where N denotes the number of reported infected, in seven European countries (in order to avoid the noise of the real data, researchers computed these rates by fitting the data for the first and second waves to the rational and the logistic formulae, respectively). Second, researchers computed the function v(t) defined as the ratio of the cumulative number of deaths to the total number of reported infected cases that occurred three weeks prior to the date that the accumulated number of deaths was computed.

The computed rate of reported infected cases in the seven European countries analyzed was larger in the second wave, which supports the suggestion that the circulating strain of the virus of the second wave was more infectious. Figure 3a presents the relevant curves for Spain, which is prototypical of all cases examined. Similarly, the computed rate of deaths was much lower, seen in Figure 3b.

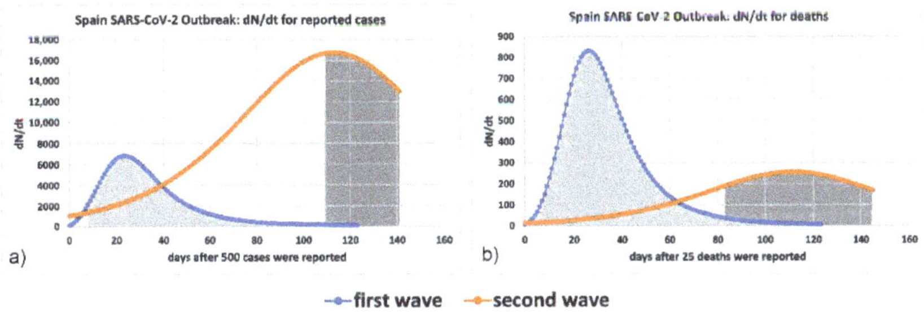

Figure 3. The rate of the (**a**) reported infected cases and (**b**) total number of deceased (dN/dt) for the first and second waves in Spain. The shaded areas indicate the lockdown periods.

For the case of Portugal, the rate of deaths can also be computed indirectly by examining the logistic and rational models. By comparing the parameters of the fitted logistic formula for Portugal (Figure 2) between the first and the second waves, it is confirmed that the rate of deaths is lower in the second wave (the parameter k is 0.0778 for the first and 0.0564 for the second, whilst the parameter N_f is 1489 and 6076).

In order to examine whether death rates were slower during the evolution of the pandemic and especially in the last half of 2020, researchers computed v(t) using the following steps. First, researchers separated the reported infected cases and the deaths for each country in the two waves and calculated their plateau. Then, in each wave, researchers computed the function v(t) by dividing the cumulative number of deaths up to a given date, by the cumulative number of reported cases 3 weeks earlier. Researchers chose the period of 3 weeks because individual infections during the last 3 weeks are not expected to greatly affect the number of deaths [51].

The graphs of v(t) for Germany, Greece, Spain, UK, Italy, Czechia, France, and Belgium are shown in Figure 4. The values of v(t) after the situation gets stabilized are shown in Table 1. These results suggest that the pathogenicity of the second Autumn/Winter wave was smaller than the first for these countries. Various factors may affect this suggestion, including increased testing, better health system capacity, earlier treatment, and increased levels of immunity in local populations. Among these factors, perhaps the increased number of testing during the second wave is of particular significance. As shown below, this effect can be quantified.

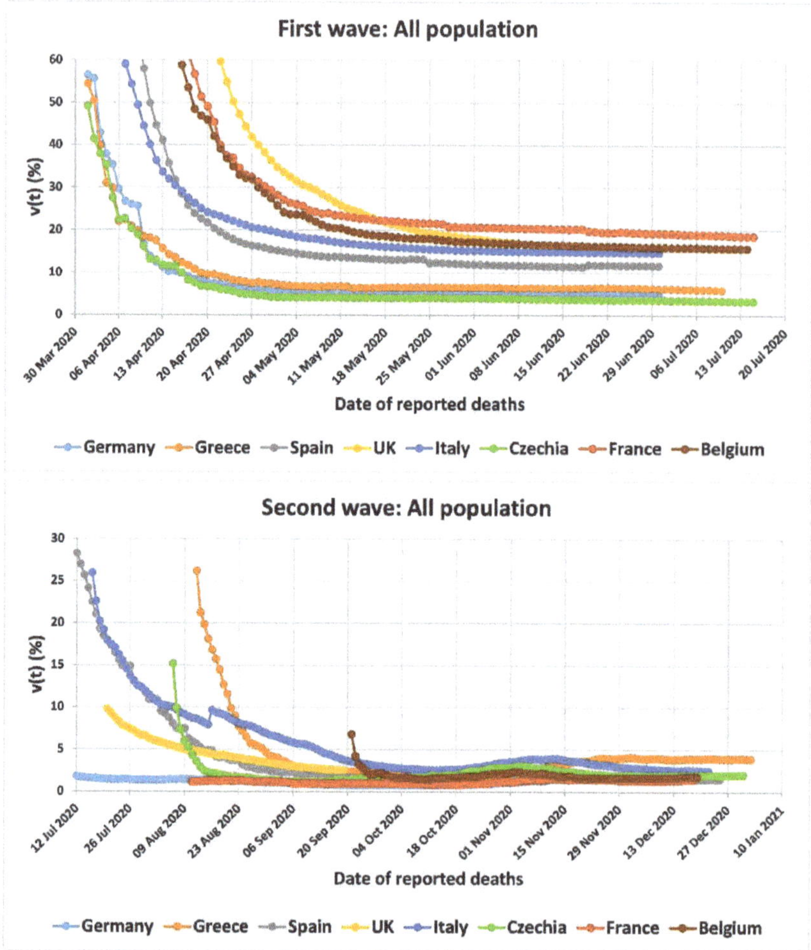

Figure 4. The function v(t) for the entire population of Germany, Greece, Spain, UK, Italy, Czechia, France, and Belgium for the first and second waves.

Table 1. Stabilization values for the function v(t) for the first and second waves, for various countries, for all population.

All Population	1st Wave		2nd Wave	
	Date	v(t) (%)	Date	v(t) (%)
Germany	30/June/2020	4.86	26/November/2020	1.50
Greece	04/July/2020	6.18	02/January/2021	3.95
Spain	30/June/2020	11.72	25/December/2020	1.49
UK	30/June/2020	15.24	19/September/2020	2.55
Italy	30/June/2020	14.77	22/December/2020	2.54
Czechia	15/July/2020	3.33	31/December/2020	2.04
France	15/July/2020	18.62	18/December/2020	1.46
Belgium	14/July/2020	15.77	19/December/2020	1.78

Indeed, let I and R denote the number of infected and reported infected individuals, and let the subscripts 1 and 2 indicate first and second wave, respectively. In the analysis that follows, the researchers assume that $I_1 = \alpha_1 R_1$ and $I_2 = \alpha_2 R_2$. Differentiating these equations with respect to time and dividing the resulting expressions, the researchers find

$$\frac{\dot{I}_2}{\dot{I}_1} = \frac{\alpha_2}{\alpha_1} \frac{\dot{R}_2}{\dot{R}_1}. \tag{5}$$

Since the number of tests increased during the second wave, $\alpha_2 < \alpha_1$.

Thus, the researchers' conclusions are valid provided that the growth of $\dot{R}_2/\dot{R}_1$ is sufficiently large so it can compensate for the decrease in α_2/α_1. Similarly, let ν^a, where the superscript 'a' denotes 'actual,' be defined by $v^a = d/I$. Then, $v^a = v/a$, and hence:

$$\frac{v_2^\alpha}{v_1^\alpha} = \frac{\alpha_1}{\alpha_2} \frac{v_2}{v_1} \tag{6}$$

The researchers' conclusions remain valid, despite the increase in the number of tests during the second wave, provided that the decrease of v_2/v_1 is sufficiently small to compensate for the growth of α_1/α_2. The researchers have been able to find data for the ratio α_2/α_1 only for Italy and UK; these numbers are quite small, namely 1.40 and 1.65, respectively [52,53]. Researchers speculate that similar rations are valid for the other counties considered in the researchers' study. Such small ratios will yield slight modifications for the graphs in Figure 4 and the values in the Table 1, but the overall conclusions remain the same.

6. Conclusions

The researchers have reviewed different predictive models used in the collaborative efforts published in [2–8] and have emphasized that the success of the researchers' forecasting models is due to the fact that, for large time, they capture the essential behavior of a recently introduced improved mechanistic models. Of course, mathematical modelling is only suggestive and cannot provide definitive proof of the different biological behaviors of the virus. In particular, the number of deaths and the rates of confirmed cases vary significantly across countries and there is significant dependency on the testing performed, as well as significant underreporting [54]. Moreover, the index of the probability of death per case of disease (Infection Fatality Rate) also varies from country to country. This is the result of a variety of factors, including, for example, differences in testing strategies and in case ascertainment. In addition, variance in population characteristics and comorbidities among countries and continents affects the observed morbidity and mortality (e.g., age is the most significant factor associated with increased mortality). Moreover, the percentage of cases involving specific high-risk sub-populations (such as those in nursing homes [55]) varies according to country. Furthermore, differences in timing of measures adopted, as well as differences in targeted control strategies across countries (including targeting the high-risk population like the middle-aged and over), affects death rates. Relating to this observation, the health system quality and capacity widely varies across nations and continents. The saturation of medical facilities may further affect mortality rates, especially in vulnerable high-risk populations.

Researchers have also shown that the mathematical modelling tools used in the first wave, as well as variations of these tools, can be useful for the analysis of subsequent waves. The researchers have illustrated this fact by analyzing the second wave. The researchers suggest that this wave is characterized by higher transmissibility and less virulence than the first wave. However, in these connections, it should be noted that several clinical and physiological factors may affect the disease course towards a better outcome. Among these are the increasing experience of doctors treating the disease and its complications, along with early diagnosis, small hospital volumes in early stages of the second wave that allowed for better care, and the use of new antivirals and immune modulation treatments. All these effects could potentially lead to milder clinical forms of the disease [56,57]. Thus, the value of the ratio proposed herein may tend to underestimate the virulence of new strains.

In conclusion, it should be noted that it is not possible to predict the clinical effect of new mutations. For example, although the second wave apparently involved a less virulent strain than the first, the third wave was more severe. On the other hand, the omicron variant is highly transmittable but also has very low virulence.

Author Contributions: Conceptualization, A.S.F. and S.T.; methodology, A.S.F.; software, N.D. and G.A.K.; formal analysis, N.D. and G.A.K.; writing—original draft preparation, A.S.F. and S.T.; writing—review and editing, A.S.F., S.T., N.D. and G.A.K.; supervision, A.S.F. and S.T. All authors have read and agreed to the published version of the manuscript.

Funding: A.S.F. was supported by EPSRC, UK (RG79707), in the form of a senior Fellowship.

Data Availability Statement: The data presented in this study are publicly available on the various sites cited within the manuscript.

Conflicts of Interest: The authors declare no conflict of interest.

References

1. Holmdahl, I.; Buckee, C. Wrong but useful-What Covid-19 epidemiologic models can and cannot tell us. *N. Engl. J. Med.* **2020**, *383*, 303–305. [CrossRef] [PubMed]
2. Fokas, A.S.; Dikaios, N.; Kastis, G.A. Mathematical models and deep learning for predicting the number of individuals reported to be infected with SARS-CoV-2. *J. R. Soc. Interface* **2020**, *17*, 20200494. [CrossRef] [PubMed]
3. Fokas, A.S.; Dikaios, N.; Kastis, G.A. Covid-19: Predictive mathematical formulae for the number of deaths during lockdown and possible scenarios for the post-lockdown period. *Proc. R. Soc. A* **2021**, *477*, 20200745. [CrossRef] [PubMed]
4. Fokas, A.S.; Kastis, G.A. SARS-CoV-2: The Second Wave in Europe. *J. Med. Internet Res.* **2021**, *23*, e22431. [CrossRef] [PubMed]
5. Fokas, A.S.; Cuevas-Maraver, J.; Kevrekidis, P.G. A quantitative framework for exploring exit strategies from the COVID-19 lockdown. *Chaos Solitons Fractals* **2020**, *140*, 110244. [CrossRef]
6. Fokas, A.S.; Cuevas-Maraver, J.; Kevrekidis, P.G. Easing COVID-19 lockdown measures while protecting the older restricts the deaths to the level of the full lockdown. *Sci. Rep.* **2021**, *11*, 5839. [CrossRef] [PubMed]
7. Fokas, A.S.; Oberai, A.A.; Yortsos, Y.C. A novel SEIR type model exhibiting algebraic behavior. *in preparation*.
8. Luhar, M.; Oberai, A.A.; Fokas, A.S.; Yortsos, Y.C. Accounting for Super-Spreader Events and Algebraic Decay in SIR Models. *Comput. Methods Appl. Mech. Eng.* 2022, *submitted*.
9. Zhou, P.; Yang, X.-L.; Wang, X.-G.; Hu, B.; Zhang, L.; Zhang, W.; Si, H.-R.; Zhu, Y.; Li, B.; Huang, C.-L.; et al. A pneumonia outbreak associated with a new coronavirus of probable bat origin. *Nature* **2020**, *579*, 270–273. [CrossRef]
10. Hochreiter, S.; Schmidhuber, J. Long Short-Term Memory. *Neural Comput.* **1997**, *9*, 1735–1780. [CrossRef]
11. Graves, A.; Schmidhuber, J. Framewise phoneme classification with bi-directional LSTM and other neural network architectures. *Neural Netw.* **2005**, *18*, 602–610. [CrossRef] [PubMed]
12. Schuster, M.; Paliwal, K.K. Bidirectional recurrent neural networks. *IEEE Trans. Signal Process.* **1997**, *45*, 2673–2681. [CrossRef]
13. Ferguson, N.M.; Laydon, D.; Nedjati-Gilani, G.; Imai, N.; Ainslie, K.; Baguelin, M.; Ghani, A.C. Impact of Non-Pharmaceutical Interventions (NPIs) to Reduce COVID-19 Mortality and Healthcare Demand. Imperial College, London, March 2020. Available online: https://www.imperial.ac.uk/mrc-global-infectious-disease-analysis/covid-19/ (accessed on 20 March 2020).
14. Ramaswamy, H.; Oberai, A.A.; Luhar, M.; Yortsos, Y.C. Understanding the R0 of pademics. In Proceedings of the 42nd Ibero-Latin-American Congress on Computational Methods in Engineering (XLII CILAMCE) and the 3rd Pan American Congress on Computational Mechanics (III PANACM), Rio de Janeiro, Brazil, 9–12 November 2021; p. 9449.
15. Lauring, A.S.; Andino, R. Quasispecies theory and the behavior of RNA viruses. *PLoS Pathog.* **2010**, *6*, e1001005. [CrossRef] [PubMed]
16. Ghedin, E.; Sengamalay, N.A.; Shumway, M.; Zaborsky, J.; Feldblyum, T.; Subbu, V.; Spiro, D.J.; Sitz, J.; Koo, H.; Bolotov, P.; et al. Large-scale sequencing of human influenza reveals the dynamic nature of viral genome evolution. *Nature* **2005**, *437*, 1162–1166. [CrossRef]
17. Badua, C.; Baldo, K.A.T.; Medina, P.M.B. Genomic and proteomic mutation landscapes of SARS-CoV-2. *J. Med. Virol.* **2021**, *93*, 1702–1721. [CrossRef]
18. Artesi, M.; Bontems, S.; Gobbels, P.; Franckh, M.; Maes, P.; Boreux, R.; Meex, C.; Melin, P.; Hayette, M.P.; Bours, V.; et al. A Recurrent Mutation at Position 26340 of SARS-CoV-2 Is Associated with Failure of the E Gene Quantitative Reverse Transcription-PCR Utilized in a Commercial Dual-Target Diagnostic Assay. *J. Clin. Microbiol.* **2020**, *58*, e01598-20. [CrossRef]
19. Al Khatib, H.A.; Benslimane, F.M.; Elbashir, I.E.; Coyle, P.V.; Al Maslamani, M.A.; Al-Khal, A.; Al Thani, A.A.; Yassine, H.M. Within-Host Diversity of SARS-CoV-2 in COVID-19 Patients With Variable Disease Severities. *Front. Cell Infect. Microbiol.* **2020**, *10*, 575613. [CrossRef]

20. Pandit, B.; Bhattacharjee, S.; Bhattacharjee, B. Association of clade-G SARS-CoV-2 viruses and age with increased mortality rates across 57 countries and India. *Infect. Genet. Evol.* **2021**, *90*, 104734. [CrossRef]
21. Andreano, E.; Piccini, G.; Licastro, D.; Casalino, L.; Johnson, N.V.; Paciello, I.; Monego, S.D.; Pantano, E.; Manganaro, N.; Manenti, A.; et al. SARS-CoV-2 escape from a highly neutralizing COVID-19 convalescent plasma. *Proc. Natl. Acad. Sci. USA* **2021**, *118*, e2103154118. [CrossRef]
22. Amanat, F.; Strohmeier, S.; Rathnasinghe, R.; Schotsaert, M.; Coughlan, L.; García-Sastre, A.; Krammer, F. Introduction of two prolines and removal of the polybasic cleavage site lead to higher efficacy of a recombinant spike-based SARS-CoV-2 vaccine in the mouse model. *mbio* **2021**, *12*, e02648-20. [CrossRef]
23. Korber, B.; Fischer, W.M.; Gnanakaran, S.; Yoon, H.; Theiler, J.; Abfalterer, W.; Hengartner, N.; Giorgi, E.E.; Bhattacharya, T.; Foley, B.; et al. Tracking Changes in SARS-CoV-2 Spike: Evidence that D614G Increases Infectivity of the COVID-19 Virus. *Cell* **2020**, *182*, 812–827.e19. [CrossRef] [PubMed]
24. Mansbach, R.A.; Chakraborty, S.; Nguyen, K.; Montefiori, D.C.; Korber, B.; Gnanakaran, S. The SARS-CoV-2 Spike Variant D614G Favors an Open Conformational State. *Sci. Adv.* **2021**, *7*, eabf3671. [CrossRef] [PubMed]
25. Long, S.W.; Olsen, R.J.; Christensen, P.A.; Bernard, D.W.; Davis, J.J.; Shukla, M.; Nguyen, M.; Saavedra, M.O.; Yerramilli, P.; Pruitt, L.; et al. Molecular Architecture of Early Dissemination and Massive Second Wave of the SARS-CoV-2 Virus in a Major Metropolitan Area. *mBio* **2020**, *11*, e02707-20. [CrossRef] [PubMed]
26. Volz, E.; Hill, V.; McCrone, J.T.; Price, A.; Jorgensen, D.; O'Toole, Á.; Southgate, J.; Johnson, R.; Jackson, B.; Nascimento, F.F.; et al. Evaluating the Effects of SARS-CoV-2 Spike Mutation D614G on Transmissibility and Pathogenicity. *Cell* **2021**, *184*, 64–75. [CrossRef]
27. COVID-19 Situation Update for the EU/EEA, as of Week 7 2021, Updated 25 February 2021. European Center for Disease Control. Available online. https://www.ecdc.europa.eu/en/cases-2019-ncov-eueea (accessed on 1 March 2021).
28. COVID-19 Situation Worldwide, as of Week 7 2021, Updated 25 February 2021. European Center for Disease Control. Available online: https://www.ecdc.europa.eu/en/geographical-distribution-2019-ncov-cases (accessed on 1 March 2021).
29. Yurkovetskiy, L.; Wang, X.; Pascal, K.E.; Tomkins-Tinch, C.; Nyalile, T.; Wang, Y.; Baum, A.; Diehl, W.E.; Dauphin, A.; Carbone, C.; et al. Structural and Functional Analysis of the D614G SARS-CoV-2 Spike Protein Variant. *Cell* **2020**, *183*, 739–751.e8. [CrossRef]
30. Li, Q.; Wu, J.; Nie, J.; Zhang, L.; Hao, H.; Liu, S.; Zhao, C.; Zhang, Q.; Liu, H.; Nie, L.; et al. The Impact of Mutations in SARS-CoV-2 Spike on Viral Infectivity and Antigenicity. *Cell* **2020**, *182*, 1284–1294.e9. [CrossRef]
31. Plante, J.A.; Liu, Y.; Liu, J.; Xia, H.; Johnson, B.A.; Lokugamage, K.G.; Zhang, X.; Muruato, A.E.; Zou, J.; Fontes-Garfias, C.R.; et al. Spike mutation D614G alters SARS-CoV-2 fitness. *Nature* **2021**, *592*, 116–121. [CrossRef]
32. Hou, Y.J.; Chiba, S.; Halfmann, P.; Here, C.; Kuroda, M.; Dinnon, K.H., III; Leist, S.R.; Schäfer, A.; Nakajima, N.; Takahashi, K.; et al. SARS-CoV-2 D614G variant exhibits efficient replication ex vivo and transmission in vivo. *Science* **2020**, *370*, 1464–1468. [CrossRef]
33. Zhou, B.; Thao, T.T.N.; Hoffmann, D.; Taddeo, A.; Ebert, N.; Labroussaa, F.; Pohlmann, A.; King, J.; Steiner, S.; Kelly, J.N.; et al. SARS-CoV-2 spike D614G change enhances replication and transmission. *Nature* **2021**, *592*, 122–127. [CrossRef]
34. Daniloski, Z.; Jordan, T.X.; Ilmain, J.K.; Guo, X.; Bhabha, G.; tenOever, B.R.; Sanjana, N.E. The D614G mutation in SARS-CoV-2 Spike increases transduction of multiple human cell types. *eLife* **2021**, *10*, e65365. [CrossRef]
35. van Dorp, L.; Richard, D.; Tan, C.C.S.; Shaw, L.P.; Acman, M.; Balloux, F. No evidence for increased transmissibility from recurrent mutations in SARS-CoV-2. *Nat. Commun.* **2020**, *11*, 5986. [CrossRef] [PubMed]
36. Callaway, E. The coronavirus is mutating-does it matter? *Nature* **2020**, *585*, 174–177. [CrossRef] [PubMed]
37. Claro, I.M.; da Silva Sales, F.C.; Ramundo, M.S.; Candido, D.S.; Silva, C.A.M.; de Jesus, J.G.; Manuli, E.R.; de Oliveira, C.M.; Scarpelli, L.; Campana, G.; et al. Local Transmission of SARS-CoV-2 Lineage B.1.1.7, Brazil, December 2020. *Emerg. Infect. Dis.* **2021**, *27*, 970–972. [CrossRef] [PubMed]
38. Dao, M.H.; Nguyen, H.T.; Nguyen, T.V.; Nguyen, A.H.; Luong, Q.C.; Vu, N.H.P.; Pham, H.T.T.; Nguyen, T.N.T.; Thach, D.H.; Nguyen, L.V.; et al. New SARS-CoV-2 Variant of Concern Imported from the United Kingdom to Vietnam, December 2020. *J. Med. Virol.* **2021**, *93*, 2628–2630. [CrossRef] [PubMed]
39. Umair, M.; Ikram, A.; Salman, M.; Alam, M.M.; Badar, N.; Rehman, Z.; Tamim, S.; Khurshid, A.; Ahad, A.; Ahmad, H.; et al. Importation of SARS-CoV-2 Variant B.1.1.7 in Pakistan. *J. Med. Virol.* **2021**, *93*, 2623–2625. [CrossRef] [PubMed]
40. Yadav, P.D.; Nyayanit, D.A.; Sahay, R.R.; Sarkale, P.; Pethani, J.; Patil, S.; Baradkar, S.; Potdar, V.; Patil, D.Y. Isolation and characterization of the new SARS-CoV-2 variant in travellers from the United Kingdom to India: VUI-202012/01 of the B.1.1.7 lineage. *J. Travel Med.* **2021**, *28*, taab009. [CrossRef]
41. Alpert, T.; Brito, A.F.; Lasek-Nesselquist, E.; Rothman, J.; Valesano, A.L.; MacKay, M.J.; Petrone, M.E.; Breban, M.I.; Watkins, A.E.; Vogels, C.B.F.; et al. Early introductions and community transmission of SARS-CoV-2 variant B.1.1.7 in the United States. *Cell* **2021**, *184*, 2595–2604.e13. [CrossRef]
42. Firestone, M.J.; Lorentz, A.J.; Wang, X.; Como-Sabetti, K.; Vetter, S.; Smith, K.; Holzbauer, S.; Meyer, S.; Ehresmann, K.; Danila, R.; et al. First Identified Cases of SARS-CoV-2 Variant B.1.1.7 in Minnesota-December 2020–January 2021. *MMWR Morb. Mortal. Wkly. Rep.* **2021**, *70*, 278–279. [CrossRef]
43. Galloway, S.E.; Paul, P.; MacCannell, D.R.; Johansson, M.A.; Brooks, J.T.; MacNeil, A.; Slayton, R.B.; Tong, S.; Silk, B.J.; Armstrong, G.L.; et al. Emergence of SARS-CoV-2 B.1.1.7 Lineage-United States, December 29, 2020–January 12, 2021. *MMWR Morb. Mortal. Wkly. Rep.* **2021**, *70*, 95–99. [CrossRef]

44. Leung, K.; Shum, M.H.; Leung, G.M.; Lam, T.T.; Wu, J.T. Early transmissibility assessment of the N501Y mutant strains of SARS-CoV-2 in the United Kingdom, October to November 2020. *Eurosurveillance* **2021**, *26*, 2002106. [CrossRef]
45. Pfefferle, S.; Gunther, T.; Kobbe, R.; Czech-Sioli, M.; Nörz, D.; Santer, R.; Oh, J.; Kluge, S.; Oestereich, L.; Peldschus, K.; et al. SARS Coronavirus-2 variant tracing within the first Coronavirus Disease 19 clusters in northern Germany. *Clin. Microbiol. Infect.* **2021**, *27*, 130.e5–130.e8. [CrossRef] [PubMed]
46. European Centre for Disease Prevention and Control. Risk Assessment: SARS-CoV-2-Increased Circulation of Variants of Concern and Vaccine Rollout in the EU/EEA, 14th Update. Available online: https://www.ecdc.europa.eu/en/publications-data/covid-19-risk-assessment-variants-vaccine-fourteenth-update-february-2021 (accessed on 1 March 2021).
47. Mwenda, M.; Saasa, N.; Sinyang, N.; Busby, G.; Chipimo, P.J.; Hendry, J.; Kapona, O.; Yingst, S.; Hines, J.Z.; Minchella, P.; et al. Detection of B.1.351 SARS-CoV-2 Variant Strain-Zambia, December 2020. *MMWR Morb. Mortal. Wkly. Rep.* **2021**, *70*, 280–282. [CrossRef] [PubMed]
48. Munoz, M.; Patino, L.H.; Ballesteros, N.; Paniz-Mondolfi, A.; Ramírez, J.D. Characterizing SARS-CoV-2 genome diversity circulating in South American countries: Signatures of potentially emergent lineages? *Int. J. Infect. Dis.* **2021**, *105*, 329–332. [CrossRef] [PubMed]
49. Maggi, F.; Novazzi, F.; Genoni, A.; Baj, A.; Spezia, P.G.; Focosi, D.; Zago, C.; Colombo, A.; Cassani, G.; Pasciuta, R.; et al. Imported SARS-COV-2 Variant P.1 Detected in Traveler Returning from Brazil to Italy. *Emerg. Infect. Dis.* **2021**, *27*, 1249–1251. [CrossRef]
50. Collier, D.A.; De Marco, A.; Ferreira, I.; Meng, B.; Datir, R.P.; Walls, A.C.; Kemp, S.A.; Bassi, J.; Pinto, D.; Silacci-Fregni, C.; et al. Sensitivity of SARS-CoV-2 B.1.1.7 to mRNA vaccine-elicited antibodies. *Nature* **2021**, *593*, 136–141. [CrossRef]
51. Coronavirus (COVID-19) Infection Survey Technical Article: Waves and Lags of COVID-19 in England, June 2021. Available online: https://www.ons.gov.uk/peoplepopulationandcommunity/healthandsocialcare/conditionsanddiseases/articles/coronaviruscovid19infectionsurveytechnicalarticle/wavesandlagsofcovid19inenglandjune2021 (accessed on 15 August 2021).
52. Traini, M.C.; Caponi, C.; Ferrari, R.; De Socio, G.V. SARS-CoV-2 unreported cases in Italy: Analysis of serological survey and vaccination scenarios. *Infect. Dis. Model.* **2021**, *6*, 909–923. [CrossRef]
53. How Many Cases of Covid-19 Are There? A Q&A. Available online: https://www.nuffieldtrust.org.uk/news-item/how-many-cases-of-covid-19-are-there-a-q-a (accessed on 15 August 2021).
54. Campolieti, M. COVID-19 deaths in the USA: Benford's law and under-reporting. *J. Public Health* **2021**, fdab161. [CrossRef]
55. Team, E.P.H.E.; Danis, K.; Fonteneau, L.; Danis, K.; Fonteneau, L.; Georges, S.; Daniau, C.; Bernard-Stoecklin, S.; Domegan, L.; O'Donnell, J.; et al. High impact of COVID-19 in long-term care facilities, suggestion for monitoring in the EU/EEA, May 2020. *Eurosurveillance* **2020**, *25*, 2000956.
56. Horwitz, L.I.; Jones, S.A.; Cerfolio, R.J.; Francois, F.; Greco, J.; Rudy, B.; Petrilli, C.M. Trends in COVID-19 Risk-Adjusted Mortality Rates. *J. Hosp. Med.* **2021**, *16*, 90–92. [CrossRef]
57. Gandhi, M.; Rutherford, G.W. Facial Masking for Covid-19-Potential for "Variolation" as We Await a Vaccine. *N. Engl. J. Med.* **2020**, *383*, e101. [CrossRef]

encyclopedia MDPI

Entry

Trust in Science and COVID-19

Marilena Mousoulidou [1,*], Andri Christodoulou [1], Marios Argyrides [1], Michailina Siakalli [2] and Louiza Constantinou [1]

[1] Department of Psychology, Neapolis University Pafos, 2 Danais Avenue, Paphos 8042, Cyprus; andri.christodoulou@nup.ac.cy (A.C.); m.argyrides.1@nup.ac.cy (M.A.); lconstantinou@dl.mlsi.gov.cy (L.C.)
[2] Department of Economics and Business, Neapolis University Pafos, 2 Danais Avenue, Paphos 8042, Cyprus; m.siakalli@nup.ac.cy
* Correspondence: marilena.mousoulidou@nup.ac.cy

Definition: In this entry, trust in science is defined as the reliance, confidence, and dependence on science to understand scientific information. With the outbreak of, and the uncertainty surrounding the COVID-19 pandemic, turning towards science and trusting the specialized knowledge of experts is of particular importance during this period.

Keywords: trust, science, COVID-19

1. Introduction

Trust is an important construct that influences the actions of individuals, organizations, and societies. Every day, people need to make decisions, and frequently, trust plays a critical role in the decisions they undertake. It is, therefore, imperative, especially in periods of crises, for individuals to know whom and what to trust.

From December 2019, a novel SARS-CoV-2 virus broke out in China and rapidly spread across the world. Along with the virus, the fear of uncertainty concerning the future spread. On 11th March 2020, after 118,000 cases in 114 countries, the World Health Organization (WHO) declared COVID-19 a pandemic [1]. The WHO's declaration prompted clinicians, scientists, and scientific organizations worldwide to provide valuable medical and epidemiological information to control the spread of the virus. This included information about the virus' transmissibility, the severity of the disease, and preventive public health behaviors and measures. The virus was considered highly contagious [2] and therefore demanded from the public a high level of compliance to the suggested prevention guidelines. Like with other viruses in the past that entailed uncertainty, people had to turn to science to stop the spread of the virus.

This entry aims to provide a more thorough understanding of the significant role of trust in science during the COVID-19 era. It begins by defining trust in science and then discusses some within-individual factors (religion, political orientation, education, socioeconomic status, and psychological factors) that influence trust in science. The role of this trust in the accuracy of information one receives is also discussed by examining the effect of social media, misinformation, and conspiracy theories. Next, the role of trust in science in public policy and its effect on preventive behaviors (compliance to public measures and vaccination) is explored. The entry closes with some general conclusions.

Citation: Mousoulidou, M.; Christodoulou, A.; Argyrides, M.; Siakalli, M.; Constantinou, L. Trust in Science and COVID-19. *Encyclopedia* **2022**, 2, 602–616. https://doi.org/10.3390/encyclopedia2010040

Academic Editors: Stephen Bustin and Raffaele Barretta

Received: 20 February 2022
Accepted: 2 March 2022
Published: 10 March 2022

2. Importance of Trust in Science in Times of a Pandemic

Trust is a complicated concept that scholars from different disciplines have extensively researched. Generally, trust involves a willingness and belief of one person (the trustor) to place confidence and rely upon another party's (the trustee) honesty and sincerity in performing a particular action [3–5]. This action is essential for the trustor and, therefore, without controlling or monitoring the other party, is willing to take the risk and depend on the trustee. In other words, the trustor is in a vulnerable position when trusting the other party. Trust is important in many respects. It is fundamental for the development of stability, inclusiveness, and economic progress in societies, as it translates to the trustworthiness of people [6,7], is essential to the functioning of the political system [8], vital for the survival and functioning of democratic institutions [9], inherent in intimate relationships [10], important in professional business relationships [11] and negotiations [12], and is essential for science.

The expression *trust in science* is twofold, referring to (a) trust for the "insiders," which refers to the scientists who are performing science and are expected to present accurate and non-manipulated or fake results, and (b) trust for the "outsiders," where outsiders are the general public who trust the scientific experts for information about science [5,13]. In other words, trust is essential both for science communication and scientific work.

Importantly, trust in science is related to the concept of *epistemic trust*; that is, the trust in the knowledge given by scientists [5,14,15]. Specifically, epistemic trust is the trustors' inclination (because of their limited resources) to depend on and defer to the experts (trustees) [14]. Epistemic trustworthiness has been found to have three interrelated yet distinct dimensions: (a) expertise (knowledge, intelligence, and training), (b) benevolence (ethicality and responsibility), and (c) integrity (honesty, fairness, and justice) [14]. These components are critical determinants of whether a trustor considers an expert trustworthy. Though it is beyond the scope of this entry, it is worth mentioning that epistemic trust comprises two related components, *default trust* and *vigilant trust*. The former refers to the minimal trust needed for successful communication, and the latter refers to the filtering of information as trustworthy [16,17].

A person will choose to trust in science based on the answer he/she will give to the question, "why should I trust science." If the epistemic trustworthiness and its dimensions are high, the person will be more likely to trust science [5,14,18]. If the person judges scientists as having expertise, benevolence, and integrity, they are more likely to show trust in science. It is worth noting that the degree of trust shown by an individual changes depending on the situation [18]. In other words, one person can show high trust towards specific scientists who meet the concept's dimensions but low to those who do not.

Additionally, it has also been suggested that trust in science varies depending on personal stances about specific topics [5]. More analytically, when an individual decides to trust a scientist or not for a specific scientific topic, the person's decision is associated with his/her stance towards that specific topic. Knowledge about a topic is produced not solely based on trust in science but also on the individual's personal position regarding that topic [5]. Scientific topics, especially in the early stages where not much is known, may produce discussions that appear to be "controversial" since the topic is discussed from different viewpoints. Awareness of such controversies might influence the person's stance, which will eventually "modify" their trust in science [5].

It is not a surprise that trust in science has a vital role during a critical period such as a pandemic. With the uncertainty surrounding an unknown virus, people need to judge and decide what is true and false. Turning to science and trusting the knowledge given by scientists plays a crucial role in one's decision and, ultimately, one's response towards novel situations [18]. Political decisions regarding how a country should battle the spread of a virus are made based on the available scientific knowledge [19]. Moreover, for the public to follow political decisions or form an informed opinion, it is critical to trust science in terms of scientific knowledge and scientists and scientific institutions [19]. Trust in science also appears to protect society from major public health crises, such as a pandemic [20], because it is among the many factors that explain adherence to public measures to stop the spread of the virus. Multiple studies have identified that trust in science is one of the factors associated with better adherence to prevention measures [20–28]. These studies have suggested that trust in science promotes adherence and that the lower the trust in science, the lower the adherence to the prevention measures [20–28]. Additionally, it was found that trust in scientists encourages more favorable attitudes towards vaccination. [21,29].

Moreover, during a pandemic, the public needs to have accurate information regarding the virus and its protection. Research has shown that prevention behaviors of spreading the COVID-19 virus (i.e., washing hands and social distancing) are related to beliefs about the virus [21,30]. Specifically, belief formation was affected by the individual's trust in science, with those trusting scientists being more likely to believe more accurate statements about the pandemic [21,30]. This is an important finding showing the importance of trust in science for disregarding inaccurate information.

The largest global survey to date that examined people's views about science included 113 countries and territories [31]. Specifically, this survey compared participants' responses during two different periods, 2018 and 2020, and found that in comparison to 2018, there was a global nine-percentage-point increase in trust levels in science and scientists during the period of the COVID-19 pandemic. However, some significant differences can be observed when examining the regions in more detail. That is, in Russia/Caucasus/Central Asia, the trust in science level remained the same; there was an increase for East Asia, Latin America, Eastern Europe, and Southeast Asia, and a decrease for Sub-Saharan Africa, which had the lowest level of trust in science in the world [31]. Regarding trust in scientists, the results generally showed a similar pattern. The survey also examined the changes in trust levels based on people's level of scientific knowledge. The results showed an overall increase in trust in science and scientists based on their knowledge [31]. This increase was significantly higher for people who reported "some," "not much," or "nothing at all" knowledge about science, with data showing at least a 10-percentage-point increase between the two periods [31]. This indicates that trust in science during a pandemic both changes and varies across countries.

During times of crises, trust in science is often linked to political trust. This is because the political authorities are those responsible for delivering and implementing the recommendations from scientists and scientific institutions. Political trust refers to how confident people feel about their governments and the extent to which they consider their government to be fair, competent, and credible [32]. It depends on the individual's overall evaluation of his or her political institution, and therefore several components contribute to whether a person will experience trust toward the political system or agents [33]. Political trust and trust in science both play their role in a person's decision about an unknown phenomenon. People who trust scientists and scientific institutions are more likely to view their suggestions as credible and legitimate and therefore more likely to accept the political decisions, and those who trust their government are more likely to support and comply with its regulations and policies [32,34,35].

3. Within Individual Factors That Influence Trust in Science

Trust in science is influenced by many variables, such as a group's previous experience, belief system, worldview, and many others [36,37]. This part of the entry discusses five individual factors that affect trust in science. These factors are extensively discussed in the literature and have been generally found to apply to most societies.

3.1. Religion

Religion has always had a key role in societies as it is considered a cultural authority shaping perceptions and influencing the public's opinions and decisions [37]. For years, the relationship between reason (science) and faith (religion) has been debated. Traditionally, *faith* has been viewed as the opposite of *reason* [38], and therefore the two were viewed as incompatible [39]. Currently, this topic is still open for discussion. Some researchers still believe that the two are in conflict, yet others believe there will be no contradiction between the two [32] when faith is adequately understood and reason adequately employed. For instance, some argue that people who follow a religion do not do so because they are against science but instead because they interpret specific phenomena from a religious point of view [39]. Although the debate is ongoing, it appears that when people need to interpret an unknown subject, they form their opinions and decisions based on data from either religion or science [40]. The choice that the person will eventually make largely depends on the experience he or she has had with each [41].

During the early stages of the COVID-19 outbreak, though it is unclear whether it was an underestimation of the risk or lack of trust in science, various religious leaders encouraged resistance to the preventive guidelines to contain the virus that were presented by the governments. Due to the contagious nature of the virus and the disregard towards the measures by followers, there were reports of virus spreading within places of worship. For instance, in South Korea, a church refused to follow the safety protocols (i.e., wearing masks, maintaining social distance), resulting in 5000 new cases, and was identified as contributing to the local epidemic [42]. Additionally, in Trinidad and Tobago [43] and in the State of Louisiana in the USA [44], the virus could not be contained as some churches refused to cease large gatherings. The former argued that believers who stopped attending the church lacked faith [43], whereas the latter stated that COVID-19 was politically motivated [44]. Consequently, public measures were not followed.

Importantly, religious people seem to be more skeptical towards science. For example, it has been noted that religious people do not view science epistemically but rather from a moral point of view, which leads them to be more skeptical [45]. Furthermore, it has been shown that religiosity negatively affects trust in science, regardless of other factors such as society or specific religion [37]. Moreover, concerning European countries, data are available from a recent Special Eurobarometer conducted between April and May 2021 entitled "European citizens' knowledge and attitudes towards science and technology." [46]. Overall, this analysis indicated that almost one-third of respondents agreed that there was too much dependence on science and not enough on faith. However, there were considerable differences at a country level; in six countries, at least half agreed on depending too much on science with the largest proportions seen in Cyprus (68%), Bulgaria (59%) and Greece (56%) [46]. Contrarily, 13% of those in Finland and Belgium and 15% in Sweden and Ireland thought this was the case [46]. These percentages were also affected by individual factors such as education level, gender, etc. [46]. Lastly, a novel study examined the role of trust in science towards compliance with prevention guidelines during the COVID-19 pandemic. The researchers found that although religion does not directly affect public compliance, it was correlated with less trust in science, which led to lower compliance with the public measures [27].

3.2. Political Orientation

Political orientation is an important factor that was found to influence trust in science in some countries. Though politics is very complicated, political orientation is divided between the left and right parties. Left supporters are considered liberal and democratic views, and right supporters are considered those who have conservative or republican views [47]. Research has shown that Democrats, as opposed to Republicans, demonstrate higher trust in science regarding its fundamental principles (confidence, decision making, judgment, and unbiased data) [48].

Specifically, research has shown that trust in science is declining among the supporters and members of conservative political orientations [49–51]. This was mostly observed regarding global climate change matters, but it seems that it has been exacerbated by the COVID-19 pandemic. In comparison to liberals, conservatives in general have less trust in science [50]. Nonetheless, the same research indicates that there is a difference when distinguishing among "impact" and "production" scientists, with the former focusing on understanding human health and people's impact on the environment, while the latter focuses on the effects on the economy. The findings suggest that conservatives, compared to liberals, demonstrate greater trust in production scientists than in impact scientists, thus illustrating that the economy plays a key role [50]. The measures enforced by governments worldwide to prevent the spread of the virus may be considered as impact-specific scientific endeavors, with measures such as social distancing.

The COVID-19 pandemic and the public measures taken to slow down the spread of the virus have again underlined the differences between conservatives and liberals. According to recent research, conservatives tend to defy the protective measures and are less concerned about the virus than liberals [51]. Literature supports that conservatives tend to have a conspiratorial way of thinking, believing that presented facts are not, in actuality, the truth [52]. This seems to be magnified when it comes to conspiracies about COVID-19 in particular [51]. Research from the United States has shown that trust in President Trump and the state governors impacted the levels of concern about the virus in the USA, with conservatives trusting the president and federal government more and liberals trusting state governors [51]. Notably, at the same time, conservatives showed less trust in science than liberals, thus illustrating how trust in science can turn into a political issue [51].

Significantly, what seems to have affected trust in science when combined with political orientation is that, although the information about the virus comes from sources of science, governments enforce measures on a political level. In this respect trust in science interplays with trust in the political system and trust in the political authorities. One can have high trust in science, yet low trust in the political institution, which will eventually influence one's response. Results from the Special Eurobarometer show that respondents tend to agree that scientists should intervene in political debate to ensure that decisions take into account scientific evidence (68%), with fewer agreeing with the opposite statement that scientists should not intervene in political debate when decisions ignore scientific evidence (39%) [46].

Political orientation was also found to significantly impact susceptibility to misinformation, with greater susceptibility observed in conservatives than in liberals in Spain, Ireland, and Mexico [53]. Moreover, a longitudinal survey study has shown that political orientation is related to the accuracy of information people believe. Specifically, liberals were more likely to believe more accurate statements about the pandemic than conservatives [30].

It is important to note that the association of political orientation with trust in science is complicated and is much less apparent in some countries. For instance, in some countries, opposition to the elite, often found in political stances such as populism, is what influences the level of trust in science [54]. The followers of this stance hold that true knowledge comes from ordinary people and not from the elite, which are usually considered to be the ones that are wealthy or well educated [55]. A study conducted in Switzerland during the COVID-19 pandemic found that science-related populist attitudes decreased after the pandemic [55], thus indicating that the pandemic minimized the strong ideas they held about science.

3.3. Education

Education has been shown to influence general trust [56] and trust in science [57]. Education has been viewed as an essential factor for trust in science. This is largely because more educated people are arguably more able to access scientific information and understand their findings than their less-educated counterparts. Research has shown that education, in terms of traditional education and in terms of scientific knowledge, are both predictive factors of trust in science [58,59]. Moreover, in terms of analytical thinking and cognitive reflection, education is a critical factor in processing information, therefore leading people towards trust in science and the ability to distinguish it from misinformation [60,61].

There is also the suggestion that trust in science is influenced not by the level of schooling one received but rather by the education one achieved. For instance, some argue that highly educated individuals in the humanities or social sciences have lower confidence in science and even decreased trust in science [58,62]. This shows that it is not a simple causal relationship. For instance, studies found a weak association between education level and trust in science [27,63], and there is also support from research that higher education may lead to less trust in science [58]. One possible reason behind this finding is that highly educated individuals demonstrate more critical thinking and search for information before deciding whom to trust.

Importantly, there appears to be a so-called *science confidence gap* that is influenced by the person's education. This term refers to people who place great trust in scientific principles and methods but at the same time do not trust scientific institutions. Research has shown that this gap is smaller among more educated than among less educated individuals [57].

3.4. Socioeconomic Status—Poverty

To our knowledge there has been no study that directly examined the relationship between socioeconomic status and trust in science specifically. Nevertheless, numerous studies have explored trust in general and socioeconomic status. For instance, the financial status of a person, and specifically the income, appears to affect trust attitudes. It has been found that having lower income and education, as well as belonging to a minority group, is associated with low trust [64]. Moreover, a recent study has shown that people who identify themselves as members of a minority group are more likely to be susceptible to misinformation [53]. Minorities who have been discriminated against by the governments show greater distrust in institutions, which may, in turn, affect trust in science [53]. Research also indicates that the higher the household income the higher the trust of individuals and the higher the income inequality the lower the level of social trust [65]. In contrast, there have been studies showing that individuals from poorer backgrounds may be more trusting than those from higher socioeconomic backgrounds [66].

In terms of the pandemic, because public measures are mandated by politicians (governments or states), minorities tend to have lower trust, which in turn affects trust in science [67]. Finally, in the time of the COVID-19 pandemic, research shows that socioeconomic status, particularly poverty, negatively affects the implementation of restrictive measures during a pandemic [25]. Due to the work travel requirements, there is greater mobility demonstrated by these groups, and therefore this in turn increases the risk of people being exposed to the virus [25].

3.5. Personality Traits

The Big Five personality traits have been traditionally considered in psychology to influence a person's behavior. The term does not refer to five single traits, but rather to five broad categories of traits, with each including many personality characteristics [56,68]. The Big Five traits are: neuroticism (emotionally unstable, tensed, anxious), openness (insightful, intellectually curious), agreeableness (helpful, trustful, sympathetic), conscientiousness (responsible, reliable), and extraversion (talkative, outgoing, active) [68]. Research has shown that there seems to be a correlation between trust and certain personality traits. Extraversion has been found to be positively correlated with trust, as extraverted people seem to show cooperative behaviors towards other people [69,70]. Moreover, trust in strangers and friends has been found to have a positive correlation with both agreeableness and openness [68,71].

On the other hand, high levels of neuroticism are linked to lower levels of trust in others [68]. Though the research identifies the personality mentioned above traits as predictors of trust in general, no such link is noted regarding trust in science specifically. However, it can be argued that personality traits such as extraversion, openness, and agreeableness could also play an important role in trust in science.

Furthermore, according to research, people's sense of personal control over their lives positively correlates with trust [72]. This means that people who believe that they are the masters of their fate tend to show more trusting attitudes towards others than those who have a more resigned view of their lives [72]. Recent research has also shown a positive correlation between trust and social intelligence, as people who appear to exhibit high social intelligence tend to be better judges of the trustworthiness of others [73,74].

4. Accuracy of Information and Trust in Science

With the growth of digital technology, information is readily available to the public, allowing people to access scientific information like never before [14]. For instance, via the internet, people can find a lot of information within seconds [14]. On the other hand, having a lot of information available does not necessarily mean that the information is credible. During periods of pandemic, people are bombarded with enormous amounts of information. There is a lot of conflicting scientific information available, which poses a challenge to people who need to filter out the information that is not accurate. Research has shown that the information people consider accurate or not is strongly related to their level of trust in science [30]. Results from the Special Eurobarometer [46] mentioned previously showed that, overall, 86% of the respondents perceive the influence of science and technology on society as positive, a finding that is nine percentage points higher than in 2013. Even in within-country comparison, more than seven in ten respondents in every country think the influence is positive [46]. At the same time, though, when looking at individual questions, one will notice that significant variability in levels of trust in science exists from country to country. More specifically, when asked about agreeing that science and technology could improve everyone's lives but primarily improves the lives of people who are already better off, Cyprus (75%), Hungary (71%), and Bulgaria (70%) had the highest rates whereas Finland, Estonia, and the Netherlands had 9% agreeing with this statement [46]. Concerning the truthfulness of scientists, the Special Eurobarometer [46] data showed that 70% of Germans and Slovenians think scientists are truthful, but only 45% of Slovaks and 36% of Irish think this. Once again, these percentages were also affected by individual factors such as education level, gender, etc. [46]. Thus, the following section describes the relationship between trust in science and the accuracy of information by looking specifically at social media, misinformation, and conspiracy theories.

4.1. Social Media

Nowadays, people tend to rely on the internet to educate themselves on science, technology, politics or even the news around the world. Specifically, it has been noted that social media, rather than webpages or online searches, are now the main source of information for many people [75]. It has also been found that social media (such as Facebook, Instagram, Twitter, YouTube etc.) appear to relate more with trust in science when compared to traditional media or online news [19]. Research shows a positive correlation between trust in science and social media news, as long as the information extracted comes from sources, even scientists, they trust [19,76]. At the same time, however, social media can be a source of misinformation depending on the sources accessed.

The main issue with being informed via social media is the lack of verification or control over what is being published and the possibility of such sources of information being unofficial [53,77] and therefore not scientifically based. A key element of social media is that the more a post is liked, shared, or commented on, the greater its popularity and the more influential it appears to the public. Consequently, with no verification of the accuracy of the information, or the source, misinformation can be widely and continually spread.

Even though social media make science more accessible to everyone, it is hard to put a brake on the spread of misinformation on these platforms. According to research, people who want to influence others about certain scientific matters, such as vaccination, tend to use social media as a platform to be heard by the public [19]. Recent research has shown that people who are informed about COVID-19 via social media are more susceptible to misinformation than those who are informed via other sources [53]. On the other hand, via social media, it is more likely that scientific information will be spread faster and more effectively, as it allows the public to be informed directly from the source, whether it is a scientific institution or a university [19]. Fortunately, the use of social media allows scientists or scientific institutions to correct the misinformation that is being spread [78].

4.2. Misinformation

First and foremost, what needs to be highlighted is that according to cross-cultural research, trust in science is negatively correlated with susceptibility to misinformation [53]. This shows the importance of trusting scientific institutions and scientists for accurate information during a pandemic [53]. As mentioned above, social media are the main source of information for people nowadays. More often than not, people tend to trust what they read online if they believe it comes from a trustworthy source. Although a positive correlation between trust in science and social media has been found, people do not always know the difference between scientific information and misinformation [19]. Therefore, social media can be used to promote both sides. During COVID-19, people have been bombarded with information from mainstream media, online websites, and social media. The difference between mainstream media and social media (or websites) is the accuracy of published information. For example, recent data concerning the most viewed YouTube videos about COVID-19 shows that more than 25% of them had misleading content [79]. Research has shown that more than 40% of British social media users came across misinformation about COVID-19, most of them daily [80]. This would not be a problem if it was not repeated exposure, increasing the belief in such misinformation [81]. It has been shown that people who believe in fake news tend to show lower trust in science and scientists [82]. Moreover, distrust towards the government and mainstream media were predictive factors of believing misinformation as accurate [83,84].

Recent research has shown that people who score higher in numeracy tasks and show more trust in scientists are most likely not to believe misinformation about COVID-19 [53]. In addition, as mentioned above, political orientation seems to have a significant impact on susceptibility to misinformation, with conservatives being more susceptible than liberals. Finally, the same research indicates that people who believe that politicians rather than scientists can deal with the virus are most likely to believe in misinformation [53]. At this point, it has to be noted that although the majority of people consider COVID-19 misinformation as not credible, a significant amount of others do not share the same belief [53].

4.3. Conspiracy Theories

From the early stages of the pandemic, conspiracy theories have been circulating. With the rapid progression of the virus, a lot of unknown variables were at play, and as such, people needed an explanation to make sense of the events. Therefore, conspiracy theories became popular because they provided a context within which people could understand what was happening while simultaneously placing the situation's responsibility on an identifiable party.

Conspiracy theories regarding COVID-19 cover a wide range of information about the pandemic. The most common suggests that the virus was manufactured in a laboratory, is connected to the 5G network, and the governments use it to manipulate people [53,85]. Another conspiracy theory concerning vaccination claims that a microchip is contained in the vaccine to control the population [86]. A recent study has shown that people who believe in conspiracy theories about the pandemic and the virus tend to reject scientific information, affecting their compliance with public measures taken to minimize contagion [87]. Furthermore, the literature indicates that people who believe in one conspiracy theory are more vulnerable to believe in other conspiracy theories [88]. In a recent cross-cultural study, about 16% of the participants supported the trustworthiness of the 5G theory [53].

Furthermore, in the Special Eurobarometer mentioned above [46], Cyprus and Greece had the highest scores (58% and 52%, respectively) on agreeing that there is a cure for cancer and is hidden from the world, compared to Sweden's 4% and Denmark's 5%. A similar picture can be seen when asked about viruses being created in labs to control our freedom, with Cyprus, Romania, and Bulgaria having the highest scores of agreeing to this statement (53% and 52%, respectively) compared to 6% of Denmark and 7% of the Netherlands [46].

These percentages were also affected by individual factors such as education level and gender, thus further supporting the complexity of the issue [46].

5. Trust in Science and Public Policy

Aiming to reduce social interaction and limit the contagion of COVID-19, public health and social measures have been implemented worldwide. On 10th January 2020, following the outbreak of COVID-19, the WHO issued a comprehensive package addressing the management of the unknown virus and encouraged governments globally to follow the guidelines provided [89]. The guidelines were based on the transmissibility of respiratory viruses such as MERS and SARS, as not much was known about the SARS-CoV-2 virus at the time [89]. With a focus on reducing contagion of acute respiratory infections, the guidelines included: avoiding close contact with infected persons, frequent handwashing, avoiding unprotected contact with farm or wildlife animals, the practice of cough etiquette, and enhancement of standard infection prevention and control practices in health care settings. With the development of the pandemic, new data became available to scientists, and as such, new guidelines emerged.

Overall, health protection guidelines are based on scientific research, clinical trials, and experiments. Scientists and scientific institutions propose them because their research shows that they are more effective in containing the spread of the virus. Governments then follow these research-based guidelines and issue mandatory policies for the public to slow down the spread of the virus. Compliance with public measures—whether people follow and adhere to the recommended guidelines provided by governments—is related to various factors, including trust in science [20–28].

At the beginning of the COVID-19 outbreak, most governments decided that people needed to limit their face-to-face contacts to manage this situation better, so they implemented lockdowns and/or curfews. This policy led people who lived or worked in big cities to massively return to their homes in other areas of the city or villages. India was a great example of the effects of such a decision, as the curfew policy forced many workers to return to their villages, even on foot (as public transportation was over capacity), risking the spread of the virus outside the cities in areas which were not medically prepared for the COVID-19 outbreak [90].

As mentioned above, part of the public policies implemented in many countries were the lockdowns and the curfews. Therefore, public policies affected people's freedom and limited their social life. On the other hand, the success in handling this pandemic depends on the implementation of these mandates, and that requires people to trust science and have faith that their government is making the right choices, which will be applied for a limited amount of time. Research suggests that applying the government's measures is affected by people's trust in public institutions, with people trusting the institutions that they consider as more credible sources of information [22]. Subsequently, people's perception of how the government is handling a pandemic such as COVID-19 greatly affects institutional trust, as observed in the previous pandemic of Ebola [25].

6. Trust in Science and Preventive Behaviors

A theoretical model that explains how people behave and cope during extreme stressful and threatening situations is the Protection Motivation Theory [PMT] [91–93]. This model is essential since it effectively determines the individuals who will follow the recommended preventive practices in previous pandemics, such as SARs and H1N1 Influenza [94,95]. According to this model, people are guided by extrinsic and intrinsic factors when performing the desired behavior. This framework suggests two multidimensional determinants of motivation: (a) threat appraisal and (b) coping appraisal. *Threat appraisal* refers to the personal belief and perception of the individual regarding the degree of harm in contracting a disease (perceived severity) and the personal perception of one's possibility to experience harm (perceived vulnerability). *A coping appraisal* is one's belief of the effectiveness of a recommended behavior in preventing or removing the possible harm (response efficacy) and the actual costs associated with performing the recommended behavior (self-efficacy) [91–93]. Studies have shown that the PMT is effective in predicting COVID-19 preventive behavior intentions [96–98].

During periods of crisis, people need to make choices regarding unknown events, such as following public measures or getting vaccinated. Such decisions are often challenging, as people need reassurance that they are making the right choice. The current section examines how trust in science can influence the behavior of individuals by reviewing compliance to the public measures and vaccination decisiveness.

6.1. Compliance with Public Measures

Literature suggests that a complex interplay of factors influences the desire of people to undertake the recommended actions during a crisis, such as the sociodemographic characteristics, knowledge, personal responsibility, perception of personal risk or threat [99], and one's personal stance towards a scientific topic [5], among others. The above factors are tied to trust since information that is coming from trusted sources is more likely to be considered accurate and can influence one's willingness to adhere to the recommended measures [99]. Importantly, trust has been also found to be a predictor of compliance to protective measures [20–28]. Political trust, trust in government, epistemic trust, and trust in science can play a role in an individual's decision and skepticism.

People are more likely to act in accordance with the proposed guidelines if they consider COVID-19 to be a serious risk and if they exhibit trust in science. Plohl and Musil [27] found that though certain factors such as political conservatism, religiosity, conspiracy ideation, and intellectual curiosity did not directly affect compliance, they did affect trust in science, which subsequently affected compliance. Similarly, higher levels of intellectual curiosity indicated greater trust in science and greater compliance with COVID-19 prevention measures [27].

Literature has shown that trust in science is a predictor of following scientific guidelines regarding health issues [36]. Recent research regarding the COVID-19 pandemic indicates that people who have higher levels of trust in science, in terms of scientists and scientific institutions, tend to show more compliance with the public measures [53]. In a study that examined the willingness to engage in behaviors to prevent and contain the spread of the virus in 23 countries, it was found that trust in science, governments, and citizens, played a crucial role in favor of people's compliance and intention to engage in discretionary efforts, a role more significant than the threat of the virus itself [26].

6.2. Vaccination Decisiveness

Vaccination hesitancy has been a serious issue for the past few years, as it was considered a threat to public health worldwide [100]. Research about vaccination against SARS-CoV-2 estimates that if more than 10% of the population refuses to get vaccinated, it could undermine the benefits of vaccination for the whole population [101]. According to recent research, people who trust science in terms of scientists and scientific institutions are more willing to get vaccinated or advise a friend or a family member to do so [53]. As previously mentioned, the source of information is vital in how a person reacts to the COVID-19 guidelines, whether through vaccination or protective measures. Accordingly, studies have found that vaccination hesitancy is correlated with exposure to misinformation and conspiracy theories found mainly online [102,103]. Moreover, in addition to vaccination hesitancy, the prompting of others to refuse vaccination has been linked to conspiracy mentality [104].

Recent research about COVID-19 vaccinations has shown that there are two main factors, aside from trust in science, that have a more substantial causality relation with vaccination hesitancy: (a) the attitudes people have for vaccinations in general and (b) conspiracy mentality about COVID-19 [36]. Regarding the attitudes, a recent international survey with countries with low and middle income [105] showed that individuals who believed in the effectiveness of the vaccine, who had higher knowledge about COVID-19, higher education, and greater worry/fear about the virus, were more likely to accept vaccination against COVID-19 virus. On the contrary, the lower the income, the higher medical issues/chronic disease, and the more the side-effects people perceived the vaccine had, the lower the acceptance of the COVID-19 vaccine. Interestingly, vaccine decisiveness varied according to region. Asian countries with an increased perception of fear regarding the side effects, such as Thailand, Malaysia, and Bangladesh, had less vaccine acceptance, whereas for African countries, their reasoning for less vaccine acceptance was the belief that it was created to harm others [105]. It is essential to consider the factors that affect vaccination hesitancy before developing campaigns for public vaccination. These campaigns should be created according to the target group and not be generic messages [106], accounting for each country's cultural setting [105].

7. Concluding Remarks

The main goal of this entry was to explain the significant role of trust in science during the COVID-19 pandemic. The main conclusions of this entry are the following:

- Trust is a complex concept that is important in many respects.
- A specific type of trust, trust in science, is critical for overcoming the ongoing health crisis. This is because it is associated with the source of information one considers accurate, and it could influence the behavior of individuals regarding unknown events, such as compliance with public measures and vaccination decisiveness. Science is the force that guides the future of societies and the basis of policies made by governments in times of crisis.
- Many factors influence science trust, including religion, political orientation, education, socioeconomic status, and personality traits.
- Since the pandemic is not over yet, and possibly future pandemics will occur again, finding ways to improve the public's trust in science is crucial.
- Scientists and scientific institutions, and consequently governments, should aim at finding ways to help the public comprehend the information presented by scientists. This approach will eventually increase the trust in science, which will be beneficial during the COVID-19 pandemic and future crises that might be encountered.
- Based on some of the cross-country comparisons mentioned in this entry, in addition to the individual factors, each country should look more closely at their individual/unique data and adjust their chosen interventions more targeted than doing so on a national level.

Author Contributions: Conceptualization M.M., A.C., M.A., M.S. and L.C.; investigation, M.M., A.C., M.A., M.S. and L.C.; writing—original draft preparation, M.M., A.C., M.A., M.S. and L.C.; writing—review and editing M.M., A.C., M.A., M.S. and L.C.; supervision M.M., A.C., M.A. and M.S.; project administration M.M., A.C., M.A., M.S. and L.C. All authors have read and agreed to the published version of the manuscript.

Funding: This research received no external funding

Institutional Review Board Statement: Not applicable.

Informed Consent Statement: Not applicable.

Data Availability Statement: Not applicable.

Conflicts of Interest: The authors declare no conflict of interest.

Entry Link on the Encyclopedia Platform: https://encyclopedia.pub/21791.

References

1. World Health Organization, [WHO]. WHO Director-General's Opening Remarks at the Media Briefing on COVID-19 [Press Release]. Available online: https://www.who.int/director-general/speeches/detail/who-director-general-s-opening-remarks-at-the-media-briefing-on-covid-19---11-march-2020 (accessed on 20 November 2021).
2. Mohapatra, R.K.; Pintilie, L.; Kandi, V.; Sarangi, A.K.; Das, D.; Sahu, R.; Perekhoda, L. The Recent Challenges of Highly Contagious COVID-19, Causing Respiratory Infections: Symptoms, Diagnosis, Transmission, Possible Vaccines, Animal Models, and Immunotherapy. *Chem. Biol. Drug Des.* **2020**, *96*, 1187–1208. [CrossRef] [PubMed]
3. Blöbaum, B. Key Factors in the Process of Trust. On the Analysis of Trust under Digital Conditions. In *Trust and Communication in a Digitized World: Models and Concepts of Trust Research*; Blöbaum, B., Ed.; Springer International Publishing: Cham, Switzerland, 2016; pp. 3–25.
4. Cambridge Dictonary (Online). Meaning of Trust in English. Available online: https://dictionary.cambridge.org/dictionary/english/trust (accessed on 20 November 2021).
5. Hendriks, F.; Kienhues, D.; Bromme, R. Trust in Science and the Science of Trust. In *Trust and Communication in a Digitized World: Models and Concepts of Trust Research*; Blöbaum, B., Ed.; Springer International Publishing: Cham, Switzerland, 2016; pp. 143–159.
6. Rothstein, B.; Uslaner, E.M. All for All: Equality, Corruption, and Social Trust. *World Polit.* **2005**, *58*, 41–72. [CrossRef]
7. Rotter, J.B. Interpersonal Trust, Trustworthiness, and Gullibility. *Am. Psychol.* **1980**, *35*, 1–7. [CrossRef]
8. Bakir, V.; Barlow, D.M. Exploring Relationships between Trust Studies and Media Studies. In *Communication in the Age of Suspicion: Trust and the Media*; Bakir, V., Barlow, D.M., Eds.; Palgrave Macmillan UK: London, UK, 2007; pp. 9–23. [CrossRef]
9. Mishler, W.; Rose, R. What Are the Origins of Political Trust?: Testing Institutional and Cultural Theories in Post-Communist Societies. *Comp. Polit. Stud.* **2001**, *34*, 30–62. [CrossRef]
10. Blöbaum, B. Preface. In *Trust and Communication in a Digitized World: Models and Concepts of Trust Research*; Blöbaum, B., Ed.; Progress in IS; Springer International Publishing: Cham, Switzerland, 2016; pp. v–ix.
11. Blois, K.J. Trust in Business to Business Relationships: An Evaluation of Its Status. *J. Manag. Stud.* **1999**, *36*, 197–215. [CrossRef]
12. Kong, D.T.; Dirks, K.T.; Ferrin, D.L. Interpersonal Trust within Negotiations: Meta-Analytic Evidence, Critical Contingencies, and Directions for Future Research. *Acad. Manag. J.* **2014**, *57*, 1235–1255. [CrossRef]
13. Feinstein, N. Salvaging Science Literacy. *Sci. Educ.* **2011**, *95*, 168–185. [CrossRef]
14. Hendriks, F.; Kienhues, D.; Bromme, R. Measuring Laypeople's Trust in Experts in a Digital Age: The Muenster Epistemic Trustworthiness Inventory (METI). *PLoS ONE* **2015**, *10*, e0139309. [CrossRef]
15. Origgi, G. Epistemic Trust. In *Information Evaluation*; John Wiley & Sons, Ltd.: Hoboken, NJ, USA, 2013; pp. 35–54. [CrossRef]
16. Origgi, G. Is Trust an Epistemological Notion? *Episteme* **2004**, *1*, 61–72. [CrossRef]
17. Origgi, G. Epistemic Injustice and Epistemic Trust. *Soc. Epistemol.* **2012**, *26*, 221–235. [CrossRef]
18. Sulik, J.; Deroy, O.; Dezecache, G.; Newson, M.; Zhao, Y.; El Zein, M.; Tunçgenç, B. Facing the Pandemic with Trust in Science. *Humanit. Soc. Sci. Commun.* **2021**, *8*, 301. [CrossRef]
19. Huber, B.; Barnidge, M.; Gil de Zúñiga, H.; Liu, J. Fostering Public Trust in Science: The Role of Social Media. *Public Underst. Sci.* **2019**, *28*, 759–777. [CrossRef] [PubMed]
20. Sailer, M.; Stadler, M.; Botes, E.; Fischer, F.; Greiff, S. Science Knowledge and Trust in Medicine Affect Individuals' Behavior in Pandemic Crises. *Eur. J. Psychol. Educ.* **2021**, *32*, 77–112. [CrossRef]
21. Algan, Y.; Cohen, D.; Davoine, E.; Foucault, M.; Stantcheva, S. Trust in Scientists in Times of Pandemic: Panel Evidence from 12 Countries. *Proc. Natl. Acad. Sci. USA* **2021**, *118*, e2108576118. [CrossRef] [PubMed]
22. Bicchieri, C.; Fatas, E.; Aldama, A.; Casas, A.; Deshpande, I.; Lauro, M.; Parilli, C.; Spohn, M.; Pereira, P.; Wen, R. In Science We (Should) Trust: Expectations and Compliance across Nine Countries during the COVID-19 Pandemic. *PLoS ONE* **2021**, *16*, e0252892. [CrossRef] [PubMed]
23. Dohle, S.; Wingen, T.; Schreiber, M. Acceptance and Adoption of Protective Measures during the COVID-19 Pandemic: The Role of Trust in Politics and Trust in Science. *Soc. Psych. Bull.* **2020**, *15*, 1–23. [CrossRef]
24. Maloney, W.; Taskin, T. *Determinants of Social Distancing and Economic Activity during COVID-19: A Global View. Policy Research, Working Paper*; Policy Research, Working Paper No. 9242; World Bank: Washington, DC, USA, 2020.
25. Mazive, E.; Baza, G.; Xirinda, G.; Manhique, I.; Mouco, J.; Matola, S.; UNU-WIDER. *The Role of Trust and of Poverty in Compliance with Social Distancing Measures in Africa during the COVID-19 Pandemic*; WIDER Working Paper 2021; UNU-WIDER: Helsinki, Finland, 2021; Volume 2021. [CrossRef]
26. Pagliaro, S.; Sacchi, S.; Pacilli, M.G.; Brambilla, M.; Lionetti, F.; Bettache, K.; Bianchi, M.; Biella, M.; Bonnot, V.; Boza, M.; et al. Trust Predicts COVID-19 Prescribed and Discretionary Behavioral Intentions in 23 Countries. *PLoS ONE* **2021**, *16*, e0248334. [CrossRef] [PubMed]
27. Plohl, N.; Musil, B. Modeling Compliance with COVID-19 Prevention Guidelines: The Critical Role of Trust in Science. *Psychol. Health Med.* **2021**, *26*, 1–12. [CrossRef] [PubMed]
28. Stosic, M.D.; Helwig, S.; Ruben, M.A. Greater Belief in Science Predicts Mask-Wearing Behavior during COVID-19. *Pers. Individ. Dif.* **2021**, *176*, 110769. [CrossRef] [PubMed]
29. Sturgis, P.; Brunton-Smith, I.; Jackson, J. Trust in Science, Social Consensus and Vaccine Confidence. *Nat. Hum. Behav.* **2021**, *5*, 1528–1534. [CrossRef] [PubMed]

30. van Stekelenburg, A.; Schaap, G.; Veling, H.; Buijzen, M. Investigating and Improving the Accuracy of US Citizens' Beliefs About the COVID-19 Pandemic: Longitudinal Survey Study. *J. Med. Internet Res.* **2021**, *23*, e24069. [CrossRef] [PubMed]
31. Wellcome Global Monitor 2020: COVID-19. Available online: https://wellcome.org/reports/wellcome-global-monitor-covid-19/2020 (accessed on 3 January 2022).
32. Levi, M.; Stoker, L. Political Trust and Trustworthiness. *Annu. Rev. Polit. Sci.* **2000**, *3*, 475–507. [CrossRef]
33. Davies, B.; Lalot, F.; Peitz, L.; Heering, M.S.; Ozkececi, H.; Babaian, J.; Davies Hayon, K.; Broadwood, J.; Abrams, D. Changes in Political Trust in Britain during the COVID-19 Pandemic in 2020: Integrated Public Opinion Evidence and Implications. *Humanit. Soc. Sci. Commun.* **2021**, *8*, 166. [CrossRef]
34. Nadelson, L.; Jorcyk, C.; Yang, D.; Jarratt Smith, M.; Matson, S.; Cornell, K.; Husting, V. I Just Don't Trust Them: The Development and Validation of an Assessment Instrument to Measure Trust in Science and Scientists. *Sch. Sci. Math.* **2014**, *114*, 76–86. [CrossRef]
35. Oude Groeniger, J.; Noordzij, K.; van der Waal, J.; de Koster, W. Dutch COVID-19 Lockdown Measures Increased Trust in Government and Trust in Science: A Difference-in-Differences Analysis. *Soc. Sci. Med.* **2021**, *275*, 113819. [CrossRef] [PubMed]
36. Allington, D.; McAndrew, S.; Moxham-Hall, V.; Duffy, B. Coronavirus Conspiracy Suspicions, General Vaccine Attitudes, Trust and Coronavirus Information Source as Predictors of Vaccine Hesitancy among UK Residents during the COVID-19 Pandemic. *Psychol. Med. First View.* **2021**, 1–12. [CrossRef] [PubMed]
37. O'Brien, T.L.; Noy, S. Cultural Authority in Comparative Context: A Multilevel Analysis of Trust in Science and Religion. *J. Sci. Study Relig.* **2018**, *57*, 495–513. [CrossRef]
38. Swindal, J. Faith and Reason. Internet Encyclopedia of Philosophy. A Peer-Reviewed Academic Resource. Available online: https://iep.utm.edu/faith-re/ (accessed on 23 November 2021).
39. O'Brien, T.L.; Noy, S. Traditional, Modern, and Post-Secular Perspectives on Science and Religion in the United States. *Am. Sociol. Rev.* **2015**, *80*, 92–115. [CrossRef]
40. Edgell, P.; Hull, K.E. Cultural Schemas of Religion, Science, and Law in Talk About Social Controversies. *Sociol. Forum* **2017**, *32*, 298–320. [CrossRef]
41. Evans, J.H. Faith in Science in Global Perspective: Implications for Transhumanism. *Public Underst. Sci.* **2014**, *23*, 814–832. [CrossRef]
42. BBC News. Coronavirus: South Korea Church Leader Apologises for Virus Spread. *BBC News*. 2 March 2020. Available online: https://www.bbc.com/news/world-asia-51701039 (accessed on 23 November 2021).
43. Wildman, W.J.; Bulbulia, J.; Sosis, R.; Schjoedt, U. Religion and the COVID-19 Pandemic. *Relig. Brain Behav.* **2020**, *10*, 115–117. [CrossRef]
44. Griffith, J. Louisiana Pastor Defies Coronavirus Order, Draws over 1 K People to Services. Available online: https://www.nbcnews.com/news/us-news/louisiana-pastor-defies-coronavirus-order-draws-over-1-000-people-n1168501 (accessed on 22 November 2021).
45. Evans, J.H. Epistemological and Moral Conflict Between Religion and Science. *J. Sci. Study Relig.* **2011**, *50*, 707–727. [CrossRef]
46. European Commission Brussels. Special Eurobarometer 516: European Citizens' Knowledge and Attitudes towards Science and Technology—September 2021. Available online: https://europa.eu/eurobarometer/surveys/detail/2237 (accessed on 5 February 2022).
47. Dictionary.com. Why Do "Left" and "Right" Mean Liberal and Conservative? Available online: https://www.dictionary.com/e/leftright/ (accessed on 23 November 2021).
48. Funk, C.; Hefferon, M.; Kennedy, B.; Johnson, C. *Trust and Mistrust in Americans' Views of Scientific Experts*; Pew Research Center Science & Society: Washington, DC, USA, 2019.
49. Gauchat, G. Politicization of Science in the Public Sphere: A Study of Public Trust in the United States, 1974 to 2010. *Am. Sociol. Rev.* **2012**, *77*, 167–187. [CrossRef]
50. McCright, A.M.; Dentzman, K.; Charters, M.; Dietz, T. The Influence of Political Ideology on Trust in Science. *Environ. Res. Lett.* **2013**, *8*, 044029. [CrossRef]
51. Ruisch, B.C.; Moore, C.; Granados Samayoa, J.; Boggs, S.; Ladanyi, J.; Fazio, R. Examining the Left-Right Divide Through the Lens of a Global Crisis: Ideological Differences and Their Implications for Responses to the COVID-19 Pandemic. *Polit. Psychol.* **2021**, *42*, 795–816. [CrossRef] [PubMed]
52. Lamberty, P.K.; Hellmann, J.H.; Oeberst, A. The Winner Knew It All? Conspiracy Beliefs and Hindsight Perspective after the 2016 US General Election. *Pers. Individ. Differ.* **2018**, *123*, 236–240. [CrossRef]
53. Roozenbeek, J.; Schneider, C.R.; Dryhurst, S.; Kerr, J.; Freeman, A.L.J.; Recchia, G.; van der Bles, A.M.; van der Linden, S. Susceptibility to Misinformation about COVID-19 around the World. *R. Soc. Open Sci.* **2020**, *7*, 201199. [CrossRef] [PubMed]
54. Krange, O.; Kaltenborn, B.P.; Hultman, M. "Don't Confuse Me with Facts"—How Right Wing Populism Affects Trust in Agencies Advocating Anthropogenic Climate Change as a Reality. *Humanit. Soc. Sci.* **2021**, *8*, 255. [CrossRef]
55. Mede, N.G.; Schäfer, M.S. Science Related Populism Declining during the COVID-19 Pandemic: A Panel Survey of the Swiss Population before and after the Coronavirus Outbreak. *Public Underst. Sci.* **2021**, *31*, 211–222. [CrossRef] [PubMed]
56. Oskarsson, S.; Dawes, C.; Johannesson, M.; Magnusson, P.K.E. The Genetic Origins of the Relationship between Psychological Traits and Social Trust. *Twin Res. Hum. Genet.* **2012**, *15*, 21–33. [CrossRef]
57. Achterberg, P.; de Koster, W.; van der Waal, J. A Science Confidence Gap: Education, Trust in Scientific Methods, and Trust in Scientific Institutions in the United States, 2014. *Public Underst. Sci.* **2017**, *26*, 704–720. [CrossRef] [PubMed]

58. Bak, H.-J. Education and Public Attitudes toward Science: Implications for the "Deficit Model" of Education and Support for Science and Technology. *Soc. Sci. Q.* **2001**, *82*, 779–795. [CrossRef]
59. Nisbet, M.C.; Scheufele, D.A.; Shanahan, J.; Moy, P.; Brossard, D.; Lewenstein, B.V. Knowledge, Reservations, or Promise?: A Media Effects Model for Public Perceptions of Science and Technology. *Commun. Res.* **2002**, *29*, 584–608. [CrossRef]
60. De keersmaecker, J.; Roets, A. 'Fake News': Incorrect, but Hard to Correct. The Role of Cognitive Ability on the Impact of False Information on Social Impressions. *Intelligence* **2017**, *65*, 107–110. [CrossRef]
61. Guess, A.; Nagler, J.; Tucker, J. Less than You Think: Prevalence and Predictors of Fake News Dissemination on Facebook. *Sci. Adv.* **2021**, *5*, eaau4586. [CrossRef] [PubMed]
62. Fuller, S. Science Wars. In *Science Wars*; Duke University Press: New York, NY, USA, 1996; pp. 29–60. [CrossRef]
63. Wilgus, S.; Travis, J. A Comparison of Ideal-Point and Dominance Response Processes with a Trust in Science Thurstone Scale. In *Quantitative Psychology*; Wiberg, M., Culpepper, S., Janssen, R., González, J., Molenaar, D., Eds.; Springer International Publishing: Cham, Switzerland, 2019; pp. 415–428.
64. Alesina, A.; La Ferrara, E. Who Trusts Others? *J. Public Econ.* **2002**, *85*, 207–234. [CrossRef]
65. Rainer, H.; Siedler, T. Does Democracy Foster Trust? *J. Comp. Econ.* **2009**, *37*, 251–269. [CrossRef]
66. Brandt, M.J.; Wetherell, G.; Henry, P.J. Changes in Income Predict Change in Social Trust: A Longitudinal Analysis. *Polit. Psychol.* **2015**, *36*, 761–768. [CrossRef]
67. Timmermann, C. Epistemic Ignorance, Poverty and the COVID-19 Pandemic. *ABR* **2020**, *12*, 519–527. [CrossRef] [PubMed]
68. Freitag, M.; Bauer, P.C. Personality Traits and the Propensity to Trust Friends and Strangers. *Soc. Sci. J.* **2016**, *53*, 467–476. [CrossRef]
69. Hiraishi, K.; Yamagata, S.; Shikishima, C.; Ando, J. Maintenance of Genetic Variation in Personality through Control of Mental Mechanisms: A Test of Trust, Extraversion, and Agreeableness. *Evol. Hum. Behav.* **2008**, *29*, 79–85. [CrossRef]
70. LePine, J.A.; Van Dyne, L. Voice and Cooperative Behavior as Contrasting Forms of Contextual Performance: Evidence of Differential Relationships with Big Five Personality Characteristics and Cognitive Ability. *Appl. Psychol.* **2001**, *86*, 326–336. [CrossRef] [PubMed]
71. Dinesen, P.T.; Nørgaard, A.S.; Klemmensen, R. The Civic Personality: Personality and Democratic Citizenship. *Political Stud.* **2014**, *62* (Suppl. S1), 134–152. [CrossRef]
72. Uslaner, E. The roots of trust. In *The Moral Foundations of Trust*; Cambridge University Press: Cambridge, UK, 2022; pp. 76–114. [CrossRef]
73. Hiraishi, K.; Ando, J.; Ono, Y.; Hasegawa, T. General Trust and Individual Differences on the Wason Selection Task with Sharing-Rule. *Psychologia* **2004**, *47*, 226–237. [CrossRef]
74. Sturgis, P.; Read, S.; Allum, N. Does Intelligence Foster Generalized Trust? An Empirical Test Using the UK Birth Cohort Studies. *Intelligence* **2010**, *38*, 45–54. [CrossRef]
75. Brossard, D. New Media Landscapes and the Science Information Consumer. *Proc. Natl. Acad. Sci. USA* **2013**, *110* (Suppl. S3), 14096. [CrossRef] [PubMed]
76. Collins, K.; Shiffman, D.; Rock, J. How Are Scientists Using Social Media in the Workplace? *PLoS ONE* **2016**, *11*, e0162680. [CrossRef]
77. Weingart, P.; Guenther, L. Science Communication and the Issue of Trust. *JCOM* **2016**, *15*, C01. [CrossRef]
78. Vraga, E.K.; Bode, L. Using Expert Sources to Correct Health Misinformation in Social Media. *Sci. Commun.* **2017**, *39*, 621–645. [CrossRef]
79. Li, H.O.-Y.; Bailey, A.; Huynh, D.; Chan, J. YouTube as a Source of Information on COVID-19: A Pandemic of Misinformation? *BMJ Glob. Health* **2020**, *5*, e002604. [CrossRef] [PubMed]
80. OFcom, Making Communications Work for Everyone. Half of UK Adults Exposed to False Claims about Coronavirus. Available online: https://www.ofcom.org.uk/about-ofcom/latest/media/media-releases/2020/half-of-uk-adults-exposed-to-false-claims-about-coronavirus (accessed on 30 November 2021).
81. Pennycook, G.; Cannon, T.D.; Rand, D.G. Prior Exposure Increases Perceived Accuracy of Fake News. *J. Exp. Psych. Gen.* **2018**, *147*, 1865–1880. [CrossRef] [PubMed]
82. Lewandowsky, S.; Oberauer, K. Motivated Rejection of Science. *Curr. Dir. Psychol. Sci.* **2016**, *25*, 217–222. [CrossRef]
83. Kim, M.; Cao, X. The Impact of Exposure to Media Messages Promoting Government Conspiracy Theories on Distrust in the Government: Evidence from a Two-Stage Randomized Experiment. *Int. J. Commun.* **2016**, *10*, 20.
84. van der Linden, S.; Panagopoulos, C.; Azevedo, F.; Jost, J.T. The Paranoid Style in American Politics Revisited: An Ideological Asymmetry in Conspiratorial Thinking. *Polit. Psychol.* **2021**, *42*, 23–51. [CrossRef]
85. Imhoff, R.; Lamberty, P. A Bioweapon or a Hoax? The Link Between Distinct Conspiracy Beliefs About the Coronavirus Disease (COVID-19) Outbreak and Pandemic Behavior. *Soc. Psychol. Personal Sci.* **2020**, *11*, 1110–1118. [CrossRef]
86. Baines, A.; Ittefaq, M.; Abwao, M. #Scamdemic, #Plandemic, or #Scaredemic: What Parler Social Media Platform Tells Us about COVID-19 Vaccine. *Vaccines* **2021**, *9*, 421. [CrossRef] [PubMed]
87. Uscinski, J.E.; Enders, A.M.; Klofstad, C.; Seelig, M.; Funchion, J.; Everett, C.; Wuchty, S.; Premaratne, K.; Murthi, M. Why Do People Believe COVID-19 Conspiracy Theories? *HKS Misinf. Rev.* **2020**. [CrossRef]
88. Miller, J.M. Do COVID-19 Conspiracy Theory Beliefs Form a Monological Belief System? *CJPS* **2020**, *53*, 319–326. [CrossRef]

89. World Health Organization [WHO]. Listings of WHO's Response to COVID-19. Available online: https://www.who.int/news/item/29-06-2020-covidtimeline (accessed on 1 December 2021).
90. Arundhati, R. The Pandemic Is a Portal. Available online: https://www.ft.com/content/10d8f5e8-74eb-11ea-95fe-fcd274e920ca (accessed on 1 December 2021).
91. Rogers, R.W. A Protection Motivation Theory of Fear Appeals and Attitude Change1. *J. Psychol.* **1975**, *91*, 93–114. [CrossRef]
92. Hromatko, I.; Tonković, M.; Vranic, A. Trust in Science, Perceived Vulnerability to Disease, and Adherence to Pharmacological and Non-Pharmacological COVID-19 Recommendations. *Front Psychol.* **2021**, *12*, 1425. [CrossRef]
93. Lahiri, A.; Jha, S.S.; Chakraborty, A.; Dobe, M.; Dey, A. Role of Threat and Coping Appraisal in Protection Motivation for Adoption of Preventive Behavior during COVID-19 Pandemic. *Front. Public Health* **2021**, *9*, 851. [CrossRef] [PubMed]
94. Bults, M.; Beaujean, D.J.; de Zwart, O.; Kok, G.; van Empelen, P.; van Steenbergen, J.E.; Richardus, J.H.; Voeten, H.A. Perceived Risk, Anxiety, and Behavioural Responses of the General Public during the Early Phase of the Influenza A (H1N1) Pandemic in the Netherlands: Results of Three Consecutive Online Surveys. *BMC Public Health* **2011**, *11*, 2. [CrossRef] [PubMed]
95. Sadique, M.Z.; Edmunds, W.J.; Smith, R.D.; Meerding, W.J.; de Zwart, O.; Brug, J.; Beutels, P. Precautionary Behavior in Response to Perceived Threat of Pandemic Influenza. *Emerg. Infect. Dis.* **2007**, *13*, 1307. [CrossRef] [PubMed]
96. Al-Rasheed, M. Protective Behavior against COVID-19 among the Public in Kuwait: An Examination of the Protection Motivation Theory, Trust in Government, and Sociodemographic Factors. *Soc. Work Public Health* **2020**, *35*, 546–556. [CrossRef] [PubMed]
97. Kıcali, Ü.Ö.; Acar, D. An Integrated Approach to COVID-19 Preventive Behaviour Intentions: Protection Motivation Theory, Information Acquisition, and Trust. *Soc. Work Public Health* **2021**, 1–16. [CrossRef] [PubMed]
98. Kowalski, R.M.; Black, K.J. Protection Motivation and the COVID-19 Virus. *Health Commun.* **2021**, *36*, 15–22. [CrossRef] [PubMed]
99. Ahluwalia, S.C.; Edelen, M.O.; Qureshi, N.; Etchegaray, J.M. Trust in Experts, Not Trust in National Leadership, Leads to Greater Uptake of Recommended Actions during the COVID-19 Pandemic. *Risk Hazards Crisis Public Policy* **2021**, *12*, 283–302. [CrossRef] [PubMed]
100. World Health Organization [WHO]. Ten Health Issues WHO Will Tackle This Year. Available online: https://www.who.int/news-room/spotlight/ten-threats-to-global-health-in-2019 (accessed on 25 November 2021).
101. DeRoo, S.S.; Pudalov, N.J.; Fu, L.Y. Planning for a COVID-19 Vaccination Program. *JAMA* **2020**, *323*, 2458–2459. [CrossRef] [PubMed]
102. Lyons, B.; Merola, V.; Reifler, J. Not Just Asking Questions: Effects of Implicit and Explicit Conspiracy Information About Vaccines and Genetic Modification. *Health Commun.* **2019**, *34*, 1741–1750. [CrossRef] [PubMed]
103. Wilson, S.L.; Wiysonge, C. Social Media and Vaccine Hesitancy. *BMJ Glob. Health* **2020**, *5*, e004206. [CrossRef] [PubMed]
104. Chadwick, A.; Kaiser, J.; Vaccari, C.; Freeman, D.; Lambe, S.; Loe, B.S.; Vanderslott, S.; Lewandowsky, S.; Conroy, M.; Ross, A.R.N.; et al. Online Social Endorsement and COVID-19 Vaccine Hesitancy in the United Kingdom. *Soc. Media Soc.* **2021**, *7*, 20563051211008816. [CrossRef]
105. Bono, S.A.; Faria de Moura Villela, E.; Siau, C.S.; Chen, W.S.; Pengpid, S.; Hasan, M.T.; Sessou, P.; Ditekemena, J.D.; Amodan, B.O.; Hosseinipour, M.C.; et al. Factors Affecting COVID-19 Vaccine Acceptance: An International Survey among Low- and Middle-Income Countries. *Vaccines* **2021**, *9*, 515. [CrossRef] [PubMed]
106. Chou, W.-Y.S.; Budenz, A. Considering Emotion in COVID-19 Vaccine Communication: Addressing Vaccine Hesitancy and Fostering Vaccine Confidence. *Health Commun.* **2020**, *35*, 1718–1722. [CrossRef] [PubMed]

encyclopedia

MDPI

Entry

Adverse Events Profile of COVID-19 Preventative Strategies

Kunal M. Ajmera

Department of Hospital Medicine, Calvert Health Medical Center, Prince Frederick, MD 20678, USA; kunalajmera@gmail.com

Definition: The COVID-19 pandemic has caused millions of deaths and has affected most people across the world, either directly or indirectly. Many preventative and therapeutic strategies have been employed since the beginning of the pandemic. With the development of the mRNA vaccine within a year of the start of the pandemic, we are entering a new era of vaccinology, and the adverse event profile of the COVID-19 vaccine is also becoming more apparent with time. While the benefits of the vaccines and other preventative strategies certainly outweigh the risk of adverse events, prospective clinical trials are urgently needed to determine whether specific populations, including those with a personal or family history of autoimmune disease, are at higher risk of developing certain adverse events, in order to minimize risk further.

Keywords: COVID-19; COVID-19 vaccine; adverse events

Citation: Ajmera, K.M. Adverse Events Profile of COVID-19 Preventative Strategies. *Encyclopedia* **2022**, 2, 457–465. https://doi.org/10.3390/encyclopedia2010028

Academic Editors: Stephen Bustin and Raffaele Barretta

Received: 17 December 2021
Accepted: 29 January 2022
Published: 7 February 2022

1. Introduction

The severe acute respiratory syndrome coronavirus 2 (SARS-CoV-2) COVID-19 is a novel RNA β-coronavirus that has spread globally among humans since its first appearance in Wuhan, China. SARS-CoV-2 is known to affect multiple organs in the human body, including the lungs, brain, heart, pancreas, and kidneys. With constant genetic mutation in the virus spike protein resulting in the development of new strains, rises in case numbers have been observed since the start of the pandemic in different parts of the world. Most recently, with rising case numbers caused by the South African Beta variant, many countries have again imposed travel restrictions and nationwide lockdowns. Current knowledge on the safety profile of COVID-19 vaccines is from phase 1–3 randomized controlled trials conducted during the early stage of the vaccine development, and from vaccine safety surveillance programs implemented in several countries. More extensive prospective clinical trials are needed for a complete understanding of COVID-19 vaccines' adverse event profile. Growing evidence suggests autoimmunity is an independent risk factor for developing adverse events post-COVID-19 vaccination. More extensive prospective clinical trials are needed for a complete understanding of COVID-19 vaccines' adverse event profile. This review article summarizes the etiopathology of COVID-19 and some of the uncommon adverse events associated with prevention strategies (primary prevention such as vaccines and secondary prevention such as monoclonal antibodies).

2. COVID-19 Etiopathology

SARS-CoV-2 belongs to the Coronavirus family and is named after the genetically similar SARS-CoV, which caused a pandemic in 2002–2003 [1]. Since the World Health Organization (WHO) declared the start of a pandemic on 11 March 2020 [2], there have been more than 250 million confirmed cases of COVID-19 worldwide, including 5 million deaths, as of 25 November 2021 [3]. Almost 48 million cases have been registered in the US alone, and more than 750,000 people have died as of 28 November 2021 [4]. Common symptoms of infection are a sore throat, dry cough, shortness of breath, fever, chills, loss of appetite, diarrhea, and loss of taste or smell. COVID-19 spreads when either droplets and particles containing the virus from an infected person are exhaled and breathed in by another person, likely standing within six feet, or if these infected droplets and particles reach another person's eyes, nose, or mouth through coughing or sneezing. Touching the mucous membrane lining of the eyes, nose, or mouth with hands that have a virus can also facilitate virus spread. Various reports have been published that report SARS-CoV-2 as a cause of acute respiratory distress syndrome [5], new-onset diabetes [6], cardiovascular adverse events [7], rhabdomyolysis [8,9], and various neurologic complications [10]. The effects on various organs result from direct viral toxicity or indirectly via host immune responses secondary to the infection. COVID-19 exhibits its effects in two stages. The initial stage of virus entry into host cells, by the viral spike protein binding to angiotensin-converting enzyme 2 (ACE2) receptors present on host cells [11,12]. This initial phase is followed by the late stage of hyperimmune response caused by the production of cytokines such as TNF-alpha, GM-CSF, IL-1, IL-6, and interferon-phigamma. The severity of the disease also depends on the host immunity: higher hospitalization rates and more severe symptoms and fatal outcomes have been documented in patients with weak innate immunity, such as in elderly patients and those with co-morbidities such as diabetes, hypertension, obesity, and immunosuppression.

3. Prevention Strategies

3.1. Primary Prevention

Primary prevention strategies aim to prevent the occurrence of COVID-19 in individuals and comprise of the strict usage of face masks, maintaining appropriate social distancing and proper hand hygiene, and widespread vaccination against the viral agent of this disease.

The most commonly administered vaccines in the US are two mRNA vaccines [13] with more than 94% efficacy, made by Pfizer–BioNTech (BNT162b2) and Moderna (mRNA-1273), as well as one modified adenoviral vaccine with more than 65% efficacy made by Johnson and Johnson (Janssen) [14]. The messenger RNA in the mRNA vaccines possesses the genetic information required to produce surface spike proteins. Host antigen-presenting cells enable the recognition of these spike protein antigens by lymphocytes, which produce complementary antibodies. Another means by which the vaccine produces immunity is by inducing CD4+ and CD8+ T cell immune responses. Host CD4+ T cells induce the production of cytokines, whereas CD8+ T cells remove the virus from the intracellular compartment [15,16]. The Janssen vaccine is not a live viral vaccine, but instead carries a modified adenoviral vector with the genetic code for the SARS-CoV-2 spike protein antigen, which triggers an immune response and protects the host against actual viral infection [17]. Some of the other vaccines available outside the US are ChAdOx1-nCoV (non-replicating vector vaccine manufactured by Oxford and AstraZeneca), Gam-COVID-Vac (non-replicating vector vaccine manufactured by Gamaleya Research Institute), CoronaVac (inactivated vaccine manufactured by SinoVac), and BBIBP-CorV and WBIP (inactivated vaccine manufactured by Sinopharm).

Post-Vaccination Adverse Events

In general, vaccines are safe, with common adverse effects of injection site pain, redness, swelling, myalgia, fever, chills, and fatigue. There are currently no absolute contraindications for vaccination, except for a history of allergies or anaphylaxis, which may increase the recipient's risk of experiencing such an adverse event to COVID-19 vaccines. Because the mRNA vaccines are the first of their kind to be licensed for use in humans and have been available for less than a year, data on short- and long-term adverse events are currently limited. The Vaccine Adverse Event Reporting System (VAERS) database, published by the Centers for Disease Control (CDC), USA, aims to assess and report the real-world adverse event profile for these vaccines. Even though VAERS is the only way to assess adverse event profiles on a broad scale, this dataset also has limitations, including passive data collection and underreporting. Therefore, the occurrence of adverse events in real-world populations of vaccinated individuals maybe even higher.

Various case reports and case series of unusual adverse events from the vaccines have been published, some of which have proven fatal. One such adverse event is rhabdomyolysis [11,18–20]. Rhabdomyolysis is a potentially life-threatening clinical syndrome that typically results from a skeletal muscle injury, resulting in the release of toxic levels of myoglobin, electrolytes, enzymes such as, creatinine phosphokinase (CPK), aldolase, lactate dehydrogenase, and other substances into the circulating blood [21]. Common risk factors for rhabdomyolysis include viral infections such as CMV, COVID-19, excess alcohol use, heat exhaustion, over-exercising, or genetic factors [11]. According to VAERS, at least 201 vaccine recipients have experienced this adverse event (of which 110 were male, 86 female, and 5 unknown); of these, 16 individuals (12 male and 4 female) died as of 17 December 2021 [22].

Further analysis by age group reveals that all recipients who experienced this adverse event were over the age of 50. Aggressive intravenous hydration remains the primary mode of treatment for rhabdomyolysis, but this condition often progresses despite treatment, and may lead to renal failure requiring hemodialysis. It is not entirely clear why some vaccine recipients and not others develop rhabdomyolysis post-vaccination; however, currently, the available literature suggests that the presence of autoimmune conditions such as rheumatoid arthritis and the use of medications such as statins may be independent risk factors for the development of post-vaccination rhabdomyolysis [11]. The post-vaccination CPK level should be checked in a larger clinical trial to assess whether the vaccine causes an asymptomatic rise in the CPK level post-administration in all recipients and if only those with risk factors develop the symptomatic stage (i.e., rhabdomyolysis).

Post-vaccination cardiac adverse events are also well documented. As per the VAERS dataset, 2339 vaccine recipients (1113 male, 1189 female, and 37 unknown) have experienced atrial fibrillation (AF) after vaccination, as of 17 December 2021. Of these, 144 (70 female and 74 male) died from this adverse event. Upon further analysis of VAERS data [22], pre-existing cardiac disease increases the risk of cardiac adverse events. The majority of recipients who experienced this adverse event were over the age of 50. Only 175 recipients were under 50 and experienced AF post-vaccination. Overall, Pfizer–BioNTech had the highest incidence of this particular adverse event, and all three individuals below age 50 who died from this adverse event had received the Pfizer–BioNTech vaccination. One newborn age <6 months also experienced AF post-Moderna vaccine administration. AF is usually caused by ectopic foci, single-circuit reentry, or multiple-circuit reentry. Any inflammation of cardiac muscles can make the atria more vulnerable to fibrillation [23]. Typical clinical presentation is the patient displaying chest pain, shortness of breath, chest palpitations, lightheadedness, or dizziness. There is compelling evidence that dysregulated immune systems can produce autoantibodies against specific ion channels on cardiac myocytes, thus promoting cardiac arrhythmias [24]. It is not entirely clear why some patients develop new-onset atrial fibrillation post-vaccination at this time; however, it is possible that when vaccines trigger an immune reaction, a dysregulated immune system resulting from autoimmune conditions can potentially produce autoantibodies against cardiomyocytes or cardiac ion channels, leading to cardiac myocyte inflammation and cardiac arrhythmias.

Reports of post-vaccination myocarditis, pericarditis, ventricular fibrillation, ventricular flutter, and cardiac arrest have also been documented. A total of 2444 vaccine recipients experienced myocarditis, 1916 experienced pericarditis, 254 experienced ventricular tachycardia, 205 had ventricular fibrillation, and 956 experienced cardiac arrest after vaccination. Of these, 47, 13, 28, 53, and 626 vaccine recipients, respectively, died from these adverse events. The age-wise distribution shows that 1784 individuals under the age of 50 developed myocarditis, 1189 developed pericarditis, 89 developed ventricular tachycardia, 34 developed ventricular fibrillation, and 200 vaccine recipients under age 50 developed cardiac arrest. Again, no data are available regarding personal medical history, family history, home medications use, and risk factors for further analysis. The question of why some individuals experience these adverse events remains to be answered. Table 1 summarizes the data on cardiac adverse events following vaccination against COVID-19. Table 2 describes these incidences and deaths by complication and vaccine type.

Table 1. Cardiac adverse events post-COVID-19 vaccination.

Vaccine	Sex	Myocarditis	Pericarditis	Ventricular Tachycardia	Ventricular Fibrillation	Cardiac Arrest
JANSSEN	Female	23	33	07	04	34
	Male	28	47	11	15	57
	Unknown	7	8	-	-	1
MODERNA	Female	273	314	46	40	145
	Male	521	374	59	41	217
	Unknown	15	14	1	-	08
PFIZER-BioNTech	Female	460	422	63	50	211
	Male	1090	694	66	52	263
	Unknown	27	10	1	03	20
Total		**2444**	**1916**	**254**	**205**	**956**
Deaths		**47**	**13**	**28**	**53**	**626**

Table 2. Incidence and death from diabetes post-COVID-19 vaccination.

Vaccine	Sex	Event Reported	Deaths
JANSSEN	Female	268	12
	Male	211	17
	Unknown	15	1
MODERNA	Female	1560	39
	Male	998	62
	Unknown	24	1
PFIZER-BioNTech	Female	2625	41
	Male	1572	64
	Unknown	69	3
Total		7342	240

VAERS data also show that 7342 individuals have so far developed post-vaccination diabetes (Table 2) as of 17 December 2021, although the type of diabetes is not specified. In addition, 1263 recipients under 50 years of age developed diabetes as an adverse event post-vaccination. No data are available on diabetes risk factors among these individuals, such as the family history of diabetes, personal history of obesity, or the presence of prediabetes. It also does not specify whether this adverse event was short-lived or whether these vaccine recipients required longer-term dietary modification, oral hypoglycemic agents, or insulin treatment. Autoimmunity has an acceptable role in the development of diabetes, among many others. Dysfunctional immune responses can trigger the production of tumor necrosis factor (TNF)-α and other pro-inflammatory cytokines, and the production of autoantibodies against the pancreas, resulting in dysregulated insulin production and sensitivity and insulin-dependent diabetes mellitus (IDDM) [25,26]. There have been reports of people who tested positive for glutamic acid decarboxylase (GAD)-65 antibody (an autoantibody against the pancreas) developing diabetes following COVID-19 infection [27]. These findings support the role of autoimmunity in the development of post-COVID-19 diabetes. The role of autoimmunity in the development of new-onset diabetes post-COVID-19 vaccination should be explored.

There have also been 673 documented cases of post-vaccination renal failure (285 females and 379 males), including 227 deaths; 6688 documented cases of stroke (3894 female, 2661 males, and 133 unknown), including 379 deaths; 2542 documented cases of respiratory failure (1153 females and 1371 males), including 806 deaths; 238 documented cases of liver failure (115 females, 117 males, and 6 unknown) including 79 deaths; 1090 documented cases of thrombocytopenia (591 females and 471 males), including 119 deaths; and

462 documented cases of hypothyroidism (425 female, 31 male, and 6 unknown) including 7 deaths after vaccination against COVID-19 [22]. Hypothyroid as an adverse event was seen to be the highest in females receiving Pfizer–BioNTech. Table 3 summarizes the complete adverse event profile. Seventy-four recipients under age 50 developed renal failure, 1413 developed stroke, 214 developed respiratory failure, 48 developed liver failure, 311 developed thrombocytopenia, and 142 recipients under age 50 developed hypothyroidism. The role of autoimmunity has been well-documented in developing thrombocytopenia, cerebrovascular accident (CVA), hypothyroidism, and liver and renal failure [28–32]. In autoimmune conditions, the immune system, upon stimulation with the vaccine, can potentially produce autoantibodies against blood vessels resulting in vasculitis/stroke, thyroid tissue resulting in hypothyroidism, hepatocytes, or platelets resulting in liver failure and thrombocytopenia. Heme protein deposition in renal tubules from autoimmune hemolysis is a well-known cause of autoimmune renal failure [32]. Whether these adverse events are short- or long-term remains to be seen. There are no data on whether these individuals had any risk factors for these conditions, such as personal or family history of autoimmune disorders, history of hypertension, COPD (chronic obstructive pulmonary disease), tobacco use, alcohol use, antiplatelet medications, hepatitis, or fatty liver.

Table 3. Other major adverse events post-COVID-19 vaccination.

Vaccine	Renal Failure	CVA (Stroke)	Respiratory Failure	Liver Failure	Thrombocyto-Penia	Hypothroid
JANSSEN	68	816	267	31	177	28
MODERNA	272	2567	903	80	344	40
PFIZER-BioNTech	333	3305	1372	127	569	389
Total	673	6688	2542	238	1090	462
Deaths	227	379	806	79	119	7

3.2. Secondary Prevention

Secondary prevention strategies for COVID-19 aim to reduce the impact of the disease in individuals who already have it by attenuating progression to later disease stages, using passive immunotherapy with monoclonal antibodies (mAbs). For high-risk, mild-to-moderate, non-hospitalized cases of COVID-19, the US Food and Drug Administration (FDA) approved emergency use of the mAb cocktails casirivimab/imdevimab (REGN-COV2; approved in November 2020) and bamlanivimab/etesevimab (approved on February 2021) [33,34]. Additionally, dexamethasone, remdesivir, and tocilizumab have also been used as a means of secondary prevention for different indications. For example, remdesivir is an antiviral and is the only Food and Drug Administration-approved medicine used in treating hospitalized COVID-19 patients. Systemic corticosteroids such as dexamethasone are standard of care in all COVID-19 patients requiring supplemental oxygen, as it suppresses the cytokine storm induced by the hyperactive immune system [35]. Tocilizumab prevents IL-6, which is involved in the late hyper-inflammatory stage caused by COVID-19 infection [36], by antagonizing IL-6 receptors.

mAbs are particularly useful in the early stages of COVID-19 infection. They bind to the viral spike protein and block viral entry into host cells, thereby preventing viral replication and reducing viral load, which reduces the risk of disease progression to the cytokine-mediated hyperinflammatory phase [37,38]. mAbs are generally safe. The most common adverse events of REGN-COV2 are allergic reactions immediately post-infusion, such as fever/chills, dyspnea, hives, and itching. Some minor local side effects such as bruising, pain, or soreness at the injection site are commonly reported. However, one case report published recently documented life-threatening gastrointestinal (GI) bleeding after infusion with REGN-COV2, requiring admission to an intensive care unit, massive blood transfusion, and urgent hemicolectomy [39]. The pathology report for this individual did not indicate a bleeding site, but showed a viable colon and terminal ileum with diverticulosis. GI bleeding is a well-known side effect of long-term tocilizumab treatment, primarily due to its anti-IL-6 receptor activity, as this receptor is involved in enterocyte proliferation in the GI tract [40,41]. However, the individual in this case study did not have any prior risk factors such as a history of GI bleeding or receipt of antiplatelet or anticoagulant medications. It remained unclear why this patient developed the fatal GI bleed following mAB infusion.

4. Conclusions and Prospects

The development of mRNA vaccines with more than 94% efficacy in less than one year is a highly significant medical achievement. With widespread vaccination still taking place, and the efficacy of the vaccines against new mutated strains of the virus continuously being assessed, it is vital to record and examine their associated adverse event profiles.

Based on this review, it is evident that these adverse events occur equally in both males and females and across all types of vaccines, except for the incidence rate for the development of hypothyroid, which is seen more in females than males. In addition, the older population aged >50 years is at the highest risk for developing severe adverse events for most adverse events, except for the incidence of myocarditis and pericarditis, which was seen to be slightly higher in the younger populations than in the recipients aged >50 years.

Some questions remain to be answered. Prospective clinical trials are required to determine whether the personal history of autoimmune conditions is an independent risk factor for the development of adverse events. Interestingly, the adverse events profile of vaccines is almost identical to the adverse event of actual COVID-19 infection. No other vaccines have had so much of a broad-spectrum adverse events potential in the past. Adjuvant polyethylene glycol used in mRNA vaccines has never been used before in human vaccines. The adjuvants play an essential role in enhancing the desired immune response [42,43]. Adjuvant-induced autoimmune response (ASIA) is also an equally well-known phenomenon, and the role of PEG in inducing an autoimmune reaction to vaccine certainly needs to be explored. Currently, no guidelines are available for vaccination in patients with autoimmune disorders. It is yet to be determined whether certain adverse events generally occur after the first dose itself or only after the second dose. Whether the second dose of the vaccine should be administered at the recommended interval after the first dose in those with autoimmune conditions or if the interval between two doses should be extended to minimize adverse events needs to be looked into. People with known risk factors should be advised to watch for potential adverse events. Having this understanding will also give potential vaccine recipients a chance to decide if they would like to receive the vaccine or not after understanding the risks vs. benefits. The collection of more information on risk factors from prospective studies, such as personal or family histories of autoimmune conditions, co-morbidities, and medications, will help identify patients at greater risk of developing certain adverse events, for whom measures could be taken to mitigate the risk. For example, it may be appropriate to advise short, temporary breaks from medications or substance use, such as statins or alcohol, post-vaccination against COVID-19 to minimize the risk of adverse events such as rhabdomyolysis. Vaccine recipients with risk factors such as obesity or a family history of diabetes should be educated on symptoms of new-onset diabetes such as polyuria, polydipsia, polyphagia, or weight loss, so as to prevent complications from uncontrolled blood sugar levels such as diabetic ketoacidosis. Vaccine recipients with a known underlying cardiac disorder should be advised to watch for symptoms like chest pain, palpitation, or shortness of breath and to seek immediate medical attention in such a case. Knowing about such symptoms would help vaccine recipients seek timely medical attention to minimize the risk of developing complications and further death.

While the benefits of vaccination outweigh the risks and adverse events in the global population, more work is urgently needed to help minimize potentially serious adverse events in high-risk groups.

5. Summary

- The severe acute respiratory syndrome coronavirus 2 (SARS-CoV-2) COVID-19 is a novel RNA β-coronavirus that has caused millions of deaths and has affected most people across the world, either directly or indirectly.
- Primary prevention of the disease is mainly possible due to the rapid advancement of the vaccines, whereas secondary prevention mostly aims at identifying the disease in the early stages and preventing the advancement of the disease with the help of the monoclonal antibodies, or through the use of the interleukin-6 (IL-6), such as tocilizumab.
- With global mass vaccination, we are also learning more about adverse events related to vaccines and other preventative strategies.
- Vaccines and other measures to counter this deadly condition are safe in general and the benefits certainly outweigh the harms. However, growing evidence suggests autoimmunity as an independent risk factor in the development of a higher incidence of various adverse events post-COVID-19-vaccination. It is of utmost importance to develop guidelines regarding COVID-19 vaccination such as the total number of required doses including booster doses, duration between two doses, and post-vaccination monitoring in this group.

Funding: The author has not declared receiving any grant/funding for this research from any funding agency in the public, commercial, or not-for-profit sectors.

Institutional Review Board Statement: This research did not involve humans or animals.

Informed Consent Statement: This research did not involve humans or animals.

Conflicts of Interest: The author reports no conflict of interest (financial or non-financial) in this work.

Entry Link on the Encyclopedia Platform: https://encyclopedia.pub/20419.

References

1. Ksiazek, T.G.; Erdman, D.; Goldsmith, C.S.; Zaki, S.R.; Peret, T.; Emery, S.; Tong, S.; Urbani, C.; Comer, J.A.; Lim, W.; et al. A novel coronavirus associated with severe acute respiratory syndrome. *N. Engl. J. Med.* **2003**, *348*, 1953–1966.
2. Domenico, C.; Vanelli, M. WHO declares COVID-19 a pandemic. *Acta Bio Med. Atenei Parm.* **2020**, *91*, 157.
3. WHO Coronavirus (COVID-19) Dashboard. Available online: https://covid19.who.int/ (accessed on 3 December 2021).
4. COVID Data Tracker. United States COVID-19 Cases, Deaths, and Laboratory Testing (NAATs) by State, Territory, and Jurisdiction. Available online: https://covid.cdc.gov/covid-data-tracker (accessed on 3 December 2021).
5. Xia, B.; Shen, X.; He, Y.; Pan, X.; Liu, F.L.; Wang, Y.; Yang, F.; Fang, S.; Wu, Y.; Duan, Z.; et al. SARS-CoV-2 envelope protein causes acute respiratory distress syndrome (ARDS)-like pathological damages and constitutes an antiviral target. *Cell Res.* **2021**, *31*, 847–860. [CrossRef] [PubMed]
6. Ajmera, K.M. COVID-19 and Its Association with New-Onset Diabetes. *Arch. Clin. Med. Case Rep.* **2021**, *5*, 855–861. [CrossRef]
7. Spinoni, E.G.; Mennuni, M.; Rognoni, A.; Grisafi, L.; Colombo, C.; Lio, V.; Renda, G.; Foglietta, M.; Petrilli, I.; D'Ardes, D. Contribution of atrial fibrillation to in-hospital mortality in patients with COVID-19. *Circ. Arrhythmia Electrophysiol.* **2021**, *14*, e009375. [CrossRef]
8. Buckholz, A.P.; Kaplan, A.; Rosenblatt, R.E.; Wan, D. Clinical Characteristics, Diagnosis, and Outcomes of 6 Patients With COVID-19 Infection and Rhabdomyolysis. *Mayo Clin. Proc.* **2020**, *95*, 2557–2559. [CrossRef]
9. Valente-Acosta, B.; Moreno-Sanchez, F.; Fueyo-Rodriguez, O.; Palomar-Lever, A. Rhabdomyolysis as an initial presentation in a patient diagnosed with COVID-19. *BMJ Case Rep.* **2020**, *13*, e236719. [CrossRef]
10. Alquisiras-Burgos, I.; Peralta-Arrieta, I.; Alonso-Palomares, L.A.; Zacapala-Gómez, A.E.; Salmerón-Bárcenas, E.G.; Aguilera, P. Neurological Complications Associated with the Blood-Brain Barrier Damage Induced by the Inflammatory Response During SARS-CoV-2 Infection. *Mol. Neurobiol.* **2021**, *58*, 520–535. [CrossRef]
11. Ajmera, K.M. Fatal case of rhabdomyolysis post-covid-19 vaccine. *Infect. Drug Resist.* **2021**, *14*, 3929. [CrossRef]
12. Zheng, Y.-Y.; Ma, Y.-T.; Zhang, J.-Y.; Xie, X. COVID-19 and the cardiovascular system. *Nat. Rev. Cardiol.* **2020**, *17*, 259–260. [CrossRef]
13. Meo, S.A.; Bukhari, I.A.; Akram, J.; Meo, A.S.; Klonoff, D.C. COVID-19 vaccines: Comparison of biological, pharmacological characteristics and adverse effects of Pfizer/BioNTech and moderna vaccines. *Eur. Rev. Med. Pharmacol. Sci.* **2021**, *25*, 1663–1669. [PubMed]
14. Livingston, E.H.; Malani, P.N.; Creech, C.B. The Johnson & Johnson Vaccine for COVID-19. *AMA* **2021**, *325*, 1575.

15. Priya, S.A.D.; Kavitha, S.; Venugopal, P.; Sriram, D.K.; George, M. Can mRNA Vaccines Turn the Tables During the COVID-19 Pandemic? Current Status and Challenges. *Clin. Drug Investig.* **2021**, *41*, 499–509.
16. Pfizer and BioNTech Provide Data from German Phase 1/2 Study Further Characterizing Immune Response Following Immunization with Lead COVID-19 Vaccine Candidate BNT162b2. Pfizer. Available online: https://www.pfizer.com/news/press-release/press-release-detail/pfizer-and-biontech-provide-data-german-phase-12-study (accessed on 20 February 2021).
17. Centers for Disease Control and Prevention (CDC). Understanding Viral Vector COVID-19 Vaccines. Available online: https://www.cdc.gov/coronavirus/2019-ncov/vaccines/different-vaccines/viralvector.html (accessed on 3 December 2021).
18. Nassar, M.; Chung, H.; Dhayaparan, Y.; Nyein, A.; Acevedo, B.J.; Chicos, C.; Zheng, D.; Barras, M.; Mohamed, M.; Alfishawy, M. COVID-19 vaccine induced rhabdomyolysis: Case report with literature review. *Diabetes Metab. Syndr.* **2021**, *15*, 102170. [CrossRef] [PubMed]
19. Mack, M.; Nichols, L.; Guerrero, D.M. Rhabdomyolysis secondary to COVID-19 vaccination. *Cureus* **2021**, *13*, e15004. [CrossRef]
20. Tan, A.; Stepien, K.M.; Narayana, S.T.K. Carnitine palmitoyltransferase II deficiency and post-COVID vaccination rhabdomyolysis. *QJM Int. J. Med.* **2021**, *114*, 596–597. [CrossRef]
21. Zager, R.A. Rhabdomyolysis and myohemoglobinuric acute renal failure. *Kidney Int.* **1996**, *49*, 314–326. [CrossRef]
22. United States Department of Health and Human Services (DHHS), Public Health Service (PHS), Centers for Disease Control (CDC)/Food and Drug Administration (FDA), Vaccine Adverse Event Reporting System (VAERS) 1990—12/10/2021, CDC WONDER On-Line Database. Available online: http://wonder.cdc.gov/vaers.html (accessed on 16 December 2021).
23. Nattel, S.; Burstein, B.; Dobrev, D. Atrial remodeling and atrial fibrillation: Mechanisms and implications. *Circ. Arrhythmia Electrophysiol.* **2008**, *1*, 62–73. [CrossRef]
24. Lazzerini, P.E.; Capecchi, P.L.; Laghi-Pasini, F.; Boutjdir, M. Autoimmune channelopathies as a novel mechanism in cardiac arrhythmias. *Nat. Rev. Cardiol.* **2017**, *14*, 521–535. [CrossRef]
25. Scheen, A.J. Pathophysiology of type 2 diabetes. *Acta Clin. Belg.* **2003**, *58*, 335–341. [CrossRef]
26. Greenberg, A.S.; McDaniel, M.L. Identifying the links between obesity, insulin resistance, and beta-cell function: Potential role of adipocyte-derived cytokines in the pathogenesis of type 2 diabetes. *Eur. J. Clin. Investig.* **2002**, *32* (Suppl. S3), 24–34. [CrossRef] [PubMed]
27. Marchand, L.; Pecquet, M.; Luyton, C. Type 1 diabetes onset triggered by COVID-19. *Acta Diabetol.* **2020**, *57*, 1265–1266. [CrossRef] [PubMed]
28. Parikh, N.S.; Merkler, A.E.; Iadecola, C. Inflammation, autoimmunity, infection, and stroke: Epidemiology and lessons from therapeutic intervention. *Stroke* **2020**, *513*, 711–718. [CrossRef] [PubMed]
29. Chong, B.H.; Ho, S.J. Autoimmune thrombocytopenia. *J. Thromb. Haemost.* **2005**, *3*, 1763–1772. [CrossRef]
30. Weetman, A.P. Autoimmune thyroid disease. *Autoimmunity* **2004**, *37*, 337–340. [CrossRef] [PubMed]
31. Stravitz, R.T.; Lefkowitch, J.H.; Fontana, R.J.; Gershwin, M.E.; Leung, P.S.C.; Sterling, R.K.; Manns, M.P.; Norman, G.L.; Lee, W.M.; Acute Liver Failure Study Group. Autoimmune acute liver failure: Proposed clinical and histological criteria. *Hepatology* **2011**, *53*, 517–526. [CrossRef] [PubMed]
32. Qian, Q.; Nath, K.A.; Wu, Y.; Daoud, T.M.; Sethi, S. Hemolysis and acute kidney failure. *Am. J. Kidney Dis.* **2010**, *56*, 780–784. [CrossRef]
33. Deb, P.; Molla, M.M.A.; Saif-Ur-Rahman, K.M. An update to monoclonal antibody as therapeutic option against COVID-19. *Biosaf. Health* **2021**, *3*, 87–91. [CrossRef]
34. NIH. Anti-SARS-CoV-2 Monoclonal Antibodies—COVID 19 Treatment. 2020. Available online: https://www.covid19treatmentguidelines.nih.gov/anti-sars-cov-2-antibody-products/anti-sars-cov-2-monoclonal-antibodies/ (accessed on 3 December 2021).
35. The RECOVERY Collaborative Group. Dexamethasone in hospitalized patients with Covid-19—Preliminary report. *N. Engl. J. Med.* **2020**, *7*, 17.
36. Pettit, N.N.; Nguyen, C.T.; Mutlu, G.M.; Wu, D.; Kimmig, L.; Pitrak, D.; Pursell, K. Late onset infectious complications and safety of tocilizumab in the management of COVID-19. *J. Med. Virol.* **2021**, *93*, 1459–1464. [CrossRef]
37. Baum, A.; Fulton, B.O.; Wloga, E.; Copin, R.; Pascal, K.E.; Russo, V.; Giordano, S.; Lanza, K.; Negron, N.; Ni, M.; et al. Antibody cocktail to SARS-CoV-2 spike protein prevents rapid mutational escape seen with individual antibodies. *Science* **2020**, *369*, 1014–1018. [CrossRef] [PubMed]
38. Both, L.; Banyard, A.C.; van Dolleweerd, C.; Wright, E.; Ma, J.K.; Fooks, A.R. Monoclonal antibodies for prophylactic and therapeutic use against viral infections. *Pediatr. Pol.* **2013**, *88*, T15–T23. [CrossRef] [PubMed]
39. Ajmera, K.M.; Heather, W. Spontaneous Lower Gastrointestinal Bleeding Following Casirivimab/Imdevimab Treatment for COVID-19 Infection: A Case Presentation and Short Literature Review. *Arch. Clin. Biomed. Res.* **2021**, *5*, 756–762.
40. Mauro, A.; De Grazia, F.; Lenti, M.V.; Penagini, R.; Frego, R.; Ardizzone, S.; Savarino, E.; Radaelli, F.; Bosani, M.; Orlando, S.; et al. upper gastrointestinal bleeding in COVID-19 inpatients: Incidence and management in a multicenter experience from Northern Italy. *Clin. Res. Hepatol. Gastroenterol.* **2021**, *45*, 101521. [CrossRef]

41. Rojo, M.; Cano-Valderrama, O.; Picazo, S.; Saez, C.; Gómez, L.; Sánchez, C.; Sanz-Ortega, G.; Torres, A.J. Gastrointestinal Perforation after Treatment with Tocilizumab: An Unexpected Consequence of COVID-19 Pandemic. *Am. Surg.* **2020**, *86*, 565–566. [CrossRef] [PubMed]
42. Watad, A.; Sharif, K.; Shoenfeld, Y. The ASIA syndrome: Basic concepts. *Mediterr. J. Rheumatol.* **2017**, *28*, 64–69. [CrossRef] [PubMed]
43. Chung, Y.H.; Beiss, V.; Fiering, S.N.; Steinmetz, N.F. COVID-19 vaccine frontrunners and their nanotechnology design. *ACS Nano* **2020**, *14*, 12522–12537. [CrossRef] [PubMed]

encyclopedia

MDPI

Entry

Domestic Violence against Women and COVID-19

Constantina Zamba *, Marilena Mousoulidou and Andri Christodoulou

Department of Psychology, Neapolis University Pafos, 2, Danae Avenue, Paphos 8042, Cyprus; marilena.mousoulidou@nup.ac.cy (M.M.); andri.christodoulou@nup.ac.cy (A.C.)
* Correspondence: k.zamba@nup.ac.cy

Definition: Domestic violence against women is defined as harmful behavior that occurs within a home and it involves aggressive and violent conduct towards women. Since the outbreak of the COVID-19 pandemic, and following the restrictions imposed to combat the pandemic (lockdowns, staying at home, isolation), domestic violence against women has increased worldwide. The current entry presents existing knowledge and discusses issues important for public awareness.

Keywords: domestic violence; violence against women; COVID-19; pandemic; lockdown

1. Introduction and History of Domestic Violence

According to Carl Rogers, *"The strongest force of our universe is not overriding power, but love"* [1] (p. 204). Domestic violence is not a new phenomenon [2]. Unfortunately, domestic violence has existed since the dawn of human civilization. Additionally, even today, in some cultures and belief systems, and regardless of the existing human rights, domestic violence within families or towards women, is still encountered [2]. It has been reported that 1 in 3 women have been subject to gender-based violence by their intimate partner or by a non-partner at least once in their lifetime in different regions [3].

Domestic violence against women is not a new phenomenon [4]. It is a multidimensional and complex phenomenon that many have attempted to explain throughout the years [5–7]. It has been influenced mainly by the views of Christian and Judeo cultural and ideological beliefs, law, and Greek philosophy that purported patriarchy—male-dominant behavior which views the male as a superior figure [8]. During the Roman era and under Roman law, a woman was considered to be the property of her husband to do with as he pleased (abuse, beat or kill) as a way of demonstrating who was in control in the home [9]. According to some religions, during the 15th century the husband had the right to judge a woman for the way she behaved and acted [9]. At this stage, domestic violence against women was not evident or yet defined, as a man beating his wife was considered to be an indication that he cared about his wife's soul [9]. During the 15th century in the United Kingdom, a man had the right to be abusive towards his wife in order to maintain discipline in his home and family [9]. All these stereotypes and beliefs were carried over from generation to generation for centuries, making it extremely difficult to prevent these views on gender-based violence [5,10]. Colonial (patriarchal) institutions benefited by the inequality between genders and colonization (power, control, and patronage) as men were further empowered to abuse women [10,11]. This brutality broke down the confidence of many women, and their sense of self, and as a result women were victimized for years [10]. During the 16th and 17th century, women who disobeyed their husbands were still punished [8,11]. For instance, during 1711–1713 in London, it was reported that a man named Antony Pitts beat, kicked, and locked-up his wife, because she disobeyed his order [8].

A new era has begun since 1960, whereby domestic violence against women became more well-known to the media as more cases started being revealed [12]. Additionally, starting in the 1970s, in some States, men were banned from having the right to beat their wife as a stricter enforcement of laws against violence was observed [12,13]. In the 1970s,

Citation: Zamba, C.; Mousoulidou, M.; Christodoulou, A. Domestic Violence against Women and COVID-19. *Encyclopedia* **2022**, 2, 441–456. https://doi.org/10.3390/encyclopedia2010027

Academic Editors: Stephen Bustin and Raffaele Barretta

Received: 16 December 2021
Accepted: 31 January 2022
Published: 6 February 2022

2 to 4 million women still reported abusive behavior by their partners annually [9]. A major change in communities and in many societies began after 1970, when the Women's Movement raised awareness on domestic violence against women. The definition of domestic violence changed form, and laws appeared to be more evident in theory and practice after 1973 [14]. The term "domestic violence", after the Women's Movement, was first used in 1973 without yet being clearly defined [14].

Between 1975 and 1978, 170 shelters for abused women opened worldwide [9,14]. In the U.S. in 1978, more than 300 shelters were established to prevent domestic violence against women. Finally, during the end of the 1970s, domestic violence was defined and considered as a crime as many interventions were justified by the Criminal Justice System of the USA [15]. After the 1980s, emergency hotline services also became more visible, as well as legislation reform, new government programs and policies, and emergency support for women who were victims of domestic violence [9]. Since 1980, more legislation was enacted in different countries demonstrating the massive need to prevent domestic violence against women, a continuous battle that requires further progress [12]. During the 19th century, violence against women from their partners began to be understood [16]. As a social phenomenon, it began to be recognized. Sometimes it was implicitly accepted, and at other times, this phenomenon was ignored completely.

Laws against domestic violence and police interventions became a reality during the 20th century; in fact, convictions and arrests started taking place [16]. It is important to note, however, that since incidents of domestic violence are not always physical and apparent there are reported cases that are not convicted. For instance, the reporting of shouting in a neighbor's house might not be recorded as a notifiable crime [17].

However, since the outbreak of the COVID-19 pandemic, statistical data shows a rapid increase in cases of domestic violence against women [18]. This mainly stemmed from the implications of the restrictions imposed due to the pandemic, such as staying at home and quarantining [19]. Staying at home during COVID-19 is a method used for safety, but not every home felt safe. Domestic violence is a social phenomenon that pervades all cultures, countries, and societies, regardless of demographics, traditions, socioeconomic class, education, and health. Nowadays, it is recognized as a direct or indirect crime. This phenomenon seems to affect the entirety of society [20]. This entry will present an overview of domestic violence in crisis situations and domestic violence's association with COVID-19. It will mainly outline the types of domestic violence, the cycle of abuse, the role of the victim and perpetrator, as well as the effects, after-effects, challenges, and interventions.

2. Defining Domestic Violence, Pandemics, and COVID-19

2.1. *Definition of Domestic Violence*

There are numerous definitions of *Domestic Violence*, also referred to as "Domestic abuse" and "Controlling behavior" and it is defined as any form of behavior that uses control and power on a person without their permission and occurs amongst members under the same household [21]. Abuse can occur in many different types of relationships, such as couples living together, separated, married, dating, as well as in any other type of human relationship and not just between intimate partners. However, the most common form of abuse worldwide is "violence against women". *Violence against women* refers to any act of violence directed against a woman because of her gender. Violence against women is hence seen as gender-based violence [22], and is defined as a chronic syndrome characterized by physical, sexual, emotional or psychological harm in the private or public life of a woman which may include threats, acts of violence, deprivation of liberty, and coercion [23]. Violence against women can be identified in all societies to some degree, including criminal assaults within or outside the home, enforced isolation, not being allowed to contact family or friends, and many others [24].

2.2. Definition of Pandemics

A pandemic is defined as any type of disease that extends massively to large geographical areas, categorized as trans-regional, inter-regional and global [25]. Pandemics are eras of emergencies that have extreme mechanisms of spread which empirically have a spectrum of etiologies and no single accepted definition or explanation of their cause. Some of the most well-known pandemics around the world include COVID-19, HIV, cholera, the black death, influenza, AIDS, West Nile disease, plague, dengue, and obesity [26,27].

2.3. Definition of COVID-19

According to the World Health Organization [WHO], COVID-19 is defined as a disease that is infectious and is mainly caused by a virus called SARS-CoV-2 [28]. It rapidly emerged in December 2019 and continued spreading aggressively worldwide since [29]. It is believed that anyone can become infected with COVID-19 and become ill at any age. The most commonly reported symptoms include headaches, fever, tiredness, cough, loss of smell or taste, loss of appetite, sore throat, diarrhea, rash on skin, and red eyes [28]. Some more serious symptoms that people with COVID-19 experience are: chest pain, difficulty breathing, confusion, loss of speech. Therefore, most cases develop mild or moderately mild symptoms, and the majority of patients recover without being hospitalized. Unfortunately, there are cases whereby hospitalization is necessary, as people experience severe symptoms, becoming seriously ill, and needing longer periods of recovery [28]. By the 10th of December 2021, more than 267,865,289 cases of COVID-19 were reported, of which 5,285,888 died from the disease [30]. According to the WHO [28], as of 9th of December 2021, 8,158,815,265 vaccines were administered worldwide to prevent the spread of the virus [28]. Preventative measures for COVID-19 suggested by the WHO [28] are: (1) vaccination, (2) social distancing, (3) wearing a fitted mask, (4) washing hands regularly (or rubbing hands with antiseptic), (5) covering nose and mouth when sneezing and coughing, (6) choosing open places when visiting others, and (7) self-isolate when feeling unwell and stay at home until fully recovered from the virus [28].

3. Domestic Violence against Women and COVID-19

During the pandemic and lockdowns due to COVID-19, domestic violence increased dramatically [31–34]. Evidence supports that domestic and sexual violence are exacerbated due to numerous factors that stem from disasters (such as war, disease, illness, tsunami, etc.) and pandemics [3,35–41]. Previous research found an association between cases of gender-based violence and crises, with inequity worsening during such periods [32,42–45]. Evidence shows an increase in sexual violence and harassment against women when individuals attempt to procure necessary needs during a crisis, such as food, water, and firewood [32]. It was found that one of the main reasons that domestic violence increases during a virus outbreak is the breakdown and reformation of laws [19], which includes the implementation of lockdowns. Such periods of forced proximity between partners increases the time spent together, and impedes victims of domestic violence from "escaping" their home (such as going to work or to social events) [46,47]. Additionally, due to the fact that social services and police have different emergencies and priorities during a pandemic, victims of domestic abuse may not be as well supported as they were before the pandemic. Similarly, perpetrators are not dealt with in the same manner as they would have been prior to a crisis; therefore, there is a lack of immediate punishment or restrictions [40]. It is worth noting that there have been reports showing that interpersonal ineffectiveness and violence within families increase rapidly during crisis situations [48]. Consequently, the need to increase support for victims has been emphasized, which might minimize violence when people are asked to quarantine or stay at home for longer periods during a crisis [32].

Research focusing on the association between the COVID-19 pandemic and domestic violence is still developing. Previous periods of crisis can provide an indication of what could be expected. Research suggests that intimate partner violence increased in previous disasters, for example, during the Earthquake in Haiti in 2007 [46], during the tsunami in

Asia in 2004 [32], and during Hurricane Katrina in 2005 [46]. Specifically, after the tsunami in Sri Lanka, violence against women and sexual abuse were proven to have an increase in cases [32]. Some outbreaks of previous viruses or diseases, such as Cholera, Nipah, and Ebola caused a huge increase in incidents of domestic violence against women [49,50]. In Africa, when the disease of Ebola began to spread, cases of sexual assault, rape, and violence against women increased as well [51]. Furthermore, crisis situations and domestic violence against women are interlinked [51] due to the many effects and circumstances that occur in people's lives either externally or internally.

Existing evidence supports that COVID-19 has also led to an increase in intimate partner violence, especially towards women [3], or has at least made it more common [52]. Since the outbreak of the pandemic, authorities, governments, and various organizations have begun to warn the public about the possible impacts it will have on areas such as domestic violence [53]. The transmissibility of the virus led many countries to declare mandatory lockdowns to reduce deaths and the further spread of the virus [53]. A global economic crisis ensued, and the circumstances of this crisis triggered many incidents of domestic violence. The stress and discomfort of people began to appear during the lockdowns [54] as people were asked to spend more time at home [55] which had a massive impact on their lives, especially on their psychological well-being. People were asked to confine themselves at home and stay away from family members, friends, schools, and even their workplace in some cases [55]. The latter has severely impacted families as it increased isolation, unemployment, and financial insecurity. All of these factors can escalate domestic violence both by men with a history of abusive behavior, as well as by those without [55].

In addition, domestic violence has become more prevalent during the COVID-19 pandemic [31] due to the increase in drug use [56], unemployment [57], criminal activity [58,59], educational difficulties [60], psychological difficulties [31], and isolation [46,47]. A drastic change in people's everyday life occurred during the pandemic as individuals had to deal with economic uncertainty, mental health problems, well-being difficulties, and negative feelings such as loneliness and anxiety [32]. Moreover, there is ongoing research for global information with regard to the association between domestic violence and COVID-19 worldwide [33,61–78].

3.1. Statistical Data and Percentages of Domestic Violence against Women during COVID-19

Statistical data were gathered, by country, to identify the effect COVID-19 had on domestic violence against women. In Albania, more than 245 cases were reported up to March 2020 [76]. In Argentina, more than 1280 reports were made for violence within families [62]. In Australia, an increase of 40% in calls made by victims asking for immediate help [70] was reported and there was a 75% rise in online searches for "Domestic Violence: How to get help" [71]. In Belgium, there was a 70% increase in calls during the first 16 weeks following the first lockdown [64] by victims. In Canada, 55,000 calls were made to Women's Domestic Helplines, 11,630 of which were never answered due to the massive number of calls received [74].

Inadequate funding for shelters, helplines, staff salaries, and other operating costs in such a hectic period during the pandemic was also a limitation in preventing domestic violence against women in many countries [66]. In China, 90% of reports were related to domestic violence [78]. In Colombia, 225% increase in cases were recorded during the first lockdown [69]. In Cyprus, a 30% increase was observed in helpline calling centers during the announcement of the first restrictions and the first lockdown [79]. In Fiji, 500 calls were made by women in April 2020 alone [63] and 1000 reports of violence against women were recorded by the Ministry [68]. In France, a 36% rise in domestic violence was identified by the police in Paris [71]. India reported 587 cases of domestic violence in only March and April of 2020 [75]. Israel reported a 35% increase in domestic violence from March until May 2020 [77].

For many countries, there is no information available regarding domestic violence against women. Additionally, with the continuation of the pandemic and the associated challenges, updated statistics are continuously available. An increase in domestic violence against women has been noted in countries such as the Netherlands, New Zealand, Pakistan, Russia, Singapore, Spain, Tunisia, Turkey, United Kingdom, United States, and Venezuela [40]. Worth mentioning is the fact that the opposite effect was also observed in some countries. For instance, in Denmark there was a rise in homelessness by men who reported experiencing conflicts during the pandemic crisis [73]. Some countries, such as Switzerland and Italy, announced that there was a decrease in calls reporting domestic violence at the beginning of this crisis, which could have been caused by the fact that women might have found it difficult to ask for help during the first lockdown [67]. Additionally, in Germany, at the beginning of the pandemic, domestic violence against women was reported to be 28% lower than during the period of 2018–2019 [61].

3.2. Types of Domestic Violence and Their Association with COVID-19

If the general, the public were asked about the types of violence they associate with domestic violence, and the majority of the respondents would most probably answer that they associate physical violence with domestic violence [80]. Physical abuse is the most recognizable form of abuse as it is clearly the most visible one [81]. It is likely the only abusive behavior we all know. However, it is not the only type of abuse [82]. There are several types, and each type affects people differently. As expected, some types of abuse are perceived to be riskier to an individual than others [83]. Nevertheless, no type of abuse should be regarded as more important than the other. Some of the most common forms of abuse against women include: physical, sexual, psychological, verbal, financial, spiritual, and emotional [84]. The person using abusive behavior would use control and gender privilege to commit any of the aforementioned types [85]. All those types escalated during COVID-19, mainly due to lockdowns and isolation [86]. Recent research concluded that from all the different types of abuse, the psychological one appeared to be the one most frequently reported by victims during COVID-19 [87]. 50% of women reported experiencing verbal/psychological abuse, 40% sexual abuse, and 36% physical abuse [87]. Additionally, 90% of women that experienced abuse during the first lockdown stated that they did not ask for help, and 73% of victims that experienced domestic violence before COVID-19 stated that they also experienced abuse during the first lockdown [88]. There is a lack of research on the types of abuse victims of domestic violence experience the most frequently during COVID-19. This information would have allowed researchers to focus on a particular type of domestic violence. Whether common or not, prevention of all types should be sought.

4. The Effects of COVID-19 in Domestic Violence against Women

Previous pandemics, such as swine flu, influenza, as well as the current COVID-19 pandemic, were found to have many psychological effects on people [72]. Domestic violence against women during COVID-19 has affected women in various ways including experiences of chronic pain, sleep disturbances, changes in everyday life routine, depression symptoms, post-traumatic stress disorder, other types of abuse, brain injuries, sexual diseases, substance abuse and many other psychological symptoms, such as avoidance, anxiety, hyperarousal, low mood, re-experiencing trauma. [72,89–94]. It is clear that the multitude of effects domestic violence has on its victims is exacerbated during periods of crisis. According to the United Nations, there are several reasons why domestic violence incidents against women did not show an increase at the start of the pandemic, yet have increased as the pandemic progressed [40]. During the lockdowns, many women lost their jobs or had to work from home, they provided home schooling for their children, and those who lost their jobs became more financially dependent on their partners. Financial dependence on partners is identified as one of the factors that can increase domestic violence against women [95] as it makes it harder for the victim to leave the perpetrator. During lockdowns, individuals also reported experiencing higher levels of distress and depression symptoms [96]. Women coping with mental health difficulties before COVID-19, or who were abused during COVID-19, reported having severe symptoms of stress, depression, and anxiety [96]. Additionally, women abused before and during the pandemic were at a higher risk for mental health-related difficulties [96].

In addition, alcohol sales increased during the lockdowns [97,98], and evidence shows that alcoholism tends to increase the incidence of domestic violence against women [99]. Additionally, closed proximity to male partners during quarantine gives very little to no freedom to women, which can also lead to more domestic violence at home [40]. The fact that many men lost their jobs and income during COVID-19, altered the power dynamics in many homes. Some male figures were left feeling unable to serve the role of provider for their families, which in turn made them experience inadequacy and emasculation [100,101]. Those negative feelings experienced by men were also shown to increase domestic violence against women [101]. Additionally, law enforcement was overwhelmed with new demands during COVID-19, and because of the minimal training and lack of preparation, this resulted in the reduced protection of women who experienced domestic violence by their partners [102]. This also led the victims to become hesitant to report the abuse, and led perpetrators to feel more in control and to continue the abuse. An increase in domestic homicides was also identified since the start of the pandemic [103]. Suicides were also linked to domestic violence and the pandemic [103]. Homicides and suicides illustrate the seriousness of domestic violence during COVID-19, as many women lost their lives due to this aggressive social phenomenon.

4.1. The Role of the Victim

Most victims tend to believe that abuse befalls everyone, that it is unavoidable and difficult to escape [104]. Victims feel that they are being betrayed by their intimate partner every time an abusive behavior occurs. This betrayal, accompanied with the experience of some type of abuse, causes emotional pain to the victim, and often physical injuries as well. In addition, the victim's psychological well-being and health deteriorates [105]. In particular, victims often experience some of the following: (1) live in fear and constant worry about their safety and safety of others, (2) experience loss of self-worth and low self-confidence, (3) dependency on their abuser emotionally and financially, (4) difficulty to end their marriage, (5) daily experience of danger, (6) fear of the unknown if they leave the abuser, (7) passive behavior to protect themselves and others from the experience of more abuse [104].

As mentioned earlier, some countries reported that there was no increase in domestic violence against women. According to the United Nations, this was mainly due to three reasons [40]. Firstly, the women were stuck in the same home as the abuser, which made it more difficult for the victim to escape and reach out for support. Secondly, the women felt uncertain and hesitant to ask for help as they did not know what to expect during lockdowns. Thirdly, domestic violence against women was not the only priority for social services and law enforcement during the pandemic and lockdowns [40]. Victims of domestic violence might have felt abandoned during the pandemic and their assistance options were reduced [104,106]. Additionally, many of the victims might have had to stay with their abuser during quarantines which might have caused them further distress. In cases in which victims were able to access support at a shelter home during lockdowns, the newness of the shelter home added an extra source of insecurity [104,106]. Victims of domestic violence also might have been scared to leave their homes and visit a police station to report domestic violence or visit a hospital to treat their injuries as they feared contracting the virus [106]. Undoubtedly, domestic violence victims have had to face several difficulties during the pandemic.

4.2. The Role of the Perpetrator

Perpetrators demonstrate abusive and aggressive behavior, which may vary in frequency; there are those whose behavior is exhibited more frequently and those who display the behavior on rarer occasions. Abusers usually act compulsively and their behavior can inflict serious emotional and/or physical injuries [104]. Some men with abusive behavior find satisfaction from the suffering of the victim, and abusers can be diagnosed with various personality disorders, aggressive patterns, sociopathic tendencies, and psychological or psychiatric problems [107]. However, perpetrators are not always diagnosed, as most abusers report intense anger and feelings of remorse and guilt after an outburst [104]. Some abusers use aggressive and controlling behavior to achieve what they want. Perpetrators sometimes act in a premeditated fashion and at other times they act compulsively. For a perpetrator, personal gain is more important than what could happen to the victim [104]. Evidence shows that abusers are aware of the impact that their actions could have on a victim but act abusively nonetheless [104,105].

During the pandemic, several studies illustrated that lockdowns gave greater control, power, and freedom to perpetrators to abuse their victims [20,108]. Especially during lockdowns, abusers found it easier to enforce their tactics on their victims since they now had access to any conversation the victims had, access to their social media, their phones, and generally, access to their lives [104]. Additionally, the fact that victims had limited support options during the pandemic, accentuated the power that perpetrators felt over their victims. [109]. The increase in the power and control of the perpetrators, increases the risk of domestic violence against women.

4.3. The Cycle of Violence/Abuse

The cycle of violence identifies three stages (honeymoon period, tension building, and explosive phase), and illustrates that the perpetrator is not always abusive towards a victim [110,111]. This on/off abusive behavior by the perpetrator is what entices victims to stay. A sense of care and love wrongly convinces the victim that there is a good period as well as the honeymoon period. The honeymoon phase usually occurs at the beginning of the relationship. Abusers can highly manipulate their victims, giving them a false belief of security, love, and safety [110]. During this period, there is no sign of violent behavior, and perpetrators often behave in a way that makes their victims desire and appreciate them.

The tension-building phase is usually the time when the victim notices the tension in the relationship and some negative traits of the abuser, such as anger, jealousy, and irritation [110]. At this stage, the victim begins to feel fearful, humiliated, embarrassed, and angry. However, at this stage the perpetrator tries to act 'normal', sometimes trying to explain how they feel, but always nurturing the victim [110]. Lastly, the explosive phase is when the abusive behavior escalates. During this phase, victims may experience emotional, sexual, verbal, physical, or other types of abuse. At this stage, perpetrators have full control and power over the victim and the victim feels frightened, numb, helpless, and trapped [110]. This stage is always followed with apologies and promises for better behavior in the future. The cycle of abuse is experienced repeatedly in many domestic violence cases. During COVID-19, abusers found an opportunity to exercise more coercive control over their victims [112], thus maintaining the tension-building and explosive phases longer than usual.

5. Interventions for the Prevention of Domestic Violence against Women during COVID-19

The rise of domestic violence against women during COVID-19 emphasizes the challenges faced globally and the need for immediate action. The early detection of domestic violence is the first step to intervention. Early detection often occurs by health care professionals during routine check-ups, as research has shown that victims often complain of various symptoms (chronic pain, back pain, headaches, among others) requiring medical attention [113]. However, early detection involves everyone, including health, social and mental health care professionals, people who work in criminal justice settings and abuse services, police officers, victims of violence, and the general public among others [114]. Awareness of the signs of domestic violence and reporting such an awareness to the appropriate agency is important for both professionals and the general public. Evidence suggests that multi-disciplinary interventions can minimize the shadow of domestic violence [115]. Some interventions suggested in related research include (1) reform or development of regulations and laws, (2) development of educational programs, (3) development of new shelters, (4) improvement of mental health support, (5) development of face-to-face solutions, (6) creation of virtual solutions, and (7) creation of new escape plans [115].

5.1. Reform or Development of Regulations and Laws

The reform and development of regulations and laws can further improve the prevention of domestic violence against women. A possible way is through the development of a national registration system for abusers that would allow people to investigate whether their partner has a history of abusive behavior [115]. Thus, reducing the potential dangers faced by victims. This database could also provide valuable insight for future cases and could potentially improve the prevention of domestic violence. A national registration system for domestic violence was created in July of 2020 and it is currently being used in China [116]. In some countries, after victims report domestic violence, due to threats and fear for their lives, they drop the charges. New legislation that would accelerate the court action process and at the same time ensure the continuation of the investigation, regardless of whether the victim has recanted the charges, will further prevent the recurrence of domestic violence [19]. It is important, once a report is filed by victims, for police and social services to demand immediate court action according to the assessed risk [19].

5.2. Development of Educational Programs

Educating individuals about domestic violence, the different types of violence, how to seek help and gather support, is important in acknowledging this social phenomenon and preventing it [117,118]. Many non-governmental associations and government organizations are developing psycho-educational programs to inform the public about domestic violence. These psycho-educational programs are available for different communities, such as schools, businesses, companies, universities, among others. Psycho-educational campaigns could inform more women that might be experiencing abuse on how to acknowledge abuse and seek help from the appropriate services [115]. Raising awareness about domestic violence can help both victims and perpetrators seek support and minimize their engagement within the abusive environment. Educating different communities could also help to prevent women from experiencing domestic violence in the future. Changing norms, values, and prejudices towards gender-based violence is a goal that should be relentlessly pursued.

5.3. Development of New Shelters

The essentials that a domestic violence victim requires at a time of crisis are: access to medical support, food, psychological support, social support, and shelter [119]. The opening of more women's shelters that provide the essentials above is vital during times of crises (such as in pandemics and lockdowns). During COVID-19, and especially during lockdowns, many shelters were at full capacity and struggled to accommodate the massive number of domestic violence cases [120–123]. More shelter support services would help to accommodate the higher number of domestic violence victims during crises.

5.4. Mental Health Support and Solutions

Whilst the COVID-19 crisis remains, restrictions such as social distancing and lockdowns will continue to exist. The barrier of social distancing and the inability for in-person interaction due to restrictions, indicate some of the reasons domestic violence victims face difficulties in getting support. The inadequate mental health support services offered during lockdowns can have a great impact on domestic violence cases. During COVID-19, the lack of mental health support was evident, and many people were placed on waiting lists in order to receive support from a psychologist, psychiatrist, or other mental health professionals; something that was also noticed during previous crises [124–127]. Research however suggests, that technology-based interventions can benefit victims that experience domestic violence and can reduce symptoms of anxiety, low mood, and depression, and reduce exposure to abusers [128,129]. Findings suggest that technological interventions and approaches have the potential for better outcomes than face-to-face interventions [130].

Many countries have helplines and virtual help solutions for victim support [131]. There is evidence that online silent services are very effective as victims can ask for help without being easily noticed by the perpetrator [131]. In the UK, statistical data gathered from the "Respect Helpline", which is a helpline that deals with domestic abuse, showed that 581% of victims gathered support through Respects' website, 185% through email, and 97% gathered support through Respects' helpline [132]. Another empowering service is the ad hoc online platform which provides support to victims that are in immediate need. The ad hoc service is already used in France, Norway, Italy, Germany, and Spain, providing in one website, all the resources that a victim of domestic violence needs [115,133]. Developing such platforms worldwide is very important in preventing domestic violence, as these systems were shown to be very effective [134]. During COVID-19, domestic violence helplines, reported that some requests were delayed due to the massive number of victims' requests [135]. More professionals and staff need to be hired to support these services and victims of domestic violence. Governments in different countries need to develop further online help-seeking services and telephone helplines to minimize the effort and time victims need to find or request help [134]. Victims' immediate access to resources and information is another prevention method for domestic violence.

Women tend to find it easier to share information about domestic violence when they are using online support rather than in-person [136]. However, it is crucial that the victim is separated from the abuser when receiving mental health support online as the sharing of domestic violence incidents in front of the abuser can escalate the abuse [115]. Advancing technology-based interventions globally, and offering mental health support worldwide would be beneficial for preventing domestic violence against women [137]. Creating a global mental health system that connects many experts in mental health, would allow victims of domestic violence to receive support promptly [138]. Governments and organizations would have more control of domestic violence cases and would be better equipped to prevent abuse against women and children.

5.5. Real-Time Solutions

During lockdowns, victims of domestic violence only had access to businesses that were essential for survival, mainly supermarkets and pharmacies [115]. Those businesses created a valuable outlet and perhaps their only opportunity to seek help. Some governments established silent mechanisms, such as coded messages, sounds, and alarm buttons and signals, to assist women that experienced abuse to be able to ask for help without being noticed by the abuser [139–141]. Many countries, such as Norway, Spain, the Netherlands, France, and Italy have already created a coded message, namely "Mask 19", that abused women can use to seek help for domestic violence [140,142,143]. In the UK, the code-word "ANI", meaning "Action Needed Immediately", is used by victims of domestic violence in order to request help [144]. With the use of the code-word police or social services are notified, without attracting the attention of the perpetrator [140,144]. It is worth noting that many countries do not yet have coded messages for domestic violence. The use of coded messages could potentially help to reduce domestic violence incidents. For example, training staff of global chain restaurants and coffee shops, in recognizing coded messages could ensure the notification of the appropriate services (police, social services). Additionally, creating one global code message for seeking help could eliminate potential confusion and allow individuals to be cognizant of the meaning of the message and the actions they should undertake.

5.6. Escape Plans

A need to develop new escape plans for victims of domestic violence is highly recommended in times of crisis. More professionals need to be trained and educated on escape plans and risk assessment. Additionally, sound collaborations between services and professionals in multidisciplinary teams, has been found to be more effective for victims when planning escape plans [115]. This is because it is hard for a victim of domestic violence to leave when the perpetrator is at home [83]. A lack of detailed escape plans can place the victim at higher risk, as an escape from the perpetrator can be very dangerous [83]. Victims usually feel more settled when they can obtain some supplies and important documents before they escape. Some important things that domestic violence victims are asked to have access to when planning an escape plan are: bank account details, copies of important documents for victim and children, clothes, house keys, and a phone without tracking settings [145]. Special protection programs for victims need further development in order to ensure the anonymity of the victim for safety purposes [146]. Additionally, the fact that some domestic violence victims are not able to prepare an escape plan, leads to a need for more support during the process after escaping. Some victims are not able to gather some essentials before leaving their home, and services or volunteers in shelters can support these victims and their children by providing these necessities. Creating shelters that not only provide safety but also, psychological support, food, clothing, phone, access to important documents, is vital.

6. Conclusions

- The pandemic resulted in an increase in incidents of domestic violence against women worldwide.
- Domestic violence affects everyone in the society and especially women.
- During the COVID-19 pandemic, restrictions led to grater isolation, financial dependency, insecurity, and passivity of the victim.
- The pandemic period, the perpetrators power and control over the victims was increased.
- The tension-building and explosive phases of the cycle of violence were prolonged.
- It is evident that there is a lack of psychological and practical interventions that could promote mental health and well-being, during the COVID-19 pandemic, particularly for domestic violence victims.
- New multidisciplinary teams and interventions can be established for victims of domestic violence, which may further encourage movements to globally minimize domestic violence tendencies.
- In the context of COVID-19, more research on domestic violence in times of crisis needs to be conducted. Such research should focus on identifying possible solutions, raising awareness of the problem and the resources available to combat the problem, and on the development of new interventions to help the victims.

Author Contributions: Conceptualization C.Z., M.M. and A.C.; investigation, C.Z., M.M. and A.C.; writing—original draft preparation, C.Z., M.M. and A.C.; writing—review and editing C.Z., M.M. and A.C.; supervision C.Z., M.M. and A.C.; project administration C.Z., M.M. and A.C. All authors have read and agreed to the published version of the manuscript.

Funding: This research received no external funding.

Institutional Review Board Statement: Not applicable.

Informed Consent Statement: Not applicable.

Data Availability Statement: Not applicable.

Conflicts of Interest: The authors declare no conflict of interest.

Entry Link on the Encyclopedia Platform: https://encyclopedia.pub/20416

References

1. Rogers, R.C. *A Way of Being*; Houghton Mifflin: Boston, MA, USA, 1980; ISBN 0-395-75530-1.
2. Fader, S. A History of Domestic Violence: How Much Have Things Changed? BetterHelp. Available online: https://www.betterhelp.com/advice/domestic-violence/a-history-of-domestic-violence-how-much-have-things-changed/ (accessed on 9 November 2021).
3. Hunter, J. WHO: 1 in 3 Women Affected by Physical or Sexual Violence. Available online: https://aoav.org.uk/2013/1-in-3-women-to-be-affected-by-physical-or-sexual-violence/ (accessed on 10 November 2021).
4. Fulu, E.; Miedema, S. Violence Against Women: Globalizing the Integrated Ecological Model. *Violence Against Women* **2015**, *21*, 1431–1455. [CrossRef] [PubMed]
5. National Research Council. *Understanding Violence Against Women*; Crowell, N.A., Burgess, A.W., Eds.; The National Academies Press: Washington, DC, USA, 1996. [CrossRef]
6. Miller, S.L. Expanding the Boundaries: Toward a More Inclusive and Integrated Study of Intimate Violence. *Violence Vict.* **1994**, *9*, 183–199. [CrossRef]
7. O'Toole, L.L.; Schiffman, J.R.; Sullivan, R. Preface: Conceptualizing Gender Violence. In *Gender Violence, 3rd Edition: Interdisciplinary Perspectives*; O'Toole, L.L., Schiffman, J.R., Sullivan, R., Eds.; New York University Press: New York, NY, USA, 2007; pp. xi–xvi. [CrossRef]
8. Fox, V.C. Historical Perspectives on Violence Against Women. *J. Int. Women's Stud.* **2002**, *4*, 15–34.
9. National Library of Medicine. Domestic Violence in the 1970s. Available online: https://circulatingnow.nlm.nih.gov/2015/10/15/domestic-violence-in-the-1970s/ (accessed on 2 November 2021).
10. Nicholls, T. Concerning Violence against Women: A Fanonian Analysis of Colonizing the Female Body. *E-Cad. CES* **2012**, *16*. [CrossRef]
11. Breines, I.; Connell, R.; Eide, I. Unesco. In *Male Roles, Masculinities and Violence*; UNESCO Pub.: Paris, France, 2000.
12. Davis, J. Domestic Abuse. In *School of Law Enforcement Supervision Session XVII*; Cabot Police Department: Cabot, AR, USA, 2014.
13. Swisher, K.; Wekesser, C. (Eds.) *Violence Against Women*; Greenhaven Press: San Diego, CA, USA, 1994.
14. Rudnick Law. A Brief History & Overview of Domestic Violence. Available online: https://www.rudnicklaw.com/blog/history-domestic-violence/ (accessed on 24 November 2021).
15. Erez, E. Domestic violence and the criminal justice system: An overview. *Online J. Issues Nurs.* **2002**, *7*, 4.
16. Johnson, R. Changing Attitudes About Domestic Violence. *J. Law Order* **2002**, *50*. 60–62, 64, 65.
17. Elkin, M. Domestic abuse and the criminal justice system, England and Wales—Office for National Statistics. Available online: https://www.ons.gov.uk/peoplepopulationandcommunity/crimeandjustice/articles/domesticabuseandthecriminaljusticesystemengla november2019 (accessed on 26 January 2022).
18. World Health Organization [WHO]. Levels of Domestic Violence Increase Globally, including in the Region, as COVID-19 Pandemic Escalates. Available online: http://www.emro.who.int/violence-injuries-disabilities/violence-news/levels-of-domestic-violence-increase-as-covid-19-pandemic-escalates.html (accessed on 23 January 2022).
19. European Parliament. *Tackling Violence against Women and Domestic Violence in Europe—The Added Value of the Istanbul Convention and Remaining Challenges*; Think Tank; European Parliament: Brussels, Beligium, 2020.
20. Repucci, S.; Slipowitz, A. Democracy under Lockdown: The Impact of COVID-19 on the Global Struggle for Freedom. Available online: https://freedomhouse.org/report/special-report/2020/democracy-under-lockdown (accessed on 27 December 2021).
21. United Nations. What Is Domestic Abuse? Available online: https://www.un.org/en/coronavirus/what-is-domestic-abuse (accessed on 14 December 2021).
22. Perrin, N.; Marsh, M.; Clough, A.; Desgroppes, A.; Yope Phanuel, C.; Abdi, A.; Kaburu, F.; Heitmann, S.; Yamashina, M.; Ross, B.; et al. Social Norms and Beliefs about Gender Based Violence Scale: A Measure for Use with Gender Based Violence Prevention Programs in Low-Resource and Humanitarian Settings. *Confl. Health* **2019**, *13*, 6. [CrossRef]
23. World Health Organization [WHO]. *Domestic Violence: A Priority Public Health Issue in the Western Pacific Region*; Regional Office for the Western Pacific: Manila, Philippine, 1998.
24. Hegarty, K.; Roberts, G. How common is domestic violence against women? The definition of partner abuse in prevalence studies. *Aust. New Zealand J. Public Health* **1998**, *22*, 49–54. [CrossRef]
25. Taubenberger, J.K.; Morens, D.M. Pandemic Influenza—Including a Risk Assessment of H5N1. *Rev. Sci. Tech.* **2009**, *28*, 187–202. [CrossRef]
26. Morens, D.M.; Folkers, G.K.; Fauci, A.S. What Is a Pandemic? *J. Infect. Dis.* **2009**, *200*, 1018–1021. [CrossRef]
27. United Nation Women. The Shadow Pandemic: Violence against Women during COVID-19. UN Women—Europe and Central Asia. Available online: https://eca.unwomen.org/en/news/in-focus/in-focus-gender-equality-in-covid-19-response/violence-against-women-during-covid-19?fbclid=IwAR2VF8TfTPkkzusNRWLxjk4luVRCpwg4p4H0xsTjW35QTUHj0lCCXQPk8zE (accessed on 10 December 2021).
28. World Health Organization [WHO]. Coronavirus disease—(COVID-19). Available online: https://www.who.int/westernpacific/health-topics/coronavirus (accessed on 28 November 2021).
29. Anastasiades, E.; Argyrides, M.; Mousoulidou, M. Misinformation about COVID-19: Psychological Insights. *Encyclopedia* **2021**, *1*, 1200–1214. [CrossRef]

30. Worlds Health Organisation [WHO]. WHO Coronavirus (COVID-19) Dashboard. Available online: https://covid19.who.int (accessed on 27 November 2021).
31. World Health Organization [WHO]. WHO Health Emergency Dashboard. Available online: https://extranet.who.int/publicemergency (accessed on 27 November 2021).
32. Mittal, S.; Singh, T. Gender-Based Violence During COVID-19 Pandemic: A Mini-Review. *Front. Glob. Women's Health* **2020**, *1*, 4. [CrossRef] [PubMed]
33. International Federation of Red Cross and Red Crescent Societies. *World Disasters Report 2015*; IFRC Campaigns: Lyon, France, 2020.
34. New Zealand Family Violence Clearinghouse (NZFVC). Preventing and responding to family, whānau and sexual violence during COVID-19. Available online: https://nzfvc.org.nz/COVID-19/preventing-responding-violence-COVID-19 (accessed on 30 November 2021).
35. Buttell, F.P.; Carney, M.M. Examining the Impact of Hurricane Katrina on Police Responses to Domestic Violence. *J. Traumatol.* **2009**, *15*, 6–9. [CrossRef]
36. Enarson, E.; Chakrabarti, P.G.D. *Women, Gender and Disaster: Global Issues and Initiatives*; SAGE Publications India Pvt Ltd.: New Dheli, India, 2009.
37. Peterman, A.; Potts, A.; O'Dennell, M.; Thompson, K.; Shah, N.; Oertelt-Prigione, S.; Van Gelder, N. *Pandemics and Violence against Women and Children*; Centrer for Global Development: Washington, DC, USA, 2020.
38. Rescue Organisation. Everything on Her Shoulders: Rapid Assesment on Gender and Violence against Women and Girls in the Ebola Outbreak in Beni, DRC. International Rescue Committee: New York, NY, USA,, 2019.
39. Schumacher, J.A.; Coffey, S.F.; Norris, F.H.; Tracy, M.; Clements, K.; Galea, S. Intimate Partner Violence and Hurricane Katrina: Predictors and Associated Mental Health Outcomes. *Violence Vict.* **2010**, *25*, 588–603. [CrossRef] [PubMed]
40. United Nation Peacekeeping Force in Cyprus (UNFICYP). DOMESTIC VIOLENCE and COVID-19. Available online: https://unficyp.unmissions.org/domestic-violence-and-covid-19 (accessed on 30 November 2021).
41. Weitzman, A.; Behrman, J.A. Disaster, Disruption to Family Life, and Intimate Partner Violence: The Case of the 2010 Earthquake in Haiti. *Sociol. Sci.* **2016**, *3*, 167–189. [CrossRef]
42. Dobson, N. From under the Mud-Pack: Women and the Charleville Floods. *Macedon Dig.* **1994**, *9*, 11–13. [CrossRef]
43. Enarson, E.; Fordham, M. From Women's Needs to Women's Rights in Disasters. *Glob. Environ. Change Part B Environ. Hazards* **2011**, *3*, 133–136. [CrossRef]
44. Fothergill, A.; Peek, L.A. Poverty and Disasters in the United States: A Review of Recent Sociological Findings. *Natural Hazards* **2004**, *32*, 89–110. [CrossRef]
45. Palermo, T.; Peterman, A. Undercounting, Overcounting and the Longevity of Flawed Estimates: Statistics on Sexual Violence in Conflict. *Bull. World Health Organ.* **2011**, *89*, 924–925. [CrossRef]
46. Campbell, A.M. An Increasing Risk of Family Violence during the COVID-19 Pandemic: Strengthening Community Collaborations to Save Lives. *Forensic Sci. Int.* **2020**, *2*, 100089. [CrossRef]
47. Usta, J.; Murr, H.; El-Jarrah, R. COVID-19 Lockdown and the Increased Violence Against Women: Understanding Domestic Violence During a Pandemic. *Violence Gend* **2021**, *8*, 133–139. [CrossRef]
48. UNESCO. 11th Global Summit of National Ethics/Bioethics Committees. Available online: https://en.unesco.org/events/11th-global-summit-national-ethicsbioethics-committees (accessed on 28 November 2021).
49. Davies, S.E.; Bennett, B. A Gendered Human Rights Analysis of Ebola and Zika: Locating Gender in Global Health Emergencies. *Int. Aff.* **2016**, *92*, 1041–1060. [CrossRef]
50. Onyango, A.M.; Resnick, K.; Davis, A.; Shah, R.R. Gender-based violence among adolescent girls and young women: A neglected consequence of the west african ebola outbreak. In *Pregnant in the Time of Ebola: Women and Their Children in the 2013-2015 West African Epidemic*; Schwartz, D.A., Anoko, J.N., Abramowitz, S.A., Eds.; Springer International Publishing: Cham, Switzerland, 2019; pp. 121–132.
51. Yasmin, S. The Ebola Rape Epidemic No One's Talking About:When the Outbreak Hit West Africa, Fevers Spiked—And So Did Rates of Teenage Pregnancy. Available online: https://foreignpolicy.com/2016/02/02/the-ebola-rape-epidemic-west-africa-teenage-pregnancy/ (accessed on 20 November 2021).
52. Kluger, J. Domestic Violence is a Pandemic within the COVID-19 Pandemic. Available online: https://time.com/5928539/domestic-violence-covid-19/ (accessed on 14 November 2021).
53. Perez-Vincent, S.M.; Carreras, E.; Gibbons, M.A.; Murphy, T.E.; Rossi, M. *COVID-19 Lockdowns and Domestic Violence: Evidence from Two Studies in Argentina*; Inter-American Development Bank: Washington, DC, USA, 2020. [CrossRef]
54. Card, D.; Dahl, G.B. Family Violence and Football: The Effect of Unexpected Emotional Cues on Violent Behavior*. *Q. J. Econ.* **2011**, *126*, 103–143. [CrossRef] [PubMed]
55. Piquero, A.R.; Jennings, W.G.; Jemison, E.; Kaukinen, C.; Knaul, F.M. Domestic Violence during the COVID-19 Pandemic—Evidence from a Systematic Review and Meta-Analysis. *J. Crim. Justice* **2021**, *74*, 101806. [CrossRef]
56. Engel, L.; Farley, E.; Tilley, J. *COVID-19 and Opioid Use Disorder*; Council on Criminal Justice: Washington, DC, USA, 2020; Volume 11.
57. Fana, M.; Torrejón Pérez, S.; Fernández-Macías, E. Employment Impact of COVID-19 Crisis: From Short Term Effects to Long Terms Prospects. *J. Ind. Bus. Econ.* **2020**, *47*, 391–410. [CrossRef]

58. Eisner, M.; Nivette, A. Violence and the Pandemic: Urgent Questions for Research. In *HFG Research and Policy in Brief*; Harry Frank Guggenheim Foundation: New York, NY, USA, 2020.
59. Rosenfeld, R.; Lopez, E. Pandemic, Social Unrest, and Crime in U.S. Cities. *Counc. Crim. Justice* **2021**, *33*, 72–82. [CrossRef]
60. OECD. *Lessons for Education from COVID-19: A Policy Maker's Handbook for More Resilient Systems*; Organisation for Economic Co-operation and Development: Paris, France, 2020.
61. Väter ohne Rechte. Frauenorganisationen fürchten um Geld. Available online: https://www.vaeter-ohne-rechte.at/frauenorganisationen-fuerchten-um-geld/ (accessed on 15 December 2021).
62. Argentina, C.-C.S.d.J.d.l.N. La Oficina de Violencia Doméstica Recibió Denuncias Que Comprenden a 1623 Personas afectadas. Available online: http://www.ovd.gov.ar/ovd/verNoticia.do?idNoticia=4307 (accessed on 21 November 2021).
63. Banerjee, S. Coronavirus Lockdown. Pune Zilla Parishad Plans Tough Action to Check Domestic Violence. In *The Hindu*; Pune: Chennai, India, 2020.
64. Belga. Zeventig Procent Meer Oproepen over Geweld Bij Hulplijn 1712 Sinds Lockdown. Available online: https://www.hln.be/nieuws/zeventig-procent-meer-oproepen-over-geweld-bij-hulplijn-1712-sinds-lockdown~{}a669952e/ (accessed on 15 December 2021).
65. Boserup, B.; McKenney, M.; Elkbuli, A. Alarming Trends in US Domestic Violence during the COVID-19 Pandemic. *Am. J. Emerg. Med.* **2020**, *38*, 2753–2755. [CrossRef]
66. CBC News. COVID-19 Exacerbated Violence Against Women. Frontline Workers Want Essential Service Funding. Available online: https://www.cbc.ca/news/canada/british-columbia/covid-intimate-partner-violence-1.5830614 (accessed on 15 December 2021).
67. European Emergency Number Association. *COVID-19: Impact on Mental Health and Domestic Violence*; European Emergency Number Association: Brussels, Belgium, 2020.
68. Fiji Women's Crisis Centre. A "Dangerous" Rise in Domestic Violence in Fiji. Available online: https://www.rnz.co.nz/international/pacific-news/426844/a-dangerous-rise-in-domestic-violence-in-fiji (accessed on 15 December 2021).
69. Janetsky, M. Violence against Women up Amid Latin America COVID-19 Lockdowns. Available online: https://www.aljazeera.com/features/2020/4/20/violence-against-women-up-amid-latin-america-covid-19-lockdowns (accessed on 23 November 2021).
70. Johnston, K. COVID-19 Coronavirus: Domestic Violence is the Second, Silent Epidemic Amid Lockdown. Available online: https://www.nzherald.co.nz/nz/covid-19-coronavirus-domestic-violence-is-the-second-silent-epidemic-amid-lockdown/5ZUPUGT2MBITLISTC4RVGOCK24/ (accessed on 21 November 2021).
71. Kottasova, I.; Donato, D.V. Women Are Using Code Words at Pharmacies to Escape Domestic Violence. *CNN*. Available online: https://edition.cnn.com/2020/04/02/europe/domestic-violence-coronavirus-lockdown-intl/index.html (accessed on 15 December 2021).
72. Mak, I.W.C.; Chu, C.M.; Pan, P.C.; Yiu, M.G.C.; Chan, V.L. Long-Term Psychiatric Morbidities among SARS Survivors. *Gen. Hosp. Psychiatry* **2009**, *31*, 318–326. [CrossRef]
73. Olsen, M. Kø til Mandecenter: Familier Kortslutter efter Ugers Hjemmeisolation. *Politiken.dk*. Available online: https://politiken.dk/forbrugogliv/art7749751/Familier-kortslutter-efter-ugers-hjemmeisolation(accessed on 25 November 2021).
74. Owe, B. 'Back to square one': Calls to domestic violence lines jump again as coronavirus surges—National. *Globalnews.ca*. Available online: https://globalnews.ca/news/7398324/coronavirus-canada-gender-based-violence/(accessed on 22 November 2021).
75. Rukmini, S. Locked down with Abusers: India Sees Surge in Domestic Violence. Available online: https://www.aljazeera.com/news/2020/4/18/locked-down-with-abusers-india-sees-surge-in-domestic-violence (accessed on 25 November 2021).
76. United Nations Development Program. Amidst Coronavirus Pandemic, UNDP Rings the Alarm on Domestic Violence—UNDP in Europe and Central Asia. Available online: https://www.eurasia.undp.org/content/rbec/en/home/stories/coronavirus-pandemic-albania-domestic-violence.html. (accessed on 25 November 2021).
77. Yaron, L. More Women Die by Suicide as the Coronavirus Crisis Ushers in Rise in Domestic Violence. Available online: https://www.haaretz.com/israel-news/.premium-suicide-cases-linked-to-rise-in-domestic-violence-in-wake-of-coronavirus-crisis-1.8835250 (accessed on 22 January 2022).
78. Zhang, W. Domestic Violence Cases Surge During COVID-19 Epidemic. Available online: https://www.sixthtone.com/news/1005253/https%3A%2F%2Fwww.sixthtone.com%2Fnews%2F1005253%2Fdomestic-violence-cases-surge-during-covid-19-epidemic (accessed on 22 November 2021).
79. Association for the Prevention and Handling of Violence in the Family [SPAVO]. 2021 Statistics. Available online: https://domviolence.org.cy/statistika/ (accessed on 24 January 2022).
80. Arizona Coalition to End Sexual and Domestic Violence. Types of Domestic Violence. Available online: https://www.acesdv.org/domestic-violence-graphics/types-of-abuse/ (accessed on 25 January 2022).
81. Doorways. Types of Domestic Violence. Available online: https://www.doorwaysva.org/our-work/education-advocacy/the-facts-about-domestic-violence/types-of-domestic-violence/ (accessed on 25 January 2022).
82. Rakovec-Felser, Z. Domestic Violence and Abuse in Intimate Relationship from Public Health Perspective. *Health Psychol. Res.* **2014**, *2*, 1821. [CrossRef]
83. Davies, J. *Victim-Defined Safety Planning: A Summary*; National Resource Center on Domestic Violence (NRCDV): Harrisburg, PA, USA, 2017.

84. Association for the Prevention and Handling of Violence in the Family [SPAVO]. About Domestic Violence—Association for the Prevention and Handling of Violence in the Family. Available online: https://domviolence.org.cy/en/themata-endooikogeniakis-vias/ (accessed on 25 January 2022).
85. Baugher, A.; Gazmararian, J. Masculine Gender Role Stress and Violence: A Literature Review and Future Directions. *Aggress. Violent Behav.* **2015**, *24*, 107–112. [CrossRef]
86. Evans, M.L.; Lindauer, M.; Farrell, M.E. A Pandemic within a Pandemic—Intimate Partner Violence during COVID-19. *N. Engl. J. Med.* **2020**, *383*, 2302–2304. [CrossRef] [PubMed]
87. United Nation Women. COVID-19 and Violence against Women: What the Data Tells Us. Available online: https://www.unwomen.org/en/news-stories/feature-story/2021/11/covid-19-and-violence-against-women-what-the-data-tells-us (accessed on 25 January 2022).
88. Lausi, G.; Pizzo, A.; Cricenti, C.; Baldi, M.; Desiderio, R.; Giannini, A.M.; Mari, E. Intimate Partner Violence during the COVID-19 Pandemic: A Review of the Phenomenon from Victims' and Help Professionals' Perspectives. *Int. J. Environ. Res. Public Health* **2021**, *18*, 6204. [CrossRef]
89. Reissman, B.D.; Watson, J.P.; Klomp, W.R.; Tanielian, L.T.; Prior, D.S. Pandemic Influenza Preparedness: Adaptive Responses to an Evolving Challenge. *J. Homel. Secur. Emerg. Manag.* **2006**, *3*, 1–28. [CrossRef]
90. Zhang, J.; Lu, H.; Zeng, H.; Zhang, S.; Du, Q.; Jiang, T.; Du, B. The Differential Psychological Distress of Populations Affected by the COVID-19 Pandemic. *Brain Behav. Immun.* **2020**, *87*, 49–50. [CrossRef] [PubMed]
91. Campbell, J.C. Health Consequences of Intimate Partner Violence. *Lancet* **2002**, *359*, 1331–1336. [CrossRef]
92. National Institute of Justice. *Violence Against Women: Identifying Risk Factors, Research in Brief*; National Institute of Justice: Washington, DC, USA, 2004.
93. Jackson, H.; Philp, E.; Nuttall, R.L.; Diller, L. Traumatic Brain Injury: A Hidden Consequence for Battered Women. *Prof. Psychol. Res. Pract.* **2002**, *33*, 39–45. [CrossRef]
94. Walker, L.E.A. Battered-Woman Syndrome. In *The Encyclopedia of Clinical Psychology*; John Wiley & Sons, Ltd.: Hoboken, NJ, USA, 2015; pp. 1–4. [CrossRef]
95. Arthur, C.; Clark, R. Determinants of Domestic Violence: A Cross-National Study. *Int. J. Sociol. Fam.* **2009**, *35*, 147–167.
96. Sediri, S.; Zgueb, Y.; Ouanes, S.; Ouali, U.; Bourgou, S.; Jomli, R.; Nacef, F. Women's Mental Health: Acute Impact of COVID-19 Pandemic on Domestic Violence. *Arch. Womens Ment. Health* **2020**, *23*, 749–756. [CrossRef]
97. Polakovic, G. Pandemic Drives Alcohol Sales—and Raises Concerns about Substance Abuse. Available online: https://news.usc.edu/168549/covid-19-alcohol-sales-abuse-stress-relapse-usc-experts/ (accessed on 20 November 2021).
98. Henson, S. Survey Shows Drug & Alcohol Use Increase During COVID-19 Pandemic. Available online: https://www.therecoveryvillage.com/drug-addiction/news/drug-alcohol-use-rising-during-covid/ (accessed on 15 November 2021).
99. Field, A.C.; Caetano, R.; Nelson, S. Alcohol and Violence Related Cognitive Risk Factors Associated with the Perpetration of Intimate Partner Violence. *J. Fam. Violence* **2004**, *19*, 249–253. [CrossRef]
100. Schneider, D.; Harknett, K.; McLanahan, S. Intimate Partner Violence in the Great Recession. *Demography* **2016**, *53*, 471–505. [CrossRef]
101. Bradbury, J.C.; Isham, L. The Pandemic Paradox: The Consequences of COVID-19 on Domestic Violence. *J. Clin. Nurs.* **2020**, *29*, 2047–2049. [CrossRef]
102. UNISEF GBViE Helpdesk. Emergency Reponses to Public Health Outbreaks. Available online: https://www.sddirect.org.uk/media/1617/health-responses-and-gbv-short-query-v2.pdf (accessed on 19 November 2021).
103. Bates, L.; Hoeger, K.; Stoneman, J.M.; Whitaker, A. *Domestic Homicides and Suspected Victim Suicides During the COVID-19 Pandemic 2020–2021*; Home Office: London, UK, 2021.
104. Fuller, R. *Domestic Violence: Characteristics of Abusers and Victims*; New York Behavioral Health: New York, NY, USA, 2015.
105. Thompson, M.P.; Simon, T.R.; Saltzman, L.E.; Mercy, J.A. Epidemiology of Injuries among Women after Physical Assaults: The Role of Self-Protective Behaviors. *Am. J. Epidemiol.* **1999**, *150*, 235–244. [CrossRef] [PubMed]
106. Fielding, S. In Quarantine with an Abuser: Surge in Domestic Violence Reports Linked to Coronavirus. *The Guardian*, 3 April 2020.
107. Stroshine, S.M.; Robinson, A. The Decision to End Abusive Relationships: The Role of Offender Characteristics. *J. Crim. Justice Behav.* **2003**, *30*, 97–117. [CrossRef]
108. Gearin, M.; Knight, B. Family Violence Prepetrators Using COVID-19 as "a Form of Abise We Have Not Experienced Before". *ABC News*, 28 March 2020.
109. Van Gelder, N.; Peterman, A.; Potts, A.; O'Donnell, M.; Thompson, K.; Shah, N.; Oertelt-Prigione, S. COVID-19: Reducing the Risk of Infection Might Increase the Risk of Intimate Partner Violence. *EClinicalMedicine* **2020**, *21*, 100348. [CrossRef] [PubMed]
110. Astrid Burke Psychotherapy. Understanding Intimate Partner Violence Part II: Disrupting the Cycle of Abuse. Available online: https://www.astridburke.com/blog-posts/understanding-intimate-partner-violence-part-ii-disrupting-the-cycle-of-abuse (accessed on 28 November 2021).
111. Ghani, A.M. Figure 2: The Cycle of Violence in Domestic Violence Relationship. Available online: https://www.researchgate.net/figure/The-cycle-of-violence-in-domestic-violence-relationship_fig4_334537790 (accessed on 28 November 2021).
112. Battered Women's Justice Project. *Coercive Control during COVID-19: New Tactics*. Battered Women's Justice Project. Available online: https://www.bwjp.org/news/covid-coercive-control-wheel-combined.pdf (accessed on 15 November 2021).

113. Di Franco, M.; Martines, G.F.; Carpinteri, G.; Trovato, G.; Catalano, D. Domestic Violence Detection amid the COVID-19 Pandemic: The Value of the WHO Questionnaire in Emergency Medicine. *QJM Int. J. Med.* **2021**, *114*, 637–641. [CrossRef] [PubMed]
114. National Institute for Health and Care Excellence [NICE]. Domestic Violence and Abuse: Multi-Agency Working. Available online: https://www.nice.org.uk/guidance/ph50 (accessed on 3 December 2021).
115. Su, Z.; McDonnell, D.; Roth, S.; Li, Q.; Šegalo, S.; Shi, F.; Wagers, S. Mental Health Solutions for Domestic Violence Victims amid COVID-19: A Review of the Literature. *Glob. Health* **2021**, *17*, 67. [CrossRef]
116. Express Web Desk. Chinese City Launches Database for Couples Considering Marriage to Check If Partner Has Domestic Abuse History. Available online: https://indianexpress.com/article/world/chinese-city-launches-database-for-couples-considering-marriage-to-check-if-partner-has-domestic-abuse-history-6474157/ (accessed on 29 November 2021).
117. McCleary-Sills, J.; Namy, S.; Nyoni, J.; Rweyemamu, D.; Salvatory, A.; Steven, E. Stigma, Shame and Women's Limited Agency in Help-Seeking for Intimate Partner Violence. *Glob. Public Health* **2016**, *11*, 224–235. [CrossRef]
118. Francis, L.; Loxton, D.; James, C. The Culture of Pretence: A Hidden Barrier to Recognising, Disclosing and Ending Domestic Violence. *J. Clin. Nurs.* **2017**, *26*, 2202–2214. [CrossRef]
119. Maslow, A.H. A Theory of Human Motivation. *Psychol. Rev.* **1943**, *50*, 370–396. [CrossRef]
120. Taub, A. A New COVID-19 Crisis: Domestic Abuse Rises Worldwide. *The New York Times*, 6 April 2020.
121. Townsend, M. Revealed: Surge in Domestic Violence during COVID-19 Crisis. *The Observer*, 12 April 2020.
122. Thompson, A. Nation's Largest Hotel Chain Shelters Domestic Abuse Survivors. Available online: https://www.smh.com.au/national/nsw/nation-s-largest-hotel-chain-shelters-domestic-abuse-survivors-20200406-p54hl5.html (accessed on 26 January 2022).
123. Slakoff, D.C.; Aujla, W.; PenzeyMoog, E. The Role of Service Providers, Technology, and Mass Media When Home Isn't Safe for Intimate Partner Violence Victims: Best Practices and Recommendations in the Era of COVID-19 and Beyond. *Arch. Sex. Behav.* **2020**, *49*, 2779–2788. [CrossRef]
124. Xiang, Y.-T.; Ng, C.H.; Yu, X.; Wang, G. Rethinking Progress and Challenges of Mental Health Care in China. *World Psychiatry* **2018**, *17*, 231–232. [CrossRef] [PubMed]
125. Hu, X.; Rohrbaugh, R.; Deng, Q.; He, Q.; Munger, K.F.; Liu, Z. Expanding the Mental Health Workforce in China: Narrowing the Mental Health Service Gap. *Psychiatr. Serv.* **2017**, *68*, 987–989. [CrossRef] [PubMed]
126. Xu, X.; Li, X.-M.; Xu, D.; Wang, W. Psychiatric and Mental Health Nursing in China: Past, Present and Future. *Arch. Psychiatr. Nurs.* **2017**, *31*, 470–476. [CrossRef] [PubMed]
127. Caron, C. 'Nobody Has Openings': Mental Health Providers Struggle to Meet Demand. *The New York Times*, 17 February 2021.
128. Emezue, C.; Bloom, T.L. PROTOCOL: Technology-Based and Digital Interventions for Intimate Partner Violence: A Meta-Analysis and Systematic Review. *Campbell Syst. Rev.* **2021**, *17*, e1132. [CrossRef]
129. Ford-Gilboe, M.; Varcoe, C.; Scott-Storey, K.; Perrin, N.; Wuest, J.; Wathen, C.N.; Case, J.; Glass, N. Longitudinal Impacts of an Online Safety and Health Intervention for Women Experiencing Intimate Partner Violence: Randomized Controlled Trial. *BMC Public Health* **2020**, *20*, 260. [CrossRef]
130. Cohen, J.A.; Mannarino, A.P.; Jankowski, K.; Rosenberg, S.; Kodya, S.; Wolford, G.L. A Randomized Implementation Study of Trauma-Focused Cognitive Behavioral Therapy for Adjudicated Teens in Residential Treatment Facilities. *Child Maltreat* **2016**, *21*, 156–167. [CrossRef]
131. United Nations Population Fund [UNFPA]. Silent Solutions Available to Quarantined Survivors of Domestic Violence. Available online: https://www.unfpa.org/news/silent-solutions-available-quarantined-survivors-domestic-violence (accessed on 11 December 2021).
132. United Nations. UN Supporting 'Trapped' Domestic Violence Victims during COVID-19 Pandemic. Available online: https://www.un.org/en/coronavirus/un-supporting-%E2%80%98trapped%E2%80%99-domestic-violence-victims-during-covid-19-pandemic (accessed on 12 December 2021).
133. Elks, S.; Davies, S. Coronavirus Codewords: Help or Hindrance in Domestic Abuse? *Reuters*, 15 April 2020.
134. Hallsworth, M. Rethinking Public Health Using Behavioural Science. *Nat. Hum. Behav.* **2017**, *1*, 612. [CrossRef]
135. EuroMed Rights. *COVID-19 and the Increase in Domestic Violence against Women. Cases of Jordan, Italy, Morocco and Tunisia*. EuroMed Rights. Available online: https://euromedrights.org/wp-content/uploads/2020/07/Domestic-violence-amid-COVID19-EuroMed-Rights.pdf (accessed on 20 November 2021).
136. Nguyen-Feng, V.N.; Romano, F.N.; Frazier, P. Emotional Abuse Moderates Efficacy of an Ecological Momentary Stress Management Intervention for College Students. *J. Couns. Psychol.* **2019**, *66*, 461–472. [CrossRef]
137. Medecins Sans Frontieres Doctors Without Borders. Discover How We Respond to Emergencies and Manage Our Global Network. Available online: https://www.doctorswithoutborders.org/who-we-are/how-we-work (accessed on 15 November 2021).
138. Su, Z.; McDonnell, D.; Ahmad, J. The Need for a Disaster Readiness Mindset: A Key Lesson from the Coronavirus Disease 2019 (COVID-19) Pandemic. *Infect. Control. Hosp. Epidemiol.* **2021**, 1–2. [CrossRef]
139. World Health Organization [WHO]. The Rrise and Rise of Interpersonal Violence—An Unintended Impact of the COVID-19 Response on Families. Available online: https://www.euro.who.int/en/health-topics/Life-stages/pages/news/news/2020/6/the-rise-and-rise-of-interpersonal-violence-an-unintended-impact-of-the-covid-19-response-on-families (accessed on 9 December 2021).

140. Ertan, D.; El-Hage, W.; Thierrée, S.; Javelot, H.; Hingray, C. COVID-19: Urgency for Distancing from Domestic Violence. *Eur. J. Psychotraumatol.* **2020**, *11*, 1800245. [CrossRef]
141. Leidner, R. *Fast Food, Fast Talk: Service Work and the Routinization of Everyday Life*; University of California Press: Berkeley, CA, USA, 1993.
142. SafeLives. SafeLives Position Paper on the use of a Code Word (ANN - Action Needed Now) for Domestic Abuse Victims During COVID-19. Available online: https://safelives.org.uk/sites/default/files/resources/Domestic%20Abuse%20Code%20Word%20during%20Covid%2019%20-%20SafeLives%20position%20paper%20summary.pdf (accessed on 2 December 2021).
143. Dutch News. Ministry Introduces Code Word "Masker 19" for Domestic Abuse. Available online: https://www.dutchnews.nl/news/2020/05/ministry-introduces-code-word-masker-19-for-domestic-abuse/ (accessed on 23 January 2022).
144. UK Government. Domestic abuse: How to Get Help. Available online: https://www.gov.uk/guidance/domestic-abuse-how-to-get-help (accessed on 9 December 2021).
145. Goodkind, J.R.; Sullivan, C.M.; Bybee, D.I. A Contextual Analysis of Battered Women's Safety Planning. *Violence Against Women* **2004**, *10*, 514–533. [CrossRef]
146. Victim Connect Resource Center. Address Confidentiality. Available online: https://victimconnect.org/learn/address-confidentiality/ (accessed on 23 January 2022).

encyclopedia

MDPI

Entry

Secondary Education and COVID-19

Michailina Siakalli [1,*], Marilena Mousoulidou [2,*], Andri Christodoulou [2], Angela Savvidou [2] and Kyriaki Kouppa [2]

[1] Department of Economics and Business, Neapolis University Pafos, 2 Danaes Avenue, Paphos 8042, Cyprus
[2] Department of Psychology, Neapolis University Pafos, 2 Danaes Avenue, Paphos 8042, Cyprus; andri.christodoulou@nup.ac.cy (A.C.); a.savvidou.1@nup.ac.cy (A.S.); k.koupa@nup.ac.cy (K.K.)
* Correspondence: m.siakalli@nup.ac.cy (M.S.); marilena.mousoulidou@nup.ac.cy (M.M.)

Definition: Secondary education is the second stage of formal education and traditionally begins after primary school, usually about age 11 to 13. The COVID-19 pandemic caused immeasurable changes to the educational system which inevitably greatly impacted secondary education. The current entry describes the changes in secondary education imposed by the pandemic and explores the accompanying challenges.

Keywords: secondary education; COVID-19; challenges

Citation: Siakalli, M.; Mousoulidou, M.; Christodoulou, A.; Savvidou, A.; Kouppa, K. Secondary Education and COVID-19. *Encyclopedia* **2022**, 2, 409–427. https://doi.org/10.3390/encyclopedia2010025

Academic Editors: Stephen Bustin and Raffaele Barretta

Received: 14 December 2021
Accepted: 31 January 2022
Published: 2 February 2022

1. Introduction

The COVID-19 pandemic is an unprecedented crisis. What sets it apart from past health and other crises is that the SARS-CoV-2 virus, because of its high transmissibility, spread worldwide within a short period of time. As of 15 November 2021, there have been over 249 million positive cases and over 5 million deaths documented [1]. As COVID-19 was a novel virus, aside from its transmissibility, nothing was yet known regarding its effects and containment. Therefore, efforts focused on how past epidemics were combated, with social and physical distancing identified as the most successful measure [2,3]. Consequently, countries primarily employed this measure in school settings as a way to prevent the spread [4]. This ultimately led to the complete or partial closing of schools. Contrary to previous outbreaks, where education was disrupted for a short time, COVID-19 was the only pandemic that led to a large-scale and prolonged disruption of education [5].

It is worth noting how education was affected in previous crises. For instance, during the severe acute respiratory syndrome (SARS) outbreak in China in 2003, some governments chose to proceed with school closures as a way to prevent the disease from spreading. SARS's symptoms were similar to those of COVID-19, and it was identified as the first serious transmissible disease to occur in the 21st century [6]. School closures ranged from three weeks in Singapore [7] to over two months in China [8]. Other prevention measures that were applied included class cancellation strategies among upper secondary school and college students [9], mandatory temperature monitoring in primary and lower secondary schools [10,11], and suspension of other child-related activities, such as sports, to prevent large gatherings that could spread the disease [7].

In general, it was found that school closure as a prevention technique did not make a notable difference in the SARS outbreak [12]. This was the case mainly due to the low transmission rate that was reported in educational settings and the low occurrence of the infection in children [8,12,13]. The transmission of SARS among children could be accounted for primarily by households, acquaintances, and relations outside of the school setting [12]. A challenge that occurred from school closures for working parents, especially for those that were healthcare workers, was the additional childcare needs that emerged and the lack of sufficient resources to satisfy them [14,15].

Influenza A (H1N1) was another pandemic of the 21st century. Specifically, it occurred in 2009 in Mexico, and it spread worldwide, with the fatality number reaching 18,449 by

August 2010 [16]. Through the outbreak, school closures in various countries lasted a month or less [17,18]. In some countries, effective alternatives to complete school closures were used. For example, restricting students in one classroom with one main teacher was found to be an effective preventive measure [19,20].

Furthermore, during the Middle East respiratory syndrome (MERS) outbreak in 2015 in South Korea, following 186 confirmed cases and 38 deaths [21], a large number of schools were closed on a national scale. However, school closures were only for 10 days as health experts considered this measure unnecessary [22,23]. Nevertheless, preventive procedures were implemented in educational settings, such as temperature monitoring, which raised concerns from educators. This was because the teachers reported that they did not have the appropriate training to handle and implement such procedures, feared the associated stigma for students that did not meet the temperature criteria, and had an increased workload [24].

Notably, the largest impact on education was experienced during the Ebola virus disease (EVD) outbreak in West Africa between the years 2014 and 2016 [25,26]. During this outbreak, the countries that were most exposed to the virus were Guinea, Liberia, and Sierra Leone, with 28,610 cases and 11,308 deaths documented [25]. In 2014, the rapid transmissibility of EVD led to school closures in the three countries that lasted seven to nine months, causing the loss of a whole academic year [27]. This resulted in serious educational setbacks caused by the expanding learning gaps. Additionally, a large increase in school dropouts was noted, especially in secondary school students from low-income households [28].

Likewise, other crises have affected the educational process. For example, earthquakes have inflicted physical damage on educational institutes, which has led to learning being disrupted and students being deprived of their educational rights. However, in many cases, the learning process was restored relatively quick with the use of remote teaching methods, such as online learning [29,30]. With human life loss and educational resources demolished, natural disasters have a negative impact on academic achievement of secondary school students and often lead to class repetition [31]. The financial loss caused by natural disasters often causes students to drop out of school and join the workforce so they can contribute to the household income [32]. Moreover, in countries prone to natural disasters, there is reduced investment in education [33], and the restoration of the educational process highlights the necessity for rapid reactions to students' needs [34].

On 11 March 2020, COVID-19 was declared a pandemic by the World Health Organization (WHO, Geneva, Switzerland) [35]. In an effort to prevent the rapid spread of the virus SARS-CoV-2 that causes COVID-19, governments suspended the normal operation of schools. From early on, China and Mongolia had taken the initiative to close schools as a preventive measure. Following the WHO's announcement proclaiming COVID-19 as a global pandemic in March, a total number of 109 countries ensued with school closures, and by April 2020, this increased to 151 countries [36]. Reports estimate that 99% of the student population was affected [37]. School closures varied from partially open to complete closure due to COVID-19. Fully closed schools included pre-primary to upper secondary level educational institutions, where at least 80% of their enrolled student population was affected. Partially open schools were of three types: (a) schools that were open for some grade levels or age groups only, (b) open in certain areas only, and (c) open with reduced in-person class time. For most countries, complete or partial school closures lasted for over 21 weeks [36]. Yet, some countries set criteria which allowed them to avoid closing all of their schools. For example, they set a cut-off for class sizes (e.g., Iceland), closed only certain levels of schools (e.g., only upper secondary schools in Sweden switched to distance learning), or reorganized their academic year to reduce the loss of instruction time (e.g., Korea, Lithuania, Australia) [38]. It is worth noting, however, that school closures do not imply cessation of education, but rather the transformation and adaptation of the mode of teaching.

It appears that educational institutes and systems were unprepared to handle a disaster of such an extent [5]. Therefore, the unfamiliar territory in the educational context amplified the concerns of schools, educators, and students, who were called to swiftly adapt to a new reality [39].

2. Education in the Era of COVID-19

COVID-19 has been a global crisis, forcing countries to rethink how education could be accomplished despite school closures. Though the use of digital technology was not new in education, since the outbreak, it has become the primary modality. This was to ensure the continuity of education while containing the SARS-CoV-2 virus. The following section explores how education was modified during the period of the pandemic.

2.1. Distance Education

Distance education received great popularity from many countries during school closures, as a shift from face-to-face to remote teaching was emerging. Alternative education arrangements included online teaching through digital platforms, launching educational radio or television programs, and delivering learning packages with printed resources such as worksheets and textbooks to students [5]. The digital platforms enabled teachers to educate in actual time through virtual meeting programs and provided students with learning materials to utilize in their own time [40]. Furthermore, some countries were able to use pre-existing remote learning platforms that allowed students to revise the subject content from the beginning of the year by providing digital books and worksheets, and online activities [41]. Other countries such as Mexico further supported their students using television programs [42]. Nevertheless, digital platforms were most popular in developed countries, whereas other means of remote learning, such as radio and television broadcasts, were employed by developing countries.

2.2. Hybrid Learning Model

Many governments chose to re-open schools once the pandemic was in recession and the transmission risk decreased. During such times, schools further developed the hybrid approach to learning, also known as "blended learning". The hybrid method is a combination of conventional classroom-based instruction and online education [43]. In the hybrid educational approach, teachers make use of technologies designed for online teaching to enhance or substitute sections of the classroom-based instruction [44]. The instruction is provided through online platforms and in classroom, intermittently, providing the advantage of personalized teaching with the flexibility and ease of online formats [44–46]. Moreover, it offers possibilities that facilitate creativity, critical thinking, and skill development [47,48]. Even though there is limited research focusing on the effect of hybrid learning on secondary school students, it has been found to be an effective instructional method [45,49,50]. Whether used independently or combined with other teaching methods, it results in elevated student achievement [51].

In the context of the COVID-19 pandemic, hybrid education was utilized and developed further due to necessity. It was applied to avoid the congregation of large groups of students, lowering the risk of virus transmission while maintaining interactive lessons. The hybrid method combines synchronous learning such as in-person meetings through online platforms, such as Microsoft Teams, and asynchronous learning, such as assignments, pre-recorded lessons, and group projects [52]. It gives teachers the chance to provide students with reading material and enriched resources. It also affords students the freedom and flexibility to study the available material independently, and to conduct online class discussions through discussion boards [53].

The rotation model of hybrid learning has also been used during the pandemic in secondary schools. In this type of learning, teachers organized student attendance in alternation with distance learning, with different groups of students receiving classroom-based instruction on certain days of the week, and online schooling the rest [54]. In general, hybrid learning has been found to be a suitable educational approach during the COVID-19 pandemic [55]. Recent studies aimed to determine the effectiveness of the instructional modalities, with findings suggesting that the hybrid and classroom-based models offer more instructional time, cover more material, and facilitate better student achievement, as opposed to distance learning [56].

A possible disadvantage of hybrid learning is the reduced in-class instruction time, which ultimately disrupts the conventional way of teaching [40]. Validation, accreditation, and recognition of skills and knowledge produced through hybrid learning need to be integrated for hybrid education to be considered as effective and efficient as conventional modes of learning [57].

2.3. *Synchronous or Asynchronous Learning*

With remote education, student learning can take place in a synchronous or asynchronous setting. There is evidence of both types being used in secondary education since the start of the pandemic [58–60]. Learning in a synchronous setting involves real-time student–teacher communication. This allows for an immediate response, such as real-time lessons that take place through virtual meeting platforms and discussions in online forums, which is an advantage compared to purely online courses. A possible disadvantage of synchronous learning is its lack of flexibility [34]. On the other hand, a possible disadvantage of an asynchronous setting is that instantaneous feedback is not available, and student learning occurs independently, such as by utilizing uploaded learning material or learning through educational television or radio programs [61]. A benefit of asynchronous learning is convenience, where students can learn in a flexible manner and work at their own pace [34].

2.4. *Student Assessment*

Student assessment is a vital part of the educational system. It provides not only a great insight into students' progress but also feedback with regard to the teaching quality students receive, and the possible improvements that could be implemented. Assessment has also been found to impact students' motivation [62]. Because of the pandemic, the way students are assessed was impacted, with concerns raised about whether examinations are the appropriate method [63]. Currently, to our knowledge, three main approaches were used for assessing students in secondary education, namely, the cancellation of examinations, the suspension of examinations, or the transformation of examinations to an online format [64]. Moreover, a popular online learning evaluation method during the COVID-19 era was e-assessments (electronic assessments), whereby technology is used to deliver assessments and feedback through digital platforms [65].

Assessment methods have also been impacted in other ways. For instance, both in conventional and online assessments, some countries decreased the number of exams by excluding some subjects, while others reduced the learning content that students needed to cover for exams or altered the exam format by lowering the number of questions in the exam paper [64]. In addition, some schools switched to a reliable alternative to examinations [66], where students' learning was evaluated based solely on teacher assessment or teacher assessment combined with previous exam performance [64]. Lastly, there were countries which decided to assess secondary school students' learning based entirely on the feedback of homework and assignments that students completed in the current school year [67].

3. Challenges in Education during COVID-19

The sudden shift in in-person education to partly or fully remote education was challenging for teachers, students, and parents, as it required their swift adaptation. Educators were called to use alternative teaching methods that required the use of technological means, such as computers, laptops, phones, televisions, and radios, as well as digital expertise. This transitional phase has been described as a stressful period for a lot of educators [54,68]. Even though they coped with it and were able to transfer teaching to a digital form with their technological knowledge, this was not without its challenges [54]. The difficulties that arose involved the use of digital platforms, the communication with students, and the assessment and handling of students' reduced attention and understanding [54]. In this part of the paper, the challenges experienced in education are explored.

3.1. Digital Competence

Teachers' lack of digital skill and knowledge has been a main obstacle in the changes implemented in the educational system due to the COVID-19 pandemic. Information and communications technology (ICT) skills have become essential to teachers in order to cope with their new job requirements [40]. Teachers have been reporting a strong need for training in utilizing ICT for education, even before the pandemic [69]. The ICT skills in the educational setting include basic computer skills, knowledge regarding the use of computers to seek, access, and share information, and use of computers as a learning device [70]. During the COVID-19 outbreak, teachers have utilized ICT in remote learning mainly by uploading resources to online platforms [71]. There seemed to be a lack of digital knowledge among teachers, especially in education-related tools, that made the transition to technology-based remote teaching a great challenge for them [67,72].

3.2. Remote Education

The COVID-19 pandemic demanded shifting to remote or hybrid structures, with several challenges arising for students who were required to swiftly adjust to the educational changes. The first problem was students' limited skills in digital technology, since it was difficult for students who lacked those skills to be able to participate in online classes [5,73,74]. Another difficulty was the accessibility to digital devices. Without a digital device, participation in an online class for students was impractical. Another challenge was internet connectivity. On the one hand, internet access is vital for participating in online meetings, and on the other hand, good connectivity is essential for avoiding interruptions that inevitably disrupt the learning process. To prevent these challenges, students had to have access to high-speed internet connectivity and digital devices, which was a burden itself since it required financial investment [73].

Other reported challenges for students were the lack of understanding because of inadequate explanations offered by teachers, confusion with regard to the activities students were expected to complete due to the lack of teacher–student interaction, and the insufficient feedback provided by teachers. Consequently, elevated stress levels, as well as motivation decline, were experienced by students [41].

3.3. Increased Workload

In a short timeframe, the swift shift to alternative teaching methods burdened teachers with additional obligations for which they were not adequately prepared [5]. Consequently, educators' workload increased considerably [54]. The limited digital abilities of educators contributed substantially to the increased workload they reported [72]. Teachers' effort to deal with digital difficulties and simultaneously effectively educate and interact with students also led to increased stress and workloads [54].

Likewise, new challenges arose for teachers who utilized hybrid learning during this period. The demands of simultaneously interacting with classroom students and students who were virtually attending the class were an extra burden for teachers [54]. Studies showed that for educators, remote teaching caused decreased engagement with students, since they adopted a passive teaching approach with limited interaction, increased anxiety levels, and signs of burnout [68,71].

3.4. Academic Performance

From the early stages of the COVID-19 pandemic, there have been reports of a decrease in educational engagement [68]. This could be explained by the influence of health-related and financial concerns (e.g., limited resources to cover educational needs) that led to low levels of motivation and increased levels of anxiety [5]. Since academic achievement has been repeatedly associated with student engagement [75], the observed educational disengagement during the COVID-19 pandemic is a matter of concern.

Moreover, learning losses and related declines in academic performance for secondary school students have been reported [76,77]. According to studies, the learning losses can be primarily attributed to the alternative educational methods implemented for remote learning, and the associated challenges [77]. For instance, in an analysis by Lichand and colleagues [77], it was found that learning losses could be attributed to remote learning, irrespective of other changes caused by the pandemic itself, such as the economic and health consequences. Note, however, that there are studies that provided alternate evidence with regard to students' academic performance. For example, learning loss was not observed in secondary school students in Belgium [78], and students' grades remained stable in Sweden [54]. There have also been reports that the use of alternative assessment methods increases students' scores and passing rates [64].

Furthermore, there have been reports that the physical closure of schools resulted in less time spent in learning, which affects performance and appears to lead to learning losses. For instance, Di Pietro and colleagues [79] reported the results of the School Barometer that examined the school situation in Germany, Austria, and Switzerland, between the months of March and April 2020. This survey showed that students' weekly learning decreased between 4 and 8 h during the 2020 COVID-19 lockdown, compared to when schools were open, with one in five students reporting that they were studying less than 9 h per week.

Disasters amplify social inequalities [37], and as such, it is not a surprise that there have been reports of disparities during the pandemic [5,76]. There have been reports that pandemic-related challenges led to the expansion of the achievement gap between students from low-income, middle-income, and high-income households [80]. Nevertheless, there is also contradicting evidence reporting that no such differences can be observed [81], and that social disparities are greater for primary school students [82,83].

3.5. Daily Routines

Research suggests that having a daily routine can balance the adverse effects of stress exposure during periods of crisis [84–86]. The transformation of education due to the COVID-19 crisis greatly impacted the daily routines of students, teachers, and parents alike. Students had to adapt quickly to a new unstructured daily schedule that involved coping with the requirements of online/digital education, such as attending classes from home, studying from home, being evaluated from home, and interacting with classmates and teachers from home. Because of the many and sudden changes that took place, the structure of the week was lost, and students were responsible for finding ways to organize their own time schedule and allocate their time to studying, completing other responsibilities at home, playing, and performing other activities they enjoy.

Allocating their time to fit in online learning was particularly challenging, especially for primary and young secondary school students who have not fully developed self-management and self-motivation skills [87]. The daily routines of secondary students were also affected by the lack of traditional invigilation/supervision. Learning and studying via online means were difficult since they demanded autonomous learning from students who had to reschedule their daily routines and find ways to learn and master self-control and independent work [88]. For teachers, online supervision was challenging and very different from the supervision in a physical classroom. Likewise, for parents, the difficulty stemmed from the combination of child supervision and teleworking [88].

Developing and implementing a regular routine are also very important for students' mental health. Research has shown that, especially during times that schools are closed, the disruption of daily routines might negatively impact adolescents' mental health [89]. The high amount of time students were spending at home influenced their normal sleeping, eating, and exercising patterns [90–93]. The WHO [94], as early as 18 March 2020, published guidelines to help the public deal with the psychological distress caused by the pandemic. One guideline was directed to the carers of children, denoting the importance of stay-at-home routines and performing activities such as exercises, hobbies, and schoolwork for children who spent most of their time at home [94].

Routines also appear to be important for adolescents with prior mental health problems, risking a relapse for those who missed their regular school routines due to the closing of schools [95]. Interesting results were obtained from surveys conducted by the UK charity organization YoungMinds [93,96–98] in different time periods during the pandemic (March 2020, summer 2020, autumn 2020, and February 2021). The organization examined adolescents and young adults aged between 13 and 25 with a history of mental health needs. The results showed that many participants considered that maintaining routines, such as taking part in exercise or dance classes, was a coping strategy for managing their mental health, something that was not possible during March 2020 due to the lockdown [93]. A similar finding was also observed in the surveys that followed, with the most recent one, in February 2021, showing that 45% of participants responded that having a routine was helpful during periods of lockdown [98]. Results from March 2020 and February 2021 [93,98] also showed that spending a lot of time at home, loss of routine, and isolation can have a negative impact on their mental health. Loss of routine was considered by some participants as a negative coping strategy, leading them to overthink self-harmful behaviors [93,98].

For adolescents, peer relationships are of great importance, since they provide emotional and social support [99–101]. Not engaging with friends, and in extra-curricular activities, leads some students to experience boredom [95]. Therefore, finding ways to reform their routine and to interact with their friends, especially during periods of lockdown, was very important. Research suggests that adolescents found ways to adapt by reconstructing their routines and incorporating video calls for communicating and spending time with their friends [102].

The normal daily routines of teachers and parents were also affected due to home confinement, with a significant increase in daily stressors [92,103]. Teachers had to transform a workplace in their house for teleworking, create new teaching routines to cope with online education, combine all these with household chores, and, for those with children, find ways to manage teaching, parenting, and caregiving simultaneously. Parents faced similar problems because of the many changes in their daily routines, such as home schooling, teleworking, and caregiving [92,103].

3.6. Career-Related Plans

The COVID-19 pandemic also seems to be affecting students' future career-related plans. During this period, there has been uncertainty regarding future education and occupation, which, in turn, has led to an increased demand for career guidance, especially for high school students [104,105]. The SARS-CoV-2 virus outbreak caused changes in the job market, which, in turn, altered the attraction of various professions. This caused confusion in secondary school-age children with respect to their career orientation [105].

Moreover, secondary school students' engagement is found to predict enrollment in higher education institutes, with lower engagement being associated with a decreased possibility of registration [106]. As previously noted, during the COVID-19 pandemic, educational disengagement for secondary school students has been observed [68], and the school dropout risk has substantially risen [57,77]. This increase has been associated with remote learning methods, student disengagement, and financial and health-related concerns [57,77]. In general, in secondary school-age children, pessimism regarding their future career seems to prevail [107].

3.7. *Socio-Economic Factors*

The COVID-19 pandemic has led to a global economic crisis. Unemployment and poverty rates substantially increased, and economies endured declines with limited prospects of recovery in the subsequent years [108]. The closure of entire economic sectors and the enforcement of preventive measures, such as lockdowns, have brought about a drop in worldwide economic activity [108]. Consequently, this effect on the educational system has been noted at both a country-wide and an individual level.

3.7.1. Country/System Level

Due to the aforementioned economic crisis, schools' capacity to educate effectively, as well as students' ability to learn, has been restricted. Therefore, in most countries, governments have taken steps to support alternative education, such as distance learning, and COVID-19-related modifications to the educational system. Such support measures include financial support, provision of digital equipment, and staff acquisition and training [40]. For example, in the United States, an emergency fund was initiated to support primary and secondary schools [109]. In the United Kingdom, the government financed schools to cover COVID-19-associated costs, such as added cleaning costs, and free meal arrangements for students that could not attend [110]. The government in Italy provided schools with the necessary equipment, staff, and training to facilitate distance learning and lent digital devices to students from low-income families [111]. Lastly, the government in Estonia recruited services to distribute learning materials, such as worksheets and textbooks, to students' households during physical school closures [40].

In other countries whose resources are limited to provide such large-scale support, the majority of the population does not have access to technological devices (e.g., phones, computers) to deliver or receive education through online platforms. Therefore, in such cases, governments utilized different strategies, such as launching educational television and radio programs [108].

3.7.2. Individual Level

The catastrophe experienced by the global economy caused by the pandemic has also affected the population at an individual level. The increased unemployment and poverty rates are of concern to both parents and students [112]. Remote learning has proven to be a challenging education alternative for many families, especially those coming from low-income households [113–115]. In particular, a major challenge for students from low-income families is the limited access they have to digital devices and connectivity [5,80], which, as stated earlier, are essential elements for remote education.

Moreover, studies indicate that there is an increase in parental worry regarding children's academic performance in families with a lower income [116]. In many cases, students need further instruction, and parents need to assist them with their academic obligations. This poses a challenge, especially for working parents with low levels of education [113]. Generally, it appears that students who come from low-income families have a higher need for additional education-related resources and instruction [116]. Consequently, during the pandemic, the inequality gap in educational opportunity and achievement has expanded [5,80].

4. Psychological Insights

Populations' mental health has been greatly affected because of the pandemic. Numerous studies documented increases in anxiety, depression, and stress symptoms in the general population since COVID-19 spread worldwide [117–122]. In line with pre-pandemic research, it appears that younger people and people with a history of mental health problems are those who are at greater risk [117,123]. It is well documented that periods of extreme situations, such as quarantine and social isolation, negatively impact people [124,125]. Therefore, it is not a surprise that during the pandemic, studies related social isolation to symptoms of depression and anxiety [124]. In addition, since the start of the outbreak, there have been increased cases of suicidal attempts [126,127], which appears to be associated with the limited social contact and feelings of loneliness the population is experiencing [128]. This section explores how the mental health of secondary school students, parents, and educators has been affected during the pandemic.

4.1. Mental Health of Students

Among those who were significantly impacted during the COVID-19 outbreak were primary school-age and secondary school-age children, who had to face great adjustments with regard to their learning. This had led to the development or enhancement of emotional difficulties, and a decrease in their overall well-being [117]. Specifically, an increase in anxiety and depression symptomatology has been found in secondary school-age children [101,129–131]. This contributes to the decline noted in their school-related motivation and might explain the lower student engagement levels observed [68]. In addition, traumatic stress symptoms, as well as increased anger, have also been observed during the pandemic period [124]. There are many factors that could explain the emotional difficulties and the decrease in the well-being of students due to the closures and uncertainty surrounding the pandemic. Some attributable factors include self-isolation, limited social interactions and peer experiences, loss of daily routine, boredom, uncertainty for the future, economic concerns, disease-related fear, family stress, lack of physical activity, lack of resources, and disease-associated stigma [93,95–98,117,124].

Importantly, more attention needs to be placed on student mental health problems, since they interfere with critical elements for academic success, such as memory, concentration, and motivation [132]. This is in accordance with pre-pandemic research reporting that anxiety and depression negatively impact student learning and academic performance [133], such as difficulty in concentrating and carrying out school-related activities [134]. The possible impact of the reported psychological problems arising since the start of the outbreak can already be seen from the documented motivation, engagement, and learning losses [68,76,77]. Lastly, mental health difficulties could also explain the increase in education losses which, in turn, might lead to lower enrollment in higher educational institutions.

4.2. Mental Health of Parents

The mental health of parents has also been affected during this period. Studies showed that life adjustments and COVID-related challenges led to anxiety and depression in parents [117,119,120]. Economic concerns, role variations, health and safety worries, and loss of daily routines have been found to be related to an increase in anxiety and fatigue levels [117,118,122]. With the introduction of alternative learning methods, parents had to adopt the role of supplementary teacher, which was found to be associated with elevated psychological distress and anxiety for parents of primary and secondary school students [116,135]. Furthermore, stressors such as financial concerns and social isolation impacted family relations [136], which increases the likelihood of child abuse [137]. Conflicts within the family appear to impact the mental health of parents. For instance, in a study that examined the mental health of parents of primary, secondary, and tertiary students in China, Wu et al. [116] found that compared to harmonious families, parents with family conflicts had higher levels of depression, anxiety, and stress. It is worth noting that maladaptive family functioning has also been found to be related to the development of psychological problems in secondary school-age children [138]. Lastly, in line with findings from previous pandemics, such as H1N1, pandemic-related stress experienced by parents was identified as a contributing factor to the increase in children's mental health problems [139,140]. Highly anxious parents may overestimate the danger of external factors and, as such, act with hypervigilance and overprotection in many cases. This, in turn, facilitates worry and anxious responses from their children [141].

4.3. Mental Health of Educators

Amongst the many changes that took place during the outbreak of the pandemic were work-related adjustments that educators had to make. With remote teaching being introduced, educators were forced to immediately adapt to the new system [5]. The alternative teaching methods placed extra pressure on educators, generated more work-related obligations, and increased their workload [54]. In concordance with previous findings, technology use and technical competence caused higher levels of stress in educators [54,72,142]. Importantly, studies found signs of burnout (e.g., fatigue) in educators [68,71,143], which, according to research, could be attributed to teleworking [144]. Accordingly, work-related stress during teleworking seems to be higher for educators with children [144]. Moreover, during this period, there have been indications of a decline in educators' quality of life [145], as well as signs of depressive symptoms [146]. Worth noting, however, is the finding that during distance education, there has been a decline in educators' anxiety that is related to classroom-based student management. These mental health difficulties experienced by educators are important as they influence educators' engagement in the classroom, due to the more passive teaching approach [68,71].

5. A Positive Viewpoint?

Emergencies can create a setting where modifications to practices are more easily obtained and are applied in an accelerated pace [34]. With the challenges and ambivalence surrounding the pandemic, it is often difficult to consider a positive effect of such situations. Nonetheless, research shows that some pandemic-related changes to education have proven to be beneficial in the long run regardless of socio-economic status. As reviewed before, countries, regardless of their socio-economic status, took initiatives to adapt to the physical school closures and continued to provide education to students [40,42,110,111]. The following are some of the positive effects that have been found.

5.1. Educational System Evolvement

The outbreak crisis made the value of schools and educators evident [5] and acted as an opportunity to reconsider the future of education [54]. Regardless of the initial hesitancy of educational organizations concerning the transition from conventional teaching methods to remote learning, many benefits were identified. These include overall flexibility as it is student centered, time and location flexibility, variety in material and lesson format [147], greater accessibility [148], improvement in communication and interaction between student and educator through the use of tools such as videoconferences, email, chats, and forums [149,150], and adapted lessons based on the learning objectives and the needs of the learner [151]. E-learning allows plan flexibility, and students can adopt their own pace of learning, which subsequently decreases school-related anxiety and facilitates skill development [73]. Accordingly, the pandemic positively impacted the attitudes of teachers and students regarding distance education and promoted the development of various approaches and skills [104].

5.2. Skill Development

In general, the educational challenges that emerged from physical school closures and alternative learning methods facilitated various skills in students and teachers. For instance, it has been documented that in the context of hybrid learning, student critical thinking flourished [53,73]. Moreover, education outside of the school environment offered the opportunity for independence to be developed in students, allowing self-reflection and focus outside of peer influence and pressure [152]. The unconventional educational methods enabled innovation and creativity in both educators and students [153], possibly due to the exploration of new learning methodologies in a different educational context [154]. Creativity is considered a vital ability in students [155] and has played a key role in managing the pandemic-related difficulties [156]. Lastly, research has shown that the greater the creativity demonstrated by students, the less anxiety they experienced [154].

5.3. Benefit to Relationships

Since the start of the pandemic, the nature of many relationships has changed. Part of this could be because it mobilized people to reconsider their life, to set priorities, and to recognize or re-evaluate their values. However, most of the changes can be attributed to the pandemic-related impacts, such as physical school closure, social isolation, and alternative educational practices. For example, the parent–child daily interaction time has increased since the start of the outbreak [157,158], which has provided the opportunity for quality face-to-face interaction [158]. The quality of the parent–child relationship is significant since it can act as a protective factor of emotional difficulties experienced by secondary school-age children during the pandemic [159]. Furthermore, the increased parental participation in the educational process (e.g., remote learning, aiding in arising learning challenges) can improve the parent–child relationship [5].

The collaboration between teachers and parents to ensure that students receive the best possible education with the new mode of teaching improved the parent–teacher relationship [28]. Moreover, teacher–student relationships were modified, since the health crisis pushed teachers towards an approach with more emphasis on student well-being [160]. For instance, an increase in teacher support and reassurance was documented during the virus outbreak [161]. Therefore, this could further facilitate student adjustment, well-being, and academic achievement [162,163]. According to Chamizo-Nieto and colleagues [163], it would be interesting to examine whether this will last in the post-COVID-19 period.

6. Concluding Remarks

The COVID-19 pandemic forced numerous changes to education. Those who were mostly impacted by these changes were educators and students, who had to quickly adapt to the new reality. The adaptation to remote formats of learning, physical school closures, and the implementation of social and physical distance measures restricted the regular learning process. Although technology is not new in educational settings, the pandemic forced learning to become fully digitalized. This caused more challenges for everyone involved in secondary education. This entry described the alterations that took place, the challenges that arose, and the impact on students', parents', and educators' mental health and ended with some positive outcomes that surfaced because of the new way of learning. The pandemic is not over yet, and therefore the educational system is still in constant alert. However, as compared to the start of the pandemic outbreak, the educational system is now more prepared to combat the challenges, but there are still unknown paths yet to be discovered.

Specifically, the main conclusions of this entry are the following:

- The pandemic resulted in educational changes and disrupted the regular learning process.
- The mode of teaching became primarily digitized/virtual to reduce the transmissibility of the virus which affected all parties involved (students, teachers, parents).

- Several challenges for students, teachers, and parents emerged. These included the use of digital platforms and digital competence, increased workload, the loss of daily routines, changes in career-related plans, and socio-economic impacts.
- The new mode of learning impacted students', teachers', and parents' mental health.
- Possible beneficial changes due to the pandemic, such as the evolvement of the educational system and skill development, were discussed. However, the long-term effects are still unknown.
- The educational system adapted to the several challenges that arose due to the pandemic. However, since the pandemic is ongoing, any accompanying current and unforeseen challenges will need to be addressed, with special attention given to the impact on all parties involved (students, educators, and parents).

Author Contributions: Conceptualization, M.S., M.M., A.C., A.S. and K.K.; investigation, M.S., M.M., A.C., A.S. and K.K.; writing—original draft preparation, M.S., M.M., A.C., A.S. and K.K.; writing—review and editing, M.S., M.M., A.C., A.S. and K.K.; supervision, M.S., M.M. and A.C.; project administration, M.S., M.M., A.C., A.S. and K.K. All authors have read and agreed to the published version of the manuscript.

Funding: This research received no external funding.

Institutional Review Board Statement: Not applicable.

Informed Consent Statement: Not applicable.

Data Availability Statement: Not applicable.

Conflicts of Interest: The authors declare no conflict of interest.

Entry Link on the Encyclopedia Platform: https://encyclopedia.pub/20415.

References

1. World Health Organization [WHO]. Weekly Epidemiological Update on COVID-19—9 November 2021. Available online: https://www.who.int/publications/m/item/weekly-epidemiological-update-on-covid-19---9-November-2021 (accessed on 15 November 2021).
2. Bin Nafisah, S.; Alamery, A.H.; Al Nafesa, A.; Aleid, B.; Brazanji, N.A. School Closure during Novel Influenza: A Systematic Review. *J. Infect. Public Health* **2018**, *11*, 657–661. [CrossRef]
3. Viner, R.M.; Russell, S.J.; Croker, H.; Packer, J.; Ward, J.; Stansfield, C.; Mytton, O.; Bonell, C.; Booy, R. School Closure and Management Practices during Coronavirus Outbreaks Including COVID-19: A Rapid Systematic Review. *Lancet Child Adolesc. Health* **2020**, *4*, 397–404. [CrossRef]
4. Ferguson, N.; Laydon, D.; Nedjati Gilani, G.; Imai, N.; Ainslie, K.; Baguelin, M.; Bhatia, S.; Boonyasiri, A.; Cucunuba Perez, Z.; Cuomo-Dannenburg, G. *Report 9: Impact of Non-Pharmaceutical Interventions (NPIs) to Reduce COVID19 Mortality and Healthcare Demand*; Imperial College London: London, UK, 2020. [CrossRef]
5. Reimers, F.M. Learning from a Pandemic. The Impact of COVID-19 on Education Around the World. In *Primary and Secondary Education During COVID-19: Disruptions to Educational Opportunity During a Pandemic*; Reimers, F.M., Ed.; Springer International Publishing: Cham, Switzerland, 2022; pp. 1–37. [CrossRef]
6. World Health Organization [WHO]. Severe Acute Respiratory Syndrome (SARS). Available online: https://www.who.int/westernpacific/health-topics/severe-acute-respiratory-syndrome (accessed on 16 November 2021).
7. Chan, K.P. Control of Severe Acute Respiratory Syndrome in Singapore. *Environ. Health Prev. Med.* **2005**, *10*, 255–259. [CrossRef] [PubMed]
8. Pang, X.; Zhu, Z.; Xu, F.; Guo, J.; Gong, X.; Liu, D.; Liu, Z.; Chin, D.P.; Feikin, D.R. Evaluation of Control Measures Implemented in the Severe Acute Respiratory Syndrome Outbreak in Beijing, 2003. *JAMA* **2003**, *290*, 3215–3221. [CrossRef] [PubMed]
9. Huang, C.; Liu, X.; Sun, S.; Li, S.C.; Deng, M.; He, G.; Zhang, H.; Wang, C.; Zhou, Y.; Zhao, Y.; et al. Insights into the Transmission of Respiratory Infectious Diseases through Empirical Human Contact Networks. *Sci. Rep.* **2016**, *6*, 31484. [CrossRef] [PubMed]
10. Chng, S.Y.; Chia, F.; Leong, K.K.; Kwang, Y.P.; Ma, S.; Lee, B.W.; Vaithinathan, R.; Tan, C.C. Mandatory Temperature Monitoring in Schools during SARS. *Arch. Dis. Child.* **2004**, *89*, 738. [CrossRef]
11. Tan, C.C. SARS in Singapore-Key Lessons from an Epidemic. *Ann. Acad. Med. Singap.* **2006**, *35*, 345–349.

12. Wong, G.W.K.; Li, A.M.; Ng, P.C.; Fok, T.F. Severe Acute Respiratory Syndrome in Children. *Pediatric Pulmonol.* **2003**, *36*, 261–266. [CrossRef]
13. Peiris, J.; Lai, S.; Poon, L.; Guan, Y.; Yam, L.; Lim, W.; Nicholls, J.; Yee, W.; Yan, W.; Cheung, M.; et al. Coronavirus as a Possible Cause of Severe Acute Respiratory Syndrome. *Lancet* **2003**, *361*, 1319–1325. [CrossRef]
14. DiGiovanni, C.; Conley, J.; Chiu, D.; Zaborski, J. Factors Influencing Compliance with Quarantine in Toronto During the 2003 SARS Outbreak. *Biosecurity Bioterrorism Biodefense Strategy Pract. Sci.* **2004**, *2*, 265–272. [CrossRef]
15. O'Sullivan, T.L.; Amaratunga, C.; Phillips, K.P.; Corneil, W.; O'Connor, E.; Lemyre, L.; Dow, D. If Schools Are Closed, Who Will Watch Our Kids? Family Caregiving and Other Sources of Role Conflict among Nurses during Large-Scale Outbreaks. *Prehospital Disaster Med.* **2009**, *24*, 321–325. [CrossRef] [PubMed]
16. World Health Organization. Regional Office for the Eastern Mediterranean. Pandemic (H1N1) 2009—Update 112. Available online: https://www.who.int/emergencies/disease-outbreak-news/item/2010_08_06-en (accessed on 17 November 2021).
17. Cauchemez, S.; Van Kerkhove, M.D.; Archer, B.N.; Cetron, M.; Cowling, B.J.; Grove, P.; Hunt, D.; Kojouharova, M.; Kon, P.; Ungchusak, K.; et al. School Closures during the 2009 Influenza Pandemic: National and Local Experiences. *BMC Infect. Dis.* **2014**, *14*, 207. [CrossRef] [PubMed]
18. Wu, J.T.; Cowling, B.J.; Lau, E.H.Y.; Ip, D.K.M.; Ho, L.-M.; Tsang, T.; Chuang, S.-K.; Leung, P.-Y.; Lo, S.-V.; Liu, S.-H.; et al. School Closure and Mitigation of Pandemic (H1N1) 2009, Hong Kong. *Emerg. Infect. Dis.* **2010**, *16*, 538–541. [CrossRef] [PubMed]
19. Markel, H.; Lipman, H.B.; Navarro, J.A.; Sloan, A.; Michalsen, J.R.; Stern, A.M.; Cetron, M.S. Nonpharmaceutical Interventions Implemented by US Cities During the 1918–1919 Influenza Pandemic. *JAMA* **2007**, *298*, 644–654. [CrossRef]
20. Yen, M.-Y.; Chiu, A.W.-H.; Schwartz, J.; King, C.-C.; Lin, Y.E.; Chang, S.-C.; Armstrong, D.; Hsueh, P.-R. From SARS in 2003 to H1N1 in 2009: Lessons Learned from Taiwan in Preparation for the next Pandemic. *J. Hosp. Infect.* **2014**, *87*, 185–193. [CrossRef]
21. Korea Disease Control and Prevention Agency (KDCA). Middle East Respiratory Syndrome (MERS). Available online: https://www.kdca.go.kr/contents.es?mid=a30329000000 (accessed on 16 November 2021).
22. Ha, K.-M. A Lesson Learned from the MERS Outbreak in South Korea in 2015. *J Hosp. Infect.* **2016**, *92*, 232–234. [CrossRef]
23. World Health Organization. *Middle East Respiratory Syndrome Coronavirus (MERS CoV): Summary of Current Situation, Literature Update and Risk Assessment*; World Health Organization: Geneva, Switzerland, 2015. Available online: https://apps.who.int/iris/handle/10665/179184 (accessed on 16 November 2021).
24. Lee, I.S.; Yoon, J.H.; Hong, E.J.; Kim, C.Y. Schools' Response to MERS(MERS-CoV) Outbreak: Schools' Discretionary Response in Absence of Control Tower. *J. Korean Soc. Sch. Health* **2015**, *28*, 188–199. [CrossRef]
25. World Health Organization [WHO]. Ebola Virus Disease. Available online: https://www.who.int/news-room/fact-sheets/detail/ebola-virus-disease (accessed on 17 November 2021).
26. Shultz, J.M.; Espinel, Z.; Espinola, M.; Rechkemmer, A. Distinguishing Epidemiological Features of the 2013–2016 West Africa Ebola Virus Disease Outbreak. *Disaster Health* **2016**, *3*, 78–88. [CrossRef]
27. Wongani, G.T. Lessons from Ebola: How to Reach the Poorest Children when Schools Reopen. UNICEF Connect, 15 June 2020. Available online: https://blogs.unicef.org/blog/lessons-from-ebola-how-to-reach-the-poorest-children-when-schools-reopen/ (accessed on 17 November 2021).
28. Smith, W.C. Consequences of School Closure on Access to Education: Lessons from the 2013–2016 Ebola Pandemic. *Int. Rev. Educ.* **2021**, *67*, 53–78. [CrossRef]
29. Barboni, L. From Shifting Earth to Shifting Paradigms: How Webex Helped Our University Overcome an Earthquake. CISCO, Upshot by Influitive. 2019. Available online: https://upshotstories.com/stories/from-shifting-earth-to-shifting-paradigms-how-webex-helped-our-university-overcome-an-earthquake (accessed on 25 November 2021).
30. Todorova, N.; Bjorn-Andersen, N. University Learning in Times of Crisis: The Role of IT. *Account. Educ.* **2011**, *20*, 597–599. [CrossRef]
31. Onigbinde, L. The Impacts of Natural Disasters on Educational Attainment: Cross-Country Evidence from Macro Data. Master's Thesis, University of San Francisco, San Francisco, CA, USA, 2018.
32. Kousky, C. Impacts of Natural Disasters on Children. *Future Child.* **2016**, *26*, 73–92. [CrossRef]
33. Cuaresma, J.C. Natural Disasters and Human Capital Accumulation. *World Bank Econ. Rev.* **2010**, *24*, 280–302. [CrossRef]
34. Bojović, Ž.; Bojović, P.D.; Vujošević, D.; Šuh, J. Education in Times of Crisis: Rapid Transition to Distance Learning. *Comput. Appl. Eng. Educ.* **2020**, *28*, 1467–1489. [CrossRef]
35. World Health Organization [WHO]. WHO Director-General's Opening Remarks at the Media Briefing on COVID-19 [Press Release]. 11 March 2020. Available online: https://www.who.int/director-general/speeches/detail/who-director-general-s-opening-remarks-at-the-media-briefing-on-covid-19---11-March-2020 (accessed on 22 November 2021).
36. United Nations Educational, Scientific and Cultural Organization [UNESCO]. COVID-19, Education: From disruption to recovery. Available online: https://en.unesco.org/covid19/educationresponse (accessed on 22 November 2021).
37. Reddy, V.; Soudien, C.; Winnaar, L. Disrupted Learning during COVID-19: The Impact of School Closures on Education Outcomes in South Africa. *HSRC Rev.* **2020**, *18*, 10–12.

38. Organisation for Economic Co-operation and Development [OECD]. Country Education Responses to the Coronavirus (COVID-19) Pandemic. Available online: https://www.oecd.org/education/country-education-responses-coronavirus.htm (accessed on 16 November 2021).
39. Rasiah, R.; Kaur, H.; Guptan, V. Business Continuity Plan in the Higher Education Industry: University Students' Perceptions of the Effectiveness of Academic Continuity Plans during Covid-19 Pandemic. *Appl. Syst. Innov.* **2020**, *3*, 51. [CrossRef]
40. Schleicher, A. The Impact of COVID-19 on Education Insights from Education at a Glance. Organisation for Economic Co-operation and Development [OECD]. 2020. Available online: https://www.oecd.org/the-impact-of-covid-19-on-education-insights-education-at-aglance-2020.pdf (accessed on 21 November 2021).
41. Hammerstein, S.; König, C.; Dreisörner, T.; Frey, A. Effects of COVID-19-Related School Closures on Student Achievement-A Systematic Review. *Front. Psychol.* **2021**, *12*, 4020. [CrossRef] [PubMed]
42. Vázquez, M.C.O. Mexico's COVID-19 Distance Education Program Compels a Re-Think of the Country's Future of Education. *Brookings* **2020**. Available online: https://www.brookings.edu/blog/education-plus-development/2020/04/21/mexicos-covid-19-distance-education-program-compels-a-re-think-of-the-countrys-future-of-education/ (accessed on 10 December 2021).
43. The Glossary of Education Reform. Blended Learning Definition. Great Schools Partnership. Available online: https://www.edglossary.org/blended-learning/ (accessed on 19 November 2021).
44. Maxwell, C. What Blended Learning Is- and Isn't. Available online: https://www.blendedlearning.org/what-blended-learning-is-and-isnt/ (accessed on 19 November 2021).
45. Lamport, M.A.; Hill, R.J. Impact of Hybrid Instruction on Student Achievement in Post-Secondary Institutions: A Synthetic Review of the Literature. *J. Instruct. Res.* **2012**, *1*, 49–58. [CrossRef]
46. O'Byrne, W.I.; Pytash, K.E. Hybrid and blended learning: Modifying pedagogy across path, pace, time, and place. *J. Adolesc. Adult Lit.* **2015**, *59*, 137–140. [CrossRef]
47. Barrón-Estrada, M.L.; Zatarain-Cabada, R.; Zatarain-Cabada, R.; Reyes García, C.A. A Hybrid Learning Compiler Course. In *Hybrid Learning*; Tsang, P., Cheung, S.K.S., Lee, V.S.K., Huang, R., Eds.; Springer: Berlin/Heidelberg, Germany, 2010; pp. 229–238. [CrossRef]
48. Garrison, D.R.; Kanuka, H. Blended Learning: Uncovering Its Transformative Potential in Higher Education. *Internet High. Educ.* **2004**, *7*, 95–105. [CrossRef]
49. Bernard, R.M.; Borokhovski, E.; Schmid, R.F.; Tamim, R.M.; Abrami, P.C. A Meta-Analysis of Blended Learning and Technology Use in Higher Education: From the General to the Applied. *J. Comput. High. Educ.* **2014**, *26*, 87–122. [CrossRef]
50. McFarlin, B.K. Hybrid Lecture-Online Format Increases Student Grades in an Undergraduate Exercise Physiology Course at a Large Urban University. *Adv. Physiol. Educ.* **2008**, *32*, 86–91. [CrossRef] [PubMed]
51. Means, B.; Toyama, Y.; Murphy, R.; Bakia, M.; Jones, K. *Evaluation of Evidence Based Practices in Online Learning: A Meta-Analysis and Review of Online Learning Studies*; US Department of Education: Washington, DC, USA, 2009; p. 93.
52. Su, F. Blended Learning Pedagogy in Higher Education. In *Encyclopedia of Educational Innovation*; Peters, M.A., Heraud, R., Eds.; Springer: Singapore, 2019; pp. 1–6. [CrossRef]
53. Ariawan, S.; Malang, S. Building Critical Thinking in Covid-19 Pandemic Era: Impossible or I Am Possible? *Int. Res. J. Adv. Sci. Hub* **2020**, *2*, 127–130. [CrossRef]
54. Nilsberth, M.; Liljekvist, Y.; Olin-Scheller, C.; Samuelsson, J.; Hallquist, C. Digital Teaching as the New Normal? Swedish Upper Secondary Teachers' Experiences of Emergency Remote Teaching during the COVID-19 Crisis. *Eur. Educ. Res. J.* **2021**, *20*, 442–462. [CrossRef]
55. Prilipsky, R.E.; Zaeva, M.A. A Hybrid System for Building a Personal Knowledge Base. *Procedia Comput. Sci.* **2020**, *169*, 96–99. [CrossRef]
56. Kaufman, J.H.; Diliberti, M.K. *Divergent and Inequitable Teaching and Learning Pathways During (and Perhaps beyond) the Pandemic: Key Findings from the American Educator Panels Spring 2021 COVID-19 Surveys*; RAND Corporation: Santa Monica, CA, USA, 2021. [CrossRef]
57. United Nations. Policy Brief: Education during COVID-19 and beyond. 2020. Available online: https://www.un.org/sites/un2.un.org/files/sp_policy_brief_covid-19_and_education_august_2020.pdf (accessed on 21 November 2021).
58. Barlovits, S.; Jablonski, S.; Milicic, G.; Ludwig, M. Diastance Learning in Mathematics Education: Synchronous and Asynchronous Learning with MathicityMap@Home. In *EDULEARN21 Proceedings*; IATED: Online Conference, 2021; pp. 10179–10189. Available online: https://library.iated.org/view/BARLOVITS2021DIS (accessed on 10 December 2021).
59. Moorhouse, B.L.; Wong, K.M. Blending Asynchronous and Synchronous Digital Technologies and Instructional Approaches to Facilitate Remote Learning. *J. Comput. Educ.* **2021**. [CrossRef]
60. Ryan, M.P. An Analysis of Fully Synchronous Pandemic Secondary Education. In *Handbook of Research on Emerging Pedagogies for the Future of Education: Trauma-Informed, Care, and Pandemic Pedagogy*; Bozkurt, A., Ed.; IGI Global: Hershey, PA, USA, 2021; pp. 250–268. [CrossRef]

61. Fabriz, S.; Mendzheritskaya, J.; Stehle, S. Impact of Synchronous and Asynchronous Settings of Online Teaching and Learning in Higher Education on Students' Learning Experience During COVID-19. *Front. Psychol.* **2021**, *12*, 4544. [CrossRef]
62. Rust, C.; O'Donovan, B.; Price, M. A Social Constructivist Assessment Process Model: How the Research Literature Shows Us This Could Be Best Practice. *Assess. Eval. High. Educ.* **2005**, *30*, 231–240. [CrossRef]
63. Cairns, R. Exams Tested by Covid-19: An Opportunity to Rethink Standardized Senior Secondary Examinations. *Prospects* **2020**, *51*, 331–345. [CrossRef]
64. Bai-Yun, C. The Effects of COVID-19 on International Secondary Assessment. 2020. Available online: https://www.naric.org.uk/downloads/The%20Effects%20of%20COVID=19%20on%20International%20Secondary%20Assessment%20-%20UK%20NARIC.pdf (accessed on 29 November 2021).
65. Abduh, M.Y.M. Full-Time Online Assessment during COVID-19 Lockdown: EFL Teacher's Perception. *Asian EFL J.* **2021**, *28*, 26–46.
66. Rimfeld, K.; Malanchini, M.; Hannigan, L.J.; Dale, P.S.; Allen, B.; Hart, S.A.; Plomin, R. Teacher Assessments during Compulsory Education Are as Reliable, Stable and Heritable as Standardized Test Scores. *J. Child. Psychol. Psychiatry* **2019**, *60*, 1278–1288. [CrossRef] [PubMed]
67. Farhana, Z.; Tanni, S.A.; Shabnam, S.; Chowdhury, S.A. Secondary Education during Lockdown Situation Due to COVID-19 Pandemic in Bangladesh: Teachers' Response on Online Classes. *JEP* **2020**, *11*, 97–102. [CrossRef]
68. Lavonen, J.; Salmela-Aro, K. Experiences of Moving Quickly to Distance Teaching and Learning at All Levels of Education in Finland. In *Primary and Secondary Education during COVID-19: Disruptions to Educational Opportunity during a Pandemic*; Reimers, F.M., Ed.; Springer International Publishing: Cham, Switzerland, 2022; pp. 105–123. [CrossRef]
69. Organisation for Economic Co-operation and Development [OECD]. *TALIS 2018 Results (Volume I): Teachers and School Leaders as Lifelong Learners*; TALIS, OECD Publishing: Paris, France, 2019.
70. Comi, S.L.; Argentin, G.; Gui, M.; Origo, F.; Pagani, L. Is It the Way They Use It? Teachers, ICT and Student Achievement. *Econ. Educ. Rev.* **2017**, *56*, 24–39. [CrossRef]
71. Tartavulea, C.V.; Albu, C.N.; Albu, N.; Dieaconescu, R.I.; Petre, S. Online Teaching Practices and the Effectiveness of the Educational Process in the Wake of the COVID-19 Pandemic. *Amfiteatru Econ.* **2020**, *22*, 920–936. [CrossRef]
72. Portillo, J.; Garay, U.; Tejada, E.; Bilbao, N. Self-Perception of the Digital Competence of Educators during the COVID-19 Pandemic: A Cross-Analysis of Different Educational Stages. *Sustainability* **2020**, *12*, 10128. [CrossRef]
73. Adesina, E.M.; Orija, J.I. Benefits and Challenges of Online Learning in the Era of COVID-19. In Proceedings of the 2nd International Conference, The Federal Polytechnic, Ilaro, Nigeria, 10–11 November 2020.
74. Priyadarshini, A.; Bhaumik, R. E-Readiness of Senior School Learners to Online Learning Transition amid COVID-19 Lockdown. *Asian J. Distance Educ.* **2020**, *15*, 244–256.
75. Lei, H.; Cui, Y.; Zhou, W. Relationships between Student Engagement and Academic Achievement: A Meta-Analysis. *SBP J.* **2018**, *46*, 517–528. [CrossRef]
76. Donnelly, R.; Patrinos, H.A. Learning Loss during Covid-19: An Early Systematic Review. *Prospects* **2021**. [CrossRef]
77. Lichand, G.; Dória, C.A.; Neto, O.L.; Cossi, J. The Impacts of Remote Learning in Secondary Education during the Pandemic in Brazil. 2021. Available online: https://ssrn.com/abstract=3841775 (accessed on 30 January 2022).
78. Maldonado, J.E.; De Witte, K. The Effect of School Closures on Standardised Student Test Outcomes. *Br. Educ. Res. J.* **2021**. [CrossRef]
79. Di Pietro, G.; Biagi, F.; Dinis Mota Da Costa, P.; Karpinski, Z.; Mazza, J. *The Likely Impact of COVID-19 on Education: Reflections Based on the Existing Literature and Recent International Datasets*; EUR 30275 EN; Publications Office of the European Union: Luxembourg, 2020; ISBN 978-92-76-19937-3. [CrossRef]
80. Goudeau, S.; Sanrey, C.; Stanczak, A.; Manstead, A.; Darnon, C. Why Lockdown and Distance Learning during the COVID-19 Pandemic Are Likely to Increase the Social Class Achievement Gap. *Nat. Hum. Behav.* **2021**, *5*, 1273–1281. [CrossRef]
81. Kuhfeld, M.; Tarasawa, B.; Johnson, A.; Ruzek, E.; Lewis, K. *Learning during COVID-19: Initial Findings on Students' Reading and Math Achievement and Growth*; Brief, NWEA; 2020. Available online: https://eric.ed.gov/?id=ed505824 (accessed on 30 January 2022).
82. Engzell, P.; Frey, A.; Verhagen, M.D. Learning Loss Due to School Closures during the COVID-19 Pandemic. *Proc. Natl. Acad. Sci. USA* **2021**, *118*, e2022376118. [CrossRef] [PubMed]
83. Schult, J.; Mahler, N.; Fauth, B.; Lindner, M.A. Did Students Learn Less during the COVID-19 Pandemic? Reading and Mathematics Competencies Before and After the First Pandemic Wave. *PsyArXiv Preprints* **2021**. [CrossRef]
84. Goodwin, R.; Sugiyama, K.; Sun, S.; Aida, J.; Ben Ezra, M. Psychological Distress after the Great East Japan Earthquake: Two Multilevel 6-Year Prospective Analyses. *Br. J. Psychiatry* **2020**, *216*, 144–150. [CrossRef] [PubMed]
85. Hou, W.K.; Lai, F.T.; Ben-Ezra, M.; Goodwin, R. Regularizing Daily Routines for Mental Health during and after the COVID-19 Pandemic. *J. Glob. Health* **2020**, *10*, 020315. [CrossRef] [PubMed]

86. Parks, V.; Drakeford, L.; Cope, M.R.; Slack, T. Disruption of Routine Behaviors Following the Deepwater Horizon Oil Spill. *Soc. Nat. Resour.* **2018**, *31*, 277–290. [CrossRef]
87. Xiao, C.; Li, Y. Analysis on the Influence of the Epidemic on the Education in China. In Proceedings of the 2020 International Conference on Big Data and Informatization Education (ICBDIE), Zhangjiajie, China, 23–25 April 2020; pp. 143–147. [CrossRef]
88. Cheng, X.; Pellegrini, M.; Zhou, L.; Cheung, A.C.K. Not Only Survival but Stronger: The Impact of Alarming Invader of SARS-CoV-2 on Global Education. *Sci. Insights Educ. Front.* **2020**, *7*, 835–860. [CrossRef]
89. Galea, S.; Merchant, R.M.; Lurie, N. The Mental Health Consequences of COVID-19 and Physical Distancing: The Need for Prevention and Early Intervention. *JAMA Intern Med.* **2020**, *180*, 817–818. [CrossRef]
90. Altena, E.; Baglioni, C.; Espie, C.A.; Ellis, J.; Gavriloff, D.; Holzinger, B.; Schlarb, A.; Frase, L.; Jernelöv, S.; Riemann, D. Dealing with Sleep Problems during Home Confinement Due to the COVID-19 Outbreak: Practical Recommendations from a Task Force of the European CBT-I Academy. *J. Sleep Res.* **2020**, *29*, e13052. [CrossRef]
91. Becker, S.P.; Gregory, A.M. Editorial Perspective: Perils and Promise for Child and Adolescent Sleep and Associated Psychopathology during the COVID-19 Pandemic. *J. Child. Psychol. Psychiatr.* **2020**, *61*, 757–759. [CrossRef]
92. Muñoz-Fernández, N.; Rodríguez-Meirinhos, A. Adolescents' Concerns, Routines, Peer Activities, Frustration, and Optimism in the Time of COVID-19 Confinement in Spain. *J. Clin. Med.* **2021**, *10*, 798. [CrossRef]
93. YoungMinds. Covid Impact on Young People with Mental Health Needs Survey 1: March 2020. Available online: https://www.youngminds.org.uk/media/xq2dnc0d/youngminds-coronavirus-report-march2020.pdf (accessed on 20 January 2022).
94. World Health Organization [WHO]. Regional Office for the Eastern Mediterranean. Mental Health and Psychosocial Considerations during the COVID-19 Outbreak. Available online: https://www.who.int/publications-detail-redirect/WHO-2019-nCoV-MentalHealth-2020.1 (accessed on 18 January 2022).
95. Lee, J. Mental Health Effects of School Closures during COVID-19. *Lancet Child Adolesc. Health* **2020**, *4*, 421. [CrossRef]
96. YoungMinds. Covid Impact on Young People with Mental Health Needs Survey 2: Summer 2020. Available online: https://www.youngminds.org.uk/media/04apxfrt/youngminds-coronavirus-report-summer-2020.pdf (accessed on 20 January 2022).
97. YoungMinds. Covid Impact on Young People with Mental Health Needs Survey 3: Autumn 2020—Return to School. Available online: https://www.youngminds.org.uk/media/0h1pizqs/youngminds-coronavirus-report-autumn-2020.pdf (accessed on 20 January 2022).
98. YoungMinds. Covid Impact on Young People with Mental Health Needs Survey 4: February 2021. Available online: https://www.youngminds.org.uk/media/esifqn3z/youngminds-coronavirus-report-jan-2021.pdf (accessed on 20 January 2022).
99. Brown, B.B.; Larson, J. Peer Relationships in Adolescence. In *Handbook of Adolescent Psychology*; Lerner, R.M., Steinberg, L., Eds.; John Wiley & Sons, Ltd.: Hoboken, NJ, USA, 2009; pp. 74–103. [CrossRef]
100. Ellis, W.E.; Zarbatany, L. Understanding Processes of Peer Clique Influence in Late Childhood and Early Adolescence. *Child Dev. Perspect.* **2017**, *11*, 227–232. [CrossRef]
101. Ellis, W.E.; Dumas, T.M.; Forbes, L.M. Physically Isolated but Socially Connected: Psychological Adjustment and Stress among Adolescents during the Initial COVID-19 Crisis. *Can. J. Behav. Sci.* **2020**, *52*, 177–187. [CrossRef]
102. Buzzi, C.; Tucci, M.; Ciprandi, R.; Brambilla, I.; Caimmi, S.; Ciprandi, G.; Marseglia, G.L. The Psycho-Social Effects of COVID-19 on Italian Adolescents' Attitudes and Behaviors. *Ital. J. Pediatrics* **2020**, *46*, 69. [CrossRef]
103. Sahu, P. Closure of Universities Due to Coronavirus Disease 2019 (COVID-19): Impact on Education and Mental Health of Students and Academic Staff. *Cureus* **2020**, *12*, e7541. [CrossRef]
104. Ananiadou, K.; Borbély-Pecze, T.; Hooley, T.; Jürges, A.; Kadletz, F.; Katayama, H.; Kettunen, J.; Kraatz, S.; Harrison, C.M.; Mann, A.; et al. *Career Guidance Policy and Practice in the Pandemic: Results of a Joint International Survey. European Commission*; Publication Office of the European Commission: Luxembourg, 2021. [CrossRef]
105. Mann, A.; Denis, V.; Percy, C. Career Ready?: How Schools Can Better Prepare Young People for Working Life in the Era of COVID-19. In *OECD Education Working Papers*; OECD Publishing: Paris, France, 2020. [CrossRef]
106. Fraysier, K.; Reschly, A.; Appleton, J. Predicting Postsecondary Enrollment with Secondary Student Engagement Data. *J. Psychoeduc. Assess.* **2020**, *38*, 882–899. [CrossRef]
107. Prince's Trust. Pandemic Highlights "Aspiration Gap" as Young People Lose Hope. Available online: https://www.princes-trust.org.uk/about-the-trust/news-views/aspiration-gap-research (accessed on 22 November 2021).
108. OECD Economic Outlook. *Organisation for Economic Co-Operation and Development*; OECD Publishing: Paris, France, 2021.
109. Elementary and Secondary School Emergency Relief [ESSER]. Coronavirus Aid, Relief, and Economic Security (CARES) Act. Available online: https://www.nj.gov/education/esser/cares/ (accessed on 22 November 2021).
110. Department of Education. School Funding: Exceptional Costs Associated with Coronavirus (COVID-19) for the Period from March to July 2020. Available online: https://www.gov.uk/government/publications/coronavirus-covid-19-financial-support-for-schools/school-funding-exceptional-costs-associated-with-coronavirus-covid-19-for-the-period-march-to-july-2020 (accessed on 21 November 2021).

111. UNICEF; Università Cattolica. 1 in 3 Italian Families Unable to Support Children's Remote Learning during the Lockdown. Available online: https://www.unicef-irc.org/article/2109-1-in-3-italian-families-unable-to-support-childrens-remote-learning-during-the-lockdown-unicef-and-università-cattolica.html (accessed on 21 November 2021).
112. Kalil, A.; Mayer, S.; Shah, R. *Impact of the COVID-19 Crisis on Family Dynamics in Economically Vulnerable Households*; University of Chicago, Becker Friedman Institute for Economics: Chicago, IL, USA, 2020.
113. Azevedo, J.P.; Hasan, A.; Goldemberg, D.; Geven, K.; Iqbal, S.A. Simulating the Potential Impacts of COVID-19 School Closures on Schooling and Learning Outcomes: A Set of Global Estimates. *World Bank Res. Obs.* **2021**, *36*, lkab003. [CrossRef]
114. Cullinane, C.; Montacute, R. *Research Brief: April 2020: COVID-19 and Social Mobility Impact Brief#1: School Shutdown*; Sutton Trust: London, UK, 2020.
115. Kosaretsky, S.; Zair-Bek, S.; Kersha, Y.; Zvyagintsev, R. General Education in Russia During COVID-19: Readiness, Policy Response, and Lessons Learned. In *Primary and Secondary Education during Covid-19: Disruptions to Educational Opportunity During a Pandemic*; Reimers, F.M., Ed.; Springer International Publishing: Cham, Switherland, 2022; pp. 227–261. [CrossRef]
116. Wu, M.; Xu, W.; Yao, Y.; Zhang, L.; Guo, L.; Fan, J.; Chen, J. Mental Health Status of Students' Parents during COVID-19 Pandemic and Its Influence Factors. *Gen. Psychiatr.* **2020**, *33*, e100250. [CrossRef]
117. Gruber, J.; Prinstein, M.J.; Clark, L.A.; Rottenberg, J.; Abramowitz, J.S.; Albano, A.M.; Aldao, A.; Borelli, J.L.; Chung, T.; Davila, J.; et al. Mental Health and Clinical Psychological Science in the Time of COVID-19: Challenges, Opportunities, and a Call to Action. *Am. Psychol.* **2021**, *76*, 409–426. [CrossRef]
118. Horesh, D.; Brown, A.D. Traumatic Stress in the Age of COVID-19: A Call to Close Critical Gaps and Adapt to New Realities. *Psychol. Trauma Theory Res. Pract. Policy* **2020**, *12*, 331–335. [CrossRef] [PubMed]
119. Hyland, P.; Shevlin, M.; McBride, O.; Murphy, J.; Karatzias, T.; Bentall, R.P.; Martinez, A.; Vallières, F. Anxiety and Depression in the Republic of Ireland during the COVID-19 Pandemic. *Acta Psychiatr. Scand.* **2020**, *142*, 249–256. [CrossRef] [PubMed]
120. Özdin, S.; Bayrak Özdin, Ş. Levels and Predictors of Anxiety, Depression and Health Anxiety during COVID-19 Pandemic in Turkish Society: The Importance of Gender. *Int. J. Soc. Psychiatry* **2020**, *66*, 504–511. [CrossRef] [PubMed]
121. Salari, N.; Hosseinian-Far, A.; Jalali, R.; Vaisi-Raygani, A.; Rasoulpoor, S.; Mohammadi, M.; Rasoulpoor, S.; Khaledi-Paveh, B. Prevalence of Stress, Anxiety, Depression among the General Population during the COVID-19 Pandemic: A Systematic Review and Meta-Analysis. *Glob. Health* **2020**, *16*, 57. [CrossRef]
122. Shevlin, M.; McBride, O.; Murphy, J.; Miller, J.G.; Hartman, T.K.; Levita, L.; Mason, L.; Martinez, A.P.; McKay, R.; Stocks, T.V.A.; et al. Anxiety, Depression, Traumatic Stress and COVID-19-Related Anxiety in the UK General Population during the COVID-19 Pandemic. *BJPsych Open* **2020**, *6*, e125. [CrossRef]
123. Nock, M.K.; Kessler, R.C. Prevalence of and Risk Factors for Suicide Attempts versus Suicide Gestures: Analysis of the National Comorbidity Survey. *J. Abnorm. Psychol.* **2006**, *115*, 616–623. [CrossRef]
124. Brooks, S.K.; Webster, R.K.; Smith, L.E.; Woodland, L.; Wessely, S.; Greenberg, N.; Rubin, G.J. The Psychological Impact of Quarantine and How to Reduce It: Rapid Review of the Evidence. *Lancet* **2020**, *395*, 912–920. [CrossRef]
125. Cacioppo, S.; Grippo, A.J.; London, S.; Goossens, L.; Cacioppo, J.T. Loneliness: Clinical Import and Interventions. *Perspect. Psychol. Sci.* **2015**, *10*, 238–249. [CrossRef]
126. Bhuiyan, A.K.M.I.; Sakib, N.; Pakpour, A.H.; Griffiths, M.D.; Mamun, M.A. COVID-19-Related Suicides in Bangladesh Due to Lockdown and Economic Factors: Case Study Evidence from Media Reports. *Int. J. Ment. Health Addict.* **2020**, *19*, 2110–2115. [CrossRef]
127. Dsouza, D.D.; Quadros, S.; Hyderabadwala, Z.J.; Mamun, M.A. Aggregated COVID-19 Suicide Incidences in India: Fear of COVID-19 Infection Is the Prominent Causative Factor. *Psychiatry Res.* **2020**, *290*, 113145. [CrossRef]
128. Calati, R.; Ferrari, C.; Brittner, M.; Oasi, O.; Olié, E.; Carvalho, A.F.; Courtet, P. Suicidal Thoughts and Behaviors and Social Isolation: A Narrative Review of the Literature. *J. Affect. Disord.* **2019**, *245*, 653–667. [CrossRef] [PubMed]
129. Marques de Miranda, D.; da Silva Athanasio, B.; Sena Oliveira, A.C.; Simoes-e-Silva, A.C. How Is COVID-19 Pandemic Impacting Mental Health of Children and Adolescents? *Int. J. Disaster Risk Reduct.* **2020**, *51*, 101845. [CrossRef] [PubMed]
130. Jiao, W.Y.; Wang, L.N.; Liu, J.; Fang, S.F.; Jiao, F.Y.; Pettoello-Mantovani, M.; Somekh, E. Behavioral and Emotional Disorders in Children during the COVID-19 Epidemic. *J. Pediatrics* **2020**, *221*, 264–266.e1. [CrossRef] [PubMed]
131. Magson, N.R.; Freeman, J.Y.A.; Rapee, R.M.; Richardson, C.E.; Oar, E.L.; Fardouly, J. Risk and Protective Factors for Prospective Changes in Adolescent Mental Health during the COVID-19 Pandemic. *J. Youth Adolesc.* **2021**, *50*, 44–57. [CrossRef] [PubMed]
132. Orgilés, M.; Morales, A.; Delvecchio, E.; Mazzeschi, C.; Espada, J.P. Immediate Psychological Effects of the COVID-19 Quarantine in Youth from Italy and Spain. *Front. Psychol.* **2020**, *11*, 2986. [CrossRef]
133. McArdle, J.; Hamagami, F.; Chang, J.Y.; Hishinuma, E.S. Longitudinal Dynamic Analyses of Depression and Academic Achievement in the Hawaiian High Schools Health Survey Using Contemporary Latent Variable Change Models. *Struct. Equ. Modeling* **2014**, *21*, 608–629. [CrossRef]

134. Humensky, J.; Kuwabara, S.A.; Fogel, J.; Wells, C.; Goodwin, B.; Voorhees, B.W.V. Adolescents With Depressive Symptoms and Their Challenges With Learning in School. *J. Sch. Nurs.* **2010**, *26*, 377–392. [CrossRef]
135. Davis, C.R.; Grooms, J.; Ortega, A.; Rubalcaba, J.A.-A.; Vargas, E. Distance Learning and Parental Mental Health During COVID-19. *Educ. Res.* **2021**, *50*, 61–64. [CrossRef]
136. Westrupp, E.M.; Bennett, C.; Berkowitz, T.; Youssef, G.J.; Toumbourou, J.W.; Tucker, R.; Andrews, F.J.; Evans, S.; Teague, S.J.; Karantzas, G.C.; et al. Child, Parent, and Family Mental Health and Functioning in Australia during COVID-19: Comparison to Pre-Pandemic Data. *Eur. Child Adolesc. Psychiatry* **2021**. [CrossRef]
137. Brown, S.M.; Doom, J.R.; Lechuga-Peña, S.; Watamura, S.E.; Koppels, T. Stress and Parenting during the Global COVID-19 Pandemic. *Child Abuse Negl.* **2020**, *110 Pt 2*, 104699. [CrossRef]
138. McLaughlin, K.A.; Greif Green, J.; Gruber, M.J.; Sampson, N.A.; Zaslavsky, A.M.; Kessler, R.C. Childhood Adversities and First Onset of Psychiatric Disorders in a National Sample of US Adolescents. *Arch. Gen. Psychiatry* **2012**, *69*, 1151–1160. [CrossRef] [PubMed]
139. Spinelli, M.; Lionetti, F.; Pastore, M.; Fasolo, M. Parents' Stress and Children's Psychological Problems in Families Facing the COVID-19 Outbreak in Italy. *Front. Psychol.* **2020**, *11*, 1713. [CrossRef] [PubMed]
140. Sprang, G.; Silman, M. Posttraumatic Stress Disorder in Parents and Youth after Health-Related Disasters. *Disaster Med. Public Health Prep.* **2013**, *7*, 105–110. [CrossRef]
141. Aktar, E.; Nikolić, M.; Bögels, S.M. Environmental Transmission of Generalized Anxiety Disorder from Parents to Children: Worries, Experiential Avoidance, and Intolerance of Uncertainty. *Dialogues Clin. Neurosci.* **2017**, *19*, 137–147. [CrossRef] [PubMed]
142. Dragano, N.; Lunau, T. Technostress at Work and Mental Health: Concepts and Research Results. *Curr. Opin. Psychiatry* **2020**, *33*, 407–413. [CrossRef]
143. Stachteas, P.; Stachteas, C. The Psychological Impact of the COVID-19 Pandemic on Secondary School Teachers. *Psychiatriki* **2020**, *31*, 293–301. [CrossRef]
144. Palumbo, R. Let Me Go to the Office! An Investigation into the Side Effects of Working from Home on Work-Life Balance. *Int. J. Public Sect. Manag.* **2020**, *33*, 771–790. [CrossRef]
145. Lizana, P.A.; Vega-Fernadez, G.; Gomez-Bruton, A.; Leyton, B.; Lera, L. Impact of the COVID-19 Pandemic on Teacher Quality of Life: A Longitudinal Study from before and during the Health Crisis. *Int. J. Environ. Res. Public Health* **2021**, *18*, 3764. [CrossRef]
146. Ozamiz-Etxebarria, N.; Berasategi Santxo, N.; Idoiaga Mondragon, N.; Dosil Santamaría, M. The Psychological State of Teachers During the COVID-19 Crisis: The Challenge of Returning to Face-to-Face Teaching. *Front. Psychol.* **2021**, *11*, 3861. [CrossRef]
147. Dhawan, S. Online Learning: A Panacea in the Time of COVID-19 Crisis. *J. Educ. Technol. Syst.* **2020**, *49*, 5–22. [CrossRef]
148. Al-Dosari, H. Faculty Members and Students Perceptions of E-Learning in the English Department: A Project Evaluation. *J. Soc. Sci.* **2011**, *7*, 291. [CrossRef]
149. Adnan, M.; Anwar, K. Online Learning amid the COVID-19 Pandemic: Students' Perspectives. *J. Pedagog. Sociol. Psychol.* **2020**, *2*, 45–51. [CrossRef]
150. Coman, C.; Țîru, L.G.; Meseșan-Schmitz, L.; Stanciu, C.; Bularca, M.C. Online Teaching and Learning in Higher Education during the Coronavirus Pandemic: Students' Perspective. *Sustainability* **2020**, *12*, 10367. [CrossRef]
151. Suresh, M.; Priya, V.V.; Gayathri, R. Effect of E-Learning on Academic Performance of Undergraduate Students. *Drug Invent. Today* **2018**, *10*, 1797–1800.
152. Ariebowo, T. Autonomous Learning during COVID-19 Pandemic: Students' Objectives and Preferences. *J. Foreign Lang. Teach. Learn. (Online)* **2021**, *6*, 56–77. [CrossRef]
153. Yustina, Y.; Syafii, W.; Vebrianto, R. The Effects of Blended Learning and Project-Based Learning on Pre-Service Biology Teachers' Creative Thinking through Online Learning in the Covid-19 Pandemic. *J. Pendidik. IPA Indones.* **2020**, *9*, 408–420. [CrossRef]
154. Patston, T.J.; Kennedy, J.; Jaeschke, W.; Kapoor, H.; Leonard, S.N.; Cropley, D.H.; Kaufman, J.C. Secondary Education in COVID Lockdown: More Anxious and Less Creative—Maybe Not? *Front. Psychol.* **2021**, *12*, 391. [CrossRef]
155. Kupers, E.; Lehmann-Wermser, A.; McPherson, G.; van Geert, P. Children's Creativity: A Theoretical Framework and Systematic Review. *Rev. Educ. Res.* **2019**, *89*, 93–124. [CrossRef]
156. Kapoor, H.; Kaufman, J.C. Meaning-Making Through Creativity During COVID-19. *Front. Psychol.* **2020**, *11*, 3659. [CrossRef]
157. Uzun, H.; Karaca, N.H.; Metin, Ş. Assesment of Parent-Child Relationship in Covid-19 Pandemic. *Child. Youth Serv. Rev.* **2021**, *120*, 105748. [CrossRef]
158. Vaterlaus, J.M.; Shaffer, T.; Patten, E.V.; Spruance, L.A. Parent-Child Relationships and the COVID-19 Pandemic: An Exploratory Qualitative Study with Parents in Early, Middle, and Late Adulthood. *J. Adult Dev.* **2021**, *28*, 251–263. [CrossRef] [PubMed]
159. Janssens, J.J.; Achterhof, R.; Lafit, G.; Bamps, E.; Hagemann, N.; Hiekkaranta, A.P.; Hermans, K.S.F.M.; Lecei, A.; Myin-Germeys, I.; Kirtley, O.J. The Impact of COVID-19 on Adolescents' Daily Lives: The Role of Parent-Child Relationship Quality. *J. Res. Adolesc.* **2021**, *31*, 623–644. [CrossRef] [PubMed]
160. Hamilton, L.S.; Grant, D.; Kaufman, J.H.; Diliberti, M.K.; Schwartz, H.L.; Hunter, G.P.; Setodji, C.M.; Young, C.J. *COVID-19 and the State of K–12 Schools: Results and Technical Documentation from the Spring 2020 American Educator Panels COVID-19 Surveys*; RAND Corporation: Santa Monica, CA, USA, 2020. [CrossRef]
161. Daniel, S.J. Education and the COVID-19 Pandemic. *Prospects* **2020**, *49*, 91–96. [CrossRef] [PubMed]

162. Lan, X.; Scrimin, S.; Moscardino, U. Perceived Parental Guan and School Adjustment among Chinese Early Adolescents: The Moderating Role of Interdependent Self-Construal. *J. Adolesc.* **2019**, *71*, 18–27. [CrossRef] [PubMed]
163. Chamizo-Nieto, M.T.; Arrivillaga, C.; Rey, L.; Extremera, N. The Role of Emotional Intelligence, the Teacher-Student Relationship, and Flourishing on Academic Performance in Adolescents: A Moderated Mediation Study. *Front. Psychol.* **2021**, *12*, 695067. [CrossRef]

encyclopedia

Entry

COVID-19 and Psychological Impact

Nereida Bueno-Guerra

Department of Psychology, Comillas Pontifical University (Campus Cantoblanco), 28049 Madrid, Spain; nbguerra@comillas.edu

Definition: The worldwide mental health burden associated to COVID-19. The psychological symptoms associated to COVID-19 can originate from three different sources: lockdowns, pandemic life and virus infection (both COVID-19 and post COVID-19 condition). Within the psychological symptoms it can be found: anxiety, depression, post-traumatic stress, fatigue and cognitive impairment (i.e., 'brain fog', mental slowness, deficits in attention, executive functioning, working memory, learning, articulation, and/or psychomotor coordination). Plus, two psychological conditions associated to the COVID-19 pandemic have been coined so far by the World Health Organization: pandemic fatigue and post COVID-19 condition. The increase of psychological symptoms both in the general population and in frontline workers (especially health-care workers) generates an unprecedented number of psychological patients and it challenges national mental health systems.

Keywords: mental health; SARS-CoV-2; COVID-19; lockdown; frontline workers; pandemic fatigue; post COVID-19 condition; anxiety; depression; stress

Citation: Bueno-Guerra, N. COVID-19 and Psychological Impact. *Encyclopedia* **2022**, 2, 400–408. https://doi.org/10.3390/encyclopedia2010024

Academic Editors: Stephen Bustin and Raffaele Barretta

Received: 6 January 2022
Accepted: 25 January 2022
Published: 2 February 2022

1. Introduction

The COVID-19 pandemic officially declared in March 2020 [1] is both "an epidemiological and psychological crisis" [2]. Aside from the harmful physical effects that the sickness may cause in infected patients, three collateral factors contribute to an unprecedented worldwide mental health burden in both infected and non-infected people: preventive isolation measures taken worldwide (i.e., lockdowns), drastic changes in daily life (i.e., deceased relatives, overflowed frontline workers, social distancing, curfews) and COVID-19 and post COVID-19 related psychological symptoms. The purpose of the present manuscript is to summarize the most up-to-date accumulated knowledge so far (5 January 2022) about the psychological impact of each factor (see Table 1 at the end of this entry for a brief summary of its content).

Importantly, given the overwhelming number of studies, a broad vision has been prioritized by selecting systematic reviews, meta-analysis and longitudinal research over transversal or nation-specific studies, whenever possible. However, this strategy does not ensure the provision of causal or relational knowledge given the fact that most of the studies conducted and published so far are cross-sectional (i.e., measuring a specific population group in a specific point of time) rather than longitudinal (i.e., gathering several measures of a specific population group along a period of time) or prospective (i.e., starting the data collection before the pandemic outbreak, which may count as a baseline, and continuing afterwards, to allow for comparisons), and therefore, even systematic reviews may be biased in their conclusions.

In those cases where the broad vision also implied citing a vast number of studies, due to space restrictions, two selection criteria were applied: chronological order of publication (first-year pandemic stage: March to December 2020 and late pandemic stage: from January 2021 on) to illustrate any potential longitudinal tendency and the affiliation of the authors (citing at least one study per continent, if any) to illustrate any potential cross-cultural difference. Despite the efforts invested to avoid a Western vision of COVID-19 and its psychological impact, this entry may lack cultural diversity due to the low publication rate of low-income countries.

Table 1. Brief summary of sources and symptoms of psychological impact related to COVID-19.

Lockdowns	Pandemic Life	COVID-19 Infection
Not alarmingly affected global population but suicide vigilance is recommended	Global increase in the rates of anxiety, depression and post-traumatic disorders	COVID-19 infection: cognitive impairment and fatigue
Vulnerable subgroups: autism, pregnancy, homeless	Vulnerable subgroups: OCD, depression	Post COVID-19 condition (3 months after infection): cognitive impairment and fatigue over 2 months
Risk contexts: domestic violence, intrafamilial child abuse	Front-line workers more exposed, especially health-care workers	Post-intensive care syndrome in intensive care unit survivors: cognitive impairment and mental health problems
Pandemic fatigue: demotivation to follow preventive measures	Abundance of cross-sectional rather than longitudinal and prospective studies, preventing causal knowledge	Both patients and their relatives (current carers) may be at risk of psychological impact

2. Lockdowns

The characterization of COVID-19 as a "pandemic" by the World Health Organization (WHO) in March 2020 [1] entailed several nationwide public health measures, among which unprecedented lockdowns in recent decades took place. Lockdowns can be defined as the confinement of specific or general groups of population imposed by a certain authority during a given time aiming to reduce the spread of some disease as well as to attenuate the hospital pressure created by the above-average healthcare demands that the disease causes (the so-called "buy time" measure [3]) [4]. During the lockdowns, the confined population's outdoor movements and activities are restricted, which usually entails a general closure of non-essential businesses and establishments. Therefore, the psychological wellbeing associated with the maintenance of rewarding events (such as relative visits, trips or outdoor leisure time) or routines (such as going to school/work or shopping) can be dramatically reduced.

The psychological impact that the lockdowns might cause in the population had no previous modern referent because there are no historical records of previous simultaneous worldwide strict confinements during the last century. Most resembling lockdowns might be the public actions taken during the two influenza pandemics across the XX century, however, they were not regularly adopted nationwide; varied in intensity—from lazarettos to border closures—and did not happen coordinately with other nations or in an instant-globalized Internet based world; see [5] for a revision of quarantines since Middle Age times. There is also little evidence of prior measurements of the psychological impact of more than three months of confinement. The closest study available was a rapid review published some days before the pandemic characterization listing the evidence about the psychological impact of recent regional quarantines of a maximum of 21 days caused by SARS, Ebola, H1N1 influenza and Middle East respiratory syndrome [6]. They found that symptoms were "wide-ranging, substantial and can be long-lasting" (p. 919) and provided six suggestions to ameliorate them: keeping the lockdowns as short as possible, giving a lot of information, providing adequate supplies, reducing boredom and improving communication, paying especial attention to health-care workers and appealing to altruism.

After COVID-19 lockdowns, research about the psychological impact concluded that, fortunately, the lockdowns themselves seemed not to have contributed to produce significant psychological impact in the general population: a recent metanalysis found that their magnitude was "small and highly heterogeneous, suggesting that lockdowns do not have uniformly detrimental effects on mental health and that most people are psychologically resilient to their effects" [7] (abstract). Indeed, suicide rates did not rise during house confinement, as a time-series analysis from 21 countries showed [8]. However, optimism should not prevent further strategies, because the return after lockdowns can have a rebound effect and some authors suggest remaining cautious and vigilant, especially with regards to suicide [9,10]. Moreover, even when at a general level the psychological impact of lockdowns was low, for certain vulnerable sectors of population it was severe, such as children and adolescents [11], subjects with autism spectrum [12], pregnant women [13], homeless people [14], people in poverty, migrants and refugees [13], to name a few. As a future lesson, researchers suggest that using common psychological impact measures in different samples would benefit further cross-cultural comparison, i.e., [6] (see Section 3, "Pandemic life", for a list of the most used instruments to measure each disorder).

Behaviours with associated negative psychological consequences changed during lockdowns, especially those related to addiction. Whereas a metanalysis about alcohol consumption revealed that the average intake did not vary significantly, it did within subsamples with some previous mental health/alcohol-related risk factors [15] or those who were already chronic/excessive consumers, as a four-year longitudinal study showed [16]. The same happened to gambling: although bets decreased across countries, in some subsamples problematic gambling was increased [17]. This evidence shows that people with previous vulnerable factors should be especially protected in times of significant life adversity, such as an international emergency health crisis. Furthermore, crimes that cause relevant psychological impact, such as domestic violence, intrafamilial sexual abuse, production and demand for child sexual exploitation material, online-grooming and cyberbullying increased worldwide during lockdowns because the confinement led to permanent contact between offenders and victims as well as to higher rates of unsupervised Internet connection between children. In this sense, there is evidence of a worldwide increase in domestic violence cases, as systematic reviews report [18,19], as well as an increase of calls to domestic violence helplines [20] so that more than fifty countries integrated prevention and response to violence against women and girls into COVID-19 response plans, as the United Nations Data Platform shows [21]. Multiple international voices raised concern about the need for child protection at home due to the high risk of violence against them, i.e., [22] and data showed that child sexual exploitation material demand raised [23].

The return to regular life after lockdown has been associated with the folk syndrome coined "cabin fever", describing "a combination of anxiety, lassitude, irritability, moodiness, boredom, depression, or feeling of dissatisfaction in response to confinement, bad weather, routine, isolation, or lack of stimulation" [24]. However, this popular syndrome has no correspondent official nosologic entity. Indeed, according to the WHO, the unique psychological impact officially recognized as being related to COVID-19 measures is "pandemic fatigue". Pandemic fatigue describes "demotivation to follow recommended protective behaviours emerging gradually over time and affected by a number of emotions, experiences and perceptions, such as complacency, alienation and hopelessness. It is an expected and natural response to a prolonged public health crisis—not least because the severity and scale of the COVID-19 pandemic have called for the implementation of invasive measures with unprecedented impacts on the daily lives of everyone, including those who have not been directly affected by the virus itself" [25] (pp. 4–7).

3. Pandemic Life

Living life during the COVID-19 pandemic entails adapting to different preventive measures and both the interpersonal and financial consequences of the virus spread. Meta-analyses reviewing the impact that the COVID-19 pandemic has had on mental health mostly focus on three disorders: anxiety, depression and post-traumatic stress. These studies usually differentiate the sample evaluated between the general population and frontline workers since the latter have been more exposed to contagion, traumatic images and have experienced an overwhelming workload. Within the different jobs considered among frontline workers, health care workers have been the most studied professional group so far. Next, there is a summary of the accumulated knowledge about anxiety, depression and post-traumatic stress across three different sections and within each section there is specific mention of studies with samples of health care workers.

3.1. Anxiety

During the COVID-19 pandemic, different national preventive measures and international recommendations have been applied: from general closure of non-essential businesses and establishments to time restricted openings, curfews and travel restrictions; from mandatory vaccination to some population sectors and face mask use to periodic handwashing and ventilation. This situation forces people to flexibly adapt to new scenarios, remain alert about the spread of the virus and sometimes lose previous income levels. Moreover, the news remains the main source of information for the general population, usually updating daily about new virus variants, preventive measures, legal changes or providing data on the economic impact and death and incidence rates. This situation helps people to be informed as well as makes them constantly alert about the spread of the virus. Consequently, the modification of regular civil life under the feeling of uncertainty, the constant need to be alert, the economic instability with large-scale job loss and the permanent information about contagions and death, within this new uncontrollable situation, may contribute to the emergence of anxiety disorders.

A study reviewing research that provided the pre- and post COVID-19 prevalence of mental health burden across 204 countries reported that after one year of the COVID-19 pandemic, there was a 25.6% global increase of the prevalence of anxiety disorders, namely, an additional 76.2 million (64.3 to 90.6) estimated cases [26]. Even when there are countries lacking data, these numbers reveal a high global psychological impact that can potentially impact mental care systems. With regards to health care workers, systematic reviews and meta-analysis found that this professional sector had a higher level of anxiety compared to general population (24% [27] (November, 2020), 34.4% [28] (December 2020) from 8.5% to 13% [29] (January 2021)) and, in all cases, the level of anxiety was constantly higher in Western rather than Asian professionals [30] (May 2021), whereas other authors suggested higher rates in Middle-Eastern professionals [31] (March 2021).

The most at-risk of suffering from anxiety disorders (both onset or increasing pre-existing symptoms) are people with obsessive-compulsive symptoms, such as concerns about becoming contaminated themselves, fear of unknowingly spreading contamination and causing harm to others, overestimation of threats and tendencies to seek reassurance by excessive searching for news on COVID-19 [32]. Unfortunately, for all of them, living surrounded by necessary guidelines and signage on hygienic measures about how to prevent the virus spread, such as periodic handwashing, can reinforce their obsessive ideas. Moreover, doomscrolling, or spending an excessive amount of screen time devoted to the absorption of negative news [33], may also approach high rates within the pandemic.

Finally, and for further research purposes, the instruments employed to measure anxiety in the meta-analysis and systematic reviews are, in alphabetical order: DASS-21: Depression Anxiety Stress Scale; GAD: General Anxiety Disorder; HADS: Hospital Anxiety and Depression Scale; HAMA: Hamilton Anxiety Rating Scale.

3.2. Depression

During the COVID-19 pandemic, the number of contagions and deaths has constantly increased, varying periodically from curve deflations to exponential peaks. This situation has led people to lose loved ones, or even suffer COVID-19 health issues themselves with long-term sequelae. The pandemic has also led to the reduction of rewarding activities and fueled negative further perspectives about the future due to financial loss, recurrent new contagion waves and difficulties to schedule prevalence-dependent massive outdoor activities (e.g., weddings, music concert), which may contribute to depressive mood.

Within the aforementioned study reviewing research that provided the pre- and post COVID-19 prevalence of mental health burden across 204 countries after one year of the COVID-19 pandemic, it is reported that there is a 27.6% global increase of the prevalence of depressive disorders, namely, an additional 53.2 million (44.8 to 62.9) estimated cases [26]. With regards to health care workers, systematic reviews and meta-analysis found that this professional sector had a higher level of depression compared to the general population: 25% [27] (November, 2020), 31.8% [28] (December, 2020), from 9.5% to 12.2% [29] (January 2021) and 23% [30] (May 2021).

A revision of the psychological consequences for relatives caused by losing loved ones after being in an intensive care unit (ICU), which is the treatment of choice for severe COVID-19 patients, estimated that "the number of cases of complicated grief following COVID-19 deaths may virtually reach the number of overall COVID-19 deaths" [34] (p. 3). Therefore, one of the most at-risk groups of suffering from depression may be those who lost relatives because of COVID-19 disease. In addition, despite the rates of suicide seeming to decreas during the first months of the pandemic [8], the research community suggests being vigilant with these groups of the population [9].

Finally, and for further research purposes, the instruments employed to measure depression in the meta-analysis and systematic reviews are, in alphabetical order: CES-D: Center for Epidemiologic Studies Depression Scale; DASS: Depression Anxiety Stress Scale; HADS: Hospital Anxiety and Depression Scale and HAMD: Hamilton Depression Rating Scale.

3.3. *Post-Traumatic Stress*

The population has witnessed (first-hand or through public information) both COVID-19 related dramatic images, such as accumulated coffins of COVID-19 deceased patients, intubated patients and threatening behaviours, such as actions specifically associated to situations of emergency conducted by peers (i.e., non-perishable stockpiling, panic buying). All this together with the constant threat of being infected may be strong enough to meet the criteria for traumatic events, given their uniqueness and because witnesses may feel their life is at risk.

Indeed, meta-analysis conducted early after the pandemic characterization found that one-in-four adults [35] or a similar 20% (95% CI: 14–25%, $p < 0.001$) [36] experienced significant traumatic stress due to the COVID-19 pandemic. Importantly, the pandemic is almost two years long already and the persistence of the stressor is associated with the chronicity of the disorder and with its comorbidity with psychiatric diagnosis. Therefore, the number of people in the population at risk of developing further psychiatric and psychological needs is high.

With regards to health care workers, systematic reviews and meta-analysis found that this professional sector had a higher level of post-traumatic stress compared to the general population: 13% (Krishnamoorthy, November, 2020), 11.4% [28] (December, 2020), 21% [31] (March 2021) or two in every ten healthcare workers [37] (March 2021).

Finally, and for further research purposes, the instruments employed to measure post-traumatic symptoms in the meta-analysis and systematic reviews are, in alphabetical order: IES-R: Impact of Event Scale-Revised; PSS: Perceived Stress Scale; PTSD-SS: Self-Assessment Scale for Post-Traumatic Stress Disorder; PTSS: Post-Traumatic Stress Syndrome.

4. COVID-19 and Post COVID-19 Psychological Symptoms

The COVID-19 infection may spread to the nervous system and cause cognitive impairment in patients, in consonance with reports about previous viral epidemics that found neurological disorders and cognitive alterations after infection [38]. These psychological consequences are not only restricted to the aforementioned disorders such as depression, anxiety and post-traumatic stress (meta-analysis show that infected patients reported anxiety, depression [39,40] and about three in every ten experienced PTSD symptoms [37]) but also expand to alterations in basic cognitive procedures.

Indeed, an analysis of more than 80 thousand participants supported the hypothesis that COVID-19 has a multi-domain impact on human cognition [41]. Importantly, a cohort study of almost 500 participants informed that negative cognitive performance appears to be associated to some COVID-19 symptoms: "headache, anosmia and dysgeusia constituted the main risk factors for cognitive impairment related with attention, memory and executive function [whereas] the need for oxygen therapy and diarrhea were also associated with memory, attention and executive function deficits" [42] (abstract). A systematic review found that studies reported cognitive deficits, fatigue at follow-up and sleep disturbances, concluding that infected patients are "at risk of psychiatric sequelae but the symptoms generally improve over time" [39].

Unfortunately, the remission of symptoms from COVID-19 infection can also persist [41]. Following a Delphi methodology, namely, including patients, experts and physicians in the working team, the WHO has developed the definition for "post COVID-19 condition": "Post COVID-19 condition occurs in individuals with a history of probable or confirmed SARS-CoV-2 infection, usually 3 months from the onset of COVID-19 with symptoms and that last for at least 2 months and cannot be explained by an alternative diagnosis. Common symptoms include fatigue, shortness of breath, cognitive dysfunction but also others and generally have an impact on everyday functioning. Symptoms may be new onset following initial recovery from an acute COVID-19 episode or persist from the initial illness. Symptoms may also fluctuate or relapse over time" [43].

A meta-analysis found the proportion of individuals experiencing fatigue 12 or more weeks following COVID-19 diagnosis was 0.32 (95% CI, 0.27, 0.37; $p < 0.001$; n = 25,268; I2 = 99.1%), whereas the proportion of individuals exhibiting cognitive impairment was 0.22 (95% CI, 0.17, 0.28; $p < 0.001$; n = 13,232; I2 = 98.0) 12 or more weeks following COVID-19 diagnosis [44] (December, 2021). The cognitive impairment included: 'brain fog', mental slowness (i.e., increase in time needed to perform tasks such as reading/writing documents), deficits in attention (i.e., difficulty in concentrating), executive functioning and working memory (i.e., forgetfulness, spatial memory dysfunctions), learning (i.e., difficulties in learning new skills or procedures), articulation (i.e., difficulties forming words; feeling lost for words), and/or psychomotor coordination [40,44]. So far, the literature is scarce, and the heterogeneity of samples and procedures preclude generalization, however, the recognition of the post COVID condition by WHO should encourage further investigation since the quality of life of the people affected may be reduced.

Importantly, survivors of intensive care units (ICUs) may also experience post-intensive care syndrome (PICS) some months after discharge, which may include a vast array of symptoms collectively grouped into physical impairment, cognitive impairment and mental health problems. Since COVID-19 can entail ICU hospitalization, a recent review has warned about the prevalence of symptoms associated to PICS in COVID-19 patients, reaching high rates of psychological impact: 20–57% pertaining to cognitive impairments and 6–60% pertaining to mental health problems after 1–6 months after discharge [45]. Therefore, further research in the psychological impact of COVID-19 may also consider the study of PICS in discharged COVID-19 patients as well as in their relative carers.

5. Conclusions and Prospects

The rapid fluctuation and emergence of variants of the virus as well as the astonishing rhythm of publication of new COVID-19 related studies makes this entry easily out-of-date. However, there is some solid unperishable data (see Table 1).

Across this entry, the psychological impact associated with COVID-19 has been related to three aspects: experiencing lockdowns, living in a pandemic or getting infected. With regards to COVID-19 lockdowns, these measures have not alarmingly and globally affected the population, except for certain vulnerable subgroups and victims of crimes committed at home. However, the absence of global, alarming symptoms after lockdowns should not prevent further vigilance after release, especially with regards to suicide. Demotivation to follow preventive measures during a prolonged public health crisis has been coined "pandemic fatigue".

With regards to living in the COVID-19 pandemic, there is evidence of a global increase in the rates of anxiety, depression and post-traumatic disorders in the general population. Certain subgroups are more at risk of suffering from anxiety (i.e., OCD patients) or depression (i.e., complicated grief). The worst mental health burden is globally found in health care workers.

With regards to COVID-19 infection, the most prevalent psychological symptoms are associated with cognitive impairment and fatigue. Plus, post COVID-19 condition is a term coined to describe the onset or persistence of fatigue, shortness of breath and cognitive dysfunction for 2 months, usually 3 months after having been infected. The cognitive impairment of post COVID-19 condition includes: 'brain fog', mental slowness, deficits in attention, executive functioning and working memory, learning, articulation and/or psychomotor coordination. Furthermore, in COVID-19 patients discharged from ICU the prevalence of cognitive impairment and mental health problems as part of a broader PICS is high, therefore, psychological and medical follow-ups should be considered and these symptoms further investigated.

Finally, it is important to note that most of the studies included in the systematic reviews commented on so far followed a cross-sectional methodology, namely, they described the mental state of the population in their samples at a certain point of time, therefore not allowing causal or longitudinal knowledge to be provided, but inferential. These studies are relevant because they are descriptive of an unprecedented health crisis in recent history. However, it is also very informative to look at longitudinal studies because they can provide baseline levels (before the pandemic outbreak) to be compared to pandemic levels, so that the potential significant differences found can be less doubtlessly attributed to the effects of the pandemic. These studies are scarce because they imply both a periodic interest in monitoring the mental health of the population and some reserved budget devoted to the assessment task. In this respect, official national reports about mental health are one eligible piece of evidence, since they provide longitudinal data at different waves in large samples and they are usually freely available (e.g., see UK report about mental distress: it increased from 18.9% (95% CI 17.8–20.0) in 2018–2019 to 27.3% (26.3–28.2) in April, 2020) [46]. In addition, prospective studies collecting data at several points during a certain period can be very informative. Concretely, by measuring the mental health during different moments along the COVID-19 pandemic period, the potential long-term psychological symptoms, or cumulative consequences of certain subgroups of the population, such as health care workers, can be revealed (e.g., this study [47] collected data during three COVID-19 waves: April–May 2020, December 2020 and April–May 2021 and was able to conclude that there was an elevated frequency of anxiety, an increasing prevalence of depression and active thoughts of leaving their jobs in Italian health workers). Thus, the methodology of the studies is crucial to carefully conclude about the psychological impact related to COVID-19 depending on our interest (i.e., describing, comparing, foreseeing). Indeed, future studies about psychological impact should consider these interests to look for previous data (and produce longitudinal data) or to propose different measurement points (and produce repeated cross-sectional data).

Funding: This research received no external funding.

Data Availability Statement: Not applicable.

Acknowledgments: I would like to acknowledge all those researchers that, in times of adversity, despite their own psychological impact, took the time to continue building new knowledge. It is thanks to all of them that this entry can be written. Plus, I would also like to thank to two anonymous reviewers and to María Jesús Maldonado Belmonte and Ángela Bernardo Álvarez for their comments on an earlier version of this manuscript.

Conflicts of Interest: The author declares no conflict of interest.

Entry Link on the Encyclopedia Platform: https://encyclopedia.pub/19030.

References

1. WHO. Director-General's Opening Remarks at the Media Briefing on COVID-19-11 March 2020. Available online: https://www.who.int/director-general/speeches/detail/who-director-general-s-opening-remarks-at-the-media-briefing-on-covid-19-11-march-2020 (accessed on 5 January 2022).
2. APA. Psychological Impact of COVID-19. Available online: https://www.apa.org/topics/covid-19/psychological-impact (accessed on 5 January 2022).
3. WHO TEAM. Coronavirus Disease (COVID-19): Herd Immunity, Lockdowns and COVID-19. Available online: https://www.who.int/news-room/questions-and-answers/item/herd-immunity-lockdowns-and-covid-19 (accessed on 5 January 2022).
4. CDCP: Centers for Disease Control and Prevention. Quarantine and Isolation. Available online: https://www.cdc.gov/quarantine/quarantineisolation.html (accessed on 5 January 2022).
5. Tognotti, E. Lessons from the History of Quarantine, from Plague to Influenza A. *Emerg. Infect. Dis.* **2013**, *19*, 254–259. [CrossRef]
6. Brooks, S.K.; Webster, R.K.; Smith, L.E.; Woodland, L.; Wessely, S.; Greenberg, N.; Rubin, G.J. The psychological impact of quarantine and how to reduce it: Rapid review of the evidence. *Lancet* **2020**, *395*, 912–920. [CrossRef]
7. Prati, G.; Mancini, A.D. The psychological impact of COVID-19 pandemic lockdowns: A review and meta-analysis of longitudinal studies and natural experiments. *Psychol. Med.* **2021**, *51*, 201–211. [CrossRef]
8. Pirkis, J.; John, A.; Shin, S.; DelPozo-Banos, M.; Arya, V.; Analuisa-Aguilar, P.; Appleby, L.; Arensman, E.; Bantjes, J.; Baran, A.; et al. Suicide trends in the early months of the COVID-19 pandemic: An interrupted time-series analysis of preliminary data from 21 countries. *Lancet Psychiatry* **2021**, *8*, 579–588. [CrossRef]
9. Botchway, S.; Fazel, S. Remaining vigilant about COVID-19 and suicide. *Lancet Psychiatry* **2021**, *8*, 552–553. [CrossRef]
10. John, A.; Pirkis, J.; Gunnell, D.; Appleby, L.; Morrissey, J. Trends in suicide during the covid-19 pandemic. *BMJ* **2020**, *371*, m4352. [CrossRef] [PubMed]
11. Panchal, U.; de Pablo, G.S.; Franco, M.; Moreno, C.; Parellada, M.; Arango, C.; Fusar Poli, P. The impact of COVID-19 lockdown on child and adolescent mental health: Systematic review. *Eur. Child Adolesc. Psychiatry* **2021**, 1–27. [CrossRef]
12. Latzer, I.T.; Leitner, Y.; Karnieli-Miller, O. Core experiences of parents of children with autism during the COVID-19 pandemic lockdown. *Autism* **2021**, *25*, 1047–1059. [CrossRef]
13. Fan, S.; Guan, J.; Cao, L.; Wang, M.; Zhao, H.; Chen, L.; Yan, L. Psychological effects caused by COVID-19 pandemic on pregnant women: A systematic review with meta-analysis. *Asian J. Psychiatry* **2020**, *56*, 102533. [CrossRef]
14. Naik, S.S.; Gowda, G.S.; Shivaprakash, P.; Subramaniyam, B.A.; Manjunatha, N.; Muliyala, K.P.; Reddi, V.S.K.; Kumar, C.N.; Math, S.B.; Gangadhar, B.N. Homeless people with mental illness in India and COVID-19. *Lancet Psychiatry* **2020**, *7*, e51–e52. [CrossRef]
15. Acuff, S.F.; Strickland, J.C.; Tucker, J.A.; Murphy, J.G. Changes in alcohol use during COVID-19 and associations with contextual and individual difference variables: A systematic review and meta-analysis. *Psychol. Addict. Behav.* **2021**. [CrossRef] [PubMed]
16. Alladio, E.; Visintin, L.; Lombardo, T.; Testi, R.; Salomone, A.; Vincenti, M. The Impact of COVID-19 Pandemic and Lockdown on Alcohol Consumption: A Perspective from Hair Analysis. *Front. Psychiatry* **2021**, *12*, 632519. [CrossRef] [PubMed]
17. Sachdeva, V.; Sharma, S.; Sarangi, A. Gambling behaviors during COVID-19: A narrative review. *J. Addict. Dis.* **2021**, 1–9. [CrossRef] [PubMed]
18. Kourti, A.; Stavridou, A.; Panagouli, E.; Psaltopoulou, T.; Spiliopoulou, C.; Tsolia, M.; Sergentanis, T.N.; Tsitsika, A. Domestic Violence During the COVID-19 Pandemic: A Systematic Review. *Trauma Violence Abus.* **2021**. [CrossRef]
19. Piquero, A.R.; Jennings, W.G.; Jemison, E.; Kaukinen, C.; Knaul, F.M. Domestic violence during the COVID-19 pandemic-Evidence from a systematic review and meta-analysis. *J. Crim. Justice* **2021**, *74*, 101806. [CrossRef]
20. UN. The Shadow Pandemic: Violence against Women during COVID-19. Available online: https://www.unwomen.org/en/news/in-focus/in-focus-gender-equality-in-covid-19-response/violence-against-women-during-covid-19 (accessed on 5 January 2022).
21. UNDP. COVID-19 Global Gender Response Tracker. Available online: https://data.undp.org/gendertracker/ (accessed on 5 January 2022).
22. UNICEF. COVID-19 and Its Implications for Protecting Children Online. Available online: https://www.unicef.org/sites/default/files/2020-04/COVID-19-and-Its-Implications-for-Protecting-Children-Online.pdf (accessed on 5 January 2022).
23. EU Commissioner EU Commissioner. Opening Statement by Commissioner Johansson on "Schengen, Migration and Asylum Policy and the EU Security Strategy in the Context of COVID-19" at the European Parliament Committee on Civil Liberties, Justice and Home Affairs. Available online: https://ec.europa.eu/commission/commissioners/2019-2024/johansson/announcements/opening-statement-commissioner-johansson-schengen-migration-and-asylum-policy-and-eu-security_en (accessed on 5 January 2022).
24. Crawford, P. Editorial Perspective: Cabin fever–the impact of lockdown on children and young people. *Child Adolesc. Ment. Health* **2021**, *26*, 167–168. [CrossRef]
25. WHO. *Pandemic Fatigue–Reinvigorating the Public to Prevent COVID-19: Policy Framework for Supporting Pandemic Prevention and Management*; Licence: CC BY-NC-SA 3.0 IGO; WHO Regional Office for Europe: Copenhagen, Denmark, 2020. Available online: https://apps.who.int/iris/handle/10665/337574 (accessed on 5 January 2022).

26. Santomauro, D.F.; Herrera, A.M.M.; Shadid, J.; Zheng, P.; Ashbaugh, C.; Pigott, D.M.; Abbafati, C.; Adolph, C.; Amlag, J.O.; Aravkin, A.Y.; et al. COVID-19 Mental Disorders Collaborators. Global prevalence and burden of depressive and anxiety disorders in 204 countries and territories in 2020 due to the COVID-19 pandemic. *Lancet* **2021**, *398*, 1700–1712. [CrossRef]
27. Krishnamoorthy, Y.; Nagarajan, R.; Saya, G.K.; Menon, V. Prevalence of psychological morbidities among general population, healthcare workers and COVID-19 patients amidst the COVID-19 pandemic: A systematic review and meta-analysis. *Psychiatry Res.* **2020**, *293*, 113382. [CrossRef]
28. Batra, K.; Singh, T.P.; Sharma, M.; Batra, R.; Schvaneveldt, N. Investigating the Psychological Impact of COVID-19 among Healthcare Workers: A Meta-Analysis. *Int. J. Environ. Res. Public Health* **2020**, *17*, 9096. [CrossRef]
29. Neto, R.M.D.S.; Benjamim, C.J.R.; Carvalho, P.M.D.M.; Neto, M.L.R. Psychological effects caused by the COVID-19 pandemic in health professionals: A systematic review with meta-analysis. *Prog. Neuro-Psychopharmacol. Biol. Psychiatry* **2020**, *104*, 110062. [CrossRef]
30. Danet, A.D. Impacto psicológico de la COVID-19 en profesionales sanitarios de primera línea en el ámbito occidental. Una revisión sistemática. *Med. Clin.* **2021**, *156*, 449–458. [CrossRef] [PubMed]
31. Li, Y.; Scherer, N.; Felix, L.; Kuper, H. Prevalence of depression, anxiety and post-traumatic stress disorder in health care workers during the COVID-19 pandemic: A systematic review and meta-analysis. *PLoS ONE* **2021**, *16*, e0246454. [CrossRef] [PubMed]
32. Shafran, R.; Coughtrey, A.; Whittal, M. Recognising and addressing the impact of COVID-19 on obsessive-compulsive disorder. *Lancet Psychiatry* **2020**, *7*, 570–572. [CrossRef]
33. Soroka, S.; Fournier, P.; Nir, L. Cross-national evidence of a negativity bias in psychophysiological reactions to news. *Proc. Natl. Acad. Sci. USA* **2019**, *116*, 18888–18892. [CrossRef]
34. Gesi, C.; Carmassi, C.; Cerveri, G.; Carpita, B.; Cremone, I.M.; Dell'Osso, L. Complicated Grief: What to Expect After the Coronavirus Pandemic. *Front. Psychiatry* **2020**, *11*, 489. [CrossRef]
35. Cooke, J.E.; Eirich, R.; Racine, N.; Madigan, S. Prevalence of posttraumatic and general psychological stress during COVID-19: A rapid review and meta-analysis. *Psychiatry Res.* **2020**, *292*, 113347. [CrossRef]
36. Zhang, L.; Pan, R.; Cai, Y.; Pan, J. The Prevalence of Post-Traumatic Stress Disorder in the General Population during the COVID-19 Pandemic: A Systematic Review and Single-Arm Meta-Analysis. *Psychiatry Investig.* **2021**, *18*, 426–433. [CrossRef]
37. Salehi, M.; Amanat, M.; Mohammadi, M.; Salmanian, M.; Rezaei, N.; Saghazadeh, A.; Garakani, A. The prevalence of post-traumatic stress disorder related symptoms in Coronavirus outbreaks: A systematic-review and meta-analysis. *J. Affect. Disord.* **2021**, *282*, 527–538. [CrossRef]
38. Ritchie, K.; Chan, D.; Watermeyer, T. The cognitive consequences of the COVID-19 epidemic: Collateral damage? *Brain Commun.* **2020**, *2*, fcaa069. [CrossRef]
39. Schou, T.M.; Joca, S.; Wegener, G.; Bay-Richter, C. Psychiatric and neuropsychiatric sequelae of COVID-19—A systematic review. *Brain Behav. Immun.* **2021**, *97*, 328–348. [CrossRef]
40. Vanderlind, W.M.; Rabinovitz, B.B.; Miao, I.Y.; Oberlin, L.E.; Bueno-Castellano, C.; Fridman, C.; Jaywant, A.; Kanellopoulos, D. A systematic review of neuropsychological and psychiatric sequalae of COVID-19: Implications for treatment. *Curr. Opin. Psychiatry* **2021**, *34*, 420–433. [CrossRef] [PubMed]
41. Hampshire, A.; Trender, W.; Chamberlain, S.R.; Jolly, A.E.; Grant, J.E.; Patrick, F.; Mazibuko, N.; Williams, S.C.; Barnby, J.M.; Hellyer, P.; et al. Cognitive deficits in people who have recovered from COVID-19. *EClinicalMedicine* **2021**, *39*, 101044. [CrossRef] [PubMed]
42. Almeria, M.; Cejudo, J.C.; Sotoca, J.; Deus, J.; Krupinski, J. Cognitive profile following COVID-19 infection: Clinical predictors leading to neuropsychological impairment. *Brain Behav. Immun. Health* **2020**, *9*, 100163. [CrossRef] [PubMed]
43. WHO. A Clinical Case Definition of Post COVID-19 Condition by a Delphi Consensus, 6 October 2021. Available online: https://www.who.int/publications/i/item/WHO-2019-nCoV-Post_COVID-19_condition-Clinical_case_definition-2021.1 (accessed on 5 January 2022).
44. Ceban, F.; Ling, S.; Lui, L.M.; Lee, Y.; Gill, H.; Teopiz, K.M.; Rodrigues, N.B.; Subramaniapillai, M.; Di Vincenzo, J.D.; Cao, B.; et al. Fatigue and cognitive impairment in Post-COVID-19 Syndrome: A systematic review and meta-analysis. *Brain Behav. Immun.* **2021**, *101*, 93–135. [CrossRef] [PubMed]
45. Nakanishi, N.; Liu, K.; Kawakami, D.; Kawai, Y.; Morisawa, T.; Nishida, T.; Sumita, H.; Unoki, T.; Hifumi, T.; Iida, Y.; et al. Post-Intensive Care Syndrome and Its New Challenges in Coronavirus Disease 2019 (COVID-19) Pandemic: A Review of Recent Advances and Perspectives. *J. Clin. Med.* **2021**, *10*, 3870. [CrossRef] [PubMed]
46. Pierce, M.; Hope, H.; Ford, T.; Hatch, S.; Hotopf, M.; John, A.; Kontopantelis, E.; Webb, R.; Wessely, S.; McManus, S.; et al. Mental health before and during the COVID-19 pandemic: A longitudinal probability sample survey of the UK population. *Lancet Psychiatry* **2020**, *7*, 883–892. [CrossRef]
47. Magnavita, N.; Soave, P.M.; Antonelli, M. A One-Year Prospective Study of Work-Related Mental Health in the Intensivists of a COVID-19 Hub Hospital. *Int. J. Environ. Res. Public Health* **2021**, *18*, 9888. [CrossRef]

encyclopedia

Systematic Review

Dental Patients' Perspective on COVID-19: A Systematic Review

Stefano Salgarello , Elisabetta Audino, Paolo Bertoletti, Matteo Salvadori and Maria Luisa Garo *

Department of Medical and Surgery Specialties, Dental School, University of Brescia, Radiological Sciences and Public Health, 25123 Brescia, Italy; stefano.salgarello@unibs.it (S.S.); bettaz92@gmail.com (E.A.); paolobertoletti1993@gmail.com (P.B.); salvaz.dori@gmail.com (M.S.)
* Correspondence: marilu.garo@gmail.com; Tel.: +39-030-383424

Definition: The COVID-19 epidemic has changed patients' approach to dental treatments. While dentists worldwide have shown an excellent level of adaptability to face the new challenges presented by the unprecedented situation due to the rapid spread of COVID-19, dental patients have witnessed a sudden suspension of elective treatments and a slow resumption of dental care activities after several national lockdowns. In addition, the general climate of anxiety and fear due to the high COVID-19 risk and the high level of mortality has influenced the perception and attitudes of people towards dental activity, inducing many dental patients to avoid appointments to the dentist if not highly urgent. We present an overview of the current state of knowledge about dental patients' perception, perspective, attitude, and expectations towards a full resumption of regular dental treatments.

Keywords: perception; dental patient; dental treatment; safety; COVID-19

Citation: Salgarello, S.; Audino, E.; Bertoletti, P.; Salvadori, M.; Garo, M.L. Dental Patients' Perspective on COVID-19: A Systematic Review. *Encyclopedia* **2022**, 2, 365–381. https://doi.org/10.3390/encyclopedia2010022

Academic Editors: Stephen Bustin and Raffaele Barretta

Received: 17 January 2022
Accepted: 26 January 2022
Published: 1 February 2022

1. Introduction

Since the beginning of the COVID-19 pandemic, dental professionals have been exposed to a high level of anxiety and stress due to several changes that have affected dentistry in many ways. To date, many international and national guidelines and recommendations are available to support dentists in their everyday dental activities [1,2]. In addition, many studies have investigated dentists' perceptions, problems, attitudes, and expectations worldwide to understand how dentists have faced the unprecedented situation due to the COVID-19 outbreak [3–5].

The management of the emergencies and urgencies in public and private dental clinics during the various national lockdown, the handling of COVID-19 patients in need of urgent dental treatments, the optimization of the personal protective equipment (PPE), and the appropriate approach to resume the regular dental activity with a high level of safety for dental staff and patients have been deeply analyzed [6–10].

In the first COVID-19 outbreak period, many countries adopted prudential measures to reduce the risk of contagion, such as suspending elective dental treatments and recommending executing only non-postponable dental treatments. However, after the first waves of COVID-19, the need to restart private and public dental activities has become the first and foremost goal of many dental professionals [11].

2. Synthesis

From the end of 2020, the availability of COVID-19 vaccines has supported a complete restart of dental activity, allowing the medical staff to resume their work with a certain level of safety and confidence [12,13].

Therefore, if, on the one hand, COVID-19 has created an unprecedented situation for all health services, on the other hand, this is also an unknown situation for patients, who have to handle fear of COVID-19 contagion and discomfort situations due to the suspension of planned dental treatments [14,15].

In this context, the psychological consequence of COVID-19 should not be neglected [16]. As emerged in a recent Chinese study, people living in a pandemic can suffer from different levels of psychological distress, experiencing increased fear of becoming infected [17]. In dentistry, this higher level of stress and anxiety can be translated into a series of ugly behaviors, such as avoidance of dental appointments, treatment delays, and adoption of therapies based on their experience and common sense without the support of their dentists [18].

This work aimed to review the current literature about the role of COVID-19 in the perceptions, perspectives, attitudes, and expectations of patients toward dental treatments and the risk of COVID-19 infection within dental clinics.

2.1. Methods

A systematic review of the current literature was performed following PRISMA (Preferred Reporting Items for Systematic Reviews and Meta-Analyses) guidelines [19]. On the basis of the inclusion criteria, we selected original studies reporting dental patients' perceptions or perspectives during the COVID-19 pandemic and their attitudes and expectations about the safe restart of dental clinics and dental offices activities.

PubMed and Web of Science databases were searched using the following search terms: (COVID-19 [Title/Abstract]) AND (dental patient [Title/Abstract]) AND (perspective or perception [Title/Abstract]).

The search strategy was carried out from September to October 2021, without time and language restriction. First, the resultant citations were screened by title, followed by abstracts and then full texts. In addition to the initial search, references in the selected sources were checked manually, and further studies were included if relevant.

Additionally, hand searches were performed to identify possible articles other than those found in the electronic databases. Two reviewers (MLG and EA) performed the first (title/abstract screening) and second (full-text assessment) steps of the search process. Any disagreement was discussed and then solved by consensus.

All original peer-reviewed research publications were considered. Inclusion criteria for eligible studies were: (1) studies carried out on COVID-19 impact in dentistry; (2) studies reporting dental patients' perceptions, perspectives, or attitudes toward dental treatment during the COVID-19 pandemic; (3) studies analyzing dental patients' anxiety or fear.

Data extraction was organized in tables containing the following information:

- Study characteristics: first author, year, country.
- Study design, period, and setting.
- Sample size and patients' characteristics (gender and age).
- Types of dental emergency/urgency.
- Questionnaire structure.
- Main outcomes.

No numerical information was extracted from the figures reported in the study publications.

The risk of bias was assessed through the CHERRIES (*Checklist for Reporting Results of* Internet E-Surveys) or SUrge (*SUrvey Reporting GuidelinE*), as suggested by Weir et al. [20].

Given the lack of a validated checklist to evaluate the surveys, we adapted the CHERRIES checklist for web-based surveys and SUrge for self-administered surveys non-online administered. For both checklists, we applied the following procedure. For each checklist item, we assigned a value of 1 if the topic was reported in the study, and a value of 0 if it was not registered. Each survey's final score was determined by calculating the sum of all valid items divided by their number. Low-, moderate-, or high-quality studies were assessed according to the following evaluation: final score < 35% = low quality; 35% $\leq$ final score < 75% = moderate quality; final score $\geq$ 75% = high quality.

2.2. Study Selection

The literature search identified 205 studies. After removing duplicates and screening titles and abstracts, 15 full-text studies were reviewed. Ten studies between 2020 and 2021 met the inclusion and exclusion criteria. A flow diagram of the search strategy results is presented in Figure 1.

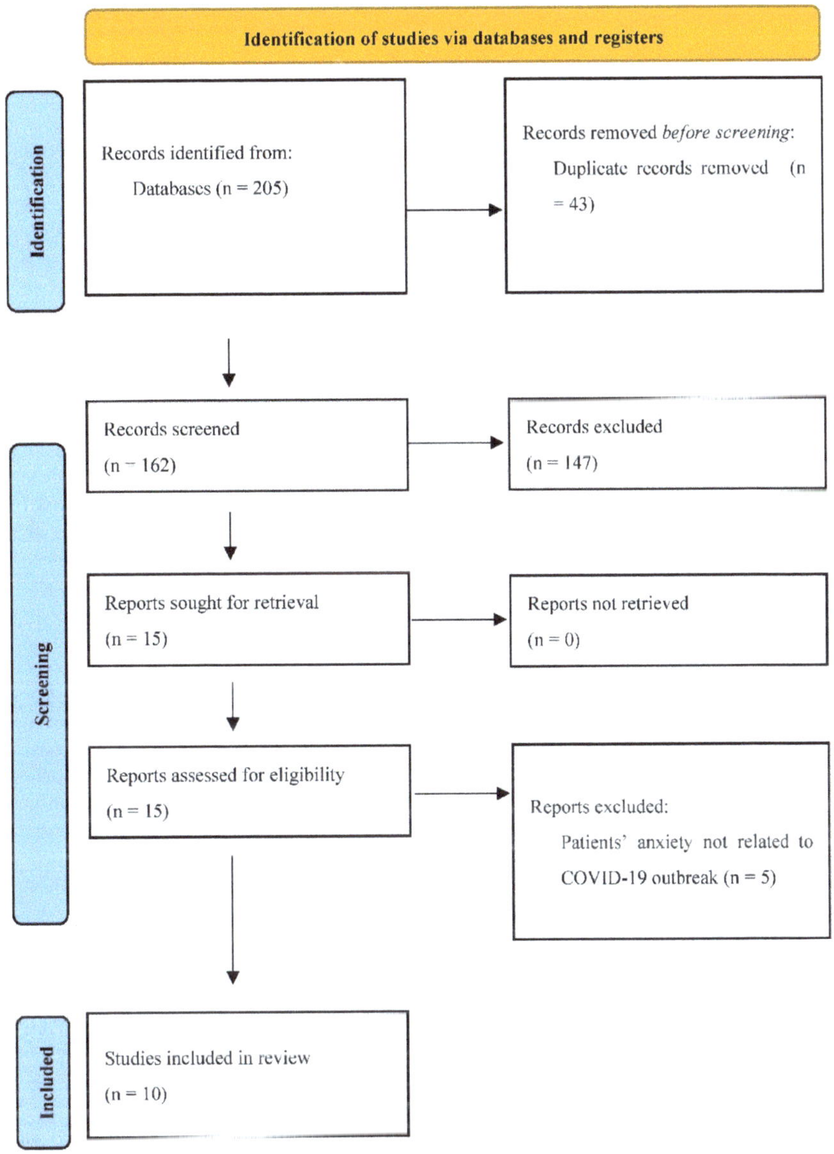

Figure 1. PRISMA Flow chart.

2.3. Risk of Bias

Given the lack of a specific tool for evaluating bias in surveys, we assessed the risk of bias using two checklists. The overall risk of bias assessment of the included studies is presented in Tables S1 and S2 in Supplementary Materials. Five studies reported a moderate level of bias [21–25], while the remaining five studies showed low quality [26–30].

In surveys administered through online platforms (Table S1 in Supplementary Materials), all studies reported the survey design describing the target population or sample frame. For IRB approval and informed consent process, IRB approval was obtained by seven out of eight studies [21–24,26,29,30], informed consent was obtained by four studies [22,25,28,29], and data protection was reported by only one study [22], while it was not applicable by four surveys [21,23,27,29]. Development and pre-testing were performed by only two studies [22,30]. For the recruitment process and description of the sample having access to the questionnaire, a closed survey was applied by all studies; only one indicated that the contact mode was not through the Internet [21], while advertising to announce the survey was carried out only by Moffat et al. [22]. All surveys were administered through the web or by email; six out of eight surveys described the context [21–24,28,30], and only two studies were not mandatory surveys [28,30]. Only one study used incentives [22], although this item was applicable for only two studies [21,22]. The timeframe was identified in five studies [21–24,28]. All included studies did not report the number of items, number of screens, and completeness check, while review steps were only adopted by Peloso et al. [29]. The unique visitor ID was assessed by two surveys [21,29], while none of the studies reported view rate, participation rate, and completion rate. For preventing multiple entries from the same individual, i.e., using cookies, IP check, log file analysis, and registration, no precautions were adopted by all surveys. Information about the handling of incomplete questionnaires was not described. Statistical corrections were adopted by five studies [21–24,28].

Two studies were evaluated through SUrge [25,27]. Although with slight differences, both studies lacked information regarding many items. Mainly, neither study reported the procedures used to develop, pre-test, and validate the new survey, sample size calculation and its representativeness, the type of contact, and incentives. Furthermore, the statistical analysis did not provide information about non-response error, response rate, and handling of missing data. In addition, neither study reported considerations about the non-response rate and possible differences in respondents' samples and discussed the external validity of the findings. The complete results of risk of bias for both studies are reported in Table S2 (Supplementary Materials).

2.4. Study Characteristics

We provide a descriptive summary of the study design, period, setting, sample size, gender, age, types of dental emergency/urgency treated during the period of interest, and the questionnaire structure in Table 1. We included a total of 10 studies: 2 carried out in Brazil [26,29], 2 in the U.S.A. [22,25], 1 in Spain [21], Turkey [27], Italy [28], Saudi Arabia [23], China [24], and Nigeria [30], respectively.

Table 1. Studies characteristics.

Study	Country	Study Design	Period	Setting	Sample Size	Gender	Age	Types of Dental Emergency/Urgency	Questionnaire Structure	Main Outcomes
Cotrin et al. (2020) [26]	Brasil	Survey	NR *	Private Dental Clinics	354	231 females and 123 males	35.49 ± 13.93	Orthodontic treatments	• Socio-Demographics • Quarantine • Level of anxiety (NRS): 0 no anxiety—10 extreme anxiety	• 78.2% go out just when needed; 13% not leave home; 8.8% go out as usual without respecting the quarantine • Feelings about COVID-19: 44.7% is calm; 23.4% is afraid; 22.9% is anxious; 5.6% is indifferent; 3.4% is in panic • Level of anxiety: 4.98 ± 2.42 • Dental appointment attendance: 60.2% would go to an appointment; 25.1% would go only in case of urgency/emergency; 14.7% would not go • Females more anxious, afraid, and in panic than men in relation to quarantine and the COVID-19 pandemic • Males were more willing to go a dental appointment than females • Males were more concerned about a delay in treatment than females • PPE fundamental: surgical mask (88.7%), medical head cap (81.1%), lab coat (55.9%), face shield (55.1%) • Good practices: avoiding crossing other patients at reception (78%), PPE for patients (35%), alcohol gel available at reception (91.8%)

Table 1. *Cont.*

Study	Country	Study Design	Period	Setting	Sample Size	Gender	Age	Types of Dental Emergency/Urgency	Questionnaire Structure	Main Outcomes
Moffat et al. (2020) [22]	USA	Survey	May 2020	Web-survey through Amazon Mechanical Turk (MTurk)	452	198 females, 250 males, and 4 NR	40 years	None	• Socio-Demographics • Perceived susceptibility to contract COVID-19 during dental appointments • Attitudes and beliefs regarding the risk of contracting COVID-19 during dental appointments • Events that need to occur for patients to feel comfortable returning to the dental office	• Concerned about contracting COVID-19 from dental professionals (3.7 ± 1.7) and other patients in the dental office (3.3 ± 1.8) • Aware of the government recommendations to dental professionals for appropriate dental treatment during the COVID-19 outbreak (3.8 ± 1.9) • Trust that dental offices follow government recommendations to dental professionals for appropriate dental treatment during the COVID-19 outbreak (2.2 ± 1.2) • Concerned that visiting dental providers will cause a shortage in PPE available for healthcare providers fighting COVID-19 (4.5 ± 1.9) • The risk of getting COVID-19 in the dental office outweighs the risk of me not getting necessary dental treatment completed (3.6 ± 1.7)
Peloso et al. (2020) [29]	Brazil	Survey	NR *	Private Dental Clinics	595	412 females and 183 males	38.21 ±13.94	74.3% orthodontic18.4% oral rehabilitation7.3% restorative or other	• Socio-Demographics • Presence of symptoms related to COVID-19 • Dental treatments received during the quarantine • Contacts with own dentist to schedule an appointments • Willing to go to dentist for an emergency • Concerns about attending a dental appointment • PPE used by dentist and in the dental office	• Concerned about attending a dental appointment included the risk of getting infected and/or contaminating the family (18.5%) • 5% afraid because dentists are a group at high risk of contamination • Dental treatments can wait (20.2%) • Females more anxious and afraid than males • Males more willing to go a dental appointment • Females not worried about how quarantine might affect their dental treatment • More anxious, afraid, or panicked would attend an appointment in the case of emergency (47.1%, 46.4%, and 62.5%) • Importance of disposable lab coat (63.9%), disposable mask (67.4%), having alcohol gel at reception (85.4%), avoiding close contact with other patients at reception (63.5%), having PPE for patients (41.8%)

Table 1. *Cont.*

Study	Country	Study Design	Period	Setting	Sample Size	Gender	Age	Types of Dental Emergency/Urgency	Questionnaire Structure	Main Outcomes
Arqub et al. (2021) [25]	USA	Survey	July–October 2020	Dental Clinic	154	95 females and 59 males	29.30 ± 12.01	Orthodontic treatments	• Socio-Demographics • Physiological aspects relevant to clinical orthodontics • Emergencies • Preferences regarding the urgency on following up treatment during the pandemic and preferred communication means • Patients' insight on postponing or discontinuing treatment, schedules appointment intervals due to safety concerns • Clinic facilities, screening protocols, pretesting for COVID-19 • Phycological symptoms (Kessler Psychological Distress Scale)	• Extremely pleased with the restrictive protocols at the clinic (80.51%) and the idea that telephone and pre-clinical appointment screening is an effective tool to prevent the spread of infection (68%) • Useful tools: pretesting patients (81.81%), the staff, and orthodontists (85.06%) during the pandemic • Dentist should wear full PPE and N95 mask (45.5%)

Table 1. *Cont.*

Study	Country	Study Design	Period	Setting	Sample Size	Gender	Age	Types of Dental Emergency/Urgency	Questionnaire Structure	Main Outcomes
Gonzales-Olmo et al. (2021) [21]	Spain	Survey—Repeated measures design (before and after Spain lockdown)	March–June 2020	Web-survey addressed to community of Madrid	961	559 females and 402 males	38.4 ± 16.1	None	• Socio-Demographics • Perceived vulnerability to disease (PVD) • Scale of fear of COVID-19 • Structured questions about avoidance behavior towards the dental clinic • Question covering whether the participant had been ill with COVID-19	• Significantly higher scores on T1 than T0, both in infectability ($p < 0.01$) and in aversion to germs ($p < 0.01$) • Significant positive correlation between COVID-19 fear scale and the subscales of infectability and germ aversion in T0 and T1 ($p < 0.01$) • Strong positive association between fear of COVID-19 in T1 and aversion to germs in T0 ($p < 0.01$) • Higher score for women for infectability and germ aversion in T1 ($p < 0.01$) • Those who contracted COVID-19 reported a higher COVID fear score ($p < 0.01$) • 30.9% afraid of going to the dentist because of the possibility of contagion with COVID-19, although 56.3% continues to go to the dentist • 23.5% would go to the dentist because they had not finished their treatments, but 42.5% would not start esthetic, orthodontic, or implant treatments • 43.7% would not go to the dentist, 24.5% for fear of COVID-19, 16% because of financial problems, 3.2% for other reasons—more than half would maintain this decision until the disease is eradicated or an effective treatment is found • 20.7% would not go to the dentist even in case of gum problems; 20.2% would not go even if they suspected cavities; 16.3% would not go even if filling or teeth were fractured • Dentist avoidance: high perceived infectability (OR = 4.21, 95%CI: 2.87–5.64), high fear of COVID-19 (OR = 5.18, 95%CI: 2.96–9.4), older than 60 years (OR = 7.63, 95%CI:3.56–15.35)

Table 1. *Cont.*

Study	Country	Study Design	Period	Setting	Sample Size	Gender	Age	Types of Dental Emergency/Urgency	Questionnaire Structure	Main Outcomes
Karagözoğlu et al. (2021) [27]	Turkey	Survey	NR	Dentistry Faculty	300	145 females and 155 males	18–38: 53%, 39–59: 31.7%; 60–80: 15.3%	Patients receiving dental treatment	• Socio-Demographics • COVID-19 and patient-related questions • Spielberg's STAT-S anxiety scale	• Mean anxiety score: 43.38 ± 8.34 • Higher anxiety score in those who think that COVID-19 can be transmitted through dental treatment ($p < 0.001$), would not seek dental treatment if their condition was not urgent ($p < 0.003$), think that dentists have a high risk of contamination, thought that dentist can transmit COVID-19 during dental treatment, and believe they could be infected by the other patients in the waiting area • Lower anxiety score in those who thought that adequate measures were taken in the dental unit ($p < 0.001$), the measures taken by dentists while treating patients were sufficient, feel safe because healthcare professionals received the COVID-19 vaccine, and would have had the dental treatment safely if vaccinated
Martina et al. (2021) [28]	Italy	Survey	May–November 2020	Web Survey	1566	852 females, 698 males, 16 NR	18–29: 31.3%30–39: 29.8%40–49: 18.3%; 50–59: 10.6%; 60–69: 6.8%; >70.3%	Orthodontic care	• Socio-Demographics • Anxiety over going to the dentist • Presence of TMD symptoms • Orthodontic treatment and the perception of the risk of continuing orthodontic treatment	• 55.3% believed that there is a greater risk of contracting COVID-19 at a dental practice • Men less afraid to go to a dentist clinic • Younger people less scared to go to a dental clinic than people over 40 ($p < 0.001$) • Higher level of anxiety was associated with a fear of going to a dental practice • 79.5% thought than in the dental practice there was a greater risk of contracting COVID-19 • For 84.6%, COVID-19 increased the fear of going to the dentist

Table 1. *Cont.*

Study	Country	Study Design	Period	Setting	Sample Size	Gender	Age	Types of Dental Emergency/Urgency	Questionnaire Structure	Main Outcomes
Nazir et al. (2021) [23]	Saudi Arabia	Survey	June–July 2020	Scientific research unit at the College of Dentistry	606	246 females and 360 males	30.49 ± 12.01	Patients receiving dental treatment	• Socio-Demographics • Dental Fear Survey (DFS) and Modified Dental Anxiety Scale (MDAS) • Dental attendance patterns • Visiting a dental office in case of emergency during the COVID-19 pandemic	• Higher DFS in females (41.17 ± 17.94) than in males (37.65 ± 20.34) ($p = 0.029$)
Quan et al. (2021) [24]	China	Survey	February–March 2020	Dental Clinic	1078	786 females and 292 males	22.59 ± 8.28	Orthodontic patients	• Socio-Demographics • Self-management ability of oral health and compliance and cooperation • Orthodontic problems and emergencies during the pandemic • Risk perception about the COVID-19 pandemic • Self-Rating Anxiety Scale	• Patients who faced orthodontic problems: 55.1% contacted their attending doctor; 33.3% thought the problem was tolerable and did not take any measure; 23.1% indicated they could solve it by themselves according to their experiences or common sense. • Difficulties of orthodontic follow-up visits: 67.9% worried about the risk of infection

Table 1. Cont.

Study	Country	Study Design	Period	Setting	Sample Size	Gender	Age	Types of Dental Emergency/Urgency	Questionnaire Structure	Main Outcomes
Umeh et al. (2021) [30]	Nigeria	Survey		Public and private dental facilities	304	221 females and 83 males	35.6	Orthodontic patients receive treatment	• Socio-Demographics • Perception of COVID-19 risk in orthodontic treatment • Knowledge about COVID-19 infection • Risk perception and attitude toward the COVID-19 infection	• Orthodontic patients were severely (40.8%) or moderately (30.6%) vulnerable to contracting the disease but were willing regardless to carry on with their orthodontic treatment during the pandemic (72.4%) • Fear of contracting the virus during a routine appointment: 39.8% • Missed routine appointment: 27.3% • Increased treatment time: 35.5% • Increase in cost of treatment: 8.6% • Patients have a significant role in infection control in the orthodontic practice setting (81.3% social distancing in the clinic, 82.9% temperature screening before entering the clinic; 69.7%; asked relevant screening question; 78.9% limiting child's company; 80.9%; wearing facemasks in the clinic; 88.5% handwashing in the dental clinic)

Studies were carried out in 2020–2021: Quan et al. from February to March 2020, Gonzales et al. from March to June 2020, Moffat et al. in May 2020, Martina et al. from May to November 2020, Arqub from July to October 2020, and Nazir et al. from June to July 2020. Two studies [26,29] did not report the period of questionnaire administration but referred to that period being before the COVID-19 peak in Brazil: we presume before June 2020. Respondents were chosen in different settings: for four studies in public dental clinics or however related to academic scientific research units [24,26,28,29], three studies administered the questionnaires through private dental clinics [21,23,27], and two through web-survey addressed to local communities [21,22]. Only one study distributed the questionnaires to public and private dental clinics [30].

Six thousand three hundred and seventy (6370) patients were included in the studies. Three thousand seven hundred and forty-five (3745) respondents were female (female-male ratio 1.44). The mean age varied between 22.59 ± 8.28 [24] and 40 years [22]. Two studies reported age ranges instead of mean age [27,28], showing a high prevalence of young people (18–38 years) and a mild prevalence of older people (older than 60 years). Six studies involved mainly patients with orthodontic problems [21,23,24,27,29,30], two studies involved patients who received dental treatments after the COVID-19 outbreak [23,27], and the other two studies involved respondents who did not necessarily receive dental treatments after the COVID-19 outbreak [21,22].

All questionnaires were structured to gather data about socio-demographic questions (e.g., age, gender, education background, ethnicity, income, and city of residence). Three investigated COVID-19 and patient-related problems such as quarantine, COVID-19 symptoms, and COVID-19 infection [21,23,26]. Six studies investigated patients' anxiety toward dental treatments through different validated or not-validated psychometric scales [21,23–27]. Nine studies investigated the risk perceptions, attitudes, avoidance behaviors, and beliefs toward the COVID-19 infection during dental treatments [21–26,28–30]. Five studies investigated protocols and procedures adopted by dental clinics to safeguard patients and allow them to feel comfortable about returning to the dental offices [22,25,26,29,30]. One study analyzed preferences regarding the urgency of following up treatments during the pandemic and preferred communication methods with the dentist [25]. Gonzales et al. only investigated possible reasons to avoid dental treatments [21].

2.5. *Anxiety, Risk Perception, and Attitudes toward Dental Treatments during the Pandemic*

Cotrin et al. [26], in a survey carried out presumably from March to June 2020, including 354 Brazilian respondents, reported a high level of anxiety (4.98 ± 2.42) among quarantine patients, with a substantial prevalence among females. Feelings about COVID-19 ranged from a relaxed (44.7%) or indifferent (5.6%) attitude to feelings of pain (3.4%), fear (23.4%), or anxiety (22.9%). Males were more willing to go to a dental appointment and more concerned about the delay in dental treatments due to COVID-19 restrictions. Dental appointment attendance continued to represent an important factor in everyday life, because 60.2% of the respondents would go to dental appointments for elective treatments. In comparison, only 25.1% of them would go only in case of urgency or emergency. About 15% of the respondents would not go to a dental appointment due to fear of contagion.

The same level of anxiety and fear emerged in Gonzales et al. study [21], which involved people living in Madrid. In an accurate comparison of the attitudes and perceptions of people toward dental treatment during the Spanish lockdown (March–June 2020), they showed that 30.9% of the respondents were afraid of going to the dentist because of the possibility of contagion with COVID-19. However, 56.3% of them continued to go to the dentist. More than 23% of the respondents decided to continue to go to the dentist because the planned dental treatment was not finished. The fear of COVID-19 impacted the start of new dental treatments such as orthodontics or implants: 42.5% of the Spanish respondents reported no intention to start a new treatment because of financial problems (16%) or fear of COVID-19 (24.5%). More than half of the interviewees would not go to the dentist until the disease was eradicated or an effective treatment was found. About 21% of the respondents stated they would not go to the dentist even in case of gum problems, 20.2% would not go even if they suspected cavities, and 16.3% would not go even if filling or teeth were fractured. The probability of dental avoidance due to the fear of COVID-19 infection was equal to 84% (OR = 5.18, 95%CI: 2.96–9.4) and increased to 88% in people older than 60 years (OR = 7.63, 95%CI: 3.56–15.35). Comparing infectability perception and aversion to germs at the beginning and at the end of the Spanish lockdown, Gonzales et al. showed an increase in the score of perceived vulnerability to disease, with a significant positive correlation between COVID-19 fear scale and infectability perception or aversion to germs in the post-lockdown period ($p < 0.01$).

In a study involving 300 patients who received dental treatments after the COVID-19 outbreak, Karagözoğlu et al. [27] reported a high level of anxiety (43.38 ± 8.34), especially in those who thought that COVID-19 could be transmitted through dental treatment ($p < 0.001$). Moreover, they showed that dental clinics were considered places with a high risk of contamination, given the close contact with dentists and other patients. Patients who would not seek dental treatment if their condition was not urgent also showed a higher level of anxiety ($p < 0.003$). On the contrary, a lower anxiety score was reported in patients who thought that adequate measures were taken in the dental unit ($p < 0.001$) and the measures taken by the dentists while treating patients were sufficient. A lower level of anxiety was also registered in patients who felt safe because healthcare professionals received the COVID-19 vaccine.

In a large study conducted in China involving 1078 orthodontic patients, Quan et al. [24] reported some difficulties for follow-up visits in 67.9% of respondents because of the risk of COVID-19 infection. However, during the pandemic crisis, 55.1% of the respondents contacted their attending doctors; on the contrary, 33.3% did not take any measure, and 23.1% even preferred to solve the problem according to their experience or common sense.

Two studies [23,25] did not report a significant level of dental anxiety related to the COVID-19 outbreak. However, Nazir et al. registered a higher level of dental fear among females (41.17 ± 17.94) than among males (37.65 ± 20.34) ($p = 0.029$).

In an American survey conducted in May 2020 through Amazon Mechanical Turk, Moffat et al. [22] interviewed 448 people. Many concerns were reported about contracting COVID-19 from dental professionals (3.7 ± 1.7) and other patients (3.3 ± 1.8) in the dental offices. However, the risk of getting COVID-19 in a dental office overweighed the risk of not getting necessary dental treatments.

Peloso et al. [29] in their study about patients' perceptions in private dental clinics, that involved 595 Brazilians, showed that some interviewees were concerned about attending dental appointments because of the possibility of getting infected and/or of contaminating their family (18.5%), sometimes because dentists were considered at high risk of contamination. About 47% and 63% of the respondents reported increased feelings of anxiety, fear, or pain when the dental appointment was not postponable because of an emergency. About 20% of the respondents said that dental treatment could wait. In this study also, females were more worried about COVID-19 infection and less willing to go to dental appointments than males.

In a large study conducted on 1566 Italian orthodontic patients interviewed after the Italian lockdown (March–May 2020), Martina et al. [28] showed that 55.3% of the respondents believed there was a greater risk of COVID-19 infection during dental treatments. Furthermore, for 84.6% of patients, COVID-19 increased the fear of going to the dentist. Younger people and males were less scared to go to the dentist, while females and people older than 40 showed a high level of fear.

In a Nigerian survey conducted from 2020 until 2021 in public and private dental facilities involving 304 orthodontic patients, Umeh et al. [30] showed that people perceived themselves severely or moderately vulnerable to contracting COVID-19 (40.8% and 30.5%, respectively) but were willing to carry on with their dental treatments during the pandemic (72.4%). However, approximately 40% of the interviewees reported a certain level of fear of contracting the virus during dental appointments. In addition, the patients perceived the increase in treatment time and cost.

2.6. Protocols and Procedures for COVID-19 Infection Control in the Dental Setting

Five studies investigated the patients' perception of protocols and procedures adopted in dental clinics to reduce the risk of COVID-19 infection [22,25,26,29,30].

Two studies [26,29], both carried out in Brazil, showed that wearing PPE improved patients' confidence in dental professionals. In Cotrin et al. [26], more than 80% of the patients reported reduced anxiety and fear when dentists wore surgical masks and medical head caps during dental treatments; over half of the respondents reported a positive reduction of fear when dentists and medical staff wore face shields. In addition, some safety procedures, such as alcohol gel for patients and avoidance of crossing patients in the waiting areas, showed a positive effect in reducing the fear of COVID-19 infection in dental offices. The same trend, although with some percentage reductions, also emerged in Peloso et al. [29]

Moffat et al. [22] focused on patients' confidence and awareness about the appropriate use of government recommendations within dental offices. The respondents reported low levels of trust that dental offices follow government recommendations to dental professionals during the COVID-19 pandemic (2.2 ± 1.2). At the same time, they perceived themselves as aware of the government recommendation to dental professionals for appropriate dental treatments during the COVID-19 outbreaks (3.8 ± 1.9).

In Arqub et al. [25], approximately 80% of the respondents believed that pretesting patients and medical staff during the pandemic reduced patients' fear of COVID-19 infection in dental offices; wearing full PPE or N95 masks by dentists during dental treatments helped to increase patients' trust in the safety of dental treatments.

Finally, Umeh et al. [30] reported that patients attributed a crucial role to many safety procedures to access dental offices: social distancing, temperature screening before access, relevant screening questions, limiting the number of adults accompanying a child, wearing facemasks, and handwashing were found to play a crucial role in enhancing patients' trust.

3. Current Status

This work aimed to understand dental patients' perspectives, perceptions, attitudes, and expectations toward dental treatments after the first year of the COVID-19 pandemic. In the last two years, many studies have investigated the role of dentists in reducing COVID-19 risk infection and resuming their daily activity keeping a high level of safety [31]. Although dental professionals have been considered at high risk due to the close contact with patients' mouth and the upper respiratory tract [2] and the use of aerosol-generating procedures [32–35], many recommendations and guidelines have provided support to restart dental activity safely.

For the patients, returning to good oral health habits without increasing the risk of COVID-19 infection, and therefore returning to routine dental care, is very important as it provides extensive benefits to the population [22].

Many encouraging findings have emerged from our work. Patients are aware of the recommendation to reduce the risk of contagion and stringently follow them. Social distancing, handwashing with alcohol gel, wearing face masks, and avoiding close contact with other patients were perceived as safe procedures to access dental clinics. The same positive perception emerged when dentists wore all PPE and used N95 or FFP2 masks or face shields during dental treatments. The adoption of these procedures by dentists was not considered a hindrance to dental treatments. Still, it was an appropriate medical staff's behavior to assure the optimal resumption of elective dental treatments. Assurances of public health officials and institutions of the safety restart of routine dental care have also been reported as determinants in enhancing trust in this resumption [22].

About anxiety and fear of COVID-19 infection during dental treatments, we observed an increased sense of pain and nervousness during the first COVID-19 outbreak. Due to stringent lockdowns, people closed in their homes suffered a higher level of anxiety [17], which necessarily had repercussions on behaviors and perceptions toward dental treatments. This perception should be considered as multifactorial. While a high level of dental anxiety was observed after confinement in different studies, with a prevalence ranging from 27.2 to 38.7% [36,37], it should be observed that dental treatments require patients to avoid, albeit for a short time, the use of personal protection, like masks and social distancing, tools that continue to be indicated as the first and essential barriers to prevent infection, even now that vaccines are available in many countries and large populations have already received two vaccine doses [38].

Females demonstrated a significantly higher dental anxiety and fear than males. This can be partly explained as the consequence of females' higher level of anxiety toward dental treatments [39,40] and, in the last two years, toward the COVID-19 pandemic [41]. During the COVID-19 pandemic, males were more willing to attend a dental appointment, while females were strongly prevented from going to the dentist by their fear of infection, and a natural aversion to germs made them prefer to postpone non-urgent dental appointments [21].

About the behaviors of younger people, we report different findings. In Cotrin et al., the younger showed a higher level of anxiety and depressive symptoms toward dental treatments than older people [26]. On the contrary, Martina et al. reported a higher level of fear among younger people than among people over 40 years [28]. These contrasting results should be due to the different times of observation. During the evolution of the COVID-19 pandemic, scientific evidence has proved a higher risk of infection for older people that could have translated in a significant growing attention of the adults to avoid situations that could increase the risk of contagion. Thus, dentist avoidance emerged as a protective measure during quarantine, especially for patients who perceive a high risk of infection, are afraid of COVID-19, and are older than 60 years [21].

This study has several limitations. First, significant heterogeneity among the included studies was observed, preventing us from determining a quantitative prevalence of dental anxiety associated with the COVID-19 pandemic. Second, the sample sizes varied from hundreds of patients to more than 1500. Thus, in some cases, the sample size could not be representative of the reference population. Third, some studies reported dental anxiety and fear of patients not needing dental care and who would not schedule dental care at that time, so that the lack of a concrete need could have altered the perception. Fourth, the prevalence of COVID-19 infection and mortality in the interviewed area was not considered. Finally, all included studies had a cross-sectional design and were executed by adopting a self-reported questionnaire that, in some cases, used not-validated tools for psychometric measurements.

4. Conclusions and Prospects

The dental profession has always faced complex challenges related to viral pandemics. However, as demonstrated during the COVID-19 outbreak, dentists have promptly responded to new scenarios, improving safety. According to the COVID-19 guidelines, dentists change their workflows patterns or re-configure their clinic settings to ensure safety. Many precautions consist in increasing the use of protective materials and/or in prolonging the treatment time. If, on the one hand, these behaviors assure high safety standards for patients and dental treatments, on the other hand, they increase the cost of dental treatments. To reduce the impact of such new costs, some dentists have added significant charges for PPE to their bills, especially in the case of aerosol-generating procedures. In these cases, the cost of safety is entirely absorbed by patients who may be induced to go to the dentist only in cases of urgency. On the contrary, the lack of national policies to reduce the impact of the cost related to the proper application of the recommended guidelines, also in private dental offices, can increase the pressure on dentists and may set the stage for increased errors to avoid a significant rise of patients' cost.

How to prevent such negative scenarios? These issues spotlight the need for shared national policies to reduce the negative impact of the COVID-19 crisis. As done in many countries to support national and local economies, in the new normalcy of dentistry after the COVID-19 outbreak, sharing costs among patients, dentists, and national policies may help restore the regular dental activity, helping patients not to renounce dental treatments.

In conclusion:

- The availability of vaccines for the population and the awareness of patients about recommended guidelines to prevent COVID-19 contagion support a safe and lasting resumption of routine dental activities
- Communication with patients about adopted precautions in dental clinics plays a fundamental role in reducing patients' dental anxiety and fear related to the risk of COVID-19 infection within dental clinics.
- Compliance with dentist appointments should be encouraged, helping patients rediscover the confidential relationship of trust with their dentist and return to regular dental visits.
- Identifying economic policies to support the current financial pressure due to the high cost of dental treatments may speed up the return to normalcy for dentists and patients.

Supplementary Materials: The following supporting information can be downloaded at: https://www.mdpi.com/article/10.3390/encyclopedia2010022/s1. Table S1: Risk of bias-CHERRIES Checklist. Table S2: Risk of bias-SUrge Checklist.

Author Contributions: Conceptualization, S.S. and M.L.G.; methodology, M.L.G. and E.A.; software, M.L.G. and P.B.; validation, S.S., M.L.G., E.A., and M.S.; writing—original draft preparation, M.L.G., E.A., and P.B.; writing—review and editing, S.S. and M.S.; supervision, M.L.G. and E.A.; project administration, M.L.G. All authors have read and agreed to the published version of the manuscript.

Funding: This research received no external funding.

Informed Consent Statement: Not Applicable.

Conflicts of Interest: The authors declare no conflict of interest.

Abbreviations

DFS	Dental Fear Survey
MDAS	Modified Dental Anxiety Scale
MTurk	Mechanical Turk
NRS	Numerical Rating Scale
PPE	Personal Protective Equipment
PVD	Perceived Vulnerability to disease
TMD	Temporomandibular Disorders

References

1. American Dental Association. ADA Recommending Dentists Postpone Elective Procedures. Available online: https://www.ada.org/en/publications/ada-news/2020-archive/march/ada-recommending-dentists-postpone-elective-procedures (accessed on 29 October 2021).
2. Center for Disease Control and Prevention, SARS-CoV-2 and Transmission. Available online: https://www.cdc.gov/coronavirus/2019-ncov/science/science-briefs/sars-cov-2-transmission.html (accessed on 29 October 2021).
3. Bakaeen, L.G.; Masri, R.; AlTarawneh, S.; Garcia, L.T.; AlHadidi, A.; Khamis, A.H.; Hamdan, A.M.; Baqain, Z.H. Dentists' knowledge, attitudes, and professional behavior toward the COVID-19 pandemic: A multisite survey of dentists' perspectives. *J. Am. Dent. Assoc.* **2021**, *152*, 16–24. [CrossRef] [PubMed]
4. Beltran-Aguilar, E.; Benzian, H.; Niederman, R. Rational perspectives on risk and certainty for dentistry during the COVID-19 pandemic. *Am. J. Infect. Control.* **2021**, *49*, 131–133. [CrossRef] [PubMed]
5. Salgarello, S.; Salvadori, M.; Mazzoleni, F.; Salvalai, V.; Francinelli, J.; Bertoletti, P.; Lorenzi, D.; Audino, E.; Garo, M.L. Urgent Dental Care During Italian Lockdown: A Cross-sectional Survey. *J. Endod.* **2021**, *47*, 204–214. [CrossRef] [PubMed]

6. Ball, M.; Akintola, D.; Harrington, Z.; Djemal, S. Emergency dental care triage during the COVID-19 pandemic. *Br. Dent. J.* **2021**, 1–5. [CrossRef] [PubMed]
7. Eggmann, F.; Haschemi, A.A.; Doukoudis, D.; Filippi, A.; Verna, C.; Walter, C.; Weiger, R.; Zitzmann, N.U.; Bornstein, M.M. Impact of the COVID-19 pandemic on urgent dental care delivery in a Swiss university center for dental medicine. *Clin. Oral Investig.* **2021**, *25*, 5711–5721. [CrossRef] [PubMed]
8. Ostrc, T.; Pavlovic, K.; Fidler, A. Urgent dental care on a national level during the COVID-19 epidemic. *Clin. Exp. Dent. Res.* **2021**, *7*, 271–278. [CrossRef] [PubMed]
9. Pajpani, M.; Patel, K.; Bendkowski, A.; Stenhouse, P. Rapid response: Activity from a hospital based Urgent Dental Care Centre during the COVID-19 pandemic. *Br. J. Oral Maxillofac. Surg.* **2020**, *58*, e98–e103. [CrossRef]
10. Walter, E.; von Bronk, L.; Hickel, R.; Huth, K.C. Impact of COVID-19 on Dental Care during a National Lockdown: A Retrospective Observational Study. *Int. J. Environ. Res. Public Health* **2021**, *18*, 7963. [CrossRef]
11. Salgarello, S.; Salvadori, M.; Mazzoleni, F.; Francinelli, J.; Bertoletti, P.; Audino, E.; Garo, M.L. The New Normalcy in Dentistry after the COVID-19 Pandemic: An Italian Cross-Sectional Survey. *Dent. J.* **2021**, *9*, 86. [CrossRef]
12. American Dental Association. ADA 'Strongly' Encouraging Dental Professionals to be Vaccinated for COVID-19. Available online: https://www.ada.org/en/publications/ada-news/2021-archive/july/ada-strongly-encouraging-dental-professionals-to-be-vaccinated (accessed on 29 October 2021).
13. Zigron, A.; Dror, A.A.; Morozov, N.G.; Shani, T.; Haj Khalil, T.; Eisenbach, N.; Rayan, D.; Daoud, A.; Kablan, F.; Marei, H.; et al. COVID-19 Vaccine Acceptance Among Dental Professionals Based on Employment Status During the Pandemic. *Front Med.* **2021**, *8*, 618403. [CrossRef]
14. Menhadji, P.; Patel, R.; Asimakopoulou, K.; Quinn, B.; Khoshkhounejad, G.; Pasha, P.; Garcia Sanchez, R.; Ide, M.; Kalsi, P.; Nibali, L. Patients' and dentists' perceptions of tele-dentistry at the time of COVID-19. A questionnaire-based study. *J. Dent.* **2021**, *113*, 103782. [CrossRef] [PubMed]
15. Yavan, M.A. Effects of the COVID-19 pandemic on new patient visits for orthodontic treatment: A comparison of 2020 and the previous 3 years. *J. World Fed. Orthod.* **2021**, *10*, 127–131. [CrossRef] [PubMed]
16. Guo, H.; Zhou, Y.; Liu, X.; Tan, J. The impact of the COVID-19 epidemic on the utilization of emergency dental services. *J. Dent. Sci.* **2020**, *15*, 564–567. [CrossRef] [PubMed]
17. Huang, Y.; Zhao, N. Generalized anxiety disorder, depressive symptoms and sleep quality during COVID-19 outbreak in China: A web-based cross-sectional survey. *Psychiatry Res.* **2020**, *288*, 112954. [CrossRef] [PubMed]
18. Lei, L.; Huang, X.; Zhang, S.; Yang, J.; Yang, L.; Xu, M. Comparison of Prevalence and Associated Factors of Anxiety and Depression Among People Affected by versus People Unaffected by Quarantine During the COVID-19 Epidemic in Southwestern China. *Med. Sci. Monit.* **2020**, *26*, e924609. [CrossRef]
19. Moher, D.; Liberati, A.; Tetzlaff, J.; Altman, D.G.; Group, P. Preferred reporting items for systematic reviews and meta-analyses: The PRISMA statement. *PLoS Med.* **2009**, *6*, e1000097. [CrossRef]
20. Weir, K.R.; Ailabouni, N.J.; Schneider, C.R.; Hilmer, S.N.; Reeve, E. Considerations for systematic reviews of quantitative surveys: Learnings from a systematic review of the patients' Attitudes Towards Deprescribing questionnaire. *Res. Soc. Adm. Pharm.* **2021**, *18*, 2345–2349. [CrossRef]
21. Gonzalez-Olmo, M.J.; Delgado-Ramos, B.; Ortega-Martinez, A.R.; Romero-Maroto, M.; Carrillo-Diaz, M. Fear of COVID-19 in Madrid. Will patients avoid dental care? *Int. Dent. J.* **2022**, *72*, 76–82. [CrossRef]
22. Moffat, R.C.; Yentes, C.T.; Crookston, B.T.; West, J.H. Patient Perceptions about Professional Dental Services during the COVID-19 Pandemic. *JDR Clin. Trans. Res.* **2021**, *6*, 15–23. [CrossRef]
23. Nazir, M.; Almulhim, K.S.; AlDaamah, Z.; Bubshait, S.; Sallout, M.; AlGhamdi, S.; Alhumaid, J. Dental Fear and Patient Preference for Emergency Dental Treatment Among Adults in COVID-19 Quarantine Centers in Dammam, Saudi Arabia. *Patient Prefer. Adherence* **2021**, *15*, 1707–1715. [CrossRef]
24. Quan, S.; Guo, Y.; Zhou, J.; Zhang, G.; Xing, K.; Mei, H.; Li, J. Orthodontic emergencies and mental state of Chinese orthodontic patients during the COVID-19 pandemic. *BMC Oral Health* **2021**, *21*, 477. [CrossRef] [PubMed]
25. Arqub, S.A.; Voldman, R.; Ahmida, A.; Kuo, C.L.; Godoy, L.D.C.; Nasrawi, Y.; Al-Khateeb, S.N.; Uribe, F. Patients' perceptions of orthodontic treatment experiences during COVID-19: A cross-sectional study. *Prog. Orthod.* **2021**, *22*, 17. [CrossRef] [PubMed]
26. Cotrin, P.; Peloso, R.M.; Oliveira, R.C.; de Oliveira, R.C.G.; Pini, N.I.P.; Valarelli, F.P.; Freitas, K.M.S. Impact of coronavirus pandemic in appointments and anxiety/concerns of patients regarding orthodontic treatment. *Orthod. Craniofac. Res.* **2020**, *23*, 455–461. [CrossRef] [PubMed]
27. KaragÖZoĞLu, İ.; Parlar ÖZ, Ö. Investigation of the patients' perception on dental treatment and their anxiety levels during the COVID-19 pandemic process. *J. Health Sci. Med.* **2021**, *4*, 710–715. [CrossRef]
28. Martina, S.; Amato, A.; Faccioni, P.; Iandolo, A.; Amato, M.; Rongo, R. The perception of COVID-19 among Italian dental patients: An orthodontic point of view. *Prog. Orthod.* **2021**, *22*, 11. [CrossRef]
29. Peloso, R.M.; Pini, N.I.P.; Sundfeld Neto, D.; Mori, A.A.; Oliveira, R.C.G.; Valarelli, F.P.; Freitas, K.M.S. How does the quarantine resulting from COVID-19 impact dental appointments and patient anxiety levels? *Braz. Oral Res.* **2020**, *34*, e84. [CrossRef]
30. Umeh, O.D.; Utomi, I.L.; Isiekwe, I.G.; Aladenika, E.T. Impact of the coronavirus disease 2019 pandemic on orthodontic patients and their attitude to orthodontic treatment. *Am. J. Orthod. Dentofac. Orthop.* **2021**, *159*, e399–e409. [CrossRef]

31. Ather, A.; Patel, B.; Ruparel, N.B.; Diogenes, A.; Hargreaves, K.M. Coronavirus Disease 19 (COVID-19): Implications for Clinical Dental Care. *J. Endod.* **2020**, *46*, 584–595. [CrossRef]
32. Lanmark 360. Survey of COVID-19 Dental Patients' Perceptions and Attitudes Toward Returning to Dental Practices. Available online: https://lanmark360.com/research/Lanmark360-Dental-Patients-COVID-19-Survey-Results.pdf (accessed on 29 October 2021).
33. Innes, N.; Johnson, I.G.; Al-Yaseen, W.; Harris, R.; Jones, R.; Kc, S.; McGregor, S.; Robertson, M.; Wade, W.G.; Gallagher, J.E. A systematic review of droplet and aerosol generation in dentistry. *J. Dent.* **2021**, *105*, 103556. [CrossRef]
34. Peng, X.; Xu, X.; Li, Y.; Cheng, L.; Zhou, X.; Ren, B. Transmission routes of 2019-nCoV and controls in dental practice. *Int. J. Oral Sci.* **2020**, *12*, 9. [CrossRef]
35. Zimmermann, M.; Nkenke, E. Approaches to the management of patients in oral and maxillofacial surgery during COVID-19 pandemic. *J. Craniomaxillofac. Surg.* **2020**, *48*, 521–526. [CrossRef] [PubMed]
36. Mazza, C.; Ricci, E.; Biondi, S.; Colasanti, M.; Ferracuti, S.; Napoli, C.; Roma, P. A Nationwide Survey of Psychological Distress among Italian People during the COVID-19 Pandemic: Immediate Psychological Responses and Associated Factors. *Int. J. Environ. Res. Public Health* **2020**, *17*, 3165. [CrossRef] [PubMed]
37. Roy, D.; Tripathy, S.; Kar, S.K.; Sharma, N.; Verma, S.K.; Kaushal, V. Study of knowledge, attitude, anxiety & perceived mental healthcare need in Indian population during COVID-19 pandemic. *Asian J. Psychiatr.* **2020**, *51*, 102083. [CrossRef] [PubMed]
38. Our World in Data, Coronavirus (COVID-19) Vaccinations. Available online: https://ourworldindata.org/covid-vaccinations (accessed on 15 October 2021).
39. Jeddy, N.; Nithya, S.; Radhika, T.; Jeddy, N. Dental anxiety and influencing factors: A cross-sectional questionnaire-based survey. *Indian J. Dent. Res.* **2018**, *29*, 10–15. [CrossRef]
40. Lin, C.S.; Wu, S.Y.; Yi, C.A. Association between Anxiety and Pain in Dental Treatment: A Systematic Review and Meta-analysis. *J. Dent. Res.* **2017**, *96*, 153–162. [CrossRef]
41. Wang, C.; Pan, R.; Wan, X.; Tan, Y.; Xu, L.; Ho, C.S.; Ho, R.C. Immediate Psychological Responses and Associated Factors during the Initial Stage of the 2019 Coronavirus Disease (COVID-19) Epidemic among the General Population in China. *Int. J. Environ. Res. Public Health* **2020**, *17*, 1729. [CrossRef]

encyclopedia

MDPI

Entry

Asymptomatic Patients and Immune Subjects

Sheila Veronese * and Andrea Sbarbati

Department of Neurosciences, Biomedicine and Movement Sciences, Verona University, 10 Sq. L.A.Scuro, 37134 Verona, Italy; andrea.sbarbati@univr.it
* Correspondence: sheila.veronese@univr.it

Definition: An asymptomatic patient is someone who contracts a disease but shows no symptoms. An immune subject is a person who is free from virus infection. Both of these categories of people experience the limitations of government imposed by a pandemic situation, with one important difference. Probably only the first subjects contribute, in spite of themselves, to the spread of the disease and to the contagion of the people most susceptible to the virus. This implies that their detection is essential to limit infections. Therefore, knowing the characteristics of these people and those immune to the virus can be extremely useful in mitigating the effects of the disease and/or defeating it.

Keywords: natural immunity; asymptomatic subjects; sickle cell disease; obesity; population density; age; gender

1. Introduction

The spread of a disease in a country can depend on the effectiveness of the measures put in place to contain it and on the characteristics of the health system of the country itself. In the case of COVID-19, a disease resulting from a new virus, the whole world reacted by taking drastic measures, such as repeated total lockdowns during peaks of contagion.

The analysis of the data on infections, hospitalizations, and deaths showed that the virus has had very different effects from country to country. Overall, an immediate attempt was made to identify and protect the people who could be at increased risk of contracting this disease. It was quickly realized that the most severe forms of COVID-19 affected people over the age of 60 and/or with health conditions, such as lung or heart disease, diabetes, or conditions affecting the immune system [1]. However, country-to-country differences emerged on the groups of people at greatest risk.

This is the case, for example, of people with diabetes, who were listed in second place in the top 10 groups of people at risk of developing severe and life-threatening forms of COVID-19 by the European Union's European Center for Disease Prevention and Control (ECDC) of the European Union [2], while they ranked eighth among people who could be most at risk of serious illness by the Centers for Disease Control and Prevention (CDC) of the United States of America [3].

It should be emphasized that the containment measures adopted by the different countries have been different. The peaks of contagion occurred at different times, resulting in non-coincident lockdown periods in adjacent countries. The same political choices of the moment of initiation of the individual lockdowns, of their duration, and of the number of people authorized to continue essential work activities could have influenced both the contagion and mortality rates. The health protocols implemented in the various hospitals could also have played a decisive role in this regard.

These considerations lead to the conclusion that people with a certain pathology could be more at risk in some countries than in others. However, there may be other pre-existing factors that may have made some people more or less susceptible to the disease than others, leading to the development of mild forms of infection. Furthermore, it should

Citation: Veronese, S.; Sbarbati, A. Asymptomatic Patients and Immune Subjects. *Encyclopedia* **2022**, *2*, 109–126. https://doi.org/10.3390/encyclopedia2010008

Academic Editor: Stephen Bustin

Received: 15 November 2021
Accepted: 7 January 2022
Published: 11 January 2022

not be forgotten that, as with all viruses, even for SARS-CoV-2 there can be people who are immune.

Immune subjects have undergone all forms of containment, to no effect, but this can be considered an acceptable price given the gravity of the situation.

Patients who have developed mild forms of COVID-19, paucisymptomatic or asymptomatic, are instead those who have probably contributed, in spite of themselves, to the spread of the disease and to the contagion of the most susceptible people.

Perhaps early characterization of both of these two groups of subjects could have mitigated the effects of SARS-CoV-2 and could, however, still be useful in explaining its spread dynamics.

Taking all these considerations into account, we analyzed the contagion and mortality data from Italy, relating to the first wave of infections, in order to identify which people were less susceptible to the virus. The characteristics of these people were then also observed on a global scale to understand whether the data found for Italy were general or specific for this country.

2. Italy

2.1. First Wave of Infections

Why Italy? Because Italy is the first country in Europe where SARS-CoV-2 spread. Probably also for this reason it is the country that has suffered the greatest damage, presenting both a diffusion rate and a mortality rate among the highest, both in the European continent and in the whole world [4].

Italy is divided in three parts: north, center, and south. These areas are not geographically divided, and there is a high mobility between the different regions, both for business reasons and for tourism factors. The first generalized lockdown in Italy took place in the period of 11 March–3 May 2020 [5,6]. Although the characteristics of this country did not hinder the spread of SARS-CoV-2, the first wave of COVID-19 in the various Italian areas was not homogeneous, and there was a greater spread and aggression, especially in the north compared to southern Italy (Table 1).

Table 1. Epidemiological data in northern and southern Italy.

Northern Italy	No. [1] of Cases	No. [1] of Deaths	Infections in the Total Population [in %]	Southern Italy	No. [1] of Cases	No. [1] of Deaths	Infections in the Total Population [in %]
Aosta Valley	1223	146	0.973	Abruzzo	3662	472	0.279
Emilia-Romagna	31,094	4458	0.697	Apulia	5119	555	0.127
Friuli Venezia Giulia	3651	348	0.300	Basilicata	505	28	0.090
Liguria	10,683	1571	0.689	Calabria	1408	97	0.072
Lombardy	98,545	16,857	0.980	Campania	5976	442	0.103
Piedmont	32,440	4143	0.745	Molise	511	23	0.167
Trentino-South Tyrol	7925	697	0.739	Sardinia	1859	134	0.113
Veneto	22,190	2107	0.452	Sicily	4091	286	0.082
Total	260,407	30,327	0.697 ± 0.232		23,131	2037	0.129 ± 0.067
Deaths [in %]		11.65				8.81	

[1] No., number. COVID-19 data available as of 25 August 2020 [4].

From the beginning of the pandemic to 25 August 2020, the date of full resumption of socio-economic activities, keeping the prevention measures active, the spread of the disease was more than ten times higher in the north than in the south (mean = 0.697, sd = 0.232, min = 0.300, max = 0.980 in the north vs. mean = 0.129, sd = 0.067, min = 0.072, max = 0.279 in the south) (Figure 1a). The death rate was 15 times higher in the north than in the south, with the death-to-infection ratio higher in the north (Figure 1b) [4].

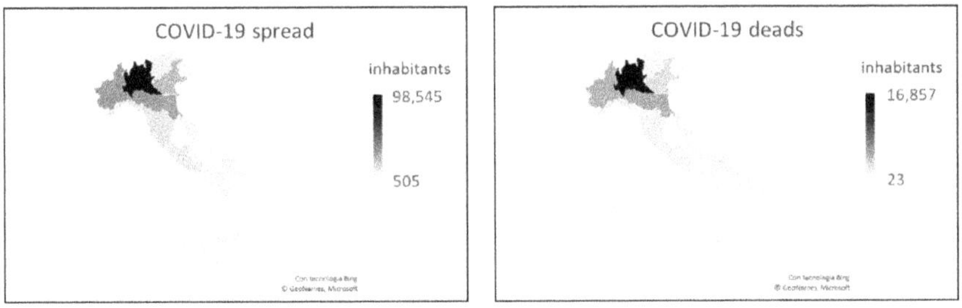

(a) (b)

Figure 1. COVID-19 data as of 25 August 2020. (**a**) Number of cases. (**b**) Number of deaths. Both graphs show the greatest severity in northern Italy, particularly in the Lombardy region.

What caused these differences?

Northern and southern Italy have different demographic and socio-economic characteristics.

Compared to the south, the north has a higher number of inhabitants (27,746,113 vs. 20,597,424) and a greater population density (202 vs. 140 inhabitants/km^2) (Figure 2). There is no doubt that, in the areas with the highest population density, the contagion is more widespread, even if protection and prevention measures are adopted.

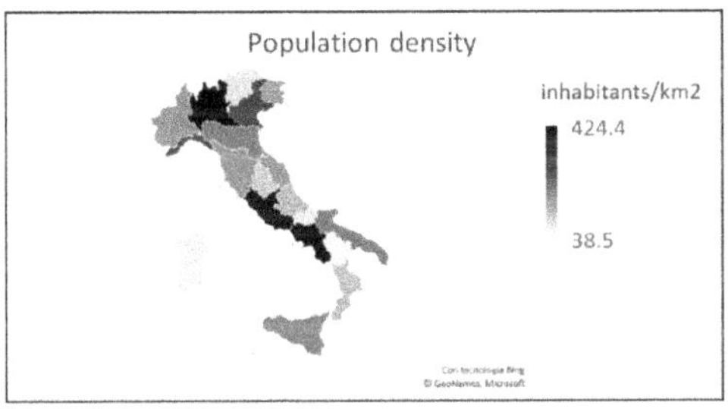

Figure 2. Italian population density (updated to 2019). Some regions of central-southern Italy have a high population density which, in reality, is linked to the presence of large urban centers (such as Rome in Lazio and Naples in Campania).

Furthermore, in percentage terms, the population is older in the north than in the south [7]. The greater number of inhabitants and the difference in age distribution mean that in the north there are 2.2 million more inhabitants aged > 64 years (Figure 3). Given the greater susceptibility to SARS-CoV-2 of people aged > 60 years, these data are compatible with the greater severity highlighted in northern Italy [4], even if they are not sufficient to explain the huge gap between the two areas.

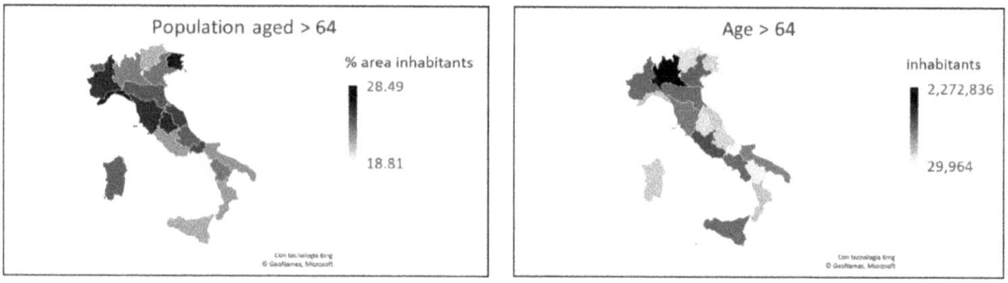

(a) (b)

Figure 3. Distribution of the Italian population aged > 64 in percentage (**a**) and absolute (**b**) terms (updated to 2019).

Another peculiarity of COVID-19 in Italy concerns the gender difference. It quickly emerged that although infections affected men and women at the same rate [8], the death rate was lower for the latter [9]. These data have been tracked over time and were still valid as of 17 September 2021.

The national percentage distribution of the male and female population indicates homogeneity throughout the territory, with a presence of only 2.63% more females than males. These data, however, mainly concern the population > 64 years, in which there are 2.97% more women than men. This percentage is higher in the north than in the south (3.20% vs. 2.53%) and implies that, in the north compared to the south, there are 1.3 million more women than men and a total of 0.9 million more women than men aged > 64 years [7] (Figure 4).

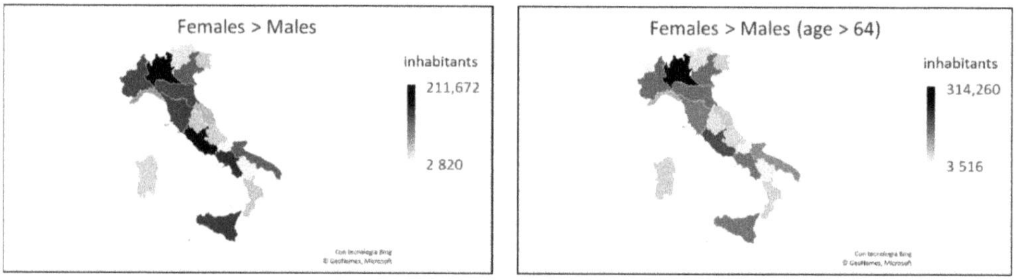

(a) (b)

Figure 4. Distribution of the male and female populations in Italy, overall (**a**) and only for the age group > 64 years (**b**) (updated to 2019).

The graphs in Figure 4 are similar to the graphs in Figure 1 on SARS-CoV-2 prevalence and COVID-19 mortality. This seems to be in contrast to the higher male mortality figure because where there are more females, fewer deaths should be expected. Given that the number of infections is equally distributed between the sexes, although the number of females is greater, can it be assumed that females are less susceptible than males to contracting the virus, and therefore female mortality is lower than male mortality?

Another characteristic aspect of Italy is food, and there is a clear difference between north and south in terms of culinary culture, a difference which is reflected in weight problems. From the Italian population, 46.3% have weight problems. Furthermore, 35.4% of people have a body mass index (BMI) within the limits of overweight (BMI = 25–29.9 kg/m^2), and 10.7% are obese (BMI > 30 kg/m^2). The population of northern Italy appears to be in better physical condition than that of the south. Compared to the national value, all the southern regions except Sardinia have a higher percentage of problems, while all the northern regions present lower values [10].

The figure worsens considering only the adult population (>18 years). The regions of northern Italy have lower overweight percentages than the regions of southern Italy, excluding Sardinia. This trend is also valid for the data relating to obesity, with the exception of Veneto, Friuli-Venezia Giulia, and Emilia-Romagna, which have obesity rates similar to those of the southern regions (Figure 5).

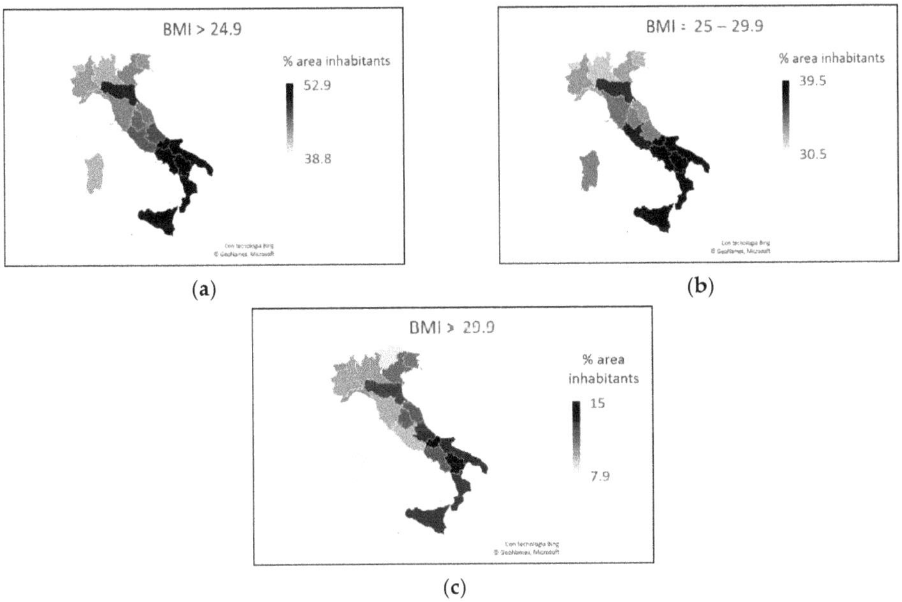

Figure 5. (**a**) Total percentages of weight problems in the individual regions, considering the adult population only. (**b**) Percentage of overweight adults in the various regions. (**c**) Percentage of obese adults in the various regions.

Overweight rates increase as people reach 74. From the age of 75, the trend reverses and rates decrease. The number of overweight males is greater than the number of overweight females, and over 64 years of age, the difference (overweight males—overweight females) is 12%. Obesity rates also increase with people's age up to 64 years. From the age of 65, the trend changes and rates fall. Males are more obese than females up to 74 years of age. From the age of 75, the percentage of obese males and females is the same [10].

Comparing data on the prevalence and death rates of COVID-19 with data on BMI, an almost surprising inverse relationship emerges. During the first phase of the infection in Italy, COVID-19 was more prevalent and more lethal in areas where the population had lower BMI rates. People aged > 74, for whom overweight rates decline, and people aged > 64, for whom obesity rates decline, were the most affected by the virus and had the worst disease outcomes. Does this mean that excess visceral adipose tissue may be a protective factor against SARS-CoV-2?

However, males aged > 64 with more weight problems than females had higher mortality rates. Can excess visceral fat protect a person from contracting the disease, but aggravate symptoms if he/she becomes infected?

The last two aspects that we consider, looking for a correlation with COVID-19 in Italy, are the blood group and the pathological states related to the levels of iron in the blood in the different geographical areas.

A link between blood groups and susceptibility to COVID-19 has already been described, and blood group A was more susceptible to the disease than group O, which appears to be more immune [11]. These data are in line with what has already been demonstrated for other diseases, such as Helicobacter pylori and norovirus infections, and for cholera and malaria [12,13]. In his work, Anstee (2010) states that protection against these infectious diseases derives from the inheritance of polymorphisms in the genes that encode and regulate the expression of ABH and Lewis antigens in body secretions [12]. Cooling (2015) highlighted the possible protective mechanisms deriving from the gene polymorphism of blood groups [13].

In Italy, the most common blood group is group A. North and south differ in the diffusion rate of group A, which is double in the north compared to the south (Table 2) [14]. This evidence could help explain COVID-19′s lower southern spread.

Table 2. Distribution of blood groups in Italy.

Blood Group	Northern Italy	Southern Italy
A [in %]	44	19
O [in %]	40	41

Another aspect seems to be linked to the greater spread of SARS-CoV-2 in the north and less in the south: pathologies related to iron levels in the blood. Southern Italy is part of the thalassemia prevalence area [15,16], and in general, anemia is more common here than in northern Italy [17,18]. Thalassemia is present in the north almost exclusively in southern Veneto and northern Emilia-Romagna, up to 20% of population [15,16,19]. Of the people with anemia, 80% are of predominantly Sicilian origin and from Southern Italy [17].

Figure 6a,b show, respectively, the distribution of thalassemia and anemia in the different areas of Italy. Figure 6c represents the distribution of hemochromatosis in Italy.

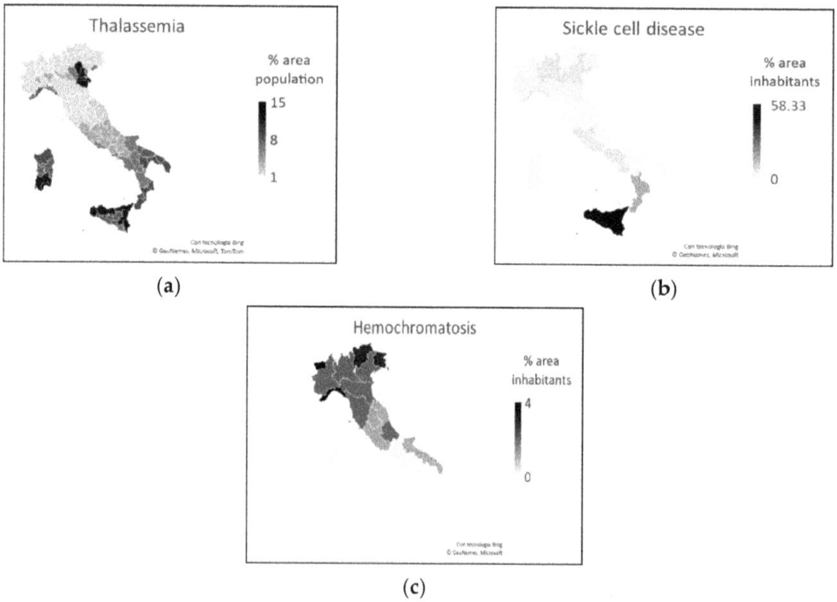

Figure 6. (**a**) Thalassemia distribution. (**b**) Anemia distribution. (**c**) Hemochromatosis distribution.

Hemochromatosis and other iron overload diseases are more common in the north than in southern Italy. In particular, the spread of these diseases decreases from north to south [20–27].

There is a clear similarity between Figures 1 and 6 of the areas where COVID-19 had the least impact and the areas with the highest rates of people with thalassemia and anemia.

That similarity is also present between areas where COVID-19 had a significant impact and areas with higher percentages of people with iron overload disease.

How can these data be explained? Why is the amount of iron in the blood important for SARS-CoV-2?

In the rest of the chapter, we will explore the complex aspect of anemic forms, and as regards iron overload diseases, we can hypothesize that they can favor the contagion and negative outcome of COVID-19 because they are generally associated with other diseases, such as diabetes, hepatic dysfunction, and cardiac dysfunction [26,27], which are all morbidities considered risk factors for the development of severe forms of COVID-19 [1–3].

2.2. 17 September 2021

After the first wave of infections, there were two more waves of COVID-19 in Italy until 17 September 2021 [28–31], and SARS-CoV-2 has continued to mutate [32]. Did the considerations made on the basis of the analysis of the data relating to the first wave remain valid over time?

Figure 7 presents the situation of infections and the number of deaths in Italy, as of 17 September 2021, after three waves of infections, with relative lockdowns, and after 6 months from the start of the vaccination campaign.

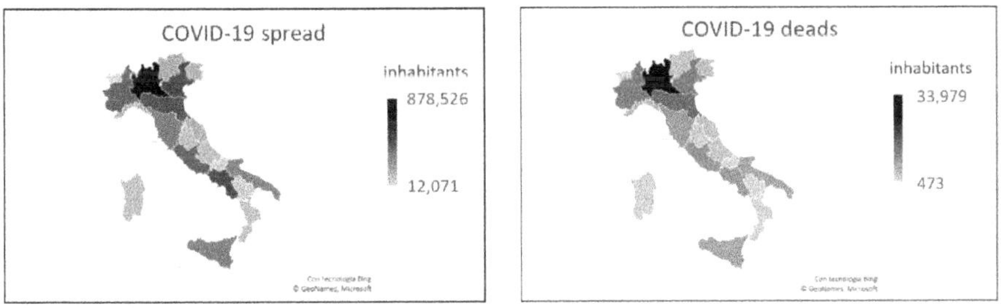

(a) (b)

Figure 7. COVID-19 data as of September 17, 2021. (**a**) Number of cases. (**b**) Number of deaths. Both graphs show that Lombardy and northern Italy continue to be the areas most affected by this disease.

In some regions of southern Italy, such as Campania, Apulia, and Sicily, the levels of contagion have increased significantly, reaching similar percentages to some regions of northern Italy. However, if we compare the number of infections and deaths with respect to the total population of the different areas, we note that northern Italy continues to be more affected than southern Italy [4]. Furthermore, the number of deaths among patients seems to show a lower aggressiveness of the virus in the south (Table 3).

The disease spread model reflects the percentages of population density, especially considering the large cities of southern Italy. There is also a notable similarity between Figure 7 and Figures 3b and 4, with regards to the age and sex characteristics of the population. The considerations inherent to these two aspects are therefore confirmed, as are those related to BMI, blood groups, and diseases related to the concentration of iron in the blood. It should be noted, in particular, that in the regions of southern Italy that have reached a number of infections similar to that of the northern regions, both the percentage of infections in the total population and the percentage of deaths (in the total population, and in the total of infections) are lower than the same variables in the north (Table 4).

Table 3. Epidemiological data in northern and southern Italy.

Northern Italy	No. [1] of Cases	No. [1] of Deaths	Infections in the Total Population [in %]	Southern Italy	No. [1] of Cases	No. [1] of Deaths	Infections in the Total Population [in %]
Aosta Valley	12,071	473	9.61	Abruzzo	80,556	2535	6.14
Emilia-Romagna	419,717	13,427	9.41	Apulia	266,881	6764	6.63
Friuli Venezia Giulia	112,817	3813	9.28	Basilicata	29,708	607	5.28
Liguria	111,775	4395	7.21	Calabria	81,857	1369	4.20
Lombardy	878,526	33,979	8.73	Campania	452,471	7853	7.80
Piedmont	376,475	11,742	8.64	Molise	14,437	495	4.72
Trentino-South Tyrol	124,259	2557	11.59	Sardinia	74,619	1624	4.55
Veneto	464,283	11,736	9.47	Sicily	291,964	6673	5.84
Total	2,499,923	82,122	9.24 ± 1.22		1,292,493	27,920	5.65 ± 1.20
Deaths/cases [in %]		3.25 ± 0.68				2.38 ± 0.63	

[1] No., number. COVID-19 data available on 17 September 2021 [4].

Table 4. Spread and mortality in the regions of southern Italy with the highest number of infections.

	% Cases/Population	% Deads/Population	% Deads/Cases
Apulia	6.63	0.17	2.53
Campania	7.80	0.14	1.74
Sicily	5.84	0.13	2.29

COVID-19 data available on 17 September 2021 [4].

3. What Can Be Concluded by Observing the Italian Situation?

From the data considered, it seems to emerge that, in Italy, despite the spread occurring throughout the national territory, the highest rates of contagion occurred in areas with greater population density, where there was also a greater number of elderly people. In the areas of southern Italy, less affected by the first wave, the spread took place in the later stages. However, the number of infections and mortality rates indicate a lower severity of the disease. An excess of visceral fat accumulation, within the limits of overweight (not obese), seems to have mitigated the effects of the disease. This is also the case with the presence of thalassemia and forms of anemia, while iron overload diseases appear to have worsened the outcome of the disease.

4. Rest of the World

Extending the research done for a small country to the rest of the world may seem pretentious. Each country has its own peculiarities that can tip the balance, in this case, in the number of infections and in the number of deaths from COVID-19.

Given that the aspects examined for Italy are general socio-demographic aspects, the extension of the survey is possible and may prove useful.

The spread of the COVID-19 pandemic to the rest of the world has not been uniform. As of 17 September 2021, American states have been particularly affected, both in terms of the number of infected and the number of deaths. To this date, the United States and Brazil alone accounted for 27.71% of cases and 26.95% of deaths worldwide. Both of these countries had a higher contagion rate than Italy (12.72% for USA and 9.99% for Brazil vs. 7.83% for Italy), and while Brazil had approximately the same rate of lethality (Brazil 2.79%

vs. Italy 2.81%), the United States had a much lower lethality rate than Italy (only 1.60%) [4]. What made the difference?

India, the second country in the world for the number of infections, had an infection rate of 2.43% and a lethality rate of 1.33% [4]. This means that despite the large number of infections and deaths linked to the total number of inhabitants of this country, the virus here seems to have failed to spread and manifest itself in a serious manner. Given the situation in this country, however, it is necessary to use the conditional because it is not possible to be sure that all cases have actually been registered.

The values, however, underline how the pandemic has evolved extremely differently on the American and Asian continents.

Considering African countries, the lowest number of infections in the world was recorded here, despite this continent presenting the highest mortality rate compared to the rest of the world (2.52% vs. 2.05%). The latter figure is undoubtedly linked to health problems and the very low level of assistance available on this continent. It is striking that South Africa alone, the most European of African countries, accounts for 35.32% of infections and 41.83% of deaths on its continent. If the data relating to this country are added to the data relating to Morocco and Tunisia, two other countries that have numerous interactions with Europe, we obtain that the three countries alone represent 55.17% of infections and 60.47% of deaths in Africa [4].

The question arises whether the virus in the first variant that spread in Europe was more aggressive and lethal than the one that arrived in Africa at a later time. There is also the possibility that not all cases from the latter continent are known, and, therefore, it is only possible to estimate the severity of COVID-19 in Africa. There is also, however, the possibility that the population here actually contracted the virus less and developed less severe forms of the disease.

The number of infected and deceased people is shown in Figure 8.

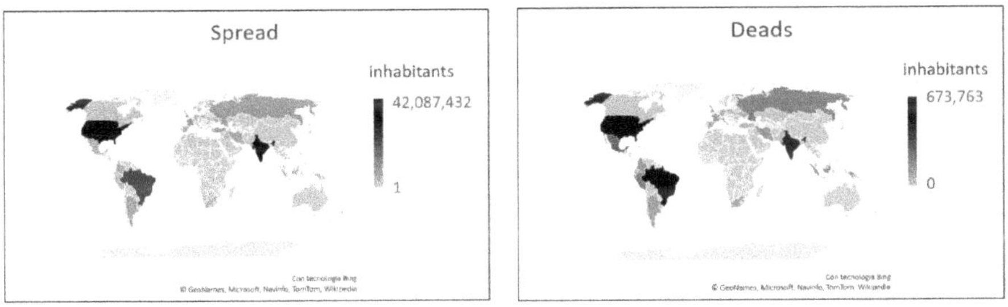

(a) (b)

Figure 8. COVID-19 data as of 17 September 2021. (**a**) Number of cases. (**b**) Number of deaths. Both graphs show the extremely variability in the diffusion and severity of this disease.

Considering the population density in the world, the highest values are recorded in Europe and Asia. The areas of the world with the lowest population density are Russia, Canada, and some African states (Figure 9) [33,34].

In terms of gender and age of the population, overall, there are a total of 51.6 million more males than females in the world. Up to the age of 54, there are more males than females (143.9 million). Over the age of 54, the trend reverses with 92.3 million more women than men. There are more males than females in Asia and in many North African states, considering both the overall population and the population aged > 64 [35]. People live longer in European countries, Canada, Oceania, and Japan than in African countries [33], and mean age values align with survival rates [33,35]. From this it follows that, in these countries, there are more people aged > 64 years (Figure 10).

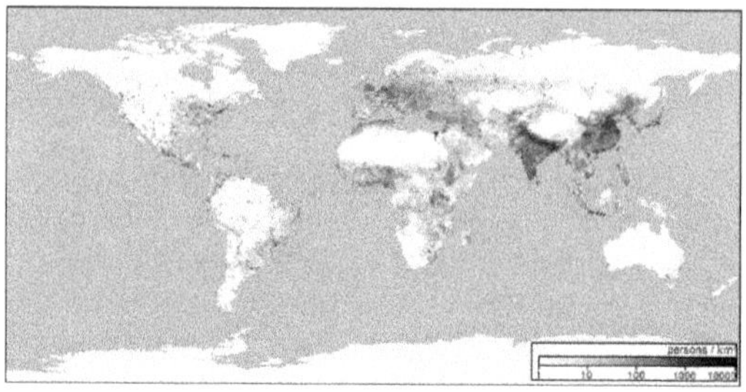

Figure 9. World population density (updated to 2000) [34].

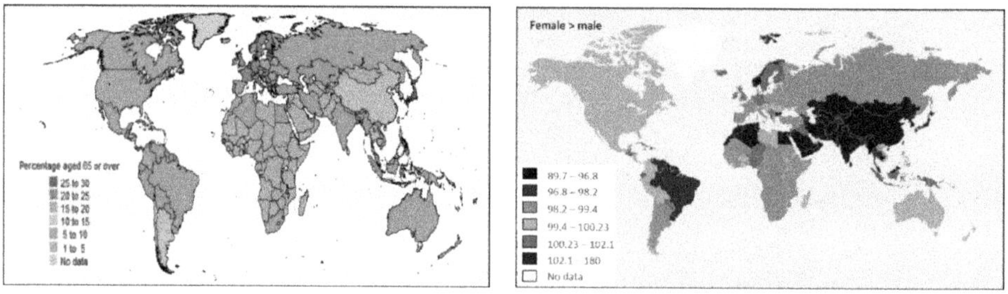

(a) (b)

Figure 10. (**a**) Distribution of the World population aged > 65 as a percentage. (**b**) Distribution of the male and female population in the World [33].

The statistics on the age of the population in Italy and in the rest of the world are in line with the spread of COVID-19, which is lower in countries where the average age is lower (e.g., Africa) [33,35]. A different trend is found only in South Asia, where the spread is high compared to Europe [4], despite the average age of the Asian population being lower than that of the European population [33]. However, the death rate in Asia is lower than in Europe [4].

The fact that in the world there is a greater presence of women aged > 64 years compared to males, and that the number of infections is the same between males and females, while it should be higher for women (who are in greater numbers), supports the hypothesis that women are more immune or develop COVID-19 more frequently than males in asymptomatic or paucisymptomatic forms, forms that are not detected. Data on the higher death rate for males than for females [36] seem to confirm a tendency for females to develop less severe forms of the disease.

Analyzing data on the weight of the population in the world, the obesity rate is highest in the United States and Saudi Arabia. The problem of obesity is more relevant in the American states, in Europe, in Australia, and in the countries of the Mediterranean area. Problems of malnutrition, on the other hand, are more common in Africa and in the countries of South Asia [37] (Figure 11).

While in Italy the number of infections and deaths seems to indicate excess weight as a protective factor against SARS-CoV-2, the data in the rest of the world do not seem to match. It should be noted that the number of cases of serious and morbid obesity is much lower in Italy than in many other countries of the world [38]. In the United States, where the obesity problem is most severe [37], obesity is listed among the top eight risk factors for COVID-19 [3]. In Europe, where obesity problems, although present, are less prominent than in America, obesity ranks eleventh on the list of risk factors [2]. The spread could affect more obese people in countries where there are actually more obese people. Obesity could, therefore, become a risk factor only when it exceeds a certain degree, such as to induce other pathological states, as it is easier for people aged > 60 years to develop these [39]. There is little data on the impact of obesity on COVID-19 severity [40].

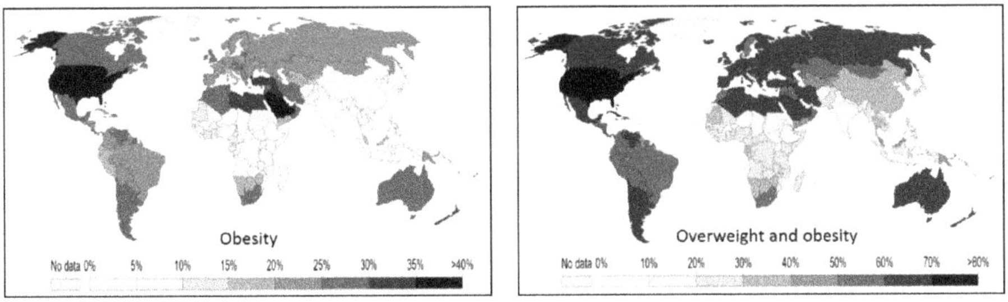

(a) (b)

Figure 11. (**a**) Percentages of obese adults in various countries. (**b**) Percentages of overweight adults by country [37].

As far as haematological characteristics are concerned, blood group O is the most widespread in the world and is found, in particular, in America, Africa, and eastern Russia. Group A is more common in Europe, Australia, and the far north of America. Group B is the least widespread in the world and is found in Asia, Eastern Europe, and, to a lesser extent, Africa (Figure 12) [41].

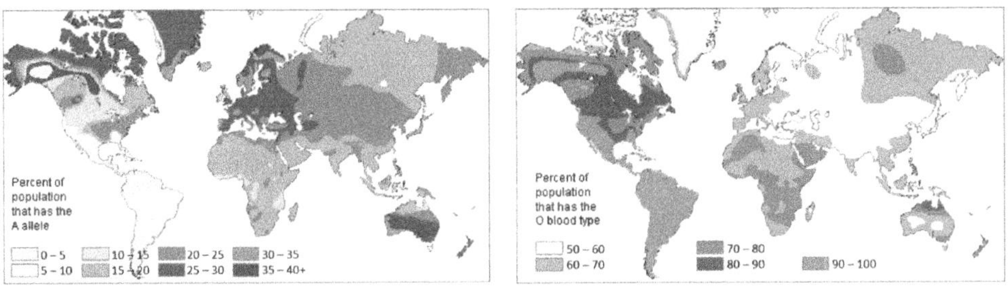

(a) (b)

Figure 12. (**a**) Distribution of blood group A. (**b**) Distribution of blood group O [41].

In Italy, the different distribution of blood groups between north and south confirms the greater susceptibility to COVID-19 in people with blood type A compared to people with blood type O. The prevalence of blood group O and not A in Chinese, American, and African populations seems to explain why, despite the high number of infections, the mortality rate is relatively low [42].

All the considerations made so far do not explain why SARS-CoV-2 affects more men and older people. The data relating to the incidence of hemochromatosis in northern Italy and anemia and thalassemia in the south seem to answer this question [15–17,19,21–27]. In Europe, the countries of the Mediterranean area, where anemic forms prevail among the population [43,44], record lower mortality rates than the countries of Northern Europe, where iron overload diseases are more frequent (Figure 13) [23–27].

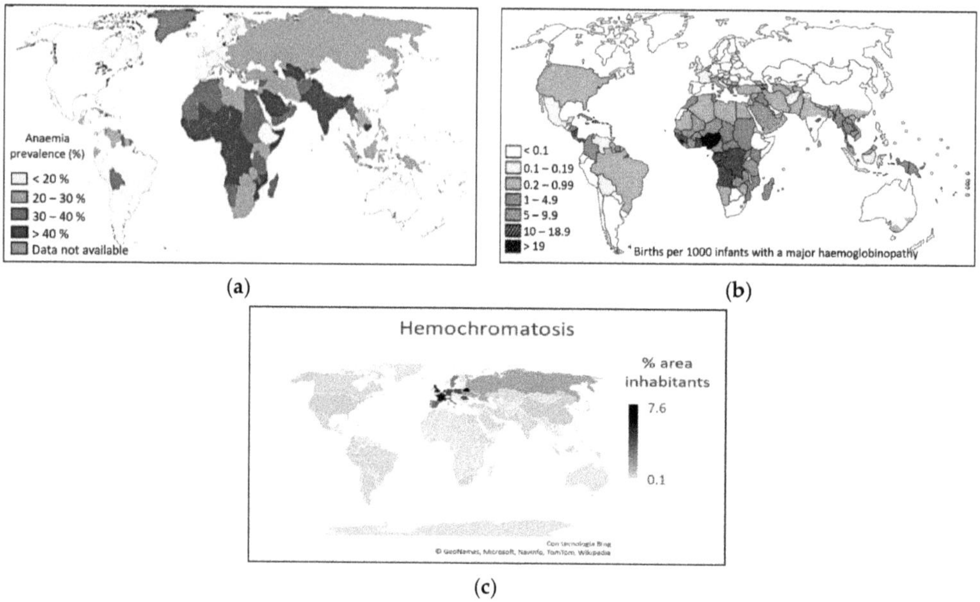

Figure 13. (**a**) Anemia distribution [42–44]. (**b**) Thalassemia distribution [45]. (**c**) Hemochromatosis distribution [23–27,42,46].

This is despite the fact that the rates of contagion among the population are sometimes higher in the countries of the Mediterranean area than in the countries of northern Europe [4]. Here, on the other hand, hemochromatosis and iron overload diseases are more frequent [46]. For these diseases, the incidence decreases progressively in non-Hispanic whites, Native Americans, blacks, Pacific Islanders, up to Asians, in which they are practically absent [47]. Conversely, Asians, particularly from the south-east; Africans; and populations of the eastern Mediterranean area are more prone to diseases such as thalassemia and forms of anemia [42–45]. Even in American countries, data on blood group distribution [41] and incidence of iron overload disease [25] and forms of anemia [43,44] appear to be related to a reduced death rate from COVID-19 [4].

Hemochromatosis causes excessive absorption of iron by the intestine, resulting in the accumulation of this metal in other organs and tissues. Males show much more frequent and more severe symptoms than women, with the first manifestations of the disease between the ages of 40 and 50. In women, before menopause, the clinical picture is ten times less frequent than in men due to the loss of iron during menstruation and during pregnancy. Therefore, women develop signs and symptoms of hemochromatosis-related organ damage approximately 10 years after men [48]. This could really be linked to the greater severity of COVID-19 in males, more prone to pathological forms linked to the accumulation of iron in the body.

Extremely interesting is the relationship that seems to exist between the levels of iron present in people's blood, both in terms of deficiency and in terms of excess, and the severity of COVID-19. Many viruses have been shown to hijack cells for replication, and efficient replication requires an iron-filled host [49,50]. Indeed, iron-filled cells turn out to be good sites for viruses. Conditions such as hemochromatosis or iron overload disease, in which the serum iron level is increased, compromise host defenses and increase susceptibility to various infectious diseases [50]. In populations where the incidence of hemochromatosis is high, a virus such as SARS-CoV-2 could find a perfect environment to live in, causing the disease to spread widely. In thalassemic and anemic subjects, on the other hand, the proliferation of the virus would be more difficult, in the former due to cyclic blood transfusions (15–20 days) associated with chelating agents (to eliminate the abnormal accumulation of iron in the organs) which is commonly used as a therapy and causes blood purification [42], and in the latter due to the absence of iron.

The data in the literature seem to confirm these observations [51,52]. However, anemic patients are not immune to COVID-19 and, if infected, their picture is immediately severe [53]. On the other hand, the inflammatory state induced by SARS-CoV-2 [54], which worsens with the duration of the disease [55], is often accompanied by systemic hypoferritinemia [56,57]. This obviously strongly compromises an already anemic patient.

The particular link between COVID-19 and blood, and the iron contained in it, really seems to explain why women have a lower death rate than men, but also why children are less affected than adults. In fact, in children, the rates of anemia are very high [43,44]. It is, however, mandatory to use the conditional, since this disease can be defined in many ways, except simple, the greater or lesser mortality in a country is not attributable to a single factor.

It should be emphasized that the resistance of anemic subjects to COVID-19 has been observed by other researchers. Particular attention was paid to sickle cell disease (SCD), which we analyze below.

5. Sickle Cell Disease and COVID-19

There are several forms of anemia dependent on different causes. There may be anemia due to excess bleeding, such as in the case with pregnancy and breastfeeding, some surgeries, and trauma. There may be sickle cell anemia and hemolytic anemias due to excessive destruction of red blood cells. There can be aplastic anemias due to reduced or impaired production of red blood cells and hemoglobin, as in the case of nutritional deficiencies (iron, vitamin B12, and folic acid) or diseases (which induce poor absorption of iron, vitamin B12, and folic acid), such as Crohn's disease or celiac disease.

SCD is particular because it is a genetic disease. If people with SCD were truly immune to COVID-19, then we would have a favorable genetic condition against this disease. Some genetic diseases are known to show resistance to some infectious diseases [58], and in this case, the term heterozygous advantage is used. SCD already presents the heterozygous advantage over falciparum malaria [59,60]. Could it be that it also has this advantage against COVID-19?

We analyzed the data available in literature on the incidence and lethality of COVID-19 for subjects with SCD. We performed a literature search on the PubMed database, considering all the works published from the beginning of the pandemic until March 2021, one year after the diffusion of COVID-19 in Italy. For the research, we used the terms "sickle cell," "COVID-19," and "SARS-CoV-2." Non-English articles, articles that did not contain patient numbers, and articles for which full text could not be obtained were excluded. With the literature research, we identified ninety-two articles, and, applying the exclusion criteria, we selected 43 articles. Among these, 28 studies were single case or case reports with a limited number of patients ($\leq$10 patients).

Of particular interest is the study of de Sanctis et al. [51], conducted on 9499 patients with hemoglobinopathies, followed in 17 centers in 10 different countries. Only 13 patients contracted SARS-CoV-2, with an incidence of 0.14%. Other studies in adults [61–64] and children [62,64,65] showed a favorable outcome of COVID-19, with milder clinical presentations than the general population had [61–63,66]. The published data are such as to raise the question of whether SCD really increases the risk of SARS-CoV-2 infection [67] or, conversely, may be a protective factor against COVID-19 [62,68–70].

Opinions contrary to the previous observations were found in Minniti et al. [71], and Panepinto et al. [72], which reported a worsening of the course of COVID-19 in patients with SCD, and in three other studies [73–75], which reported no differences in either symptomatology or outcome between subjects with and without SCD from COVID-19.

Possible factors that may play a role in the adaptation of the immune response of SCD patients to COVID-19 were well elucidated in Azerad et al. [68], and citations in other articles are summarized in Table 5.

Table 5. Factors that may play a role in adapting the immune response of SCD patients to COVID-19.

Factors	References
Host response adaptation with parasite sequestration and cytoadhesion to the endothelium.	[69]
High plasma interferon-α concentrations and type I interferon signature by neutrophils.	[70]
Formation of a fibrin trap for pathogenic invaders that promotes the immune elector cell recruitment.	[71]
Role of erythrocytes in the immune response.	[72]
The biomechanical characteristics of the cell membrane prevent the virus-host cell adhesion.	[73]

Unfortunately, it is not possible to perform a statistical analysis because some articles are mini-reviews where there are duplicate values.

The lack of data is, however, compatible with a very low incidence of SARS-CoV-2 in patients with SCD. This value could actually indicate a lower susceptibility of these patients to contract the virus, although the causes of this lower propensity are not yet certain. However, this value could only be linked to greater prevention and protection of these subjects, followed in national reference centers, which often have tightened the health protocols necessary for patient care and adopted forms of remote monitoring and support through applications of telemedicine. The same patients, aware of their fragility, have adopted more careful behaviors and have correctly used individual protection tools (for example face masks) since the beginning of the COVID-19 pandemic. These attentions have undoubtedly contributed to a lower incidence of SARS-CoV-2 in these subjects.

Regarding the lower severity of COVID-19, in Table 5, we have summarized some of the hypotheses that have already been formulated to explain this finding, but further studies are needed to clarify this aspect. In fact, to date, the data present in the literature are mainly statistical or hypothetical.

6. Conclusions

There is no doubt that until September 2021, women and especially children had a lower susceptibility to SARS-CoV-2 and developed COVID-19 less severely than men. The causes of this are unclear. All these subjects can fall into the category of asymptomatic or paucisymptomatic subjects. None of these individuals are truly immune to COVID-19.

There are multiple factors that determine susceptibility to a virus and the severity of a disease. In this chapter, we have analyzed various socio-demographic aspects. Two unexpected factors that deserve further investigation are the correlation with body fat and the amount of iron in the blood. Evidence related to SCD also indicates that genetics play a role, perhaps not a secondary one.

Undoubtedly, it is the overlap of the aspects considered in this chapter and of many other socio-demographic aspects that determine the consequences of the COVID-19 in people affected.

7. Highlights

- SARS-CoV-2 has spread more to areas with higher population density and an older population.
- Although women and men had the same infection rate, the former developed less severe forms of COVID-19.

- Children appear to be immune to SARS-CoV-2 and/or manifest COVID-19 predominantly in asymptomatic and paucisymptomatic forms.
- In Italy, an excess of visceral fat accumulation, within the limits of overweight or mildly obese, seems to have mitigated the outcome of COVID-19.
- Worldwide, excess visceral fat in non-mild forms of obesity appears to have worsened the outcome of COVID-19, possibly due to obesity-related conditions.
- Worldwide, the presence of thalassemia and forms of anemia appear to have mitigated the effects of COVID-19.
- Worldwide, iron overload diseases appear to have worsened the outcome of COVID-19.

Author Contributions: Conceptualization, S.V. and A.S.; investigation, S.V. and A.S.; writing—original draft preparation, S.V. and A.S.; writing—review and editing, S.V. and A.S. All authors have read and agreed to the published version of the manuscript.

Funding: This research received no external funding.

Data Availability Statement: The data presented in this study are publicly available on the various Internet sites cited in the work. The links are present in the references.

Conflicts of Interest: The authors declare no conflict of interest.

Entry Link on the Encyclopedia Platform: https://encyclopedia.pub/19257.

References

1. World Health Organization. COVID-19: Vulnerable and High Risk Groups. Available online: https://www.who.int/westernpacific/emergencies/covid-19/information/high-risk-groups (accessed on 8 September 2021).
2. ECDPC-European Centre for Disease Prevention and Control. COVID-19 Surveillance Report. Updated 2 September 2021. Available online: https://covid19-surveillance-report.ecdc.europa.eu/#5_risk_groups_most_affected (accessed on 8 September 2021).
3. CDC-Centers for Disease Control and Prevention, U.S. Department of Health and Human Service. Underlying Medical Conditions Associated with High Risk for Severe COVID-19: Information for Healthcare Providers. Updated 13 May 2021. Available online: https://www.cdc.gov/coronavirus/2019-ncov/hcp/clinical-care/underlyingconditions.html (accessed on 8 September 2021).
4. Lab24, Il Sole 24 Ore. Coronavirus in Italy: Updated Map and Case Count. 2021. Available online: https://lab24.ilsole24ore.com/coronavirus/en/ (accessed on 9 September 2021).
5. "Coronavirus, Conte: "In Italia Fino al 25 Marzo Chiusi i Negozi Tranne Alimentari e Farmacie. Sui Trasporti Possibili Riduzioni. Effetti tra 14 Giorni"" [Coronavirus, Conte: "In Italy until March 25, Shops Except Food and Pharmacies are Closed. Possible Reductions on Transport. Effects for 14 Days"]. La Repubblica (In Italian). Available online: https://www.repubblica.it/politica/2020/03/11/news/coronavirus_conte_italia_governo_misure-250988471/?ref=RHPPTP-BL-I250988111-C12-P1-S1.12-T1 (accessed on 11 March 2020).
6. "Italy Extends Lockdown until May 3rd Despite Pressure from Business". The Local.it. 2020. Available online: https://www.thelocal.it/20200410/italy-set-to-extend-lockdown-until-early-may/ (accessed on 11 April 2020).
7. UrbiStat, S.r.l. Maps, Analysis and Statistics about the Resident Population. 2019. Available online: https://ugeo.urbistat.com/AdminStat/it/it/demografia/dati-sintesi/italia/380/1 (accessed on 13 September 2021).
8. The COVID-19 Task Force of the Department of Infectious Diseases and the IT Service, Italian Higher Institute of Health. COVID-19 Integrated Surveillance Data in Italy. 2021. Available online: https://www.epicentro.iss.it/en/coronavirus/sars-cov-2-dashboard (accessed on 13 September 2021).
9. COVID-19 Surveillance Group, Italian Higher Institute of Health. Characteristics of COVID-19 Patients Dying in Italy. Report Based on Available Data on 21 July 2021. Available online: https://www.epicentro.iss.it/en/coronavirus/bollettino/Report-COVID-2019_21_july_2021.pdf (accessed on 13 September 2021).
10. Osservatorio Nazionale Sulla Salute Nelle Regioni Italiane. Rapporto Osservasalute 2020. Fumo, Alcol, Alimentazione, Eccesso Ponderale e Prevenzione. Updated 17 May 2021. Available online: https://www.osservatoriosullasalute.it/osservasalute/rapporto-osservasalute-2020 (accessed on 13 September 2021).
11. Severe Covid-19 GWAS Group; Ellinghaus, D.; Degenhardt, F.; Bujanda, L.; Buti, M.; Albillos, A. Genomewide association study of severe Covid-19 with respiratory failure. *N. Engl. J. Med.* **2020**, *383*, 1522–1534. [CrossRef] [PubMed]
12. Anstee, D.J. The relationship between blood groups and disease. *Blood* **2010**, *115*, 4635–4643. [CrossRef]
13. Cooling, L. Blood groups in infection and host susceptibility. *Clin. Microbiol. Rev.* **2015**, *28*, 801–870. [CrossRef]
14. AVIS Comunale Forlì. I Gruppi Sanguigni. Available online: https://www.avisforli.it/gruppi-sanguigni-avis-forli_34c18.html (accessed on 13 September 2021).
15. Mento, C.; Piraino, B.; Rizzo, A.; Vento, R.; Rigoli, L.; Moschella, E.; Salpietro, C.; Settineri, S. Affective control and life satisfaction in thalassemics. *Int. J. Psychol. Res.* **2015**, *8*, 90–97. [CrossRef]

16. Associazione PieraCutino. La Talassemia in Cifre. Available online: http://www.pieracutino.it/la-talassemia-in-cifre/ (accessed on 13 September 2021).
17. Russo-Mancuso, G.; Romeo, M.A.; Guardabasso, V.; Schilirò, G. Survey of sickle cell disease in Italy. *Haematologica* **1998**, *83*, 875–881.
18. Russo, G.; De Franceschi, L.; Colombatti, R.; Rigano, P.; Perrotta, S.; Voi, V.; Palazzi, G.; Fidone, C.; Quota, A.; Graziadei, G.; et al. Current challenges in the management of patients with sickle cell disease—A report of the Italian experience. *Orphanet. J. Rare Dis.* **2019**, *14*, 120. [CrossRef] [PubMed]
19. Del Senno, L.; Pirastu, M.; Barbieri, R.; Bernardi, F.; Buzzoni, D.; Marchetti, G.; Perrotta, C.; Vullo, C.; Kan, Y.W.; Conconi, F. beta (+)-Thalassaemia in the Po river delta region (northern Italy): Genotype and beta globin synthesis. *J. Med. Genet.* **1985**, *22*, 54–58. [CrossRef]
20. Serre, J.L. *Diagnostic Techniques in Genetics*; John Wiley & Sons: Hoboken, NJ, USA, 2007.
21. Piperno, A.; Sampietro, M.; Pietrangelo, A.; Arosio, C.; Lupica, L.; Montosi, G.; Vergani, A.; Fraquelli, M.; Girelli, D.; Pasquero, P.; et al. Heterogeneity of hemochromatosis in Italy. *Gastroenterology* **1998**, *114*, 996–1002. [CrossRef]
22. De Gobbi, M.; D'Antico, S.; Castagno, F.; Testa, D.; Merlini, R.; Bondi, A.; Camaschella, C. Screening selected blood donors with biochemical iron overload for hemochromatosis: A regional experience. *Haematologica* **2004**, *89*, 1161–1167.
23. Lucotte, G.; Dieterlen, F. A European allele map of the C282Y mutation of hemochromatosis: Celtic versus Viking origin of the mutation? *Blood Cells Mol. Dis.* **2003**, *31*, 262–267. [CrossRef]
24. Distante, S.; Robson, K.J.; Graham-Campbell, J.; Arnaiz-Villena, A.; Brissot, P.; Worwood, M. The origin and spread of the HFE-C282Y haemochromatosis mutation. *Hum. Genet.* **2004**, *115*, 269–279. [CrossRef]
25. Ulvik, R.J. Hereditary haemochromatosis through 150 years. *Tidsskr. Nor. Legeforen.* **2016**, *136*, 2017–2021. [CrossRef] [PubMed]
26. Arthritis Research. Type 1 Haemochromatosis. Available online: https://www.arthritisresearch.us/haemolytic-anaemia/type-1-haemochromatosis.html (accessed on 13 September 2021).
27. TeamHaem. Case 71–Summary. Available online: https://teamhaem.com/2017/01/27/case-71-summary/ (accessed on 13 September 2021).
28. Tondo, L. Italy at a Crossroads as Fears Grow of Covid-19 Second Wave. The Guardian. 2020. Available online: https://www.theguardian.com/world/2020/aug/19/italy-at-a-crossroads-as-fears-grow-of-covid-19-second-wave (accessed on 20 August 2020).
29. Boffey, D.; Carroll, R.; Connolly, K.; Giuffrida, A.; Henley, J.; Jones, S.; Oltermann, P.; Rankin, J.; Smith, H.; Walker, S.; et al. As Covid Cases Rise Again, How Are Countries in Europe Reacting? The Guardian. 2020. Available online: https://www.theguardian.com/world/2020/sep/23/as-covid-cases-rise-again-how-are-countries-in-europe-reacting (accessed on 24 September 2020).
30. BBC News. Covid-19: Italy Returns to Strict Lockdown for Easter. 2021. Available online: https://www.bbc.com/news/world-europe-56621342 (accessed on 4 April 2021).
31. Kington, T. A Year after COVID-19 Slammed Italy, a Third Wave Is Making It Deja vu All Over Again. Los Angeles Time. 2021. Available online: https://www.latimes.com/world-nation/story/2021-03-19/italy-deja-vu-year-after-coronavirus-first-hit (accessed on 20 March 2021).
32. DeSimone, D.C. COVID-19 Variants: What's the Concern?-What's the Concern about the New COVID-19 Variants? Are They More Contagious? Mayo Foundation for Medical Education and Research (MFMER). FAQ-20505779. 2021. Available online: https://www.mayoclinic.org/diseases-conditions/coronavirus/expert-answers/covid-variant/faq-20505779 (accessed on 10 September 2021).
33. UN—United Nations, Department of Economic and Social Affairs, Population Division. World Population Prospects 2019. Online Edition. Rev. 1. Available online: https://population.un.org/wpp/Download/Standard/Population/ (accessed on 24 September 2021).
34. NEO—NASA Earth Observations. Population Density. Available online: https://neo.sci.gsfc.nasa.gov/view.php?datasetId=SEDAC_POP (accessed on 24 September 2021).
35. CIA—Central Intelligence Agency—United States of America. The World Factbook. Available online: https://www.cia.gov/the-world-factbook/ (accessed on 24 September 2021).
36. UN Women—United Nations Women. COVID-19: Emerging Gender Data and Why It Matters. Available online: https://data.unwomen.org/resources/covid-19-emerging-gender-data-and-why-it-matters (accessed on 24 September 2021).
37. Ritchie, H.; Roser, M. Obesity. Published Online at OurWorldInData.org. Available online: https://ourworldindata.org/obesity (accessed on 24 September 2021).
38. NCD-RisC—Non-Communicable Disease-Risk Factor Collaboration. Adult Body-Mass Index. Available online: http://ncdrisc.org/data-visualisations-adiposity.html (accessed on 24 September 2021).
39. Seidu, S.; Gillies, C.; Zaccardi, F.; Kunutsor, S.K.; Hartmann-Boyce, J.; Yates, T.; Singh, A.K.; Davies, M.J.; Khunti, K. The impact of obesity on severe disease and mortality in people with SARS-CoV-2: A systematic review and meta-analysis. *Endocrinol. Diabetes Metab.* **2020**, *4*, e00176. [CrossRef] [PubMed]
40. Peres, K.C.; Riera, R.; Martimbianco, A.L.C.; Ward, L.S.; Cunha, L.L. Body Mass Index and Prognosis of COVID-19 Infection. A Systematic Review. *Front. Endocrinol.* **2020**, *11*, 562. [CrossRef]

41. O'Neil, D. Modern Human Variation: An Introduction to Contemporary Human Biological Diversity. Distribution of Blood Types. Available online: https://www2.palomar.edu/anthro/vary/vary_3.htm (accessed on 24 September 2021).
42. Modell, B.; Darlison, M. Global epidemiology of haemoglobin disorders and derived service indicators. *Bull. World Health Organ.* **2008**, *86*, 480–487. [CrossRef] [PubMed]
43. WHO—World Health Organization. The Global Prevalence of Anaemia in 2011. Available online: https://apps.who.int/iris/bitstream/handle/10665/177094/9789241564960_eng.pdf (accessed on 24 September 2021).
44. Benoist, B.; McLean, E.; Egll, I.; Cogswell, M. Worldwide Prevalence of Anaemia 1993–2005: WHO Global Database on Anaemia. Available online: http://apps.who.int/iris/bitstream/handle/10665/43894/9789241596657_eng.pdf?sequence=1 (accessed on 24 September 2021).
45. WHO—World Health Organization. Global Distribution of Haemoglobin Disorders, in Terms of Births of Affected Infants per 1000 Births. Available online: https://www.who.int/genomics/public/Maphaemoglobin.pdf (accessed on 10 January 2022).
46. Adams, D.M.; Reboussin, J.C.; Barton, C.E.; McLaren, C.E.; Eckfeldt, J.H.; McLaren, G.D.; Dawkins, F.W.; Acton, R.T.; Harris, E.L.; Gordeuk, V.R.; et al. Hemochromatosis and iron-overload screening in a racially diverse population. *N. Engl. J. Med.* **2005**, *352*, 1769–1778. [CrossRef]
47. Zacharski, L.R.; Ornstein, D.L.; Woloshin, S.; Schwartz, L.M. Association of age, sex, and race with body iron stores in adults: Analysis of NHANES III data. *Am. Heart J.* **2000**, *140*, 98–104. [CrossRef] [PubMed]
48. Powell, L.W.; Seckington, R.C.; Deugnier, Y. Haemochromatosis. *Lancet* **2016**, *388*, 706–716. [CrossRef]
49. Drakesmith, H.; Prentice, A. Viral infection and iron metabolism. *Nat. Rev. Microbiol.* **2008**, *6*, 541–552. [CrossRef]
50. Khan, F.A.; Fisher, M.A.; Khakoo, R.A. Association of hemochromatosis with infectious diseases: Expanding spectrum. *Int. J. Infect. Dis.* **2007**, *11*, 482–487. [CrossRef]
51. de Sanctis, V.; Canatan, D.; Corrons, J.L.V.; Karimi, M.; Daar, S.; Kattamis, C.; Soliman, A.T.; Wali, Y.; Alkindi, S.; Huseynov, V.; et al. Preliminary data on COVID-19 in patients with hemoglobinopathies: A multicentre ICET-A study. *Mediterr. J. Hematol. Infect. Dis.* **2020**, *12*, e2020046. [CrossRef] [PubMed]
52. Motta, I.; Migone De Amicis, M.; Pinto, V.M.; Balocco, M.; Longo, F.; Bonetti, F.; Ciancesin, B.; Graziadei, G.; Cappellini, M.D.; De Franceschi, L.; et al. SARS-CoV-2 infection in beta thalassemia: Preliminary data from the Italian experience. *Am. J. Hematol.* **2020**, *95*, E198–E199. [CrossRef] [PubMed]
53. Mendy, A.; Apewokin, S.; Wells, A.A.; Morrow, A.L. Factors associated with hospitalization and disease severity in a racially and ethnically diverse population of COVID-19 patients. *MedRxiv* **2020**. [CrossRef]
54. Huang, I.; Pranata, R.; Lim, M.A.; Oehadian, A.; Alisjahbana, B. C-reactive protein, procalcitonin, D-dimer, and ferritin in severe coronavirus disease-2019: A meta-analysis. *Ther. Adv. Respir. Dis.* **2020**, *14*, 1753466620937175. [CrossRef] [PubMed]
55. Zhou, F.; Yu, T.; Du, R.; Fan, G.; Liu, Y.; Liu, Z.; Xiang, J.; Wang, Y.; Song, B.; Gu, X.; et al. Clinical course and risk factors for mortality of adult inpatients with COVID-19 in Wuhan, China: A retrospective cohort study. *Lancet* **2020**, *395*, 1054–1062. [CrossRef]
56. Litton, E.; Lim, J. Iron metabolism: An emerging therapeutic target in critical illness. *Crit. Care.* **2019**, *23*, 81–88. [CrossRef]
57. Northrop-Clewes, C.A. *The Interpretation of Indicators of Iron Status during an Acute Phase Response. Annex 4 in Assessing the Iron Status of Populations*, 2nd ed.; WHO: Geneva, Switzerland, 2007. Available online: https://www.who.int/publications/i/item/9789241596107 (accessed on 10 January 2022).
58. Withrock, I.C.; Anderson, S.J.; Jefferson, M.A.; McCormack, G.R.; Mlynarczyk, G.S.A.; Nakama, A.; Lange, J.K.; Berg, C.A.; Acharya, S.; Stock, M.L.; et al. Genetic diseases conferring resistance to infectious diseases. *Genes Dis.* **2015**, *2*, 247–254. [CrossRef]
59. Allison, A.C. Polymorphism and natural selection in human populations. *Cold Spring Harb. Symp. Quant. Biol.* **1964**, *29*, 137–149. [CrossRef] [PubMed]
60. Gong, L.; Parikh, S.; Rosenthal, P. Biochemical and immunological mechanisms by which sickle cell trait protects against malaria. *Malar. J.* **2013**, *12*, 317–325. [CrossRef]
61. Al Yazidi, L.S.; Al Hinai, Z.; Al Waili, B.; Al Hashami, H.; Al Reesi, M.; Al Othmani, F.; Al Noobi, B.; Al Tahir, N.; Elsidig, N.; Al Barwani, I.; et al. Epidemiology, characteristics and outcome of children hospitalized with COVID-19 in Oman: A multicenter cohort study. *Int. J. Infect. Dis.* **2021**, *104*, 655–660. [CrossRef]
62. Arlet, J.B.; de Luna, G.; Khimoud, D.; Odièvre, M.H.; de Montalembert, M.; Joseph, L.; Chantalat-Auger, C.; Flamarion, E.; Bartolucci, P.; Lionnet, F.; et al. Prognosis of patients with sickle cell disease and COVID-19: A French experience. *Lancet Haematol.* **2020**, *7*, e632–e634. [CrossRef]
63. Balanchivadze, N.; Kudirka, A.A.; Askar, S.; Almadhoun, K.; Kuriakose, P.; Fadel, R.; Dabak, V. Impact of COVID-19 infection on 24 patients with sickle cell disease. One center urban experience, Detroit, MI, USA. *Hemoglobin* **2020**, *44*, 284–289. [CrossRef]
64. McCloskey, K.A.; Meenan, J.; Hall, R.; Tsitsikas, D.A. COVID-19 infection and sickle cell disease: A UK centre experience. *Br. J. Haematol.* **2020**, *190*, e57–e58. [CrossRef]
65. Vilela, T.S.; Braga, J.A.P.; Loggetto, S.R. Hemoglobinopathy and pediatrics in the time of COVID-19. *Hematol. Transfus. Cell Ther.* **2020**, *43*, 87–100. [CrossRef]
66. Chakravorty, S.; Padmore-Payne, G.; Ike, F.; Tshibangu, V.; Graham, C.; Rees, D.; Stuart-Smith, S. COVID-19 in patients with sickle cell disease-a case series from a UK Tertiary Hospital. *Haematologica* **2020**, *105*, 2691–2693. [CrossRef]
67. Menapace, L.A.; Thein, S.L. COVID-19 and sickle cell disease. *Haematologica* **2020**, *105*, 2501–2504. [CrossRef]

68. Azerad, M.A.; Bayoudh, F.; Weber, T.; Minon, J.M.; Ketelslegers, O.; Hoyoux, M.; Ren, X.; Kaye, O.; De Marneffe, N.; Fraipont, V.; et al. Sickle cell disease and COVID-19: Atypical presentations and favorable outcomes. *EJHaem* **2020**, *1*, 338–341. [CrossRef] [PubMed]
69. Hussain, F.A.; Njoku, F.U.; Saraf, S.L.; Molokie, R.E.; Gordeuk, V.R.; Han, J. COVID-19 infection in patients with sickle cell disease. *Br. J. Haematol.* **2020**, *189*, 851–852. [CrossRef]
70. Justino, C.C.; Campanharo, F.F.; Augusto, M.N.; Morais, S.C.; Figueiredo, M.S. COVID-19 as a trigger of acute chest syndrome in a pregnant woman with sickle cell anemia. *Hematol. Transfus. Cell Ther.* **2020**, *42*, 212–214. [CrossRef]
71. Minniti, C.P.; Zaidi, A.U.; Nouraie, M.; Manwani, D.; Crouch, G.D.; Crouch, A.S.; Callaghan, M.U.; Carpenter, S.; Jacobs, C.; Han, J.; et al. Clinical predictors of poor outcomes in patients with sickle cell disease and COVID-19 infection. *Blood Adv.* **2021**, *5*, 207–215. [CrossRef] [PubMed]
72. Panepinto, J.A.; Brandow, A.; Mucalo, L.; Yusuf, F.; Singh, A.; Taylor, B.; Woods, K.; Payne, A.B.; Peacock, G.; Schieve, L.A. Coronavirus disease among persons with sickle cell disease, United States, March 20–May 21, 2020. *Emerg. Infect. Dis.* **2020**, *26*, 2473–2476. [CrossRef] [PubMed]
73. Alkindi, S.; Elsadek, R.A.; Al-Madhani, A.; Al-Musalhi, M.; AlKindi, S.Y.; Al-Khadouri, G.; Al Rawahi, B.; Al-Ruqeishi, S.; Al-Yazeedi, J.; Wali, Y.A.; et al. Impact of the coronavirus 2019 (COVID-19) on vasooclusive crisis in patients with sickle cell anaemia. *Int. J. Infect. Dis.* **2021**, *106*, 128–133. [CrossRef] [PubMed]
74. Singh, A.; Brandow, A.M.; Panepinto, J.A. COVID-19 in individuals with sickle cell disease/trait compared with other Black individuals. *Blood Adv.* **2021**, *5*, 1915–1921. [CrossRef] [PubMed]
75. Tezol, O.; Unal, S. Anxiety level and clinical course of patients with sickle cell disease during the COVID-19 outbreak. *Arch. Pediatr.* **2021**, *28*, 136–140. [CrossRef] [PubMed]

encyclopedia MDPI

Entry

Molecular Aspects of Spike–ACE2 Interaction

Luigi De Masi [1,*], Maria Antonia Argenio [2], Deborah Giordano [2] and Angelo Facchiano [2,*]

[1] National Research Council (CNR), Institute of Biosciences and BioResources (IBBR), Via Università 133, 80055 Portici, Italy

[2] National Research Council (CNR), Institute of Food Sciences (ISA), Via Roma 64, 83100 Avellino, Italy; maria.antonia.argenio@gmail.com (M.A.A.); deborah.giordano@isa.cnr.it (D.G.)

* Correspondence: luigi.demasi@ibbr.cnr.it (L.D.M.); angelo.facchiano@isa.cnr.it (A.F.)

Definition: A new betacoronavirus (CoV-2) is responsible for the pandemic of severe acute respiratory syndrome (SARS) that began in China at the end of 2019, today known as COronaVIrus Disease 2019 (COVID-19). Subsequent studies confirmed the human angiotensin-converting enzyme 2 (hACE2) as the main cell receptor of spike trimeric glycoprotein, located on the viral envelope, mediating the CoV-2 invasion into the host cells through the receptor-binding domain (RBD) of the spike. Computational analysis of the known experimental 3D structures of spike–ACE2 complexes evidenced distinguishing features in the molecular interactions at the RBD-cell receptor binding interface between CoV-2 and previous CoV-1. The spike represents a key target for drug design as well as an optimal antigen for RNA/viral vector vaccines and monoclonal antibodies in order to maximize prevention and therapy of COVID-19.

Keywords: COVID-19; SARS; coronavirus; CoV-1; CoV-2; viral spike protein; receptor-binding domain (RBD); human ACE2; binding interface

Citation: De Masi, L.; Argenio, M.A.; Giordano, D.; Facchiano, A. Molecular Aspects of Spike–ACE2 Interaction. *Encyclopedia* **2022**, *2*, 96–108. https://doi.org/10.3390/encyclopedia2010007

Academic Editor: Stephen Bustin

Received: 20 November 2021
Accepted: 5 January 2022
Published: 10 January 2022

1. Introduction

A pneumonia outbreak of unknown origin first emerged in Wuhan, Hubei province of China, during the last months of 2019 [1–3]. The etiologic agent was identified by the Coronaviridae Study Group of the International Committee on Taxonomy of Viruses (CSG-ICTV) as an unknown positive-strand RNA betacoronavirus (CoV-2) [4], the seventh coronavirus known to infect humans, designated as severe acute respiratory syndrome coronavirus 2 (SARS-CoV-2). It emerged as highly transmissible from human to human, and was related to SARS-CoV-1 of 2002 with 82% genome identity. Based on the established practices and studies of phylogeny, it was defined as being of probable zoonotic origin [5–8]. The new disease, named the CoronaVIrus Disease 2019 (COVID-19), rapidly spread worldwide due to human-to-human contacts, and the World Health Organization (WHO) declared global pandemic status in March 2020. There is high variability in disease severity, with asymptomatic and paucisymptomatic cases of COVID-19, while severe cases can evolve towards a life-threatening SARS. CoV-2 showed a death rate lower than that of CoV-1, although with pronounced geographical variability [1,9,10]. This suggests that the molecular interactions between the host receptor and the coronavirus variants play an important role in successful infection. However, different host proteins play the roles of receptors/interactors in coronavirus infection, with consequences in comorbidities [11].

Recent researches on infectious capacity of this novel coronavirus established that human angiotensin converting enzyme 2 (hACE2), a homodimer protein attached to cell membrane and exposed at the external environment, is a host receptor for CoV-2 as for CoV-1 in 2002 [12–23]. Also known as ACEH (ACE homologue), hACE2 belongs to the angiotensin-converting enzyme family of peptidyl dipeptidases (zinc-dependent metalloprotease) and it is homologous to human angiotensin-converting enzyme 1 (hACE1), but with a broader substrate specificity. While hACE1 generates the vasoconstrictor peptide angiotensin 2 (AT_2), hACE2 can lower blood pressure by catalyzing the cleavage of angiotensin 1 (AT_1) (inactive decapeptide precursor of AT_2) into AT1–9 (vasodilator), and AT_2 (vasoconstrictor octapeptide) into the vasodilator AT1–7 [21]. Both hACE1 and hACE2 are AT_1-converting enzymes and regulators of blood pressure that have counterbalance roles by acting on vasoactive peptides from the renin-angiotensin-aldosterone system (RAAS). In the bloodstream, the renin protease secreted from the kidneys cleaves the angiotensinogen (AGT) secreted by the liver to form AT_1, which in turn generates AT_2 or AT1–9 from the actions of hACE1 and hACE2, respectively. AT_2 is cleaved by multiple enzymes, most importantly hACE2, to form AT1–7. AT_2 also forms AT_4 via the action of aminopeptidases (APs), both AT_2 and AT_4 act via AT_1 receptors. As hACE2 opposes the actions of AT_2, it has a key role in the RAAS. Therefore, there is a beneficial effect in hypertension and cardiovascular diseases when AT_2 concentration decreases.

Although hACE2 is hijacked by some coronaviruses, its primary physiological role is in the hydrolysis of AT_1 and AT_2, peptide hormones that control vasoconstriction and blood pressure [21]. It is a type I membrane protein primarily expressed in the lungs, heart, kidneys, liver, and small intestine, while its decreased expression is associated with cardiovascular diseases. The monomer of hACE2 consists of an N-terminal peptidase domain (PD) and a C-terminal collectrin-like domain that ends with a transmembrane alpha helix and an approximately 40-residue intracellular segment. Collectrin is a renal protein without catalytic domain and has no similarity with hACE1. Thus, hACE2 may have evolved as a chimera between the ACE-like domain and the collectrin domain. The PD of hACE2 is responsible for processing AT_1 to produce AT1–9, which is then processed by other enzymes to become AT1–7, or directly to cleave AT_2 to give AT1–7. In contrast with hACE1, hACE2 does not hydrolyze bradykinin and is not inhibited by hACE1 inhibitors (ACE-I). At the onset of the pandemic, the use over time of ACE-I has been postulated to increase susceptibility to COVID-19 in patients with hypertension [24]. RAAS-inhibition can upregulate the expression of the hACE2 receptor, so the therapeutic treatment with ACE-I might promote the infection. However, to date, no evidence exists that RAAS inhibitors can increase the host's susceptibility to COVID-19.

The trimeric glycoprotein spike of coronaviruses is anchored in the envelope of the characteristic virion, and many copies of these macromolecules give the likeness of a crown, "corona" in Latin, the word used for the name of these viruses. The spike mediates the recognition of the host hACE2 receptor throughout its receptor-binding domain (RBD), corresponding to the 318–510 sequence region of CoV-2. One of the three spike chains exposes RBD in a structural conformation easy to reach by the hACE2 receptor. So, the spike directly binds with its RBD to the host receptor hACE2-PD, exploiting hACE2 to carry on the infection of the human host (Figure 1).

The specific amino acid sequence of this spike portion plays a key role in conferring to CoV-2 the ability to infect humans, being known as responsible for the species specificity [6,9,25]. Following infection, the ligand-receptor interaction occurs, the complex spike–ACE2 is formed, and spike is cleaved into two fragments by serine proteases, such as transmembrane protease serine 2 (TMPRSS2): the N-terminal S1 fragment containing the RBD bound to ACE2–PD, and the C-terminal S2 fragment responsible for the membrane fusion of the virus with the host cell [13]. Therefore, the molecular interaction and the stable binding between spike RBD and ACE2-PD are propaedeutic to the invasion of host cells by CoV-2. The S1 fragment of CoV-2 has a sequence portion with around 70% shared amino acid identity with the corresponding sequence of CoV-1, while the S2 fragment shares 99% identity with the corresponding sequence of CoV-1 [5]. More particularly, inside the S1 fragment, RBD shows high sequence identity between the two coronaviruses with the exception of its C-terminal region, which is involved in the direct binding with the hACE2 receptor [5]. Therefore, spike RDB is under selective pressure to evade host immune response. This aspect would explain the high mutation frequency observed in spike RBD. Thus, anticoronavirus antibodies (Ab) designed against the core domain of spike RBD and the S2 fragment should be potentially effective with a broad spectrum versus genetic variants of spike [26]. Novel spikes may likely increase the virulence by evading the host immunity within species and enabling host-switches by altering cross-species receptor recognition. Additionally, the spike has been identified as a critical recombination hotspot [5,27]. Therefore, it is very likely that the sequence variability of the spike, as well as of the hACE2 host receptor, may modulate virion intake and consequent disease severity. Consequently, the spike represents an optimal target for the development of RNA/viral vector vaccines, monoclonal Ab, diagnostics, and therapies [9,26]. Moreover, spike RBD can be extremely useful for in silico function predictions based on structure, also as a result of mutations, in the interactions with neutralizing Ab and hACE2 [9,15,26].

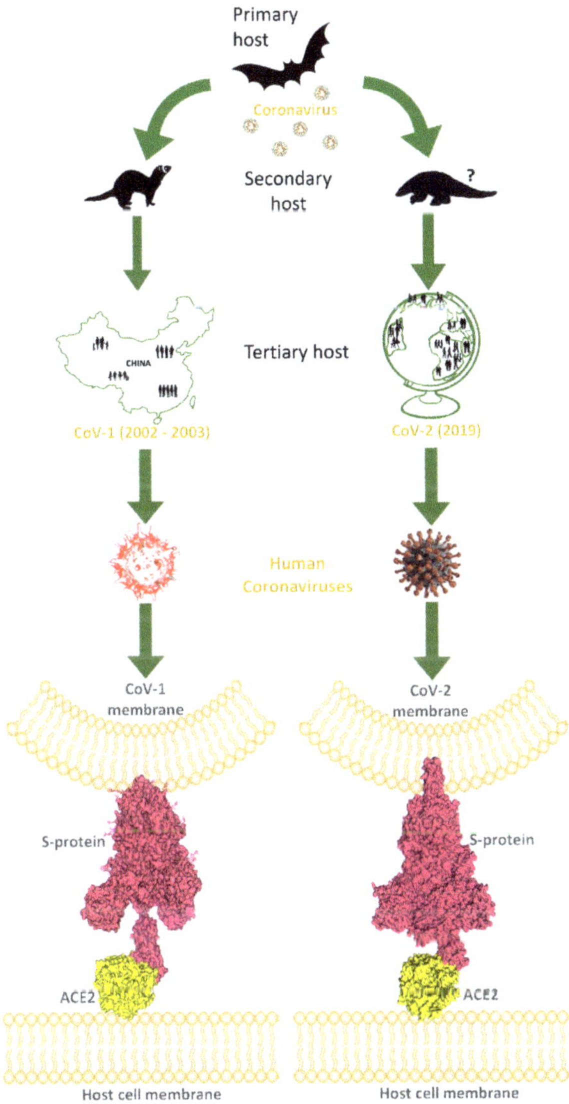

Figure 1. This image explains how coronaviruses spread from bats, as primary hosts, to humans, as tertiary hosts, showing complex spike–ACE2 interactions. Both originated from bats, considered natural reservoirs of SARS-like coronaviruses, CoV-1 and CoV-2 infected the human population via

intermediate animal hosts in which viruses underwent an adaptation, exploiting their rapid evolution ability. In the case of CoV-1 (left side of the image), the intermediate host was identified in the masked palm-civets and, by subsequent mutations, CoV-1 became able to jump into humans (tertiary host) and led to the epidemic outbreak that emerged in China and spread in few other countries, to a lower extent, from the end of 2002 to 2003 July. For CoV-2 (right side of the image), the intermediate host is still uncertain, but was probably pangolin, from which CoV-2-related coronaviruses have been isolated. However, after the rapid evolution of these viruses in the secondary hosts, CoV-2 became able to infect the human population causing the COVID pandemic in 2019. Human coronaviruses can interact by the RBD of their trimeric spike glycoproteins, exposed on the membrane of viral envelope, with hACE2 proteins, expressed on the surface of host cells. At the bottom of the image, these interactions are visible for hACE2 and the CoV-1 spike (PDB code: 6CS2; left side, in yellow and magenta surfaces, respectively), and for hACE2 interacting with the CoV-2 spike (PDB codes: 7SBO, 7C8D; right side, in yellow and magenta surfaces, respectively).

CoV-2 is being spread much more rapidly than CoV-1. Although many studies have been carried out, it has not yet been definitely established whether the interaction of spike–hACE2 is stronger with CoV-1 or CoV-2, and how this aspect can be put in relation with their different infectivity levels. The computational studies in the literature seem to report conflicting results. Preliminary in silico analysis predicted the free energy values of binding between the spike RBD (CoV-1 and CoV-2) and hACE2. First molecular docking simulations between the spike RBD of CoV-1 and hACE2 showed that their interaction is energetically favored with respect to CoV-2, which nevertheless showed a significant binding affinity to hACE2 [7]. Further in silico researches by molecular modeling and docking showed low binding energy in the CoV-2 spike–ACE2 complex as compared to CoV-1 [6]. Based on the structure of the CoV-2 spike experimentally solved in the prefusion conformation and on the kinetics of this interaction quantified by surface plasmon resonance, another study evidenced that the CoV-2 spike binds to hACE2 with higher affinity (10- to 20-fold) than the spike of CoV-1 [20]. In the same study, many differences at molecular level were evidenced when the spikes of CoV-1 and CoV-2 interacted with hACE2. In this regard, the spike of CoV-2 uses the hACE2 receptor less efficiently than the spike of the CoV-1 strain of 2002, but more efficiently than the CoV-1 strain of 2003 [18,25]. The CoV-2 mutations located in the spike-RBD region likely cause higher infectivity and lower pathogenicity than CoV-1 of 2002 with around 10% mortality rate [15,18,27]. Although the genome of CoV-2 has 82% nucleotide identity with CoV-1, and the spike of CoV-2 shares about 76% sequence identity with that of CoV-1 [5], the free energy of binding between the spike and hACE2 is comparable for CoV-2 and CoV-1 [17]. These results are compatible with the fact that the CoV-2 spike-RBD residues at the spike–ACE2 interface may have evolved in extremely complex ways from different common ancestors. Overall, the results of these studies differ on how the structural peculiarities between the two coronaviruses in the binding of spike to hACE2 can differently stabilize the ligand–receptor interactions of the complex spike–ACE2.

Several other proteins have been investigated for the potential activity as receptor or interactor of the spikes of coronaviruses, including CoV-2. TMPRSS2 is a serine protease upregulated by androgen hormones; it is involved in the infection process of many viruses, including coronaviruses, acting on the spike and hACE2, and facilitating virus–cell membrane fusion [13,28]. Another receptor/interactor of the spike is neuropilin-1 (NRP1), a cell-surface receptor for vascular endothelial growth factor 165 (VEGF-165) and semaphorins. NRP1 binds furin-cleaved substrates, and is implicated in CoV-2 infectivity [29–31]. Other receptors or interactors of coronaviruses, and potentially of CoV-2, are also known. Dipeptidyl peptidase 4 (DDP4) is a glycoprotein membrane receptor involved in T-cell activation, with peptidase activity, and it is known as the MERS receptor [32]. Another serine protease, TMPRSS11D, cleaves and activates the spike of human coronavirus 229E (HCoV-229E), facilitating its cell entrance [33]. The C-type lectin domain family

4 member M (CLEC4M) is a membrane protein, known as an attachment receptor for hepatitis C virus (HCV), Ebola virus, human coronavirus 229E, and CoV-1 [34]. Many of these receptors are involved in several pathologies, and more in particular in the main COVID-19 comorbidities, thus suggesting that tissue expression of these proteins may be related to the epidemiological features of COVID-19 patients [11]. Moreover, several studies have proposed sialic acids on the host cell surface as possible co-receptors, acting as a further attachment mechanism that facilitates CoV-2 to enter the cell [35].

To discover potential molecular targets, as there are only a few functional therapeutic agents and several vaccines are currently available, a more in-depth understanding of the molecular interaction mechanisms underlying the initial steps of infection is required. In fact, massive interventions were directed against the first CoV-2 that appeared in 2019, but the emergence of its genetic variants, above all related to spike mutations, presents new challenges based on their high transmissibility and putting in doubt the efficacy of the first vaccines. Therefore, more recent studies have set out to investigate the structural interactions at the chain–chain interface in the spike–ACE2 complexes of crystallographic structures of both CoV-1 and CoV-2 available in the Protein Data Bank (PDB), the single worldwide repository of information about the 3D structural data of biological macromolecules [36]. Structures of the claw-like ACE2-PD in complex with the RBD or spike have revealed the molecular details of their interaction. On the one hand, these studies showed what specific amino acid residues are involved in ligand–receptor binding and how they interact at the spike–ACE2 interface. On the other hand, they allowed to evidence interesting structural characteristics, and differences between CoV-1 and CoV-2. Therapy and prevention of COVID-19 could benefit from these findings, because the spike is a key target for designing therapeutic agents and a viral antigen for optimal vaccine and monoclonal Ab development.

2. Spike–ACE2 Interactions

2.1. Analysis of the Interaction of hACE2 with the Spikes from CoV-1 and CoV-2

The amino acid sequences of RBDs from CoV-1 and CoV-2 spikes present approximately 60% of identical amino acids [37]. Sequence differences between CoV-1 and CoV-2 are mainly present in two regions of RBD, i.e., from position 430 to 462 and from position 470 to 503 (CoV-2 numbering). The X-ray crystallographic structures of hACE2 in complex with the CoV-2 or CoV-1 spike have been solved and made available to the scientific community by means of the PDB archive [36]. These complex structures have been investigated in detail to find what amino acids are responsible for molecular interaction. It has been shown that 29 and 33 amino acid residues of spikes from CoV-2 and CoV-1 interact with 32 and 33 residues of receptor hACE2, respectively, at least in one of the complex structures [37]. Most of the spike amino acids involved in the binding interface are located in correspondence of the RBD regions differing between the spikes from CoV-2 and CoV-1. In more detail, out of 29 interacting amino acids of the CoV-2 spike, 23 residues interact with the receptor in all investigated complexes (Figure 2). Similarly, out of 33 amino acids of the CoV-1 spike, 23 residues interact with hACE2 in all investigated complexes.

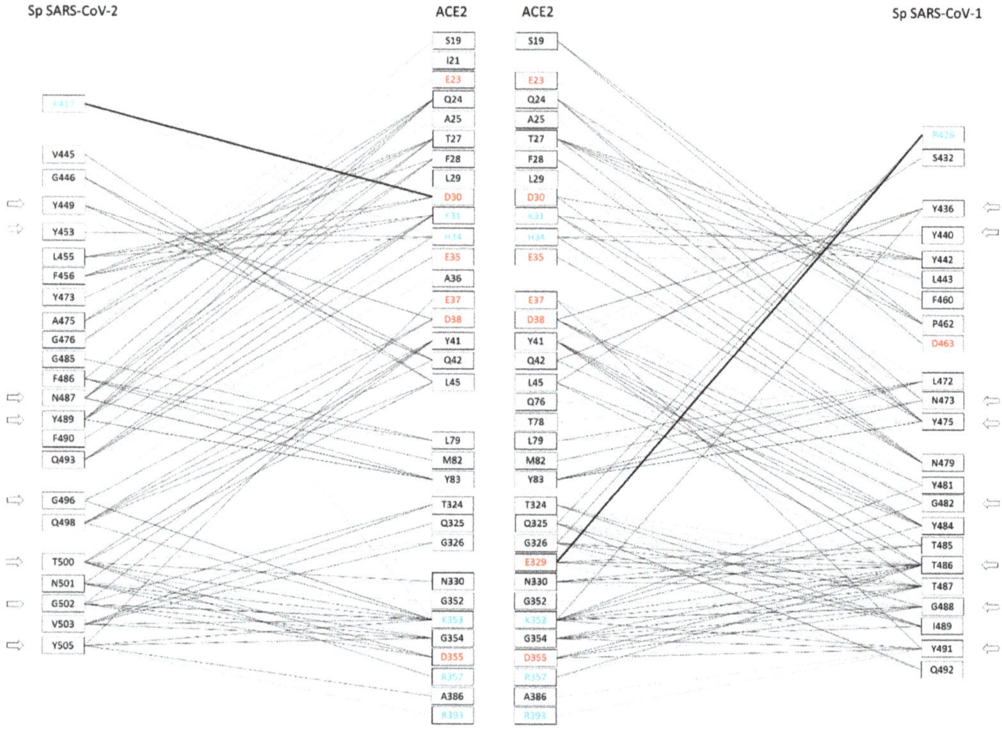

Figure 2. Amino acid residues of the spikes of CoV-2 and CoV-1 interacting with hACE2 at the binding interface, and vice versa (adapted from Giordano et al. 2021 [37]). The amino acids are color-coded: red = negatively charged residues; cyan = positively charged residues. The side arrows indicate the relative positions of the eight amino acid residues conserved to CoV-2 and CoV-1 spikes. The network of interactions between hACE2 and CoV-2/CoV-1 spikes (presented side-by-side) is restricted to H-bond and generic interactions (thin lines) and salt-bridges (large lines).

Therefore, these interactions may be particularly relevant for the virus-specific recognition modes of the hACE2 protein. By comparing the two sets of 23 amino acids from CoV-2 and CoV-1, it was possible to identify 19 residues that have a correspondence in the two aligned spike sequences for all analyzed complexes. Out of these residues, eight are identical in both sequences: Y449, Y453, N487, Y489, G496, T500, G502, and Y505 (numbers referred to the CoV-2 spike). These identical residues that interact with the cell receptor in all complexes may have a key function in the binding of CoV-2/CoV-1 spikes with hACE2. Their conservation in the two coronaviruses suggests that functional constraints may have protected them from evolutionary pressure, despite their localization in the two regions of the RBDs with higher sequence variability (position 430–462 and 470–503, see as mentioned above), or very close for Y505. The importance of such observation is related to determining important conserved epitopes of spikes exploitable for maximizing Ab elicitation upon vaccination, above all in the cases of spike variants [26,38]. Nevertheless, the other 15 residues were also notable, being specific to each spike and involved in the interactions of all available spike–ACE2 complexes. Out of 15 residues, there are other 11 amino acids from each spike that, although not identical to each other, correspond in the sequence position and interact with hACE2 (for details, see Table 1 in [37]). In most cases, the conservation of their chemical interactions with hACE2, similarly to what was observed for the eight amino acids already listed, could point out conserved functional features. At last, four amino acid residues of the CoV-2 spike, i.e., K417, G446, G485, and F490, make peculiar interactions with hACE2. The most interesting interaction is related to the residue K417, which binds D30 of hACE2 by H-bond and salt bridge interactions (see Figure 3).

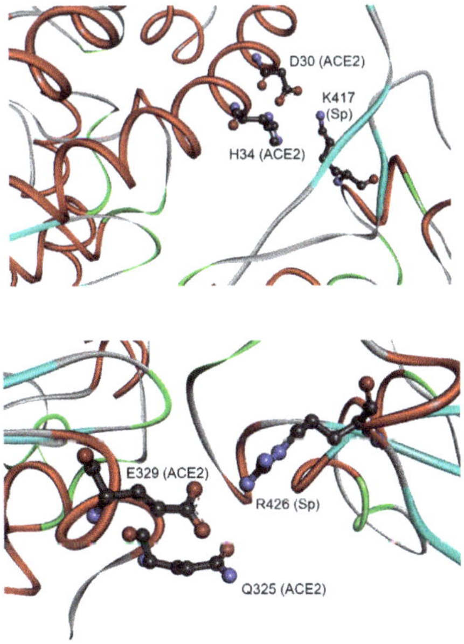

Figure 3. Molecular view of the peculiar interactions formed by CoV-2 K417 and CoV-1 R426 residues of the spike (adapted from Giordano et al., 2021 [37]). The upper panel shows the interaction of CoV-2 spike–K417 with ACE2-D30 and H34; both proteins are represented as backbone ribbons, with helix regions in red, beta-strand regions in cyan, and turns in green. The lower panel shows the interaction of CoV-1 spike–R426 with ACE2-Q325 and E329, with proteins drawn similarly to the upper panel.

This represents an important structural difference in the binding to hACE2 of the CoV-2 spike in comparison to the spike of CoV-1. For this last protein, the four peculiar residues that interact with hACE2 are Y481, R426, T485, and Q492. Also in this case, one of them, i.e., the residue R426, forms an H-bond and salt bridge with one residue of hACE2, i.e., E329, and in addition an H-bond with Q325. The discriminative target residues on hACE2 for the interaction of K417 of the CoV-2 spike and R426 of the CoV-1 spike suggest different modes of binding to the receptor in the two coronaviruses.

2.2. Different Regions of hACE2 Interact with Spikes of CoV-1 and CoV-2

While hACE2 has a negatively charged binding surface, spike RBDs are overall positively charged, forming the complex spike–ACE2 by attractive forces [39]. This is also in agreement with the observation that the spike RBD is recognized mainly by polar amino acid residues located into the extracellular PD of hACE2 [20,21]. At the same time, peculiar different amino acid residues and salt bridge/H-bond positions utilized by the spikes of CoV-1 and CoV-2 allow them to bind differently with hACE2 [39]. The binding interface between hACE2 and CoV-2 spike has been investigated by experimental methods since the first half of 2020, and three models of complexes were deposited in the PDB archives. These structures have been studied by several authors in order to analyze in detail the molecular interaction of the spike with the human protein recognized as the main cellular receptor. Looking at the interface from the hACE2 side, 33 amino acid residues interact with CoV-1 and 32 residues with CoV-2, respectively (as mentioned above), with 30 of them being in common.

In Figure 4, the sequence of the hACE2 region that interacts with the spike is shown, putting in evidence the amino acids that interact with spikes from both CoV-1 and CoV-2. In fact, despite the high similarity between the spikes of the two coronaviruses, it has been reported that they interact with hACE2 by creating peculiar interactions, although in the context of similar structures. In particular, the unique salt bridge observed with the spike of CoV-2 involves hACE2 D30, while the unique salt bridge observed with the spike of CoV-1 involves hACE2 E329. Similarly, a peculiar H-bonds network binds the spike from CoV-2 to the N-terminal region of hACE2, while in the case of the spike from CoV-1 a distinctive network is formed with the central region of the hACE2 sequence. The amino acids of hACE2 that interact only with the CoV-2 spike are I21 and A36, while Q76, T78, and E329 interact only with the CoV-1 spike.

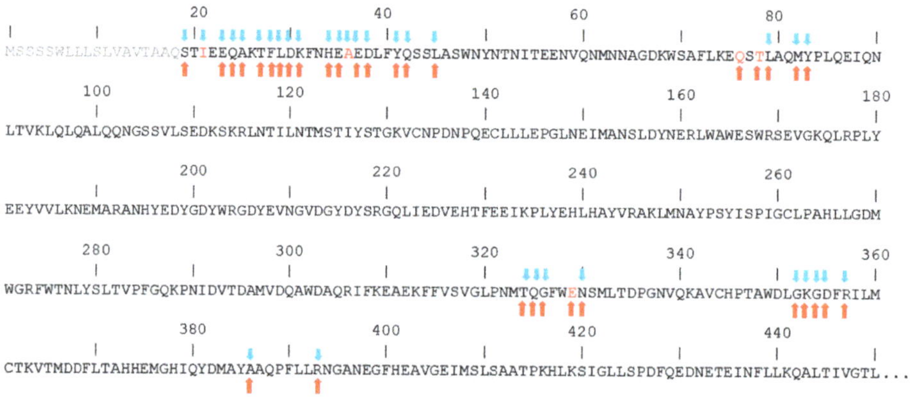

Figure 4. Interaction of hACE2 amino acids with the spikes of CoV-2 (blue arrows) and CoV-1 (red arrows). Amino acid letters in red indicate unique interaction. Segment 1–18 of the sequence is shown in grey because it is not present in the experimental structures.

Further surface interactions concern hydrophobic contacts as reported in the literature (see Figure 12 of [12] and Supplementary Table S1 of [37]). In particular evidence, hydrophobic interactions are formed by two tyrosine residues conserved in both coronaviruses, i.e., Y489 and Y505 of CoV-2, corresponding to Y475 and Y491 of CoV-1. The conservation of these two tyrosines suggests that their aromatic rings may represent important interaction points with hACE2. It is also interesting to note the peculiar presence of the aromatic rings of F456 and F486 at the surface in the case of CoV-2, corresponding in CoV-1 to L443 and L472, respectively. These two phenylalanine residues of CoV-2 form stacking interactions with the aromatic residues F28 and Y83 at the ACE2 surface, whereas in the case of CoV-1 the two leucine residues have also hydrophobic contacts with ACE2 residues, but evidently do not give rise to aromatic interactions.

The analysis of the complex binding network on the ligand–receptor surfaces revealed that both the spikes interact with hACE2 in correspondence with the N-terminal region (residues 19–83) and central sequence region (residues 324–393). The N-terminal region forms discriminative interactions with CoV-2, as the salt bridge between D30 of hACE2 and K417 of spike. The central region, which also includes the residues 345–346 responsible for the substrate binding [40], has peculiar interactions with CoV-1, as the H-bonds and salt bridge of hACE2 Q325 and E329 with R426 of the spike. These differences observed at the surface of the interaction with the hACE2 receptor show that the two spikes differentially bind to the two districts on the surface of hACE2, with potential consequences for the mechanisms of infection and virulence.

2.3. Structural Predictions of CoV-2 Mutations on the Spike–ACE2 Binding

The modulation of the interactions of the spike on the two surface regions of hACE2 could be related to the different infection ability, also including the CoV-2 variants. A structural comparison of the amino acids at the chain–chain interface can be used to design solutions effective against the binding to the receptor hACE2 of the CoV-2 spike and its mutational variants.

With regard to the mutations of the spike RBD, four CoV-2 major lineages were identified [41–43]: Alpha (B.1.1.7) with the mutation N501Y, first detected in the UK; Beta (B.1.351, in South Africa) and Gamma (P.1, in Brazil) with the three identical mutations K417N, E484K, and N501Y (as in Alpha); and Delta (B.1.617, in India) with the mutations L452R and T478K. Among the spike mutational events, K417 was found to be critical in the binding to hACE2. K417 binds to D30 of hACE2 by salt bridge and H-bond interactions, so the K417N mutation might impair the bond for hACE2 of the Beta and Gamma variants by loss of the positively charged K417. Contrarily, spike N501 interacts with hACE2 by the residue Y41 by H-bond (as the later-mentioned T487 of the CoV-1 spike), and the N501Y mutation in the Alpha, Beta, and Gamma variants, might both maintain the H-bond and add an aromatic interaction by introducing a tyrosine side chain, thus reinforcing the binding to hACE2. However, the sterical hindrance of the tyrosine might introduce perturbations at the chain–chain interface. In fact, recently, simulations of molecular dynamics performed on this mutation showed a reduced binding affinity of the B.1.1.7 spike for hACE2, as the residue Y501 restructured the chain–chain interface conformation of the spike–ACE2 complex by decreasing the linear interaction energy between RBD and hACE2 [44]. It is important to note that the other CoV-2 spike substitutions, i.e., E484K, L452R, and T478K, could have been selected—as these sites include amino acids that are not involved in relevant interactions in wild-type coronavirus. Interestingly, these three mutations introduce three further positive charges on the spike, with a possible gain of charge–charge interaction with the hACE2 surface, in agreement with the investigations by Xie et al. [39] already mentioned above. The gain of additional positive charges on the mutated spikes may create further attractive charge interactions that increase the binding affinity of spike to the hACE2 receptor. However, the double mutation observed in Beta and Gamma variants (i.e., K417N and E484K) removed the interaction couples D30-K417 and K31-E484 based on opposite charges. Anyway, their close spatial proximity on hACE2 suggests that in that region the positive side chain of K417 on the CoV-2 surface might be preserved at least in the opposite-charge couple D30-K484.

In November 2021, a variant of concern named Omicron (B.1.1.529 in South Africa) was classified by the WHO [42]. Although studies on this new variant are rapidly appearing, for now it is difficult to define a clear state of the art. This new variant presents a large number of modifications in the spike. Out of these, about half of amino acid substitutions occur within the RBD and thus may affect the interaction with hACE2 and neutralizing Ab. There are cases in common with previous variants, and novel occurrences. In particular evidence, K417N was also observed in Beta and Gamma variants; S477N in Iota variant; E484A was not observed in previous variants, although E484 was substituted by lysine in many variants; N501Y was also present in Alpha, Beta, and Gamma variants.

However, the precise structural impact of known mutations within the RBD on the binding stability of the spike with hACE2 needs yet to be investigated thoroughly [44].

2.4. Mutagenesis Studies on the Spike–ACE2 Interface from Previous SARS Outbreaks

The first human coronavirus (CoV-1), identified as the etiological agent of atypical pneumonia (successively named SARS), originated in late 2002 in Guangdong Province of China. Within a short time, CoV-1 spread worldwide, affecting more than 8000 individuals and being responsible for over 700 deaths during the first outbreak in 2002–2003 [9]. Infected wildlife animals, traded in the live animal markets in China, were suspected as most likely to be the source of CoV-1 human infections (Figure 1). Masked palm-civets (*Paguma larvata* Hamilton-Smith, 1827) and raccoon dogs (*Nyctereutes procyonoides* Gray, 1834) were considered the most important viral carriers, intermediate hosts that boost the spread of the virus from the natural reservoir to humans. In fact, the probable wildlife reservoirs of coronaviruses and SARS-like coronaviruses in China are horseshoe bats (*Rhinolophus* genus Lacépède, 1799). Coronaviruses were likely subjected to an impressive selective pressure during animal-to-human transmission. The spike is a key determinant in the coronavirus–host interaction and this is also the case in interspecies transmission. It was shown that a few alterations of amino acid residues in the spike lead to changes in viral susceptibility in animal and human hosts. Spikes from the coronavirus of palm-civets and from two human outbreaks were compared by Li and colleagues [9]. The affinity of the spike for hACE2 was the determinant for viral infectivity and disease severity. The spike from the severe 2002 outbreak bound hACE2 more efficiently than the spike from the mild 2003 outbreak and from the virus of palm-civets. The low affinity of the spike from the virus of palm-civets was complemented by mutagenizing to the earlier severe outbreak the amino acid residues K479N and S487T. Moreover, the double mutation from human coronavirus to palm-civet virus N479/T487→K479/S487 inhibited interaction with hACE2. Two facing residues of positively charged lysine, K479 in the spike from the palm-civet virus and K31 in hACE2 (Figure 4), repulsively interfered with the formation of the complex spike–ACE2. The K479–K31 repulsive effect is absent in the infection of palm-civets, as they have the polar residue T31 in their ACE2. The residues N479 and T487 of the CoV-1 spike correspond to the residues Q493 and N501 of CoV-2 spike, respectively, both identified in a recent in silico analysis as interacting with hACE2 [37]. These last findings confirmed results on CoV-1, suggesting the hypothesis of a key role for Q493 and N501 of CoV-2 spike in the high-affinity binding to hACE2. Indeed, Q493 interacts with the hACE2 residues K31 and H35. In addition, K31 interacts with the residue E484 of the CoV-2 spike and other two residues upstream of Q493 (F490 and L492). In the same way, mutagenesis analysis of position 487 showed the key role of a threonine in increasing the affinity for human and non-human ACE2. It corresponds to the residue N501 of CoV-2, subject to the N501Y mutation in the Alpha, Beta, and Gamma variants. In silico analysis showed that N501 interacts with the residue hACE2 Y41 (similarly present in palm-civet and rat ACE2), which in turn interacts with two residues upstream of N501 (Q498 and T500). Altogether, these findings indicate that variations of the CoV-2 spike in the sites 493 and 501 (479 and 487 in CoV-1 spike) are compatible with the binding of novel coronavirus to the human receptor by the recognition of the K31 and Y41 residues [9,37]. These mutational hotspots may be elements predictive in the risk assessment of new coronavirus variants/lineages [43,44]. The same in silico analysis also evidenced the presence of peculiar interactions by R426 of the CoV-1 spike [37], not mutagenized in that study [9], as well as K417 of CoV-2 spike corresponding to V404 of the CoV-1 spike, unknown at that time. Notably, these interactions concern the CoV-2 spike K417 with hACE2 D30, and the CoV-1 spike R426 with hACE2 E329 (Figure 3). These residues are not conserved in mouse and rat ACE2, where the same positions are occupied by N30 and A/T329 [45]. These facts contribute to explain why both the coronaviruses are unable to hijack murine ACE as a cell receptor.

To better understand the coronavirus spillover from animal species to humans, Li et al. (2005) [9] also carried out mutagenesis studies, creating chimeras of hACE2 with palm-civet and rat ACE2. The low affinity for hACE2 of the spike from the palm-civet virus was complemented by altering hACE2 to the palm-civet counterpart in the residues at the positions 31–40 and K353. Moreover, the alterations to the human counterpart of the residues NFS→MYP (position 82–84) and H353K convert rat ACE2, whose wild type does not bind the CoV-1 spike, to an effective cell receptor. The mutations K31D and Y41A on hACE2 interfered with CoV-1 spike interaction, as well as the mutations D355A and R357A downstream of K353. These results allowed localization of the CoV-1 spike-binding domain above the cleft of the catalytic pocket of hACE2 [9]. The results by Li et al. (2005) [9] can be partially applied to the spike–hACE2 interaction of CoV-2, as shown by in silico analysis of experimental complexes [37]. In fact, the region of hACE2 from position 19 to 45 is also interacting with the CoV-2 spike with more interactions than CoV-1 (Figures 2 and 4). Further interacting regions are located at the sequence position 76–83 of hACE2 with Y83, at 324–330, and at 352–357 with three amino acid residues (K353, D355, and R357) important for the binding to CoV-1 spike but less so to the CoV-2 spike [37]. Moreover, the same in silico analysis identified the residues Q325 and E329 interacting with R426 of the CoV-1 spike. However, the mutagenesis of Q325P and E329T to the corresponding residues of rat ACE2 did not show the effects on its binding to the CoV-1 spike [9]. Since the CoV-1 spike has more interactions than CoV-2 within the hACE2 portion 325–357, these could balance the mutagenesis and justify its limited effect.

3. Conclusions and Prospects

Different interactions of the spikes from CoV-1 and CoV-2 with hACE2 can be responsible for the high spread from human to human of the novel coronavirus. The molecular interactions at the chain–chain interface of the spike–ACE2 complex are extremely decisive for the coronavirus attack to human cells. The understanding of the underpinning mechanism of action as well as possible interaction differences, as in the case of spike variants, are essential for developing innovative strategies to fight the pandemic. The in silico analysis on the experimentally determined spike–ACE2 complexes defined which and how residues interact at the ligand–receptor interface at molecular level. These studies evidenced peculiar differences between CoV-1 and CoV-2 with potential health implications. The spike from CoV-2 binds to the hACE2 differently from the spike of CoV-1, and this may contribute to the different contagiousness, regardless of high or low molecular affinity. The complex network of the interactions at the binding interface between hACE2 and the spike showed strong interactions of CoV-2 spike with the N-terminal region of hACE2, while the CoV-1 spike mainly had interactions with the central region of hACE2. Further studies are still needed to unveil the detailed molecular basis of virus–cell recognition, consequent cell invasion, cell–cell transmission, human-to-human spread, and the pathogenesis of CoV-2, as well as to optimize diagnostic, antiviral, and vaccination strategies. Unfortunately, coronaviruses are an example of the evolution of animal viruses into deadly human pathogens. From now on, it is of paramount importance that we watch over wildlife as a strategy for the prevention and control for infectious diseases.

Author Contributions: Conceptualization, L.D.M. and A.F.; investigation, L.D.M., M.A.A., D.G. and A.F.; writing—original draft preparation, L.D.M., D.G. and A.F.; writing—review and editing, L.D.M. and A.F. All authors have read and agreed to the published version of the manuscript.

Funding: D.G. is a PostDoc supported within the project "CIR01_00017—"CNRBiOmics—CENTRO NAZIONALE DI RICERCA IN BIOINFORMATICA PER LE SCIENZE "OMICHE"—RAFFORZAMENTO DEL CAPITALE UMANO"—CUP B56J20000960001. D.G. and A.F. activity is part of the Italian node of ELIXIR, the research infrastructure for life-science data.

Conflicts of Interest: The authors declare no conflict of interest.

Entry Link on the Encyclopedia Platform: https://encyclopedia.pub/19190.

References

1. She, J.; Jiang, J.; Ye, L.; Hu, L.; Bai, C.; Song, Y. 2019 novel coronavirus of pneumonia in Wuhan, China: Emerging attack and management strategies. *Clin. Transl. Med.* **2020**, *9*, 19. [CrossRef] [PubMed]
2. Wu, F.; Zhao, S.; Yu, B.; Chen, Y.M.; Wang, W.; Song, Z.G.; Hu, Y.; Tao, Z.W.; Tian, J.H.; Zhang, Y.Z.; et al. A new coronavirus associated with human respiratory disease in China. *Nature* **2020**, *579*, 265–269. [CrossRef] [PubMed]
3. Zhu, N.; Zhang, D.; Wang, W.; Li, X.; Yang, B.; Song, J.; Zhao, X.; Huang, B.; Shi, W.; Lu, R.; et al. A Novel Coronavirus from Patients with Pneumonia in China, 2019. *N. Engl. J. Med.* **2020**, *382*, 727–733. [CrossRef]
4. International Committee on Taxonomy of Viruses (ICTV). Available online: https://talk.ictvonline.org (accessed on 22 July 2021).
5. Chan, J.F.-W.; Kok, K.H.; Zhu, Z.; Chu, H.; To, K.K. W.; Yuan, S.; Yuen, K. Y. Genomic characterization of the 2019 novel human-pathogenic coronavirus isolated from a patient with atypical pneumonia after visiting Wuhan. *Emerg. Microbes Infect.* **2020**, *9*, 221–236. [CrossRef] [PubMed]
6. He, J.; Tao, H.; Yan, Y.; Huang, S.Y.; Xiao, Y. Molecular Mechanism of Evolution and Human Infection with SARS-CoV-2. *Viruses* **2020**, *12*, 428. [CrossRef] [PubMed]

7. Xu, X.; Chen, P.; Wang, J.; Feng, J.; Zhou, H.; Li, X.; Zhong, W.; Hao, P. Evolution of the novel coronavirus from the ongoing Wuhan outbreak and modeling of its spike protein for risk of human transmission. *Sci. China Life Sci.* **2020**, *63*, 457–460. [CrossRef]
8. Zhong, N.S.; Zheng, B.J.; Li, Y.M.; Poon, L.L.M.; Xie, Z.H.; Chan, K.H.; Li, P.H.; Tan, S.Y.; Chang, Q.; Xie, J.P.; et al. Epidemiology and cause of severe acute respiratory syndrome (SARS) in Guangdong, People's Republic of China, in February, 2003. *Lancet* **2003**, *362*, 1353–1358. [CrossRef]
9. Li, W.; Zhang, C.; Sui, J.; Kuhn, J.H.; Moore, M.J.; Luo, S.; Wong, S.K.; Huang, I.C.; Xu, K.; Vasilieva, N.; et al. Receptor and viral determinants of SARS-coronavirus adaptation to human ACE2. *EMBO J.* **2005**, *24*, 1634–1643. [CrossRef]
10. Rabi, F.A.; Al Zoubi, M.S.; Kasasbeh, G.A.; Salameh, D.M.; Al-Nasser, A.D. SARS-CoV-2 and Coronavirus Disease 2019: What We Know So Far. *Pathogens* **2020**, *9*, 231. [CrossRef]
11. Facchiano, A.; Facchiano, F.; Facchiano, A. An investigation into the molecular basis of cancer comorbidities in coronavirus infection. *FEBS Open Bio* **2020**, *10*, 2363–2374. [CrossRef]
12. Hatmal, M.M.; Alshaer, W.; Al-Hatamleh, M.A.I.; Hatmal, M.; Smadi, O.; Taha, M.O.; Oweida, A.J.; Boer, J.C.; Mohamud, R.; Plebanski, M. Comprehensive Structural and Molecular Comparison of Spike Proteins of SARS-CoV-2, SARS-CoV and MERS-CoV, and Their Interactions with ACE2. *Cells* **2020**, *9*, 2638. [CrossRef]
13. Hoffmann, M.; Kleine-Weber, H.; Schroeder, S.; Krüger, N.; Herrler, T.; Erichsen, S.; Schiergens, T.S.; Herrler, G.; Wu, N.H.; Nitsche, A.; et al. SARS-CoV-2 Cell Entry Depends on ACE2 and TMPRSS2 and Is Blocked by a Clinically Proven Protease Inhibitor. *Cell* **2020**, *181*, 271–280. [CrossRef]
14. Li, W.; Moore, M.J.; Vasilieva, N.; Sui, J.; Wong, S.K.; Berne, M.A.; Somasundaran, M.; Sullivan, J.L.; Luzuriaga, K.; Greenough, T.C.; et al. Angiotensin-converting enzyme 2 is a functional receptor for the SARS coronavirus. *Nature* **2003**, *426*, 450–454. [CrossRef] [PubMed]
15. Li, F.; Li, W.; Farzan, M.; Harrison, S.C. Structure of SARS coronavirus spike receptor-binding domain complexed with receptor. *Science* **2005**, *309*, 1864–1868. [CrossRef] [PubMed]
16. Song, W.; Gui, M.; Wang, X.; Xiang, Y. Cryo-EM structure of the SARS coronavirus spike glycoprotein in complex with its host cell receptor ACE2. *PLoS Pathog.* **2018**, *14*, e1007236. [CrossRef] [PubMed]
17. Othman, H.; Bouslama, Z.; Brandenburg, J.T.; da Rocha, J.; Hamdi, Y.; Ghedira, K.; Srairi-Abid, N.; Hazelhurst, S. Interaction of the spike protein RBD from SARS-CoV-2 with ACE2: Similarity with SARS-CoV, hot-spot analysis and effect of the receptor polymorphism. *Biochem. Biophys. Res. Commun.* **2020**, *527*, 702–708. [CrossRef]
18. Wan, Y.; Shang, J.; Graham, R.; Baric, R.S.; Li, F. Receptor Recognition by the Novel Coronavirus from Wuhan: An Analysis Based on Decade-Long Structural Studies of SARS Coronavirus. *J. Virol.* **2020**, *94*, e00127-20. [CrossRef]
19. Wang, Q.; Zhang, Y.; Wu, L.; Niu, S.; Song, C.; Zhang, Z.; Lu, G.; Qiao, C.; Hu, Y.; Yuen, K.Y.; et al. Structural and Functional Basis of SARS-CoV-2 Entry by Using Human ACE2. *Cell* **2020**, *181*, 894–904. [CrossRef]
20. Wrapp, D.; Wang, N.; Corbett, K.S.; Goldsmith, J.A.; Hsieh, C.-L.; Abiona, O.; Graham, B.S.; McLellan, J.S. Cryo-EM Structure of the 2019-nCoV Spike in the Prefusion Conformation. *Science* **2020**, *367*, 1260–1263. [CrossRef]
21. Yan, R.; Zhang, Y.; Li, Y.; Xia, L.; Guo, Y.; Zhou, Q. Structural basis for the recognition of SARS-CoV-2 by full-length human ACE2. *Science* **2020**, *367*, 1444–1448. [CrossRef]
22. Kirchdoerfer, R.N.; Wang, N.; Pallesen, J.; Wrapp, D.; Turner, H.L.; Cottrell, C.A.; Corbett, K.S.; Graham, B.S.; McLellan, J.S.; Ward, A.B. Stabilized coronavirus spikes are resistant to conformational changes induced by receptor recognition or proteolysis. *Sci. Rep.* **2018**, *8*, 15701. [CrossRef] [PubMed]
23. Lan, J.; Ge, J.; Yu, J.; Shan, S.; Zhou, H.; Fan, S.; Zhang, Q.; Shi, X.; Wang, Q.; Zhang, L.; et al. Structure of the SARS-CoV-2 spike receptor-binding domain bound to the ACE2 receptor. *Nature* **2020**, *581*, 215–220. [CrossRef]
24. Fang, L.; Karakiulakis, G.; Roth, M. Are patients with hypertension and diabetes mellitus at increased risk for COVID-19 infection? *Lancet Respir. Med.* **2020**, *8*, e21. [CrossRef]
25. Xu, J.; Zhao, S.; Teng, T.; Abdalla, A.E.; Zhu, W.; Xie, L.; Wang, Y.; Guo, X. Systematic Comparison of Two Animal-to-Human Transmitted Human Coronaviruses: SARS-CoV-2 and SARS-CoV. *Viruses* **2020**, *12*, 244. [CrossRef] [PubMed]
26. Ahmed, S.F.; Quadeer, A.A.; McKay, M.R. Preliminary Identification of Potential Vaccine Targets for the COVID-19 Coronavirus (SARS-CoV-2) Based on SARS-CoV Immunological Studies. *Viruses* **2020**, *12*, 254. [CrossRef] [PubMed]
27. Graham, R.L.; Baric, R.S. Recombination, reservoirs, and the modular spike: Mechanisms of coronavirus cross-species transmission. *J. Virol.* **2010**, *84*, 3134–3146. [CrossRef] [PubMed]
28. Shirato, K.; Kawase, M.; Matsuyama, S. Wild-type human coronaviruses prefer cell-surface TMPRSS2 to endosomal cathepsins for cell entry. *Virology* **2018**, *517*, 9–15. [CrossRef]
29. Cantuti-Castelvetri, L.; Ojha, R.; Pedro, L.D.; Djannatian, M.; Franz, J.; Kuivanen, S.; van der Meer, F.; Kallio, K.; Kaya, T.; Anastasina, M.; et al. Neuropilin-1 facilitates SARS-CoV-2 cell entry and infectivity. *Science* **2020**, *370*, 856–860. [CrossRef] [PubMed]
30. Daly, J.L.; Simonetti, B.; Klein, K.; Chen, K.E.; Williamson, M.K.; Antón-Plágaro, C.; Shoemark, D.K.; Simón-Gracia, L.; Bauer, M.; Hollandi, R.; et al. Neuropilin-1 is a host factor for SARS-CoV-2 infection. *Science* **2020**, *370*, 861–865. [CrossRef]
31. Mayi, B.S.; Leibowitz, J.A.; Woods, A.T.; Ammon, K.A.; Liu, A.E.; Raja, A. The role of Neuropilin-1 in COVID-19. *PLoS Pathog.* **2021**, *17*, e1009153. [CrossRef]

32. Raj, V.S.; Mou, H.; Smits, S.L.; Dekkers, D.H.; Müller, M.A.; Dijkman, R.; Muth, D.; Demmers, J.A.A.; Zaki, A.; Fouchier, R.A.M.; et al. Dipeptidyl peptidase 4 is a functional receptor for the emerging human coronavirus-EMC. *Nature* **2013**, *495*, 251–254. [CrossRef] [PubMed]
33. Zumla, A.; Chan, J.; Azhar, E.I.; Hui, D.S.; Yuen, K.Y. Coronaviruses—Drug discovery and therapeutic options. *Nat. Rev. Drug Discov.* **2016**, *15*, 327–347. [CrossRef] [PubMed]
34. Li, H.; Tang, N.L.; Chan, P.K.; Wang, C.Y.; Hui, D.S.; Luk, C.; Kwok, R.; Huang, W.; Sung, J.J.-Y.; Kong, Q.-P.; et al. Polymorphisms in the C-type lectin genes cluster in chromosome 19 and predisposition to severe acute respiratory syndrome coronavirus (SARS-CoV) infection. *J. Med. Genet.* **2008**, *45*, 752–758. [CrossRef] [PubMed]
35. Sun, X.L. The Role of Cell Surface Sialic Acids for SARS-CoV-2 Infection. *Glycobiology* **2021**, *31*, 1245–1253. [CrossRef] [PubMed]
36. Protein Data Bank (PDB). Available online: https://www.rcsb.org (accessed on 22 July 2021).
37. Giordano, D.; De Masi, L.; Argenio, M.A.; Facchiano, A. Structural Dissection of Viral Spike-Protein Binding of SARS-CoV-2 and SARS-CoV-1 to the Human Angiotensin-Converting Enzyme 2 (ACE2) as Cellular Receptor. *Biomedicines* **2021**, *9*, 1038. [CrossRef] [PubMed]
38. Walls, A.C.; Park, Y.J.; Tortorici, M.A.; Wall, A.; McGuire, A.T.; Veesler, D. Structure, Function, and Antigenicity of the SARS-CoV-2 Spike Glycoprotein. *Cell* **2020**, *181*, 281–292. [CrossRef]
39. Xie, Y.; Karki, C.B.; Du, D.; Li, H.; Wang, J.; Sobitan, A.; Teng, S.; Tang, Q.; Li, L. Spike proteins of SARS-CoV and SARS-CoV-2 utilize different mechanisms to bind with human ACE2. *Front. Mol. Biosci.* **2020**, *7*, 591873. [CrossRef]
40. Towler, P.; Staker, B.; Prasad, S.G.; Menon, S.; Tang, J.; Parsons, T.; Ryan, D.; Fisher, M.; Williams, D.; Dales, N.A.; et al. ACE2 X-ray structures reveal a large hinge-bending motion important for inhibitor binding and catalysis. *J. Biol. Chem.* **2004**, *279*, 17996–18007. [CrossRef]
41. PANGO Lineages: Latest Epidemiological Lineages of SARS-CoV-2. Available online: https://cov-lineages.org (accessed on 22 July 2021).
42. CoVariants. Available online: https://covariants.org (accessed on 22 July 2021).
43. Rambaut, A.; Holmes, E.C.; O'Toole, Á.; Hill, V.; McCrone, J.T.; Ruis, C.; du Pleiss, L.; Pybus, O.G. A dynamic nomenclature proposal for SARS-CoV-2 lineages to assist genomic epidemiology. *Nat. Microbiol.* **2020**, *5*, 1403–1407. [CrossRef]
44. Socher, E.; Conrad, M.; Heger, L.; Paulsen, F.; Sticht, H.; Zunke, F.; Arnold, P. Mutations in the B.1.1.7 SARS-CoV-2 Spike Protein Reduce Receptor-Binding Affinity and Induce a Flexible Link to the Fusion Peptide. *Biomedicines* **2021**, *9*, 525. [CrossRef] [PubMed]
45. Nesci, S. SARS-CoV-2 first contact: Spike–ACE2 interactions in COVID-19. *Chem. Biol. Drug Des.* **2021**, *98*, 207–211. [CrossRef]

encyclopedia

MDPI

Entry

Limbic Encephalitis Associated with COVID-19

Natalia A. Shnayder [1,2,*], Timur K. Sirbiladze [1,*], Irina V. Demko [2], Marina M. Petrova [2] and Regina F. Nasyrova [1,3]

[1] Institute of Personalized Psychiatry and Neurology, Shared Core Facilities, V. M. Bekhterev National Medical Research Centre for Psychiatry and Neurology, 192019 Saint Petersburg, Russia; nreginaf77@gmail.com
[2] Shared Core Facilities "Molecular and Cell Technology", V. F. Voino-Yasenetsky Krasnoyarsk State Medical University, 660022 Krasnoyarsk, Russia; demko64@mail.ru (I.V.D.); stk99@yandex.ru (M.M.P.)
[3] International Centre for Education and Research in Neuropsychiatry, Samara State Medical University, 443099 Samara, Russia
* Correspondence: naschnaider@yandex.ru (N.A.S.); t.sirbiladze96@gmail.com (T.K.S.); Tel.: +7-(812)-670-02-2078-14 (N.A.S. & T.K.S.)

Definition: Limbic encephalitis (LE) is an inflammatory disease of the brain, in which lesion is anatomically limited in structures of the limbic system. In some cases, LE can start with symptoms of limbic dysfunction with further involvement of other regions of the brain. Classic LE syndrome includes such symptoms as the development of personality disorders, depression, sleep disorders, epileptic seizures, hallucinations and cognitive disorders (short-term and long-term memory impairment). The information of clinical examination, electroencephalogram (EEG), magnetic resonance imaging (MRI) and cerebrospinal fluid studies (CSF) suggest the diagnosis of LE in most patients with Coronavirus Disease 2019 (COVID-19).

Keywords: limbic system; limbic encephalitis; COVID-19; neurological complication

Citation: Shnayder, N.A.; Sirbiladze, T.K.; Demko, I.V.; Petrova, M.M.; Nasyrova, R.F. Limbic Encephalitis Associated with COVID-19. *Encyclopedia* **2022**, *2*, 26–35. https://doi.org/10.3390/encyclopedia2010003

Academic Editor: Stephen Bustin

Received: 3 November 2021
Accepted: 17 December 2021
Published: 22 December 2021

1. History of Limbic Encephalitis

Limbic encephalitis (LE) was first described in 1960 by Brierley et al. [1]. Later, in 1968, Corsellis et al. suggested the term "Limbic Encephalitis" [2]. For the next few decades, LE was considered a rare autoimmune disease strictly associated with cancer [3]. However, the development of neuroimaging and antineuronal antibodies detection methods demonstrated that LE can be divided in to two main variants: the first variant is LE, associated with paraneoplastic antibodies or cancer (typical LE), and the second variant is LE, without paraneoplastic antibodies or cancer (atypical LE) [4,5]. Studies in the following years showed that LE can be associated with variative antigen localization and different antibodies [6]. Other studies showed that most patients with LE are found to have antibodies to neuronal cell-surface antigens [7]. These antigens can be expressed in different regions of the central nervous system (CNS), and the limbic system (especially hippocampal formation) is known as one of the common localizations, followed by the cerebellum.

Now, LE is known as a relatively frequent autoimmune disorder of CNS [6,8]. Typical LE syndrome includes such symptoms as the development of personality disorders, depression, sleep disorders, epileptic seizures, hallucinations and cognitive disorders [7,8].

2. Para-Infectious Variants of Limbic Encephalitis

Alongside para-neoplastic LE, para-infectious LE [9] should be distinguished. It is primarily associated with production of antibodies to *Herpesviridae* family viruses, especially antibodies to *Herpes simplex virus-1* (HSV-1). However, other members of this family (*Varicella zoster*, *Cytomegalovirus*, etc.) are almost never associated with neuroimaging changes typical to LE. An exception to this is *Human herpesvirus 6* (HHV-6), which is considered as a possible cause of LE symptoms in patients with immunosuppression [6]. Due to chronic persistence of HSV-1 and HHV-6 in CNS, the pathological process in para-infectious LE is characterized not only by direct virus invasion but also by the production of specific autoantibodies, produced as result of cross presentation mechanisms [9].

Since 2019, increasing interest and attention have being given to the features of clinical presentation of COVID-19, caused by *Severe Acute Respiratory Syndrome Coronavirus-2* (SARS-CoV-2). At this time, there is growing data, confirming the direct impact of SARS-CoV-2 on the limbic system of the brain and its immune-mediated damage [10–12]. According to the neuroimaging data, pathologic changes of the limbic system associated with COVID-19 can be both unilateral or bilateral (more common). Those changes are frequently found bilateral in the olfactory cortex, hippocampal formation, insula, right cingulate gyrus, left Rolandic operculum and left Heschl's gyrus. Studies showed the correlation between neuroimaging findings and clinical manifestations, typical to LE associated with SARS-CoV-2. Thus, neuroimaging changes in hippocampal formation, right cingulate gyrus, left Rolandic operculum, and left Heschl's gyrus correlated with cognitive disorders (memory impairment), while odor perception impairment (central hyposmia or anosmia) correlated with pathologic changes in mediobasal region of the temporal lobe (hippocampus) and the right cingulate gyrus [10]. In addition, the possible damage to the limbic system is testified by a number of case reports describing COVID-19 as a possible factor, provoking interictal and ictal epileptiform activity in temporal localization according to EEG, including seizures as the onset of CNS damage in children and adult patients with COVID-19 [13–15]. In addition, there are a number of studies describing COVID-19 patients with the development of such symptoms as cognitive disorders, personality disorders, anxiety-depressive disorders and, sometimes, aggressive behavior with psychosis [16,17]. This combined gives strong evidence of possible LE associated with SARS-CoV-2. Interestingly, these symptoms, typical for LE, have been described not only in patients in the acute phase of COVID-19 but also in the late recovery period [18,19]

Furthermore, cases of LE associated with the asymptomatic course of COVID-19 have been described. These cases show that neurological manifestations of COVID-19 are not always a reflection of the severe course of the disease. Because of that, an additional examination to exclude COVID-19 in patients with symptoms of limbic dysfunction may be considerable [20]. Due to the absence of viral RNA or specific antibodies in cerebrospinal fluid (CSF), it might be the case that damage of the limbic system in COVID-19 patients is primarily associated with the autoimmune response, induced by SARS-CoV-2. Therefore, the nature of this pathological process may be described as para-infectious, and high-field Magnetic Resonance Imaging (MRI) of limbic structures can be considered as an important method of intravital diagnosis of para-infectious LE associated with SARS-CoV-2 [20,21].

Given all this, it is reasonable to expect a SARS-CoV-2-associated LE to become a new multidisciplinary challenge in neurology and psychiatry practice. In addition, it seems to be the case that with the spread of the COVID-19 pandemic, the frequency of para-infectious LE associated with SARS-CoV-2 may exceed the frequency of LE associated with *Herpesviruses*, which makes this a topic of high concern requiring more studies.

Neuroanatomy of Limbic System and COVID-19

According to the data of previous studies, SARS-CoV-2 can be the cause of demyelinating processes, neurodegeneration and other changes associated with brain aging and neurodegenerative diseases [22]. However, only few clinical cases and thematic reviews describe the features of neurological changes in the acute phase of COVID-19, while the long-term consequences in COVID-19 patients are even less described [23].

Brain lesions caused by SARS-CoV-2 are variative. Among all possible targets, the involvement of the limbic system and limbic dysfunction caused by COVID-19 seems to be the most important one. The reason of such importance is explained by the fact that limbic dysfunction can cause not only personality disorders and behavioral changes (including schizoaffective disorders) but also lead to severe social disadaptation as a result. In the following section, we will discuss structures of the limbic system, which are primarily affected in COVID-19 patients (Table 1; Figure 1).

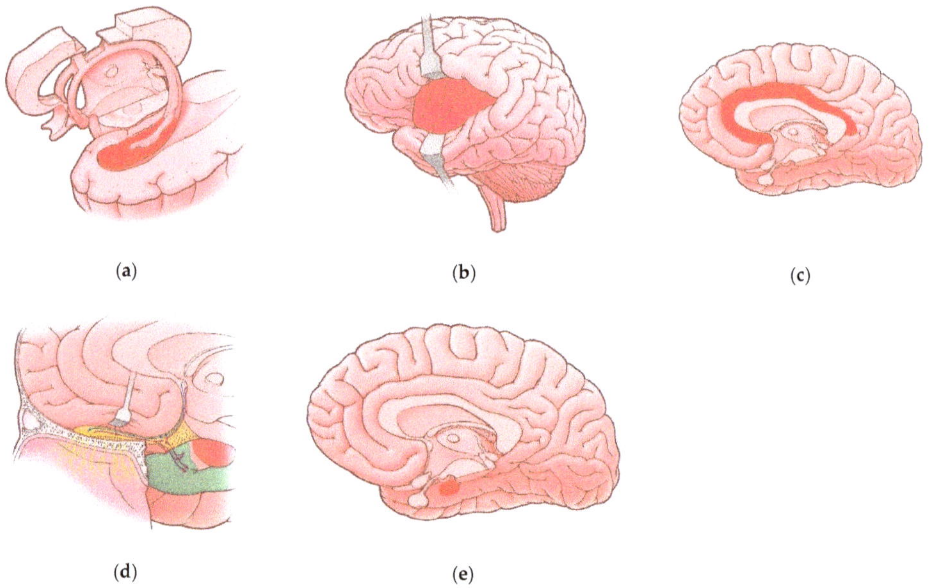

Figure 1. Regions of the limbic system affected in COVID-19 patients: (**a**) Hippocampus; (**b**) insula; (**c**) cingulate gyrus; (**d**) olfactory cortex—red-colored region represents uncus and green-colored region represents parahippocampal gyrus, red and blue lines represent olfactory pathways; (**e**) Amygdala (projection).

The hippocampus (hippocampal formation) is a complex structure of the brain located in the mesial region of the temporal lobe. The hippocampus plays a significant role in learning processes and memory. In addition, it is involved in the development of emotional and behavioral reactions and spatial orientation. Lesions of this region can lead to memory impairment, decreased learning ability, anxiety-depressive disorders, schizoaffective disorders and seizure onset [24]. According to studies, COVID-19-associated hippocampal lesions can feature with focal ictal and interictal epileptiform activity, mnestic process disturbances, impairment of episodic memory and consciousness impairment [10,25].

The amygdala (amygdaloid bodies) is a structure of the brain, represented by a nuclei formation, which is located in the anteromedial region of the temporal lobes. Functions of this structure include the development of adaptive reactions to emotionally significant events (especially threatening one), involvement in memory processes, face recognition [26,27] and also in olfactory perception [28]. Despite the available neuroimaging data showing changes in the amygdala of patients with COVID-19, the corresponding clinical features are still not characterized enough. However, some authors noticed a correlation between neuroimaging changes in the amygdala and possible vulnerability to depressive disorders in COVID-19 patients [29].

The insula is a region of the cerebral cortex that lies deep in the lateral sulcus. Due to numerous connections with other brain regions and structures, the insula takes part in variative processes: gustatory stimuli analysis, development of emotional reactions, empathy, evaluation of risk, attention control (recognition of a "new" stimuli), interoception, autonomic nervous system regulation, involvement in vestibular, auditory stimuli analysis and pain perception [30]. Damage to the insula can cause the impairment of gustatory perception (dysgeusia and ageusia), changes in emotional behavior (apathy, increased anxiety, decreased empathy) and memory impairment [31]. As for features accompanying changes in this region in COVID-19 patients, some case reports describe possible courses presenting disturbances in pain perception and interoception [32].

The cingulate gyrus is a part of the limbic system, known to be responsible for the development and processing of emotions, education and involved in memory processes. Pathological changes in the cingulate gyrus can lead to the development of depressive disorders, personality disorders and schizoaffective disorders (including psychosis) [33]. The involvement of this region is frequently described in patients with COVID-19, manifesting as the development of anxiety and depressive disorders, confusion and attention and short-term memory disturbances [10,23].

The olfactory cortex is a group of structures in the brain, including the olfactory nucleus, the olfactory bulb, the frontal and temporal parts of piriform cortex, partially the amygdala, the entorhinal cortex and the parahippocampal gyrus. Functionally, this region is responsible not only for the analysis of olfactory stimuli but also takes part in memory processes and the development of certain emotional or social reactions [34,35]. Pathological processes in the olfactory cortex can cause olfactory perception impairment, memory consolidation disturbances and trigger focal epileptiform activity-focal sensory or psychosensory epileptic seizures (olfactory hallucinations) [35,36]. COVID-19 is known to induce the altered olfactory perception as both an acute or long-lasting symptom. Altered olfactory perception in COVID-19 patients is known to manifest as an acute symptom as well as a long-term persisting condition. Moreover, these alterations are variative: hyposmia—decreased perception of odors; anosmia—complete absence of odor perception; parosmia—distorted perception of common odors; and phantosmia—the sensation of smell in the absence of its source. Due to frequent negative characteristic of altered smell (malodorant, fetid smell), olfactory perception distortions can have a significant impact on quality of life in patients with COVID-19 [37–39].

Parosmia can be associated with central or peripheral lesions, caused by SARS-CoV-2, because COVID-19 can affect both the olfactory bulb and the cortical centers of the olfactory analisator [38]. In addition, paradoxical regrowth of new olfactory axons can prolong the parosmia in patients after COVID-19. However, studies suggest olfactory training as an effective method of improving olfactory function in patients with COVID-19-associated persistent parosmia [40].

In comparison, Araújo et al. (2021) suggest a death of olfactory neurons and neurodegeneration in the olfactory bulb to be a primary cause of persistent olfactory dysfunction in patients after COVID-19 [41]. Thus, studies of the brain using 18F-FDG-PET showed hypometabolism in the left orbitofrontal cortex, which correlated with olfactory bulb edema in MRI [37,38]. In addition, persistent anosmia can present as a single symptom in COVID-19 patients, therefore, it should be considered as a possible marker for this infection [42].

Damage of the olfactory cortex attributed to COVID-19 generally leads to olfactory disturbances (hyposmia and anosmia) [10], but the frequency and intensity of those symptoms are variative in patients, even if age and the severity of COVID-19 are comparable. Thus, the frequency of olfactory dysfunction in COVID-19 patients can range from 15% to 98% [43–45]. However, it is reasonable to mention that specifics of used methods of interviewing patients and information gathering can have significant influence, potentially causing this variety.

The real cause for this phenomenon is not fully understood yet. Perhaps hyposmia or anosmia persisting after COVID-19 can be considered as a marker of limbic dysfunction and LE in general. In the long-term perspective, persisting anosmia can have an impact on the quality of patients' lives, also possibly accompanied with the development of depression [46,47], anxiety [48], problems with socialization [49,50], cognitive impairment [49,51,52] and anorexia with related complications [48].

Moreover, Pirker-Kees et al. (2021) demonstrated that olfactory dysfunction can be associated with cognitive impairment, even in patients with mild COVID-19 [53]. In addition, since previous studies [54] showed correlation between olfactory dysfunction and cognitive impairment with neuroimaging changes in the limbic system, altered olfactory perception presumably can be considered as marker of limbic system involvement in patients with mild and subclinical COVID-19.

Table 1. Regions of the limbic system affected in COVID-19 patients.

Region of Limbic System	Associated Manifestations in COVID-19 Patients	References
Hippocampus	Memory impairment Impaired Consciousness Seizures	[10,25]
Insula	Pain perception disturbances Interoception disturbances	[32]
Cingulate gyrus	Anxiety disorders Depressive disorders Cognitive impairments (brain fog) Impaired episodic memory Attention disturbances	[23]
Olfactory cortex	Olfactory dysfunction (hyposmia, anosmia)	[10,41]
Amygdala	Vulnerability to depressive disorders	[29]

3. Discussion

Given all this, para-infectious LE, associated with SARS-CoV-2, meets the definition of autoimmune LE according to Graus' criteria [55]:

(1) Subacute onset (rapid progression of less than 3 months) of working memory deficits (short-term memory loss), altered mental status or psychiatric symptoms associated with limbic system involvement;
(2) At least one of the following:
   - New focal CNS findings, seizures not explained by a previously known seizure disorder;
   - CSF pleocytosis (white blood cell counts of more than five cells per mm3);
   - MRI features suggestive of encephalitis;
(3) Reasonable exclusion of alternative causes.

When all three criteria are met, a diagnosis of LE can be made.

Therefore, analyzed studies [10,21,23,25,32] show that para-infectious LE, associated with SARS-CoV-2, can be considered as an independent disease, which should be studied more because the possible consequences for patients and society are unclear, while the frequency and prognosis of this disease still need to be clarified. Interestingly, it is possible for para-infectious LE, associated with SARS-CoV-2 to occur in patients with respiratory system involvement, as well as in patients with no respiratory symptoms [10], including single cases of isolated attack on the limbic system [20]. In the majority of described clinical cases, the most common neurological symptoms of this disease were: cognitive impairment; focal and generalized tonic-clonic seizures, including the development of status epilepticus; neuropsychiatric symptoms (olfactory and visual hallucinations, short-term memory loss, anxiety-depressive disorders, socialization problems); and olfactory dysfunction [10,21,23,25,32]. The presence of ictal or (more common) interictal abnormal activity located in the temporal lobe in electroencephalography (EEG) should be considered as a significant factor [13]. According to MRI, damage of the limbic system in COVID-19, in most cases, was bilateral in the form of T2-weighted imaging (T2) and Fluid attenuated inversion recovery (FLAIR) hyperintensity. Moreover, contrasting with gadolinium increased the frequency of those findings [10,20].

MR-spectroscopy with evaluation markers such as peak of N-acetylaspartate (NAA), Choline (Cho), Creatine (Cr), Lactate (Lac), Glutamate–Glutamine complex (Glx) and Myoinositol (MI) can become a promising method for diagnosing neurodegenerative and neuroinflammatory processes in para-infectious LE associated with SARS-CoV-2 [56] (Table 2).

Table 2. Brain metabolites used for magnetic resonance spectroscopy in patients with limbic encephalitis [56].

Metabolite	Commentary
N-acetylaspartate (NAA) Chemical Shift = 2.02	It is a derivative of amino acids synthesized in neurons and further transported along axons. A reliable marker of the viability of neurons, axons and dendrites.
Choline (Cho) Chemical Shift = 3.22	It is part of cell membranes and cholinergic synaptic endings of neurons and takes part in lipid metabolism.
Creatine (Cr) Chemical shift = 3.02; 3.94	The main marker of energy processes in astrocytes and neurons. It is formed during the conversion of the high-energy compound Adenosine triphosphate to Adenosine diphosphate. In the brain tissue, the signal intensity in many cases remains constant, even with pathological changes.
Lactate (Lac) Chemical Shift = 1.33	It is not detected in normal brain tissue. It is contained in the cerebrospinal fluid (0.9 mmol/L). Indicator of anaerobic glycolysis.
Glutamate-Glutamine Complex (Glx) Chemical shift = 2.1–2.5	Astrocyte marker and neurotoxin, respectively. Glutamine (2-aminopentanamide 5 oxic acid) is the 1 of the 20 standard amino acids that make up the protein. Excitatory neurotransmitter.
Myoinositol (MI) Chemical Shift = 3.56	Myelin degradation product. The concentration rises in multiple sclerosis and decreases in tumors. It rises in the center of the epileptogenic focus and decreases in the tissues adjacent to it.

An interesting fact is that in most patients with SARS-CoV-2, serological tests on autoimmune panels, including autoantibodies against intracellular, synaptic and surface antigens previously described in LE of a different etiology, were negative [21]. According to this fact, some authors consider the development of SARS-CoV-2-associated para-infectious LE caused by secondary hyperinflammatory syndrome with a massive release of proinflammatory cytokines and chemokines in the limbic system of the brain [21,57,58]. Taken together, these facts explain the scientific and clinical interest in studying the role of pro-inflammatory cytokines, including interleukin-1-beta (IL-1), interleukin-6 (IL-6) and tumor necrosis factor-alpha (TNF-α), in the development of para-infectious LE associated with SARS-CoV-2, as overexpression of these cytokines has been described in previous studies of drug resistant para-infectious temporal lobe epilepsy [59–63] and also in cognitive disorders including shot-term and long-term memory [64] and Alzheimer's type dementia [65].

The overexpression of proinflammatory cytokines can be genetically determined [66], which can explain the high risk of developing para-infectious LE associated with SARS-CoV-2 in patients with an unfavorable genetic profile. In addition, the autoimmune mechanisms of LE associated with SARS-CoV-2 is unlikely to be associated with the production of antineuronal autoantibodies, provoked by the virus and possible molecular mimicry [21]. However, we should admit that the number of questions about the problem of LE associated with SARS-CoV-2 highly exceeds the number of answers we currently have.

4. Limitations

The publications that we have analyzed over the past two years show a small number of reports of clinical cases of SARS-CoV2-associated LE yet. However, the number of cases will increase with the growth of publications and research on this important problem of neurology and psychiatry. Currently, a study of the frequency of occurrence of this disease in Russia and in the world has been launched. The results of new studies may be analyzed in the future.

Probably, there are any other factors (age, gender, specific underlying pathological conditions, etc.) likely related to the involvement of the limbic system in patients with COVID-19 and post-COVID-19 syndrome. This is a very interesting and important question. We agree that the study of these factors (environmental, non-genetic and genetic) is of undoubted scientific and clinical interest. Other recent literature concerning autoimmune encephalitis and SARS-CoV2 are discussed, and the difference between SARS-CoV2-associated autoimmune encephalitis and LE is also very important [67]. However, this topic is currently insufficiently studied, despite its high relevance. We are studying these factors, but so far, the duration of the study is short, so today we cannot give a definite answer to this question.

There are summary ideas and the available knowledge about SARS-CoV2-associated LE in this entry paper. However, the requirements for the entry paper do not allow us to consider the proposed mechanisms of SARS-CoV2′s effects on the limbic system in more detail.

This entry paper demonstrates that the number of confirmed cases of SARS-CoV2-associated LE has been increasing over the past year. This may be due to a new strain of this virus or antigenic mimicry. In addition, the authors' own clinical experience shows that in the last three months alone, four cases of this disease were identified. They all require separate reports.

The general limitations are that there are currently more questions about LE associated with SARS-CoV-2 than answers.

5. Conclusions

Concluding, we should mention that the number of publications dedicated to para-infectious LE associated with SARS-CoV-2 is currently limited. However, the high tropism of SARS-CoV-2 to the structures of the limbic system of the brain, with the possibility of isolated lesions of these areas in children and adults without respiratory symptoms of COVID-19, and the high number of new cases of this infection in population worldwide indicates the importance of this interdisciplinary problem in neurology and psychiatry. In addition, the development of an autoimmune process in the CNS is also possible after the respiratory symptoms was resolved, as the long-term consequence in patients with the pulmonary form of COVID-19. In patients with a high risk of developing para-infectious LE associated with SARS-CoV-2, the diagnostic algorithm in the acute and subacute periods should include analysis of CSF, EEG monitoring and brain MRI. In patients with asymptomatic or mild COVID-19 (without respiratory symptoms) and long-term consequences of COVID-19 (long-COVID-19), the diagnostic algorithm should include neuropsychological testing, brain MRI, EEG and serological testing (evaluating the pro-inflammatory cytokines and antibodies to SARS-CoV-2 IgG). This algorithm can help in the risk assessment and early diagnosis of para-infectious LE associated with SARS-CoV-2; moreover, it gives information for consideration in treatment planning. An important but controversial issue is the acceptability of revaccination against COVID-19 in patients with high risk of developing para-infectious LE or patients with this disease.

Future research on biomarkers for the risk of developing para-infectious LE associated with SARS-CoV-2 and its severity is necessary to expand our knowledge about this new immune-mediated CNS disease and its possible consequences for patients and society.

Author Contributions: Conceptualization, N.A.S.; methodology, I.V.D. and R.F.N.; software, T.K.S.; validation, N.A.S., T.K.S. and R.F.N.; formal analysis, T.K.S.; investigation, N.A.S. and T.K.S.; resources, T.K.S.; data curation, T.K.S.; writing—original draft preparation, N.A.S. and T.K.S.; writing—review and editing, M.M.P. and R.F.N.; visualization, T.K.S.; supervision, N.A.S.; project administration, R.F.N. All authors have read and agreed to the published version of the manuscript.

Funding: This research received no external funding.

Institutional Review Board Statement: Not applicable.

Informed Consent Statement: Not applicable.

Acknowledgments: The authors appreciate Polina S. Kulagina for her help in preparing the figures.

Conflicts of Interest: The authors declare no conflict of interest.

Entry Link on the Encyclopedia Platform: https://encyclopedia.pub/18652.

References

1. Brierley, J.B.; Corsellis, J.A.N.; Hierons, R. Subacute encephalitis of later adult life. Mainly affecting the limbic areas. *Brain* **1960**, *83*, 357–368. [CrossRef]
2. Corsellis, J.A.; Goldgerg, G.J.; Norton, A.R. "Limbic encephalitis" and its association with carcinoma. *Brain* **1968**, *91*, 481–496. [CrossRef] [PubMed]
3. Bakhelt, A.M.; Kennedy, P.G.; Behan, P.O. Paraneoplastic limbic encephalitis: Clinico-pathological correletions. *J. Neurol. Neurosurg. Psychiatry* **1990**, *53*, 1084–1088. [CrossRef] [PubMed]
4. Gultekin, S.H.; Rosenfeld, M.R.; Voltz, R.; Eichen, J.; Posner, J.B.; Dalmau, J. Paraneoplastic limbic encephalitis: Neurological symptoms, immunological findings and tumor association in 50 patients. *Brain* **2000**, *123*, 1481–1494. [CrossRef]
5. Vitaliani, R.; Mason, W.; Ances, B.; Zwerdling, T.; Jiang, Z.; Dalmau, J. Paraneoplastic encephalitis, psychiatric symptoms, and hypoventilation in ovarian teratoma. *Ann. Neurol.* **2005**, *58*, 594–604. [CrossRef]
6. Tüzün, E.; Dalmau, J. Limbic encephalitis and variants: Classification, diagnosis and treatment. *Neurologist* **2007**, *13*, 261–271. [CrossRef] [PubMed]
7. Wagner, J.; Witt, J.A.; Helmstaedter, C., Malter, M.P.; Weber, B.; Elger, C.E. Automated volumetry of the mesiotemporal structures in antibody-associated limbic encephalitis. *J. Neurol. Neurosurg. Psychiatry* **2014**, *86*, 735–742. [CrossRef] [PubMed]
8. Shnayder, N.A.; Dmitrenko, D.V.; Dykno, Y.A.; Ezhikova, V.V. Paraneoplastic limbic encephalitis in neurological and oncological practice. *Russ. J. Oncol.* **2013**, *1*, 49–57.
9. Shnayder, N.A.; Panina, Y.S.; Dmitrenko, D.V.; Krjzhanovskaya, S.V.; Molgachev, A.A. Parainfectious limbic encephalitis associated with herpes viridae viruses. *Probl. Women Health* **2014**, *9*, 58–69.
10. Lu, Y.; Li, X.; Geng, D.; Mei, N.; Wu, P.Y.; Huang, C.C.; Jia, T.; Zhao, Y.; Wang, D.; Xiao, A.; et al. Cerebral Micro-Structural Changes in COVID-19 Patients–An MRI-based 3-month Follow-up Study. *EClinicalMedicine* **2020**, *25*, 100484. [CrossRef] [PubMed]
11. Bridwell, R.; Long, B.; Gottlieb, M. Neurologic complications of COVID-19. *Am. J. Emerg. Med.* **2020**, *38*, 1549.e3–1549.e7. [CrossRef]
12. Paterson, R.W.; Brown, R.L.; Benjamin, L.; Nortley, R.; Wiethoff, S.; Bharucha, T.; Jayaseelan, D.L.; Kumar, G.; Raftopoulos, R.E.; Zambreanu, L.; et al. The emerging spectrum of COVID-19 neurology: Clinical, radiological and laboratory findings. *Brain* **2020**, *143*, 3104–3120. [CrossRef] [PubMed]
13. Kurd, M.; Hashavya, S.; Benenson, S.; Gilboa, T. Seizures as the main presenting manifestation of acute SARS-CoV-2 infection in children. *Seizure* **2021**, *92*, 89–93. [CrossRef] [PubMed]
14. Sohal, S.; Mansur, M. COVID-19 Presenting with Seizures. *IDCases* **2020**, *20*, e00782. [CrossRef] [PubMed]
15. Santos de Lima, F.; Issa, N.; Seibert, K.; Davis, J.; Wlodarski, R.; Klein, S.; El Ammar, F.; Wu, S.; Rose, S.; Warnke, P.; et al. Epileptiform activity and seizures in patients with COVID-19. *J. Neurol. Neurosurg. Psychiatry* **2021**, *92*, 565–566. [CrossRef]
16. Machhi, J.; Herskovitz, J.; Senan, A.M.; Dutta, D.; Nath, B.; Oleynikov, M.D.; Blomberg, W.R.; Meigs, D.D.; Hasan, M.; Patel, M.; et al. The Natural History, Pathobiology, and Clinical Manifestations of SARS-CoV-2 Infections. *J. Neuroimmune Pharmacol.* **2020**, *15*, 359–386. [CrossRef]
17. Troyer, E.A.; Kohn, J.N.; Hong, S. Are we facing a crashing wave of neuropsychiatric sequelae of COVID-19? Neuropsychiatric symptoms and potential immunologic mechanisms. *Brain Behav. Immun.* **2020**, *87*, 34–39. [CrossRef]
18. Carroll, E.; Neumann, H.; Aguero-Rosenfeld, M.E.; Lighter, J.; Czeisler, B.M.; Melmed, K.; Lewis, A. Post-COVID-19 inflammatory syndrome manifesting as refractory status epilepticus. *Epilepsia* **2020**, *61*, e135–e139. [CrossRef]
19. Wu, Y.; Xu, X.; Chen, Z.; Duan, J.; Hashimoto, K.; Yang, L.; Liu, C.; Yang, C. Nervous system involvement after infection with COVID-19 and other coronaviruses. *Brain Behav. Immun.* **2020**, *87*, 18–22. [CrossRef] [PubMed]
20. Zambreanu, L.; Lightbody, S.; Bhandari, M.; Hoskote, C.; Kandil, H.; Houlihan, C.F.; Lunn, M.P. A case of limbic encephalitis associated with asymptomatic COVID-19 infection. *J. Neurol. Neurosurg. Psychiatry* **2020**, *91*, 1229–1230. [CrossRef]
21. Pizzanelli, C.; Milano, C.; Canovetti, S.; Tagliaferri, E.; Turco, F.; Verdenelli, S.; Nesti, L.; Franchi, M.; Bonanni, E.; Menichetti, F.; et al. Autoimmune limbic encephalitis related to SARS-CoV-2 infection: Case-report and review of the literature. *Brain Behav. Immun. Health* **2021**, *12*, 100–210. [CrossRef] [PubMed]
22. Dinakaran, D.; Manjunatha, N.; Naveen Kumar, C.; Suresh, B.M. Neuropsychiatric aspects of COVID-19 pandemic: A selective review. *Asian J. Psychiatry* **2020**, *53*, 102–188. [CrossRef] [PubMed]
23. Hugon, J.; Msika, E.F.; Queneau, M.; Farid, K.; Paquet, C. Long COVID: Cognitive complaints (brain fog) and dysfunction of the cingulate cortex. *J. Neurol.* **2021**, *18*, 1–3. [CrossRef] [PubMed]
24. Anand, K.S.; Dhikav, V. Hippocampus in health and disease: An overview. *Ann. Indian Acad. Neurol.* **2012**, *15*, 239–246.
25. Moriguchi, T.; Harii, N.; Goto, J.; Harada, D.; Sugawara, H.; Takamino, J.; Ueno, M.; Sakata, H.; Kondo, K.; Myose, N.; et al. A first case of meningitis/encephalitis associated with SARS-Coronavirus-2. *Int. J. Infect. Dis.* **2020**, *94*, 55–58. [CrossRef] [PubMed]

26. Adolphs, R.; Tranel, D.; Hamann, S.; Young, A.W.; Calder, A.J.; Phelps, E.A.; Anderson, A.; Lee, G.P.; Damasio, A.R. Recognition of facial emotion in nine individuals with bilateral amygdala damage. *Neuropsychologia* **1999**, *37*, 1111–1117. [CrossRef]
27. McGaugh, J.L. The amygdala modulates the consolidation of memories of emotionally arousing experiences. *Annu. Rev. Neurosci.* **2004**, *27*, 1–28. [CrossRef]
28. Patin, A.; Pause, B.M. Human amygdala activations during nasal chemoreception. *Neuropsychologia* **2015**, *78*, 171–194. [CrossRef]
29. Zhang, S.; Cui, J.; Zhang, Z.; Wang, Y.; Liu, R.; Chen, X.; Feng, Y.; Zhou, J.; Zhou, Y.; Wang, G. Functional connectivity of amygdala subregions predicts vulnerability to depression following the COVID-19 pandemic. *J. Affect. Disord.* **2021**, *297*, 421–429. [CrossRef]
30. Uddin, L.Q.; Nomi, J.S.; Hébert-Seropian, B.; Ghaziri, J.; Boucher, O. Structure and Function of the Human Insula. *J. Clin. Neurophysiol.* **2017**, *34*, 300–306. [CrossRef]
31. Di Stefano, V.; De Angelis, M.V.; Montemitro, C.; Russo, M.; Carrarini, C.; di Giannantonio, M.; Brighina, F.; Onofrj, M.; Werring, D.J.; Simister, R. Clinical presentation of strokes confined to the insula: A systematic review of literature. *Neurol. Sci.* **2021**, *42*, 1697–1704. [CrossRef]
32. Coen, M.; Kaiser, C.; Naimi, R.; Uginet, M.; Hentsch, L.; Serratrice, J.; Allali, G. Beyond silent hypoxemia: Does COVID-19 can blunt pain perception? Comment on The neuroinvasive potential of SARS CoV2 may play a role in the respiratory failure of COVID 19 patients. *J. Med. Virol.* **2021**, *93*, 1915–1916. [CrossRef] [PubMed]
33. Leech, R.; Sharp, D.J. The role of the posterior cingulate cortex in cognition and disease. *Brain A J. Neurol.* **2014**, *137*, 12–32. [CrossRef] [PubMed]
34. Zhou, G.; Lane, G.; Cooper, S.L.; Kahnt, T.; Zelano, C. Characterizing functional pathways of the human olfactory system. *Elife* **2019**, *24*, e47177. [CrossRef]
35. Takehara-Nishiuchi, K. Entorhinal cortex and consolidated memory. *Neurosci. Res.* **2014**, *84*, 27–33. [CrossRef] [PubMed]
36. Vaughan, D.N.; Jackson, G.D. The piriform cortex and human focal epilepsy. *Front. Neurol.* **2014**, *5*, 259. [CrossRef] [PubMed]
37. Guedj, E.; Campion, J.Y.; Dudouet, P.; Kaphan, E.; Bregeon, F.; Tissot-Dupont, H.; Guis, S.; Barthelemy, F.; Habert, P.; Ceccaldi, M.; et al. 18F-FDG brain PET hypometabolism in patients with long COVID. *Eur. J. Nucl. Med. Mol. Imaging* **2021**, *48*, 2823–2833. [CrossRef]
38. Yousefi-Koma, A.; Haseli, S.; Bakhshayeshkaram, M.; Raad, N.; Karimi-Galougahi, M. Multimodality Imaging With PET/CT and MRI Reveals Hypometabolism in Tertiary Olfactory Cortex in Parosmia of COVID-19. *Acad. Radiol.* **2021**, *28*, 749–751. [CrossRef]
39. Xydakis, M.S.; Albers, M.W.; Holbrook, E.H.; Lyon, D.M.; Shih, R.Y.; Frasnelli, J.A.; Pagenstecher, A.; Kupke, A.; Enquist, L.W.; Perlman, S. Post-viral effects of COVID-19 in the olfactory system and their implications. *Lancet Neurol.* **2021**, *20*, 753–761. [CrossRef]
40. Makaronidis, J.; Firman, C.; Magee, C.G.; Mok, J.; Balogun, N.; Lechner, M.; Carnemolla, A.; Batterham, R.L. Distorted chemosensory perception and female sex associate with persistent smell and/or taste loss in people with SARS-CoV-2 antibodies: A community based cohort study investigating clinical course and resolution of acute smell and/or taste loss in people. *BMC Infect. Dis.* **2021**, *21*, 221. [CrossRef]
41. Araújo, L.; Arata, V.; Figueiredo, R.G. Olfactory Disorders in Post-Acute COVID-19 Syndrome. *Sinusitis* **2021**, *5*, 116–122. [CrossRef]
42. Mehraeen, E.; Behnezhad, F.; Salehi, M.A.; Noori, T.; Harandi, H.; SeyedAlinaghi, S. Olfactory and gustatory dysfunctions due to the coronavirus disease (COVID-19): A review of current evidence. *Eur. Arch. Otorhinolaryngol.* **2021**, *278*, 307–312. [CrossRef] [PubMed]
43. Borsetto, D.; Hopkins, C.; Philips, V.; Obholzer, R.; Tirelli, G.; Polesel, J.; Boscolo-Rizzo, P. Self-reported alteration of sense of smell or taste in patients with COVID-19: A systematic review and meta-analysis on 3563 patients. *Rhinology* **2020**, *58*, 430–436. [CrossRef] [PubMed]
44. Carrillo-Larco, R.M.; Altez-Fernandez, C. Anosmia and dysgeusia in COVID-19: A systematic review. *Wellcome Open Res.* **2020**, *13*, 594. [CrossRef] [PubMed]
45. Costa, K.V.T.D.; Carnaúba, A.T.L.; Rocha, K.W.; Andrade, K.C.L.; Ferreira, S.M.S.; Menezes, P.L. Olfactory and taste disorders in COVID-19: A systematic review. *Braz. J. Otorhinolaryngol.* **2020**, *86*, 781–792. [CrossRef]
46. Hur, K.; Choi, J.S.; Zheng, M.; Shen, J.; Wrobel, B. Association of alterations in smell and taste with depression in older adults. *Laryngoscope Investig. Otolaryngol.* **2018**, *3*, 94–99. [CrossRef]
47. Kohli, P.; Soler, Z.M.; Nguyen, S.A.; Muus, J.S.; Schlosser, R.J. The Association Between Olfaction and Depression: A Systematic Review. *Chem. Senses* **2016**, *41*, 479–486. [CrossRef]
48. Croy, I.; Nordin, S.; Hummel, T. Olfactory disorders and quality of life–an updated review. *Chem. Senses* **2014**, *39*, 185–194. [CrossRef] [PubMed]
49. Valsamidis, K.; Printza, A.; Constantinidis, J.; Triaridis, S. The Impact of Olfactory Dysfunction on the Psychological Status and Quality of Life of Patients with Nasal Obstruction and Septal Deviation. *Int. Arch. Otorhinolaryngol.* **2020**, *24*, e237–e246. [CrossRef]
50. Schablitzky, S.; Pause, B.M. Sadness might isolate you in a non-smelling world: Olfactory perception and depression. *Front. Psychol.* **2014**, *5*, 45. [CrossRef]
51. Nordin, S.; Brämerson, A. Complaints of olfactory disorders: Epidemiology, assessment and clinical implications. *Curr. Opin. Allergy Clin. Immunol.* **2008**, *8*, 10–15. [CrossRef]

52. Ahmedy, F.; Mazlan, M.; Danaee, M.; Abu Bakar, M.Z. Post-traumatic brain injury olfactory dysfunction: Factors influencing quality of life. *Eur. Arch. Oto-Rhino-Laryngol.* **2020**, *277*, 1343–1351. [CrossRef] [PubMed]
53. Pirker-Kees, A.; Platho-Elwischger, K.; Hafner, S.; Redlich, K.; Baumgartner, C. Hyposmia Is Associated with Reduced Cognitive Function in COVID-19: First Preliminary Results. *Dement. Geriatr. Cogn. Disord.* **2021**, *50*, 68–73. [CrossRef]
54. Dintica, C.S.; Marseglia, A.; Rizzuto, D.; Wang, R.; Seubert, J.; Arfanakis, K.; Bennett, D.A.; Xu, W. Impaired olfaction is associated with cognitive decline and neurodegeneration in the brain. *Neurology* **2019**, *92*, e700–e709. [CrossRef] [PubMed]
55. Graus, F.; Titulaer, M.J.; Balu, R.; Benseler, S.; Bien, C.G.; Cellucci, T.; Cortese, I.; Dale, R.C.; Gelfand, J.M.; Geschwind, M.; et al. A clinical approach to diagnosis of autoimmune encephalitis. *Lancet Neurol.* **2016**, *15*, 391–404. [CrossRef]
56. Solomatova, E.S.; Shnayder, N.A.; Molgachev, A.A.; Dmitrenko, D.V.; Strotskaya, I.G. Magnetic resonance spectroscopy of the brain in the diagnosis of temporal lobe epilepsy. *Neurol. Neuropsychiatry Psychosom.* **2018**, *10*, 51–55. [CrossRef]
57. Mehta, P.; McAuley, D.F.; Brown, M.; Sanchez, E.; Tattersall, R.S.; Manson, J.J. HLH Across Speciality Collaboration UK. COVID-19: Consider cytokine storm syndromes and immunosuppression. *Lancet* **2020**, *395*, 1033–1034. [CrossRef]
58. Perrin, P.; Collongues, N.; Baloglu, S.; Bedo, D.; Bassand, X.; Lavaux, T.; Gautier-Vargas, G.; Keller, N.; Kremer, S.; Fafi-Kremer, S.; et al. Cytokine release syndrome-associated encephalopathy in patients with COVID-19. *Eur. J. Neurol.* **2021**, *28*, 248–258. [CrossRef]
59. Popova, T.E.; Shnayder, N.A.; Petrova, M.M.; Nikolaeva, T.Y.; Kantimirova, E.A.; Isaeva, N.V.; Shnayder, V.A.; Panina, Y.S.; Dyuzhakova, A.V.; Dyuzhakov, S.K. Herpesvirus-associated central and peripheral nervous system involvement: Two clinical cases. *Neurol. Neuropsychiatry Psychosom.* **2015**, *7*, 28–34. [CrossRef]
60. Shnayder, N.A.; Panina, Y.S.; Popova, T.E. A clinical case of pseudotumorous chronic parainfectious limbic encephalitis. *Neurol. Neuropsychiatry Psychosom.* **2014**, *6*, 49–54. [CrossRef]
61. Shnayder, N.A.; Kantzalakova, N.I., Krijanovskaya, S.V.; Panina, Y.S. Perceived ways of diagnostic help optimisation to patients with symptomatic epilepsy on chronic herpesvirus encephalitis. *Epilepsy Paroxysmal Cond.* **2015**, *7*, 6–17. [CrossRef]
62. Lorigados Pedre, L.; Morales Chacón, L.M.; Pavón Fuentes, N.; Robinson Agramonte, M.L.A.; Serrano Sánchez, T.; Cruz-Xenes, R.M.; Díaz Hung, M.L.; Estupiñán Díaz, B.; Báez Martín, M.M.; Orozco-Suárez, S. Follow-Up of Peripheral IL-1β and IL-6 and Relation with Apoptotic Death in Drug-Resistant Temporal Lobe Epilepsy Patients Submitted to Surgery. *Behav. Sci.* **2018**, *8*, 21. [CrossRef]
63. Na, K.S.; Jung, H.Y.; Kim, Y.K. The role of pro-inflammatory cytokines in the neuroinflammation and neurogenesis of schizophrenia. *Prog. Neuropsychopharmacol. Biol. Psychiatry* **2014**, *48*, 277–286. [CrossRef] [PubMed]
64. Hansen, N. Long-term memory dysfunction in limbic encephalitis. *Front. Neurol.* **2019**, *10*, 330. [CrossRef] [PubMed]
65. Ng, A.; Tam, W.W.; Zhang, M.W.; Ho, C.S.; Husain, S.F.; McIntyre, R.S.; Ho, R.C. IL-1β, IL-6, TNF- α and CRP in Elderly Patients with Depression or Alzheimer's disease: Systematic Review and Meta-Analysis. *Sci. Rep.* **2018**, *8*, 12050. [CrossRef] [PubMed]
66. Panina, Y.S.; Dmitrenko, D.V.; Shnayder, N.A.; Egorova, E.V.; Usoltseva, A.A. Association of carriers of single nucleotide polymorphisms rs1143634 and rs16944 in gene Il-1B and rs6265 in gene BDNF with temporal lobe epilepsy. *Neurol. Neuropsychiatry Psychosom.* **2019**, *11*, 46–51. [CrossRef]
67. Sanchez, C.V.; Theel, E.; Binnicker, M.; Toledano, M.; McKeon, A. Autoimmune encephalitis after SARS-CoV-2 infection: Case frequency, findings, and outcomes. *Neurology* **2021**, *97*, e2262–e2268. [CrossRef]

encyclopedia

MDPI

Entry

The Increase in Addiction during COVID-19

Theodoros Daglis

Postdoctoral Research Fellow, Laboratory of Theoretical & Applied Economics, School of Applied Mathematics & Physics, Zografou Campus, National Technical University of Athens, Heroon Polytechneiou 9, 15780 Athens, Greece; theodagl4@gmail.com

Definition: The increase in addiction during COVID-19 is a condition that emerged as an aftermath of COVID-19-related events, for instance, fear of the spread of COVID-19, self-abstention from many activities, and restrictions established by the lockdown measures. This condition includes substance addictions such as drugs and alcohol but also behavioral addictions such as gambling, gaming, pornography, and smartphone and internet misuse.

Keywords: COVID-19; addiction; oppression

1. Introduction

COVID-19 has negatively affected society in many ways. The COVID-19 pandemic has caused in individuals the fear of contagion, leading to self-abstention from many social activities. Additionally, the lockdown measures limited even more citizens' activities, since only some of them were allowed, leading to even more oppression, with a physical and psychological aftermath [1]. In such difficult and prolonged periods, social and emotional closeness with relatives, colleagues, and friends are necessary [2], to adequately confront the difficult period without self-destructive practices.

Isolation can affect negatively individuals, rendering them lonely and abandoned, creating a vicious cycle of withdrawal and isolation [2]. In such cases of continuous and acute oppression, many people try to find alleviation in anti-stress behaviors. The problem is that some anti-stress behaviors are not healthy, since they may have a severe and long-term negative impact on individuals. To be more precise, many people resort to addictive practices, such as excessive gaming, gambling, illegal substances, alcohol consumption, etc. [3], since the aforementioned have a direct and short-run stress relief result, but the long-run consequences of these behaviors have a serious and negative impact on health, perpetuating a negative non-ending situation, which is termed as addiction.

Even though COVID-19 had unprecedented effects on society, many researchers in the past had highlighted the effect of crises on human behavior. There are many pieces of evidence, unveiling that the oppression caused by economic, financial, and other crises and also by unemployment make people more vulnerable to addictive behaviors [4]. In this context, it is very important to understand social phenomena that have a major impact on human societies, concealing also a probable biological or even genetic tendency of humans to addiction. A thorough examination of this specific field of study is imperative.

The present entry provides an extensive literature review for the main findings regarding addiction during COVID-19. Furthermore, the entry describes empirically the academic interest for the subject of "addiction" over the years, points out alternative investigations for this specific field of study, and, finally, concludes with some probable measures that can be taken to face such social phenomena.

2. The Addiction

"Addiction" as a term originally referred to substances and, more precisely, to drugs. In the past, the literature focused mainly on three types of substance use: (a) occasional

Citation: Daglis, T. The Increase in Addiction during COVID-19. *Encyclopedia* **2021**, *1*, 1257–1266. https://doi.org/10.3390/encyclopedia1040095

Academic Editor: Stephen Bustin

Received: 19 September 2021
Accepted: 22 November 2021
Published: 24 November 2021

controlled and/or social, (b) abuse or harmful use, and (c) addiction [5]. Based on the current literature, addiction is a biopsychosocial negative condition with its main characteristic being the compulsive engagement, in one or multiple rewarding stimuli, for instance, substances [6], or compulsive behaviors that do not include substances [7], leading to dependence from these stimuli, with negative consequences. In this context, addictions are categorized into two main groups, namely, chemical addictions, including the use of substances, and behavioral addictions, including compulsive behaviors that are repeated and persistent [8]. Addictions are often linked with many behavioral disorders [9], mental health problems [10], and psychological issues [11]. The case of addictions without the use of substances may include many compulsive and unhealthy practices, such as gambling, gaming, unhealthy sexual practices (addiction to sex), pornography, dangerous behaviors, cyber addiction or addiction to the internet [9], workaholism (addiction to work), addiction to shopping [7], etc.

Addictions exhibit some common attributes since they are characterized as a chronically relapsing disorder, including a compulsion to seek and take the substance or perform the addictive behavior, loss of control in limiting the intake or the action, and the emergence of negative emotional states, such as anxiety, irritability, or dysphoria when access to substance or addictive behavior is prevented [5,12]. Moreover, most of these problematic conditions stimulate certain parts of the brain, mainly through the "brain reward" system, affecting certain neurons, for instance, the dopamine neurons. To give an example, drugs affect the production, elimination, or release of certain neurotransmitters [13], impacting in this way the human brain and, subsequently, human behavior. In some cases, the motivation of addiction is the alleviation of painful feelings while, in others, the control or expression of feelings [14–16]. In general, there are many negative characteristics with addiction, but the most common is the paradox that the individual turns to a specific drug or addictive behavior to alleviate emotional pain, a condition that is later perpetuated, putting the person into a non-ending situation where they are eventually unable to get rid of this pain [5]. In some cases, cortical areas in the frontal lobe may become dysfunctional due to excessive and long-term addiction, which may change even the personality of the individual [13].

All of the aforementioned show the importance of the study of addiction and the necessity of measures to prevent such practices. We should highlight that not all people demonstrate the same tendency for various addictions. For instance, age is an important factor, since adolescents exhibit different characteristics than older ones [17]. In the same context, gender also plays a role, since, based on their gender, people are more prone to certain substances or addictive behaviors [18].

3. Addiction during COVID-19

In periods of extensive oppression, people try to alleviate the experienced pain, often with unhealthy and short-term relief practices. If these periods are prolonged, these practices can evolve into addiction, with long-run negative consequences. This is not a piece of unprecedented evidence. Many studies have already examined and shown that recessions provoke an increase in addictions. To be more precise, binge drinking, sporadic use of cannabis, and also heavy use of hypnotics and sedatives increase during economic recessions [19]. Furthermore, binge alcoholism is also related to unemployment levels [20].

Similarly, many researchers have examined the effect of COVID-19 in the increase in addictions. During the COVID-19 pandemic, an upward trend in substance addiction was evidenced [21]. As a result, the availability of the drug supply increased [22], and the co-existence of social isolation, mental health and economic distress, the disruption of health treatment services due to COVID-19 impacted even more this vulnerable population [23,24]. The aforementioned led to more deaths during the COVID-19 pandemic [25,26].

Moreover, through post-analysis from Twitter, certain topics were found to include interest over the difficulties of coping with alcoholism during the rising of the sales of alcohol and the attention to ongoing health crises (for instance, vaping and opioids), affordable telehealth services, the relationship between nicotine and COVID-19, concerns about gambling addiction, and changing patterns in substance misuse as drug availability varied [27].

Similarly, the COVID-19 crisis and the associated lockdown measures increased the risk of drinking alcohol [28]. Furthermore, depression symptoms and pandemic-related financial difficulties were associated with tobacco and cannabis use and also with substance co-use, even in the case of pregnant women [29]. On the other hand, there were disparities across the individuals, for instance, the gender, the smoker's residence (urban or rural areas), or the severity of the smoking history of the individual [30]. There was also a relation between the duration of the pandemic and cannabis consumption [31].

Food addiction also increased, which seems to be a uniquely meaningful phenotype, beyond the effects of body mass index (BMI) to identify the repercussions of the COVID-19 pandemic [32]. Many adults showed an increase in sugar in their diet during the COVID-19 era, since greater stress related to the pandemic increased sugar intake, drinking, food addiction symptoms, and drinking frequency [33]. Furthermore, exercise addiction was at significantly lower levels during the period post-lockdown, while eating disorder symptomology scores and leisure-time exercise significantly increased during the post-COVID-19 lockdown period [34].

COVID-19 was found to be correlated also with internet addiction [35], depression, and anxiety, with many implications [3,36], especially psychosocial ones [37]. In this context, problematic internet use and internet gaming disorders increased during the pandemic, since people and mainly young individuals, especially those limited at home, resorted to excessive gaming [38]. Furthermore, individuals infected with COVID-19 were at a higher risk for internet gaming disorder and internet addiction [39]. Moreover, a minor increase in pornography viewing was evidenced, especially during the lockdown measures [40], in addition to an increase in the misuse of social networks [41]. More analytically, problematic social media use increased during COVID-19 [42] and was linked with psychological distress and insomnia [43], and a high prevalence rate of social media addiction (SMA) was evidenced [44].

Similarly, during COVID-19, the neuroticism of individuals affected cellphone addiction through online social anxiety, while extraversion affected cellphone addiction through cyber danger beliefs [45]. There was a negative effect of COVID-19 in the problematic use of smartphones from young persons, with a negative impact on their psychological and physical health [1]. A mediator between COVID-19-related exposure and post-traumatic stress disorder (PTSD) symptoms seems to be problematic smartphone use, and, in the same context, daytime sleepiness was found to partially mediate the associations between problematic smartphone use and PTSD [46]. However, the indirect association between perceived stress and mobile phone addiction can be moderated by self-control [47]. COVID-19 phobia and COVID-19 news exposure are substantial determinants of consumers' smartphone addiction, which in turn affect mobile shopping frequency, and social influence plays an important role in moderating mobile shopping frequency for individuals who seem to experience smartphone addiction [48].

The COVID-19 pandemic has affected online trading [49] and online gambling, which is considered an addictive stress reliever [50], associated with suicide attempts in young men and women, especially when trying to cope with anxiety, life satisfaction, impulsivity, and other factors [51]. For those that showed an increase in gambling behavior, there was frequently an association with problem gambling and not simply gambling behaviors [52].

There are also alternative examinations regarding the addictive behaviors and, more precisely, gambling and excess gaming activities, for instance, through the financial investigation. The rationale is that the COVID-19-related events have made people more prone to addictive behaviors, increasing the revenues of the corresponding companies that are engaged with these activities, causing the investors to turn to these companies' stocks as they are more profitable [53]. These approaches investigated global phenomena, and data were more easily available.

Many other factors affect individuals differently, playing a significant role in the case of addiction. For instance, there is a difference concerning gender and employment regarding drug consumption [31]. There were found in many individuals symptoms of clinical anxiety and depression, while depression and anxiety symptoms that were associated with the previous trauma exposure, distress and isolation, female gender, alcohol use, and income reduction increased during COVID-19 [54]. Racial-ethnic minorities undergo a greater financial burden and also greater direct adverse effects of COVID-19, including being more concerned about contracting COVID-19, not being able to get a COVID-19 test, and knowing someone who had died from COVID-19 [55]. The cases of a report of child abuse increased during COVID-19, while there is also a differentiation with pre-COVID-19 respective reports since those during COVID-19 seemed to be more emotional or sexual than other types of abuse [56], which are conditions that may lead to addictions as well.

On the other hand, not only has COVID-19 led to an increase in addictions but also many addictions led to an increase in the risk of getting sick with COVID-19. To be more precise, the frequency of risk factors was high for people that are characterized as multi-users, who are also susceptible to worse COVID-19 prognosis [57]. Addicted people are facing many difficulties in accessing healthcare services, rendering them even more vulnerable to drugs by illegal means [26]. A difficulty in the access to the health services that was evidenced, due to treatment disruptions during the COVID-19 pandemic, made matters worse, including reduced access to harm-reduction services, opioid agonist treatment, medical professionals, withdrawal management and treatment services, shelters and housing, and food banks [58]. This decrease in the service capacity resulted in the deterioration of health issues and risky substance-use behaviors among people who use drugs. On the other hand, opioid agonist treatment take-home "carries" cited greater access and also more prescription deliveries [58].

Policymakers shifted to more inclusive approaches of co-production of recommendations. The barriers to adoption and implementation that emerged, as a result of the new regulations, included stigma, lack of integration, and overcriminalization [59]. All of the aforementioned affected negatively substance users, and the available help diminished.

Summing up, COVID-19 is related to many addictions that increased during the pandemic. Most of them include internet addiction, gaming, gambling, various drugs, alcohol, and pornography. We should note that even if this phenomenon is of global origin, not all countries and regions exhibit the same magnitude and characteristics. For instance, countries with severe government budgets also decreased the funds in the various health programs, and, similarly, those that have the highest rate of unemployment are those whose citizens are more prone to adverse consequences of crises [4]. So, not all people were affected in the same way and severity by COVID-19-related events.

As stated above, addictions are mainly categorized into two groups: chemical and behavioral addictions [8]. Based on this distinction, we summarize the literature review findings in Table 1. We should note that, in the DSM-5, only gambling addiction and internet gaming addiction are categorized as behavioral addictions [60]. However, many researchers include in the behavioral addictions many other problematic behaviors, such as food addiction, pornography addiction, social network addiction, etc. [7], which we also included in our study for completeness reasons.

Table 1. Literature review summary regarding the addictions during COVID-19.

Addiction	Type of Addiction	References
Drugs	Chemical	[21–29]
Alcohol	Chemical	[21,27–29,33,54]
Tobacco/vaping	Chemical	[21,30]
Marijuana/cannabis	Chemical	[21,31]
Internet	Behavioral	[3,35–37,39]
Smartphone	Behavioral	[1,45–48]
Gaming	Behavioral	[38,39,53]
Gambling and trading	Behavioral	[49–53]
Food and drinking	Behavioral	[32–34]
Pornography	Behavioral	[40]
Social networks	Behavioral	[41–44]

4. Scientometric Empirical Evidence

The scientific interest for specific subjects can be derived and investigated by many methods. A direct method is to examine the research volume produced each year for a specific subject by academia. In this way, we may have an overview of the total academic interest for this specific subject, unveiling the importance of this subject for the research community and society as well. More precisely, by searching the term "addiction" on the ScienceDirect page (https://www.sciencedirect.com/ (accessed on 13 September 2021)), and the PubMed page (https://pubmed.ncbi.nlm.nih.gov/ (accessed on 16 November 2021)), we illustrated the academic interest regarding this research field. In Figure 1, we may infer that, in 2018, the scientific works in the ScienceDirect page regarding addiction decreased. On the other hand, in 2019, they increased significantly, and, in 2020, they continued to increase even more. As for the respective scientific works in the PubMed page, there was an upward trend in almost all years, especially the most recent ones, and, more precisely, in 2020, there was an important increase of approximately 15%. The aforementioned evidence shows the importance of this specific field of study, namely, addiction during the COVID-19 pandemic.

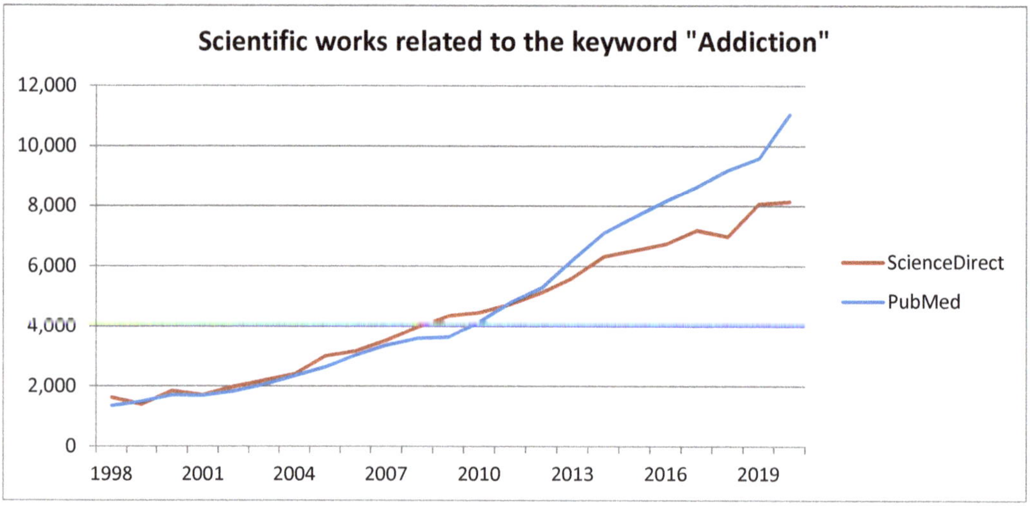

Figure 1. Plot of addiction related research works.

5. Conclusions

The present entry provided an extended literature review for addiction during COVID-19, which is a problematic and important social case that emerged from COVID-19-related events. Based on the literature, during COVID-19, many addictions increased, some of them being substance and alcohol abuse, misuse of the internet, excessive gaming, gambling, pornography, and many others. The present entry contributes to the literature by summarizing and commenting on the literature's findings, highlighting a multifaceted and global problem, which is the increase in multiple addictions during COVID-19, including evidence that most studies do not point out, since most of them are limited in specific addictions, disregarding the overall picture.

In general, in the case of addiction, many factors internal and external can co-exist affecting one another, causing many health and social problems to the individuals. This means that addiction is a multidimensional problem and does not emerge out of nowhere. An important cause for this increase is the oppression caused by the pandemic itself. The fact that during COVID-19, in multiple categories, emergency department psychiatric chief complaint prevalence increased, in comparison with the pre-COVID-19 era [61], shows that the COVID-19 pandemic has impacted significantly human psychology, leading to the search for ways to alleviate this pain, some of which may lead to severe addiction, with an even worse aftermath for the individuals. More precisely, the COVID-19 anxiety and worry, the daily stress, the degradation of the social and health support systems, the anxiety sensitivity of each individual, the probable existence of chronic diseases or psychological problems are all related to certain health and addictive behaviors that also affected the aforementioned [62]. On the other hand, some specific characteristics (e.g., ability to be resilient) can block such problematic cases; for instance, higher sensitivity is not necessarily a vulnerability factor, besides what most would expect, even during the COVID-19 pandemic, if resilience can be enhanced [63]. This evidence shows the importance of interconnection among the various factors that affect individuals.

Furthermore, another cause for the increase in addictions during COVID-19 is the vulnerability of specific individuals to such unhealthy practices. Not all people were affected in the same way and magnitude by COVID-19-related events, since many factors such as gender, income [54], and racial-ethnic minorities [55] are known to play a significant role. Besides the increase in addictive behaviors due to COVID-19, many addictive behaviors also led to an increase in the risk of getting sick with COVID-19 [57], and people with addictions are at higher risk of multimorbidity and mortality during COVID-19 [21]. This fact shows the importance of the protection of these people who may be in jeopardy. Young people seem to be more affected by technological addiction, for instance, misuse of their smartphone [1] and social media [41] and excessive gaming [38]. Moreover, some results concerning the impact of the COVID-19 on addictive behaviors had some heterogeneity; for instance, COVID-19 had a differential impact on opioid overdoses in certain US states [64], implying that further and more thorough research is needed to have a whole picture.

The social [65] and psychological [66] impacts of COVID-19 for the individuals are of great concern and should not be overseen, since COVID-19 has affected in numerous ways the individuals, for instance, their behavior, or even the way home attachment is perceived by individuals [67]. This can be justified by an increase in domestic violence and unhealthy lifestyle behaviors evidenced during the COVID-19 pandemic [68]. All of these led to a further increase in addictions.

Even though the problem is of great magnitude, it is important to have some lessons from the pandemic itself. In cases that physical touch is difficult, for instance, during lockdown measures, telemedicine could be better utilized, since, during the pandemic, health services were provided very effectively [69]. This fact shows that even in cases of emergency, some actions can help so that the impact will be less intense.

Moreover, the government can play an important role. First, increasing the government budgets for health and other social benefits could alleviate the psychological pain from individuals, so that they will not turn to unhealthy practices. Second, the governmental and local institutions could construct appropriate places for outdoor activities, such as swimming and running facilities, since these activities have been shown to affect human psychology positively [70], and render them available free of charge so that more people could have access to them. Finally, many associations could promote athletic activities for the social good, highlighting the positive effects on health.

Furthermore, the COVID-19 pandemic showed that more can be done regarding technological progress, so that people can have access to education and other important activities, as well. Many new tools and interactive teaching methods emerged during the COVID-19 era since there was a need for their utilization in education [71]. Such cases were the virtual laboratories (VLs) that were based on the use of virtual reality (VR), making it feasible and also facilitating the teaching and learning process in a wide range of training activities [71]. As for video games, even though there are drawbacks, for instance, a decrease in sleep duration, an increase in obesity, vision problems [72,73], etc., if the game's content promotes good social behaviors, they can contribute to the social good [74]. Moreover, there are also games that, apart from the social contribution, can promote physical health [75]. In the same context, since many games related to addiction and other dangerous behaviors have been constructed [76], trying to help people and especially adolescents acknowledge the importance of their choices and also the probable aftermath of such behaviors, virtual reality could be utilized in these video games, helping them communicate in a better and more realistic way the problematic conditions associated with addiction.

In conclusion, further analytical study is needed, including interpersonal (qualitative) and local-global (quantitative) studies to cross-validate and analyze the many implications that not only exist but that are also interconnected in a complex system. The case of the COVID-19 pandemic affected even more a problem that already existed and did not cause it out of nowhere.

Funding: This research received no external funding.

Institutional Review Board Statement: This research did not involve humans or animals.

Informed Consent Statement: This research did not involve humans or animals.

Conflicts of Interest: The author has no conflict of interest to declare.

Entry Link on the Encyclopedia Platform: https://encyclopedia.pub/18550.

References

1. Jin, L.; Hao, Z.; Huang, J.; Akram, H.R.; Saeed, M.F.; Ma, H. Depression and anxiety symptoms are associated with problematic smartphone use under the COVID-19 epidemic: The mediation models. *Child. Youth Serv. Rev.* **2020**, *121*, 105875. [CrossRef]
2. Ventriglio, A.; Watson, C.; Bhugra, D. Pandemics, panic and prevention: Stages in the life of COVID-19 pandemic. *Int. J. Soc. Psychiatry* **2020**, *66*, 733–734. [CrossRef]
3. Király, O.; Potenza, M.N.; Stein, D.J.; King, D.L.; Hodgins, D.C.; Saunders, J.B.; Griffiths, M.D.; Gjoneska, B.; Billieux, J.; Brand, M.; et al. Preventing problematic internet use during the COVID-19 pandemic: Consensus guidance. *Compr. Psychiatry* **2020**, *100*, 152180. [CrossRef] [PubMed]
4. Dubanowicz, A.; Lemmens, P. Chapter 8: Impact of the economic recession on addiction-prone behaviors. In *The Impact of Addictive Substances and Behaviours on Individual and Societal Well-Being*; Anderson, P., Rehm, J., Room, R., Eds.; Oxford University Press: Oxford, UK, 2015.
5. Koob, F.G.; Le Moal, M. *Neurobiology of Addiction*; Elsevier: Amsterdam, The Netherlands, 2006.
6. American Psychiatric Association. *Diagnostic and Statistical Manual of Mental Disorders*, 4th ed.; American Psychiatric Press: Washington, DC, USA, 1994.
7. Semaille, P. The new types of addiction. *Rev. Med. Brux.* **2009**, *30*, 335–357.
8. Raypole, C.; Legg, T.J. (Medically Reviewed) Types of Addiction and How They're Treated 2020. Available online: https://www.healthline.com/health/types-of-addiction#treating-behavioral-addiction (accessed on 21 November 2021).
9. Johnson, F.N. *The Multiplicities of Internet Addiction: The Misrecognition of Leisure and Learning*; Ashgate: Farnam, UK, 2009.
10. Chou, W.-P.; Lee, K.-H.; Ko, C.-H.; Liu, T.-L.; Hsiao, R.C.; Lin, H.-F.; Yen, C.-F. Relationship between psychological inflexibility and experiential avoidance and internet addiction: Mediating effects of mental health problems. *Psychiatry Res.* **2017**, *257*, 40–44. [CrossRef] [PubMed]

11. Liu, F.; Zhang, Z.; Chen, L. Mediating effect of neuroticism and negative coping style in relation to childhood psychological maltreatment and smartphone addiction among college students in China. *Child Abus. Negl.* **2020**, *106*, 104531. [CrossRef] [PubMed]
12. Koob, G.F.; Le Moal, M. Drug Abuse: Hedonic Homeostatic Dysregulation. *Science* **1997**, *278*, 52–58. [CrossRef]
13. Stoehr, D.J. *The Neurobiology of Addiction*; Chelsea House Publishers: Philadelfea, PA, USA, 2006.
14. Khantzian, E.J. The 1994 distinguished lecturer in substance abuse. *J. Subst. Abus. Treat.* **1995**, *12*, 157–165. [CrossRef]
15. Khantzian, E.J. The Self-Medication Hypothesis of Substance Use Disorders: A Reconsideration and Recent Applications. *Harv. Rev. Psychiatry* **1997**, *4*, 231–244. [CrossRef]
16. Khantzian, E.J.; Wilson, A. Substance abuse, repetition, and the nature of addictive suffering. In *Hierarchical Concepts in Psychoanalysis: Theory, Research, and Clinical Practice*; Wilson, A., Gedo, J.E., Eds.; Guilford Press: New York, NY, USA, 1993; pp. 263–283.
17. Essau, A.C. *Adolescent Addiction: Epidemiology, Assessment and Treatment (Practical Resources for the Mental Health Professional)*; Elsevier: Amsterdam, The Netherlands, 2008.
18. Charzyńska, E.; Sussman, S.; Atroszko, P.A. Profiles of potential behavioral addictions' severity and their associations with gender, personality, and well-being: A person-centered approach. *Addict. Behav.* **2021**, *119*, 106941. [CrossRef]
19. Colell, E.; Sanchez-Niubo, A.; Delclos, G.L.; Benavides, F.G.; Domingo-Salvany, A. Economic crisis and changes in drug use in the Spanish economically active population. *Addiction* **2015**, *110*, 1129–1137. [CrossRef]
20. Dávalos, M.E.; Fang, H.; French, M.T. Easing the pain of an economic downturn: Macroeconomic conditions and excessive alcohol consumption. *Health Econ.* **2011**, *21*, 1318–1335. [CrossRef]
21. Mallet, J.; Dubertret, C.; Le Strata, Y. Addictions in the COVID-19 era: Current evidence, future perspectives a comprehensive review. *Prog. Neuropsychopharmacol. Biol. Psychiatry* **2021**, *106*, 110070. [CrossRef] [PubMed]
22. Linas, B.P.; Savinkina, A.; Barbosa, C.; Mueller, P.P.; Cerdá, M.; Keyes, K.; Chhatwal, J. A clash of epidemics: Impact of the COVID-19 pandemic response on opioid overdose. *J. Subst. Abus. Treat.* **2020**, *120*, 108158. [CrossRef]
23. Cisneros, I.; Cunningham, K. COVID-19 interface with drug misuse and substance use disorders. *Neuropharmacology* **2021**, *198*, 108766. [CrossRef] [PubMed]
24. Nguyen, T.; Buxton, J.A. Pathways between COVID-19 public health responses and increasing overdose risks: A rapid review and conceptual framework. *Int. J. Drug Policy* **2021**, *93*, 103236. [CrossRef] [PubMed]
25. Slavova, S.; Rock, P.; Bush, H.M.; Quesinberry, D.; Walsh, S.L. Signal of increased opioid overdose during COVID-19 from emergency medical services data. *Drug Alcohol Depend.* **2020**, *214*, 108176. [CrossRef]
26. Dubey, M.J.; Ghosh, R.; Chatterjee, S.; Biswas, P.; Chatterjee, S.; Dubey, S. COVID-19 and addiction. *Diabetes Metab. Syndr. Clin. Res. Rev.* **2020**, *14*, 817–823. [CrossRef]
27. Glowacki, E.M.; Wilcox, G.B.; Glowacki, J.B. Identifying # addiction concerns on twitter during the COVID-19 pandemic: A text mining analysis. *Subst. Abus.* **2020**, *42*, 39–46. [CrossRef]
28. Daly, M.; Robinson, E. High-Risk Drinking in Midlife Before Versus During the COVID-19 Crisis: Longitudinal Evidence From the United Kingdom. *Am. J. Prev. Med.* **2020**, *60*, 294–297. [CrossRef]
29. Kar, P.; Tomfohr-Madsen, L.; Giesbrecht, G.; Bagshawe, M.; Lebel, C. Alcohol and substance use in pregnancy during the COVID-19 pandemic. *Drug Alcohol Depend.* **2021**, *225*, 108760. [CrossRef]
30. Yang, H.; Ma, J. How the COVID-19 pandemic impacts tobacco addiction: Changes in smoking behavior and associations with well-being. *Addict. Behav.* **2021**, *119*, 106917. [CrossRef]
31. Levy, I.; Cohen-Louck, K.; Bonny-Noach, H. Gender, employment, and continuous pandemic as predictors of alcohol and drug consumption during the COVID-19. *Drug Alcohol Depend.* **2021**, *228*, 109029. [CrossRef]
32. Schulte, E.M.; Kral, T.V.; Allison, K.C. A cross-sectional examination of reported changes to weight, eating, and activity behaviors during the COVID-19 pandemic among United States adults with food addiction. *Appetite* **2021**, *168*, 105740. [CrossRef] [PubMed]
33. Cummings, J.R.; Ackerman, J.M.; Wolfson, J.A.; Gearhardt, A.N. COVID-19 stress and eating and drinking behaviors in the United States during the early stages of the pandemic. *Appetite* **2021**, *162*, 105163. [CrossRef] [PubMed]
34. Trott, M.; Johnstone, J.; Pardhan, S.; Barnett, Y.; Smith, L. Changes in body dysmorphic disorder, eating disorder, and exercise addiction symptomology during the COVID-19 pandemic: A longitudinal study of 319 health club users. *Psychiatry Res.* **2021**, *298*, 113831. [CrossRef] [PubMed]
35. IIslam, M.S.; Sujan, M.S.H.; Tasnim, R.; Ferdous, M.Z.; Masud, J.H.B.; Kundu, S.; Mosaddek, A.S.M.; Choudhuri, M.S.K.; Kircaburun, K.; Griffiths, M.D. Problematic internet use among young and adult population in Bangladesh: Correlates with lifestyle and online activities during the COVID-19 pandemic. *Addict. Behav. Rep.* **2020**, *12*, 100311. [CrossRef] [PubMed]
36. Servidio, R.; Bartolo, M.G.; Palermiti, A.L.; Costabile, A. Fear of COVID-19, depression, anxiety, and their association with Internet addiction disorder in a sample of Italian students. *J. Affect. Disord. Rep.* **2021**, *4*, 100097. [CrossRef]
37. Ozturk, F.O.; Ayaz-Alkaya, S. Internet addiction and psychosocial problems among adolescents during the COVID-19 pandemic: A cross-sectional study. *Arch. Psychiatr. Nurs.* **2021**, *35*, 595–601. [CrossRef]
38. López-Cabarcos, M.A.; Ribeiro-Soriano, D.; Piñeiro-Chousa, J. All that glitters is not gold. The rise of gaming in the COVID-19 pandemic. *J. Innov. Knowl.* **2020**, *5*, 289–296. [CrossRef]

39. Oka, T.; Hamamura, T.; Miyake, Y.; Kobayashi, N.; Honjo, M.; Kawato, M.; Kubo, T.; Chiba, T. Prevalence and risk factors of internet gaming disorder and problematic internet use before and during the COVID-19 pandemic: A large online survey of Japanese adults. *J. Psychiatr. Res.* **2021**, *142*, 218–225. [CrossRef] [PubMed]
40. Sallie, S.N.; Ritou, V.J.E.; Bowden-Jones, H.; Voon, V. Assessing online gaming and pornography consumption patterns during COVID-19 isolation using an online survey: Highlighting distinct avenues of problematic internet behavior. *Addict. Behav.* **2021**, *123*, 107044. [CrossRef]
41. Gómez-Galán, J.; Martínez-López, J.; Lázaro-Pérez, C.; Sánchez-Serrano, J.S. Social Networks Consumption and Addiction in College Students during the COVID-19 Pandemic: Educational Approach to Responsible Use. *Sustainability* **2020**, *12*, 7737. [CrossRef]
42. Kalpana, V. Impact of social media use (SMU) on mental health during COVID-19 pandemic, Letter to the Editor. *Asian J. Psychiatry* **2021**, *63*, 102767.
43. Lin, C.Y.; Broströmb, A.; Griffithsd, M.D.; Pakpour, A.H. Investigating mediated effects of fear of COVID-19 and COVID-19 misunderstanding in the association between problematic social media use, psychological distress, and insomnia. *Internet Interv.* **2020**, *21*, 100345. [CrossRef]
44. Luo, T.; Chen, W.; Liao, Y. Social media use in China before and during COVID-19: Preliminary results from an online retrospective survey. *J. Psychiatr. Res.* **2021**, *140*, 35–38. [CrossRef] [PubMed]
45. Zhan, Z.; Wei, Q.; Hong, J.-C. Cellphone addiction during the COVID-19 outbreak: How online social anxiety and cyber danger belief mediate the influence of personality. *Comput. Hum. Behav.* **2021**, *121*, 106790. [CrossRef]
46. Hu, T.; Wang, Y.; Lin, L.; Tang, W. The mediating role of daytime sleepiness between problematic smartphone use and post-traumatic symptoms in COVID-19 home-refined adolescents. *Child. Youth Serv. Rev.* **2021**, *126*, 106012. [CrossRef]
47. Peng, Y.; Zhou, H.; Zhang, B.; Mao, H.; Hu, R.; Jiang, H. Perceived stress and Mobile phone addiction among college students during the 2019 coronavirus disease: The mediating roles of rumination and the moderating role of self-control. *Pers. Individ. Differ.* **2021**, *185*, 111222. [CrossRef]
48. Chopdar, K.P.; Paul, J.; Prodanova, J. Mobile shoppers' response to COVID-19 phobia, pessimism and smartphone addiction: Does social influence matter? *Technol. Forecast. Soc. Chang.* **2022**, *174*, 121249. [CrossRef]
49. Chiah, M.; Zhong, A. Trading from home: The impact of COVID-19 on trading volume around the world. *Financ. Res. Lett.* **2020**, *37*, 101784. [CrossRef]
50. Wardle, H.; Degenhardt, L.; Ceschia, A.; Saxena, S. The Lancet Public Health. Gambling: A neglected public health issue. *Lancet Public Health* **2021**, *6*, e2–e3. [CrossRef]
51. Wardle, H.; McManus, S. Suicidality and gambling among young adults in Great Britain: Results from a cross-sectional online survey. *Lancet Public Health* **2021**, *6*, e39–e49. [CrossRef]
52. Brodeur, M.; Audette-Chapdelaine, S.; Savard, A.C.; Kairouz, S. Gambling and the COVID-19 pandemic: A scoping review. *Prog. Neuropsychopharmacol. Biol. Psychiatry* **2021**, *111*, 110389. [CrossRef]
53. Daglis, T. The excessive gaming and gambling during COVID-19. *J. Econ. Stud.* **2021**. ahead-of-print. [CrossRef]
54. Blithikioti, C.; Nuño, L.; Paniello, B.; Gual, A.; Miquel, L. Impact of COVID-19 lockdown on individuals under treatment for substance use disorders: Risk factors for adverse mental health outcomes. *J. Psychiatr. Res.* **2021**, *139*, 47–53. [CrossRef]
55. Mistler, C.B.; Sullivan, M.C.; Copenhaver, M.M.; Meyer, J.P.; Roth, A.M.; Shenoi, S.V.; Edelman, E.J.; Wickersham, J.A.; Shrestha, R. Differential impacts of COVID-19 across racial-ethnic identities in persons with opioid use disorder. *J. Subst. Abus. Treat.* **2021**, *129*, 108387. [CrossRef]
56. Alenezi, S.; Alnamnakani, M.; Temsah, M.-H.; Murshid, R.; Alfahad, F.; Alqurashi, H.; Alonazy, H.; Alothman, M.; Aleissa, M.A. Evaluation of the impact of the COVID-19 pandemic on the reporting of maltreatment cases to the National Family Safety Program in Saudi Arabia. *Child Abus. Negl.* **2021**, *122*, 105297. [CrossRef]
57. Benzano, D.; Ornell, F.; Schuch, B.J.; Pechansky, F.; Sordi, O.A.; von Diemen, L.; Kessler, P.H.F. Clinical vulnerability for severity and mortality by COVID-19 among users of alcohol and other substances. *Psychiatry Res.* **2021**, *300*, 113915. [CrossRef] [PubMed]
58. Russell, C.; Ali, F.; Nafeh, F.; Rehm, J.; Le Blanc, S.; Elton-Marshall, T. Identifying the impacts of the COVID-19 pandemic on service access for people who use drugs (PWUD): A national qualitative study. *J. Subst. Abus. Treat.* **2021**, *129*, 108374. [CrossRef]
59. Henry, B.F.; Campbell, A.; Hunt, T.; Johnson, J.K.; Mandavia, A.D.; Chaple, M.; Arout, C.; Wu, E.; Pincus, H.A.; Nunes, E.V.; et al. COVID-19 related substance use services policy changes: Policymaker perspectives on policy development & implementation. *J. Subst. Abus. Treat.* **2021**. pre-print. [CrossRef]
60. American Psychiatric Association. *Diagnostic and Statistical Manual of Mental Disorders (DSM-5)*; American Psychiatric Publishing: Washington, DC, USA, 2013.
61. Janoczkin, A.; Kiers, S.; Edara, N.; He, P.; Li, Y. Impact of COVID-19 pandemic on emergency psychiatry-Millcreek community hospital, Erie, PA. *Compr. Psychiatry* **2021**, *110*, 152255. [CrossRef]
62. Zvolensky, M.J.; Gareya, L.; Rogersa, A.H.; Schmidtd, N.B.; Vujanovica, A.A.; Storche, E.A.; Bucknerf, J.D.; Paulusg, D.J.; Alfanoa, C.; Smitsh, J.A.J.; et al. Psychological, addictive, and health behavior implications of the COVID-19 pandemic. *Behav. Res. Ther.* **2020**, *134*, 103715. [CrossRef]
63. Limura, S. Sensory-processing sensitivity and COVID-19 stress in a young population: The mediating role of resilience. *Personal. Individ. Differ.* **2022**, *184*, 111183.

64. Root, E.D.; Slavova, S.; LaRochelle, M.; Feaster, D.J.; Villani, J.; Defiore-Hyrmer, J.; El-Bassel, N.; Ergas, R.; Gelberg, K.; Jackson, R.; et al. The impact of the national stay-at-home order on emergency department visits for suspected opioid overdose during the first wave of the COVID-19 pandemic. *Drug Alcohol Depend.* **2021**, *228*, 108977. [CrossRef]
65. Devine-Wright, P.; Pinto di Carvalho, L.; Di Masso, A.; Lewicka, M.; Manzo, L.; Williams, D. "Re-placed"—Reconsidering relationships with place and lessons from a pandemic. *J. Environ. Psychol.* **2020**, *72*, 101502. [CrossRef]
66. Meléndez, J.C.; Satorres, E.; Reyes-Olmedo, M.; Delhom, I.; Real, E.; Lora, Y. Emotion recognition changes in a confinement situation due to COVID-19. *J. Environ. Psychol.* **2020**, *72*, 101518. [CrossRef]
67. Meagher, R.B.; Cheadle, D.A. Distant from others, but close to home: The relationship between home attachment and mental health during COVID-19. *J. Environ. Psychol.* **2020**, *72*, 101516. [CrossRef]
68. Pakenham, K.I.; Landi, G.; Boccolini, G.; Furlani, A.; Grandi, S.; Tossani, E. The moderating roles of psychological flexibility and inflexibility on the mental health impacts of COVID-19 pandemic and lockdown in Italy. *J. Context. Behav. Sci.* **2020**, *17*, 109–118. [CrossRef]
69. Barney, A.; Buckelew, S.; Mesheriakova, V.; Raymond-Flesch, M. The COVID-19 Pandemic and Rapid Implementation of Adolescent and Young Adult Telemedicine: Challenges and Opportunities for Innovation. *J. Adolesc. Health* **2020**, *67*, 164–171. [CrossRef]
70. Buckley, R.C.; Brough, P.; Westaway, D. Bringing Outdoor Therapies into Mainstream Mental Health. *Front. Public Health* **2018**, *6*, 119. [CrossRef]
71. Vergara, D.; Fernández-Arias, P.; Extremera, J.; Dávila, L.P.; Rubio, M.P. Educational trends post COVID-19 in engineering: Virtual laboratories. *Mater. Today Proc.* **2021**. pre-print. [CrossRef]
72. Foti, K.E.; Eaton, D.K.; Lowry, R.; McKnight-Ely, L.R. Sufficient Sleep, Physical Activity, and Sedentary Behaviors. *Am. J. Prev. Med.* **2011**, *41*, 596–602. [CrossRef] [PubMed]
73. Straker, L.; Abbott, R.; Collins, R.; Campbell, A. Evidence-based guidelines for wise use of electronic games by children. *Ergonomics* **2014**, *57*, 471–489. [CrossRef] [PubMed]
74. Greitemeyer, T.; Mügge, D.O. Video games do affect social outcomes: A meta-analytic review of the effects of violent and prosocial video game play. *Pers. Soc. Psychol. Bull.* **2014**, *40*, 578–589. [CrossRef]
75. Williams, W.M.; Ayres, C.G. Can Active Video Games Improve Physical Activity in Adolescents? A Review of RCT. *Int. J. Environ. Res. Public Health* **2020**, *17*, 669. [CrossRef]
76. Dörner, R.; Göbel, S.; Effelsberg, W.; Wiemeyer, J. *Serious Games—Foundations. Concepts and Practice*; Springer: Berlin/Heidelberg, Germany, 2016; pp. 363–365.

encyclopedia

MDPI

Entry

Misinformation about COVID-19: Psychological Insights

Elly Anastasiades *, Marios Argyrides and Marilena Mousoulidou *

Department of Psychology, Neapolis University Pafos, 2, Danae Avenue, Paphos 8042, Cyprus; m.argyrides.1@nup.ac.cy
* Correspondence: e.loizou@nup.ac.cy (E.A.); marilena.mousoulidou@nup.ac.cy (M.M.)

Definition: While the precise conceptualization of the term misinformation remains a subject of debate, the current entry defines misinformation as any type of information which is misleading or false, regardless of intent. The COVID-19 pandemic has seen the rapid and widespread sharing of misinformation on a global scale, which has had detrimental effects on containment efforts and public health. This entry offers psychological insights to better our understanding of what makes people susceptible to believing and sharing misinformation and how this can inform interventions aimed at tackling the issue.

Keywords: misinformation; fake news; social media; COVID-19; social cognition; public health

Citation: Anastasiades, E.; Argyrides, M.; Mousoulidou, M. Misinformation about COVID-19: Psychological Insights. *Encyclopedia* **2021**, *1*, 1200–1214. https://doi.org/10.3390/encyclopedia1040091

Academic Editor: Stephen Bustin

Received: 5 October 2021
Accepted: 11 November 2021
Published: 15 November 2021

1. Introduction

December 2019 saw the emergence of SARS-CoV-2, a novel virus causing the coronavirus disease (COVID-19), which spread aggressively and rapidly across the globe. By 11 March 2020, the World Health Organization (WHO) had declared the outbreak a pandemic, and by 18 September 2021, there were over 226 million cases of COVID-19 and 4.7 million deaths reported worldwide [1]. This global crisis was paralleled by the widespread sharing of both scientific and non-scientific information surrounding COVID-19 across multiple media channels. For the first time in history, social media and technology were being used on a huge scale by public health authorities and other institutions to keep people informed, safe, and connected. Social media and technology played an essential role in the response to the pandemic, for instance, through the implementation and promotion of public health measures, the tracking and mapping of symptoms, as well as the prediction of outbreaks in real-time. At the same time, however, this same technology also facilitated the overabundant spreading of information from uninformed sources, not all of which were accurate and reliable. The global scale of the pandemic amplified this spreading as people urgently sought out and shared information in an effort to protect themselves, their families, and their communities against the virus [2].

On 15 February 2020, T.A. Ghebreyesus, the Director-General of WHO, announced the concern that the omnipresence and overabundance of often conflicting and inaccurate information posed a significant challenge for public health and was jeopardizing the response to the pandemic [3]. WHO declared that the world was facing what they termed an infodemic; "an overabundance of information, some accurate and some not, that makes it hard for people to find trustworthy sources and reliable guidance when they need it" [4] (p. 2). The COVID-19 infodemic saw the spread of information concerning the origin and cause of the virus and disease, the transmission of the virus and symptoms of the disease, available prophylactics, treatments and cures, and the impact and efficacy of interventions by public health authorities or other institutions [4]. Amongst this information was fake news, misinformation, disinformation, and conspiracy theories, which caused many to mistrust reliable sources of information and develop a distorted risk perception of the virus [5,6]. Due to this, people were less likely to adopt preventative public health behaviors, which had an adverse effect on the implementation and efficacy of containment strategies [5,7].

The management of the infodemic was soon publicly recognized by WHO as a crucial part of the response to COVID-19 [3]. On 29 June 2020, WHO held its first global infodemiology conference [8], which led to the publication of the WHO Public Health Research Agenda for Managing Infodemics [9]. In this publication, WHO identified a need for research in the field of psychology to identify factors that make people more likely to share or believe inaccurate information [9]. Understanding these factors can inform and enhance the development of innovative and creative interventions aimed at infodemic management.

This entry begins with a description of what constitutes fake news, misinformation, and disinformation, explores cases from the COVID-19 infodemic and considers the effect this has had on the societal response to the pandemic. It then goes on to explore the main psychological factors that have been found to play a role in the believability of misinformation and the role of sharing behavior. The entry ends with a description of interventions aimed at addressing misinformation.

2. Fake News, Misinformation, Disinformation, and COVID-19

The sharing of fake news is not something new. A classic example dates back to 1835 when a series of fabricated articles reporting the discovery of life and civilization on the moon was published by The Sun Newspaper in New York [10]. The mid-1890s saw a surge in fake news, when two major newspapers; W.R. Hearst's New York Journal, and J. Pulitzer's New York World competed for readers by prioritizing sensationalism over accuracy [11]. The promotion of fake news facilitated its circulation on a mass scale, a strategy which was soon adopted by other newspapers in their attempt to gain popularity. This soon came to be known as yellow journalism [11]. Another instance began in 1933, when the Nazi government founded the Reichsministerium für Volksaufklärung und Propaganda (RMVP) to enforce Nazi ideology through the spread of carefully choreographed propaganda [12]. A similar strategy was employed by the Soviet Union, with the establishment of a unit specializing in the manufacture and dissemination of disinformation in an attempt to influence political attitudes and public opinion [13]. The sharing of fake news has also played an influential role in public health issues over the years. For instance, in 1918, fake news surrounding the emergence of the H1N1 Influenza A virus led to it being coined the Spanish flu despite no evidence of it having originated from Spain at all [14]. This had significant detrimental economic and psychosocial consequences due to stigmatization [14,15].

Although the sharing of fake news is nothing new, the proliferation and democratization of social media has provided a principle conduit allowing it to spread more rapidly than ever before. With this has come accelerated growth in public and scientific interest, with the term since being referred to as a global buzzword [16,17].

2.1. *Defining Fake News, Misinformation, and Disinformation*

No consensus definition of fake news currently exists [18], although various definitions have been proposed. Fake news has been referred to as news which "aesthetically resembles actual legitimate mainstream news content but that is fabricated or extremely inaccurate" [19] (p. 389) and as "false information masquerading as verifiable truth" [20] (p. 735). Based on a review of the literature, Tandoc et al. [17] proposed a typology of fake news, defining it as news satire, news parody, fabrication, manipulation, propaganda, and advertising. A similar conceptualization was proposed by Waszak et al. [21], who added to this the idea that fake news is often irrelevant. Shu et al. [18] characterized fake news as having the intent to deceive and a verifiable lack of authenticity.

The terms misinformation and disinformation are widely used in research on fake news [16]. However, the way in which these terms are used varies. Some have used the terms to distinguish false information that is spread intentionally from that which is spread unintentionally, for example, referring to misinformation as the "inadvertent sharing of false information" and disinformation as the "deliberate creation and sharing of information known to be false" [22]. More specifically, misinformation has been referred to as the publishing of "wrong information without meaning to be wrong or having a political purpose in communicating false information", and disinformation as "manipulating and misleading people intentionally to achieve political ends" [23] (p. 24). At the same time, some have used the terms interchangeably [24,25], and others have used misinformation to mean all kinds of misleading information and disinformation to mean only that which is intentionally misleading [26,27]. In line with this, and for the purposes of this entry, the term misinformation is used to encompass all types of misleading or false information, regardless of intent.

2.2. The Role of Technology and Social Media

Advances in technology have redefined the way in which information is published, spread, and accessed [23,28]. Hardware devices, such as smartphones and tablets, are becoming more and more affordable, removing financial barriers, and allowing easier access to a variety of tools [29]. A notebook in 2001, for instance, was priced at $2200, and in 2020, a similar device was priced at just $350 [29]. As a result, the accessibility to technology is rapidly and continually increasing in what has come to be known as the democratization of technology. At the same time, technology is becoming increasingly user-friendly, providing a variety of tools in which good quality content can be easily created. Content that is of higher quality is more likely to be perceived to be from a more reliable source, and thus is more likely to be believed [30]. Using technology, such content can be instantaneously uploaded and shared online, through one of the many popular, easily accessible, free-of-charge, social media platforms, for instance. The democratization of technology therefore plays a pivotal role in the exchange and spread of misinformation.

Social media platforms, in particular, have provided an efficient, user-friendly, highly accessible tool that allows for the high-speed and cross-platform publishing and sharing of information without being vetted and at no cost [28,31]. Social media has recently been referred to as a "powerful source for fake news dissemination" [18] (p. 23). A survey carried out by the Pew Research Centre found just over half (53%) of U.S. adults get their news from social media, with Facebook, YouTube, Twitter, and Instagram being the most popular platforms of choice [32]. In addition to changing the way that news is spread, technology has also impacted the way news looks, with tweets (a written message shared on Twitter that is a maximum of 140 characters long) being considered as significant news [17]. Another critical factor to consider in the spreading of misinformation is that most social media posts are accompanied by popularity ratings (e.g., likes, shares, and comments). The more popular a post appears to be, the more attention it receives, and the more likely it is to be liked, shared, and commented on, regardless of how accurate the information is [33]. Indeed, misinformation has been found to outperform accurate information when it comes to engagement and popularity [34]. The repeated sharing of posts on and between social media platforms poses a further challenge, as it makes it more difficult for users to determine the proximate source of the information [34]. What results is an online environment with an infinitely and rapidly flowing stream of posts, some with accurate information and others with inaccurate, varying in their appearance and level of detail, with a wide range of popularity ratings and often indistinguishable sources. This makes it very challenging for people to distinguish accurate from inaccurate information.

2.3. Misinformation during the COVID-19 Pandemic

The COVID-19 pandemic provided the ideal conditions that allowed misinformation surrounding the virus to thrive; high fear, low trust, and low confidence [35]. As a result, social media platforms were inundated with shared misinformation about the virus [36–38]. For instance, it was found that over 25% of the most viewed YouTube videos relating to COVID-19 (with over 62 million views worldwide) contained misinformation [39]. Other research found that 46% of the U.K. population [40] and 48% of the U.S. population [41] reported being exposed to misinformation surrounding COVID-19, with 66% of those exposed reporting repeated exposure daily [42].

Misinformation about COVID-19 ranged from conspiracy theories that the virus was bioengineered in a lab in Wuhan, China [43], to the promotion of fake cures such as adding pepper to meals, drinking or injecting oneself with bleach, and gargling lemon and salt water [44], or that the symptoms of COVID-19 were exacerbated by the 5G cellular network [45]. Another prevailing narrative claimed the virus was being used by B. Gates to enforce a global vaccination program and surveillance regime [35]. One of the most widespread examples of COVID-19 related misinformation was Plandemic, a conspiracy film that promoted anti-scientific health advice such as to avoid wearing masks since they activate the virus [46]. Even political leaders were contributing to the spreading of fake news, despite having access to official information. For instance, both U.S. President D. Trump and Brazilian President J. Bolsonaro actively promoted hydroxychloroquine as an effective treatment against the virus despite the lack of scientific evidence on the efficacy of the drug [47]. This illustrates how the veracity of misinformation is often difficult to determine, as it is not always blatant. For instance, even though there is no conclusive evidence, hydroxychloroquine is actually being studied as a potential treatment for COVID-19 [48].

2.4. Effects of Misinformation on the Societal Response to COVID-19

The detrimental effect of misinformation surrounding the COVID-19 pandemic has been made evident by the societal response on the behavioral level [5]. Numerous events and behaviors demonstrated the extent of the believability of misinformation, with uninformed opinion and conspiracy theories often being falsely equated to scientific evidence [20]. Research has shown that believing misinformation interferes with perceptions of the seriousness of COVID-19, which causes the underestimation of the risk posed by the virus [6]. As risk perception has been found to be significantly associated with the adoption of preventative health behaviors [7], this might partially explain why so many failed to adhere to the recommended guidelines for the containment of the virus (e.g., frequent hand washing and social distancing) [49,50], and are hesitant to receive the vaccine [50,51]. An additional factor in explaining this behavior might be the increased propensity to mistrust information from expert sources that is associated with believing misinformation [50,52], leading to the adoption of avoidance behaviors over health-protective behaviors [53]. Misinformation surrounding COVID-19 has also encouraged many to try dangerous treatments with severe health consequences. For instance, the myth that COVID-19 can be cured by drinking highly concentrated alcohol led many to follow this information, resulting in over 5800 hospitalizations, 60 cases of blindness, and 800 deaths worldwide [54].

Besides influencing health behaviors, misinformation has also led to the stigmatization of various groups of people, such as the Chinese, who have faced discrimination due to biased and misleading media coverage [55]. "China Kids Stay at Home" [56] and "China is the Real Sick Man of Asia" [57] were amongst some of the headlines promoted by influential news companies worldwide. As a result, the Chinese have faced racial discrimination, unequal treatment, and social isolation, having negative psychological consequences, including stress and anxiety [58]. This discrimination was not limited to Chinese but extended to Asians more generally. For instance, between 19 March 2020, and 15 April 2020, 1497 instances of COVID-19-related discrimination against Asian-Americans were reported to the Asian Pacific Policy and Planning Council in the U.S. [59]. These included hate crimes such as the attempted murder and stabbing of a Burmese-American father, four-year-old and two-year-old because the perpetrator mistakenly assumed the family was Chinese and therefore infecting people with the virus [60]. Other acts of violence due to misinformation included the destruction of telecommunication masts and the verbal and physical abuse of telecommunication workers in the U.S., Europe, and Australasia due to the 5G conspiracy theory (cf., Jolley and Paterson [61]), as well as mob attacks [5].

3. Psychological Factors Affecting the Susceptibility to Misinformation

It should not be ignored that many were not susceptible to believing misinformation, adhering to expert-recommended guidelines, and adopting the appropriate health-preventative behaviors [7]. This begs the question of what it is that makes some people more susceptible to believing misinformation than others. Identifying such factors is important in informing interventions for addressing misinformation. This section uses psychological theory to explore what makes people susceptible to believing misinformation.

3.1. Emotionality

The rapid spread of the highly contagious SARS-CoV-2 and its associated high mortality rates meant that feelings of uncertainty and threat were rife during the COVID-19 pandemic [38]. This was exacerbated by extreme measures, such as social isolation and quarantine, aimed at containing the virus, which left many experiencing significant feelings of anger, confusion, anxiety, and stress [62]. Prolonged elevated stress-related emotions are well known to activate symptoms of depression, and this proved to be the case for many [63,64]. A systematic review and meta-analysis of research on the prevalence of stress-related emotions during the COVID-19 pandemic concluded that it had caused a significant detrimental effect on public mental health [64]. In one study, for instance, over one-third (34%) of Chinese people reported experiencing moderate to severe levels of stress or anxiety-related symptoms in response to COVID-19 [65]. The stress-related emotional response to the pandemic was deemed so significant it led to the conceptualization of COVID stress syndrome [66].

The emotional response to the COVID-19 pandemic is a crucial factor to consider for understanding the believability and spread of misinformation [38,67]. People tend to be strongly motivated to maintain a sense of control and understanding over their lives [68], and when this sense is under threat, it results in heightened feelings of anxiety [69]. In an attempt to reduce this anxiety and regain their sense of control, people "compensate with strategies that lead to greater acceptance of misconceptions" [70] (p. 3). These strategies include sense-making mechanisms, whereby information is obtained from various sources in order to make sense of a complex and unfamiliar situation, as well as having someone or something to blame and project feelings of anxiety towards [67].

Misinformation, and especially conspiracy theories, provide a narrative for people to both make sense of a situation and place the blame somewhere by explaining an event as a result of an influential individual or organization's secret attempts to achieve a sinister goal [67]. They offer an appealing solution to making sense of a situation and thus to regaining a sense of control in a way that is often clearer and simpler than that offered by accurate information. For instance, believing that China manufactured SARS-CoV-2 in a laboratory as a bioweapon offers an intelligible explanation of the origin of the virus, as well as somewhere to place the blame. The accurate account, on the other hand, which proposes that SARS-CoV-2 could have originated from the transmission of the virus from an animal to a human (a random, uncontrollable event), potentially enhances anxiety and lack of control. It has been repeatedly proven that feelings of anxiety and a lack of control foster openness to information and are a significant driving factor underlying a higher propensity to believe misinformation and conspiracy theories (see, e.g., Douglas et al. [71]).

3.2. Motivated Reasoning

On 19 April 2020, just over a month into the COVID-19 pandemic, an American protestor shouted, "This is a free country. Land of the free. Go to China if you want communism" at a nurse who was counter-protesting the lifting of quarantine measures [72]. This was one of many incidents that demonstrated how the pandemic led to the polarization of discourse and revealed deep-rooted epistemological and political positions [20]. This was largely fueled by the actions of governors and politicians, many of whom had opposing views on COVID-19 [73]. Various governors in the U.S., for instance, discounted the recommendations of health officials, failing to fully implement social distancing measures and openly discouraging the use of face masks [73]. In addition, news coverage surrounding COVID-19 was highly polarized and politicized, with politicians appearing more frequently in the news than scientists [74]. The politicization of COVID-19 was found to have had a detrimental effect on efforts to contain the virus, mainly through the spread of misinformation [75].

There is a growing body of research that links political ideology to the societal response to the pandemic [73,76,77], with political differences having been found to be the most significant factor predicting policy preferences and the adoption of health behaviors [77]. Political ideology has also been found to underlie susceptibility to believing and sharing misinformation [73], making it a crucial factor to consider in understanding the COVID-19 infodemic. The link between political ideology and the believability of misinformation can be better understood using the psychological theory of motivated reasoning or identity-protective cognition.

Motivated reasoning posits that information processing is directed so that it protects and is non-threatening to an individual's existing beliefs or identity [78]. When an individual is faced with information that conflicts with either of these, they are likely to experience cognitive dissonance, which refers to a state of mental discomfort caused by conflicting attitudes or beliefs [79]. When in cognitive dissonance, people engage in thought processes that serve to minimize this discomfort. Building on this, the theory of motivated reasoning proposes that when faced with multiple sources of polarized information, people are more likely to believe that which reinforces their pre-existing beliefs (confirmation bias) and reject those which undermine their pre-existing beliefs (disconfirmation bias) [19,73,80]. Therefore, pre-existing ideological and partisan attitudes and beliefs might prevent people from fact checking of information, and lead to higher levels of engagement with ideologically concordant information [81]. These higher levels of engagement inform the efforts of curation algorithms of social media platforms, which present the user with content which maintains their interest and maximizes engagement. As a result, people become enclosed in a filter bubble, in which they are more likely to be exposed to information that confirms their pre-existing attitudes (selective-exposure) and less likely to be exposed to diverse content [81,82]. In this way, the interaction between user engagement and algorithmic content curation contributes to the spread of misinformation, and thus presents a significant challenge in addressing the issue.

Although there is much evidence to support that political ideology is associated with believability (cf., Pennycook and Rand, [19]), it is essential to consider that this effect has been found to be smaller than that of the accuracy of the information [83]. Therefore, information that is accurate and politically discordant is more likely to be believed than misinformation that is politically concordant [19]. Since accuracy is a more significant predictor of susceptibility to misinformation than political concordance, this raises the question of why misinformation is ever believed at all. One explanation is offered by Pennycook and Rand [84], who suggest that the issue lies in whether or not people are able to accurately determine the integrity of information; therefore, that susceptibility to misinformation might actually be better explained by a lack of reasoning rather than by motivational reasoning.

3.3. Cognitive Reasoning

Dual-process theory characterizes human cognition as having two distinct thinking styles; intuitive or autonomous thinking (system 1 processing) and analytic, rational, or reflective thinking (system 2 processing) [85,86]. The distinction between the two is demonstrated through the performance on a conflict task, the intuitive, incorrect response is a result of intuitive thinking, which is speedy and effortless and requires minimal working memory resources. The correct result requires analytic thinking, which is effortful, deliberate, and requires more working memory resources. However, humans tend to instinctively avoid resource-demanding processes whenever possible [87]. According to Pennycook and Rand [84], "humans are cognitive misers, in that resource-demanding cognitive processes are typically avoided" (p. 2). This is problematic when it comes to discerning truth from falsehood, given that analytic reasoning supports sound judgment [88].

There is a growing body of research providing support for the association between analytic reasoning processes and skepticism about epistemically ambiguous information [86]. For instance, a greater tendency to engage in analytic thinking is linked to the detection of pseudo-profound bullshit [86] as well as the rejection of conspiracy theories [89], including those related to COVID-19 [90]. However, more recent research is highlighting the critical role of prior knowledge in susceptibility to misinformation. It has been shown, for example, that the association between analytic reasoning and the rejection of misinformation is significantly stronger when the information is more obviously inaccurate [84], which suggests that an individual's prior knowledge is an important factor underlying susceptibility to misinformation. This is supported by the finding that scientific reasoning has been found to be a stronger predictor of COVID-19 conspiracy theory beliefs than analytic thinking [90].

Scientific reasoning refers to having scientific knowledge and applying its "methods or principles of scientific inquiry to reasoning and problem-solving situations" [91] (p. 173). To better understand the role of scientific reasoning in the believability of misinformation, it is important to note the distinction between a belief (an attitude that is based on realistic, factual evidence), and an epistemically suspect belief (a belief which is not supported by factual evidence, and which conflicts with current knowledge) [90]. For example, the belief that methanol can cure COVID-19 conflicts with the factual evidence that methanol is toxic for human consumption. People with better scientific reasoning skills tend to hold the deep-rooted belief that scientific knowledge provides the most accurate conceptualization of the world [90]. As a result, they also tend to have beliefs which are supported by scientific evidence and therefore hold fewer epistemically suspected beliefs [92]. Therefore, it seems that having pre-exiting scientific knowledge and actually stopping to apply this knowledge to an analytical reasoning process makes people less susceptible to believing COVID-19 misinformation.

3.4. Heuristics

Cognitive psychology proposes heuristics as a thought process underlying intuitive thinking that ease the cognitive load when it comes to making judgments [93]. The word heuristic originates from the Ancient Greek word εὑρίσκω, meaning to find [93]. It refers to the process whereby an individual makes a decision based on a general rule of thumb, with very little cognitive reasoning involved [93]. Heuristics offer useful shortcuts for making a quick judgment call, however, the judgment is not guaranteed to be optimal or rational [93]. Simon [94] describes heuristics as satisficing; offering solutions that are good enough for the situation at hand, but which could be optimized. Research has shown that heuristics are used extensively in decision making in a variety of contexts (cf., Horne et al. [93]).

A recent study aimed to assess the use of heuristics in judging the veracity of COVID-19-related information [93]. Participants were shown a variety of news headlines relating to COVID-19 and were asked whether or not they believed the information and why. The researchers found that heuristics were extensively used in making judgments, and found that these fell into three broad categories; self-cognitive heuristics, content heuristics and source heuristics. Self-cognitive heuristics included heuristics based on how far the information aligned with the individual's beliefs, their previous experiences, or their pre-existing knowledge. The more these are aligned, the more likely the individual is to accept the information as accurate. It was found that people made judgments by comparing the news to beliefs such as "vaccinations are proven safe and everyone should get vaccinated", or previous experiences such as "I use the oil and it works". Content heuristics consider supporting evidence, bias, accuracy, coherency and writing style. An example of a content heuristic is "they use derogatory terms such as libtard which is an obvious sign that the article is biased". Source heuristics refer to whether the source of the information is perceived as accurate and include heuristics such as "the Chicago-Sun Times is a reputable paper".

The most commonly used heuristics were belief alignment heuristics (29%), followed by knowledge alignment heuristics (22%), with just 6% basing their judgments on perceived accuracy. These findings provide further support for the argument that a lack of cognitive reasoning, and therefore failure to accurately judge the veracity of information underlies the susceptibility to believing misinformation [84].

4. Social Media Sharing

The simple click or tap of a like or share button is all it takes for the instantaneous dissemination of information. Advances in social media technology have granted users the ability to share information across multiple platforms simultaneously. A survey carried out by the Pew Research Center found that around three-quarters (73%) of U.S. adults are multiplatform users [95]. Of Facebook users, for example, 91% also use Instagram, 90% use Twitter, 90% use LinkedIn, 89% use Pinterest, 89% use Snapchat, 85% use WhatsApp and 81% use YouTube [95]. This creates an expansive online network, allowing for the seamless sharing of information, with every single share significantly expanding its reach. If, for example, an individual with 1000 Twitter followers shared a post, which in turn was shared by just 10% of those followers (to their own network of 1,000 followers), the post will effortlessly have reached 100,000 people [96]. This illustrates how conducive social media is to the rapid spreading of information, and how sharing exacerbated the spread of misinformation that led to the COVID-19 infodemic [2]. Therefore, exploring social-media sharing behavior can enhance our understanding of the spread of misinformation during the COVID-19 pandemic.

Understanding Sharing Behavior

Shared information is often mistakenly assumed to have been shared based on the individual believing the information [19]. However, recent research has proven that this is not necessarily the case, and that information is shared for a variety of reasons [19]. In one study, for instance, participants were presented with false claims about COVID-19 and asked whether or not they would share them on social media [97]. It was found that the perception of accuracy of the statement did not play a significant role in the intention to share, with the intention to share being 91% higher than the judgment of their accuracy. These findings demonstrate that people are willing to share COVID-19 related information without being certain of its accuracy. Pennycook and Rand [19] identify three possible explanations for this disconnection between sharing intention and accuracy judgment; the preference-based account, the confusion-based account, and the inattention-based account.

Consistent with the theory of motivated reasoning [85], the preference-based account proposes that people prioritize their political identity or moral viewpoints, over accuracy and truth. From this perspective, people share misinformation, even when knowing it is inaccurate, for reasons driven by their political or moral ideology. These reasons might include virtue signaling [98], social dominance orientation [99], furthering a political agenda [77], or simply because the information is thought to be interesting [30]. However, according to Pennybrook et al. [83], just 16% of shared misinformation is driven by preference-based motives.

According to the confusion-based account, people mistakenly and genuinely believe the misinformation they share to be accurate. This perspective is supported by the findings of Pennybrook et al. [83] which showed that only one-third (33%) of shared misinformation was believed, and two-thirds (67%) was shared as a result of confusion. Based on these findings, a significant amount of information that is shared online can be explained by confusion.

The inattention-based account suggests that while people generally prefer to only share accurate information, they fail to do so due to distractions from the online social media environment. Social media environments have become an attention economy, where posts compete for user attention and provide distractions which hinder with analytic thinking processes [64]. Much content is generated and posted with the aim of capturing as much attention as possible. This often done through the posting and sharing of ideologically extreme posts with the hope of achieving high popularity ratings (likes, comments and shares). Popularity ratings have been repeatedly shown to attract more attention, regardless of information veracity [33,96]. Therefore, such an environment is likely to provide conditions which make people who engage in intuitive rather than analytic reasoning [100] especially susceptible to believing and sharing misinformation. Indeed, analytic reasoning, besides being associated with a higher tendency to reject misinformation [89], is also associated with sharing behavior that is based on more accurate judgments of information veracity [97], and the sharing of more reliable information [101]. Therefore, a lack of analytic thinking seems to be a source of misjudgments when it comes to sharing information on social media.

5. Interventions for Addressing Misinformation

Current interventions for addressing misinformation fall into four broad categories; algorithmic, corrective, legislative and psychological [102]. Algorithmic approaches use machine learning, network analysis and natural language processing to detect misinformation [18]. A ranking algorithm downranks any information that is classified as problematic, making it less likely for users to see it. Although these approaches have been implemented by social media companies including Google and Facebook, they have not been entirely effective for two main reasons. Firstly, it is not always easy to ascertain the veracity of information; the truth is not always black and white. Therefore, algorithmic approaches run the risk of false positives and unjustified censorship, which is what happened at Facebook in 2017 [103]. Secondly, misinformation evolves rapidly, as the COVID-19 infodemic has proven. Therefore, in order for algorithmic approaches to remain effective, they would need to evolve at the same pace, which is difficult given that even classifiers trained to detect misinformation were unequipped for novel claims surrounding COVID-19 [19].

Corrective approaches attempt to debunk misinformation using fact-checking and correction [104]. Fact-checking initiatives such as PolitiFact [105] and Snopes [106] check and debunk major headlines which are published on their websites. The evidence on the efficacy of fact-checking approaches is mixed, with some highlighting their efficacy in addressing misinformation, and others suggesting they could actually increase belief in misinformation [107,108]. Since it is impossible to fact-check every story, the stories which have not been checked may be mistakenly assumed to have been verified, and therefore regarded as accurate. Fact-checking and debunking approaches were not able to handle the surge of information during the COVID-19 pandemic and they are simply not scalable [109].

Some countries have adopted a legislative approach in tackling misinformation, introducing new regulation and legislation. For instance, France introduced the Fake News Law, which placed restrictions on the information media companies were allowed to publish [110]. A similar initiative was implemented in the U.K., with a specialist unit set up to counter false claims against the COVID-19 pandemic [111]. The concern with such initiatives, however, arises from granting the power for an individual organization to decide what classifies as accurate and what doesn't [102]. EUvsDisinfo (a European Union-funded group dedicated to tackling misinformation), for instance, was subject to heavy criticism, including from Dutch politicians, for infringing freedom of speech and was subsequently proposed the initiative be scrapped altogether [112].

5.1. *Psychologically-Informed Interventions for Addressing Misinformation*

The shortcomings of the approaches to addressing the sharing and spread of misinformation described above have seen scientists turn to psychology, education and the behavioral sciences in search of more effective interventions [102]. Two promising psychologically-informed approaches, namely, inoculation or prebunking, and accuracy prompts, are detailed below.

5.1.1. Inoculation

Misinformation has been described as something which "spreads through networks much like a real virus 'infecting its host' and rapidly transmitting falsehoods from one mind to another" [5] (p. 3). The non-psychological interventions described above all attempt to correct misinformation after the damage has already been done and face various difficulties in doing so. Researchers have now shifted their focus to a more proactive prebunking (i.e., preemptive bunking) or inoculation against misinformation [5,19,102,109].

This approach is based on inoculation theory, which uses an analogy from immunology [113]. Inoculation theory posits that in the same way in which vaccines work through exposure to a weakened version of a virus, preemptive exposure to weakened examples of misinformation might make people more immune, and less susceptible to believing it [113]. In what van der Linden et al. [5] term a persuasion inoculation, individuals are presented with some misinformation that has been weakened by the addition of two elements [5,102,113]. The first of these is a forewarning that the individual is about to be exposed to counter-attitudinal content (the affective basis), which is thought to elicit feelings of threat, and trigger the protection of pre-existing beliefs. The second is a preemptive refutation of counterarguments (the cognitive basis), which essentially teach and inform the user by modelling the counterarguing process. The information is weakened to the point where it doesn't actually persuade the person, but is enough to trigger protective responses such as enhanced analytical thinking [113]. Following this experience, the individual develops mental antibodies to misinformation, and will likely employ these when exposed to similar challenges in the real world, thus reducing their susceptibility to misinformation. A meta-analysis of research on inoculation theory concluded that inoculation theory is indeed effective at protecting attitudes from persuasion [114].

The Bad News Game [115] is an award-winning online browser game which puts inoculation theory into practice. It uses a simulated social media environment where the user plays the role of a misinformation creator and learns about the spreading of misinformation in an engaging way (cf., van der Linden & Roozenbeek [102] for a detailed description). Similar to this is Go Viral! [116], a practical application of inoculation theory developed by WHO in collaboration with the U.K. government, specifically aimed at inoculating people against COVID-19 misinformation. This game focuses on building resistance to three techniques used on social media to manipulate people; fearmongering, conspiracy theories and the use of fake experts. Research has shown that these games significantly improve the ability to identify and resist misinformation [102,117].

One limitation of such approaches is identified by Pennycook and Rand [84], who note that they are opt-in; people have to voluntarily choose to participate with the inoculation technique. The problem with this is that people who are low on cognitive reflection and most susceptible to misinformation (and therefore in need of inoculation), are also less likely to participate in such activities. Shorter forms of inoculation (e.g., presenting digital media literacy tips), have proven to be effective in helping people to determine news veracity [118] and these may be more scalable and have more reach.

5.1.2. Accuracy Prompts

As noted above, the inattention-based account of misinformation sharing on social media posits that people generally only want to share information that is accurate, and one of the main reasons underlying the spread of misinformation on is the failure to accurately determine its veracity prior to sharing [83,97]. Research has shown that by shifting their attention towards accuracy, people can better distinguish misinformation from accurate information [97]. Accuracy prompts encourage people to do just this by having people rate the accuracy of information prior to making a judgment about sharing it. This approach is appealing as it does not rely on software to identify and distinguish between accurate information and misinformation (as is the case with algorithmic approaches [102]). In addition, accuracy prompts are easily scalable (unlike fact-checking for instance, which is time consuming and does not cover all information [109]). Accuracy prompts provide a promising approach towards tackling misinformation in a way which preserves user autonomy and encourages them to exercise their desire to avoid sharing misinformation [83].

6. Concluding Remarks

The COVID-19 infodemic has offered a stark warning sign as to the sheer scale and detrimental effects of misinformation, highlighting the importance of understanding its spread as well as its consequences for public health and everyday life. The evidence presented in this entry has revealed a variety of factors underlying the failure to discern misinformation from truth, including values and beliefs, political ideology and scientific knowledge. Overall, however, it seems that susceptibility to misinformation is mainly due to people failing to actually stop and think about the information they are exposed to. In the chaotic online environment created by social media, intuitive reasoning trumps analytic reasoning, resulting in endless impulsive clicks and taps, mindless shares and superficially alluring popularity ratings. As a result of these findings, interventions aimed at tackling misinformation are shifting their focus from remedial approaches to preventative approaches, with creative initiatives that encourage people to think deeper before they act. Although there is still some way to go in fully understanding the spread of misinformation, the field of psychology is proving to offer valuable insights and offers promising avenues for future research.

Author Contributions: Conceptualization E.A., M.A., and M.M.; investigation, E.A., M.A., and M.M.; writing—original draft preparation, E.A., M.A., and M.M.; writing—review and editing E.A., M.A., and M.M.; supervision M.A., and M.M.; project administration E.A., M.A., and M.M. All authors have read and agreed to the published version of the manuscript.

Funding: This research received no external funding.

Conflicts of Interest: The authors declare no conflict of interest.

Entry Link: https://encyclopedia.pub/17129.

References

1. World Health Organization. WHO Coronavirus (COVID-19) Dashboard. Available online: https://covid19.who.int (accessed on 18 September 2021).
2. Tangcharoensathien, V.; Calleja, N.; Nguyen, T.; Purnat, T.; D'Agostino, M.; Garcia-Saiso, S.; Landry, M.; Rashidian, A.; Hamilton, C.; AbdAllah, A.; et al. Framework for Managing the COVID-19 Infodemic: Methods and Results of an Online, Crowdsourced WHO Technical Consultation. *J. Med. Internet Res.* **2020**, *22*, e19659. [CrossRef]
3. World Health Organisation. Munich Security Conference. Available online: https://www.who.int/dg/speeches/detail/munich-security-conference (accessed on 18 September 2021).
4. World Health Organization. Coronavirus Disease 2019 (COVID-19) Situation Report-86. Available online: https://www.who.int/docs/default-source/coronaviruse/situation-reports/20200415-sitrep-86-covid-19.pdf?sfvrsn=c615ea20_6 (accessed on 18 September 2021).
5. Van der Linden, S.; Roozenbeek, J.; Compton, J. Inoculating Against Fake News About COVID-19. *Front. Psychol.* **2020**, *11*. [CrossRef] [PubMed]
6. Krause, N.M.; Freiling, I.; Beets, B.; Brossard, D. Fact-Checking as Risk Communication: The Multi-Layered Risk of Misinformation in Times of COVID-19. *J. Risk Res.* **2020**, *23*, 1052–1059. [CrossRef]
7. Dryhurst, S.; Schneider, C.R.; Kerr, J.; Freeman, A.L.J.; Recchia, G.; van der Bles, A.M.; Spiegelhalter, D.; van der Linden, S. Risk Perceptions of COVID-19 around the World. *J. Risk Res.* **2020**, *23*, 994–1006. [CrossRef]
8. World Health Organization. 1st WHO Infodemiology Conference: How Infodemics Affect the World & How They Can Be Managed. Available online: https://www.who.int/docs/default-source/epi-win/infodemic-management/infodemiology-scientific-conference-booklet.pdf?sfvrsn=179de76a_4 (accessed on 18 September 2021).
9. World Health Organization. WHO Public Health Research Agenda For Managing Infodemics. Available online: https://www.who.int/publications/i/item/9789240019508 (accessed on 18 September 2021).
10. Gunn, J. *Alternate Worlds: The Illustrated History of Science Fiction*; A & W Visual Library: Englewood Cliffs, NJ, USA, 1975; ISBN 978-0-89104-049-1.

11. Kaplan, R.L. Yellow Journalism. In *The International Encyclopedia of Communication*; Donsbach, W., Ed.; John Wiley & Sons, Ltd.: Chichester, UK, 2008; ISBN 978-1-4051-8640-7.
12. Evans, R.J. *The Third Reich in Power*; Penguin Books: New York, NY, USA, 2006; ISBN 978-0-14-303790-3.
13. Kux, D. Soviet Active Measures and Disinformation: Overview and Assessment. *US Army War Coll. Q. Parameters* **1985**, *15*, 17.
14. Hoppe, T. "Spanish Flu": When Infectious Disease Names Blur Origins and Stigmatize Those Infected. *Am. J. Public Health* **2018**, *108*, 1462–1464. [CrossRef]
15. Basco, S.; Domènech, J.; Rosés, J.R. The Redistributive Effects of Pandemics: Evidence on the Spanish Flu. *World Dev.* **2021**, *141*, 105389. [CrossRef]
16. Farkas, J.; Schou, J. Fake News as a Floating Signifier: Hegemony, Antagonism and the Politics of Falsehood. *Javn. Public* **2018**, *25*, 298–314. [CrossRef]
17. Tandoc, E.C.; Lim, Z.W.; Ling, R. Defining "Fake News": A Typology of Scholarly Definitions. *Digit. J.* **2018**, *6*, 137–153. [CrossRef]
18. Shu, K.; Sliva, A.; Wang, S.; Tang, J.; Liu, H. Fake News Detection on Social Media: A Data Mining Perspective. *SIGKDD Explor. Newsl.* **2017**, *19*, 22–36. [CrossRef]
19. Pennycook, G.; Rand, D.G. The Psychology of Fake News. *Trends Cogn. Sci.* **2021**, *25*, 388–402. [CrossRef] [PubMed]
20. Hartley, K.; Vu, M.K. Fighting Fake News in the COVID-19 Era: Policy Insights from an Equilibrium Model. *Policy Sci.* **2020**, *53*, 735–758. [CrossRef] [PubMed]
21. Waszak, P.M.; Kasprzycka-Waszak, W.; Kubanek, A. The Spread of Medical Fake News in Social Media—The Pilot Quantitative Study. *Health Policy Technol.* **2018**, *7*, 115–118. [CrossRef]
22. Wardle, C. *Information Disorder: The Essential Glossary*; Shorenstein Center on Media, Politics, and Public Policy, Harvard Kennedy School: Harvard, MA, USA, 2018.
23. Benkler, Y.; Faris, R.; Roberts, H. *Network Propaganda: Manipulation, Disinformation, and Radicalization in American Politics*; Oxford University Press: Oxford, UK, 2018; ISBN 0-19-092364-4.
24. Floridi, L. Brave.Net.World: The Internet as a Disinformation Superhighway? *Electron. Libr.* **1996**, *14*, 509–514. [CrossRef]
25. Skinner, S.; Martin, B. Racist Disinformation on the World Wide Web: Initial Implications for the LIS Community. *Aust. Libr. J.* **2000**, *49*, 259–269. [CrossRef]
26. Keshavarz, H. How Credible Is Information on the Web: Reflections on Misinformation and Disinformation. *Infopreneurship J.* **2014**, *1*, 1–17.
27. Karlova, N.A.; Fisher, K.E. A Social Diffusion Model of Misinformation and Disinformation for Understanding Human Information Behaviour. *Inf. Res.* **2013**, *18*, 573.
28. Jewitt, R.; Dahlberg, L. The Trouble With Twittering: Integrating Social Media into Mainstream News. *Int. J. Media Cult. Politics* **2009**, *5*, 233–246. [CrossRef]
29. Karlovitz, T.J. The Democratization of Technology—And Its Limitation. In *Managing Customer Experiences in an Omnichannel World: Melody of Online and Offline Environments in the Customer Journey*; Dirsehan, T., Ed.; Emerald Publishing Limited: Bingley, UK, 2020; pp. 13–25. ISBN 978-1-80043-389-2.
30. Altay, S.; de Araujo, E.; Mercier, H. "If This Account Is True, It Is Most Enormously Wonderful": Interestingness-If-True and the Sharing of True and False News. *Digit. J.* **2021**, 1–22. [CrossRef]
31. Vosoughi, S.; Roy, D.; Aral, S. The Spread of True and False News Online. *Science* **2018**, *359*, 1146–1151. [CrossRef]
32. Pew Research Center. *News Use Across Social Media Platforms in 2020*; Pew Research Center: Washington, DC, USA, 2020.
33. Thorson, E. Changing Patterns Of News Consumption and Participation: News Recommendation Engines. *Inf. Commun. Soc.* **2008**, *11*, 473–489. [CrossRef]
34. Kang, H.; Bae, K.; Zhang, S.; Sundar, S.S. Source Cues in Online News: Is the Proximate Source More Powerful than Distal Sources? *J. Mass Commun. Q.* **2011**, *88*, 719–736. [CrossRef]
35. Shahsavari, S.; Holur, P.; Wang, T.; Tangherlini, T.R.; Roychowdhury, V. Conspiracy in the Time of Corona: Automatic Detection of Emerging COVID-19 Conspiracy Theories in Social Media and the News. *J. Comput. Soc. Sci.* **2020**, *3*, 279–317. [CrossRef] [PubMed]
36. Garfin, D.R.; Silver, R.C.; Holman, E.A. The Novel Coronavirus (COVID-2019) Outbreak: Amplification of Public Health Consequences by Media Exposure. *Health Psychol.* **2020**, *39*, 355–357. [CrossRef] [PubMed]
37. Gallotti, R.; Valle, F.; Castaldo, N.; Sacco, P.; De Domenico, M. Assessing the Risks of 'Infodemics' in Response to COVID-19 Epidemics. *Nat. Hum. Behav.* **2020**, *4*, 1285–1293. [CrossRef] [PubMed]
38. De Coninck, D.; Frissen, T.; Matthijs, K.; d'Haenens, L.; Lits, G.; Champagne-Poirier, O.; Carignan, M.-E.; David, M.D.; Pignard-Cheynel, N.; Salerno, S.; et al. Beliefs in Conspiracy Theories and Misinformation About COVID-19: Comparative Perspectives on the Role of Anxiety, Depression and Exposure to and Trust in Information Sources. *Front. Psychol.* **2021**, *12*, 646394. [CrossRef] [PubMed]
39. Li, H.O.-Y.; Bailey, A.; Huynh, D.; Chan, J. YouTube as a Source of Information on COVID-19: A Pandemic of Misinformation? *BMJ Glob. Health* **2020**, *5*, e002604. [CrossRef] [PubMed]
40. Ofcom. Half of UK Adults Exposed to False Claims about Coronavirus. Available online: https://www.ofcom.org.uk/about-ofcom/latest/features-and-news/half-of-uk-adults-exposed-to-false-claims-about-coronavirus (accessed on 19 September 2021).

41. Pew Research Center. Americans Immersed in COVID-19 News; Most Think Media Are Doing Fairly Well Covering It. Available online: https://www.journalism.org/2020/03/18/americans-immersed-in-covid-19-news-most-think-media-are-doing-fairly-well-covering-it/ (accessed on 19 September 2021).
42. Pennycook, G.; Cannon, T.D.; Rand, D.G. Prior Exposure Increases Perceived Accuracy of Fake News. *J. Exp. Psychol. Gen.* **2018**, *147*, 1865–1880. [CrossRef]
43. Andersen, K.G.; Rambaut, A.; Lipkin, W.I.; Holmes, E.C.; Garry, R.F. The Proximal Origin of SARS-CoV-2. *Nat. Med.* **2020**, *26*, 450–452. [CrossRef]
44. World Health Organization. Coronavirus Disease (COVID-19) Advice for the Public: Mythbusters. Available online: https://www.who.int/emergencies/diseases/novel-coronavirus-2019/advice-for-public/myth-busters (accessed on 19 September 2021).
45. Ahmed, W.; Vidal-Alaball, J.; Downing, J.; López Seguí, F. COVID-19 and the 5G Conspiracy Theory: Social Network Analysis of Twitter Data. *J. Med. Internet Res.* **2020**, *22*, e19458. [CrossRef]
46. Cook, J.; Van Der Linden, S.; Lewandowsky, S.; Ecker, U.K. Coronavirus, 'Plandemic'and the Seven Traits of Conspiratorial Thinking. Available online: https://theconversation.com/coronavirus-plandemic-and-the-seven-traits-of-conspiratorial-thinking-138483 (accessed on 19 September 2020).
47. Owens, B. Excitement around Hydroxychloroquine for Treating COVID-19 Causes Challenges for Rheumatology. *Lancet Rheumatol.* **2020**, *2*, e257. [CrossRef]
48. Meyerowitz, E.A.; Vannier, A.G.L.; Friesen, M.G.N.; Schoenfeld, S.; Gelfand, J.A.; Callahan, M.V.; Kim, A.Y.; Reeves, P.M.; Poznansky, M.C. Rethinking the Role of Hydroxychloroquine in the Treatment of COVID-19. *FASEB J.* **2020**, *34*, 6027–6037. [CrossRef] [PubMed]
49. Stanley, M.L.; Barr, N.; Peters, K.; Seli, P. Analytic-Thinking Predicts Hoax Beliefs and Helping Behaviors in Response to the COVID-19 Pandemic. *Think. Reason.* **2021**, *27*, 464–477. [CrossRef]
50. Freeman, D.; Waite, F.; Rosebrock, L.; Petit, A.; Causier, C.; East, A.; Jenner, L.; Teale, A.-L.; Carr, L.; Mulhall, S.; et al. Coronavirus Conspiracy Beliefs, Mistrust, and Compliance with Government Guidelines in England. *Psychol. Med.* **2020**, 1–13. [CrossRef] [PubMed]
51. Imhoff, R.; Lamberty, P. A Bioweapon or a Hoax? The Link between Distinct Conspiracy Beliefs About the Coronavirus Disease (COVID-19) Outbreak and Pandemic Behavior. *Soc. Psychol. Personal. Sci.* **2020**, *11*, 1110–1118. [CrossRef]
52. Uscinski, J.E.; Enders, A.M.; Klofstad, C.; Seelig, M.; Funchion, J.; Everett, C.; Wuchty, S.; Premaratne, K.; Murthi, M. Why Do People Believe COVID-19 Conspiracy Theories? *HKS Misinf. Rev.* **2020**. [CrossRef]
53. Lep, Ž.; Babnik, K.; Hacin Beyazoglu, K. Emotional Responses and Self-Protective Behavior Within Days of the COVID-19 Outbreak: The Promoting Role of Information Credibility. *Front. Psychol.* **2020**, *11*, 1846. [CrossRef] [PubMed]
54. Islam, M.S.; Sarkar, T.; Khan, S.H.; Mostofa Kamal, A.-H.; Hasan, S.M.M.; Kabir, A.; Yeasmin, D.; Islam, M.A.; Amin Chowdhury, K.I.; Anwar, K.S.; et al. COVID-19–Related Infodemic and Its Impact on Public Health: A Global Social Media Analysis. *Am. J. Trop. Med. Hyg.* **2020**, *103*, 1621–1629. [CrossRef]
55. Wen, J.; Aston, J.; Liu, X.; Ying, T. Effects of Misleading Media Coverage on Public Health Crisis: A Case of the 2019 Novel Coronavirus Outbreak in China. *Anatolia* **2020**, *31*, 331–336. [CrossRef]
56. Armstrong, C.; Hildebrandt, C. China Kids Stay Home. Available online: https://www.pressreader.com/australia/the-daily-telegraph-sydney/20200129/281479278389840 (accessed on 23 September 2019).
57. Mead, W.R. China Is the Real Sick Man of Asia. Available online: https://www.wsj.com/articles/china-is-the-real-sick-man-of-asia-11580773677 (accessed on 23 September 2021).
58. Zheng, Y.; Goh, E.; Wen, J. The Effects of Misleading Media Reports about COVID-19 on Chinese Tourists' Mental Health: A Perspective Article. *Anatolia* **2020**, *31*, 337–340. [CrossRef]
59. Jeung, R.; Nham, K. Incidents of Coronavirus-Related Discrimination. Available online: http://www.asianpacificpolicyandplanningcouncil.org/wp-content/uploads/CA_Report_6_30_20.pdf (accessed on 23 September 2021).
60. Tessler, H.; Choi, M.; Kao, G. The Anxiety of Being Asian American: Hate Crimes and Negative Biases During the COVID-19 Pandemic. *Am. J. Crim. Justice* **2020**, *45*, 636–646. [CrossRef] [PubMed]
61. Jolley, D.; Paterson, J.L. Pylons Ablaze: Examining the Role of 5G COVID-19 Conspiracy Beliefs and Support for Violence. *Br. J. Soc. Psychol.* **2020**, *59*, 628–640. [CrossRef] [PubMed]
62. Brooks, S.K.; Webster, R.K.; Smith, L.E.; Woodland, L.; Wessely, S.; Greenberg, N.; Rubin, G.J. The Psychological Impact of Quarantine and How to Reduce It: Rapid Review of the Evidence. *Lancet* **2020**, *395*, 912–920. [CrossRef]
63. Barzilay, R.; Moore, T.M.; Greenberg, D.M.; DiDomenico, G.E.; Brown, L.A.; White, L.K.; Gur, R.C.; Gur, R.E. Resilience, COVID-19-Related Stress, Anxiety and Depression during the Pandemic in a Large Population Enriched for Healthcare Providers. *Transl. Psychiatry* **2020**, *10*, 291. [CrossRef] [PubMed]
64. Salari, N.; Hosseinian-Far, A.; Jalali, R.; Vaisi-Raygani, A.; Rasoulpoor, S.; Mohammadi, M.; Rasoulpoor, S.; Khaledi-Paveh, B. Prevalence of Stress, Anxiety, Depression among the General Population during the COVID-19 Pandemic: A Systematic Review and Meta-Analysis. *Glob. Health* **2020**, *16*, 57. [CrossRef]
65. Qiu, J.; Shen, B.; Zhao, M.; Wang, Z.; Xie, B.; Xu, Y. A Nationwide Survey of Psychological Distress among Chinese People in the COVID-19 Epidemic: Implications and Policy Recommendations. *Gen. Psychiatry* **2020**, *33*, e100213. [CrossRef]

66. Taylor, S.; Landry, C.A.; Paluszek, M.M.; Fergus, T.A.; McKay, D.; Asmundson, G.J.G. COVID Stress Syndrome: Concept, Structure, and Correlates. *Depress. Anxiety* **2020**, *37*, 706–714. [CrossRef]
67. Šrol, J.; Ballová Mikušková, E.; Čavojová, V. When We Are Worried, What Are We Thinking? Anxiety, Lack of Control, and Conspiracy Beliefs amidst the COVID-19 Pandemic. *Appl. Cognit. Psychol.* **2021**, *35*, 720–729. [CrossRef]
68. Landau, M.J.; Kay, A.C.; Whitson, J.A. Compensatory Control and the Appeal of a Structured World. *Psychol. Bull.* **2015**, *141*, 694–722. [CrossRef]
69. Kay, A.C.; Whitson, J.A.; Gaucher, D.; Galinsky, A.D. Compensatory Control: Achieving Order Through the Mind, Our Institutions, and the Heavens. *Curr. Dir. Psychol. Sci.* **2009**, *18*, 264–268. [CrossRef]
70. Nyhan, B. Misinformation and Fact-Checking: Research Findings from Social Science. Available online: https://www.dartmouth.edu/~{}nyhan/Misinformation_and_Fact-checking.pdf (accessed on 28 September 2021).
71. Douglas, K.M.; Uscinski, J.E.; Sutton, R.M.; Cichocka, A.; Nefes, T.; Ang, C.S.; Deravi, F. Understanding Conspiracy Theories. *Political Psychol.* **2019**, *40*, 3–35. [CrossRef]
72. Armus, T.; Hassan, J. 'Go to China If You Want Communism': Anti-Quarantine Protester Clashes with People in Scrubs. Available online: https://www.washingtonpost.com/nation/2020/04/20/go-china-if-you-want-communism-anti-quarantine-protester-clashes-with-people-scrubs/ (accessed on 29 September 2021).
73. Sylvester, S.M. COVID-19 and Motivated Reasoning: The Influence of Knowledge on COVID-Related Policy and Health Behavior. *Soc. Sci. Q.* **2021**, 12989. [CrossRef]
74. Hart, P.S.; Chinn, S.; Soroka, S. Politicization and Polarization in COVID-19 News Coverage. *Sci. Commun.* **2020**, *42*, 679–697. [CrossRef]
75. Motta, M.; Stecula, D.; Farhart, C. How Right-Leaning Media Coverage of COVID-19 Facilitated the Spread of Misinformation in the Early Stages of the Pandemic in the U.S. *Can. J. Political Sci.* **2020**, *53*, 335–342. [CrossRef]
76. Harvey, J.N.; Lawson, V.L. The Importance of Health Belief Models in Determining Self-Care Behaviour in Diabetes. *Diabet. Med.* **2009**, *26*, 5–13. [CrossRef]
77. Gadarian, S.K.; Goodman, S.W.; Pepinsky, T.B. Partisanship, Health Behavior, and Policy Attitudes in the Early Stages of the COVID-19 Pandemic. *PLoS ONE* **2021**, *16*, e0249596. [CrossRef]
78. Kunda, Z. The Case for Motivated Reasoning. *Psychol. Bull.* **1990**, *108*, 480–498. [CrossRef]
79. Festinger, L. *A Theory of Cognitive Dissonance*; Stanford University Press: Redwood City, CA, USA, 1957; p. 291.
80. Freiling, I.; Krause, N.M.; Scheufele, D.A.; Brossard, D. Believing and Sharing Misinformation, Fact-Checks, and Accurate Information on Social Media: The Role of Anxiety during COVID-19. *New Media Soc.* **2021**, 146144482110114. [CrossRef]
81. Lazer, D.M.J.; Baum, M.A.; Benkler, Y.; Berinsky, A.J.; Greenhill, K.M.; Menczer, F.; Metzger, M.J.; Nyhan, B.; Pennycook, G.; Rothschild, D.; et al. The Science of Fake News. *Science* **2018**, *359*, 1094–1096. [CrossRef]
82. Spohr, D. Fake News and Ideological Polarization: Filter Bubbles and Selective Exposure on Social Media. *Bus. Inf. Rev.* **2017**, *34*, 150–160. [CrossRef]
83. Pennycook, G.; Epstein, Z.; Mosleh, M.; Arechar, A.A.; Eckles, D.; Rand, D.G. Shifting Attention to Accuracy Can Reduce Misinformation Online. *Nature* **2021**, *592*, 590–595. [CrossRef]
84. Pennycook, G.; Rand, D.G. Lazy, Not Biased: Susceptibility to Partisan Fake News Is Better Explained by Lack of Reasoning than by Motivated Reasoning. *Cognition* **2019**, *188*, 39–50. [CrossRef] [PubMed]
85. Kahneman, D. *Thinking, Fast and Slow*, 1st pbk. ed.; Farrar, Straus and Giroux: New York, NY, USA, 2013; ISBN 978-0-374-53355-7.
86. Pennycook, G.; Fugelsang, J.A.; Koehler, D.J. Everyday Consequences of Analytic Thinking. *Curr. Dir. Psychol. Sci.* **2015**, *24*, 425–432. [CrossRef]
87. Fiske, S.T.; Taylor, S.E. *Social Cognition: From Brains to Culture*, 2nd ed.; SAGE: Los Angeles, CA, USA, 2013; ISBN 978-1-4462-5814-9.
88. Kohlberg, L. Stage and sequence: The cognitive-developmental approach to socialization. In *Handbook of Socialization Theory and Research*; Goslin, D.A., Ed.; Rand McNally: Chicago, IL, USA, 1969; pp. 347–480.
89. Swami, V.; Voracek, M.; Stieger, S.; Tran, U.S.; Furnham, A. Analytic Thinking Reduces Belief in Conspiracy Theories. *Cognition* **2014**, *133*, 572–585. [CrossRef]
90. Čavojová, V.; Šrol, J.; Ballová Mikušková, E. How Scientific Reasoning Correlates with Health-Related Beliefs and Behaviors during the COVID-19 Pandemic? *J. Health Psychol.* **2020**, 135910532096226. [CrossRef]
91. Zimmerman, C. The Development of Scientific Thinking Skills in Elementary and Middle School. *Dev. Rev.* **2007**, *27*, 172–223. [CrossRef]
92. Čavojová, V.; Šrol, J.; Jurkovič, M. Why Should We Try to Think like Scientists? Scientific Reasoning and Susceptibility to Epistemically Suspect Beliefs and Cognitive Biases. *Appl. Cognit. Psychol.* **2020**, *34*, 85–95. [CrossRef]
93. Horne, B.D.; Nevo, D.; Adali, S.; Manikonda, L.; Arrington, C. Tailoring Heuristics and Timing AI Interventions for Supporting News Veracity Assessments. *Comput. Hum. Beha. Rep.* **2020**, *2*, 100043. [CrossRef]
94. Simon, H.A. Rational Choice and the Structure of the Environment. *Psychol. Rev.* **1956**, *63*, 129–138. [CrossRef]
95. Smith, A.; Anderson, M. Social Media Use in 2018. Available online: https://www.pewresearch.org/internet/2018/03/01/social-media-use-in-2018/ (accessed on 1 October 2021).
96. Brady, W.J.; Crockett, M.J.; Van Bavel, J.J. The MAD Model of Moral Contagion: The Role of Motivation, Attention, and Design in the Spread of Moralized Content Online. *Perspect. Psychol. Sci.* **2020**, *15*, 978–1010. [CrossRef] [PubMed]

97. Pennycook, G.; McPhetres, J.; Zhang, Y.; Lu, J.G.; Rand, D.G. Fighting COVID-19 Misinformation on Social Media: Experimental Evidence for a Scalable Accuracy-Nudge Intervention. *Psychol. Sci.* **2020**, *31*, 770–780. [CrossRef] [PubMed]
98. Jordan, J.J.; Rand, D.G. Signaling When No One Is Watching: A Reputation Heuristics Account of Outrage and Punishment in One-Shot Anonymous Interactions. *J. Personal. Soc. Psychol.* **2020**, *118*, 57–88. [CrossRef]
99. Lobato, E.J.C.; Powell, M.; Padilla, L.M.K.; Holbrook, C. Factors Predicting Willingness to Share COVID-19 Misinformation. *Front. Psychol.* **2020**, *11*, 566108. [CrossRef] [PubMed]
100. Kahneman, D.; Slovic, S.P.; Slovic, P.; Tversky, A. *Judgment under Uncertainty: Heuristics and Biases*; Cambridge University Press: Cambridge, UK, 1982; ISBN 0-521-28414-7.
101. Mosleh, M.; Pennycook, G.; Arechar, A.A.; Rand, D.G. Cognitive Reflection Correlates with Behavior on Twitter. *Nat. Commun.* **2021**, *12*, 921. [CrossRef]
102. Van Der Linden, S.; Rozenbeek, J. Psychological inoculation against fake news. In *The Psychology of Fake News: Accepting, Sharing, and Correcting Misinformation*; Greifeneder, R., Jaffé, M.E., Newman, E.J., Schwarz, N., Eds.; Routledge: New York, NY, USA, 2021; pp. 147–170.
103. Wakefield, J. Facebook's Fake News Experiment Backfires. Available online: https://www.bbc.com/news/technology-41900877 (accessed on 2 October 2021).
104. Zollo, F.; Bessi, A.; Del Vicario, M.; Scala, A.; Caldarelli, G.; Shekhtman, L.; Havlin, S.; Quattrociocchi, W. Debunking in a World of Tribes. *PLoS ONE* **2017**, *12*, e0181821. [CrossRef]
105. Politifact. Available online: https://www.politifact.com (accessed on 8 October 2021).
106. Snopes. Available online: https://www.snopes.com (accessed on 8 October 2021).
107. Nyhan, B.; Reifler, J. When Corrections Fail: The Persistence of Political Misperceptions. *Political Behav.* **2010**, *32*, 303–330. [CrossRef]
108. Nyhan, B.; Porter, E.; Reifler, J.; Wood, T. Taking Corrections Literally But Not Seriously? The Effects of Information on Factual Beliefs and Candidate Favorability. *SSRN J.* **2017**. [CrossRef]
109. Van Bavel, J.J.; Baicker, K.; Boggio, P.S.; Capraro, V.; Cichocka, A.; Cikara, M.; Crockett, M.J.; Crum, A.J.; Douglas, K.M.; Druckman, J.N.; et al. Using Social and Behavioural Science to Support COVID-19 Pandemic Response. *Nat. Hum. Behav.* **2020**, *4*, 460–471. [CrossRef]
110. Bremner, C. France Aims to Ban Fake News at Election Time. Available online: https://www.thetimes.co.uk/article/france-aims-to-ban-fake-news-at-election-time-jwspzjx83 (accessed on 2 October 2021).
111. BBC News Coronavirus: Unit Set up to Counter False Claims. Available online: https://www.bbc.com/news/uk-politics-51800216 (accessed on 2 October 2021).
112. Pieters, J. Dutch Politicians Want EU Anti-Fake News Watchdog Scrapped. Available online: https://nltimes.nl/2018/03/06/dutch-politicians-want-eu-anti-fake-news-watchdog-scrapped (accessed on 2 October 2021).
113. McGuire, W.J. A Vaccine for Brainwash. *Psychol. Today* **1970**, *3*, 36–64.
114. Banas, J.A.; Rains, S.A. A Meta-Analysis of Research on Inoculation Theory. *Commun. Monogr.* **2010**, *77*, 281–311. [CrossRef]
115. Bad News. Available online: www.getbadnews.com (accessed on 8 October 2021).
116. Go Viral! Available online: https://www.goviralgame.com/en/play (accessed on 8 October 2021).
117. Basol, M.; Roozenbeek, J.; Van der Linden, S. Good News about Bad News: Gamified Inoculation Boosts Confidence and Cognitive Immunity Against Fake News. *J. Cognit.* **2020**, *3*, 2. [CrossRef] [PubMed]
118. Guess, A.M.; Lerner, M.; Lyons, B.; Montgomery, J.M.; Nyhan, B.; Reifler, J.; Sircar, N. A Digital Media Literacy Intervention Increases Discernment between Mainstream and False News in the United States and India. *Proc. Natl. Acad. Sci. USA* **2020**, *117*, 15536–15545. [CrossRef] [PubMed]

encyclopedia

Entry

COVID-19 and Fake News

Javier Bustos Díaz [1,2] and Ruben Nicolas-Sans [1,2,*]

1 ESIC Business and Marketing School, Passeig Santa Eulália, 2, 08017 Barcelona, Spain; javier.bustos@esic.edu
2 Research Department, ESIC University, Avenida Juan XXIII, Pozuelo de Alarcón, 12, 28224 Madrid, Spain
* Correspondence: ruben.nicolas@esic.edu

Definition: COVID-19 can be defined as a global pandemic caused by a coronavirus that first surfaced in 2019. Fake news refers to false reports that can be found in digital media. The combination of these two concepts creates an especially mismanaged situation that can result in widespread unease among the population, to whom the news appears continuously and without quality filters.

Keywords: COVID-19; fake news; media literacy

Citation: Bustos Díaz, J.; Nicolas-Sans, R. COVID-19 and Fake News. *Encyclopedia* **2021**, *1*, 1175–1181. https://doi.org/10.3390/encyclopedia1040088

Academic Editor: Stephen Bustin

Received: 23 September 2021
Accepted: 2 November 2021
Published: 5 November 2021

1. Introduction

We live in a digital society. To put this fact into context, we must focus on the data; 48.97% of the world population uses the Internet, according to the World Bank [1]. This percentage grows exponentially if we look only at the ratio of developed countries with advanced technological infrastructures and notable levels of industrialisation, where this percentage is more than 77.42% according to the same source. The Internet has changed the way in which the world is seen and understood, but, above all, it has changed the way in which people communicate. Human relationships could not be understood today without social media, which has a penetration rate of 70% in Europe and North America [2]. In fact, according to data provided by Statista [2], in a single minute on the Internet, 69 million messages are sent from WhatsApp and Facebook Messenger, there are 5000 downloads on TikTok, 500 h of videos are uploaded onto YouTube, 197.6 million emails are sent, and there are 2 million Twitch views. In summary, society as a whole spends a large part of its time on the Internet both for leisure and for work; mankind today lives in a network society [3].

However, although leisure and connectivity are an essential part of people's daily lives, information gathering is an activity that is also carried out through these channels. The data provided by Digital News Report [4] on this question establishes that 82% of people use digital media (including social networks) as an information channel. The smartphone is the preferred device for accessing news, with 69% compared to the 49% who prefer the computer, and 18% who prefer the tablet. However, all social progress brings with it a series of consequences. In this case, although society is more interconnected than ever, it also has to face a hyperproduction of pseudo-contents [5] (contents containing intentionally false information) for which perhaps it is not prepared, and which have become a globalised problem that generated great confusion during the pandemic caused by COVID-19.

2. What Is Fake News? Towards a Definition

The Oxford Dictionary, which selected this combination of words as the word of the year in 2017 [6], defines fake news as "false reports of events, written and read on websites". Whilst it is true that this explanation can show with total clarity what fake news is, some authors go a step further and try to argue and qualify these words. In this sense, Gelfert argues that, although we understand disinformation as a type of information, fake news must be classified as a type of news. At the same time, he explains that its two most obvious characteristics are based on the type categorised as news, since fake news is presented as news, but unlike journalistic or academic information, it aims to deceive the target audience [7].

Intentionality is one of the key elements when it comes to differentiating fake news from another series of casuistry that may occur [8,9]. Within this idea it is explained that fake news should not be confused with other types of erroneous or misleading information, namely, errors by journalists or politicians, rumours or conspiracies without association to specific news articles, and entertainment-oriented formats such as satire [8].

Therefore, although we can understand fake news as being those false reports on web pages [10], we must also assume that there are, both in online press and on web portals, as well as on other information sites, a whole series of news and facts that, whether due to lack of journalistic rigour or simple human error, cannot be considered fake news.

For its part, the European Commission [11] defines this phenomenon, and explains that disinformation is "verifiably false or misleading information created, presented and disseminated for economic gain or to intentionally deceive the public". the knowledge of the agents involved in it, and the development that is spread without the intention to mislead, and often shared because the user believes it to be true.

The spread of both disinformation and misinformation can have a range of consequences, such as threatening our democracies, polarising debates, and putting the health, security, and environment of EU citizens at risk. This matter has been amplified since the spread of COVID-19 [11]. Large-scale disinformation campaigns are a major challenge for Europe and require a coordinated response from EU countries, EU institutions, social networks, news media, and EU citizens.

The Commission has developed a number of initiatives to tackle disinformation [11]:

1. The Code of Practice on Disinformation lays out a set of worldwide self-regulatory standards for industry.
2. The European Digital Media Observatory is a European hub for fact-checkers, academics, and other relevant stakeholders to support policy-makers.
3. The action plan on disinformation aims to strengthen EU capability and cooperation in the fight against disinformation.
4. The European Democracy Action Plan will develop guidelines for obligations and accountability of online platforms in the fight against disinformation.
5. The Communication on "tackling online disinformation: a European approach" is a collection of tools to tackle the spread of disinformation and ensure the protection of EU values.
6. The COVID-19 monitoring and reporting programme, carried out by signatories of the Code of Practice, acts as a transparency measure to ensure accountability in tackling disinformation.

Within the scope of fake news, there is another series of terms and concepts that are related, and yet it is not possible to find an exact definition of the phenomenon. This is the case of post-truth, which authors such as Capilla have worked on and analysed, and have concluded that, ultimately, it consists of the substitution of facts for beliefs and emotions in social discourses [12].

3. The History of Fake News

Although the term fake news is associated with the former President of the United States, Donald Trump [8,9,13], some authors point out that the dissemination of false information with a preconceived and malicious intention has existed for centuries. Regarding this fact, Salas Abad points out some of the historical moments where it can be considered that fake news was generated. In this sense, it can be remembered that Socrates already classified the sophists as transmitters of false news, or in the Middle Ages papal bulls were falsified for their own benefit [14]. On the other hand, we cannot fail to appreciate historical events that the author points out, such as the one that arose with Orson Welles' The War of the Worlds in 1938, which Salas Abad [14] compares with fake news. Following radio broadcasts of Welles' book, a great stir and social impact were generated despite the incidents being fictitious, due to the fact that the narration was so realistic that many citizens believed that an alien invasion was actually occurring.

Other authors explain that the term fake news itself appeared more than a century ago, specifically in Harper's Weekly in 1925 entitled "Fake News and the Public" [15]. In this sense, works such as the study conducted by Rodríguez-Fernández, in which fake news was collected and analysed with the objective of identifying the types of organisation in Spain most affected by fake news and the nature of the false information spread, conclude that, although the current stage of proliferation that exists within the current communication system has shown social concern for this phenomenon, it is evident that this is not a new event, and it has occurred at many moments in our recent history, especially within the political sphere as an element of electoral propaganda [16].

Finally, as mentioned at the beginning of this section, fake news has become a relevant part of the current communication system [17], which is found in both the referendum on Brexit and the election of Donald Trump in the United States, two moments of its proliferation [7].

4. Why Has Fake News Been So Successful during the Period of COVID-19?

As described in the opening paragraphs, society today is hyper-connected. For this reason, there is a rapid dissemination of information. This does not imply that all information is verified, and social networks have allowed for the dissemination of verified and unverified content, prepared by professionals and non-professionals, creating an ideal context for spreading fake news [17].

Consequently, and especially in a period of need for information such as that generated by the COVID-19 pandemic, a problem of spreading fake news with the intention of deceiving the general public has been brought about and, as described, can be found on the Internet's social networks. Its rapid dissemination is what is known as viralisation, which provides the perfect setting for fake news to spread [18].

In this new scenario, information technology and its distribution have relegated traditional media to second place; that is to say, journalism has ceased to be the guarantor of information in favour of the dissemination and speed that a retweet on Twitter or a "like" on Facebook can achieve [19]. This first factor, the decline of journalism in favour of the dissemination of social networks, has been found to be one of the decisive factors when fake news finds a media ecosystem without a gatekeeper that acts as a natural filter of information.

However, this is not the only factor. If there is a lack of journalism capable of assuming control of the flow of communication, media literacy is presented as the most solid alternative when it comes to dealing with fake news. However, the general public on many occasions do not know how to recognise false information when it is presented to them [18].

Another aspect of this new media ecosystem that has become one of the main drivers of fake news is the brevity of the exposure linked to the use of social media networks. On this issue, the new communication technologies are even supplanting those that until now were essential, for example, in the company. Thus, the use of WhatsApp has been normalised and has relegated e-mail in many aspects. In other words, as an attempt to achieve faster results, less is being written [20].

On the other hand, the constant use of social networks is itself a determining factor when it comes to being a victim of fake news. This is because the time of exposure to false news, in the specific case of Facebook, can lead users to consume this type of information because of their constant, albeit accidental, consumption from the exposure [21].

Finally, a determining factor when it comes to understanding why fake news spreads so easily and, above all, acquires the status of news for those who consume it is the viral effect of social networks. That is, legitimacy based on emotional relationships between users and their political bias is acquired once they are shared by "friends" on social networks [22].

In any case, there are studies that conclusively demonstrate that the users of social networks were motivated by various factors to share news related to COVID-19. "It is their behaviour, either vigilant or ignorant when consuming and disseminating messages related to COVID-19, that contribute to fake news spreading and its grave impacts on society" [23].

Therefore, according to the conclusions of Pérez-Dasilva et al., it has become clear that, in addition to facing an economic and public health crisis, we are facing an information crisis [13].

Following this same line of argument, the work carried out by Casero Ripollés presents empirical findings that reaffirm this hypothesis and link the situation experienced as a result of COVID-19 with the increase in the search for information. "In the case of COVID-19, 92% of adults in the United States frequently accessed the news about the pandemic, registering an increase of 34% over the period prior to the health emergency" XXI [24].

Lastly, and in relation to that which was put forth in the article by Gutiérrez et al., titled "Fake news about COVID-19: a comparative analysis of six Ibero-American countries", it is shown that the percentage of fake news that reached the traditional media is almost insignificant, which reinforces the hypothesis that fact-checking journalism is a practice that does indeed help to combat the problem of fake news [25].

5. Lack of Media Literacy

Based on the problems raised, media literacy is more necessary than ever. Authors such as Fernández-García have already stated even before the proliferation of fake news that came from the COVID-19 pandemic that, "If new generations obtain their information from social networks and other online resources, they must learn to decode what they read" [26].

However, the problem of the need to promote media literacy is not linked to fake news. Indeed, we could affirm that, if it had been considered a formal element within compulsory education, we would have witnessed a decline in fake news instead of its proliferation. Based on this, it is necessary to "analyse, study and examine the contents and objectives of literacy, to adapt them to a multimodal and media system" [27].

This last idea, raised by Gutiérrez and Tyner, is argued by the authors based on the following premise: if we understand education to be the preparation of the society of tomorrow we cannot leave the environment, which is becoming more and more digital every day, out of the study. In contrast, over the last few decades, this aspect has been relegated to the background [27].

This same premise has been defended and expanded from different angles by various academics who have even proposed direct and applicable solutions in the current context. In this sense, Aguaded et al. argued for the introduction of digital and informational education under the protection of active public policy, with the purpose of creating a media-literate general public through critical, participatory, and creative training. These same authors, among other premises, proposed at the same time the introduction of programs that would allow the general public to learn under a mixture of critical training with interpretative and investigative journalism [5].

All these questions raised so far were collected by Alcolea and Reig:

> "It is a challenge to face the power of the media and to accept the rejection that the existence of a real critical vision can generate within itself. However, the vertiginous technological change, the ubiquity of disinformation and the crucial role of the knowledge of the agents involved in it, and the development of critical thinking to face up to it forces the updating of this curriculum and its periodical review, making it more necessary than ever to approach it from a structural approach that favours a critical general public and the democratic process" [28].

Finally, and in line with what has been established so far, some authors suggest that the real solution to fight against fake news consists in applying a media education clearly, directly, and under clearly defined objectives [29].

6. How to Stop Fake News in Times of COVID-19

It is evident that, although media literacy is one of the main elements in the fight against fake news, it is also true that society as a whole has been decades late in applying it. Consequently, in the short term, it seems unlikely that this is the solution. However, a series of mechanisms have been put into place that help the user of social networks to filter this kind of information, as well as companies and entities with governmental support or entirely private companies, whose objective is to constantly analyse and report fake news.

Furthermore, some studies even propose the automatic detection of fake news as a response [30]. For example, in relation to this fact, in the case of Spain, there is the "Maldito Bulo" platform whose aim is to detect false information, but others, such as Truth-o-meter, also exist. Additionally, there is another series of tools that can improve the search quality of Internet information, such as a Google Chrome extension that launches an alert when you enter an unreliable or untrustworthy website or a satirical website (when it is not known if a website is humorous). In addition, it reports how much news from that medium has been disproved up to that moment [31].

As has been established, one of the main problems when dealing with control over fake news is found in social networks. In this regard, and as Brummette et al. [32] points out, their owners and founders must be involved to be part of the solution to the problem. Based on this, a series of proposals executed by the main social networks and by the main information search engines are presented below, taken from the works of Bustos Díaz and Ruiz del Olmo:

- Facebook, Twitter, and Instagram prominently place tools to fight against fake news, evidencing the concern on the part of social networks about the spread of false news, something that undermines the credibility of the channel.
- The involvement of the large social media platforms in this matter is due to two main issues: to reduce to a minimum the possible consumption of fake news by users, while at the same time seeking to consolidate the audience of the brand and to avoid losing users and credibility. That is, brands try to prevent themselves from becoming synonymous with fake news. Therefore, it can be concluded that it is a job that has two objectives: improving the user experience and maintaining the brand image.
- Secondly, the clear commitment of all of them to use official sources of recognised prestige as means of communication, whether press, digital, radio, or television [33].
- In all of them, the elimination of susceptible or possibly misleading accounts is a constant. As far as this is concerned, within the passive tools, we can see that the news centres created by Facebook and Twitter as well as the Instagram warning for users link directly to the World Health Organisation profile [33].

Together, the three case studies highlight the importance of quality journalism—of proven news in times of crisis. In this case, the three companies have used traditional media with proven trajectories and great credibility (despite the deterioration and general precariousness of journalistic information in recent years). There is no distinction by type of media, i.e., television, radio, and press, suggesting that the information from all of them is beyond the support that each one uses [34].

7. Conclusions

This work has theoretically addressed the conceptualisation of fake news, its evolution, its history, and the reasons that have allowed its rapid dissemination during the COVID 19 pandemic. Based on this, the following conclusions can be drawn.

In the first place, as has been shown in the development of this chapter of the book, the problem of fake news is not new. What we are experiencing now as a society is only an accentuated manifestation of a negative aspect of the information that has been manifesting itself in recent times. On the other hand, the need for the application in educational terms of media literacy is evident. The solutions addressed in the section "How to stop fake news in times of COVID-19" represent a temporary and short-term solution that does not fix the underlying problem, which is the lack of capacity of today's society to identify what is fake news and what is not.

It has also been shown that society today depends more than ever on quality journalism. Until the emergence of social networks, journalism represented a social political function that had been classified as "the fourth power". This lack of filtering of information, which has traditionally been known as the gatekeeper, is what search engines and social networks are applying. However, it seems more interesting that journalism once again assumes its role within the social context: "In a media ecosystem in which lies are institutionalised with over-information and a great abundance of sources, it is necessary to verify the veracity of the news, and here lies an opportunity for journalism" [20].

The role of politicians emerges as another key aspect in the fight against fake news. In this piece of work, a fact collected by scientific literature on this subject has been reflected. Donald Trump, for example, has become a viral phenomenon, contributing on many occasions false statements about the pandemic that have confused society. Finally, the academy is making a considerable effort to analyse, understand, and comprehend this phenomenon. Based on this, it has been observed that the term "fake news" was present in 50% of the keywords of the 10 most cited articles of the Web of Science and 70% of the most cited articles of Scopus [35]. Therefore, it seems clear that the problem must be addressed jointly, using media literacy as a driver and creator of a society more prepared to deal with fake news in combination with, as the political debate becomes more serious, a more rigorous press and an academy that continues to contribute new discoveries.

In short, we are witnessing a process in which the proliferation of fake news is flooding the digital ecosystem and, therefore, creating a social problem that can lead to collective hysteria and other associated processes. Although, as defined in this text, there are tools both in the main search engines and in social networks, we cannot leave the user aside. Digitalisation implies knowing how to use technologies, but, above all, using them responsibly. To this end, it is essential, as has been argued, to work on the process of media literacy and to go deeper in terms of social implantation in order to reduce the impact of fake news on society as a whole. Despite the existing filters in social networks and the main search engines, it is clear that fake news continues to penetrate society. Therefore, the need for media literacy has become an extremely relevant issue.

Author Contributions: Conceptualisation, J.B.D.; methodology, R.N.-S.; validation, R.N.-S.; formal analysis, R.N.-S.; investigation, R.N.-S. and J.B.D.; resources, J.B.D.; data curation, R.N.-S.; writing—original draft preparation, J.B.D.; writing—review and editing, R.N.-S.; project administration, J.B.D.; funding acquisition, J.B.D. All authors have read and agreed to the published version of the manuscript.

Funding: This research was funded by ESIC Business and Marketing, grant number ESIC 1-B-2021.

Institutional Review Board Statement: Not applicable.

Informed Consent Statement: Not applicable.

Conflicts of Interest: The authors declare no conflict of interest.

Entry Link on the Encyclopedia Platform: https://encyclopedia.pub/16888.

References

1. The World Bank. Available online: https://data.worldbank.org/indicator/IT.NET.USER.ZS (accessed on 20 August 2021).
2. Statista. Available online: https://www.statista.com/ (accessed on 20 August 2021).
3. Castells, M. *La Sociedad Red: Una Visión Global*; Alianza Editorial: Madrid, Spain, 2006; ISBN 84-206-4784-5.
4. Newman, N.; Fletcher, R.; Schulz, A.; Andı, S.; Kleis Nielsen, R. *Reuters Institute Digital News Report 2020*; Reuters Institute for the Study of Journalism: Oxford, UK, 2020; ISBN 978-1-907384-75-2.
5. Aguaded, J.I.; Romero-Rodríguez, L.M. Mediamorfosis y desinformación en la infoesfera: Alfabetización mediática, digital e informacional ante los cambios de hábitos de consumo informativo. *Educ. Knowl. Soc.* **2015**, *16*, 44–57. [CrossRef]
6. Rodríguez, C. "Fake news", palabra del año del Diccionario Oxford. In *El Mundo*; El Mundo: Madrid, Spain, 2017.
7. Gelfert, A. Fake News: A Definition. *Informal Log.* **2018**, *38*, 84–117. [CrossRef]

8. Quandt, T.; Boberg, S.; Frischlich, L.; Schatto-Eckrodt, T. Fake News. In *The International Encyclopedia of Journalism Studies*; Wiley: New York, NY, USA, 2019; pp. 1–6. [CrossRef]
9. Lopez-Borrull, A.; Vives-Gràcia, J.; Badell, J.-I. Fake news, ¿amenaza u oportunidad para los profesionales de la información y la documentación? *Prof. Inf.* **2018**, *27*, 1346–1356. [CrossRef]
10. Oxford English Dictionary. Available online: https://www.oed.com/ (accessed on 20 August 2021).
11. Comisión Europea: Lucha Contra la Desinformación. Available online: https://ec.europa.eu/info/live-work-travel-eu/coronavirus-response/fighting-disinformation_es#relatedlinks (accessed on 18 October 2021).
12. Capilla, P. ¿De qué hablamos cuando hablamos de posverdad? Análisis del término en siete diarios de calidad. *Prof. Inf.* **2019**, *28*, 1–13. [CrossRef]
13. Pérez-Dasilva, J.-A.; Meso-Ayerdi, K.; Mendiguren-Galdospín, T. Fake news y coronavirus: Detección de los principales actores y tendencias a través del análisis de las conversaciones en Twitter. *Prof. Inf.* **2020**, 1–22. [CrossRef]
14. Salas Abad, C. La primera fake news de la historia. *Hist. Comun. Soc.* **2019**, *24*, 411–431. [CrossRef]
15. Lazer, D.M.; Baum, M.A.; Benkler, Y.; Berinsky, A.J.; Greenhill, K.M.; Menczer, F.; Metzger, M.J.; Nyhan, B.; Pennycook, G.; Rothschild, D.; et al. The science of fake news. *Science* **2018**, *359*, 1094–1096. [CrossRef]
16. Rodríguez-Fernández, L. Desinformación y comunicación organizacional: Estudio sobre el impacto de las fake news. *Rev. Lat. Comun. Soc.* **2019**, *74*, 1714–1728. [CrossRef]
17. Tandoc, E.C., Jr.; Ling, R.; Westlund, O.; Duffy, A.; Goh, D.; Zheng Wei, L. Audiences' acts of authentication in the age of fake news: A conceptual framework. *New Media Soc.* **2018**, *20*, 2745–2763. [CrossRef]
18. Parra Valero, P.; Oliveira, L. Fake news: Una revisión sistemática de la literatura. *Observatorio OBS* **2018**, *12*, 54–78. [CrossRef]
19. Alonso González, M. Fake News: Desinformación en la era de la sociedad de la información. *Ámbitos Rev. Int. Comun.* **2019**, *45*, 29–52. [CrossRef]
20. Romero y Olmo, J.A. Desinformación. Concepto y perspectivas. *Análisis Real Inst. Elcano* **2019**, *41*, 1–8.
21. Nelson, J.L.; Harsh, T. The small, disloyal fake news audience: The role of audience availability in fake news consumption. *New Media Soc.* **2018**, *20*, 3720–3737. [CrossRef]
22. Pangrazio, L. What's new about 'fake news'? Critical digital literacies in an era of fake news, post-truth and clickbait. *Páginas Educ.* **2018**, *11*, 6–22. [CrossRef]
23. Apuke, O.D.; Omar, B. Noticias falsas y COVID-19: Modelando los predictores del intercambio de noticias falsas entre los usuarios de las redes sociales. *Telemát. Inf.* **2021**, *56*, 101475. [CrossRef]
24. Casero-Ripollés, A. Impacto del COVID-19 en el sistema de medios. Consecuencias comunicativas y democráticas del consumo de noticias durante el brote. *Prof. Inf.* **2020**, 1–12. [CrossRef]
25. Gutiérrez-Coba, L.M.; Coba-Gutiérrez, P.; Gómez-Díaz, J.A. Noticias falsas y desinformación sobre el COVID-19: Análisis comparativo de seis países iberoamericanos. *Rev. Lat. Comun. Soc.* **2020**, *78*, 237–264. [CrossRef]
26. Fernández-García, N. Fake news: Una oportunidad para la alfabetización mediática. *Nueva Soc.* **2017**, *269*, 66–77.
27. Gutiérrez, A.; Tyner, K. Educación para los medios, alfabetización mediática y competencia digital. *Comunicar* **2012**, *19*, 31–39. [CrossRef]
28. Alcolea-Díaz, G.; Reig, R.; Mancinas-Chávez, R. Currículo de Alfabetización Mediática e Informacional de la UNESCO para profesores desde la perspectiva de la Estructura de la Información. *Comunicar* **2020**, *28*, 103–114. [CrossRef]
29. Kendall, A.; McDougall, J. Alfabetización mediática crítica en la postmodernidad. *Comunicar* **2019**, *19*, 21–29. [CrossRef]
30. Pérez-Rosas, V.; Kleinberg, B.; Lefevre, A.; Mihalcea, R. Automatic detection of fake news. *arXiv* **2017**, arXiv:1708.07104.
31. Magallón-Rosa, R. Nuevos formatos de verificación. El caso de Maldito Bulo en Twitter. *Sphera Publ.* **2018**, *1*, 41–62.
32. Brummette, J.; DiStaso, M.; Vafeiadis, M.; Messner, M. Read all about it: The politicization of "fake news" on Twitter. *J. Mass Commun. Q.* **2018**, *95*, 497–517. [CrossRef]
33. Bustos-Díaz, J.; Ruiz-del-Olmo, F.J. Comunicar en tiempos de crisis en las redes sociales. Estrategias de verificación e intermediación informativa en los casos de Facebook, Instagram y Twitter durante la COVID-19. *Hipertext Net* **2020**, *21*, 115–125. [CrossRef]
34. Bustos-Díaz, J.; Ruiz-del-Olmo, F.J. Fuentes verificadas ante las Fakes News. El caso de Facebook, Google y Microsoft frente a la desinformación durante el COVID-19. *Rev. Estilos Aprendiz.* **2020**, *13*, 7–18.
35. Alfonso, I.B.; Galera, C.G.; Calvo, S.T. El impacto de las fake news en la investigación en Ciencias Sociales. Revisión bibliográfica sistematizada. *Hist. Comun. Soc.* **2019**, *24*, 449–469. [CrossRef]

encyclopedia

MDPI

Entry

Sheet Barrier and Intubating Stylet

Phil B. Tsai [1] and Hsiang-Ning Luk [2,*]

[1] Department of Anesthesiology, Rancho Los Amigos National Rehabilitation Center, Downey, CA 90242, USA; ptsai@dhs.lacounty.gov
[2] Department of Anesthesia, Hualien Tzu-Chi Medical Center, Hualien 97002, Taiwan
* Correspondence: lukairforce@gmail.com

Definition: Coronavirus disease 2019 (COVID-19), a respiratory syndrome caused by SARS-CoV-2, can be transmitted through respiratory droplets and aerosols of droplet nuclei. Aerosol-generating medical procedures (AGMP) are needed to take care of critically ill patients but place health care providers at risk of infection. With limited supplies of personal protective equipment (PPE), barrier systems were developed to help protect health care providers during tracheal intubation. The video intubating stylet shows promise to become the preferred intubation device in conjunction with plastic sheet barriers during the COVID-19 pandemic.

Keywords: COVID-19; endotracheal intubation; tracheal intubation; video intubating stylet; plastic sheet; barrier

Citation: Tsai, P.B.; Luk, H.-N. Sheet Barrier and Intubating Stylet. *Encyclopedia* **2021**, *1*, 1058–1075. https://doi.org/10.3390/encyclopedia1040081

Academic Editor: Stephen Bustin

Received: 26 August 2021
Accepted: 19 October 2021
Published: 25 October 2021

1. Introduction

Since the first case of viral pneumonia was reported from Wuhan, China in late December of 2019, severe acute respiratory syndrome coronavirus 2 (SARS-CoV-2), the causative pathogen for the Coronavirus disease 2019 (COVID-19) pandemic, has run rampant across the world [1]. As of 30 September 2021, there have been 232,636,622 confirmed cases and 4,762,089 COVID deaths [2]. As cases grew at an alarmingly exponential rate, it was quickly identified that COVID-19 could be transmitted through respiratory droplets and even through the aerosolization of droplet nuclei [3,4]. Because of the pathology and progression of the disease towards respiratory failure, aerosol-generating medical procedures (AGMP) such as laryngoscopy, endotracheal intubation and extubation, tracheostomy, bronchoscopy and bronchoalveolar lavage, positive pressure ventilation, cardiopulmonary resuscitation with bag-valve-mask, suctioning, and nasopharyngeal aspiration and washing would be necessary to take care of patients with COVID-19 infection [5]. Healthcare providers in the fields of anesthesiology, critical care medicine, emergency medicine, and otolaryngology, because of their roles in performing AGMPs for these patients, found themselves at risk of infection.

2. The Development of Barrier Systems

Personal protective equipment (PPE) is the primary basis for prevention of infection to healthcare workers while performing their tasks. Necessary PPE during the COVID-19 pandemic includes medical-grade masks, respirators, goggles, eye shields, face shields, gowns, gloves, shoe coverings, and head coverings [6] (Figure 1). Strict donning and doffing procedures are necessary to avoid accidental contamination of other work areas and the transmission to other patients and staff in the hospital [7]. It was quickly realized that there were not sufficient stores of PPE to safely allow healthcare providers to perform daily patient care during the pandemic [8]. Industry had a hard time ramping up production in a timely manner, and global disparities existed and have continued to exist. Without adequate PPE, coupled with other factors such as a lack of available testing, especially during the early stages of the pandemic [9], the growing number of confirmed and suspected cases, as well as an overwhelming workload, frontline medical workers endured significant anxiety performing their expected duties as they worried about becoming infected, as well as transmitting the disease to family members [10]. Currently, over 18 months into the pandemic, even with the rollout of vaccines, challenges to their widespread deployment as well as the proliferation of COVID-19 variants have prevented the world from curtailing the disease [11].

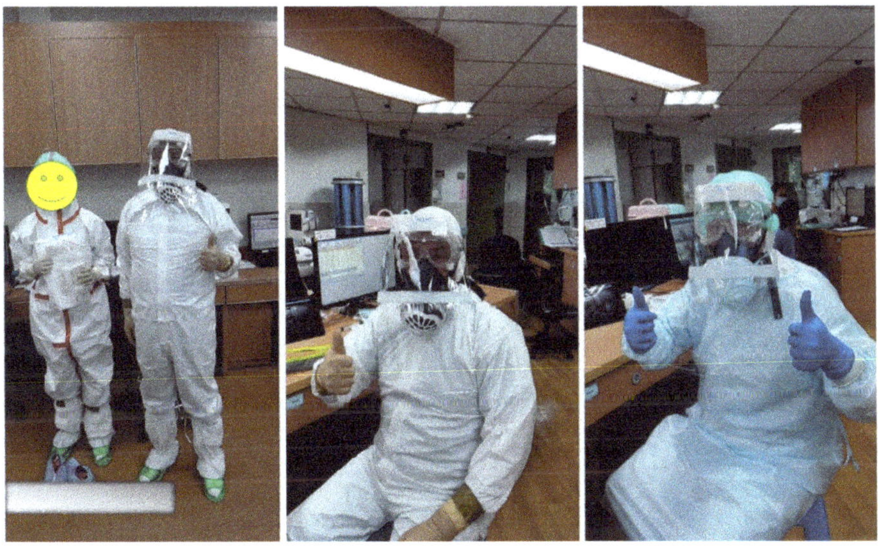

Figure 1. Examples of personal protective equipment (PPE) used by medical staff while caring for patients undergoing aerosol generating medical procedures (AGMP) during the COVID-19 pandemic.

Without adequate PPE, health care professionals quickly looked to alternative means of protection against viral transmission. One strategy was the use of a transparent physical barriers. The first reported model was designed by a Taiwanese anesthesiologist who constructed a transparent four-sided box made of plexiglass that was placed between the patient and the airway manager during tracheal intubation [12] (Figure 2A). The plans for this structure were quickly shared on social media [13], and Canneli et al. were the first to report on its use in the scientific literature [14]. Subsequently, after this idea was promoted by news and social media and the device was proliferated and distributed to some users, multiple variations of barrier devices were introduced [15–21]. These barriers were applied not just for endotracheal intubation and airway management (Figure 2B,C) but were utilized in various aspects of medical care, as well as applied to facilitate other forms of human interaction during the pandemic (Figure 3). On 1 May 2020, the United States Food and Drug Administration (FDA) issued an emergency use authorization (EUA) for protective barrier enclosures [22]. Over time, three general device types were identified: (1) rigid transparent box, (2) plastic sheet with frame, and (3) plastic sheet without frame (Figure 2).

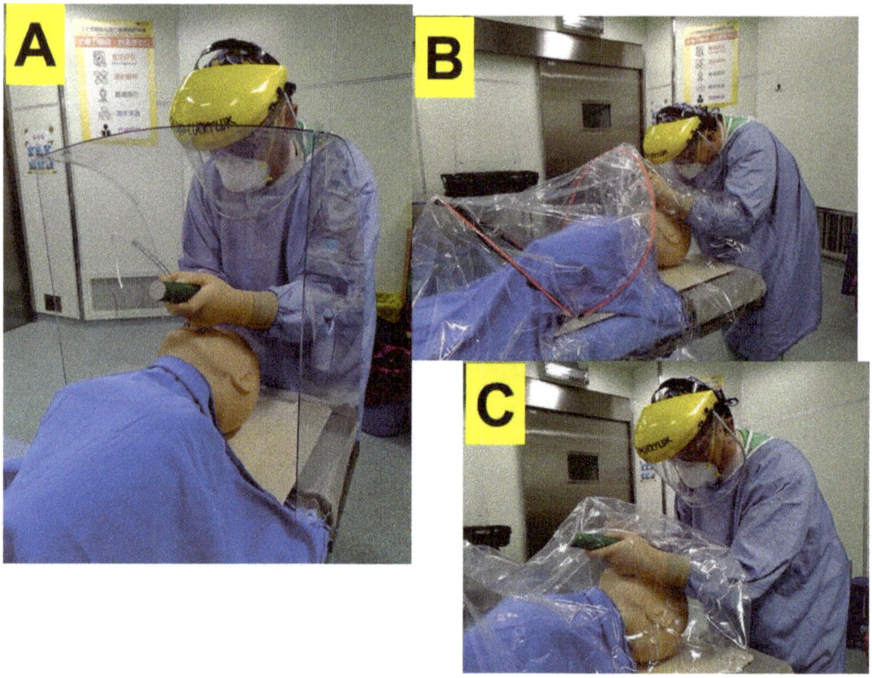

Figure 2. Various barrier systems utilized during performance of direct laryngoscopy and endotracheal intubation. (**A**) Rigid plastic box, (**B**) Plastic sheet with frame, (**C**) Plastic sheet without frame.

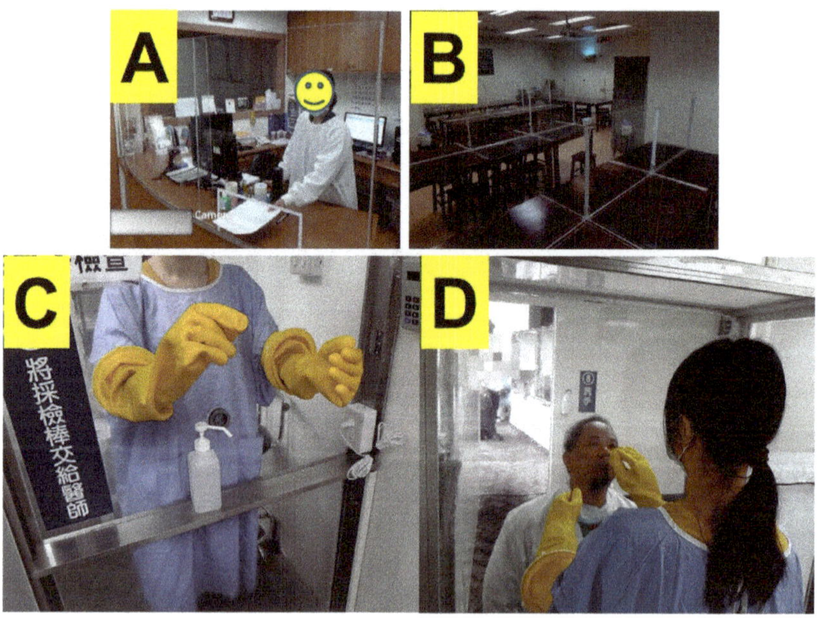

Figure 3. Various applications of transparent plastic barriers during the COVID-19 pandemic. (**A**) Front desk, (**B**) Cafeteria, (**C**,**D**) Nasopharyngeal COVID-19 testing.

Meanwhile, some airway management experts expressed their serious concerns on such a MacGyverism-style improvised medical device (e.g., the "aerosol box") and argued about the untested effectiveness and safety issues of this EUA device [23–27]. The main concerns raised against such physical barrier enclosure include the following: (1) restriction of hand movement of the intubator and assistants; (2) heavy and bulky plexiglass is difficult to carry and position or reposition in emergency situations; (3) limited for certain body habitus and positions; (4) confined space for airway maneuvering; (5) ergonomically difficult to manipulate airway equipment; (6) introducing other new risks of cross-contamination during the use, disinfection, and disposal processes; (7) increases the cognitive load of the staff and the risk of subsequent contamination; and (8) breaches in PPE due to a tear cut by the box edge. Some pointed out that such an unvalidated box design does not reduce risks (of being infected) and probably has unintended safety consequences to the airway managers, medical staff, and the patients.

3. Tracheal Intubation during the COVID-19 Pandemic

Tracheal or endotracheal intubation, the process of placing a breathing tube in the patient's airway in order to maintain patency of the airway and provide oxygenation and ventilation, is often necessary in patients with critical respiratory illness [28]. Traditionally, the intubation process involves manipulating the head and neck to align the oral, laryngeal, and pharyngeal axes, the placement of a laryngoscope into the oropharynx to retract the tongue and soft tissues of the mouth, and the introduction of an endotracheal tube (ETT), loaded onto a stylet, past the glottic opening [29]. This procedure can be performed by a single operator, but an assistant often helps with the optimization of patient positioning such as jaw lift and lip retraction, handing the ETT-mounted stylet to the intubator, removing the stylet after the ETT has passed the vocal cords, and/or inflating the cuff of the endotracheal tube.

The intubation process places the healthcare professional at risk for COVID-19 infection as during traditional direct laryngoscopy, the anesthesia provider may need to be very close to the patient's mouth in order to obtain a view of the glottis to advance the ETT (Figures 2 and 4A). During the COVID-19 pandemic, it was subsequently recommended that videolaryngoscopy be preferentially utilized for tracheal intubation [5,30,31]. The technology behind a videolaryngoscope is that a camera is placed at the tip of the device, which is projected to a monitor, either mounted on the device itself or on an independent stand. The airway manager is able to obtain a view of the patient's airway and guide the ETT through the patient's glottis without placing his or her face in close proximity to the patient's airway (Figure 4B). A recent Cochrane review had concluded that videolaryngoscopy may improve the success of tracheal intubation in adult patients, especially in difficult airways situations [32]. However, it should be noted that because of the significant increased costs of a videolaryngoscope, this device may not be available in every setting across the world.

There are many videolaryngoscopes on the market today, with regional preferences in a range of designs and costs. A subset of the videolaryngoscope is the video intubating stylet. This device is a rigid or semi-rigid stylet equipped with a camera at the tip projecting to a separate monitor (Figures 5 and 6). The ETT is mounted onto the video stylet in a similar fashion to a traditional stylet. The tip of the stylet may be designed to be malleable and anteflex. Because the camera resides within the stylet as opposed to on a separate videoscope, a laryngoscope is not necessary to perform endotracheal intubation (Figures 6 and 7). "To see is to intubate" and "to see is to believe" are the mottos of the design of a video-assisted intubating stylet, a pioneering work that could change the face of airway management [33].

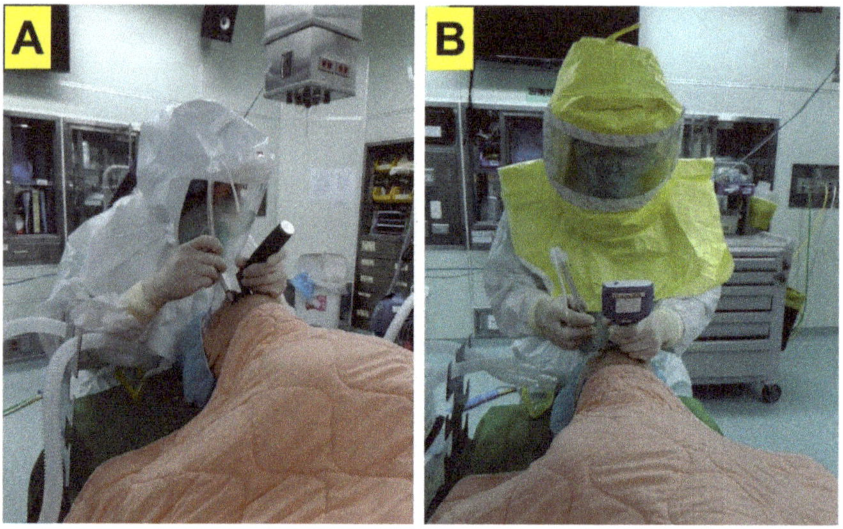

Figure 4. Proximity of the anesthesia provider to the patient's airway during: (**A**) direct laryngoscopy, (**B**) indirect laryngoscopy using a videolaryngoscope (Courtesy photos reproduced from Cell Transplantation, SAGE Journals).

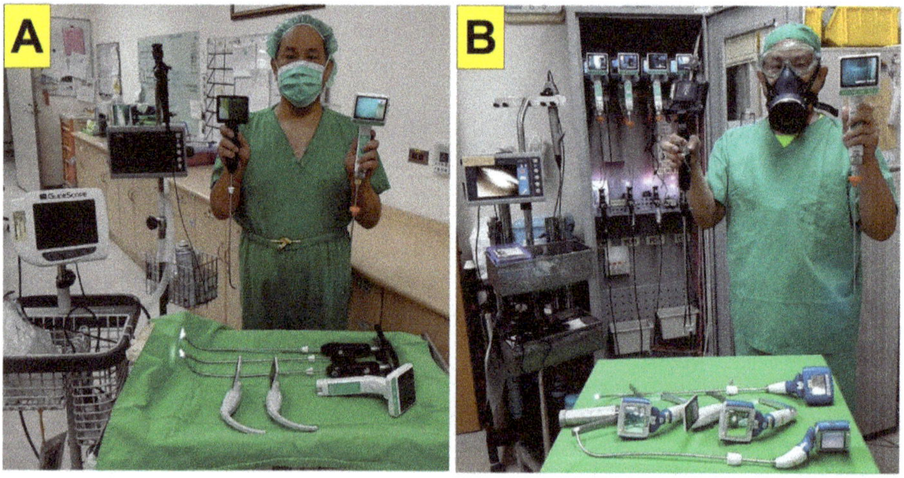

Figure 5. Prevalence of using video intubating stylet technique for tracheal intubation in Taiwan. (**A**) Department of Anesthesia in a 729-bed community hospital; (**B**) Department of Anesthesia in a 1110-bed tertiary medical Center.

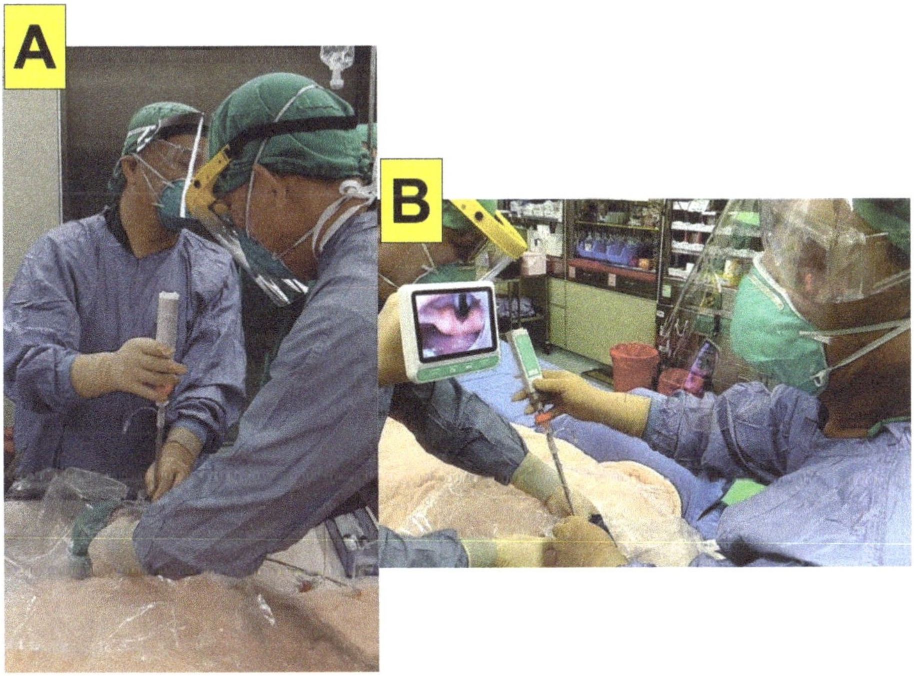

Figure 6. Real-world demonstration of endotracheal intubation utilizing the video intubating stylet and plastic sheet. A camera on the tip of the stylet captures a view of the glottis, which is projected to a separate monitor (For a demonstration video clip, see Supplementary Material). (**A**) Front view; (**B**) Side view.

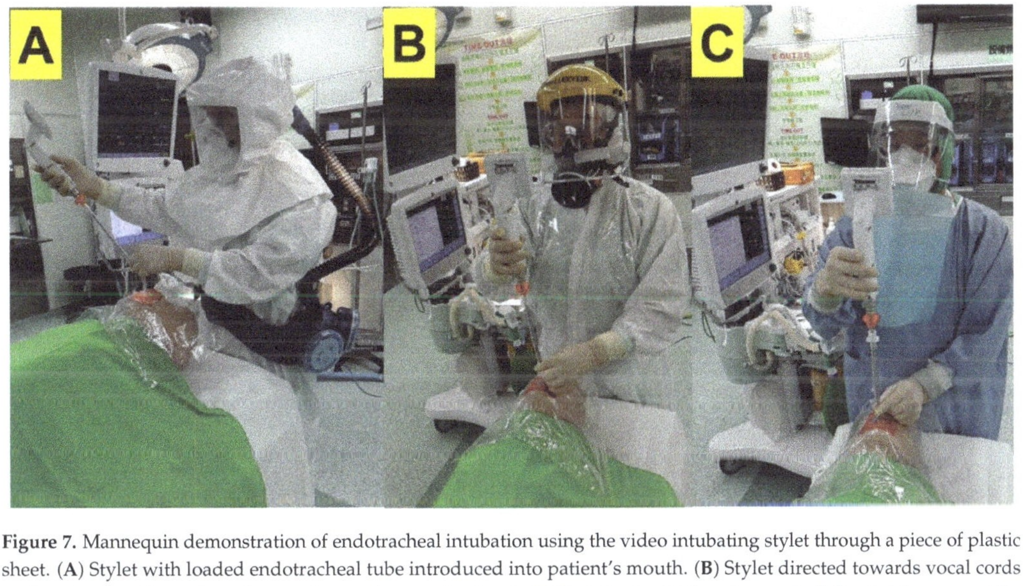

Figure 7. Mannequin demonstration of endotracheal intubation using the video intubating stylet through a piece of plastic sheet. (**A**) Stylet with loaded endotracheal tube introduced into patient's mouth. (**B**) Stylet directed towards vocal cords under visual guidance from the monitor on the proximal end. (**C**) Endotracheal tube advanced off the stylet once past the vocal cords. PPE with powered air-purifying respirator, P-100, and N-95 respirators were shown in this figure. (Courtesy photos reproduced from Asian Journal of Anesthesiology, Taiwan Society of Anaesthesiologists with permission).

A potential benefit of the intubating stylet is that it may be a more economical alternative to the videolaryngoscope. In addition, many videolaryngoscopes utilize disposal laryngoscope tips/blades, which can minimize infection but are also recurring costs. Other potential benefits of the intubating stylet include a small profile, which results in less overall patient airway manipulation, such as less opening of the mouth and less lifting of the tongue. Because of its slim profile, the video stylet is more easily sanitized compared to other videolaryngoscopes. Even prior to the COVID-19 pandemic, at many institutions, the video intubating stylet had become the preferred modality for performing tracheal intubation [34–37]. Table 1 and Figure 5 show examples of high use coverage of video-assisted intubating stylets in the departments of anesthesia in Taiwan. Moreover, among 24 medical centers in Taiwan, the departments of anesthesia in 20 of them are equipped with video-assisted intubating stylets.

Table 1. Use coverage of video-assisted intubating stylet in the Hualien Tzu-Chi Medical Center, Hualien, Taiwan.

	2016	2017	2018	2019	2020
Anesthesia Number	16,077	17,831	17,998	19,307	19,721
General Anesthesia Number	15,339	16,893	17,497	18,481	19,009
Laryngeal Mask Airway Number	5544	5134	5816	5902	5863
Endotracheal Tube Number	5953	6504	6920	6966	7418
Video Laryngoscope Number	0	0	20	100	635
Video Intubating Stylet Number	5953 **(100%)**	6504 **(100%)**	6900 **(99.7%)**	6866 **(98.6%)**	6783 **(91.4%)**

This hospital is a tertiary medical center in the east coast of Taiwan. There are 1110 beds, 1788 personnel, 20 operation rooms, 13 attending anesthesiologists, and 45 certified registered nurse anesthetists. The COVID-19 outbreak and pandemic started since December 2020.

4. Combining Barrier Systems with the Video Intubating Styletd

When incorporating a barrier system with the video stylet, the length of the intubating stylet precludes its use within a rigid barrier box (Figure 8), unless the box is drastically modified to accommodate the length of the intubating stylet. This may not be practical to manufacture, and the added height might also make the box difficult to handle as well as a safety concern to patients and medical staff. Additionally, the semi-rigid stylet is not long or flexible enough to be handled from outside the barrier box through the hand orifices at the head of the patient. It was quickly realized that the plastic sheet was the only barrier system that could be practically utilized with the video intubating stylet [38–40].

There are several ways that the plastic sheet can be utilized to protect the anesthesia provider. In its simplest unmodified form, the plastic sheet could be laid across the patient's head to function as a general barrier. The health care professional subsequently reaches under to the sheet to perform tracheal intubation (Figure 2C). Because of its malleability and transparency, other maneuvers not involving the airway itself, such as an assistant providing jaw lift, can be performed over the sheet (Figure 9). If the plastic sheet hampers the ability of the anesthesia provider to successfully intubate the patient, the sheet can be easily and rapidly removed, as opposed to the bulkier and heavier plastic box. Table 2 summarized the advantages and disadvantages of plastic sheet barriers design and aerosol box design.

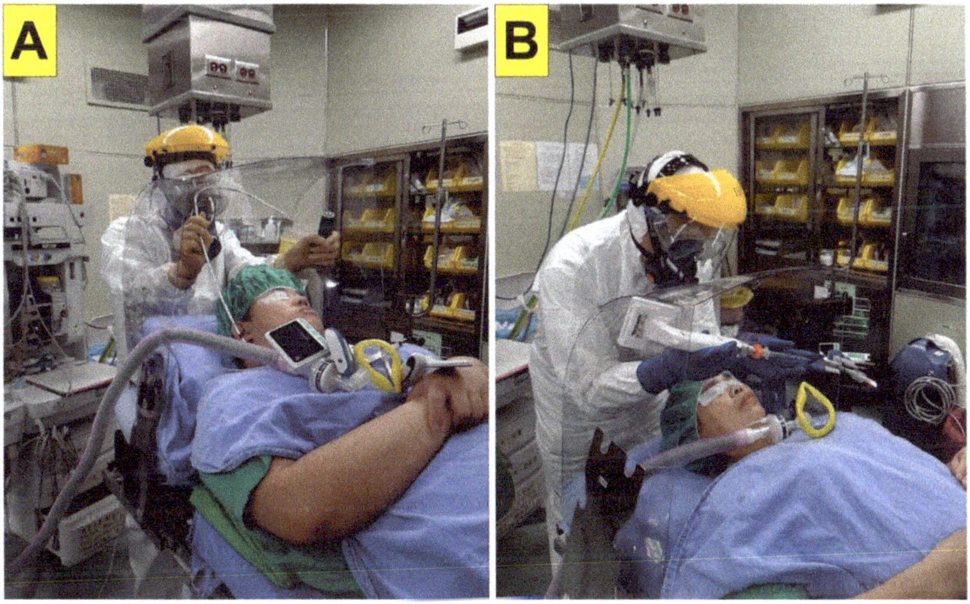

Figure 8. The plastic barrier box seriously limits the ability to perform endotracheal intubation utilizing: (**A**) the video-laryngoscope or conventional direct laryngoscope and bougie; a BMI-38 model in a ramp position; and (**B**) the video intubating stylet; a BMI-24 model in a neutral supine position. BMI: body mass index.

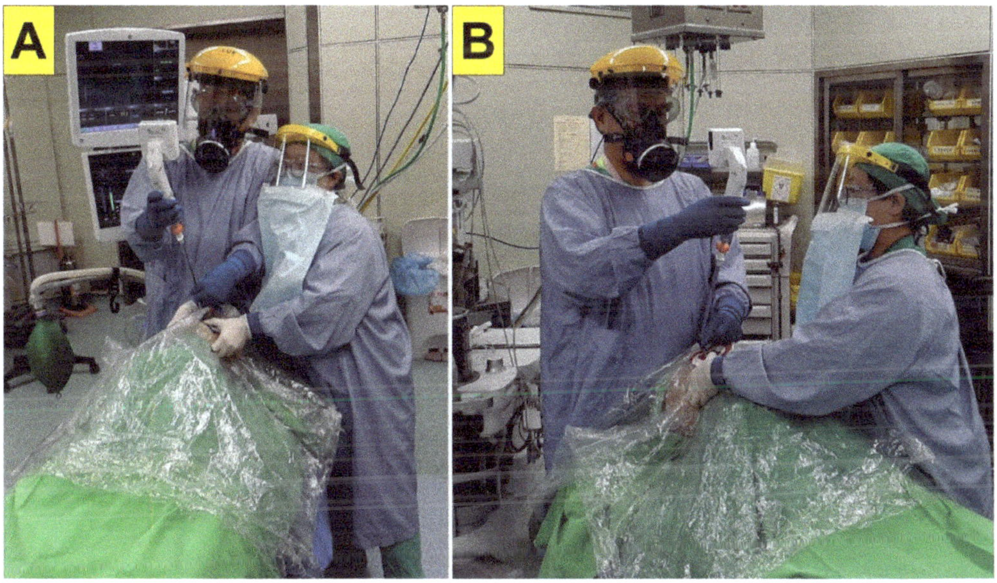

Figure 9. Endotracheal intubation utilizing a video intubating stylet with an assistant providing mouth opening and jaw lift over a plastic sheet barrier. The assistant stood either by the side of the intubator (**A**) or in the caudal direction (**B**).

Table 2. Comparison between plastic sheet and intubation box.

	Plastic Sheet	Intubation Box
Size	Small	Bulky
Weight	Light	Heavy
Texture	Soft and flexible	Hard
Space occupied	Small enough	Sizable
Need to carry, position, and reposition	Portable	Need two persons to carry and position
Set-up time and effort (carrying)	Quick and easy	More time and effort
Working location (OR, ICU, ER)	No limitation	Inconvenient at some working environment
Combative or claustrophobia patients obese patient	No issue	Could be a serious problem
Body habitus (obesity)	No added effects	Could be a serious problem
Safety distance (face-to-mouth) between intubator and patient	Safe	Safe
Kinesthetic challenges	No	Yes
Restriction of arms and hands movement (intubator's and assistant's)	Not at all	Yes
Maneuverability and dexterity	Not an issue	Could be hindered
Cause damage on PPE	Not an issue	Yes
Visibility and glaring	Transparent and clear	Could be affected
Intubation difficulties: Time to intubate/attempts/total duration/need assistance/failure	Not affected	Could be worse and risky
Difficulty manipulating airway tools (inserting laryngoscope, tube negotiation, confirmation, removal of stylet)	Not affected	Could be worse and risk
Airway visualization—Cormack Lehane score	Not affected	Could be worse
Timing tolerance of hypoxemia and hypotension	Acceptable	Low tolerance
Removal if difficult airway emergency occurred	Easy	Take time
Interference on airway manipulation	Not a problem	Could be affected
Intubating tools selection	No limits	Video laryngoscope and bougie
Cause more contamination during retrieval of the barrier	Insignificant	Potential problem
Need experience and more training	Not a problem	Needed
Learning curve	High	Could be a problem
Disposable	Yes	Not always
Workload on removal and discard and disinfection	Minimal	Annoying and difficult
Accessible and available	Yes	Not always be
Affordable	Yes	Not always be
False sense of security	Mild	Strong
Subjective feeling of difficulty on intubation	Insignificant	Notable
Mental load	Minimal	Significant
Effectiveness of aerosol prevention	Only for droplets prevention	Questionable for aerosol prevention
Safety issues on the patients	Minimal	Might cause serious problems

Any respiratory droplets and aerosols that may have been generated during intubation will settle onto the sheet or under the sheet on the patient (Figure 10), as opposed to being dispersed into the air, and there may be less risk of contamination if the sheet is carefully folded or rolled up at the end of the procedure. Additionally, there is an option to leave the sheet over the patient's head until time of extubation, thus protecting airway managers from co-infection at the end of surgery, when the patient may cough or buck at time of emergence from anesthesia. The sheet can be removed concurrently with the endotracheal tube, and so be used to collect the dirty ETT for disposal. In fact, one of the first suggested uses for the plastic sheet was not for tracheal intubation but for minimizing droplet spray during extubation [41].

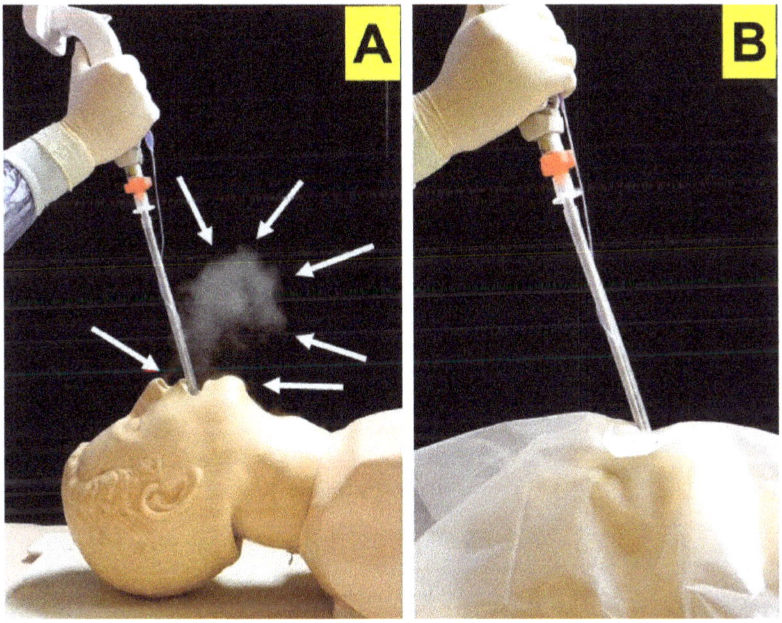

Figure 10. Mannequin demonstration of how the plastic sheet barrier prevents spread of respiratory droplets and aerosols during endotracheal intubation. (**A**) Endotracheal intubation using video intubating stylet without plastic sheet showing visible secretions (arrows) after a simulated cough. (**B**) When a plastic sheet barrier is used, secretions are contained under the sheet after a simulated cough. (Courtesy photos reproduced from Cell Transplantation [39]).

A negative aspect of simply reaching under the sheet to perform airway maneuvers is the contamination of the healthcare professional's hands and arms during the procedure. In addition, the visualization of the indirect monitor may be difficult if the screen is mounted on the videoscope itself [42]. Subsequently, plastic sheets were modified by making openings in the plastic sheet, allowing for the airway device and ETT to be passed from above the sheet or for the provider's hands to reach through [17,20] (Figures 9 and 11). Even if the monitor was affixed to the videoscope, the operator would still have an unobstructed view if the screen remained above the barrier. In order to use a videolaryngoscope with this modified plastic sheet method, either a single large opening would be made to accommodate both laryngoscope and endotracheal tube, or two smaller openings could be made in close proximity to one another. However, the larger the opening that was created into the sheet, the larger the risk for environmental contamination, defeating the purpose of using a barrier system.

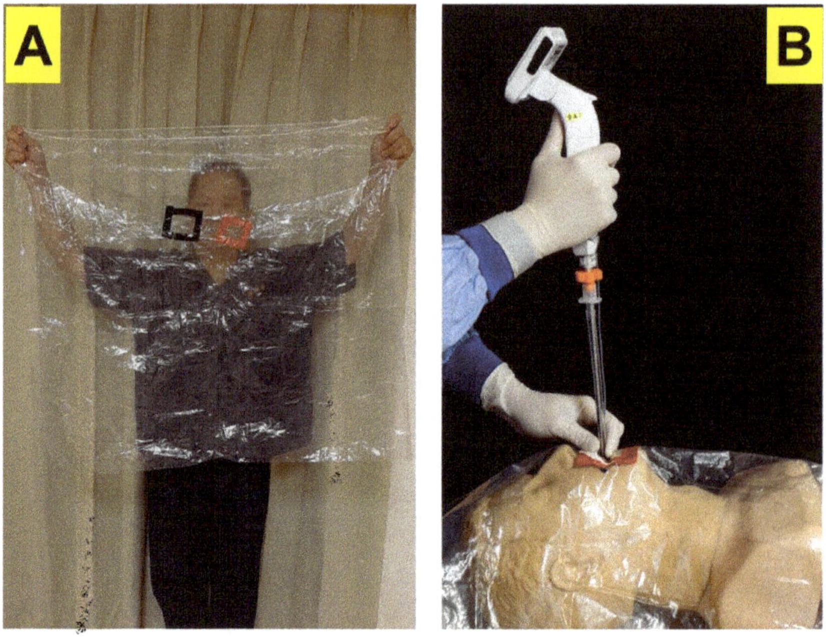

Figure 11. Modification of plastic sheet barrier with (**A**) small incisions marked by colored tape to (**B**) allow passage of intubation device from above the sheet.

The advantage of using the video intubating stylet with the plastic sheet is that because of its slim profile, only a single small opening would need to be made to allow the intubating stylet and mounted ETT to pass through (Figures 11 and 12). A single institution's protocol has been previously described in the literature, in which two small crosscuts were made into the plastic sheet with a surgical blade [38–40], (Figure 11). The purpose of the second incision was to have the ability to quickly perform mask ventilation or oral suctioning if the need arose during the intubation attempt (Figure 13). Both crosscuts were covered with transparent adhesive film, and a large bore needle was used to pierce a hole in the transparent film, minimizing the size of the defect while still making it easy to introduce the airway apparatus. As the video stylet passed through the hole, the transparent film would enlarge to accept the stylet but would also adhere to the endotracheal tube, minimizing the defect in the plastic sheet and the subsequent risk of environmental contamination.

Prefabricated plastic sheets have been produced with seam lines to allow easy removal of the plastic sheet after successful tracheal intubation (Figure 14), however, even without prefabricated sheets, a homemade sheet can be precut to facilitate its easy removal. While the plastic sheet is disposable as a medical waste, the intubating stylet is either disposable (costed from USD 50 to 100) or to be disinfected according to infection control policies and standard operating procedures adhered to local health regulations (for more detailed description, please see the reference [40]). As previously described, because the plastic sheet can also serve as protection against contamination during the extubation process, the sheet may be left over the patient's head until surgery has concluded and the ETT has been removed [17,18,41].

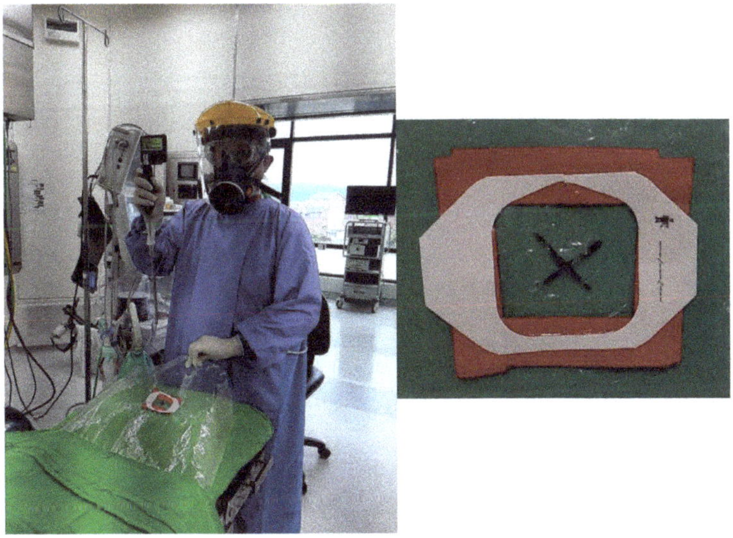

Figure 12. Only a small crosscut in the plastic sheet is needed (marked by X) to allow advancement of the video-assisted intubating stylet.

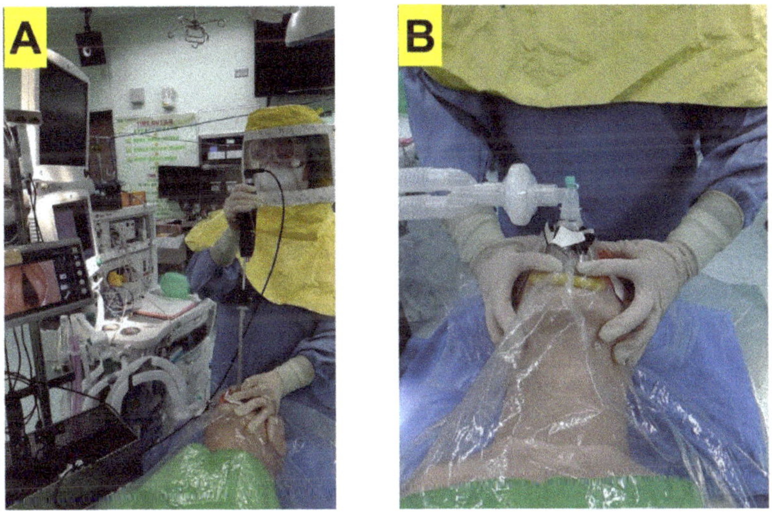

Figure 13. Two crosscuts are made into the plastic barrier sheet to allow (**A**) endotracheal intubation using a video-assisted intubating stylet, while (**B**) the second crosscut in the plastic barrier allows timely resumption of mask ventilation if the need arises during the intubation attempt. (Courtesy photo reproduced from *Asian Journal of Anesthesiology* [40] with permission).

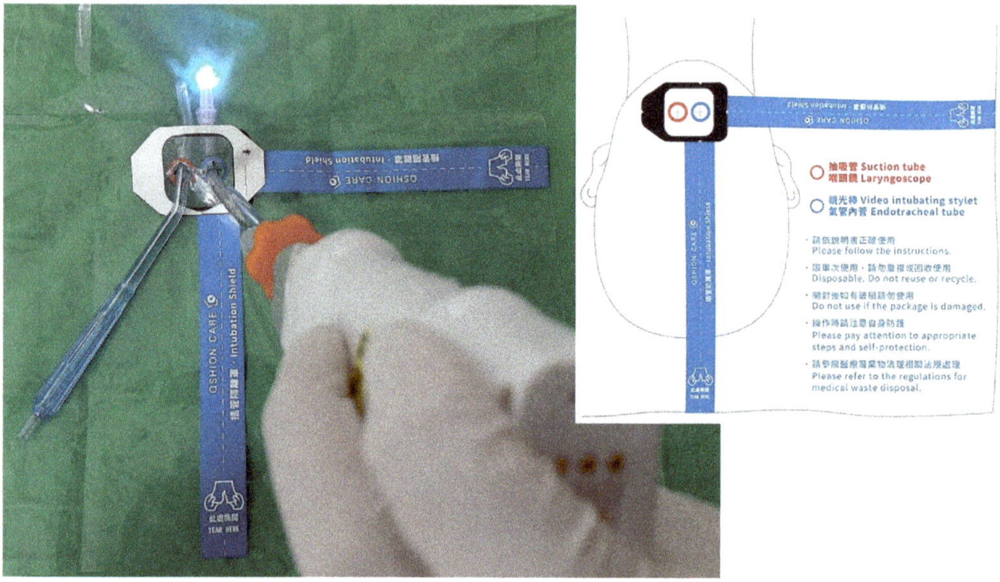

Figure 14. Prefabricated plastic sheet with areas marked by circles to guide creation of incisions for introduction of laryngoscope/suction catheter and video stylet/endotracheal tube, as well as seam lines to allow easy removal of the plastic sheet after intubation.

5. Criticisms of Barrier Methods

A recent review of the literature screened 4509 unique articles describing barrier systems and airway management, but only 123 full-text articles met the inclusion criteria [21]. Of these papers, 42% utilized a box, while 54% used a plastic sheet, further subdivided into sheets with support (32%) and without support (22%). Unfortunately, the majority of papers written on this subject have been short letters or commentaries. To date, there is not strong evidence to support the use of barrier systems, although these systems seem to have logical benefit.

Based on what has been observed and reported in the literature, a large criticism of rigid box systems has been a delay in time to intubation, with potential worsening of airway views especially in difficult intubation situations [43–45]. The rigid plastic structure limits the maneuvers an airway manager might perform to optimize the glottic view (Figures 2A and 8), and it might also hinder other staff from providing assistance during the intubation attempts. Other criticisms of the rigid box design have been environmental contamination at the open caudal end, as well as from secondary aerosolization at the time of box removal, difficulty with sanitation, and even harm to medical staff during its use [46]. Some studies concluded that plastic sheet systems do better than rigid box systems in terms of environmental exposure [47], operator ergonomics, and ease of allowing another provider to provide assistance [18]. Subsequently, on 20 August 2020, the FDA revoked the umbrella EUA for barrier devices and now recommends the concurrent use of negative pressure with these systems [48].

The use of the intubating stylet, although theoretically simpler and easier to use, has not been validated in humans. A few mannequin studies concluded that the intubating stylet was easier to use, had quicker intubation times with higher success rates compared to the traditional laryngoscope in simulated difficult airways [49,50], and a small randomized trial of patients being intubated in the lateral decubitus position suggested that the time to intubation using a video stylet was shorter compared to using a fiberoptic bronchoscope, although a greater hemodynamic response and higher incidence of sore throat was observed with the intubating stylet [51]. To date, there are sparse studies comparing the use of a video intubating stylet with a videolaryngoscope, which is currently commonly accepted as the preferred difficult airway device in the majority of the world [32].

Obesity is often associated with increased neck circumference, both of which are risk factors for difficult intubation [52], and obesity has been shown to be associated with a more severe COVID-19 course, including ICU admission and increased mortality [53,54]. COVID-19 patients in critical respiratory illness have poor respiratory reserves, and time to oxygen desaturation is rapid. A concern with using the intubating stylet in the obese patient is that it may be difficult to obtain a view of the glottis if there is significant soft tissue collapse after the induction of anesthesia. In extreme situations, jaw lift may not improve visualization of the airway. A laryngoscope, which has a wide blade to retract collapsed soft tissue structures and can facilitate maneuvering of the ETT towards the glottic opening, is typically used with the intubating stylet technique.

6. Future Directions and Conclusions

It is worthy to mention that videolaryngoscopy became a new paradigm for tracheal intubation (e.g., unanticipated and expected difficult airway management) since decades ago [32,55]. Such critical roles and increasing prevalence of videolaryngoscopy have been emerged in many clinical environments, such as emergency rooms, operating theaters, intensive care units, and wards [56–58]. Among all the intubating tools, it is interesting to note that optical (lighted and video-assisted) stylets are still not prevalent in many countries so far [59]. Such kinds of optical stylets, originally designed by Shikani [33] and later modified by Levitan [60], have been evaluated in several different clinical scenarios [61–66]. The advantages of such an airway management modality are as follows: obtaining better patient glottic view with high first-pass success rates, no need to contact any airway soft tissues and therefore causing less stimulation or tissue damages, maintaining a safe distance between the intubator from patient's mouth, high learning curve, etc.

During COVID-19 pandemic, not surprisingly, the beneficial role of videolaryngoscopy has been repeatedly advocated in several guidelines [30,31]. Meanwhile, together with videolaryngoscopy, a gum elastic bougie (GEB, also named an endotracheal tube introducer) is an effective adjunct to difficult airway management [67–71]. Therefore, both essential tools have reasonably been proposed to be included in the COVID-19 emergency tracheal intubation kit dump and tray [30,31]. However, in the real world, videolaryngoscopes and video-assisted intubating stylets might not be available in some countries and regions. In that case, the airway managers should have adequate PPE while using conventional direct laryngoscope for tracheal intubation during COVID-19 pandemic.

Although the use of a video intubating stylet in conjunction with a plastic barrier sheet may be the most efficacious method to prevent environmental contamination from droplet and aerosol exposure during AGMPs, based upon the small size of the incision in the sheet that is necessary to pass the ETT, more research is needed in this area. Plastic sheets need to be shown that they do indeed mitigate the risk of environmental exposure and health care provider co-infection during tracheal intubation and extubation. Consensus on plastic sheet modifications can help reproducibility and improve efficacy across different clinical settings and hospital situations. More randomized trials with adequate patient enrollment is necessary to investigate the following scenarios: (1) the comparison of videolaryngoscopes to video stylets in difficult airway situations, especially in morbidly obese patients; (2) the effectiveness and safety of utilizing plastic sheet barriers during airway manipulation using a variety of intubating devices; and more specifically, (3) the comparison of videolaryngoscope to the video intubating stylet in conjunction with plastic sheet barrier systems.

Nonetheless, the video intubating stylet continues to gain acceptance as an indirect video intubating device in particular regions of the world given its ease of use, short training duration, relative cost, and straightforward re-sanitation process. Plastic barrier devices have shown promise to reduce environmental contamination and hospital personnel co-infection during AGMPs such as tracheal intubation. Because of its slim profile and minimal effect to disrupt the integrity of the plastic sheet, the video intubating stylet in conjunction with the plastic sheet may indeed prove to be the preferential intubating method during the COVID-19 pandemic and beyond.

Supplementary Materials: The following are available online at https://www.mdpi.com/article/10.3390/encyclopedia1040081/s1.

Author Contributions: Conceptualization, P.B.T. and H.-N.L.; methodology, H.-N.L.; writing—original draft preparation, P.B.T.; writing—review and editing, P.B.T. and H.-N.L.; All authors have read and agreed to the published version of the manuscript.

Funding: This research received no external funding.

Institutional Review Board Statement: This article is a clinical concept paper and does not fall into the definition of "research", "human research", "clinical study", or "case report". All the presentation materials involved only mannequins, except in Figure 6 where the written informed consent was obtained from the patient before the video was taking. The authors acknowledged and complied with the guidelines of the Declaration of Helsinki-2013.

Informed Consent Statement: Written informed consent has been obtained from the patient, who cannot be identified in the Figure 6, to publish this paper.

Data Availability Statement: Not applicable.

Conflicts of Interest: The authors declare no conflict of interest.

Entry Link on the Encyclopedia Platform: https://encyclopedia.pub/16459.

References

1. Huang, C.; Wang, Y.; Li, X.; Ren, L.; Zhao, J.; Hu, Y.; Zhang, L.; Fan, G.; Xu, J.; Gu, X.; et al. Clinical features of patients infected with 2019 novel coronavirus in Wuhan, China. *Lancet* **2020**, *395*, 497–506. [CrossRef]
2. Data: WHO Coronavirus (COVID-19) Dashboard. Available online: https://covid19.who.int (accessed on 30 September 2021).
3. Yuki, K.; Fujiogi, M.; Koutsogiannaki, S. COVID-19 pathophysiology: A review. *Clin. Immunol.* **2020**, *215*, 108427. [CrossRef]
4. Hu, B.; Guo, H.; Zhou, P.; Shi, Z.L. Characteristics of SARS-CoV-2 and COVID-19. *Nat. Rev. Microbiol.* **2021**, *19*, 141–154. [CrossRef]
5. Wax, R.S.; Christian, M.D. Practical recommendations for critical care and anesthesiology teams caring for novel coronavirus (2019-nCoV) patients. *Can. J. Anaesth.* **2020**, *67*, 568–576. [CrossRef]
6. Ruskin, K.J.; Ruskin, A.C.; Musselman, B.T.; Harvey, J.R.; Nesthus, T.E.; O'Connor, M. COVID-19, personal protective equipment, and human performance. *Anesthesiology* **2021**, *134*, 518–525. [CrossRef]
7. Verbeek, J.H.; Rajamaki, B.; Ijaz, S.; Sauni, R.; Toomey, E.; Blackwood, B.; Tikka, C.; Ruotsalainen, J.H.; Kilinc Balci, F.S. Personal protective equipment for preventing highly infectious diseases due to exposure to contaminated body fluids in healthcare staff. *Cochrane Database Syst. Rev.* **2020**, *5*, CD011621.
8. Burki, T. Global shortage of personal protective equipment. *Lancet Infect. Dis.* **2020**, *20*, 785–786. [CrossRef]
9. Arnaout, R. Cooperation under pressure: Lessons from the COVID-19 swab crisis. *J. Clin. Microbiol.* **2021**, *59*, JCM0123921. [CrossRef]
10. Lai, J.; Ma, S.; Wang, Y.; Cai, Z.; Hu, J.; Wei, N.; Wu, J.; Du, H.; Chen, T.; Li, R.; et al. Factors associated with mental health outcomes among health care workers exposed to coronavirus disease 2019. *JAMA Netw. Open* **2020**, *3*, e203976. [CrossRef] [PubMed]
11. Tregoning, J.S.; Flight, K.E.; Higham, S.L.; Wang, Z.; Pierce, B.F. Progress of the COVID-19 vaccine effort: Viruses, vaccines and variants versus efficacy, effectiveness and escape. *Nat. Rev. Immunol.* **2021**, *21*, 626–636. [CrossRef] [PubMed]
12. Everington, K. Taiwanese Doctor Invents Device to Protect US Doctors against Coronavirus. 23 March 2020. Available online: https://www.taiwannews.com.tw/en/news/3902435 (accessed on 20 August 2021).
13. Lai, H.Y. Aerosol Box Protects Healthcare Providers during Endotracheal Intubation. Available online: https://sites.google.com/view/aerosolbox/home?authuser=0 (accessed on 20 August 2021).
14. Canelli, R.; Connor, C.W.; Gonzalez, M.; Nozari, A.; Ortega, R. Barrier enclosure during endotracheal intubation. *N. Engl. J. Med.* **2020**, *382*, 1957–1958. [CrossRef]
15. Fidler, R.L.; Niedek, C.R.; Teng, J.J.; Sturgeon, M.E.; Zhang, Q.; Robinowitz, D.L.; Hirsch, J. Aerosol retention characteristics of barrier devices. *Anesthesiology* **2021**, *134*, 61–71. [CrossRef] [PubMed]
16. Fried, E.A.; Zhou, G.; Shah, R.; Shin, D.W.; Shah, A.; Katz, D.; Burnett, G.W. Barrier devices, intubation, and aerosol mitigation strategies: Personal protective equipment in the time of Coronavirus Disease 2019. *Anesth. Analg.* **2021**, *132*, 38–45. [CrossRef] [PubMed]

17. Babazade, R.; Khan, E.S.; Ibrahim, M.; Simon, M.; Vadhera, R.B. Additional barrier to protect health care workers during intubation. *Anesth. Analg.* **2020**, *131*, e47–e48. [CrossRef] [PubMed]
18. Brown, H.; Preston, D.; Bhoja, R. Thinking outside the box: A low-cost and pragmatic alternative to aerosol boxes for endotracheal intubation of COVID-19 patients. *Anesthesiology* **2020**, *133*, 683–684. [CrossRef]
19. Brown, S.; Patrao, F.; Verma, S.; Lean, A.; Flack, S.; Polaner, D. Barrier system for airway management of COVID-19 patients. *Anesth. Analg.* **2020**, *131*, e34–e35. [CrossRef]
20. Emami, N.; Tanner, T.; Ogundipe, F.; Hawn, V.S.; Rubin, R.; Skae, C.C.; Shiloh, A.L.; Keene, A.B. Drape to prevent disease transmission during endotracheal intubation. *Am. J. Infect. Control* **2021**, *49*, 387–388. [CrossRef]
21. Price, C.; Ben-Yakov, M.; Choi, J.; Orchanian-Cheff, A.; Tawadrous, D. Barrier enclosure use during aerosol-generating medical procedures: A scoping review. *Am. J. Emerg. Med.* **2021**, *41*, 209–218. [CrossRef]
22. U.S. Food & Drug Administration. Emergency Use Authorization for Protective Barrier Enclosures in Response to the Evolving Coronavirus Disease 2019 (COVID-19) Pandemic. 1 May 2020. Available online: https://www.fda.gov/media/141415/download (accessed on 19 August 2020).
23. Rosenblatt, W.H.; Sherman, J.D. More on barrier enclosure during endotracheal intubation. *N. Engl. J. Med.* **2020**, *382*, e69.
24. Kovatsis, P.G.; Matava, C.T.; Payton, J.M. More on barrier enclosure during endotracheal intubation. *N. Engl. J. Med.* **2020**, *382*, e69.
25. Duggan, L.V.; Marshall, S.D.; Scott, J.; Brindley, P.G.; Grocott, H.P. The MacGyver bias and attraction of homemade devices in healthcare. *Can. J. Anaesth.* **2019**, *66*, 757–761. [CrossRef]
26. Brewster, D.J.; Begley, J.L.; Marshall, S.D. Rise and fall of the aerosol box; and what we must learn from the adoption of untested equipment. *Emerg. Med. J.* **2021**, *38*, 109–110. [CrossRef]
27. Turner, M.C.; Duggan, L.V.; Glezerson, B.A.; Marshall, S.D. Thinking outside the (acrylic) box: A framework for the local use of custom-made medical devices. *Anaesthesia* **2020**, *75*, 1566–1569. [CrossRef]
28. Berry, J.M. Conventional (laryngoscopic) orotracheal and nasotracheal intubation (single lumen tube). In *Benumof's Airway Management: Principles and Practice*, 2nd ed., Benumof, J.L., Ed.; Mosby-Elsevier: Philadelphia, PA, USA, 2007; Chapter 16; pp. 379–392.
29. Kabrhel, C.; Thomsen, T.W.; Setnik, G.S.; Walls, R.M. Videos in clinical medicine. Orotracheal intubation. *N. Engl. J. Med.* **2007**, *356*, e15. [CrossRef]
30. Cook, T.M.; El-Boghdadly, K.; McGuire, B.; McNarry, A.F.; Patel, A.; Higgs, A. Consensus guidelines for managing the airway in patients with COVID-19: Guidelines from the Difficult Airway Society, the Association of Anaesthetists, the Intensive Care Society, the Faculty of Intensive Care Medicine and the Royal College of Anaesthetists. *Anaesthesia* **2020**, *75*, 785–799.
31. Brewster, D.J.; Chrimes, N.; Do, T.B.; Fraser, K.; Groombridge, C.J.; Higgs, A.; Humar, M.J.; Leeuwenburg, T.J.; McGloughlin, S.; Newman, F.G.; et al. Consensus statement: Safe Airway Society principles of airway management and tracheal intubation specific to the COVID-19 adult patient group. *Med. J. Aust.* **2020**, *212*, 472–481. [CrossRef]
32. Lewis, S.R.; Butler, A.R.; Parker, J.; Cook, T.M.; Smith, A.F. Videolaryngoscopy versus direct laryngoscopy for adult patients requiring tracheal intubation. *Cochrane Database Syst. Rev.* **2016**, *11*, CD011136. [CrossRef]
33. Shikani, A.H. New "seeing" stylet-scope and method for the management of the difficult airway. *Otolaryngol. Head Neck Surg.* **1999**, *120*, 113–116. [CrossRef]
34. Lee, M.C.; Tseng, K.Y.; Shen, Y.C. Nasotracheal intubation in patients with limited mouth opening: A comparison between fibreoptic intubation and the Trachway®. *Anaesthesia* **2016**, *71*, 31–38. [CrossRef]
35. Yang, M.; Kim, J.A.; Ahn, H.J.; Choi, J.W.; Kim, D.K.; Cho, E.A. Double-lumen tube tracheal intubation using a rigid video-stylet: A randomized controlled comparison with the Macintosh laryngoscope. *Br. J. Anaesth.* **2013**, *111*, 990–995. [CrossRef]
36. Yoon, H.K.; Lee, H.C.; Park, J.B.; Oh, H.; Hee-Pyoung Park, H.P. McGrath MAC videolaryngoscope versus Optiscope video stylet for tracheal intubation in patients with manual inline cervical stabilization: A randomized trial. *Anesth. Analg.* **2020**, *130*, 870–878. [CrossRef]
37. Kim, J.K.; Kim, J.A.; Kim, C.S.; Ahn, H.J.; Yang, M.K.; Choi, S.J. Comparison of tracheal intubation with the Airway Scope or Clarus Video System in patients with cervical collars. *Anaesthesia* **2011**, *66*, 694–698. [CrossRef]
38. Yang, Y.L.; Huang, C.H.; Luk, H.N.; Tsai, P.B. Adaptation to the plastic barrier sheet to facilitate intubation during the COVID-19 pandemic. *Anesth. Analg.* **2020**, *131*, e97–e99. [CrossRef]
39. Luk, H.N.; Yang, Y.L.; Tsai, P.B. Application of plastic sheet barrier and video intubating stylet to protect tracheal intubators during coronavirus disease 2019 pandemic: A Taiwan experience. *Cell Transplant.* **2021**, *30*. [CrossRef]
40. Tsai, P.B.; Luk, H.N. Plastic sheet and video intubating stylet: A technical note. *Asian J. Anesthesiol.* **2021**, 1–5. [CrossRef]
41. Matava, C.T.; Yu, J.; Denning, S. Clear plastic drapes may be effective at limiting aerosolization and droplet spray during extubation: Implications for COVID-19. *Can J Anaesth* **2020**, *67*, 902–904. [CrossRef]
42. Rose, P.; Veall, J.; Chima, N.; Vowels, E.; Chitnis, S.; Flexman, A.; Tang, R. A comparison of droplet and contact contamination using 3 simulated barrier techniques for COVID-19 intubation: A quality assurance study. *CMAJ Open* **2020**, *8*, E554–E559. [CrossRef]
43. Begley, J.L.; Lavery, K.E.; Nickson, C.P.; Brewster, D.J. The aerosol box for intubation in coronavirus disease 2019 patients: An in-situ simulation crossover study. *Anaesthesia* **2020**, *75*, 1014–1021. [CrossRef]

44. Jen, T.T.H.; Gusti, V.; Badh, C.; Mehta, S.; Denomme, J.; Lockhart, S.; Shams, B.; Klaibert, B.; Chau, A. The impact of a barrier enclosure on time to tracheal intubation: A randomized controlled trial. *Can. J. Anaesth.* **2021**, *68*, 1358–1367. [CrossRef]
45. Lim, Z.J.; Ponnapa Reddy, M.; Karalapillai, D.; Shekar, K.; Subramaniam, A. Impact of an aerosol box on time to tracheal intubation: Systematic review and meta-analysis. *Br. J. Anaesth.* **2021**, *126*, e122–e125. [CrossRef]
46. Sorbello, M.; Rosenblatt, W.; Hofmeyr, R.; Greif, R.; Urdaneta, F. Aerosol boxes and barrier enclosures for airway management in COVID-19 patients: A scoping review and narrative synthesis. *Br. J. Anaesth.* **2020**, *125*, 880–894. [CrossRef]
47. Simpson, J.P.; Wong, D.N.; Verco, L.; Carter, R.; Dzidowski, M.; Chan, P.Y. Measurement of airborne particle exposure during simulated tracheal intubation using various proposed aerosol containment devices during the COVID-19 pandemic. *Anaesthesia* **2020**, *75*, 1587–1595. [CrossRef] [PubMed]
48. U.S. Food & Drug Administration. Protective Barrier Enclosures without Negative Pressure Used during the COVID-19 Pandemic May Increase Risk to Patients and Health Care Providers—Letter to Health Care Providers. 20 August 2020. Available online: https://www.fda.gov/medical-devices/letters-health-care-providers/protective-barrier-enclosures-without-negative-pressure-used-during-covid-19-pandemic-may-increase (accessed on 20 August 2021).
49. Ong, J.; Lee, C.L.; Huang, S.J.; Shyr, M.H. Comparison between the Trachway video intubating stylet and Macintosh laryngoscope in four simulated difficult tracheal intubations: A manikin study. *Tzu Chi Med. J.* **2016**, *28*, 109–112. [CrossRef]
50. Wu, M.Y.; Yiang, G.T.; Ke, J.Y.; Chen, C.S.; Lin, P.C.; Chen, Y.L. Role of Trachway versus conventional modes of intubation in difficult airway management in COVID-19 setups. *Emerg. Med. Int.* **2021**, *25*, 6614523.
51. Wahdan, A.S.; El-Refai, N.A.R.; Omar, S.H.; Abdel Moneem, S.A.; Mohamed, M.M.; Hussien, M.M. Endotracheal intubation in patients undergoing open abdominal surgery in the lateral position: A comparison between the intubating video stylet and fiberoptic intubating bronchoscopy. *Korean J. Anesthesiol.* **2021**, *74*, 234–241. [CrossRef]
52. Lundstrøm, L.H.; Møller, A.M.; Rosenstock, C.; Astrup, G.; Wetterslev, J. High body mass index is a weak predictor for difficult and failed tracheal intubation: A cohort study of 91,332 consecutive patients scheduled for direct laryngoscopy registered in the Danish Anesthesia Database. *Anesthesiology* **2009**, *110*, 266–274. [CrossRef] [PubMed]
53. Popkin, B.M.; Du, S.; Green, W.D.; Beck, M.A.; Algaith, T.; Herbst, C.H.; Alsukait, R.F.; Alluhidan, M.; Alazemi, N.; Shekar, M. Individuals with obesity and COVID-19: A global perspective on the epidemiology and biological relationships. *Obes. Rev.* **2020**, *21*, e13128. [CrossRef] [PubMed]
54. Drucker, D.J. Diabetes, obesity, metabolism, and SARS-CoV-2 infection: The end of the beginning. *Cell Metab.* **2021**, *33*, 479–498. [CrossRef]
55. Cook, T.M.; Kelly, F.E. A national survey of videolaryngoscopy in the United Kingdom. *Br. J. Anaesth.* **2017**, *118*, 593–600. [CrossRef] [PubMed]
56. Swaminathan, A.K.; Rachel Berkowitz, R.; Baker, A.; Spyres, M. Do emergency medicine residents receive appropriate video laryngoscopy training? A survey to compare the utilization of video laryngoscopy devices in emergency medicine residency programs and community emergency departments. *J. Emerg. Med.* **2015**, *48*, 613–619. [CrossRef]
57. Monette, D.L.; Brown III, C.A.; Benoit, J.L.; McMullan, J.T.; Carleton, S.C.; Steuerwald, M.T.; Eyre, A.; Pallin, D.J.; NEAR III Investigators. The impact of video laryngoscopy on the clinical learning environment of emergency medicine residents: A report of 14,313 intubations. *AEM. Educ. Train.* **2019**, *3*, 156–162. [CrossRef]
58. Ono, Y.; Tanigawa, K.; Shinohara, K.; Yano, T.; Sorimachi, K.; Inokuchi, R.; Shimada, J. Human and equipment resources for difficult airway management, airway education programs, and capnometry use in Japanese emergency departments: A nationwide cross-sectional study. *Int. J. Emerg. Med.* **2017**, *10*, 28. [CrossRef] [PubMed]
59. Liu, H.H.; Wang, Y.; Zhong, M.; Li, Y.H.; Gao, H.; Zhang, J.F.; Ma, W.H. Managing the difficult airway: A survey of doctors with different seniority in China. *Medicine* **2021**, *100*, e27181. [CrossRef]
60. Levitan, R.M. Design rationale and intended use of a short optical stylet for routine fiberoptic augmentation of emergency laryngoscopy. *Am. J. Emerg. Med.* **2006**, *24*, 490–495. [CrossRef] [PubMed]
61. Biro, P.; Bättig, U.; Henderson, J.; Seifert, B. First clinical experience of tracheal intubation with the SensaScope, a novel steerable semirigid video stylet. *Br. J. Anaesth.* **2006**, *97*, 255–261. [CrossRef]
62. Phua, D.S.; Mah, C.L.; Wang, C.F. The Shikani optical stylet as an alternative to the GlideScope® videolaryngoscope in simulated difficult intubations—A randomised controlled trial. *Anaesthesia* **2012**, *67*, 402–406. [CrossRef]
63. Cooney, D.R.; Cooney, N.L.; Wallus, H.; Wojcik, S. Performance of emergency physicians utilizing a video-assisted semi-rigid fiberoptic stylet for intubation of a difficult airway in a high-fidelity simulated patient: A pilot study. *Int. J. Emerg. Med.* **2012**, *5*, 24. [CrossRef]
64. Kok, T.; George, R.B.; McKeen, D.; Vakharia, N.; Pink, A. Effectiveness and safety of the Levitan FPS Scope™ for tracheal intubation under general anesthesia with a simulated difficult airway. *Can. J. Anaesth.* **2012**, *59*, 743–750. [CrossRef]
65. Gaszynski, T.; Pietrzyk, M.; Szewczyk, T.; Gaszynska, E. A comparison of performance of endotracheal intubation using the Levitan FPS optical stylet or Lary-Flex videolaryngoscope in morbidly obese patients. *Sci. World J.* **2014**, 207591. [CrossRef]
66. Xu, M.; Li, X.X.; Guo, X.Y.; Wang, J. Shikani optical stylet versus Macintosh laryngoscope for intubation in patients undergoing surgery for cervical spondylosis: A randomized controlled trial. *Chin. Med. J.* **2017**, *130*, 297–302. [CrossRef] [PubMed]

67. Evans, A.; Morris, S.; Petterson, J.; Hall, J.E. A comparison of the Seeing Optical Stylet and the gum elastic bougie in simulated difficult tracheal intubation: A manikin study. *Anaesthesia* **2006**, *61*, 478–481. [CrossRef] [PubMed]
68. Driver, B.; Dodd, K.; Klein, L.R.; Buckley, R.; Robinson, A.; McGill, J.W.; Reardon, R.F.; Prekker, M.E. The bougie and first-pass success in the emergency department. *Ann. Emerg. Med.* **2017**, *70*, 473–478. [CrossRef]
69. Ono, Y.; Shinohara, K.; Shimada, J.; Inoue, S.; Kotani, J. Lower maximum forces on oral structures when using gum-elastic bougie than when using endotracheal tube and stylet during both direct and indirect laryngoscopy by novices: A crossover study using a high-fidelity simulator. *BMC Emerg. Med.* **2020**, *20*, 34. [CrossRef] [PubMed]
70. Driver, B.E.; Prekker, M.E.; Klein, L.R.; Reardon, R.F.; Miner, J.R.; Fagerstrom, E.T.; Cleghorn, M.R.; McGill, J.W.; Cole, J.B. Effect of use of a bougie vs endotracheal tube and stylet on first-attempt intubation success among patients with difficult airways undergoing emergency intubation: A randomized clinical trial. *JAMA* **2018**, *319*, 2179–2189. [CrossRef] [PubMed]
71. Combes, X.; Jabre, P.; Margenet, A.; Merle, J.C.; Leroux, B.; Dru, M.; Lecarpentier, E.; Dhonneur, G. Unanticipated difficult airway management in the prehospital emergency setting: Prospective validation of an algorithm. *Anesthesiology* **2011**, *114*, 105–110. [CrossRef]

encyclopedia

MDPI

Entry

Digital Mental Health Amid COVID-19

Luke Balcombe * and Diego De Leo

Australian Institute for Suicide Research and Prevention, Department of Applied Psychology, Griffith University, Messines Ridge Road, Mount Gravatt, QLD 4122, Australia; d.deleo@griffith.edu.au
* Correspondence: lukebalcombe@gmail.com

Definition: Digital Mental Health is information and communication technology used in mental health services delivered or boosted through the Internet and related technologies, smartphone and wearable technologies as well as immersive solutions (e.g., Virtual Reality and video games). It is predominantly used as self-help services or with the assistance of a (para-)professional and/or artificial intelligence for the provision of mental health promotion as well as mental ill-health identification, prevention and intervention.

Keywords: COVID-19; digital mental health; implementation; challenges; technology; human-computer interaction; explainable artificial intelligence; integrated methodologies; efficacy; evaluation

Citation: Balcombe, L.; De Leo, D. Digital Mental Health Amid COVID-19. *Encyclopedia* **2021**, *1*, 1047–1057. https://doi.org/10.3390/encyclopedia1040080

Academic Editor: Stephen Bustin

Received: 13 July 2021
Accepted: 13 October 2021
Published: 20 October 2021

1. Introduction

1.1. Evolution of Digital Mental Health

Mental healthcare resources have been inundated during the economic and biopsychosocial recovery from COVID-19 [1,2]. Although in use since the early 2000s, an opportunity has arisen for digital mental health to fill unmet needs [3–5] and answer calls to improve the quality of and accessibility to mental health care [6–8]. It was already on a trajectory to regular practice, but COVID-19 added to demand outstripping supply of mental healthcare resources making a review of digital mental health more urgent. There has been a marked rise in the use of online self-help and telehealth interventions [9–12]. Systematic reviews found telehealth to be an effective and acceptable form of service delivery at least in the short term [13]. More generally, there are calls for higher levels of evidence, ongoing evaluation, and effective embedment [9,14–16]. A rapid meta-review found telehealth, internet-based, and app-based mobile digital interventions are well-placed to mitigate psychosocial consequences at the population level with good quality evidence on usability, safety, acceptance/satisfaction, and effectiveness [17]. Mixed levels of evidence were noted: lacking for apps having successful retention strategies; limited for mental health promotion; and lack of preliminary evidence for the long-term effects, process quality, and cost-effectiveness of digital interventions [17]. This integrative review synthesizes evidence from Scopus, ScienceDirect, CrossRef and Google Scholar searches of the challenges, systemic and practical issues, new progress, ongoing problems, and approaches of digital mental health as well as a focus on young people.

1.2. Challenges of Digital Mental Health

There is a need for rapidly deploying and efficiently integrating effective and evaluated digital solutions for users at individual, organizational, and governmental levels [6,18–20]. However, there are hindering issues in enacting a hybrid model of care e.g., the quality of digital mental health solutions needs to be better discerned and there is a need for more studies with vulnerable and at-risk populations [18]. Two systematic reviews and meta-analyses examined the effectiveness of digital mental health interventions. The first, for young adults with depression or substance misuse in low-income and middle-income countries, found moderate effectiveness when compared with control interventions [21]. The second, for anxiety and depression in perinatal patients in high-income countries, found nonspecialist providers may be effective in delivering counseling interventions [22]. However, only two online interventions were included. Further studies are required for digital intervention implementation processes to inform the optimal delivery and scale-up of these services.

There are a range of digital mental health interventions available for various mental health needs and conditions, from substance abuse recovery to suicide prevention [23]. Stronger evidence and new models of care will be necessary for higher accessibility, equity, and successful clinical implementation [5,20,24,25]. Predictive technologies (e.g., real-time machine learning algorithms) are useful for monitoring but should be deployed carefully as decision support tools [20,25,26]. On an operations level, there is the issue of integrating technology into mental health care delivery for diverse populations. The European Commission addressed organizational barriers (e.g., interoperability, and technical and legal issues) through a consortium action plan that also prioritized digital mental health research to target the most prevalent mental health problems and disorders [27]. Users need assistance to make informed decisions around the efficacy of digital mental health tools [13] as well as the intervention characteristics (e.g., convenience, suitability, reliability, user-friendliness, presentation, organizational integration, and cost). The adoption of digital tools has been hindered at the organizational and policy level—user-friendly workflows, decision models and protocols have been offered as solutions [19,28]. Suitable information, training, infrastructure, clinical guidelines, and policies may counter excessive information/workloads, ambiguous policies, mixed implementation, and a struggle to maintain systems [19,20].

2. Synthesis

2.1. *Systemic and Practical Issues*

A main barrier to equity in digital mental health interventions is that some people do not have access or skills to use digital resources [28]. There are inequities in affordable access to digital technologies for Indigenous people in Australia (63% have access to internet at home) which has a detrimental effect on cultural, social and mental health outcomes [29]. Recent efforts to implement and integrate digital mental health interventions into the United States (US) healthcare system may be helpful in reducing mental health care inequities in rural communities [30]. However, there is a lack of studies demonstrating sustainable improvements in symptoms and global functioning from specialized early intervention services [31]. Considerations other than equity include engagement, ethics, security, adaptability, and technicality [25,32]. There were mostly contextual issues noted in recent studies. An automated randomized controlled trial of an online peer-support program (Big White Wall) versus web-based information for self-management of anxiety and depression suggested a personal approach for participant engagement to explain the benefits of this novel intervention [33]. It was proposed that user engagement and satisfaction with a digital platform (Thought Spot) be related to content relevance, ease of learning, and available features [34]. The effectiveness of a digital platform with virtual coaches for cognitive behavior therapy (CBT) was explored in a qualitative study—it was important to find ways for users to be drawn to and then consistently engaged with the digital platform [35].

It was established before the current pandemic that stand-alone app-based treatments have increased affordability [36–38] but require simpler and stronger reimbursement systems [39]. ICare is an example of an adjunct online screening and intervention platform model whereby "partners will examine and compare the feasibility, acceptance, efficacy and (cost-)effectiveness, reach, and dissemination of the included online interventions" ([27], p.1). Recent adaptations of telehealth fee and reimbursement structures have yet to be evaluated for affordability. A theoretical model was applied in a patient-centered framework—using apps from the US and United Kingdom (UK) as examples—to produce country-specific estimates of the economic value of clinical improvement [40]. The new framework was proposed to help drive research priorities for digital health by explaining the factors that influence the economic value [40]. Studies have yet to establish models of mental healthcare system (cost-)effectiveness and improvement from integrating digital mental health, e.g., cohort longitudinal studies that examine scalable screening and tracking tools delivered in a hybrid model of care. Finding a balance between scalability and fidelity was noted to be important in the proposed empirical testing of a paraprofessional (peer-to-peer) digital mental health support model [41].

2.2. New Progress

Digital mental health interventions are assisting the facilitation of therapy, prediction, and prevention of mental ill-health [37,38,42–44]. The COVID-19 pandemic heightened the need to counter the medical and socio-economic effects of mental ill-health via deployment of assistive, preventative, and therapeutic solutions (e.g., internet-based data collection tools, digital platforms and apps) [13,20,45,46]. A multimethod study developed a co-designed freely available resource guide that builds on existing evidence on digital mental health tools [46]. There were safety, comfort, and flexibility noted for telehealth experiences during COVID-19, although face-to-face service delivery was still preferred [47]. There is a great opportunity for digital and data-driven tools to become prominent (e.g., machine learning algorithms and artificial intelligence (AI) platforms, the Internet of Things (IoT), digital phenotyping, and immersive solutions such as virtual reality (VR)) [25]. The resources required to guide the selection, implementation, and evaluation of machine learning algorithms and artificial intelligence (AI) platforms are available online for public use [48]. Guided adoption and integration of digital tools with clinical practice is not known to have been effectively studied.

Rapid psychological screening and tracking showed promise during COVID-19 through digital phenotyping of a telehealth platform service coupled with analysis by machine learning trained models [46]. A longitudinal observational study verified the acceptability and effectiveness of AI therapy for anxiety and depression [49]. A systematic review of the effectiveness and acceptance of technology-based psychological interventions in people with diagnosed depression found mostly positive impacts from stand-alone interventions, blended treatments, or in collaborative care trials [50]. An extensive trial of the clinical and (cost-)effectiveness of blended therapy (integration of Internet and mobile-based interventions into routine psychotherapy) is aiming for a rigorous healthcare services approach that innovates service provision while exploring mechanisms of change [51]. Technology Enabled Clinical Care (TECC) was proposed in a protocol for a longitudinal cohort study of smartphone-augmented mental health treatment primarily targeting changes in mood, anxiety, and stress [52]. The use of TECC in a System Dynamics Model may improve mental health and suicide outcomes by using technology infrastructure to quickly direct to the right mode of care as patients navigate primary and secondary mental healthcare services [53]. An informatics infrastructure (an extension of electronic health records) has advanced personalized decision-making in psychiatric care through standardized data acquisition and data access (transfer, storage, and export of clinical data) [54]. This development provides the opportunity for future studies to apply and validate real-time predictive modelling.

2.3. Ongoing Problems

Digital mental health implementation in clinical settings requires thoughtfulness and preparedness [55], along with a higher understanding of technical and medical standards, in order to increase effectiveness, validation, and user-centered design as well as to counter ethical concerns [20]. Stakeholders need an adequate infrastructure and skills-base [25,56] as well as ethical guidance in the development, deployment, and management of digital mental health solutions [20,56]. The paradoxical efforts to advance evidence and implementation of digital mental health led to the suggestion for simulation-based research [57]. Explainable Artificial Intelligence (XAI) research with predictive technologies [58] emphasized its potential to encapsulate improvement of safety and efficacy standards through stewardship and responsible innovation [25]. A narrative review on the therapeutic alliance in digital mental health interventions for those with serious mental illnesses (particularly on the psychotic spectrum or bipolar disorder) found a better understanding of human-computer interaction is required in evidence-based studies that facilitate responsible outcomes from a three-tiered approach (patient/user, mental health care practitioner, and machine) [59]. TECC is promising with regards to systematically coordinating and delivering appropriate mental health services [60]. The use of machine learning methods for statistically predicting suicide has been cautioned [61,62]. Engagement with the individual patient/user with regards to their specific problems and circumstances is preferred because the usefulness of machine learning in clinical settings is limited by an ongoing lack of information on model building, uncertain accuracy [63–65], clinical evaluation [28]. Integration of novel models of care and support for digital infrastructure/personnel require further research [25,41,59].

2.4. Approaches

Digital mental health services are available online (via desktops, mobile devices, and apps), including through web chat and peer support forums as well as by phone (e.g., calls or texts), to provide crisis support, psychotherapy, counseling, psychological treatments, health promotion, education, and prevention as well as support for recovery. A systematic review of digital mental health interventions developed for mental health practitioners during COVID-19 identified social media platforms, e-learning content, online resources, and mobile applications in 11 eligible studies [66]. However, there was a low level of empirical evaluation of these interventions (27%). Challenges and limitations related to the adoption of the reported interventions were common (55%) and greater heterogeneity is required given 45% of interventions were specific to China. A narrative review of digital psychotherapy found evidence of effectiveness for depression and anxiety disorders, of mild-to-moderate severity, from multiple randomized controlled trials and a large meta-analysis [67]. An online survey of the use of digital information and communication technologies in psychological counseling before and during a COVID-19 lockdown found overall positivity in the use of technologies and web-based interventions, with most practitioners noting approximately the same client involvement/adherence rates [68]. Interestingly, there was only a slight rise in the use of some tools (i.e., video conference, social networks, and virtual rooms), and slightly less use of others (i.e., telephone calls, emails, audio conferences, online intervention platforms, smartphone/tablet apps, online forums, and chats) [68].

A systematic review found digital interventions or counseling based on communications technologies to be as effective as face-to-face sessions [69]. Similar with traditional therapy and counseling settings, quality assurance issues that require escalation may be resolved by governing agencies or professional associations [70]. Furthermore, therapists and counselors should have computer skills and online communication competencies and should follow ethics, bylaws, rules/regulations, technological malfunction procedures and crisis procedures. A rapid review on the effectiveness of digital mental health interventions for individuals with an associated chronic disease (mental and/or physical) found web-based interventions and email had the most reports of improvement but further analyses were required before making stronger recommendations on the relevance for youth [71]. The potential for digital technologies to change clinical research and treatment is developing and a special applicability to young people experiencing mental health problems has been proposed [72]. The internet, as an information source and help-seeking promoter, as well as smartphone and wearable technologies are among promising tools. There is growing support for these approaches to be augmented in routine care especially among young people.

2.5. Digital Mental Health for Young People

Young people were the third most represented population identified in a rapid scoping review of digital mental health among at-risk groups in Asia-Pacific during COVID-19 [73]. A German longitudinal study on the mental health and coping behavior of university students before and after the onset of COVID-19 found the pandemic had a moderate overall effect [74]. A protocol for impact evaluation of an Australian digital mental health model of care for youth (headspace) outlined that there are ongoing poor mental health outcomes for young people (12–25 years of age) [75]. The Asian Pacific, German, and Australian studies found vulnerable subgroups among youth may be at high risk of negative mental health impacts. Accessibility via devices, such as smartphones and high-speed Internet, and technological literacy were noted as challenges facing Asian Pacific children and youth [73]. Significant subgroups of American youth (particularly those who live in low-income and rural areas) are also experiencing marginalization because of inadequate access to the Internet, resulting in a gap during COVID-19 which is widening pediatric mental health differences [76]. Stigmatizing attitudes, accessibility, and affordability issues are experienced by Australian youth in non-urban areas, resulting in higher self-harm, suicidal ideation, and suicide attempt rates [75]. The German study found an accumulation of negative issues (i.e., preexisting stress, anxiety, depression, overexertion, and burnout) and suggested identifying those at risk to promote mental health in significant subgroups [74].

Research on digital solutions in clinical settings proposed young people as a transformative population for mental health treatment [5]. A survey of clinicians and youth mental health service users (aged 12–25) with regards to the rapid implementation of telehealth during COVID-19 found young people were the most positively satisfied and open to its continued use [77]. The digital solutions evidence base is limited to reviews, workshops, position papers, pilot studies, trials and protocols. A scoping review of online preventive interventions for youth with emerging mental health issues noted the high incidence of common evidence-based therapies and medium incidence of a blended approach (supported by a human) [78]. The review mentioned the most common psychological symptoms and disorders in youth are heightened stress, depression, anxiety, and psychosis. The most common intervention is CBT. There were a wide range of adherence rates to digital interventions (between 27.9 and 98%). The results indicated general effectiveness, usability, and acceptability of online indicated preventive interventions for a wide range of mental health complaints, and positive mental health promotion (e.g., well-being and resilience). Future research was recommended for co-design of clinical trials based on the clinical staging model with a focus on transdiagnostic mechanisms, instruments for emerging or subclinical mental health symptoms as well as a government-backed structure for financial compensation of innovation and development.

A systematic overview of meta-analyses and systematic reviews found digital mental health interventions for young people have reasonably positive effects [79]. The evidence of effectiveness was mostly found on anxiety and depression, and to a lesser extent on stress—the main concerns are evidence-based treatment content or in-person elements that may improve engagement [79]. Only a small proportion of digital platforms are evidence-based—more needs to be known about the (cost-)effectiveness of the type of service provided, target subpopulation, and the current standard of care [79]. A systematic review also concluded there needs to be higher understanding of the (cost-)effectiveness of digital psychological interventions [80]. A randomized controlled trial is currently partly evaluating the (cost-)effectiveness of a digital alcohol moderation intervention (web app based on motivational interviewing and CBT) which was added to an existing depression treatment for young adults [81].

Innovative technologies are increasingly being used in studies on the mental health of young people. A case report on young adults with a psychotic illness found digital phenotyping via tracking on a smartphone app is a feasible way to monitor and detect patient status [82]. A proof-of-concept study with university students found early evidence that there is benefit in deploying a digital healthy-coping intervention via a chatbot for their higher levels of psychological distress [83]. There was preliminary evidence of efficacy for digital psychological interventions via games and virtual reality (VR) in children and young people [84]. A longitudinal approach to development and design as well as greater heterogeneity are required for studies evaluating digital psychological interventions [85]. A systematic review of the use of commercial off-the-shelf video games found there is efficacy for reducing stress and anxiety [86]. Video game genres included exergames, casual video games, action games, action-adventure games, and augmented reality games used on various gaming platforms, including consoles, PCs, smartphones, mobile consoles, and virtual reality systems [86]. An editorial on child and adolescent learnings of the current pandemic recommended future research designs to consider the strategic use of technology and remote learning in new educational approaches for diverse populations as well as to explain the factors that predict and improve resilience during adversity [87].

The scientific framework, methodology, and digital mental health implementation strategies for young people are marked by significant challenges including engagement, retention, fidelity, lack of personalization, and cognitive load [88]. A protocol for an evaluation study on the effectiveness of education and training of youth mental health care clinicians established that the adoption and optimization of technical solutions are integral for use in standard clinical practice [89]. The feasibility, acceptability, and initial safety profile of an online mental health service for improving help-seeking and mental health symptoms among students found: administrative barriers to uptake; time constraints for school staff to help; high drop-out rates in a series of modules; and uncertainty about improvements in help-seeking behavior and symptoms [90]. A systematic review of ethical concerns for digital mental health for young people found there is a need for better online security and data privacy as well as improved guidelines and legislation [20].

3. Conclusions and Prospects

Digital mental health is in its adolescence but there is efficacy for digital interventions at the population level. The novelty of the genre is unravelling amid COVID-19. It provides advantages for some populations: increased accessibility, acceptability, affordability, and availability of care, equity, autonomy and serviceability as well as an improved understanding of mental health. However, it is important to have in mind the disadvantages: concerns with efficacy, insufficient validation of technology, user engagement and retention issues, data security and privacy, marginalization (especially of the underserved and the unserved), and a lack of organizational readiness as well as over reliance on technology and clinical support. More needs to be known about the psychological symptoms and disorders for which it is effective. So far, the evidence of effectiveness is on common disorders (i.e., mild to moderate anxiety and depression) as well as stress. It is not yet established if some mental disorders can present more difficulties than others. Digital interventions for those with serious mental ill-health (on the psychotic spectrum and bipolar disorder) and chronic mental health conditions demonstrated significant promise despite being less established than for common disorders. Video conferences, social networks, telephone calls, and emails are common digital tools used amid COVID-19; audio conferences, smartphone/tablet apps, online intervention platforms and chats were used to a lesser extent. Clinical practitioners may use digital mental health guides; furthermore, trials are underway with TECC to help achieve faster and better quality care. Young people are a discerning population for research because of their increased use of online clinical support services. Despite the challenges of providing ethical, effective, accessible, and equitable care, digital mental health is delivering innovative ways of serving those who are isolated, lonely, and at-risk of stress, anxiety, and depression. Further research is required for reliable, valid, and replicable models of care above and beyond what is established for telehealth, digital platforms, and apps. AI technologies (especially machine learning and predictive analytics), smartphone, and wearable technologies as well as immersive solutions (VR and video games) are noteworthy prospects.

Author Contributions: Conceptualization, L.B.; investigation, L.B., writing—original draft preparation, L.B.; writing—review and editing, L.B. and D.D.L.; supervision, D.D.L.; project administration, L.B. All authors have read and agreed to the published version of the manuscript.

Funding: This research received no external funding.

Conflicts of Interest: The authors declare no conflict of interest.

Entry Link on the Encyclopedia Platform: https://encyclopedia.pub/16293.

References

1. Pirkis, J.; John, A.; Shin, S.; DelPozo-Banos, M.; Arya, V.; Analuisa-Aguilar, P.; Appleby, L.; Arensman, E.; Bantjes, J.; Baran, A.; et al. Suicide trends in the early months of the COVID-19 pandemic: An interrupted time-series analysis of preliminary data from 21 countries. *Lancet Psychiatry* **2021**, *8*, 579–588. [CrossRef]
2. Rettie, H.; Daniels, J. Coping and tolerance of uncertainty: Predictors and mediators of mental health during the COVID-19 pandemic. *Am. Psychol.* **2021**, *76*, 427–437. [CrossRef]
3. Torous, J.; Keshavan, M. COVID-19, mobile health and serious mental illness. *Schizophr. Res.* **2020**, *218*, 36–37. [CrossRef]
4. Balcombe, L.; De Leo, D. An Integrated Blueprint for Digital Mental Health Services Amidst COVID-19. *JMIR Ment. Health* **2020**, *7*, e21718. [CrossRef] [PubMed]
5. Gleeson, J.F.M.; Riper, H.; Alvarez-Jimenez, M. Editorial: Transforming Youth Mental Health Treatment Through Digital Technology. *Front. Psychiatry* **2020**, *11*, 606433. [CrossRef] [PubMed]
6. Saxena, S.; Thornicroft, G.; Knapp, M.; Whiteford, H. Resources for mental health: Scarcity, inequity, and inefficiency. *Lancet* **2007**, *370*, 878–889. [CrossRef]
7. Whittle, E.L.; Fisher, K.R.; Reppermund, S.; Lenroot, R.; Trollor, J. Barriers and Enablers to Accessing Mental Health Services for People with Intellectual Disability: A Scoping Review. *J. Ment. Health Res. Intellect. Disabil.* **2018**, *11*, 69–102. [CrossRef]
8. Rudd, B.N.; Beidas, R.S. Digital Mental Health: The Answer to the Global Mental Health Crisis? *JMIR Ment. Health* **2020**, *7*, e18472. [CrossRef] [PubMed]
9. Torous, J.; Myrick, K.J.; Rauseo-Ricupero, N.; Firth, J. Digital Mental Health and COVID-19: Using Technology Today to Accelerate the Curve on Access and Quality Tomorrow. *JMIR Ment. Health* **2020**, *7*, e18848. [CrossRef] [PubMed]
10. Guinart, D.; Marcy, P.; Hauser, M.; Dwyer, M.; Kane, J.M. Patient Attitudes Toward Telepsychiatry During the COVID-19 Pandemic: A Nationwide, Multisite Survey. *JMIR Ment. Health* **2020**, *7*, e24761. [CrossRef] [PubMed]
11. Guinart, D.; Marcy, P.; Hauser, M.; Dwyer, M.; Kane, J.M. Mental Health Care Providers' Attitudes Toward Telepsychiatry: A Systemwide, Multisite Survey During the COVID-19 Pandemic. *Psychiatr. Serv.* **2021**, *72*, 704–707. [CrossRef]
12. The Lancet Digital Health Digital tools for mental health in a crisis. *Lancet Digit. Health* **2021**, *3*, e204. [CrossRef]
13. Barnett, P.; Goulding, L.; Casetta, C.; Jordan, H.; Sheridan-Rains, L.; Steare, T.; Williams, J.; Wood, L.; Gaughran, F.; Johnson, S. Implementation of Telemental Health Services Before COVID-19: Rapid Umbrella Review of Systematic Reviews. *J. Med Internet Res.* **2021**, *23*, e26492. [CrossRef] [PubMed]
14. Whelan, P.; Stockton-Powdrell, C.; Jardine, J.; Sainsbury, J. Comment on "Digital Mental Health and COVID-19: Using Technology Today to Accelerate the Curve on Access and Quality Tomorrow": A UK Perspective. *JMIR Ment. Health* **2020**, *7*, e19547. [CrossRef] [PubMed]
15. Wind, T.R.; Rijkeboer, M.; Andersson, G.; Riper, H. The COVID-19 pandemic: The 'black swan' for mental health care and a turning point for e-health. *Internet Interv.* **2020**, *20*, 100317. [CrossRef] [PubMed]
16. Sorkin, D.H.; Janio, E.A.; Eikey, E.V.; Schneider, M.; Davis, K.; Schueller, S.M.; Stadnick, N.A.; Zheng, K.; Neary, M.; Safani, D.; et al. Rise in Use of Digital Mental Health Tools and Technologies in the United States During the COVID-19 Pandemic: Survey Study. *J. Med. Internet Res.* **2021**, *23*, e26994. [CrossRef]
17. Rauschenberg, C.; Schick, A.; Hirjak, D.; Seidler, A.; Pätzold, I.; Apfelbacher, C.; Riedel-Heller, S.G.; Reininghaus, U. Digital interventions to mitigate the negative impact of the COVID-19 pandemic on public mental health: A rapid meta-review. *PsyArXiv* **2020**. [CrossRef]
18. Balcombe, L.; De Leo, D. Psychological Screening and Tracking of Athletes and Digital Mental Health Solutions in a Hybrid Model of Care: Mini Review. *JMIR Form. Res.* **2020**, *4*, e22755. [CrossRef]

19. Ganapathy, A.; Clough, B.A.; Casey, L.M. Organizational and Policy Barriers to the Use of Digital Mental Health by Mental Health Professionals. *Telemed. e-Health* **2021**. [CrossRef]
20. Wies, B.; Landers, C.; Ienca, M. Digital Mental Health for Young People: A Scoping Review of Ethical Promises and Challenges. *Front. Digit. Health* **2021**, *3*, 697072. [CrossRef]
21. Fu, Z.; Burger, H.; Arjadi, R.; Bockting, C.L.H. Effectiveness of digital psychological interventions for mental health problems in low-income and middle-income countries: A systematic review and meta-analysis. *Lancet Psychiatry* **2020**, *7*, 851–864. [CrossRef]
22. Singla, D.R.; Lawson, A.; Kohrt, B.A.; Jung, J.W.; Meng, Z.; Ratjen, C.; Zahedi, N.; Dennis, C.-L.; Patel, V. Implementation and Effectiveness of Nonspecialist-Delivered Interventions for Perinatal Mental Health in High-Income Countries. *JAMA Psychiatry* **2021**, *78*, 498. [CrossRef] [PubMed]
23. Kozelka, E.E.; Jenkins, J.H.; Carpenter-Song, E. Advancing Health Equity in Digital Mental Health: Lessons From Medical Anthropology for Global Mental Health. *JMIR Ment. Health* **2021**, *8*, e28555. [CrossRef] [PubMed]
24. Mohr, D.C.; Lyon, A.R.; Lattie, E.G.; Reddy, M.; Schueller, S.M. Accelerating Digital Mental Health Research From Early Design and Creation to Successful Implementation and Sustainment. *J. Med. Internet Res.* **2017**, *19*, e153. [CrossRef] [PubMed]
25. Balcombe, L.; De Leo, D. Digital Mental Health Challenges and the Horizon Ahead for Solutions. *JMIR Ment. Health* **2021**, *8*, e26811. [CrossRef]
26. Schueller, S.M. Grand Challenges in Human Factors and Digital Health. *Front. Digit. Health* **2021**, *3*. [CrossRef]
27. Jacobi, C. Special issue internet interventions: Editorial "integrating technology into mental health care delivery in Europe (ICare)". *Internet Interv.* **2019**, *16*, 1–4. [CrossRef]
28. Bucci, S.; Berry, N.; Morris, R.; Berry, K.; Haddock, G.; Lewis, S.; Edge, D. "They Are Not Hard-to-Reach Clients. We Have Just Got Hard-to-Reach Services." Staff Views of Digital Health Tools in Specialist Mental Health Services. *Front. Psychiatry* **2019**, *10*, 344. [CrossRef]
29. Walker, R.; Usher, K.; Jackson, D.; Reid, C.; Hopkins, K.; Shepherd, C.; Smallwood, R.; Marriott, R. Connection to. Addressing Digital Inequities in Supporting the Well-Being of Young Indigenous Australians in the Wake of COVID-19. *Int. J. Environ. Res. Public Health* **2021**, *18*, 2141. [CrossRef]
30. Graham, A.K.; Weissman, R.S.; Mohr, D.C. Resolving Key Barriers to Advancing Mental Health Equity in Rural Communities Using Digital Mental Health Interventions. *JAMA Health Forum* **2021**, *2*, e211149. [CrossRef]
31. Lal, S.; Gleeson, J.; Rivard, L.; D'Alfonso, S.; Joober, R.; Malla, A.; Alvarez-Jimenez, M. Adaptation of a Digital Health Innovation to Prevent Relapse and Support Recovery in Youth Receiving Services for First-Episode Psychosis: Results From the Horyzons-Canada Phase 1 Study. *JMIR Form. Res.* **2020**, *4*, e19887. [CrossRef] [PubMed]
32. Borghouts, J.; Eikey, E.; Mark, G.; De Leon, C.; Schueller, S.M.; Schneider, M.; Stadnick, N.; Zheng, K.; Mukamel, D.; Sorkin, D.H. Barriers to and Facilitators of User Engagement with Digital Mental Health Interventions: Systematic Review. *J. Med. Internet Res.* **2021**, *23*, e24387. [CrossRef]
33. Morriss, R.; Kaylor-Hughes, C.; Rawsthorne, M.; Coulson, N.; Simpson, S.; Guo, B.; James, M.; Lathe, J.; Moran, P.; Tata, L.; et al. A direct to public peer support programme (Big White Wall) versus web-based information to aid self-management of depression and anxiety (The REBOOT study): Results and challenges of an automated randomised controlled trial. (Preprint). *J. Med. Internet Res.* **2020**, *23*, e23487. [CrossRef] [PubMed]
34. Shi, J.; Lo, B.; Wong, H.W.; Hollenberg, E.; Sanches, M.; Abi-Jaoudé, A.; Chaim, G.; Cleverley, K.; Henderson, J.; Johnson, A.; et al. Assessing the usability and user engagement of Thought Spot—A digital mental health help-seeking solution for transition-aged youth. *Internet Interv.* **2021**, *24*, 100386. [CrossRef] [PubMed]
35. Venning, A.; Herd, M.C.; Oswald, T.K.; Razmi, S.; Glover, F.; Hawke, T.; Quartermain, V.; Redpath, P. Exploring the acceptability of a digital mental health platform incorporating a virtual coach: The good, the bad, and the opportunities. *Health Inform. J.* **2021**, *27*, 146045822199487. [CrossRef] [PubMed]
36. Allen, N.B.; Nelson, B.W.; Brent, D.; Auerbach, R.P. Short-term prediction of suicidal thoughts and behaviors in adolescents: Can recent developments in technology and computational science provide a breakthrough? *J. Affect. Disord.* **2019**, *250*, 163–169. [CrossRef]
37. Doraiswamy, P.M.; London, E.; Varnum, P.; Harvey, B.; Saxena, S.; Tottman, S.; Campbell, S.P.; Ibanez, A.F.; Manji, H.; Al Olama, M.A.A.S.; et al. Empowering 8 Billion Minds: Enabling Better Mental Health for All via the Ethical Adoption of Technologies. *NAM Perspect.* **2019**. [CrossRef]
38. Heinsch, M.; Geddes, J.; Sampson, D.; Brosnan, C.; Hunt, S.; Wells, H.; Kay-Lambkin, F. Disclosure of suicidal thoughts during an e-mental health intervention: Relational ethics meets actor-network theory. *Ethic Behav.* **2021**, *31*, 151–170. [CrossRef]
39. Powell, A.C.; Bowman, M.B.; Harbin, H.T. Reimbursement of Apps for Mental Health: Findings from Interviews. *JMIR Ment. Health* **2019**, *6*, e14724. [CrossRef]
40. Powell, A.; Torous, J. A Patient-Centered Framework for Measuring the Economic Value of the Clinical Benefits of Digital Health Apps: Theoretical Modeling. *JMIR Ment. Health* **2020**, *7*, e18812. [CrossRef]
41. Rosenberg, B.M.; Kodish, T.; Cohen, Z.D.; Gong-Guy, E.; Craske, M.G. Design and Implementation of a Novel Peer-to-Peer Coaching Program to Support Digital Mental Health. *JMIR Ment. Health* **2021**. preprint. [CrossRef]
42. Rice, S.; Robinson, J.; Bendall, S.; Hetrick, S.; Cox, G.; Bailey, E.; Gleeson, J.F.; Alvarez-Jimenez, M. Online and Social Media Suicide Prevention Interventions for Young People: A Focus on Implementation and Moderation. *J. Can. Acad. Child Adolesc. Psychiatry = J. l'Acad. Can. Psychiatr. l'enfant l'adolesc.* **2016**, *25*, 80–86.

43. D'Alfonso, S.; Phillips, J.; Valentine, L.; Gleeson, J.; Alvarez-Jimenez, M. Moderated Online Social Therapy: Viewpoint on the Ethics and Design Principles of a Web-Based Therapy System. *JMIR Ment. Health* **2019**, *6*, e14866. [CrossRef] [PubMed]
44. Iorfino, F.; Cross, S.P.; Davenport, T.; Carpenter, J.S.; Scott, E.; Shiran, S.; Hickie, I.B. A Digital Platform Designed for Youth Mental Health Services to Deliver Personalized and Measurement-Based Care. *Front. Psychiatry* **2019**, *10*, 595. [CrossRef] [PubMed]
45. van Agteren, J.; Bartholomaeus, J.; Fassnacht, D.B.; Iasiello, M.; Ali, K.; Lo, L.; Kyrios, M. Using Internet-Based Psychological Measurement to Capture the Deteriorating Community Mental Health Profile During COVID-19: Observational Study. *JMIR Ment. Health* **2020**, *7*, e20696. [CrossRef] [PubMed]
46. Hull, T.D.; Levine, J.; Bantilan, N.; Desai, A.N.; Majumder, M.S. Analyzing Digital Evidence from a Telemental Health Platform to Assess Complex Psychological Responses to the COVID-19 Pandemic: Content Analysis of Text Messages. *JMIR Form. Res.* **2021**, *5*, e26190. [CrossRef]
47. Venville, A.; O'Connor, S.; Roeschlein, H.; Ennals, P.; McLoughlan, G.; Thomas, N. Mental health service user and worker experience of psychosocial support via telehealth through the COVID-19 pandemic: A qualitative study (Preprint). *JMIR Ment. Health* **2021**, *8*, 29671. [CrossRef]
48. Strudwick, G.; McLay, D.; Lo, B.; Shin, H.D.; Currie, L.; Thomson, N.; Maillet, É.; Strong, V.; Miller, A.; Shen, N.; et al. Development of a Resource Guide to Support the Engagement of Mental Health Providers and Patients with Digital Health Tools: Multimethod Study. *J. Med. Internet Res.* **2021**, *23*, e25773. [CrossRef]
49. Mehta, A.; Niles, A.N.; Vargas, J.H.; Marafon, T.; Couto, D.D.; Gross, J.J. Acceptability and Effectiveness of Artificial Intelligence Therapy for Anxiety and Depression (Youper): Longitudinal Observational Study. *J. Med. Internet Res.* **2021**, *23*, e26771. [CrossRef]
50. Köhnen, M.; Dreier, M.; Seeralan, T.; Kriston, L.; Härter, M.; Baumeister, H.; Liebherz, S. Evidence on Technology-Based Psychological Interventions in Diagnosed Depression: Systematic Review. *JMIR Ment. Health* **2021**, *8*, e21700. [CrossRef]
51. Baumeister, H.; Bauereiss, N.; Zarski, A.-C.; Braun, L.; Buntrock, C.; Hoherz, C.; Idrees, A.R.; Kraft, R.; Meyer, P.; Nguyen, T.B.D.; et al. Clinical and Cost-Effectiveness of PSYCHOnlineTHERAPY: Study Protocol of a Multicenter Blended Outpatient Psychotherapy Cluster Randomized Controlled Trial for Patients with Depressive and Anxiety Disorders. *Front. Psychiatry* **2021**, *12*, 660534. [CrossRef]
52. Rauseo-Ricupero, N.; Torous, J. Technology Enabled Clinical Care (TECC): Protocol for a Prospective Longitudinal Cohort Study of Smartphone-Augmented Mental Health Treatment. *JMIR Res. Protoc.* **2021**, *10*, e23771. [CrossRef]
53. Iorfino, F.; Occhipinti, J.-A.; Skinner, A.; Davenport, T.; Rowe, S.; Prodan, A.; Sturgess, J.; Hickie, I.B. The Impact of Technology-Enabled Care Coordination in a Complex Mental Health System: A Local System Dynamics Model. *J. Med. Internet Res.* **2021**, *23*, e25331. [CrossRef]
54. Blitz, R.; Storck, M.; Baune, B.T.; Dugas, M.; Opel, N. Design and Implementation of an Informatics Infrastructure for Standardized Data Acquisition, Transfer, Storage, and Export in Psychiatric Clinical Routine: Feasibility Study. *JMIR Ment. Health* **2021**, *8*, e26681. [CrossRef] [PubMed]
55. de Redon, E.; Centi, A. Realities of conducting digital health research: Challenges to consider. *Digit. Health* **2019**, *5*, 205520761986946. [CrossRef]
56. Martinez-Martin, N.; Dasgupta, I.; Carter, A.; Chandler, J.A.; Kellmeyer, P.; Kreitmair, K.; Weiss, A.; Cabrera, L.Y. Ethics of Digital Mental Health During COVID-19: Crisis and Opportunities. *JMIR Ment. Health* **2020**, *7*, e23776. [CrossRef]
57. Guo, C.; Ashrafian, H.; Ghafur, S.; Fontana, G.; Gardner, C.; Prime, M. Challenges for the evaluation of digital health solutions—A call for innovative evidence generation approaches. *NPJ Digit. Med.* **2020**, *3*, 1–14. [CrossRef] [PubMed]
58. Arrieta, A.B.; Díaz-Rodríguez, N.; Del Ser, J.; Bennetot, A.; Tabik, S.; Barbado, A.; Garcia, S.; Gil-Lopez, S.; Molina, D.; Benjamins, R.; et al. Explainable Artificial Intelligence (XAI): Concepts, taxonomies, opportunities and challenges toward responsible AI. *Inf. Fusion* **2020**, *58*, 82–115. [CrossRef]
59. Tremain, H.; McEnery, C.; Fletcher, K.; Murray, G. The Therapeutic Alliance in Digital Mental Health Interventions for Serious Mental Illnesses: Narrative Review. *JMIR Ment. Health* **2020**, *7*, e17204. [CrossRef]
60. Chekroud, A.M.; Bondar, J.; Delgadillo, J.; Doherty, G.; Wasil, A.; Fokkema, M.; Cohen, Z.; Belgrave, D.; DeRubeis, R.; Iniesta, R.; et al. The promise of machine learning in predicting treatment outcomes in psychiatry. *World Psychiatry* **2021**, *20*, 154–170. [CrossRef]
61. Mulder, R.; Newton-Howes, G.; Coid, J.W. The futility of risk prediction in psychiatry. *Br. J. Psychiatry* **2016**, *209*, 271–272. [CrossRef] [PubMed]
62. Chan, M.K.Y.; Bhatti, H.; Meader, N.; Stockton, S.; Evans, J.; O'Connor, R.C.; Kapur, N.; Kendall, T. Predicting suicide following self-harm: Systematic review of risk factors and risk scales. *Br. J. Psychiatry* **2016**, *209*, 277–283. [CrossRef] [PubMed]
63. Shatte, A.B.R.; Hutchinson, D.M.; Teague, S.J. Machine learning in mental health: A scoping review of methods and applications. *Psychol. Med.* **2019**, *49*, 1426–1448. [CrossRef] [PubMed]
64. Moon, S.J.; Hwang, J.; Kana, R.; Torous, J.; Kim, J.W. Accuracy of Machine Learning Algorithms for the Diagnosis of Autism Spectrum Disorder: Systematic Review and Meta-Analysis of Brain Magnetic Resonance Imaging Studies. *JMIR Ment. Health* **2019**, *6*, e14108. [CrossRef]
65. Graham, S.; Depp, C.; Lee, E.E.; Nebeker, C.; Tu, X.; Kim, H.-C.; Jeste, D.V. Artificial Intelligence for Mental Health and Mental Illnesses: An Overview. *Curr. Psychiatry Rep.* **2019**, *21*, 116. [CrossRef]
66. Drissi, N.; Ouhbi, S.; Marques, G.; Díez, I.D.L.T.; Ghogho, M.; Idrissi, M.A.J. A Systematic Literature Review on e-Mental Health Solutions to Assist Health Care Workers during COVID-19. *Telemed. e-Health* **2021**, *27*, 594–602. [CrossRef]

67. Weightman, M. Digital psychotherapy as an effective and timely treatment option for depression and anxiety disorders: Implications for rural and remote practice. *J. Int. Med. Res.* **2020**, *48*, 030006052092868. [CrossRef]
68. Dores, A.R.; Geraldo, A.; Carvalho, I.P.; Barbosa, F. The Use of New Digital Information and Communication Technologies in Psychological Counseling during the COVID-19 Pandemic. *Int. J. Environ. Res. Public Health* **2020**, *17*, 7663. [CrossRef]
69. Machado, D.D.B.; Laskoski, P.B.; Severo, C.T.; Bassols, A.M.; Sfoggia, A.; Kowacs, C.; Krieger, D.V.; Torres, M.B.; Gastaud, M.B.; Wellausen, R.S.; et al. A Psychodynamic Perspective on a Systematic Review of Online Psychotherapy for Adults. *Br. J. Psychother.* **2016**, *32*, 79–108. [CrossRef]
70. Dores, A.R.; Silva, R.A.; Crepulja, M.L.; Franciskovic, T.; Stevanovic, A. Ethical Aspects of the E-Tools / E-consulting with Focus on Differences from Classic Settings. In Therapy 2.0, Guidelines for Advisors, Counsellors and Therapists on the Utilization of Online Interventions. Available online: https://www.ecounselling4youth.eu/online-material/courses/files/guidelines_en.pdf (accessed on 1 October 2021).
71. Sasseville, M.; LeBlanc, A.; Boucher, M.; Dugas, M.; Mbemba, G.; Tchuente, J.; Chouinard, M.-C.; Beaulieu, M.; Beaudet, N.; Skidmore, B.; et al. Digital health interventions for the management of mental health in people with chronic diseases: A rapid review. *BMJ Open* **2021**, *11*, e044437. [CrossRef] [PubMed]
72. Cotter, J.; Bucci, S. E-mental health for young people. *Youth Mental Health* **2020**, 125–138. [CrossRef]
73. Murphy, J.K.; Khan, A.; Sun, Q.; Minas, H.; Hatcher, S.; Ng, C.H.; Withers, M.; Greenshaw, A.; Michalak, E.E.; Chakraborty, P.A.; et al. Needs, gaps and opportunities for standard and e-mental health care among at-risk populations in the Asia Pacific in the context of COVID-19: A rapid scoping review. *Int. J. Equity Health* **2021**, *20*, 1–22. [CrossRef] [PubMed]
74. Voltmer, E.; Köslich-Strumann, S.; Walther, A.; Kasem, M.; Obst, K.; Kötter, T. The impact of the COVID-19 pandemic on stress, mental health and coping behavior in German University students—A longitudinal study before and after the onset of the pandemic. *BMC Public Health* **2021**, *21*, 1–15. [CrossRef] [PubMed]
75. Piper, S.; Davenport, T.A.; LaMonica, H.; Ottavio, A.; Iorfino, F.; Cheng, V.W.S.; Cross, S.; Lee, G.Y.; Scott, E.; Hickie, I.B. Implementing a digital health model of care in Australian youth mental health services: Protocol for impact evaluation. *BMC Health Serv. Res.* **2021**, *21*, 1–9. [CrossRef] [PubMed]
76. Smith-East, M., Starks, S. COVID-19 and Mental Health Care Delivery: A Digital Divide Exists for Youth With Inadequate Access to the Internet. *J. Am. Acad. Child Adolesc. Psychiatry* **2021**, *60*, 798–800. [CrossRef] [PubMed]
77. Nicholas, J.; Bell, I.H.; Thompson, A.; Valentine, L.; Simsir, P.; Sheppard, H.; Adams, S. Implementation lessons from the transition to telehealth during COVID-19: A survey of clinicians and young people from youth mental health services. *Psychiatry Res.* **2021**, *299*, 113848. [CrossRef]
78. van Doorn, M.; Nijhuis, L.A.; Egeler, M.D.; Daams, J.G.; Popma, A.; van Amelsvoort, T.; McEnery, C.; Gleeson, J.F.; Öry, F.G.; Avis, K.A.; et al. Online Indicated Preventive Mental Health Interventions for Youth: A Scoping Review. *Front. Psychiatry* **2021**, *12*, 580843. [CrossRef]
79. Lehtimaki, S.; Martic, J.; Wahl, B.; Foster, K.T.; Schwalbe, N. Evidence on Digital Mental Health Interventions for Adolescents and Young People: Systematic Overview. *JMIR Ment. Health* **2021**, *8*, e25847. [CrossRef]
80. Bertuzzi, V.; Semonella, M.; Bruno, D.; Manna, C.; Edbrook-Childs, J.; Giusti, E.; Castelnuovo, G.; Pietrabissa, G. Psychological Support Interventions for Healthcare Providers and Informal Caregivers during the COVID-19 Pandemic: A Systematic Review of the Literature. *Int. J. Environ. Res. Public Health* **2021**, *18*, 6939. [CrossRef]
81. Schouten, M.J.E.; Dekker, J.J.M.; de Bruijn, T.Q.; Ebert, D.D.; Koomen, L.M.; Kosterman, S.L.A.; Riper, H.; Schaub, M.P.; Goudriaan, A.E.; Blankers, M. Effectiveness of a digital alcohol moderation intervention as an add-on to depression treatment for young adults: Study protocol of a multicentre pragmatic randomized controlled trial. *BMC Psychiatry* **2021**, *21*, 1–16. [CrossRef] [PubMed]
82. Wisniewski, H.; Henson, P.; Torous, J. Using a Smartphone App to Identify Clinically Relevant Behavior Trends via Symptom Report, Cognition Scores, and Exercise Levels: A Case Series. *Front. Psychiatry* **2019**, *10*, 652. [CrossRef] [PubMed]
83. Gabrielli, S.; Rizzi, S.; Bassi, G.; Carbone, S.; Maimone, R.; Marchesoni, M.; Forti, S. Engagement and Effectiveness of a Healthy Coping Intervention via Chatbot for university students: Proof-of-concept study during the COVID-19 pandemic (Preprint). *JMIR mHealth uHealth* **2021**, *9*, e27965. [CrossRef]
84. Halldorsson, B.; Hill, C.; Waite, P.; Partridge, K.; Freeman, D.; Creswell, C. Annual Research Review: Immersive virtual reality and digital applied gaming interventions for the treatment of mental health problems in children and young people: The need for rigorous treatment development and clinical evaluation. *J. Child Psychol. Psychiatry* **2021**, *62*, 584–605. [CrossRef] [PubMed]
85. Davies, E.B.; Bergin, A.D. Commentary: Let's get digital: A commentary on Halldorsson et al.'s call for more rigorous development and evaluation of immersive digital interventions for children and young people's mental health. *J. Child Psychol. Psychiatry* **2021**, *62*, 606–609. [CrossRef] [PubMed]
86. Pallavicini, F.; Pepe, A.; Mantovani, F. Commercial Off-The-Shelves Video Games for Reducing Stress and Anxiety: A PRISMA Systematic Review (Preprint). *JMIR Ment. Health* **2021**, *8*, 28150. [CrossRef] [PubMed]
87. Biel, M.G.; Hamrah, O. Editorial: Learning from the Pandemic: "Building Back Better" Through Research on Risk and Resilience with Diverse Populations. *J. Am. Acad. Child Adolesc. Psychiatry* **2021**, *60*, 445–447. [CrossRef] [PubMed]
88. Scholten, H.; Granic, I. Use of the Principles of Design Thinking to Address Limitations of Digital Mental Health Interventions for Youth: Viewpoint. *J. Med. Internet Res.* **2019**, *21*, e11528. [CrossRef]

89. Dohnt, H.C.; Dowling, M.J.; Davenport, T.A.; Lee, G.; Cross, S.P.; Scott, E.M.; Song, Y.J.C.; Hamilton, B.; Hockey, S.J.; Rohleder, C.; et al. Supporting Clinicians to Use Technology to Deliver Highly Personalized and Measurement-Based Mental Health Care to Young People: Protocol for an Evaluation Study. *JMIR Res. Protoc.* **2021**, *10*, e24697. [CrossRef]
90. O'Dea, B.; King, C.; Subotic-Kerry, M.; Achilles, M.R.; Cockayne, N.; Christensen, H. Smooth Sailing: A Pilot Study of an Online, School-Based, Mental Health Service for Depression and Anxiety. *Front. Psychiatry* **2019**, *10*, 574. [CrossRef]

encyclopedia

Entry

COVID-19 and Romantic Relationships

Octav-Sorin Candel * and Mihaela Jitaru

Faculty of Psychology and Educational Sciences, Alexandru Ioan Cuza University of Iaşi, 700554 Iaşi, Romania; jitaru.mihaela@uaic.ro

* Correspondence: candel.octav@uaic.ro

Definition: Since the beginning of 2020, the COVID-19 pandemic has impacted most people's activities and relationships. Romantic relationships are a crucial source of fulfillment and emotional safety for many individuals. However, due to the risk of illness and the social distancing norms, human interaction, even inside one's couple or family, suffered great changes. Some of these changes have the potential of disrupting people's relational or psychological well-being, but they can also have positive impacts. On the other hand, one of the most negative consequences is the growing number of intimate partner violence (IPV) incidents. Considering all these aspects, therapy would be beneficial for those affected.

Keywords: intimate partner violence; sexuality; relational satisfaction; COVID-19; lockdown effects

Citation: Candel, O.-S.; Jitaru, M. COVID-19 and Romantic Relationships. *Encyclopedia* **2021**, *1*, 1038–1046. https://doi.org/10.3390/encyclopedia1040079

Academic Editor: Stephen Bustin

Received: 16 September 2021
Accepted: 18 October 2021
Published: 20 October 2021

1. Introduction

The COVID-19 pandemic brought a number of profound alterations to people's lifestyles and relationships. While the number of cases increased during the first months of 2020, most countries imposed severe restrictions on the population. The new social distancing norms led to social isolation and separation, a situation that is likely to negatively impact the functioning of romantic relationships [1]. Early reports indicated that the population was exposed to significant stress during the pandemic, mainly due to the risks of becoming infected or losing their job [2,3].

In the context of increased stressful experiences, the quality of romantic relationships could be seriously impacted. While some couples are more vulnerable than others, researchers considered that the pandemic could harm the dyadic process for most couples [1]. This paper provides an overview of how the COVID-19 pandemic affected the creation and functioning of romantic relationships. Firstly, it concentrates on how people adapted to the social distancing norms and how they managed to find potential romantic partners under the stay-at-home orders. Secondly, it presents the most important findings related to the functioning of intimate relationships in youth and adult populations. Next, it provides some information about one of the most noteworthy concerns regarding the pandemic, namely, the potential increase in intimate partner violence [4]. Finally, it introduces some findings and recommendations related to the therapeutic process during the pandemic.

2. Online Dating during the COVID-19 Pandemic

Stay-at home orders resulted in increased levels of perceived loneliness during the early days of the pandemic [5]. This link was mitigated by relational status and living arrangements. People who were in a relationship, as well as those who were living with someone else, reported less perceived loneliness [6]. However, for those single, knowing new people and potential romantic partners became increasingly difficult given the restrictions related to social distancing. Under these conditions, online dating became an even more viable instrument in finding and selecting romantic partners [7–9]. While many individuals were already using online dating apps and other types of computer-mediated communication, the reliance on the virtual environment for romantic purposes increased during the pandemic, but the benefits of using it are not always apparent [10]. It is worth noting that the desire to meet new people did not decrease, but the safety of doing it and the negative outcomes of a potential date became more salient for those involved in online dating [11]. Missing the physicality of real contact, the ability to determine chemistry or to develop intimacy are some of the most important shortcomings that people felt while using online dating during the pandemic [10–12]. In addition, the fear of being emotionally exploited by a potential partner increased for some young women [10]. These fears are centered on the possible lack of authenticity, truthfulness, reciprocity, and accountability, especially in online dating spaces. The health status of the date also became more relevant compared to the pre-pandemic period. Thus, communication and information-seeking strategies became extremely important in reducing uncertainty during these times. Protective measures against COVID-19 infection, such as setting boundaries or directly asking about one's health status, were deployed by the individuals involved in online dating [13]. Finally, the quality of communication, especially on dating apps such as Tinder, was considered quite low [13]. Despite these drawbacks, those apprehensive of using virtual environments to communicate during the pandemic reported increased levels of relational worry and, consequently, more loneliness [14]. Thus, although not perfect, computer-mediated communication helped people during the pandemic by offering them a safer and more stable environment to meet new potential romantic partners.

3. Youths' Romantic Relationships

The social distancing measures affected the mobility of young people, with some studies showing that a large majority of adolescents engaged, at least minimally, with this norm [15]. Moreover, the pandemic was associated with mild to moderate depression and anxiety symptoms [16]. Thus, it created the premises for some important changes in the youths' romantic behaviors. Firstly, the reduced possibility of physical contact, as well as the worsening of young people's psychological state, led, for some, to a reevaluation of close relationships and of the efforts involved in their maintenance [17]. The reduction in the time spent with partners was the most important predictor for a fall in the quality of the romantic relationship during the pandemic [18]. In addition, teens, especially girls, described the maintenance process as being rather difficult due to the lack of intimacy, physical dating opportunities and psychical touch [10]. Despite these shortcomings, not all adolescents reported decreased relational quality. Some of them considered that the pandemic strengthened their relationships, but this was the case especially for those who spent significant time together with their partner [19].

The relationship between mental health and romantic relationships seems to be bidirectional. One study found that romantic relationships were the most important predictor of students' probable anxiety and also a predictor of their probable insomnia during the COVID-19 pandemic [20].

On a more positive note, young people also took advantage of modern communication methods (phone, social network sites) to keep in touch with their partners [10]. Technology use also mediated the negative relationships between self-isolation and relational quality for adolescence. While those who self-isolated more frequently reported a lower relationship quality, they also reported a higher use of technology, which led to an increase in relationship quality [21]. While stay-at-home orders and the youths' own intentions to self-isolate were hurdles in the management of romantic relationships, their communication behaviors and the adoption of new ways to communicate brought some improvements in the process.

4. Adult Romantic Relationships

The changes brought by the pandemic in areas such as couple relationships or parenting were significant. However, most studies show that the newly created situation had a rather complex array of outcomes on the functioning of couples. Some results indicated that the quality of close relationships was negatively impacted by the fear of COVID-19, depression, worry and rumination about the pandemic. When people reported higher levels on these variables, they also reported more isolation and lower abilities to reduce conflicts. Moreover, the worsening in the quality of the relationships was related to lower optimism and hope [22]. In addition, more COVID-19-related conflicts decreased the frequency of some intimate behaviors such as hugging, kissing or holding hands [23]. In the USA, there was a significant decline in marriage from 2019 to 2020 [24]. In Germany, 40% of couples reported declines in marital satisfaction during the pandemic, while only 20% considered that their satisfaction increased [25]. However, other studies showed that satisfaction remained stable during the first weeks of the pandemic and that people blamed their partners less, preferring not to attribute their negative behaviors to their internal characteristics [26]. Others found no association between quarantine and marital satisfaction, in both heterosexual and gay and lesbian couples [27,28]. Higher marital satisfaction was related to a lower impact of confinement on health, physical and emotional well-being [29].

Various psychological mechanisms could account for these conflicting results. For example, both attachment anxiety and avoidance were related to lower relational quality and family cohesion, especially when the individuals were expressing more stress [30]. In addition, people seemed to receive less partner support when their level of avoidance was higher [31]. Daily support reduced stress through enhanced gratitude [32]. Coping seems to link psychological distress and relational resilience. While negatively coping, which is positively related to distress and reduced resilience, positive coping provides protection against distress and strengthened resilience [33]. Similar associations were found in the case of relational quality [34]. In Finland, coping strategies at the relationship level (being more flexible, creating and using family time, having good family communication) were the most useful in dealing with stress [35]. In addition, the COVID-19 concerns led to more explicit stress communication, which was related to higher perceived partner dyadic coping. Thus, while the pandemic-related concerns were negatively linked to psychological well-being, they also led to improved dyadic coping, which has a protective role in well-being [36]. Resilience communication behaviors, such as creating new routines and constructing positivity together were positively related, although not directly, to the process of dyadic coping. Together, they reduce relational uncertainty, fear and anger, emotions that can decrease the level of dyadic coping. The use of humor was directly and positively related to coping [37].

On the negative side, stress was related to lower relational satisfaction only for the women with higher socioeconomic status, but not for those with lower socioeconomic status or for men [38]. Negative emotions and relational turbulence increased from before the pandemic to during the pandemic due to a decrease in partner interdependence and an increase in spousal interference [39,40]. Finally, the illness of a family member was associated with increased fear of COVID-19, anxiety, depression and stress [41] and adverse life events and perceived threat of COVID-19 affected the relational quality of same-sex couples by increasing complaint avoidance [42].

The pandemic also had an effect on the willingness to engage in a relationship. COVID-19 concerns increased the fear of being single, which, in turn, increased the importance of stability and family commitment [43]. Still, experiencing meaningful interpersonal connections during the first days of the pandemic created a context for the affirmation of the self and led to an emotional uplift [44].

Parents, compared to non-parents, were more protected against declines in marital satisfaction [25]. Moreover, there was no association between quarantine and parental burnout [27]. Still, parents felt some disruptions in their daily lives, but the division of labor in the newly created environment was not a stress source [45]. They were, however, mostly unhappy with the balance of paid and unpaid work during the pandemic [46]. The situation was more dramatic for the divorced or divorcing parents, who faced legal, financial and negotiation-related difficulties due to the pandemic [47]. Some changes were also found for the parents involved in consensual non-monogamous relationships. They spent less time with their partners when the partners were not living in the same household but more time when they were living together with the partners. In addition, some of them prioritized the more committed relationships [48].

5. Sexuality during the Pandemic

The pandemic brought important changes in people's sexual activity, although its impact was either positive or negative depending on various factors. While for some individuals, the social distancing norms meant a worsening of their sexual life, for others, spending more time with their partners lead to some improvement [49–51]. Relational status, gender and sexual orientation are, however, very important variables that should be taken into account when discussing how human sexuality was impacted by the pandemic.

Throughout the world, various studies showed that people reported less sex during the pandemic, a result that was consistent among participants from Australia, Spain, Turkey, the UK, the USA and Taiwan [7,49–54]. Women seemed to be particularly affected by the changes [55–57]. On the contrary, solo sexual activity increased, behaviors such as masturbation or using adult online sites becoming more prevalent for both men and women [7,49,50]. In addition to gender, relational status played an important role in determining the nature of the changes that happened throughout the pandemic. According to a study conducted in Turkey, the partners that spent more time together reported an increase in sexual satisfaction [50]. Similar results were found in Australia, where the participants who were single reported a more pronounced decrease in sexual activity compared to those who had a stable partner [7]. In addition, people reported having more sex with stable partners than with casual ones [7]. Finally, in Southeast Asia, one study showed no substantial differences in sexual activity before and during the pandemic in a sample of married individuals [58].

In regard to sexual orientation, some studies showed an association between being a sexual minority and decreased sex-seeking behaviors for men [53]. Others show that men having sex with men are less willing to seek casual sex but more willing to reduce the number of sexual partners or to find new ones [59,60].

Although the restrictions imposed throughout the world led to important decreases in sexual activity, some people still tried to make new additions to their sexual life. One study showed that one in five people made new additions during the pandemic by trying new sexual positions, using cybersex or watching pornography, among others [54]. In addition, the same individuals reported more sexual improvements during the same period.

Other than the demographic characteristics, multiple psychological variables are related to sexual activity. Higher risk perception of COVID-19, anxiety, stress and depression were negatively associated with the frequency of sexual activity and satisfaction [49,52,53,61]. On the contrary, those who experienced fewer disruptions in their daily lives felt more sexual desire and reported better sexual functioning [62].

In conclusion, the pandemic brought a decrease in sexual activity for most people (although some notable exceptions were present). This change was present in both the young population and in potential parents, some of whom renounced their parenthood plans [63,64]. Thus, the long-term consequences of this period should also be of particular interest given that they could impact the reproductive habits of the population.

6. Intimate Partner Violence

The restrictions imposed by the authorities due to the COVID-19 pandemic seem to also have had a significant impact on romantic conflicts and intimate partner violence (IPV) [4,65,66]. IPV encompasses any set of behaviors that lead to physical, psychological or sexual harm in an intimate relationship [67]. IPV is a product of its social context and includes physical violence (e.g., slapping, beating, etc.), psychological abuse (e.g., humiliation, threats of harm, etc.), sexual violence (any sexual coercion acts) and controlling behaviors (e.g., monitoring partner's movements, restricting access to family, friends, financial resources, education, etc.) directed against an intimate partner [67,68].

An important factor that exacerbated the impact of the lockdown on IPV is the economic stress that existed before or came along with the pandemic [69–71]. After the pandemic started, some experts were trying to bring attention to the possibility of a rapidly growing number of IPV incidents as a result of the lockdown [72–74]. In addition, recent research does indeed highlight a growing percentage of IPV incidents all over the world [4,70,75].

From the early stages of the pandemic, people reported changes in IPV, the situations involving physical and sexual violence being aggravated [76,77]. Some studies targeted the changes that appeared in the number of sexual violence incidents in romantic relationships, highlighting their increase after the start of the COVID-19 pandemic [70,77]. These changes appeared not only in heterosexual relationships but in queer couples, too [66]. The situation did not improve over time, and the reports of IPV continued to be high [4,70,75]. There are also reports that show that some countries reported fewer official incidents of IPV than before the pandemic [4], but, unfortunately, the situation might not be that good, and a lot of IPV cases might go unreported.

Before the pandemic, women were reporting more cases of psychological violence than any other type, but during it, they started experiencing even more psychological but also physical and sexual violence [70]. Inadvertently, the measures imposed to protect people from the infection with COVID-19 put in danger some categories of people. In this case, those especially endangered were those who already experienced IPV.

A specific population that was affected by the IPV incidents consists of pregnant women [78,79]. In this type of situation, there is a direct victim, but the victimization does not affect only the mother. In addition, it can become increasingly difficult for the victims to extract themselves from the situation and they may need extra support and care [78].

Throughout the research completed up to this point, there is a factor that augment the impact of lockdown on IPV and that is economic stress [69,70,75,79,80]. The changes in the household income or the dismissal of the male partner were strongly related to a higher percentage of IPV [75,80].

In conclusion, the lockdown and the economic stress that resulted from the COVID-19 pandemic had significant repercussions on couples' wellbeing. The growing number of IPV incidents should be of particular interest due to the danger that they represent to the victims [65,71]. Policy makers and those responsible for carrying them out should be especially attentive to the way that the pandemic and related effects had impacted the victims' possibility to get help and extract themselves from the dangerous situations.

7. Therapeutic Interventions

The pandemic is not a significant threat for all couples. However, most could face at least small levels of stress caused by various changes or by illness. For other couples, the problems would be more severe. Thus, therapeutic intervention would be crucial in order to help couples to face their various burdens during the pandemic. Despite this stringent need, the social distancing norms also affected the therapeutic process. One survey found out that therapists had little experience with providing online interventions for couples, but their attempts were, nevertheless, mostly successful. Still, creating a strong therapeutic alliance was considered to be more difficult under the new circumstances [81]. Using virtual couple therapy or teletherapy was recommended by various practitioners as viable and even mandatory formats in which the therapists can provide their services to those in need [82,83]. Moreover, their positive experiences encouraged couple therapists to consider virtual interventions as being very useful even after the pandemic will end [84]. Finally, practice guidance was offered for the professional that must use telehealth to work with victims of IPV [85].

8. Conclusions

The COVID-19 pandemic has a complex impact on romantic relationships from their beginning to their ending. In order to find new potential partners, people use the Internet and various communication technologies even more than before. In addition, especially among the younger individuals, the reevaluation of current relationships seems to be more important than before the pandemic. The quality of the relationship took some hits for some couples, while for others it flourished. Various demographic and psychological variables account for these differences. Although parents feel some additional burden, this might not be felt as problematic. However, those who are trying to legally end their marriage are confronted with additional problems. One crucial negative outcome is the increase in the rates of intimate partner violence and a solution for this issue is not easily approachable. While therapists experienced some difficulties due to social distancing, they also use video-chatting or teletherapy to stay in touch with their clients.

Despite the impressive number of studies that were conducted on romantic relationships during the pandemic, some shortcomings must be discussed. These studies only present a short-term image of the situation. While important, this is not enough to draw pertinent conclusions about the impact of the pandemic. Longitudinal studies with multiple yearly waves are needed to have a more complete view of how COVID-19 really impacted close relationships. In addition, not all of the studies were able to differentiate between the different stages of the COVID-19 pandemic (the start of the pandemic, the lockdown, etc.) and their distinct impact.

Author Contributions: Conceptualization, O.-S.C.; writing—original draft preparation, review and editing, O.-S.C. and M.J. All authors have read and agreed to the published version of the manuscript.

Funding: This research received no external funding.

Conflicts of Interest: The author declares no conflict of interest.

Entry Link on the Encyclopedia Platform: https://encyclopedia.pub/16297.

References

1. Pietromonaco, P.R.; Overall, N.C. Applying Relationship Science to Evaluate How the COVID-19 Pandemic May Impact Couples' Relationships. *Am. Psychol.* **2021**, *76*, 438–450. [CrossRef]
2. Crayne, M.P. The Traumatic Impact of Job Loss and Job Search in the Aftermath of COVID-19. *Psychol. Trauma* **2020**, *12*, S180–S182. [CrossRef] [PubMed]
3. Park, C.L.; Russell, B.S.; Fendrich, M.; Finkelstein-Fox, L.; Hutchison, M.; Becker, J. Americans' COVID-19 Stress, Coping, and Adherence to CDC Guidelines. *J. Gen. Int. Med.* **2020**, *35*, 2296–2303. [CrossRef]
4. Brink, J.; Cullen, P.; Beek, K.; Peters, S.A.E. Intimate Partner Violence during the Covid-19 Pandemic in Western and Southern European Countries. *Eur. J. Public Health* **2021**, ckab093. [CrossRef] [PubMed]
5. Tull, M.T.; Edmonds, K.A.; Scamaldo, K.M.; Richmond, J.R.; Rose, J.P.; Gratz, K.L. Psychological Outcomes Associated with Stay-at-Home Orders and the Perceived Impact of COVID-19 on Daily Life. *Psychiatry Res.* **2020**, *289*, 113098. [CrossRef]
6. Ray, C.D. The Trajectory and Determinants of Loneliness during the Early Months of the COVID-19 Pandemic in the United States. *J. Soc. Pers. Relat.* **2021**, *38*, 1920–1938. [CrossRef]
7. Coombe, J.; Kong, F.Y.S.; Bittleston, H.; Williams, H.; Tomnay, J.; Vaisey, A.; Malta, S.; Goller, J.L.; Temple-Smith, M.; Bourchier, L.; et al. Love during Lockdown: Findings from an Online Survey Examining the Impact of COVID-19 on the Sexual Health of People Living in Australia. *Sex. Transm. Infect.* **2021**, *97*, 357–362. [CrossRef]
8. Sepúlveda, R.; Crespo, M.; Vieira, J. Online dating em tempos de COVID-19: Práticas de uso e dinâmicas comunicacionais em transformação forçada. *Observatorio* **2021**, *15*, 76–95.
9. Wiederhold, B.K. How COVID Has Changed Online Dating-and What Lies Ahead. *Cyberpsychol. Behav. Soc. Netw.* **2021**, *24*, 435–436. [CrossRef]
10. Goldstein, A.; Flicker, S. "Some Things Just Won't Go Back": Teen Girls' Online Dating Relationships during COVID-19. *Girlhood Stud.* **2020**, *13*, 64–78. [CrossRef]
11. Winking, A.R. Online Dating Habits amid Covid-19. *Anthós* **2021**, *10*, 12.
12. Portolan, L.; McAlister, J. Jagged Love: Narratives of Romance on Dating Apps during COVID-19. *Sex. Cult.* **2021**, 1–19. [CrossRef]
13. Noland, C.M. Negotiating Desire and Uncertainty on Tinder during the COVID-19 Pandemic: Implications for the Transformation of Sexual Health Communication. *Cyberpsychol. Behav. Soc. Netw.* **2021**, *24*, 488–492. [CrossRef] [PubMed]
14. Curran, T.; Seiter, J.S. The Role of Relational Worry Due to COVID-19 in the Links between Video Chat Apprehension, Loneliness, and Adhering to CDC Guidelines. *J. Soc. Pers. Relat.* **2021**, *38*, 1869–1876. [CrossRef]
15. Oosterhoff, B.; Palmer, C.A.; Wilson, J.; Shook, N. Adolescents' Motivations to Engage in Social Distancing during the COVID-19 Pandemic: Associations with Mental and Social Health. *J. Adolesc. Health* **2020**, *67*, 179–185. [CrossRef]

16. Stavridou, A.; Stergiopoulou, A.-A.; Panagouli, E.; Mesiris, G.; Thirios, A.; Mougiakos, T.; Troupis, T.; Psaltopoulou, T.; Tsolia, M.; Sergentanis, T.N.; et al. Psychosocial Consequences of COVID-19 in Children, Adolescents and Young Adults: A Systematic Review. *Psychiatry Clin. Neurosci.* **2020**, *74*, 615–616. [CrossRef] [PubMed]
17. Goldstein, A.; Flicker, S. "It's Been a Good Time to Reflect on ... who Isn't Worth Keeping around": COVID-19, Adolescent Relationship Maintenance and Implications for Health Education. *Health Educ.* **2021**.
18. Karp, C.; Moreau, C.; Sheehy, G.; Anjur-Dietrich, S.; Mbushi, F.; Muluve, E.; Mwanga, D.; Nzioki, M.; Pinchoff, J.; Austrian, K. Youth Relationships in the Era of COVID-19: A Mixed-Methods Study among Adolescent Girls and Young Women in Kenya. *J. Adolesc. Health* **2021**, 1–8. [CrossRef]
19. Vaterlaus, J.M.; Shaffer, T.; Pulsipher, L. College Student Interpersonal and Institutional Relationships during the COVID-19 Pandemic: A Qualitative Exploratory Study. *Soc. Sci. J.* **2021**, 1–14. [CrossRef]
20. Ge, F.; Zhang, D.; Wu, L.; Mu, H. Predicting Psychological State among Chinese Undergraduate Students in the COVID-19 Epidemic: A Longitudinal Study Using a Machine Learning. *Neuropsychiatr. Dis. Treat.* **2020**, *16*, 2111–2118. [CrossRef]
21. Wright, M.F.; Wachs, S. Moderation of Technology Use in the Association between Self-Isolation during COVID-19 Pandemic and Adolescents' Romantic Relationship Quality. *Cyberpsychol. Behav. Soc. Netw.* **2021**, *24*, 493–498. [CrossRef]
22. Merolla, A.J.; Otmar, C.; Hernandez, C.R. Day-to-Day Relational Life during the COVID-19 Pandemic: Linking Mental Health, Daily Relational Experiences, and End-of-Day Outlook. *J. Soc. Pers. Relat.* **2021**, *38*, 2350–2375. [CrossRef]
23. Luetke, M.; Hensel, D.; Herbenick, D.; Rosenberg, M. Romantic Relationship Conflict Due to the COVID-19 Pandemic and Changes in Intimate and Sexual Behaviors in a Nationally Representative Sample of American Adults. *J. Sex Marital Ther.* **2020**, *46*, 747–762. [CrossRef]
24. Wagner, B.G.; Choi, K.H.; Cohen, P.N. Decline in marriage associated with the COVID-19 pandemic in the United States. *Socius* **2020**, *6*, 2378023120980328. [CrossRef]
25. Schmid, L.; Wörn, J.; Hank, K.; Sawatzki, B.; Walper, S. Changes in Employment and Relationship Satisfaction in Times of the COVID-19 Pandemic: Evidence from the German Family Panel. *Eur. Soc.* **2021**, *23* (Supp. 1), S743–S758. [CrossRef]
26. Williamson, H.C. Early Effects of the COVID-19 Pandemic on Relationship Satisfaction and Attributions. *Psychol. Sci.* **2020**, *31*, 1479–1487. [CrossRef]
27. Mousavi, S.F. Psychological Well-Being, Marital Satisfaction, and Parental Burnout in Iranian Parents: The Effect of Home Quarantine during COVID-19 Outbreaks. *Front. Psychol.* **2020**, *11*, 553880. [CrossRef] [PubMed]
28. Walsh, A.R.; Stephenson, R. Positive and Negative Impacts of the COVID-19 Pandemic on Relationship Satisfaction in Male Couples. *Am. J. Mens. Health* **2021**, *15*, 15579883211022180. [CrossRef] [PubMed]
29. Berumen, L.; Landero Hernández, R.; González Ramírez, M. Marital satisfaction and impact of confinement due to COVID-19 in Mexico. *Interacciones* **2020**, *6*, e173. [CrossRef]
30. Overall, N.C.; Chang, V.T.; Pietromonaco, P.R.; Low, R.S.T.; Henderson, A.M.E. Partners' Attachment Insecurity and Stress Predict Poorer Relationship Functioning during COVID-19 Quarantines. *Soc. Psychol. Personal. Sci.* **2021**, 194855062199297. [CrossRef]
31. Vowels, L.M.; Carnelley, K.B. Attachment Styles, Negotiation of Goal Conflict, and Perceived Partner Support during COVID-19. *Pers. Individ. Dif.* **2021**, *171*, 110505. [CrossRef]
32. Jiang, D.; Chiu, M.M.; Liu, S. Daily Positive Support and Perceived Stress during COVID-19 Outbreak: The Role of Daily Gratitude within Couples. *J. Happiness Stud.* **2021**, 1–15. [CrossRef]
33. Aydogan, D.; Kara, E.; Kalkan, E. Understanding Relational Resilience of Married Adults in Quarantine Days. *Curr. Psychol.* **2021**, 1–11. [CrossRef]
34. Randall, A.K.; Leon, G.; Basili, E.; Martos, T.; Boiger, M.; Baldi, M.; Hocker, L.; Kline, K.; Masturzi, A.; Aryeetey, R.; et al. Coping with Global Uncertainty: Perceptions of COVID-19 Psychological Distress, Relationship Quality, and Dyadic Coping for Romantic Partners across 27 Countries. *J. Soc. Pers. Relat.* **2021**, 026540752110342. [CrossRef]
35. Salin, M.; Kaittila, A.; Hakovirta, M.; Anttila, M. Family Coping Strategies during Finland's COVID-19 Lockdown. *Sustainability* **2020**, *12*, 9133. [CrossRef]
36. Donato, S.; Parise, M.; Pagani, A.F.; Lanz, M.; Regalia, C.; Rosnati, R.; Iafrate, R. Together against COVID-19 Concerns: The Role of the Dyadic Coping Process for Partners' Psychological Well-Being during the Pandemic. *Front. Psychol.* **2020**, *11*, 578395. [CrossRef] [PubMed]
37. Lillie, H.M.; Chernichky-Karcher, S.; Venetis, M.K. Dyadic Coping and Discrete Emotions during COVID-19: Connecting the Communication Theory of Resilience with Relational Uncertainty. *J. Soc. Pers. Relat.* **2021**, *38*, 1844–1868. [CrossRef]
38. Turliuc, M.N.; Candel, O.S. Not All in the Same Boat. Socioeconomic Differences in Marital Stress and Satisfaction during the Covid-19 Pandemic. *Front. Psychol.* **2021**, *12*, 635148. [CrossRef] [PubMed]
39. Knoster, K.; Howard, H.A.; Goodboy, A.K.; Dillow, M.R. Spousal Interference and Relational Turbulence during the COVID-19 Pandemic. *Commun. Res. Rep.* **2020**, *37*, 254–262. [CrossRef]
40. Goodboy, A.K.; Dillow, M.R.; Knoster, K.C.; Howard, H.A. Relational Turbulence from the COVID-19 Pandemic: Within-Subjects Mediation by Romantic Partner Interdependence. *J. Soc. Pers. Relat.* **2021**, *38*, 1800–1818. [CrossRef]
41. Koçak, O.; Koçak, Ö.E.; Younis, M.Z. The Psychological Consequences of COVID-19 Fear and the Moderator Effects of Individuals' Underlying Illness and Witnessing Infected Friends and Family. *Int. J. Environ. Res. Public Health* **2021**, *18*, 1836. [CrossRef] [PubMed]

42. Li, Y.; Samp, J.A. The Impact of the COVID-19 Pandemic on Same-Sex Couples' Conflict Avoidance, Relational Quality, and Mental Health. *J. Soc. Pers. Relat.* **2021**, *38*, 1819–1843. [CrossRef]
43. Alexopoulos, C.; Timmermans, E.; Sharabi, L.L.; Roaché, D.J.; Croft, A.; Hall, E.D.; James-Hawkins, L.; Lamarche, V.; Uhlich, M. Settling down without Settling: Perceived Changes in Partner Preferences in Response to COVID-19. *J. Soc. Pers. Relat.* **2021**, *38*, 1901–1919. [CrossRef]
44. Smallen, D. Experiences of Meaningful Connection in the First Weeks of the COVID-19 Pandemic. *J. Soc. Pers. Relat.* **2021**, 026540752110402. [CrossRef]
45. Goldberg, A.E.; McCormick, N.; Virginia, H. Parenting in a Pandemic: Work–Family Arrangements, Well-being, and Intimate Relationships among Adoptive Parents. *Fam. Relat.* **2021**, *70*, 7–25. [CrossRef]
46. Craig, L.; Churchill, B. Dual-Earner Parent Couples' Work and Care during COVID-19. *Gend. Work Organ.* **2020**, *28*, 66–79. [CrossRef]
47. Goldberg, A.E.; Allen, K.R.; Smith, J.Z. Divorced and Separated Parents during the COVID-19 Pandemic. *Fam. Process* **2021**, *60*, 866–887. [CrossRef]
48. Manley, M.H.; Goldberg, A.E. Consensually Nonmonogamous Parent Relationships during COVID-19. *Sexualities* **2021**. [CrossRef]
49. Ballester-Arnal, R.; Nebot-Garcia, J.E.; Ruiz-Palomino, E.; Giménez-García, C.; Gil-Llario, M.D. "INSIDE" Project on Sexual Health in Spain: The Impact of the Lockdown Caused by COVID-19. *Ses. Res. Social. Policy* **2020**, 1–19. [CrossRef]
50. Karagöz, M.A.; Gül, A.; Borg, C.; Erihan, İ.B.; Uslu, M.; Ezer, M.; Erbağcı, A.; Çatak, B.; Bağcıoğlu, M. Influence of COVID-19 Pandemic on Sexuality: A Cross-Sectional Study among Couples in Turkey. *Int. J. Impot. Res.* **2020**. [CrossRef]
51. Wignall, L.; Portch, E.; McCormack, M.; Owens, R.; Cascalheira, C.J.; Attard-Johnson, J.; Cole, T. Changes in Sexual Desire and Behaviors among UK Young Adults during Social Lockdown Due to COVID-19. *J. Sex Res.* **2021**, *58*, 976–985. [CrossRef]
52. Hensel, D.J.; Rosenberg, M.; Luetke, M.; Fu, T.C.; Herbenick, D. Changes in solo and partnered sexual behaviors during the COVID-19 pandemic: Findings from a US probability survey. *medRxiv* **2020**.
53. Ko, N.-Y.; Lu, W.-H.; Chen, Y.-L.; Li, D.-J.; Chang, Y.-P.; Wu, C.-F.; Wang, P.-W.; Yen, C.-F. Changes in Sex Life among People in Taiwan during the COVID-19 Pandemic: The Roles of Risk Perception, General Anxiety, and Demographic Characteristics. *Int. J. Environ. Res. Public Health* **2020**, *17*, 5822. [CrossRef] [PubMed]
54. Lehmiller, J.J.; Garcia, J.R.; Gesselman, A.N.; Mark, K.P. Less Sex, but More Sexual Diversity: Changes in Sexual Behavior during the COVID-19 Coronavirus Pandemic. *Leis. Sci.* **2021**, *43*, 295–304. [CrossRef]
55. De Oliveira, L.; Carvalho, J. Women's Sexual Health during the Pandemic of COVID-19: Declines in Sexual Function and Sexual Pleasure. *Curr. Sex. Health Rep.* **2021**, *13*, 1–13. [CrossRef]
56. Panzeri, M.; Ferrucci, R.; Cozza, A.; Fontanesi, L. Changes in Sexuality and Quality of Couple Relationship during the COVID-19 Lockdown. *Front. Psychol.* **2020**, *11*, 565823. [CrossRef]
57. Schiavi, M.C.; Spina, V.; Zullo, M.A.; Colagiovanni, V.; Luffarelli, P.; Rago, R.; Palazzetti, P. Love in the Time of COVID-19: Sexual Function and Quality of Life Analysis During the Social Distancing Measures in a Group of Italian Reproductive-Age Women. *J. Sex. Med.* **2020**, *17*, 1407–1413. [CrossRef] [PubMed]
58. Arafat, S.M.Y.; Alradie-Mohamed, A.; Kar, S.K.; Sharma, P.; Kabir, R. Does COVID-19 Pandemic Affect Sexual Behaviour? A Cross-Sectional, Cross-National Online Survey. *Psychiatry Res.* **2020**, *289*, 113050. [CrossRef]
59. Sanchez, T.H.; Zlotorzynska, M.; Rai, M.; Baral, S.D. Characterizing the Impact of COVID-19 on Men Who Have Sex with Men across the United States in April, 2020. *AIDS Behav.* **2020**, *24*, 2024–2032. [CrossRef]
60. Shilo, G.; Mor, Z. COVID-19 and the Changes in the Sexual Behavior of Men Who Have Sex With Men: Results of an Online Survey. *J. Sex. Med.* **2020**, *17*, 1827–1834. [CrossRef]
61. Balzarini, R.N.; Muise, A.; Zoppolat, G.; Gesselman, A.N.; Lehmiller, J.J.; Garcia, J.R.; Slatcher, R.B.; Mark, K. Sexual Desire in the Time of COVID-19: How COVID-Related Stressors Are Associated with Sexual Desire in Romantic Relationships. *PsyArXiv* **2021**. [CrossRef]
62. Rodrigues, D.L.; Lehmiller, J.J. COVID-19 and Sexual Desire: Perceived Fear Is Associated with Enhanced Relationship Functioning. *J. Sex. Res.* **2021**, 1–10. [CrossRef]
63. Micelli, E.; Cito, G.; Cocci, A.; Polloni, G.; Russo, G.I.; Minervini, A.; Carini, M.; Natali, A.; Coccia, M.E. Desire for Parenthood at the Time of COVID-19 Pandemic: An Insight into the Italian Situation. *J. Psychosom. Obstet. Gynaecol.* **2020**, *41*, 183–190. [CrossRef]
64. Stavridou, A.; Samiakou, C.; Kourti, A.; Tsiorou, S.; Panagouli, E.; Thirios, A.; Psaltopoulou, T.; Sergentanis, T.N.; Tsitsika, A. Sexual Activity in Adolescents and Young Adults through COVID-19 Pandemic. *Children* **2021**, *8*, 577. [CrossRef]
65. Agüero, J.M. COVID-19 and the Rise of Intimate Partner Violence. *World Dev.* **2021**, *137*, 105217. [CrossRef]
66. Walsh, A.R.; Sullivan, S.; Stephenson, R. Intimate Partner Violence Experiences during COVID-19 among Male Couples. *J. Interpers. Violence* **2021**, 8862605211005135. [CrossRef]
67. World Health Organisation. *Understanding and Addressing Violence Against Women: Intimate Partner Violence*; World Health Organisation: Geneva, Switzerland, 2012.
68. Jewkes, R. Intimate Partner Violence: Causes and Prevention. *Lancet* **2002**, *359*, 1423–1429. [CrossRef]
69. Arenas-Arroyo, E.; Fernandez-Kranz, D.; Nollenberger, N. Intimate Partner Violence under Forced Cohabitation and Economic Stress: Evidence from the COVID-19 Pandemic. *J. Public Econ.* **2021**, *194*, 104350. [CrossRef]

70. El-Nimr, N.A.; Mamdouh, H.M.; Ramadan, A.; El Saeh, H.M.; Shata, Z.N. Intimate Partner Violence among Arab Women before and during the COVID-19 Lockdown. *J. Egypt. Public Health Assoc.* **2021**, *96*, 15. [CrossRef]
71. Lyons, M.; Brewer, G. Experiences of Intimate Partner Violence during Lockdown and the COVID-19 Pandemic. *J. Fam. Violence* **2021**, 1–9. [CrossRef]
72. Buttell, F.; Ferreira, R.J. The Hidden Disaster of COVID-19: Intimate Partner Violence. *Psychol. Trauma* **2020**, *12*, S197–S198. [CrossRef]
73. Moreira, D.N.; Pinto da Costa, M. The Impact of the Covid-19 Pandemic in the Precipitation of Intimate Partner Violence. *Int. J. Law Psychiatry* **2020**, *71*, 101606. [CrossRef]
74. van Gelder, N.; Peterman, A.; Potts, A.; O'Donnell, M.; Thompson, K.; Shah, N.; Oertelt-Prigione, S.; Gender and COVID-19 Working Group. COVID-19: Reducing the Risk of Infection Might Increase the Risk of Intimate Partner Violence. *EClinicalMedicine* **2020**, *21*, 100348. [CrossRef]
75. Rayhan, I.; Akter, K. Prevalence and associated factors of intimate partner violence (IPV) against women in Bangladesh amid COVID-19 pandemic. *Heliyon* **2021**, *17*, e06619. [CrossRef]
76. Gosangi, B.; Park, H.; Thomas, R.; Gujrathi, R.; Bay, C.P.; Raja, A.S.; Seltzer, S.E.; Balcom, M.C.; McDonald, M.L.; Orgill, D.P.; et al. Exacerbation of Physical Intimate Partner Violence during COVID-19 Pandemic. *Radiology* **2021**, *298*, E38–E45. [CrossRef]
77. Jetelina, K.K.; Knell, G.; Molsberry, R.J. Changes in Intimate Partner Violence during the Early Stages of the COVID-19 Pandemic in the USA. *Inj. Prev.* **2021**, *27*, 93–97. [CrossRef]
78. Abujilban, S.; Mrayan, L.; Hamaideh, S.; Obeisat, S.; Damra, J. Intimate Partner Violence against Pregnant Jordanian Women at the Time of COVID-19 Pandemic's Quarantine. *J. Interpers. Violence* **2021**, 886260520984259. [CrossRef]
79. Muldoon, K.A.; Denize, K.M.; Talarico, R.; Boisvert, C.; Frank, O.; Harvey, A.L.J.; Rennicks White, R.; Fell, D.B.; O'Hare-Gordon, M.A.; Guo, Y.; et al. COVID-19 and Perinatal Intimate Partner Violence: A Cross-Sectional Survey of Pregnant and Postpartum Individuals in the Early Stages of the COVID-19 Pandemic. *BMJ Open* **2021**, *11*, e049295. [CrossRef]
80. Das, T.; Roy, T.B.; Roy, R. Reintegration with Family and Intimate Partner Violence (IPV) against Women among the Returnee Migrant Worker's Family during COVID-19 Induced Lockdown: A Block-Level Analysis Using Multinomial Logistic Regression Model. *Child. Youth Serv. Rev.* **2021**, *130*, 106226. [CrossRef]
81. Machluf, R.; Abba Daleski, M.; Shahar, B.; Kula, O.; Bar-Kalifa, E. Couples Therapists' Attitudes toward Online Therapy during the COVID-19 Crisis. *Fam. Process* **2021**, 12647. [CrossRef]
82. O'Reilly Treter, M.; River, L.M.; Markman, H.J. Supporting Romantic Relationships during COVID-19 Using Virtual Couple Therapy. *Cogn. Behav. Pract.* **2021**, *28*, 597–607. [CrossRef]
83. Stanley, S.M.; Markman, H.J. Helping Couples in the Shadow of COVID-19. *Fam. Process* **2020**, *59*, 937–955. [CrossRef] [PubMed]
84. Hardy, N.R.; Maier, C.A.; Gregson, T.J. Couple Teletherapy in the Era of COVID-19: Experiences and Recommendations. *J. Marital Fam. Ther.* **2021**, *47*, 225–243. [CrossRef] [PubMed]
85. Jack, S.M.; Munro-Kramer, M.L.; Williams, J.R.; Schminkey, D.; Tomlinson, E.; Jennings Mayo-Wilson, L.; Bradbury-Jones, C.; Campbell, J.C. Recognising and Responding to Intimate Partner Violence Using Telehealth: Practical Guidance for Nurses and Midwives. *J. Clin. Nurs.* **2021**, *30*, 588–602. [CrossRef] [PubMed]

encyclopedia

MDPI

Entry

Nanotechnology-Enabled COVID-19 mRNA Vaccines

Yu Gao, Kaiyun Yang, Andrew N. Shelling and Zimei Wu *

Faculty of Medical and Health Sciences, The University of Auckland, Auckland 1142, New Zealand; yu.gao@auckland.ac.nz (Y.G.); kk.yang@auckland.ac.nz (K.Y.); a.shelling@auckland.ac.nz (A.N.S.)
* Correspondence: z.wu@auckland.ac.nz; Tel.: +64-9-923-1709

Definition: COVID-19 mRNA vaccines contain synthetic mRNA sequences encoded for the Spike proteins expressed on the surface of SARS-CoV-2, and utilize the host cells to produce specific antigens that stimulate both humoral and cellular immunities. Lipid nanoparticles are essential to facilitate the intracellular delivery of the mRNA to its action site, the ribosome, to fully exert its effect.

Keywords: mRNA vaccine; lipid nanoparticles; intracellular delivery; endosome escape

1. Introduction

In December 2019, a new contagious disease, later known as the coronavirus disease-2019 (COVID-19) caused by severe acute respiratory syndrome coronavirus 2 (SARS-CoV-2), was first reported [1]. Since then, COVID-19 has rapidly spread across the globe, causing devastating medical, social, and economic consequences. In March 2020, the World Health Organisation (WHO) declared it a pandemic. There was a strong consensus that reliable vaccines are the most promising strategy to control the pandemic. Within a year after the disease outbreak, two messenger ribonucleic acid (mRNA) based vaccines became the first two vaccines to gain Emergency Use Authorisation (EUA) from the U.S. Food and Drug Administration (FDA), bringing hope to billions of people on the planet. Two mRNA vaccines, BNT162b2 (Comirnaty®) and mRNA-1273, developed by Pfizer/BioNTech and Moderna, respectively, set the milestone in scientific history as the first-ever approved mRNA vaccines and opened a new era of mRNA-based approaches to prevent various diseases [2–4]. Never before have vaccines been developed and distributed in such a short period of time. A few more mRNA-based vaccines have reached various clinical stages of development (Table 1).

The lightning-fast success of these mRNA vaccines are not only built on the extensive research in mRNA therapeutic application during the last decades, but also the major technical innovations in nanotechnology for intracellular delivery and advances in nanomedicine production. In this entry, we will first introduce the principles of the mRNA vaccines against COVID-19, followed by a detailed discussion on the roles of nanoparticles, in particular lipid nanoparticles (LNPs), in assisting the transportation of mRNA into the acting site of host cells to exert its effects. The manufacturing and storage requirements of these are also briefly outlined.

Citation: Gao, Y.; Yang, K.; Shelling, A.N.; Wu, Z. Nanotechnology-Enabled COVID-19 mRNA Vaccines. *Encyclopedia* **2021**, *1*, 773–780. https://doi.org/10.3390/encyclopedia1030059

Academic Editor: Stephen Bustin

Received: 16 July 2021
Accepted: 9 August 2021
Published: 10 August 2021

Table 1. Examples of mRNA vaccines against COVID-19 at various stages of development (updated on 4 August 2021).

Vaccine Name	Developer (s)	Formulation [5]	Stage of Development (Timeline)
CVnCoV mRNA	CureVac, Germany	LNP-mRNA	Phase IIb/III NCT 04652102 (December 2020–May 2022)
ARCT-021	Arcturus Therapeutics/Duke-NUS Medical School, USA and Singapore	LUNAR® (pH-sensitive LNP-mediated delivery of saRNA)	Phase II NCT04668339 (January 2021–April 2022) NCT04728347 (January 2021–June 2022)
LNP-nCoVsaRNA-02	Imperial College London, UK	LNP-saRNA(proprietary, cationic, PEGylated)	Phase I NCT04934111 (September 2021–August 2022)
ARCoV	PLAAMS */ Walvax Biotech, China	LNP-mRNA	Phase Ib ChiCTR2000034112 (June 2020–December 2021) ChiCTR2000039212 (October 2020–December 2021)

* PLAAMS: People's Liberation Army Academy of Military Sciences.

2. Mechanism of Action for COVID-19 mRNA Vaccines

Messenger RNA, first discovered by Brenner et al. in 1961 [6], is a single-stranded large molecule that makes a complimentary copy of one of the two DNA strands, and instructs the corresponding protein production in the ribosomes in the cytoplasm. In 1990, scientists at the University of Wisconsin demonstrated that injection of mRNA into mouse skeletal muscle resulted in persistent expression of encoded proteins, providing the first proof of the feasibility of mRNA vaccine [7]. Since then, mRNA vaccines have been researched substantially to tackle infectious disease and different types of cancer, with some reaching clinical trials [7]. The outbreak of the COVID-19 pandemic has undoubtedly sped up the approval of mRNA vaccines in human use [8].

An mRNA vaccine contains a synthetic mRNA sequence that encodes for a disease specific protein (antigen). In a SARS-CoV-2 RNA genome, there are four major viral proteins that are encoded, including the Spike, Envelope, Membrane, and Nucleocapsid proteins [8]. Among them, the Spike (S) protein attracts strong interest in vaccine development, since it is crucial for the virus to gain entry into the host cells [9]. The S protein exists as a precursor and is cleaved into two subunits, S1 and S2. The S1 subunit first binds to the host cell receptor, angiotensin converting enzyme II (ACE2) on the targeted lung cells, then sheds off, resulting in an irreversible conformational change of the S2 subunit. This structural change causes fusion of viral and cellular membranes and viral entry into the host cells, and ultimately initiates infection [9]. Both BNT162b2 and mRNA-1273 contain modified mRNA encoded for the full-length S protein with two proline substitutions (K986P and V987P) to stabilise the protein in the pre-fusion conformation [8].

Both COVID-19 mRNA vaccines are administered via intramuscular injection, where they trigger a transient localized inflammatory response, and recruit different immune cells, primarily monocytes, macrophages, and dendritic cells to the injection site via the extensive network of blood vessels [8,10]. The mRNA molecules are taken up by those recruited immune cells and utilise the ribosomes of host cells to produce S proteins. The locally transfected antigen-presenting-cells (APCs), then migrate to the draining lymph nodes and present S antigen to the B cells and T cells. Once the S antigen is recognised and internalised by B cells, it activates B cells responses and generates a neutralizing antibody. Meanwhile, different T cells are generated via different pathways [11]. After post-translational modification in the host cells, the generated S protein can be degraded in the cytoplasm into fragments, which form a complex with major histocompatibility complex class-1 molecules (MHC class 1). This complex is transported to the cell surface, and eventually enables the induction of antigen-specific CD8+ T cells (cytotoxic T cells). Alternatively, the generated S protein can be released from the host cells, and taken up by other APCs, where they are degraded in the endosomes and the fragments are loaded onto MHC class 2 molecules. The complex is then presented on the cell surface, and leads to production of antigen-specific CD4+ helper T cells, which help B cells in making antigen specific antibodies [11]. Although the B cells promoted antibody production is the primary mechanism against SARS-CoV-2, coordination of CD8+ and CD4+ T cells with the antibody response contribute significantly to enhance the protection [8].

There are two types of mRNA vaccines, non-amplifying (either conventional or base modified) or self-amplifying mRNA vaccines [12]. While non-amplifying mRNA vaccines, such as BNT162b2 and mRNA-1273 [8], only encode for the antigen that induces immune response, self-amplifying mRNA vaccines encodes for additional regions that allow them to self-replicate before protein production. Since the level of antigen expression is directly proportional to the number of mRNA delivered, non-amplifying COVID-19 mRNA vaccines require repeated administration to achieve an adequate immune response.

Compared with the conventional live attenuated, inactivated, or subunit vaccines, mRNA vaccines do not contain any infectious agents, thus are safer to administer even in an immunocompromised population [7]. Compared with DNA vaccines, mRNA vaccines do not integrate into host cell DNA, therefore, they have no potential to cause insertion-induced mutagenesis [13]. Instead, mRNA only transiently exists in the cell, and is degraded by natural cellular processes.

3. Efficacy and Safety of COVID-19 mRNA Vaccines

A total of 43,548 volunteers participated in the multinational, placebo-controlled, observer-blinded trial to study the efficacy and safety of BNT162b2 during 2020 [14]. Two doses of the vaccine (30 μg each) given 21 days apart showed an astonishing 95% efficacy at least seven days after the second dose, with similar efficacy across different age, gender, race, ethnicity, baseline body-mass index, and comorbidity groups. Similarly, a phase 3 randomized, observer-blinded, placebo-controlled trial of 30,420 participants showed that mRNA-1273 given as two doses (100 μg each), 28 days apart resulted in a 94.1% efficacy at least 14 days after the second injection [15].

The reported safety profiles of BNT162b2 and mRNA-1273 were reassuring [14,15]. In general, more participants in the vaccine group reported adverse effects than the placebo group who received saline; however, the incidence of severe adverse effects were similar. The mostly reported local adverse reaction was mild-to-moderate pain at the injection site, which usually resolved within one to two days. The most commonly reported systematic adverse reactions were fatigue and headache [14,15]. Cases of severe allergic reactions (anaphylaxis) were reported during the roll out of both mRNA vaccines [16]. Although very rare, the consequences of anaphylaxis reactions can be fatal and cause considerable fear and hesitation in the general population. Of note, the active ingredient mRNA does not cause any allergic reactions; rather, it is likely the inactive ingredients in the formulation that stimulate an unwanted immune response [16]. BNT162b2 and mRNA-1273 contain polyethylene glycol (PEG) that has been considered to induce anti-PEG antibodies. However, the link between the PEG and anaphylactic reactions to COVID-19 mRNA vaccines is yet to be established with scientific evidence [17]. Nevertheless, currently, the United States Centers for Disease Control and Prevention (CDC) advises all individuals with known severe allergic reaction to any of the components in the mRNA vaccines to avoid having the vaccines; and all other individuals should be monitored for 15 or 30 min after administration depending on the individuals previous allergic reaction to any vaccine or injectable therapy [16].

4. Mechanisms for Nanoparticle-Mediated Intracellular Delivery

4.1. The Need of Innovative Approach for Intracellular Delivery of mRNA

Despite their potential benefits, the initial development of mRNA vaccines did not attract much interest due to their intrinsic instability and the inefficient delivery into the host cells [5]. As mRNA has a large molecular size, an overall negative charge and water-loving nature, it struggles to cross the negatively charged lipid-loving cell membrane by diffusion [5]. In addition, as a self-defence mechanism, external mRNA is regarded as foreign materials by the host and is cleaved by ribonucleases (RNases) into small nucleotide units. The widely distributed RNase degrades the 'naked' mRNA outside the targeted cells and prevents it from entering into the cells. Therefore, only a small amount of mRNA is internalised via the caveolae/lipid raft-rich subdomain on the cell membrane, and subsequently accumulated in the lysosomes [18] where the majority of mRNA gets degraded. It was more recent innovations in nanotechnology for intracellular delivery that address those formidable obstacles [5] (Figure 1).

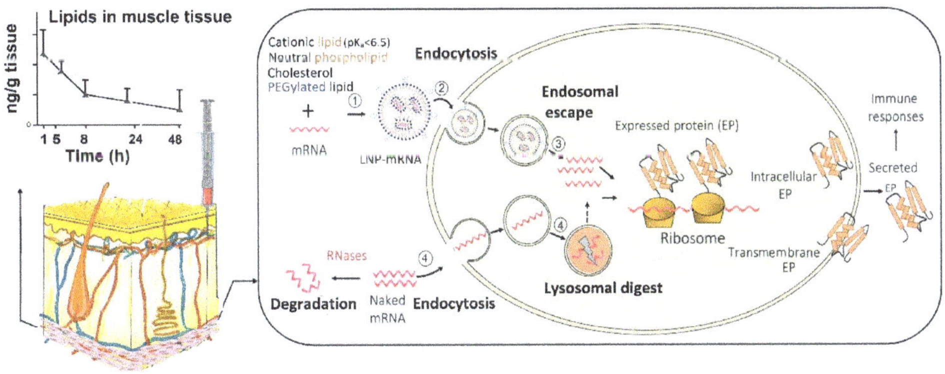

Figure 1. Uptake of mRNA-loaded lipid nanoparticles (LNPs) following intramuscular injection versus naked mRNA into the host cells and the subsequent intracellular trafficking. (1) mRNA is incorporated into LNP, which is assembled from cationic, neutral, and PEGylated lipids as well as cholesterol; (2) mRNA-loaded LNPs are internalised into the host cell; and (3) within the cell, mRNA-loaded LNPs undergo endosome escape, and release mRNA for protein synthesis. In contrast, (4) naked mRNA can be partially internalised, but the majority is degraded in lysosomes. In addition, the extracellular mRNA is cleaved by the ribonucleases (RNases) while LNPs at the injection site protect of mRNA from RNases. LNPs provide extended local tissue exposure and the pharmacokinetic profile depends on various factors such as the lipids used and particle size.

Nanoparticles are nanoscale (1–1000 nm) vesicles that have been explored as non-viral vectors for the intracellular delivery of mRNA while protecting exogenous mRNA from RNase destruction [19]. Compared with viral vectors, non-viral vectors have the advantages of less immunogenicity, easier production, and higher efficiency to carry the mRNA [20]. Versatile nano-platforms have been investigated to deliver mRNA in the body, including LNPs, polymer-based nanoparticles, polymer-lipid hybrid nanoparticles, poly-peptides, protein derivatives mRNA complexes, and gold nanoparticles [16,19]. Among these vectors, LNPs are the most commonly used due to the relative ease of large scaled manufacture, their ability to deliver the encapsulated mRNA to ribosomes (via endosome escape), and flexibility for surface modification with a ligand for specific cell targeting, for example to enhance the uptake into dendritic cells [5,18]. LNPs are versatile drug delivery systems that have been investigated to tackle various disease, including infection and cancer [21]. As LNPs consist of at least one synthetic or natural lipid layer and an aqueous, oil, solid, or amorphous core [22], hydrophilic molecules, such as mRNA, small interference RNA (siRNA) and proteins can be entrapped within the LNP aqueous core, whereas lipophilic compounds can be incorporated into the lipid layers [18]. Thus, LNPs can be co-loaded with an immunopotentiator, also known as adjuvants, to enhance the immune response of the mRNA vaccine. The choice of LNPs for mRNA vaccine delivery has shifted from traditional liposomes, lipoplexes, and cationic nanoemulsions, to more advanced solid nanoparticles and nanostructured lipid carriers [20]. LNPs were employed not only by BNT162b2 and mRNA-1273, but also by other mRNA vaccines in the development of delivery carriers, which are listed in Table 1.

4.2. Formulation Compositions of Covid-19 mRNA Vaccines

The lipids in LNPs to ferry the mRNA are usually made of four typical components (Figure 1): an ionisable cationic lipid, a PEGylated lipid, a neutral phospholipid, and cholesterol. Table 2 lists the lipid components employed in BNT162b2 and mRNA-1273, and each of these different lipids serves distinct functions:

(1) The ionisable cationic lipids show neutral or mild cationic charges at physiological pH, and become protonated (cationic) at low pH, therefore, an acid dissociation constant, or pK_a around 6.5 is ideal. At acidic environment, these lipids are able to encapsulate the negatively charged mRNA through electrostatic interactions during LNPs formation; and in the physiological environment, it becomes neutral, preventing the rapid removal of the LNPs from the circulation, and reduces toxicity. The ionisable lipid was reported to be the primary driver of immunogenicity, pharmacokinetics of the LNPs, and tissue tolerability [23]. Increased biodegradability of the ionisable lipids leads to faster elimination of lipids in muscle, spleen, and liver without necessarily compromising the immune responses as little correlation between the protein expression and immunogenicity. In addition, more biodegradable ionisable lipids are removed from the injection site faster, thus less tissue irritancy [23]. Furthermore, depending on the lipid structure, some positively charged lipid can serve as a vaccine adjuvant and stimulate the innate immune response [20]. The ionisable lipids used in BNT162b2 and mRNA-1273 are (4-hydroxybutyl)azanediyl)bis(hexane-6,1-diyl)bis(2-hexyldecanoate) (ALC-0315), and SM-102, respectively. The N:P molar ratio, defined as nitrogen (N) in the ionizable cationic lipid: phosphate (P) of the nucleotide, is approximately 6 for both vaccines [8,24].

Table 2. Lipid composition of BNT162b2 and mRNA-1273 [3,4,24].

Lipid	BNT162b2	mRNA-1273
Ionisable cationic lipid (A)	ALC-0315	SM-102
PEGylated lipid (B)	2-[(polyethylene glycol)-2000]-N,N-ditetradecylacetamide (ALC-0159)	1,2-dimyristoyl-rac-glycero3-methoxypolyethylene glycol-2000
Neutral lipid (C)	DSPC	DSPC
A:B:C:cholesterol molar ratios	46.3:1.6:9.4:42.7	50:1.5:10:38.5

(2) A PEGylated lipid consists of a hydrophilic polymer PEG conjugated to a lipid. In LNPs, the PEG chains anchored on the surface sterically stabilise the LNPs from aggregation, and prevent non-specific binding with proteins (opsonins) and removal by the reticuloendothelial system in the body [5]. However, the PEG layers could also inhibit the uptake by the targeted cells as well as interaction with the endosomal membrane, therefore, the PEG density on the LNP must be carefully tailored and are generally lower than 2% (mol) and the PEG chain length is limited to 2000.

(3) Neutral lipids are responsible for forming the backbone of the lipid layer and maintain the LNP structure. 1,2-Distearoyl-sn-glycero-3-phosphocholine (DSPC) was used in both of the currently approved COVID-19 mRNA vaccines. It is a saturated lipid with a high melting point, therefore, is able to produce a stable LNPs [20].

(4) Cholesterol in the LNP formulation acts as a stabilising agent of the particles as well as limiting non-specific LNP-protein interactions [20].

4.3. How Does LNPs Assist mRNA Delivery into the Ribosomes Inside Cells

Following intramuscular injection, LNPs provide extended local tissue exposure at the injection site [18]. A typical pharmacokinetic profile is shown in Figure 1. The pharmacokinetics of LNP vaccines depend on their particle size, surface charge, and colloidal stability of LNPs as well as the biodegradability of the ionisable cationic lipid [23]. These factors in turn determine cellular uptake and lymphatic trafficking as well as the exposure to liver and spleen [18]. LNPs smaller than 150 nm could be drained via afferent lymphatic vessels while larger LNPs are readily phagocytosed by immune cells and then trafficked to the lymph nodes. However, complexity associated with identifying the best formulation parameters as lymphatic drainage and transfection potency are not the only parameters determining the immune response.

LNPs have two major roles in mRNA delivery; mediating the uptake of mRNA into the targeted host cell and promoting the release of mRNA from endosome into the cytoplasm, thus improve the bioavailability of mRNA to ribosomes where mRNA produces proteins (antigen) (Figure 1). In addition, LNPs encapsulate the mRNA within the core, thus protecting the mRNA from being degraded by the extracellular RNases [10].

LNPs facilitate the cellular uptake of the mRNA via various endocytosis routes, for example, clathrin- and caveolae-mediated endocytosis [5,22]. The efficiency of the internalization largely depends on the selection of lipids, degree of PEGylation, particle size, and surface charge of the nanoparticles. After endocytosis, LNPs are first entrapped inside the endosomes. The ionisable cationic lipids play a crucial role in promoting the endosomal escape of mRNA. Within the acidic environment of the endosome (pH < ~6.5) the ionisable lipids become protonated. Those positively charged lipids form ion pairs with the negatively charged phospholipids in the endosome membrane, disrupt the bilayer structure and result in endosomal escape [18]. In addition, inclusion of cholesterol in the LNP structure may contribute to the fusion of the LNPs with the endosome, and promotes the release of mRNA into the cytoplasm [20]. However, the current LNPs generally have a low degree of endosome escape (<2%), and the exact mechanisms remain unclear [5]. Therefore, more research is required for further improvement.

5. Manufacturing and Stability

5.1. Manufacturing Process

The manufacturing of COVID-19 mRNA vaccines at large scale consists of three major steps. These steps include the purification of viral DNA, transcription of the DNA into mRNA, and assembly of the mRNA vaccines. Once the mRNA molecules are purified and subjected to rigorous testing, they were incorporated into the LNPs via a modified ethanol injection nanoprecipitation method [5,25]. Briefly, all oily lipid components were mixed with ethanol; and mRNA was mixed with water. The lipids and mRNA solutions were mixed in acidic buffer (pH 4–5) through a set of pumps with a highly controlled flow rate at each phase. Due to the low pH in the mixture, the lipids were positively charged, and easily came into contact with the negative charged mRNA strands via electric attraction. The lipids readily encapsulate mRNAs into the vesicles with high encapsulation efficiencies. The newly formed vaccine mixture were then neutralised to physiological pH value, filtered to remove ethanol and other impurities, and finally sterilised and frozen to be shipped across the globe [25].

5.2. Stability and Storage

As nucleic acids, all mRNA are intrinsically prone to degradation via a number of reactions, for example hydrolysis of N-glycosidic bonds (depurination) or phospho-diester bonds, oxidation of nucleobases or sugar moieties [26]. Even a small change in the structure could alter its translation performance. Both Pfizer/Biotech and Moderna's vaccines have stringent storage requirements (Table 3) and need to be thawed before administration.

Table 3. Stability and storage requirement of BNT162b2 and mRNA-1273 vaccines [3,4].

Vaccines	Un-Opened Vials			Opened Vials
	Frozen	Fridge	Abient Temperature	
BNT162b2	6 months −90–−60 °C	<5 days 2–8 °C	2 h under 30 °C	6 h 2–30 °C
mRNA-1273	6 months −25–−15 °C	<30 days 2–8 °C	≤12 h 8–25 °C	6 h 2–25 °C

6. Conclusions

The COVID-19 pandemic has ravaged the world, leaving scientists with no choice but to accelerate the development of potent and cost-effective vaccines. This milestone achievement with BNT162b2 and mRNA-1273 has opened up an exciting new era for mRNA vaccines to control communicable diseases. This would have not been possible without the break-through innovations in the nanoparticle mediated drug delivery. Nanoparticles, in particular lipid nanoparticles, help guard the mRNA to circumvent the major obstacles in cellular uptake and intracellular trafficking, and to allow the vaccines to fully elicit its immune responses.

Author Contributions: Writing—original draft preparation, Y.G.; supervision, Z.W. and A.N.S.; writing—review and editing, Z.W., A.N.S. and K.Y. All authors have read and agreed to the published version of the manuscript.

Funding: This research received no external funding.

Conflicts of Interest: The authors declare no conflict of interest.

Entry Link on the Encyclopedia Platform: https://encyclopedia.pub/14041.

Abbreviations

ACE2	Angiotensin converting enzyme II
APCs	Antigen presenting cells
CDC	Centers for Disease Control and Prevention
COVID-19	Coronavirus disease-2019
DSPC	1,2-Distearoyl-sn-glycero-3-phosphocholine
EUA	Emergency Use Authorisation
FDA	Food and Drug Administration
LNPs	Lipid nanoparticles
MHC	Major histocompatibility complex
mRNA	Messenger ribonucleic acid
PEG	Poly(ethylene glycol)
RNases	Ribonucleases
SARS-CoV-2	Severe acute respiratory syndrome coronavirus 2
WHO	World Health Organisation

References

1. Zhou, P.; Yang, X.; Wang, X.G.; Hu, B.; Zhang, L.; Zhang, W.; Si, H.R.; Zhu, Y.; Li, B.; Huang, C.L.; et al. A pneumonia outbreak associated with a new coronavirus of probable bat origin. *Nature* **2020**, *579*, 270–273. [CrossRef] [PubMed]
2. Lamb, Y.N. BNT162b2 mRNA COVID-19 vaccine: First approval. *Drugs* **2021**, *81*, 495–501. [CrossRef] [PubMed]
3. Food and Drug Administration. FDA Briefing Document: Moderna COVID-19 Vaccine. Available online: https://www.fda.gov/media/144434/download (accessed on 3 May 2021).
4. European Medicines Agency. Comirnaty: EPAR-Product Information. Available online: https://www.ema.europa.eu/en/documents/product-information/comirnaty-epar-product-information_en.pdf (accessed on 3 May 2021).
5. Wu, Z.; Li, T. Nanoparticle-mediated cytoplasmic delivery of messenger RNA vaccines: Challenges and future perspectives. *Pharm. Res.* **2021**, *38*, 473–478. [CrossRef]

6. Brenner, S.; Jacob, F.; Meselson, M. An unstable intermediate carrying information from genes to ribosomes for protein synthesis. *Nature* **1961**, *190*, 576–581. [CrossRef] [PubMed]
7. Pardi, N.; Hogan, M.J.; Porter, F.W.; Weissman, D. mRNA vaccines-a new era in vaccinology. *Nat. Rev. Drug Discov.* **2018**, *17*, 261–279. [CrossRef]
8. Verbeke, R.; Lentacker, I.; De Smedt, S.C.; Dewitte, H. The dawn of mRNA vaccines: The COVID-19 case. *J. Control. Release* **2021**, *333*, 511–520. [CrossRef]
9. Cai, Y.; Zhang, J.; Xiao, T.; Peng, H.; Sterling, S..; Walsh, R., Jr.; Rawson, S.; Rits-Volloch, S.; Chen, B. Distinct conformational states of SARS-CoV-2 spike protein. *Science* **2020**, *369*, 1586–1592. [CrossRef]
10. Zeng, C.; Zhang, C.; Walker, P.G.; Dong, Y. Formulation and delivery technologies for mRNA vaccines. In *Current Topics in Microbiology and Immunology*; Springer: Berlin/Heidelberg, Germany, 2020; pp. 1–40.
11. Wadhwa, A.; Aljabbari, A.; Lokras, A.; Foged, C.; Thakur, A. Opportunities and challenges in the delivery of mRNA-based vaccines. *Pharmaceutics* **2020**, *12*, 102. [CrossRef]
12. Blakney, A.K.; Ip, S.; Geall, A.J. An update on self-amplifying mRNA vaccine development. *Vaccines* **2021**, *9*, 97. [CrossRef]
13. Kutzler, M.A.; Weiner, D.B. DNA vaccines: Ready for prime time? *Nat. Rev. Genet.* **2008**, *9*, 776–788. [CrossRef]
14. Polack, F.; Thomas, S.; Kitchin, N.; Absalon, J.; Gurtman, A.; Lockhart, S. Safety and efficacy of the BNT162b2 mRNA COVID-19 vaccine. *N. Engl. J. Med.* **2020**, *383*, 2603–2615. [CrossRef]
15. Baden, L.R.; El Sahly, H.M.; Essink, B.; Kotloff, K.; Frey, S.; Novak, R.; Diemert, D.; Spector, S.A.; Rouphael, N.; Creech, C.B.; et al. Efficacy and safety of the mRNA-1273 SARS-CoV-2 vaccine. *N. Engl. J. Med.* **2021**, *384*, 403–416. [CrossRef] [PubMed]
16. Banerji, A.; Wickner, P.G.; Saff, R.; Stone, C.A.; Robinson, L.B.; Long, A.A.; Wolfson, A.R.; Williams, P.; Khan, D.A.; Phillips, E.; et al. mRNA vaccines to prevent COVID-19 disease and reported allergic reactions: Current evidence and suggested approach. *J. Allergy Clin. Immunol. Pract.* **2021**, *9*, 1423–1437. [CrossRef]
17. Greenhawt, M.; Abrams, E.M.; Oppenheimer, J.; Leek, T.K.V.; Mack, D.P.; Singer, A.G.; Shaker, M. The COVID-19 pandemic in 2021: Avoiding overdiagnosis of anaphylaxis risk while safely vaccinating the world. *J. Allergy Clin. Immunol. Pract.* **2021**, *9*, 1438. [CrossRef] [PubMed]
18. Reichumuth, A.M.; Oberli, M.; Jaklenec, A.; Langer, R.B.D. mRNA vaccine delivery using lipid nanoparticles. *Ther. Deliv.* **2016**, *7*, 319–334. [CrossRef] [PubMed]
19. Lorenz, C.; Fotin-Mleczek, M.; Roth, G.; Becker, C.; Dam, T.C.; Verdurmen, W.P.R.; Brock, R.; Probst, J.; Schlake, T. Protein expression from exogenous mRNA: Uptake by receptor-mediated endocytosis and trafficking via the lysosomal pathway. *RNA Biol.* **2011**, *8*. [CrossRef]
20. Aldosari, B.N.; Alfagih, I.M.; Almurshedi, A.S.; Hinrichs, J. Lipid nanoparticles as delivery systems for RNA-based vaccines. *Pharmaceutics* **2021**, *13*, 206. [CrossRef]
21. Mitchell, M.J.; Billingsley, M.M.; Haley, R.M.; Wechsler, M.E.; Peppas, N.A.; Langer, R. Engineering precision nanoparticles for drug delivery. *Nat. Rev. Drug Discov.* **2021**, *20*, 101–124. [CrossRef]
22. Li, B.; Zhang, X.; Dong, Y. Nanoscale platforms for messenger RNA delivery. *Wiley Interdiscip. Rev. Nanomed. Nanobiotechnol.* **2018**, *11*, 1530. [CrossRef]
23. Hassett, K.J.; Benenato, K.E.; Jacquinet, E.; Lee, A.; Woods, A.; Yuzhakov, O.; Himansu, S.; Deterling, J.; Geilich, B.M.; Ketova, T.; et al. Optimization of lipid nanoparticles for intramuscular administration of mRNA vaccines. *Mol. Ther. Nucleic Acids* **2019**, *15*, 1–11. [CrossRef]
24. Schoenmaker, L.; Witzigmann, D.; Kulkarni, J.A.; Verbeke, R.; Kersten, G.; Jiskoot, W.; Crommelin, D.J.A. mRNA-lipid nanoparticle COVID-19 vaccines: Structure and stability. *Int. J. Pharm.* **2021**, *601*, 120586. [CrossRef] [PubMed]
25. Corbett, K.S.; Edwards, D.K.; Leist, S.R.; Abiona, O.M.; Boyoglu-Barnum, S.; Gillespie, R.A.; Himansu, S.; Schäfer, A.; Ziwawo, C.T.; DiPiazza, A.T.; et al. SARS-CoV-2 mRNA vaccine design enabled by prototype pathogen preparedness. *Nature* **2020**, *586*, 567–571. [CrossRef] [PubMed]
26. Crommelin, D.J.A.; Anchordoquy, T.J.; Volkin, D.B.; Jiskoot, W.; Mastrobattista, E. Addressing the cold reality of mRNA vaccine stability. *J. Pharm. Sci.* **2021**, *110*, 997–1001. [CrossRef] [PubMed]

encyclopedia

MDPI

Entry

COVID-19: Evidenced Health Disparity

Ayodeji Iyanda [1,*], Kwadwo Boakye [2] and Yongmei Lu [1]

1 Department of Geography, Texas State University, San Marcos, TX 78666, USA; yl10@txstate.edu
2 School of Biological and Population Health Sciences, Oregon State University, Corvallis, OR 97331, USA; boakyek@oregonstate.edu
* Correspondence: aei11@txstate.edu

Definition: Health disparity is an unacceptable, unjust, or inequitable difference in health outcomes among different groups of people that affects access to optimal health care, as well as deterring it. Health disparity adversely affects disadvantaged subpopulations due to a higher incidence and prevalence of a particular disease or ill health. Existing health disparity determines whether a disease outbreak such as coronavirus disease 2019, caused by the severe acute respiratory syndrome coronavirus 2 (SARS-CoV-2), will significantly impact a group or a region. Hence, health disparity assessment has become one of the focuses of many agencies, public health practitioners, and other social scientists. Successful elimination of health disparity at all levels requires pragmatic approaches through an intersectionality framework and robust data science.

Keywords: health disparity; intersectionality; data science; machine learning; public health; GIS

Citation: Iyanda, A.; Boakye, K.; Lu, Y. COVID-19: Evidenced Health Disparity. *Encyclopedia* **2021**, *1*, 744–763. https://doi.org/10.3390/encyclopedia1030057

Academic Editor: Stephen Bustin

Received: 11 June 2021
Accepted: 2 August 2021
Published: 5 August 2021

1. Introduction

The coronavirus disease 2019 (COVID-19) outbreak caused by severe acute respiratory syndrome coronavirus 2 (SARS-CoV-2) was declared a pandemic by the World Health Organization on 11 March 2020 due to its growing prevalence, particularly its increase in morbidity and mortality over a wide geographic area [1], and has since generated considerable attention. The infection rate varies across geographic areas, indicating spatial and regional disparities. Evidence of regional and within-country variations in coronavirus infection and mortality has been well documented [1–5]. Shortly after the first outbreak in Wuhan, China, several other American and European countries exhibited clusters of COVID-19 infections. Not long after, the United States became a significant hotspot of COVID-19 morbidity and mortality. Figure 1 highlights the 7-day average cumulative cases of COVID-19 in five countries: the United States, Canada, Germany, the Netherlands, and Nigeria. Recently, when the distribution of COVID-19 vaccination became more accessible in most communities in the United States, the daily hospitalization cases due to infection and related death decreased significantly [6–9]. However, overwhelming evidence indicates differences in infection and associated death rates across different populations [2,3].

The recent COVID-19 pandemic revealed many things ranging from the possibilities of remote learning/working, virtual recruitment, and service delivery such as telemedicine. The pandemic has further shown additional evidence of health disparity in our society, particularly in health outcomes and access to health care systems. As a background for this paper, Figure 2 shows the intersection between structural inequality as the root cause of health disparity, public health, and data science. We believe that the adoption of intersectionality and data science approaches would help foster data-driven interventions in addressing health disparities.

Health disparity is an important theme that has generated much interest from different domains as well as a significant public health debate that must not be overlooked in any society and in chronicling the health outcomes of COVID-19, particularly in the United States. This entry paper examines the concept of health disparity within the intersection of public policy, public health, and data science (Figure 2). Furthermore, this contribution explores the definition of health disparity and determinants of health regarding COVID-19 from different countries, with specific emphasis on high-income countries with diverse populations such as the United States and the United Kingdom. For example, the United States has the most extensive published papers on health disparity, mainly from racial and ethnic, social class, gender, and sexual orientation angles, and serves as a reference point for research on racial and health disparity.

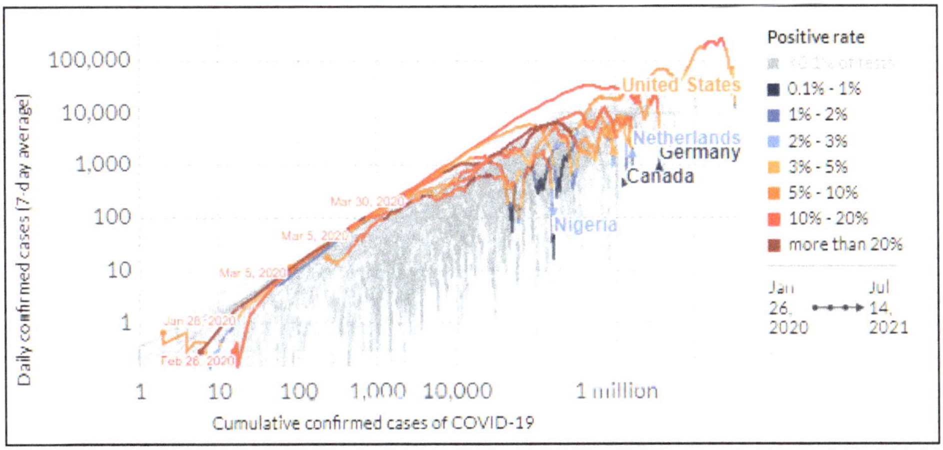

Figure 1. Cumulative confirmed global cases of COVID-19 (data source: www.Ourworldindata.org accessed 13 July 2021, Ritchie et al. [10]).

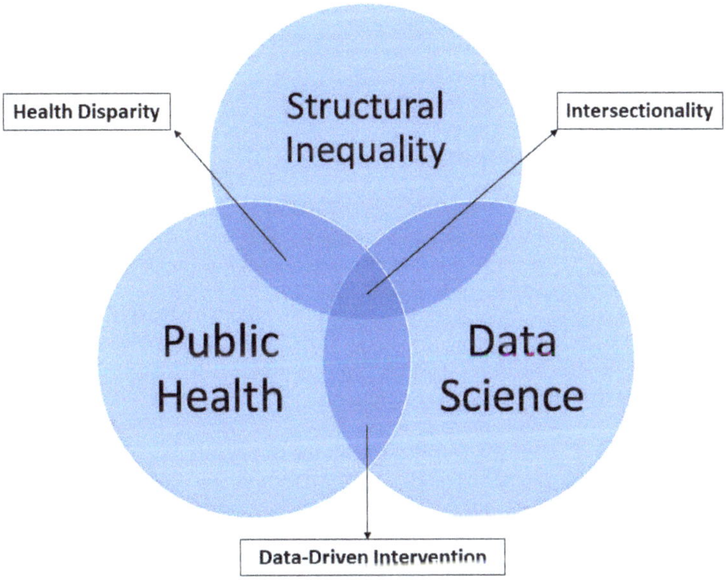

Figure 2. The intersection between structural inequality, public health, and data science.

In addition, this paper provides a general overview of the implication(s) of health disparities for achieving viable public health policies. Considering different approaches to measuring health disparity, this study presents how the field of public health and other allied (health) disciplines could leverage the power of data science such as geographic information science/systems (GIS), machine learning, and artificial intelligence to help solve some of the societal issues including the current COVID-19 pandemic. In addition, this paper contributes to the field of spatial epidemiology and public health by showing how data science and intersectionality frameworks can be fused to improve general/public health. Finally, this paper concludes with some expert-based recommendations toward reducing health disparity.

2. Defining Health Disparity

Health disparity is a ubiquitous phrase in most health writeups found on the pages of printed and digital media, journals, and reports from governmental and non-governmental organizations, as well as in discussions among health professionals, policymakers, and the general public. However, the conceptualization and determination of health disparity vary by geographic location. Table 1 presents the various but similar definitions of health disparity and health inequality as used within and outside the United States. For instance, in the United States, health disparity determines whether health, broadly used, differs by comparing different health outcomes among various population groups and subpopulations of interest. In contrast, the terms "health inequality" and "health inequity" are frequently used outside the United States. For example, the World Health Organization consistently uses the term "inequity," which connotes the differences in health that are unnecessary and avoidable but unfair and unjust [11].

Generally, health disparity refers to a higher burden of illness, injury, disability, or mortality experienced by one group relative to another. Determining which health situations could be considered unfair or unjust depends on the place and time of examination. However, the widely used measure hinges on the degree of choice involved. Essentially, any strive toward attaining equity and health is "not to eliminate all health differences so that everyone has the same level and quality of health, but to reduce or eliminate those which result from factors considered to be both avoidable and unfair" [12]. This prompts the question, what is avoidable and/or unavoidable health inequality? However, the answer to this question is beyond the scope of this article (for additional readings, see: Braveman [11,13]; also Whitehead [12]).

The National Institute of Minority Health Disparities' (NIMHD) definition [14] of health disparity highlights health differences among different populations, emphasizing disadvantaged populations. According to the legislation that birthed the NIMHD, what defines health disparity includes several factors characterized by poorer health outcomes, indicated by the overall disease incidence, prevalence, morbidity, mortality, or survival in the population compared with the general population. The NIMHD recognizes health disparity populations as racial/ethnic minorities, socioeconomically disadvantaged populations, underserved rural populations, and sexual and gender minorities.

Similarly, the United Kingdom's National Health Service describes adversely affected populations within the "Inclusion Health" framework. Inclusion health refers to "a number of groups of people who are not usually well provided for by health care services and have poorer access, experiences and health outcomes. The definition covers people who are homeless and rough sleepers, vulnerable migrants (e.g., refugees and asylum seekers), sex workers, and those from the Gypsy, Roma and Traveller communities" [15]. Nevertheless, inclusion health or each of the compositions of people affected by health disparity could be examined in more detail based on how they have been impacted by COVID-19 if and when detailed health data are available. The related findings could help inform better intervention policies to reduce health disparity among different population groups.

Table 1. Different definitions of health disparity and health inequality.

Organization, Country	Definition
National Institute of Minority Health Disparities [14]	A health difference, determined on the basis of one or more health outcomes that adversely affect disadvantaged populations.
Healthy People 2020 [16]	A particular type of health difference closely linked with social, economic, and environmental disadvantages.
Centers for Disease Control and Prevention [17]	Preventable differences in the burden of disease, injury, violence, or opportunities to achieve optimal health experienced by socially disadvantaged racial, ethnic, and other population groups and communities.
Institute of Medicine [18]	A health service disparity between population groups is determined as differences in treatment or access not justified by differences in the health status or preferences of the groups.
National Health Service [15]	Unfair and avoidable differences in health across the population and between different groups within society.

Compared to the NIMHD's definition of health disparity that centers on disadvantaged populations, Healthy People 2020's definition is more expansive. Healthy People 2020's definition of health disparities underscores social, economic, and environmental resources differentiation. Hence, health disparities adversely affect groups of people who have systematically experienced greater obstacles to health based on their racial or ethnic group, religion, socioeconomic status, gender, age, mental health, cognitive, sensory, or physical disability, sexual orientation or gender identity, geographic location, or other characteristics historically linked to discrimination or exclusion [19]. Similarly, England's National Health Service defines health inequality as unfair and avoidable differences in health across the population and between different groups within society (Table 1). Carter-Porkras and Baquet [20] presented other definitions of health disparity within the United States context. For example, the Taskforce on Black and Minority Health, Department of Health and Human Services, in 1985, used excess deaths (excess death is referred to as the difference between the number of deaths observed in minority populations and the number of deaths which would have been expected if the minority population had the same age- and sex-specific death rate as the non-minority population) of six key health indicators. These health indicators are cancer, cardiovascular disease and stroke, cirrhosis, diabetes, homicide and unintentional injuries, and infant mortality.

The Institute of Medicine differentiates health disparity between minority and non-minority groups based on clinical appropriateness, needs, and patient preferences; discrimination at the individual patient–provider level that results from biases, prejudices, stereotyping, and uncertainty in clinical communication and decision making; and, lastly, the operation of health care system functions. The American Medical Association (AMA) also recognizes health disparities in health care systems.

In 2000, the United States Department of Health and Human Services launched Healthy People 2010, which had two goals: (1) to improve the overall health status of Americans and (2) to eliminate racial and ethnic health care disparities. The AMA was deemed fit to promote this agenda. In 2004, the association established the Commission to End Health Care Disparities, while the National Medical Association was established to address gaps in health care. As part of this agenda to eliminate racial and ethnic health care disparity, the AMA strives to promote diversity by increasing the share of physicians through its policies and advocacy work and therefore proposed immigration reform as a means to eliminate health care disparities, prioritized access to care for patients with disabilities, and proposed its intent to tackle unequal treatment [21]. Hence, closing health disparities requires an intersectional approach and bold and unapologetic political willingness.

3. Intersectionality Framework and Health Disparity

Although several studies [22–25] have underscored the importance of intersectionality in adverse health outcomes, such as the current COVID-19 pandemic, its application is scarce. The adoption of intersectionality in health analysis, intervention, and policy could reduce health disparity. According to Kimberly Crenshaw [26], "intersectionality is a lens through which one can see where power comes and collides, where it locks and intersect." Intersectionality is accepting that different people have unique experiences of discrimination and privilege at different stages in their lifetime. Scholars have employed an intersectionality framework to examine the experiences of individuals belonging to different marginalized groups. Some of the indicators that should be considered in order to achieve intersectionality include race, ethnicity, gender identity, class, languages, skin color, neurodiversity, religions, (dis)ability, sexuality, mental health, age, ecological systems (neighborhood, school, office, rural–urban, local, and federal policies), education, citizenship and immigration status, housing, and body size (this list could go on). The intersectionality framework could be helpful in transformative health disparity research, especially in understanding disparity in COVID-19 health outcomes.

Furthermore, the intersectionality framework posits that inequality is experienced through multiple contexts, and it should not be examined from a single standpoint. For example, the intersectionality framework could help us understand why Black women are more likely to die through childbirth than White women (maternal mortality disparity) or why there is a high rate of incarceration or racially profiled crimes among Black men or Black adolescents/youth. Within the current COVID-19 pandemic context, we could continue to ask questions about whether more older Black, Hispanic, and Asian women were infected or died of COVID-19 and why? These are the questions intersectionality will help shed some light on if applied.

Using the intersectionality approach, Sekalala et al. [24] analyzed the intersection between age and sex to determine vaccination prioritization based on human rights needs. In addition, Eaves and Falconer Al-Hindi [23], in a short article published in Dialogues in Human Geography, claimed that "geographical research that is designed, conducted, and analyzed within an intersectional framework generates better geographical scholarship". Hence, researchers should consider how the concept of intersectionality could reveal more disparity by intersecting some of these indicators. Unfortunately, as seen in Table 2, this concept has received limited attention in the study of COVID-19.

3.1. COVID-19 Disparity

Regarding disparity in COVID-19 outcomes, it is evident that the disease has exacerbated health inequality. The health impacts of COVID-19 are unevenly distributed, particularly for underrepresented racial and ethnic minorities and migrants [27–29]. Figure 3 shows the pattern and distribution of COVID-19 deaths based on the 2017 population density per square kilometer for some selected countries. It is worth emphasizing that the pandemic did not cause health disparity in that some minority ethnic groups died at a significantly higher proportion; it only shed more light on the longstanding health disparity in various countries [30–33]. Existing data on infections, hospitalizations, and deaths reveal significant variation among and within regions and communities [27,28,34–36], prompting questions about health inequality and disparity; they have also stirred curiosity to know which populations are at higher risk and why the risk is higher for one group than others [27]. The within-country health determinants may explain this variation among the countries of the world. This type of question is what proponents of social, health and environmental justice have been pursuing before the outbreak of the COVID-19 pandemic.

Table 2. Common variable of interest, intersectionality framework, and data analytical techniques in COVID-19 research.

Study	Location	Health Outcomes	Intersectionality Framework	Common Variables of Interest								Data Analytical Techniques		
			Violence	Health Care	Public Policies	Mobility	Racial/ Ethnic Heterogeneity	Sociodemographic	Environmental Injustice	Health Disparity	Geographic/ Temporal Disparity	GIS/Spatial Statistics	AI, Machine, and Deep Learning	Aspatial
Chaudhuri et al., 2021	UK	Age-adjusted COVID-19 morality					x	x		x	x	SAR		OLS
Iyanda et al., 2020	Global	COVID-19 outbreak		x	x			x		x	x	MGWR		OLS
Iyanda et al., 2021	USA	COVID-19 case fatal ratio					x	x		x	x	GWR		Poisson
Louis-Jean et al., 2020	USA	COVID-19					x	x						
Allen Et al., 2020	USA	COVID-19 confirmed cases, deaths					x	x	x	x	x	Thematic mapping		OLS
Abedi et al., 2020	USA	COVID-19 infection rate				x	x	x		x	x	Map overlay		OLS, Pearson correlation, Forest Plot
Chen et al., 2020	China	COVID-19 Mortality rate							x			Remote sensing		Difference-in-Difference
Adams, 2020	Canada	COVID-19			x	x			x		x			Polynomial regression
Lippi et al., 2020	Italy	COVID-19 infection							x		x			Pearson's correlation
Berman & Ebisu, 2020	USA	COVID-19 infection			x				x		x			*t*-test
Travaglio et al., 2021	UK/England	COVID-19 mortality							x	x	x	Heatmap		GLM, BLR
Arimiyaw et al., 2020	SSA region	COVID-19			X				x					
Fattorini & Regoli, 2020	Italy	COVID-19							x	x	x	Thematic mapping		Pearson's correlation
Bashir et al., 2020	Germany	COVID-19 confirmed cases, deaths, recoveries							x	x				wavelet transform coherence; correlation
Bashir et al., 2020	California, USA	COVID-19 confirmed cases, deaths							x	x	x	Thematic mapping		Spearman's/ Kendall correlation
Chakraborty, 2021	USA	COVID-19 incidence rate					x	x	x	x	x	LISA		OLS, GEE
Terrel & James, 2020	Louisiana, USA	COVID-19 deaths					x	x	x	x	x			Spearman correlation; Shapiro-Wilks's test
Martinez Dy & Jayawarna, 2020	UK	COVID-19 impacts					x	x						
Krzysztofowicz & Osińska-Skotak, 2021	Poland	COVID-19 vaccination										Thiessen Polygon		

Table 2. *Cont.*

Study	Location	Health Outcomes	Intersectionality Framework	Common Variables of Interest									Data Analytical Techniques		
				Violence	Health Care	Public Policies	Mobility	Racial/ Ethnic Heterogeneity	Sociodemographic	Environmental Injustice	Health Disparity	Geographic/ Temporal Disparity	GIS/Spatial Statistics	AI, Machine, and Deep Learning	Aspatial
Bachtiger et al., 2020	Generalized	COVID-19			x									x	
Punn et al., 2020	Global	COVID-19 confirmed cases, death, recovery												x	
Cavaljal et al., 2018	Philippines	Dengue												x	
Alimadadi et al., 2020	Generalized	COVID-19												x	
Kushwaha et al., 2020		COVID-19										x		x	
Pinter et al., 2020	Hungary	COVID-19												x	
Li et al., 2021	Multi-country							x	x			x		x	
Kuo & Fu, 2021	USA	COVID-19 infection												x	
Mollalo et al., 2018	Iran	Sandfly; Cutaneous leishmaniasis											x	x	Pearson's correlation
Mele & Magazzino, 2020	India	COVID-19												x	
Biana, 2020	Philippines	COVID-19		x		x			x		x	x			
Sonu et al., 2021	USA	COVID-19	x	x							x				
Wilson et al., 2020	USA	COVID-19		x				x		x	x				
Reicher & Stott, 2020	UK, USA, France	COVID-19		x							x				
Corpuz 2021	Philippines	COVID-19		x		x					x				
Njoku et al., 2021	USA	COVID-19		x		x		x			x				
Joseph-Salisbury et al., 2021	UK	COVID-19		x		x		x							
Gibson et al., 2021	USA	COVID-19		x		x		x							
Coyne & Yatsyshina, 2020	Generalized	COVID-19		x		x									
Bailey et al., 2020	Generalized	COVID-19		x		x		x			x				
Elias et al., 2021	Generalized														

OLS ordinary least squares; GEE general estimating equation; BLR binomial linear regression; LISA local indication of spatial autocorrelation/association; SAR spatial autoregressive; GWR geographically weighted regression; MGWR multiscale GWR; GIS geographic information systems; AI artificial intelligence.

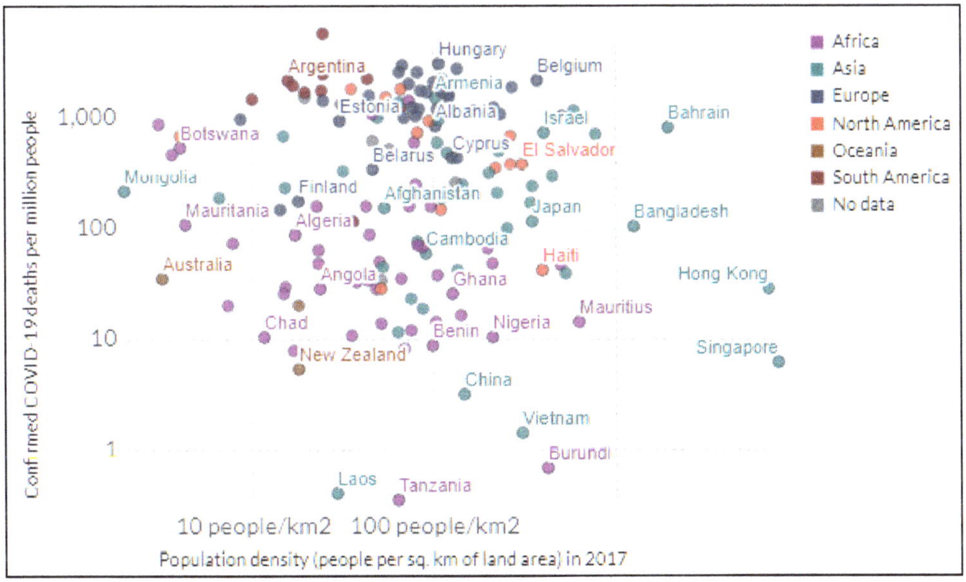

Figure 3. COVID-19 deaths versus population density based on data from 22 January to 14 July; time 20:03 London time. (data source: www.ourworldindata.org/Coronavirus-death accessed 13 July 2021; Ritchie et al., [10]). Note: countries with a < 1 million population are excluded from the visualization.

3.2. *COVID-19 and Environmental Injustice*

The advent of COVID-19 adds "icing on top of the cake" of environmental justice research that has been in progress for several decades, particularly in the United States. For example, in a roundtable discussion [37], Robert Billard referred to the COVID-19 pandemic as "a heat-seeking missile that is targeting the most vulnerable populations, and the bull's-eye is actually the environmental justice communities, the communities that are the poorest, that are the most polluted, that are the sickest when it comes to comorbidity, and the result of this heat-seeking missile called COVID-19 is a death bomb." In addition, many studies situate research on COVID-19 health disparity within the broader framework of environmental injustice [38–48]. These studies examine environmental variables such as air pollution in different geographic locations from countries in North America through Africa to Europe (e.g., Germany, Italy, and Britain).

Several studies allude to the reduction in air pollutants (e.g., $PM_{2.5}$, NO_2, O_3) from the reduced human mobility due to lockdowns [38,40,49], and several others indicate a correlation between the COVID-19 burden and environmental pollution [50,51], particularly in economically disadvantaged communities and areas with a high concentration of people of color [35,47,52–56]. For example, Chakraborty [54], using the local indicator of spatial association, showed convergence between the COVID-19 incidence rate and the respiratory risk from hazardous air pollutants across counties in the United States. Additionally, his study indicated that being Black and living in socioeconomically deprived neighborhoods increased the COVID-19 incidence, supporting a similar study from the United Kingdom [34].

Mackey et al.'s [28] systematic review of 37 cohort and cross-sectional studies and 15 ecological studies, for example, showed that African American/Black and Hispanic populations experience disproportionately higher rates of COVID-19 infection, hospitalization, and coronavirus disease-related mortality compared with non-Hispanic White populations, but not higher case fatality rates. In addition, the Atlantic, a COVID-19 dashboard that tracks infection and deaths by race/ethnicity across the United States, shows evidence of health disparity [57]. For example, Alabama, where 27% of the population is Black or African American, had a higher infection rate (29%) and the number of deaths (31%) for its Black people compared to its White population.

Chaudhuri et al.'s [34] work on the interaction of ethnicity and socioeconomic deprivation on COVID-19 mortality in the United Kingdom showed that Black, Asian, and Minority Ethnic (BAME) populations are at higher risk of developing COVID-19 and likely to experience severe health-related outcomes compared to White British populations. Relying on disaggregated ethnicity data, the England study [34] reported that the age-adjusted COVID-19 mortality rate was higher in minority neighborhoods in the highest deprivation quartile, with a high concentration of Black-African (regression coefficient, β 2.86; 95% CI 1.08–4.64), Black-Caribbean (β 9.66: 95% CI 5.25–14.06), and Bangladeshi (β 1.95: 95% CI 1.14–2.76) populations.

Using a combination of statistical and geographic information system techniques, Iyanda and colleagues [1] used 356 days of COVID-19 cases and deaths data to examine disease fatality in the United States (Table 2). They showed that African American/Black and Hispanic populations experienced disproportionately higher case fatality rates in the rural counties with a higher share of minority populations. Their findings corroborate earlier data by the Centers for Disease Control and Prevention that show that Black and Hispanic communities are three and two times more likely to be infected and die from COVID-19, and other sources have shown similar racial/ethnic disparities [35,36,53,54,57,58]. These results reinforce how structural racism may have shaped the distribution of social determinants of health and promotes social risk factors. More interestingly, action within the health care system has been hampered by a lack of understanding of how to abate the impact of institutional and structural racism on influencing minority health [59].

3.3. COVID-19 and Incidence of Violence

Table 2 presents ten studies examining different forms of violence (e.g., police brutality, riots, shooting), mostly during COVID-19. In addition to the institutional violence, environmental injustice, and segregationist and discriminatory laws that faced, majorly, the minorities and immigrants in most countries is the COVID-19 pandemic which stretches structural racism in many countries [30,37,60–65]. It has become common knowledge that "pandemics always follow the fault line of society" [33]—structural or institutional racism. Research indicates that racism and xenophobia increased during the coronavirus outbreak due to the increasing nationalism and populism [30]. For example, Gibson et al. [66] chronicled institutional responses to protests and outbreaks of violence due to the deaths of several African Americans, including Ahmaud Arbery, Breonna Taylor, and George Floyd, amidst the global COVID-19 pandemic in 2020. Similar to the experience of the violence of the #BlackLivesMatter movement in the United States, there were violence outbreaks in the United Kingdom due to longtime racism. Within the Philippine context, Corpuz [62] called to end the police brutality of Filipinos, which was exacerbated during the coronavirus outbreak. Biana [67] argued that the outcome in health disparity could be related to a matter of class. For example, being Black in the United States is considered a risk factor for disease vulnerability, while being poor in the Philippines means "to be neglected and be reduced to nothing." This assertion might as well explain the excess infections and deaths from COVID-19 in different geographies.

4. Determinants of Health Disparities

According to Healthy People 2020, several powerful and complex relationships exist between biology or genetic compositions, individual behavior, socioeconomic status, the physical environment, discrimination, racism, literacy levels [16], and non-pharmaceutical policies that influence the susceptibility, exposure, transmission, infection, recovery, and fatality rate of COVID-19 and the probability of receiving timely as well as adequate health care.

Common health determinant factors in developed and developing countries include the availability of or lack of access to high-quality education, nutritious food, decent and safe housing, affordable and dependable public transportation, culturally and socially sensitive health care providers, health insurance, and clean water and air. Several studies have examined how the COVID-19 pandemic affects some of these factors, including air quality, business, nutrition, and health care services [68–71]. In addition, available data indicate that a more significant proportion of racial and ethnic minorities depend on government assistance programs such as SNAP. Moreover, most of them have no health insurance, a critical barrier to access adequate health care, particularly during a pandemic. Research such as the work of Chakraborty [54] in the United States and Iyanda et al. [1] global ecological study highlight the importance of health insurance during the COVID-19 pandemic. Thus, it is not surprising that COVID-19 only shows the evidenced health disparity that has existed for decades in most countries.

4.1. Social and Structural Determinants of Health

Social determinants of health are the non-medical factors that influence health outcomes, and they are generally the conditions in which people are born, grow, work, live, and age, and the broader set of forces and systems shaping the conditions of daily life [72]. COVID-19 has exhibited various characteristics based on some of the previously highlighted conditions. As evidenced by the existing data, the disparities in COVID-19 morbidity and mortality in the United States were deepened mainly by structural factors such as racism [73–77]. There are different nomenclatures of structural racism. Online dictionaries describe it as societal racism, state racism, covert racism, systemic racism, and institutional racism. Irrespective of the adopted nomenclature of racism, it has significant implications on health and health outcomes.

Structural, institutional, and systemic racism synonymously refer to structures with procedures or processes that disadvantage people of color, particularly African Americans. An excellent example of structural racism is the "redlining" policies that discriminated against Black communities regarding the opportunity to secure loans [78]. Since housing is a critical determinant of health, discriminatory housing policies play a critical role in the health conditions of the group of people being discriminated against. For example, breast, colorectal, cervical, and lung cancers, as well as birth outcomes and asthma, have been shown to correlate with redlining policy [79–84]. In addition, housing congestion and overcrowding are major underlying factors for the diffusion of infectious diseases such as COVID-19. Therefore, the authors adopt structural racism in this article, which is more prevalent and favored in health research.

4.2. Structural Racism

Structural racism is how societies foster discrimination through mutually reinforcing inequitable systems. It is usually embedded through laws within society or different levels of an organization. For example, during the peak of the COVID-19 outbreak in the United States in 2020, more racial and ethnic minorities were infected and died more than their White counterparts. COVID-19 impacted more Blacks or African Americans and Hispanics than any other racial and ethnic group in the United States. Studies on COVID-19 focusing on geographic disparity in the infection, death, and case fatality rates show that Black/African Americans living in inner cities with a high population density were at high risk [85]. In addition, research on the rural–urban disparity of COVID-19 case fatality ratio in the United States indicates that Blacks in rural counties were disproportionately burdened [27]. These disparities are inherently linked with racial and housing segregation, intergenerational poverty, and structural racism [74].

Historically, African Americans had the least access to health care in the United States due to their inability to access health insurance, mainly because of the low income and low employment rate among this subpopulation [73,75,76]. In addition, African Americans were more impacted because they have limited access to single-family homes due to historical institutional discriminatory policies (e.g., redlining and FHA policies) that force them to converge in mostly the poorest, densely populated inner-city spaces [78]. Similar experiences exist for Black, Asian, and Minority Ethnic (BAME) groups in the

United Kingdom [34,86–89] and indigenous populations around the world [90–93]. Generally, minorities are disproportionately overrepresented in neighborhoods of concentrated poverty [94], which is detrimental to mental and physical health and wellbeing. Consequently, during the lockdown, the recommendations to maintain social distancing were less realistic for them and their communities.

4.3. Age and Gender Disparity

Globally, senior adults aged 65 and above are more likely to die from COVID-19 complications than other age groups, and more males than females were infected and died from the disease. What research has not readily shown is age disparity in minority groups. In addition, the observed sex and gender differences in COVID-19-related health outcomes could be explained by the sex- and gender-based medicine (SGBM) model that incorporates how biological sex and the socio-cultural aspects of gender affect health and illness [95]. Previous epidemiological research on similar respiratory infectious diseases such as the 2003 severe acute respiratory syndrome (SARS) and the 2012 Middle East respiratory syndrome (MERS) outbreaks show evidence of sex and gender disparities. Age-based research on COVID-19 also demonstrates age group disparity of COVID-19 infection and death rates within the United States context, and several examples are available globally. Sadly, despite the United States having some of the highest coronavirus cases and deaths, comprehensive age- and sex-specific data concerning patients in the United States are not currently available to the community of researchers to effectively inform health policy.

4.4. Case Study of COVID-19

COVID-19, as a peculiar case study, could help us better understand racism, structural racism, inter-racism, and equity. A deep understanding of equity matters because it helps us better understand how resources are distributed according to the underlying structure. For example, in the case of COVID-19, we could go back and analyze the distribution of PPE, hospital beds, access to care and services, and, now, the distribution of COVID-19 vaccines by race and ethnicity, age groups, and gender and sexual orientation. We can then ask whether minority communities that are most impacted receive the required care and can access vaccines as needed. Existing data on vaccine distribution at the county level indicate that counties identified as the most vulnerable and most impacted received fewer vaccines [96], indicating the existing health disparity by geography, social class, and racial and ethnic groups.

5. Implication for Achieving Global and Sustainable Health

The variances in the definition of health disparity have significant policy implications in obtaining the desired health outcomes, particularly for reaching global health goals such as the United Nations' Sustainable Development Goals and other multilateral agencies (e.g., World Health Organization and World Bank). Figure 4 presents a snapshot of global disparity in the distribution of coronavirus vaccination. A stark difference exists between developed and less developed regions. For example, the dose per 100 people varies between 4.2 in Africa and 78 in North America. Most of the prominent multilateral organizations are all part of the United Nations, intending to improve the health and wellbeing of all global citizens. Since its creation in 1945, the United Nations has provided a common platform where all the world's nations can gather together, discuss common problems such as historical pandemics and epidemics, and find shared solutions that benefit humanity.

Although some multilateral agencies do not directly seek to improve global health, they are essential mechanisms to promote healthy living. A good reference, in this case, is the World Bank, whose goal is to alleviate poverty at all levels by providing loans, credits, and grants to developing/emerging countries toward improving the standard of living of citizens in developing nations. Additional goals include implementing various development projects such as education, health care, agriculture, environmental and natural resource management, infrastructure, and other relevant projects toward general improved wellbeing. For example, at the onset of the COVID-19 pandemic, the World Bank highlighted 34 health indicators referred to as the "World Bank Indicators of Interest to the COVID-19 Outbreak," partly to investigate the global disparities and drivers of COVID-19 (see [1]). Despite the fact that the United States is an active player and frontline contributor in helping to fight global health issues and other socioeconomic matters, the COVID-19 pandemic hit hard on the "World's Police" country [97] and makes it the global hotspot of COVID-19 infection and mortality.

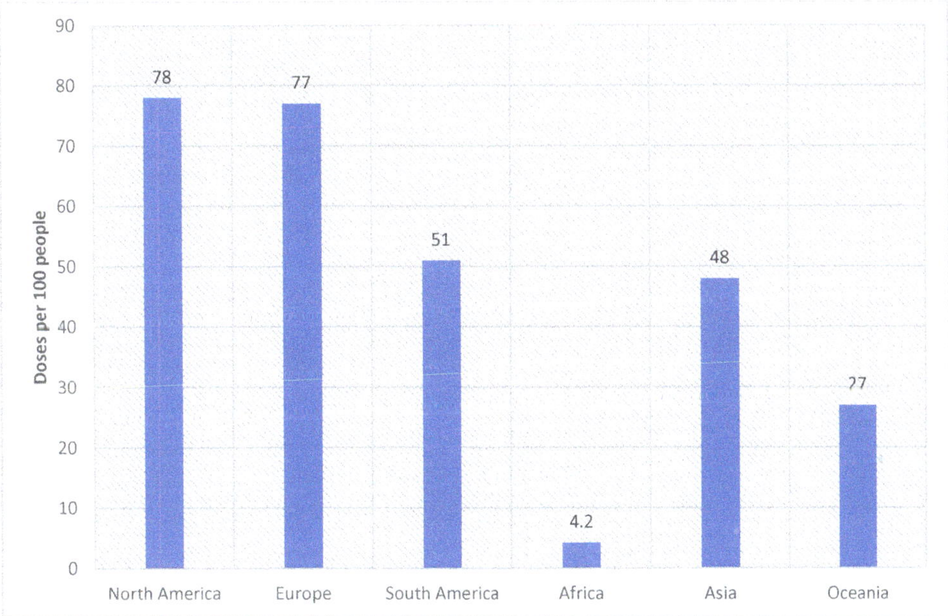

Figure 4. The global disparity in the COVID-19 vaccination doses per 100 people (data source: The New York Times [98]).

The United States Centers for Disease Control and Prevention (CDC) developed a social vulnerability index (SVI) for determining the impact of the COVID-19 community infection rate and morbidity and mortality rates. Briefly, social vulnerability refers to the potential adverse effects on communities caused by external stress on human health, including natural/human-caused disasters and disease outbreaks. Therefore, a pragmatic effort towards reducing social vulnerability can have a longtime effect on decreasing human exposure, suffering, and economic loss. Based on the CDC's SVI, counties in the United States were categorized into low to high social vulnerability [96].

Typically, neighborhoods in the highest social vulnerability tertile should be prioritized for distributing COVID-19 vaccines to quickly curtail the excess COVID-19-related morbidity and mortality, which will eventually address two common health issues—equality and equity. To address inequality, a similar allocation of health resources such as the supply of COVID-19 vaccines should be supplied proportionately based on the population across different jurisdictions or health regions. Likewise, the issue of equity can be addressed by prioritizing communities most affected by the pandemic. Nevertheless, the two issues of equity and inequality should be judiciously managed to avoid inter-racial and political conflicts.

6. Measuring Health Disparity

To monitor trends in health disparities in federally funded programs, Section 4302 of the Patient Protection and Affordable Care Act (ACA) suggests the need to improve data collection to reveal any evidence of health disparity [99]. However, a comprehensive and accurate measure of health disparity has become a significant question among public health researchers. Compared to the measure of inequities, which are relatively easy to characterize, assessing health disparities or disparities in health conditions is not easy. Generally, the effort toward measuring health disparity has one main goal: to help inform transformative policies and provide justice. Health disparity assessment requires a sufficient understanding of health disparities and consistent measurement and variables that shape them. Consequently, several approaches have been used to measure health disparities. For example, disparities can be measured relative to a standard such as a Healthy People target [100].

Researchers have measured health disparities in absolute and relative terms for better comparisons across populations, geographic areas, and indicators [101,102]. Pairwise comparisons measure health disparity when the goal is to improve the health status of a particular group or population [103]. More specifically, the absolute measure of health disparity can determine the arithmetic difference between a group rate and a reference category. In contrast, a relative measure expresses the simple difference from the reference point as a percentage of the reference point [102]. Health disparities can also be measured relative to the total population represented by the domain of groups, using graphical displays over time and finding the ratio between the highest and lowest rates [104,105].

Nevertheless, these measures vary in terms of magnitude and the opposite direction in which these magnitudes can occur due to temporal changes [101]. In addition to measuring disparity in absolute or relative terms, several issues have been associated with measuring health disparities [102]. For example, researchers could choose to measure health disparity between groups in a pairwise manner or in a summary fashion, weighting groups according to size or in terms of favorable or adverse events [102]. The most common issue with measuring health disparity is the selection of a reference point from which to measure disparity. Selecting the best measure depends on the research question at hand, as this can affect the magnitude and direction of disparities measured at a point in time [102].

7. The Role of Geospatial and Machine Learning Techniques in Health Disparity

Since the global outbreak of COVID-19, several attempts have been made to investigate factors driving the variability of COVID-19 infection, mortality rates, and case-fatality rates/ratios at different geographic scales using different approaches. One well-known technique that has gained substantial popularity in public health and epidemiology research of infectious and noninfectious diseases is the use of geographic information systems (GIS). GIS has become an essential tool for revealing spatial disparity and distribution and understanding the change in disease patterns. Furthermore, to complement medical interventions, epidemiologists are keen on discovering the origin and diffusion rate of diseases using geospatial techniques for appropriate health intervention and preventing a future outbreak. Of the 40 selected studies in Table 2, 9 highlighted the application of machine and deep learning and artificial intelligence (ML/DL/AI), and 11 used spatial and aspatial techniques to study COVID-19, reinforcing the importance of innovative technologies in disease epidemiology.

7.1. *GIS and Health Data Linkage*

The integration of spatial and nonspatial data, as well as linking census data with electronic health data to create a database that can be queried for meaningful insight in supporting health policies, is possible through the application of GISs. Geographers, spatial epidemiologists, and other spatial scientists are at the forefront in marshaling the power of GISs using spatially encoded data such as mobility data to estimate and explain COVID-19 transmission patterns in the United States and beyond. Another contribution of the use of GISs to COVID-19 studies and health disparity investigation, in general, is its capacity to empower the linkage of health outcomes (morbidity or mortality) with socioeconomic, cultural, infrastructure, and environmental data at the aggregate level (different scales) to support the ecological investigation of the possible correlation between health disparity and socioecological factors (see, for example, [1]).

Undeniably, we are currently in the era of "big data," and the use of GISs has helped governmental and non-governmental agencies handle these enormous data that keep pouring near real-time. Based on the insights gained from manipulating and analyzing the available data, policymakers, and health agencies developed non-pharmaceutical interventions such as total or partial lockdown, travel bans for nonessential workers within a country, and international travel restrictions. What we have found is that the degree of implementation of various non-pharmaceutical measures and the level of the effective reproduction number (R_t) at the time of the intervention correspond to the suppression rate of COVID-19 in the United States, that is, the average number of people each infected person can spread the virus to [27].

Moving forward, geographically focusing on policies that will eliminate the most critical determinants of health, structural racism and poverty, is crucial to reducing health disparity among racial/ethnic groups. In this regard, persistent recognition of spatial data and scientists/geographers and their tools, such as GISs, would continue to be relevant in measuring and untangling health disparities.

7.2. Disease Epidemiology, Machine Learning, and Artificial Intelligence

Apart from GIS techniques, other sophisticated data analytics techniques such as machine learning (ML), deep learning (DL), and artificial intelligence (AI) are available to help mitigate several impacts of COVID-19. The field of machine learning is both broad and deep and is constantly evolving. ML is an innovative technique that has extensive applications in prediction. The adoption of machine learning in disease epidemiology provides more accurate and useful features than a traditional explicitly calculation-based method. Furthermore, ML algorithms can analyze the risk factors considering age, social habits, location, and environmental factors. ML is essentially used for predicting future events based on available data.

Interestingly, some GIS interfaces have built-in ML algorithms that can smoothly carry out some health-based analyses. For example, ArcGIS Pro, a proprietary GIS software by ESRI [17], has built-in ML techniques and DL algorithms, e.g., a forest-based classification and regression embedded in ArcGIS Pro based on the traditional random forest (RF) technique. It is important to note that RF is a supervised learning and classification algorithm that consists of many decision trees. In a technical term, the RF techniques use bagging and feature randomness when building each tree to create an uncorrelated forest of trees whose prediction is more accurate than any individual tree. In other words, RF makes a prediction based on random samples drawn from different chunks of data (forest) to obtain optimal outcomes compared to relying on a single sample (single tree). An excellent example of how ML and AI have been used in disease surveillance is the contact tracing of COVID-19 infection. In addition, using machine learning, data scientists interlink several forms of data such as environmental, population, and mobility data with health data to predict infection, death, or fatality rates [106–108].

Punn et al. [109] used a series of ML and DL techniques such as support vector regression (SVR), polynomial regression (PR), deep neural networks (DNNs), and recurrent neural networks (RNNs) to predict the total number of confirmed, recovered, and death cases worldwide. Similarly, Pinter et al. [110] used hybrid machine learning techniques, an adaptive network-based fuzzy inference system (ANFIS), and a multi-layered perceptron-imperialist competitive algorithm (i.e., MLP-ICA) to predict time series of individuals infected with COVID-19 and mortality rates in Hungary. The authors opine that ML techniques could be more useful in epidemiological modeling than the standard susceptible-infected-resistant (SIR)-based models.

Finally, coupled with geospatial techniques, ML, DL, and AI are powerful tools to identify health disparities, especially in the era of "big data." Hence, these techniques need to be constantly applied to identify populations at high risk and transmission patterns among communities and predict death rates, other possible abnormalities, and second-order impacts emanating from COVID-19 [111]. In addition, the accrued benefits of these innovative technologies would help public health experts avert unnecessary excesses in hospitalization and deaths from preventable diseases and asking the right questions [109–114].

8. Conclusions and Prospects

Health disparity is not a new challenge, nor is it going away easily without systematic and intersectional treatment. The COVID-19 pandemic provides a stage to reveal and re-examine the health disparities we have been facing in all aspects of public health, including health outcomes (infection, hospitalization, fatality, and various health complications), health care, and disease prevention (vaccine). Evidence of health disparities across different population groups manifested through all critical stages of the COVID-19 pandemic, from susceptibility to exposure, infection, and recovery or death.

The intersectionality approach can be used as a lens to understand the power structure and dynamics in a society that are central to the various social, political, and infrastructural issues leading to or sustaining health disparity. Treatment for health disparities calls for systematic tackling of these issues that place minority groups in disadvantaged positions for health and health services. Identifying the disadvantaged populations and communities and developing and implementing community-centered and place-based policies and practices to elevate the disadvantaged is core to reducing and eventually eliminating health disparity.

The continuous development of GIS and data science has greatly enabled our capabilities to promptly integrate and process unprecedently voluminous data to reveal health issues and disease patterns of particular challenges to specific populations or communities. As a result, community-centered and population-targeting health prevention and health service initiatives can be designed accordingly. We have seen some of these technologies being adopted to guide and optimize the distribution and administration of COVID-19 vaccines [115]. For example, a study in Flint and Genesee County, Michigan, investigated disparities in COVID-19 death using a GIS-based approach. Racial and location disparities detection resulted in public health interventions leading to prevention, testing, treatment, and vaccination rollout. With the world being interconnected and knitted together more than ever before, there is no room to leave any communities or population groups out to suffer from health disparity. As it sings in the song *We're All in This Together*, "Together together, come on let's do this right."

Author Contributions: Conceptualization, A.I.; investigation, A.I.; resources, A.I.; writing—original draft preparation, A.I., K.B., and Y.L.; writing—review and editing, A.I., K.B., and Y.L.; visualization, A.I.; and supervision, Y.L. All authors have read and agreed to the published version of the manuscript.

Funding: This research received no external funding.

Institutional Review Board Statement: Not applicable.

Informed Consent Statement: Not applicable.

Data Availability Statement: Data and literature were sourced from Google Scholar. The list of works is available in the References section.

Acknowledgments: Not applicable.

Conflicts of Interest: The authors declare no conflict of interest.

Entry Link on the Encyclopedia Platform: https://encyclopedia.pub/13863.

References

1. Iyanda, A.E.; Adeleke, R.; Lu, Y.; Osayomi, T.; Adaralegbe, A.; Lasode, M.; Chima-Adaralegbe, N.J.; Osundina, A.M. A retrospective cross-national examination of COVID-19 outbreak in 175 countries: A multiscale geographically weighted regression analysis (January 11–June 28, 2020). *J. Infect. Public Health* **2020**, *13*, 1438–1445. [CrossRef]
2. John Hopkins Coronavirus Research Center. Available online: https://coronavirus.jhu.edu/map.html (accessed on 23 June 2021).
3. Kandi, V.; Thungaturthi, S.; Vadakedath, S.; Gundu, R.; Mohapatra, R.K. Mortality Rates of Coronavirus Disease 2019 (COVID-19) Caused by the Novel Severe Acute Respiratory Syndrome Coronavirus-2 (SARS-CoV-2). *Cureus* **2021**, *13*, e14081.

4. Onder, G.; Rezza, G.; Brusaferro, S. Case-Fatality Rate and Characteristics of Patients Dying in Relation to COVID-19 in Italy. *JAMA* **2020**, *323*, 1775–1776. [CrossRef] [PubMed]
5. Chaudhry, R.; Dranitsaris, G.; Mubashir, T.; Bartoszko, J.; Riazi, S. A country level analysis measuring the impact of government actions, country preparedness and socioeconomic factors on COVID-19 mortality and related health outcomes. *EClinicalMedicine* **2020**, *25*, 100464. [CrossRef]
6. Christie, A. Decreases in COVID-19 Cases, Emergency Department Visits, Hospital Admissions, and Deaths Among Older Adults Following the Introduction of COVID-19 Vaccine—United States, September 6, 2020–May 1, 2021. *Morb. Mortal. Wkly. Rep.* **2021**, *70*, 858–864. Available online: https://www.cdc.gov/mmwr/volumes/70/wr/mm7023e2.htm (accessed on 16 July 2021). [CrossRef] [PubMed]
7. Moghadas, S.M.; Vilches, T.N.; Zhang, K.; Wells, C.R.; Shoukat, A.; Singer, B.H.; Meyers, L.A.; Neuzil, K.M.; Langley, J.M.; Fitzpatrick, M.C.; et al. The impact of vaccination on COVID-19 outbreaks in the United States. *Clin. Infect. Dis.* **2021**, ciab079. [CrossRef] [PubMed]
8. Reuters. UK Coronavirus Vaccines Have Weakened Link between Infections and Death, Says Scientist. 2021. Available online: https://www.reuters.com/world/uk/uk-coronavirus-vaccines-have-weakened-link-between-infections-death-says-2021-06-27/ (accessed on 16 July 2021).
9. World Health Organization. Vaccine Efficacy, Effectiveness and Protection. 2021. Available online: https://www.who.int/news-room/feature-stories/detail/vaccine-efficacy-effectiveness-and-protection (accessed on 16 July 2021).
10. Roser, M.; Ritchie, H.; Ortiz-Ospina, E.; Hasell, J. Coronavirus Pandemic (COVID-19). Available online: https://ourworldindata.org/coronavirus (accessed on 10 August 2020).
11. Braveman, P.A.; Kumanyika, S.; Fielding, J.; LaVeist, T.; Borrell, L.; Manderscheid, R.; Troutman, A. Health Disparities and Health Equity: The Issue Is Justice. *Am. J. Public Health* **2011**, *101*, S149–S155. [CrossRef]
12. Whitehead, M. The concepts and principles of equity and health. *Health Promot. Int.* **1991**, *6*, 217–228. [CrossRef]
13. Braveman, P.; Gruskin, S. Defining equity in health. *J. Epidemiol. Community Health* **2003**, *57*, 254–258. [CrossRef]
14. National Institute of Minority Health and Health Disparity. National Minority Health and Health Disparities Research Framework. NIMHD. 2021. Available online: https://www.nimhd.nih.gov/about/overview/ (accessed on 16 July 2021).
15. The National Health Service. Health Inequalities. 2021. Available online: https://www.nhs.uk/ (accessed on 15 July 2021).
16. Office of Disease Prevention and Health Promotion. Determinants of Health: Healthy People 2020. 2020. Available online: https://www.healthypeople.gov/2020/about/foundation-health-measures/Determinants-of-Health#policymaking (accessed on 28 February 2021).
17. Center for Disease Control and Prevention. Health Disparities. 2019. Available online: https://www.cdc.gov/aging/disparities/index.htm (accessed on 16 July 2021).
18. Nelson, A. Unequal treatment: Confronting racial and ethnic disparities in health care. *J. Natl. Med. Assoc.* **2002**, *94*, 666–668.
19. Rubin, I.L.; Geller, R.J.; Martinuzzi, K.; Gitterman, B.A.; Wells, L.; Garfinkel, W.; Coles, C.D.; Merrick, J. Children's environmental health disparities: The costs and benefits of breaking the cycle. *Int. J. Child Health Hum. Dev.* **2016**, *9*, 419–430.
20. Carter-Pokras, O.; Baquet, C. What is a "health disparity"? *Public Health Rep.* **2002**, *117*, 426–434. [CrossRef]
21. American Medical Association. Reducing Disparities in Health Care. 2019. Available online: https://www.ama-assn.org/delivering-care/patient-support-advocacy/reducing-disparities-health-care (accessed on 16 June 2021).
22. Dy, A.M.; Jayawarna, D. Bios, mythoi and women entrepreneurs: A Wynterian analysis of the intersectional impacts of the COVID-19 pandemic on self-employed women and women-owned businesses. *Int. Small Bus. J. Res. Entrep.* **2020**, *38*, 391–403. [CrossRef]
23. Eaves, L.; Al-Hindi, K.F. Intersectional geographies and COVID-19. *Dialogues Hum. Geogr.* **2020**, *10*, 132–136. [CrossRef]
24. Sekalala, S.; Perehudoff, K.; Parker, M.; Forman, L.; Rawson, B.; Smith, M. An intersectional human rights approach to prioritising access to COVID-19 vaccines. *BMJ Glob. Health* **2021**, *6*, e004462. [CrossRef] [PubMed]
25. Bowleg, L. We're Not All in This Together: On COVID-19, Intersectionality, and Structural Inequality. *Am. J. Public Health* **2020**, *110*, 917. [CrossRef] [PubMed]
26. Crenshaw, K. Demarginalizing the intersection of race and sex: A Black feminist critique of antidiscrimination doctrine, feminist theory, and antiracist politics. In *University of Chicago Legal Forum*; Routledge: London, UK, 1989.
27. Mackey, K.; Ayers, C.K.; Kondo, K.K.; Saha, S.; Advani, S.M.; Young, S.; Spencer, H.; Rusek, M.; Anderson, J.; Veazie, S.; et al. Racial and ethnic disparities in COVID-19–related infections, hospitalizations, and deaths: A systematic review. *Ann. Intern. Med.* **2021**, *174*, 362–373. [CrossRef]
28. Iyanda, A.E.; Boakye, K.A.; Lu, Y.; Oppong, J.R. Racial/Ethnic Heterogeneity and Rural-Urban Disparity of COVID-19 Case Fatality Ratio in the USA: A Negative Binomial and GIS-Based Analysis. *J. Racial Ethn. Health Disparities* **2021**, 1–14. [CrossRef]
29. Moore, J.T.; Ricaldi, J.N.; Rose, C.E.; Fuld, J.; Parise, M.; Kang, G.J.; Driscoll, A.K.; Norris, T.; Wilson, N.; Rainisch, G.; et al. Disparities in Incidence of COVID-19 Among Underrepresented Racial/Ethnic Groups in Counties Identified as Hotspots During June 5–18, 2020—22 States, February–June 2020. *Morb. Mortal Wkly. Rep.* **2020**, *69*, 1122–1126. Available online: https://www.ncbi.nlm.nih.gov/pmc/articles/PMC7439982/ (accessed on 14 July 2021). [CrossRef]
30. Elias, A.; Ben, J.; Mansouri, F.; Paradies, Y. Racism and nationalism during and beyond the COVID-19 pandemic. *Ethn. Racial Stud.* **2021**, *44*, 783–793. [CrossRef]

31. Patel, J.; Nielsen, F.; Badiani, A.; Assi, S.; Unadkat, V.; Patel, B.; Ravindrane, R.; Wardle, H. Poverty, inequality and COVID-19: The forgotten vulnerable. *Public Health* **2020**, *183*, 110–111. [CrossRef]
32. Patel, P.; Hiam, L.; Sowemimo, A.; Devakumar, D.; McKee, M. Ethnicity and COVID-19. *BMJ* **2020**, *369*, m2282. Available online: https://www.bmj.com/content/369/bmj.m2282 (accessed on 13 July 2021). [CrossRef]
33. Gravlee, C.C. Systemic racism, chronic health inequities, and COVID-19: A syndemic in the making? *Am. J. Hum. Biol.* **2020**, *32*, e23482. [CrossRef]
34. Louis-Jean, J.; Cenat, K.; Njoku, C.V.; Angelo, J.; Sanon, D. Coronavirus (COVID-19) and Racial Disparities: A Perspective Analysis. *J. Racial Ethn. Health Disparities* **2020**, *7*, 1039–1045. [CrossRef]
35. Abedi, V.; Olulana, O.; Avula, V.; Chaudhary, D.; Khan, A.; Shahjouei, S.; Li, J.; Zand, R. Racial, Economic, and Health Inequality and COVID-19 Infection in the United States. *J. Racial Ethn. Health Disparities* **2020**, *8*, 732–742. [CrossRef] [PubMed]
36. Chaudhuri, K.; Chakrabarti, A.; Lima, J.M.; Chandan, J.S.; Bandyopadhyay, S. The interaction of ethnicity and deprivation on COVID-19 mortality risk: A retrospective ecological study. *Sci. Rep.* **2021**, *11*, 11555. [CrossRef]
37. Wilson, S.M.; Bullard, R.; Patterson, J.; Thomas, S.B. Environmental Justice Roundtable on COVID-19. *Environ. Justice* **2020**, *13*, 56–64. [CrossRef]
38. Zhanga, R.; Lib, H.; Khannaa, N. The Environmental Injustice of the COVID-19 Pandemic: Evidence from New York State. 2020. Available online: https://www.researchgate.net/publication/343441430_The_Environmental_Injustice_of_the_COVID-19_Pandemic_Evidence_from_New_York_State (accessed on 16 July 2021).
39. Bashir, M.F.; Jiang, B.; Komal, B.; Bashir, M.A.; Farooq, T.H.; Iqbal, N.; Bashir, M. Correlation between environmental pollution indicators and COVID-19 pandemic: A brief study in Californian context. *Environ. Res.* **2020**, *187*, 109652. [CrossRef] [PubMed]
40. Bashir, M.F.; Benghoul, M.; Numan, U.; Shakoor, A.; Komal, B.; Bashir, M.A.; Bashir, M.; Tan, D. Environmental pollution and COVID-19 outbreak: Insights from Germany. *Air Qual. Atmos. Health* **2020**, *13*, 1385–1394.
41. Mollalo, A.; Sadeghian, A.; Israel, G.D.; Rashidi, P.; Sofizadeh, A.; Glass, G.E. Machine learning approaches in GIS-based ecological modeling of the sand fly Phlebotomus papatasi, a vector of zoonotic cutaneous leishmaniasis in Golestan province, Iran. *Acta Trop.* **2018**, *188*, 187–194. [CrossRef] [PubMed]
42. Fattorini, D.; Regoli, F. Role of the chronic air pollution levels in the COVID-19 outbreak risk in Italy. *Environ. Pollut.* **2020**, *264*, 114732. [CrossRef]
43. Arimiyaw, A.W.; Abass, K.; Morgan, A.K. Minimizing the long-term impact of COVID-19 on environmental pollution in Sub-Saharan Africa. *Sustain. Sci. Pract. Policy* **2021**, *17*, 82–85. [CrossRef]
44. Travaglio, M.; Yu, Y.; Popovic, R.; Selley, L.; Leal, N.S.; Martins, L.M. Links between air pollution and COVID-19 in England. *Environ. Pollut.* **2021**, *268*, 115859. [CrossRef] [PubMed]
45. Berman, J.D.; Ebisu, K. Changes in U.S. air pollution during the COVID-19 pandemic. *Sci. Total Environ.* **2020**, *739*, 139864. [CrossRef]
46. Lippi, G.; Sanchis-Gomar, F.; Henry, B.M. Association between environmental pollution and prevalence of coronavirus disease 2019 (COVID-19) in Italy. *MedRxiv* **2020**, preprint. [CrossRef]
47. Brandt, E.B.; Beck, A.F.; Mersha, T.B. Air pollution, racial disparities, and COVID-19 mortality. *J. Allergy Clin. Immunol.* **2020**, *146*, 61–63. Available online: https://www.ncbi.nlm.nih.gov/pmc/articles/PMC7204717/ (accessed on 14 July 2021). [CrossRef]
48. Adams, M.D. Air pollution in Ontario, Canada during the COVID-19 State of Emergency. *Sci. Total Environ.* **2020**, *742*, 140516. [CrossRef] [PubMed]
49. Chen, K.; Wang, M.; Huang, C.; Kinney, P.L.; Anastas, P.T. Air pollution reduction and mortality benefit during the COVID-19 outbreak in China. *Lancet Planet. Health* **2020**, *4*, e210–e212. [CrossRef]
50. Comunian, S.; Dongo, D.; Milani, C.; Palestini, P. Air Pollution and COVID-19: The Role of Particulate Matter in the Spread and Increase of COVID-19's Morbidity and Mortality. *Int. J. Environ. Res. Public Health* **2020**, *17*, 4487. [CrossRef] [PubMed]
51. Copat, C.; Cristaldi, A.; Fiore, M.; Grasso, A.; Zuccarello, P.; Signorelli, S.S.; Conti, G.O.; Ferrante, M. The role of air pollution (PM and NO_2) in COVID-19 spread and lethality: A systematic review. *Environ. Res.* **2020**, *191*, 110129. [CrossRef]
52. Dey, T.; Dominici, F. COVID-19, Air Pollution, and Racial Inequity: Connecting the Dots. *Chem. Res. Toxicol.* **2020**, *34*, 669–671. [CrossRef]
53. Allen, O.; Brown, A.; Wang, E. Socioeconomic Disparities in the Effects of Pollution on Spread of COVID-19: Evidence from US Counties. *J. Econ. Behav. Stud.* **2021**, *12*, 33–42. [CrossRef]
54. Chakraborty, J. Convergence of COVID-19 and chronic air pollution risks: Racial/ethnic and socioeconomic inequities in the U.S. *Environ. Res.* **2021**, *193*, 110586. [CrossRef] [PubMed]
55. Millett, G.A.; Jones, A.T.; Benkeser, D.; Baral, S.; Mercer, L.; Beyrer, C.; Honermann, B.; Lankiewicz, E.; Mena, L.; Crowley, J.S.; et al. Assessing differential impacts of COVID-19 on black communities. *Ann. Epidemiol.* **2020**, *47*, 37–44. [CrossRef]
56. Terrell, K.A.; James, W. Racial Disparities in Air Pollution Burden and COVID-19 Deaths in Louisiana, USA, in the Context of Long-Term Changes in Fine Particulate Pollution. *Environ. Justice* **2020**. [CrossRef]
57. The Atlantic. Racial Data Dashboard. The COVID Tracking Project. Available online: https://covidtracking.com/race/dashboard (accessed on 10 June 2021).
58. Cheng, K.J.G.; Sun, Y.; Monnat, S.M. COVID-19 Death Rates Are Higher in Rural Counties with Larger Shares of Blacks and Hispanics. *J. Rural Health* **2020**, *36*, 602–608. [CrossRef]

59. Godsil, R.D.; Tropp, L.R.; Goff, P.A.; Powell, J.A. Addressing implicit bias, racial anxiety, and stereotype threat in education and health care. *Sci. Equal.* **2014**, *1*, 14.
60. Sonu, S.; Marvin, D.; Moore, C. The Intersection and Dynamics between COVID-19, Health Disparities, and Adverse Childhood Experiences. *J. Child Adolesc. Trauma* **2021**, 1–10. [CrossRef]
61. Reicher, S.; Stott, C. On order and disorder during the COVID-19 pandemic. *Br. J. Soc. Psychol.* **2020**, *59*, 694–702. [CrossRef]
62. Corpuz, J.C.G. 'Pandemic within a pandemic': A call to end police brutality. *J. Public Health* **2021**. [CrossRef]
63. Njoku, A.; Ahmed, Y.; Bolaji, B. Police brutality against Blacks in the United States and ensuing protests: Implications for social distancing and Black health during COVID-19. *J. Hum. Behav. Soc. Environ.* **2020**, *31*, 262–270. [CrossRef]
64. Coyne, C.J.; Yatsyshina, Y. Pandemic Police States. *Peace Econ. Peace Sci. Public Policy* **2020**, *26*. Available online: https://www.degruyter.com/document/doi/10.1515/peps-2020-0021/html (accessed on 12 July 2021). [CrossRef]
65. Bailey, J.; Flynn, A.; Henry, N. Pandemics and systemic discrimination: Technology-facilitated violence and abuse in an era of COVID-19 and antiracist protest. In *The Emerald International Handbook of Technology Facilitated Violence and Abuse*; Emerald Publishing Limited: Bingley, UK, 2021; pp. 787–797. [CrossRef]
66. Gibson, A.N.; Chancellor, R.L.; Cooke, N.A.; Dahlen, S.P.; Patin, B.; Shorish, Y.L. Struggling to breathe: COVID-19, protest and the LIS response. *Equal. Divers. Incl. Int. J.* **2020**, *40*, 74–82. [CrossRef]
67. Biana, H.T. The Matter of Class: COVID-19 in the Philippines. *Soc. Ethics Soc. J. Appl. Philos.* **2020**, *6*, 17–36.
68. Naja, F.; Hamadeh, R. Nutrition amid the COVID-19 pandemic: A multi-level framework for action. *Eur. J. Clin. Nutr.* **2020**, *74*, 1117–1121. [CrossRef]
69. Gautam, S. The Influence of COVID-19 on Air Quality in India: A Boon or Inutile. *Bull. Environ. Contam. Toxicol.* **2020**, *104*, 724–726. [CrossRef]
70. Ming, W.; Zhou, Z.; Ai, H.; Bi, H.; Zhong, Y. COVID-19 and Air Quality: Evidence from China. *Emerg. Mark. Financ. Trade* **2020**, *56*, 2422–2442. [CrossRef]
71. Zangari, S.; Hill, D.; Charette, A.T.; Mirowsky, J.E. Air quality changes in New York City during the COVID-19 pandemic. *Sci. Total Environ.* **2020**, *742*, 140496. [CrossRef]
72. World Health Organization. *Commission on Social Determinants of Health—CSDH*; WHO: Geneva, Switzerland, 2008.
73. Bin Tan, S.; Desouza, P.; Raifman, M. Structural Racism and COVID-19 in the USA: A County-Level Empirical Analysis. *J. Racial Ethn. Health Disparities* **2021**, 1–11. [CrossRef]
74. Egede, L.E.; Walker, R.J. Structural racism, social risk factors, and COVID-19—A dangerous convergence for Black Americans. *N. Engl. J. Med.* **2020**, *383*, e77. [CrossRef]
75. Zalla, L.C.; Martin, C.L.; Edwards, J.K.; Gartner, D.R.; Noppert, G.A. A Geography of Risk: Structural Racism and COVID-19 Mortality in the United States. *Am. J. Epidemiol.* **2021**, kwab059. [CrossRef]
76. Yearby, R.; Mohapatra, S. Law, structural racism, and the COVID-19 pandemic. *J. Law Biosci.* **2020**, *7*, lsaa036. [CrossRef] [PubMed]
77. Krieger, N. Enough: COVID-19, structural racism, police brutality, plutocracy, climate change—And time for health justice, democratic governance, and an equitable, sustainable future. *Am. J. Public Health* **2020**, *110*, 1620–1623. [CrossRef]
78. Rothstein, R. *The Color of Law: A Forgotten History of How Our Government Segregated America*; Liveright Publishing: New York, NY, USA, 2017.
79. Nardone, A.; Casey, J.A.; Morello-Frosch, R.; Mujahid, M.; Balmes, J.R.; Thakur, N. Associations between historical residential redlining and current age-adjusted rates of emergency department visits due to asthma across eight cities in California: An ecological study. *Lancet Planet. Health* **2020**, *4*, e24–e31. [CrossRef]
80. Nardone, A.L.; Casey, J.A.; Rudolph, K.E.; Karasek, D.; Mujahid, M.; Morello-Frosch, R. Associations between historical redlining and birth outcomes from 2006 through 2015 in California. *PLoS ONE* **2020**, *15*, e0237241. [CrossRef]
81. Huggins, J.C. A cartographic perspective on the correlation between redlining and public health in Austin, Texas–1951. *Cityscape* **2017**, *19*, 267–280.
82. Beyer, K.M.; Zhou, Y.; Matthews, K.; Bemanian, A.; Laud, P.W.; Nattinger, A. New spatially continuous indices of redlining and racial bias in mortgage lending: Links to survival after breast cancer diagnosis and implications for health disparities research. *Health Place* **2016**, *40*, 34–43. [CrossRef]
83. Krieger, N.; Wright, E.; Chen, J.T.; Waterman, P.D.; Huntley, E.R.; Arcaya, M. Cancer Stage at Diagnosis, Historical Redlining, and Current Neighborhood Characteristics: Breast, Cervical, Lung, and Colorectal Cancers, Massachusetts, 2001–2015. *Am. J. Epidemiol.* **2020**, *189*, 1065–1075. [CrossRef] [PubMed]
84. Collin, L.J.; Gaglioti, A.H.; Beyer, K.M.M.; Zhou, Y.; Moore, M.A.; Nash, R.; Switchenko, J.M.; Miller-Kleinhenz, J.M.; Ward, K.C.; McCullough, L.E. Neighborhood-Level Redlining and Lending Bias Are Associated with Breast Cancer Mortality in a Large and Diverse Metropolitan Area. *Cancer Epidemiol. Biomark. Prev.* **2020**, *30*, 53–60. [CrossRef] [PubMed]
85. Price-Haywood, E.G.; Burton, J.; Fort, D.; Seoane, L. Hospitalization and Mortality among Black Patients and White Patients with COVID-19. *N. Engl. J. Med.* **2020**, *382*, 2534–2543. [CrossRef] [PubMed]
86. Abuelgasim, E.; Saw, L.J.; Shirke, M.; Zeinah, M.; Harky, A. COVID-19: Unique public health issues facing Black, Asian and minority ethnic communities. *Curr. Probl. Cardiol.* **2020**, *45*, 100621. [CrossRef]
87. Mamluk, L.; Jones, T. The impact of COVID-19 on black, Asian and minority ethnic communities. *Natl. Inst. Health. Res. NHR Rep.* **2020**, *20*, 1–10.

88. Aldridge, R.W.; Lewer, D.; Katikireddi, S.V.; Mathur, R.; Pathak, N.; Burns, R.; Fragaszy, E.B.; Johnson, A.M.; Devakumar, D.; Abubakar, I.; et al. Black, Asian and Minority Ethnic groups in England are at increased risk of death from COVID-19: Indirect standardisation of NHS mortality data. *Wellcome Open Res.* **2020**, *5*, 88. [CrossRef] [PubMed]
89. Phiri, P.; Delanerolle, G.; Al-Sudani, A.; Rathod, S. COVID-19 and Black, Asian, and Minority Ethnic Communities: A Complex Relationship Without Just Cause. *JMIR Public Health Surveill.* **2021**, *7*, e22581. [CrossRef] [PubMed]
90. Power, T.; Wilson, D.; Best, O.; Brockie, T.; Bearskin, L.B.; Millender, E.; Lowe, J. COVID-19 and Indigenous Peoples: An imperative for action. *J. Clin. Nurs.* **2020**, *29*, 2737–2741. [CrossRef] [PubMed]
91. Ibarra-Nava, I.; Flores-Rodriguez, K.G.; Ruiz-Herrera, V.; Ochoa-Bayona, H.C.; Salinas-Zertuche, A.; Padilla-Orozco, M.; Salazar-Montalvo, R.G. Ethnic disparities in COVID-19 mortality in Mexico: A cross-sectional study based on national data. *PLoS ONE* **2021**, *16*, e0239168. [CrossRef]
92. Palamim, C.V.C.; Ortega, M.M.; Marson, F.A.L. COVID-19 in the Indigenous Population of Brazil. *J. Racial Ethn. Health Disparities* **2020**, *7*, 1053–1058. [CrossRef] [PubMed]
93. Argoty-Pantoja, A.; Robles-Rivera, K.; Rivera-Paredez, B.; Salmerón, J. COVID-19 fatality in Mexico's indigenous populations. *Public Health* **2021**, *193*, 69–75. [CrossRef]
94. Wurth, E. The health of the "forgotten" of Washington, DC: An analysis of gentrification, concentrated poverty and health. In *Donald T. Campbell Social Science Research Prize*; Paper 22; Lehigh University: New York, NY, USA, 2004.
95. Madsen, T.E.; Bourjeily, G.; Hasnain, M.; Jenkins, M.; Morrison, M.F.; Sandberg, K.; Tong, I.L.; Trott, J.; Werbinski, J.L.; McGregor, A. Sex-and gender-based medicine: The need for precise terminology. *Gend. Genome* **2017**, *1*, 122–128. [CrossRef]
96. Hughes, M.M. County-Level COVID-19 Vaccination Coverage and Social Vulnerability—United States, December 14, 2020–March 1, 2021. *Morb. Mortal Wkly. Rep.* **2021**, *70*, 431–436. Available online: https://www.cdc.gov/mmwr/volumes/70/wr/mm7012e1.htm (accessed on 29 April 2021). [CrossRef]
97. Lebovic, S. Why is America the world's police? *Boston Review*. 19 October 2020. Available online: http://bostonreview.net/politics/sam-lebovic-stephen-wertheim-tomorrow-the-world (accessed on 16 June 2021).
98. The New York Times. Covid World Vaccination Tracker. 2021. Available online: https://www.nytimes.com/interactive/2021/world/covid-vaccinations-tracker.html (accessed on 16 July 2021).
99. Medicaid and CHIP Payment and Access Commission. Comments on the U.S. Department of Health and Human Services Report to Congress on Improving the Identification of Health Care Disparities in Medicaid and CHIP [Internet]. MACPAC. 2015. Available online: https://www.macpac.gov/publication/macpac-comments-on-nov-2015-hhs-disparities-data-report/ (accessed on 16 July 2021).
100. US Department of Health and Human Services: USDHHS—Google Scholar. Available online: https://scholar.google.com/scholar_lookup?title=With+understanding+and+improving+health+and+objectives+for+improving+health&publication_year=2000& (accessed on 18 May 2021).
101. Moonesinghe, R.; Beckles, G.L. Measuring health disparities: A comparison of absolute and relative disparities. *PeerJ* **2015**, *3*, e1438. [CrossRef]
102. Keppel, K.; Pamuk, E.; Lynch, J.; Carter-Pokras, O.; Mays, V.; Pearcy, J.; Schoenbach, V.; Weissman, J.S.; Kim, I. Methodological issues in measuring health disparities. *Vital Health Stat.* **2005**, *2*, 1–16.
103. Penman-Aguilar, A.; Talih, M.; Huang, D.; Moonesinghe, R.; Bouye, K.; Beckles, G. Measurement of Health Disparities, Health Inequities, and Social Determinants of Health to Support the Advancement of Health Equity. *J. Public Health Manag. Pract.* **2016**, *22* (Suppl. 1), S33–S42. [CrossRef]
104. Talih, M. Examining socioeconomic health disparities using a rank-dependent Rényi index. *Ann. Appl. Stat.* **2015**, *9*, 992–1023. [CrossRef] [PubMed]
105. Talih, M. A reference-invariant health disparity index based on Rényi divergence. *Ann. Appl. Stat.* **2013**, *7*, 1217–1243. [CrossRef] [PubMed]
106. Mele, M.; Magazzino, C. Pollution, economic growth, and COVID-19 deaths in India: A machine learning evidence. *Environ. Sci. Pollut. Res.* **2020**, *28*, 2669–2677. [CrossRef] [PubMed]
107. Kuo, C.-P.; Fu, J.S. Evaluating the impact of mobility on COVID-19 pandemic with machine learning hybrid predictions. *Sci. Total Environ.* **2021**, *758*, 144151. [CrossRef]
108. Li, M.; Zhang, Z.; Cao, W.; Liu, Y.; Du, B.; Chen, C.; Liu, Q.; Uddin, N.; Jiang, S.; Chen, C.; et al. Identifying novel factors associated with COVID-19 transmission and fatality using the machine learning approach. *Sci. Total Environ.* **2021**, *764*, 142810. [CrossRef]
109. Punn, N.S.; Sonbhadra, S.K.; Agarwal, S. COVID-19 epidemic analysis using machine learning and deep learning algorithms. *MedRxiv* **2020**, preprint. [CrossRef]
110. Pinter, G.; Felde, I.; Mosavi, A.; Ghamisi, P.; Gloaguen, R. COVID-19 Pandemic Prediction for Hungary; A Hybrid Machine Learning Approach. *Mathematics* **2020**, *8*, 890. [CrossRef]
111. Kushwaha, S.; Bahl, S.; Bagha, A.K.; Parmar, K.S.; Javaid, M.; Haleem, A.; Singh, R.P. Significant Applications of Machine Learning for COVID-19 Pandemic. *J. Ind. Integr. Manag.* **2020**, *5*, 453–479. [CrossRef]
112. Carvajal, T.M.; Viacrusis, K.M.; Hernandez, L.F.T.; Ho, H.T.; Amalin, D.M.; Watanabe, K. Machine learning methods reveal the temporal pattern of dengue incidence using meteorological factors in metropolitan Manila, Philippines. *BMC Infect Dis.* **2018**, *18*, 183. [CrossRef] [PubMed]

113. Alimadadi, A.; Aryal, S.; Manandhar, I.; Munroe, P.B.; Joe, B.; Cheng, X. Artificial intelligence and machine learning to fight COVID-19. *Physiol. Genom.* **2020**, *52*, 200–202. [CrossRef] [PubMed]
114. Bachtiger, P.; Peters, N.S.; Walsh, S.L. Machine learning for COVID-19—Asking the right questions. *Lancet Digit. Health* **2020**, *2*, e391–e392. [CrossRef]
115. Krzysztofowicz, S.; Osińska-Skotak, K. The Use of GIS Technology to Optimize COVID-19 Vaccine Distribution: A Case Study of the City of Warsaw, Poland. *Int. J. Environ. Res. Public Health* **2021**, *18*, 5636. [CrossRef] [PubMed]

encyclopedia

MDPI

Entry

Air Quality during Covid-19 Lockdown

Gabriele Donzelli [1,2,*], Lorenzo Cioni [3], Mariagrazia Cancellieri [4], Agustin Llopis-Morales [1] and María Morales-Suárez-Varela [1,5]

1 Department of Preventive Medicine and Public Health, Food Sciences, Toxicology, and Legal Medicine, School of Pharmacy, University of Valencia, Avenida Vicente Andres Estellés s/n, Burjassot, 46100 Valencia, Spain; allomo3@alumni.uv.es
2 Department of Health Sciences, University of Florence, Viale GB Morgagni 48, 50134 Florence, Italy
3 Scuola Normale Superiore, Piazza dei Cavalieri 7, 56126 Pisa, Italy; lorenzo.cioni@sns.it
4 Hygiene and Public Health Unit, Department of Public Health, AUSL Imola, Viale Giovanni Amendola 2, 40026 Bologna, Italy; m.cancellieri@ausl.imola.bo.it (M.C.); Maria.M.Morales@uv.es (M.M.-S.-V.)
5 Biomedical Research Consortium in Epidemiology and Public Health Network (CIBERESP), Avenida Monforte de Lemos, 3-5. Pabellón 11. Planta 0, 28029 Madrid, Spain
* Correspondence: gadon@alumni.uv.es

Definition: Air pollution exposure is one of the greatest risks to health worldwide. It is estimated to be responsible for about 4.2 million deaths around the world every year owing to many serious diseases such as heart disease, stroke, acute and chronic respiratory diseases, and lung cancer. The WHO guideline limits are exceeded in several areas around the world, and it is estimated that about 90% of the world's population is exposed to high air pollution levels, especially in low- and middle-income countries. The COVID-19 pandemic has forced governments to implement severe mobility restriction measures to limit the spread of the virus. This represented a unique opportunity to study the impact of mobility on urban air quality. Several studies which have investigated the relations between the quality of the air and such containment measures have shown the significant reduction of the main pollutants in the urban environment so to encourage the adoption of new approaches for the improvement of the quality of air in the cities. The aims of this entry are both a brief analysis and a discussion of the results presented in several papers to understand the relationships between COVID-19 containment measures and air quality in urban areas.

Keywords: Covid-19; lockdown; air pollution

Citation: Donzelli, G.; Cioni, L.; Cancellieri, M.; Llopis-Morales, A.; Morales-Suárez-Varela, M. Air Quality during Covid-19 Lockdown. *Encyclopedia* **2021**, *1*, 519–526. https://doi.org/10.3390/encyclopedia1030043

Academic Editor: Stephen Bustin

Received: 23 June 2021
Accepted: 28 June 2021
Published: 1 July 2021

1. Introduction

Air pollution is a mixture of particles and gases whose sources and composition vary spatially and temporally. Air pollution in the environment derives both from anthropogenic and natural sources. While natural sources contribute mainly to air pollution in not anthropized regions (e.g., forest fires and dust storms), the contributions from human activities from anthropized regions far exceed the ones from natural sources [1].

The major anthropogenic sources of air pollution are [1]:

- Combustion of fuel in vehicle engines
- Heat and power plants
- Industrial facilities
- Waste incineration facilities
- Residential activities such as cooking, heating, and lighting with energy produced with the use of polluting fuels

The uncontrolled expansion of urban areas owing to the need to favor the then-nascent automotive industry represents one of the major factors for the acceleration of pollutants' emissions and diffusion.

Short- or long-term exposures to ambient air pollution represent high risks of both morbidity and mortality and contribute heavily to the global burden of disease. The most dangerous air pollutants are particulate matter (PM), nitrogen dioxide (NO_2), ozone (O_3), and sulfur dioxide (SO_2).

The main problem with most ambient air-polluting emissions is that, even if they derive from localized point sources, their effects are not confined to limited areas. In fact, it has been demonstrated that pollutants can travel long distances in a matter of days under favorable meteorological conditions. Therefore, health and air quality in remote areas can be affected by windblown dust, which contains high levels of particles, bacteria, and fungal spores, from desert regions like Mongolia, Africa, China, and Central Asia. Since air pollutants cross national borders over time, it seems clear that it is necessary to address this problem by adopting both global and local control policies to reduce emissions.

It is estimated that about 7 million individuals die worldwide each year due to high air pollution exposure. Ambient air pollution exposure is one of the greatest risks to health worldwide. It is estimated to be responsible for about 4.2 million deaths around the world every year owing to many serious diseases such as heart disease, stroke, acute and chronic respiratory diseases, and lung cancer. From an economic point of view, the total welfare loss in 2013 amounts to more than US$5 trillion in total welfare. According to the WHO, there is already ample evidence that children are more vulnerable to air pollution because they breathe more often, taking in more pollutants, and their nose and mouth are closer to the ground, which is where some pollutants are present in higher concentrations [2]. It is estimated that about 90% of the world's population is exposed to high air pollution levels, especially in low- and middle-income countries. [3]. WHO guideline values (Table 1) are set for the protection of health and are generally stricter than the comparable politically agreed-upon government standards [4]. WHO guidelines apply globally and are based on expert evaluation of current scientific evidence for the following pollutants: particulate matter (PM), ozone (O_3), nitrogen dioxide (NO_2), sulfur dioxide (SO_2) [5]. Most sources of outdoor air pollution are well beyond the control of both individuals and local authorities and require concerted actions from national and regional level policy-makers working in sectors like transports, energy productions, waste management, urban planning, industry, and agriculture [6].

Table 1. WHO air quality guidelines.

	Guideline Levels (μg/m^3)	
$PM_{2.5}$	1 year	10
	24 h (99th percentile)	25
PM_{10}	1 year	20
	24 h (99th percentile)	50
NO_2	1 year	40
	1 h	200
O_3	8 h, daily maximum	100
SO_2	24 h	20
	10 min	500

The set of mobility restrictive measures to limit the spread of COVID-19 imposed by the governments gave a unique opportunity to improve our understanding of the impact of mobility on air pollution in urban areas. Most governments have tried to contain the diffusion of COVID-19 through lockdowns, quarantines, and curfews, which have restricted people's movement, but for indispensable needs such as buying foods, work, and health-related issues. Moreover, all non-essential industries in most countries have been shut down, and people's movements were further restricted by imposing requirements for citizens to provide a signed justification to the authorities to be able to move both between and within cities. The effect of the lockdown on mobility was very relevant, and several studies have measured how lockdowns have modified mobility patterns at both country and local scales. For example, lockdown measures in France caused a 65% reduction in a countrywide number of displacements and were particularly effective in reducing work-related short-range mobility, especially during rush hours, and long-range recreational trips [7]. Another study highlighted that the adoption of strong and severe measures for the containment of the spreading of COVID-19 during the period from March to April 2020 generated a significant reduction in private vehicle trips in the city of Rome (−64.6% during the lockdown) [8]. Community Mobility Reports, which were created with aggregated, anonymized sets of data from users who have turned on the Location History setting from their Google Account, provide useful information for the researchers who want to study the relationship between air pollutants levels and lockdown measures. These Community Mobility Reports aim at providing insights into what has changed in response to the policies aimed at contrasting COVID-19. The reports chart movement trends over time by geography across different categories of places such as retail and recreation, groceries and pharmacies, parks, transit stations, workplaces, and residential [9]. Several studies used human mobility data collected from Google (at country-scale) mobility reports to examine the status of improved air quality in world cities due to COVID-19 that led to a temporary reduction in anthropogenic emissions [10]. For example, the analysis of the changes in air quality during the COVID-19 lockdown in Singapore used human mobility trends from Google [11], as well as a study that found empirical evidence for a relation between global vehicle transportation declines and the reduction of ambient NO_2 exposure [12].

This entry aims at obtaining a broad perspective on the impact of lockdown measures during the COVID-19 pandemic on the air quality in urban environments. For this purpose, we discussed the results reported by several studies in order to better understand the relationships between COVID-19 lockdown measures, the levels of the major pollutants in urban environments, and possibly identify which sectors contribute most to determining the levels of the pollutants. We included in this entry the following pollutants: $PM_{2.5}$, PM_{10}, NO_2, O_3, SO_2.

2. Association between Air Quality and Covid-19 Lockdown Measures

2.1. Particulate Matter

With the term Particulate Matter (PM), we denote a mixture of liquid droplets and solid particles that can be found in the air. PM is not a pollutant by itself but a complex and dynamic combination of compound particles with biological and chemical origins. The main components of PM are primarily sulfites, ammonia, nitrates, sodium chloride, mineral dust, black carbon, and water. Particles with an aerodynamic diameter less than 10 microns (PM_{10}) and fine particles of less than 2.5 microns width ($PM_{2.5}$) represent the greatest risks for health owing to their capability of penetrating human lungs and so enter into their bloodstream. Ambient PM, especially $PM_{2.5}$ [13], can also absorb poisonous pollutants, such as heavy metals, polycyclic aromatic hydrocarbons (PAHs), and VOCs. The main sources of PM include both diesel and petrol engines, the combustion of solid fuels such as coal, lignite, heavy oil, and biomass for the production of energy, as well as many other industrial activities such as building, mining, manufacture of cement, ceramic, and bricks, and smelting. Globally, 25% of urban ambient air pollution from $PM_{2.5}$ derives from traffic, 15% from industrial activities, 20% from domestic fuel burning, 22% from unspecified sources of human origin, and 18% from natural dust and salt [14]. Solutions for the sustainable reduction of ambient PM from traffic, industrial activities, and biomass burning should urgently be designed and implemented to reduce the air pollution in cities and the substantial disease burden it causes.

The comparative analysis of the PM_{10} and $PM_{2.5}$ concentrations were carried out in several studies between normal mobility and lockdown periods. One of these studies [15] analyzed $PM_{2.5}$ changes in the 50 most polluted capital cities in the world. The levels of air pollutants were collected from the air quality monitoring stations, which are provided by local environmental agencies. Overall, an average decrease of 12% of the $PM_{2.5}$ levels was observed. The highest decrease was observed in the African continent, followed by the American (22%) and the Asian (16%). In the European cities, in which we have an overall better air quality in normal times, only a reduction of 5% has been observed. A similar study carried out a comparative analysis of the variation in the PM_{10} and $PM_{2.5}$ levels of 12 cities from countries highly affected by COVID-19 [16]. The values of concentrations were collected from 162 air quality stations distributed in 12 selected cities. The concentration of $PM_{2.5}$ and PM_{10} were reduced by 20% and 34%, respectively, due to restrictions on anthropogenic emission sources during the lockdown. Other studies have focused on the study of the effects of Covid-19 lockdown measures on small–medium cities. For example, Donzelli et al. (2020) [17] studied the association between the mobility restrictions during the COVID-19 lockdown and the air pollutants levels recorded in three Italian cities, Florence, Pisa, and Lucca. For these aims, the authors also made use of meteorological data on rainfall, wind speed, temperature, relative humidity, and solar irradiance for the lockdown period and the same period of the preceding years. In fact, meteorological parameters have an important role in determining air pollution concentrations, so the authors decided to include these parameters in the analysis. Specifically for particulate matter, it is known that PM levels decrease with an increase in precipitation rate, wind speed, and temperature [18]. No evidence of a direct relationship was observed between the lockdown measures implemented by the Italian government and a reduction of PM in such cities, except in areas characterized by heavy vehicular traffic. This result is in line with the above-mentioned study, in which it was observed that the reductions in a European country of $PM_{2.5}$ are much smaller than in more heavily polluted areas of the planet. Moreover, the study of Dantas et al. (2020) [19] reported an increase in the PM_{10} concentrations in two air quality monitoring stations of the city of Rio de Janeiro, Brazil.

2.2. Nitrogen Dioxide

The main sources of nitrogen dioxide from human activities are constituted by power generation, traffic, and industry. It represents a relevant precursor of both ozone and particulate matter. Respiratory infections, as well as reduced lung function and growth and symptoms of bronchitis and asthma, can increase in people who are exposed to this type of pollutant. In addition, it is well known that nitrogen dioxide exposure is linked with higher morbidity and mortality rates related to cardiovascular and respiratory diseases.

Several studies have proved a reduction of the nitrogen dioxide (NO_2) concentrations during the lockdown period when confronted with the years or months before the lockdown. In general, reductions of concentrations in NO_2 are much more marked than those of PM, up to reaching reductions greater than 50% [20]. It is also possible to evaluate such reductions of concentrations using Tropospheric NO_2 vertical column density (VCD) from the TROPOspheric Monitoring Instrument (TROPOMI) [21]. This instrument has been used by Bassani et al. (2021) [22] for the evaluation of changes in the concentrations of NO_2 in Rome before and during the lockdown. The authors have observed reductions of 50%, 34%, and 20% at urban traffic, urban background, and rural background stations, respectively. Similarly, Donzelli et al. (2021) [23], nitric oxide levels were significantly reduced in seven air monitoring stations placed in the city of Valencia, Spain. Considerable NO_2 concentration variations between before and during the lockdown have been shown by several studies, like Mahato et al. (2020) [24], in which a reduction of 52.68% is documented. These results are also consistent with those presented in the paper of Baldasano (2020) [25], in which it was observed a significant decrease in NO_2 concentrations in Madrid and Barcelona of 62% and 50%, respectively. Another article adopted a machine learning technique so as to analyze the effect of the COVID-19 lockdown measures on main air pollutant levels from January to April 2020 in six Chinese megacities with different lockdown durations. The authors have estimated that the lockdown measures reduced ambient NO_2 concentrations by 36–53% during the most restrictive periods [26]. The concentration of NO_2 also showed a significant reduction of about 30% in the Gujarat state of western India, which has several cities characterized by poor air quality due to the presence of power plants, transportations, street dust, construction and brick kilns, and outdoor waste incineration, [27].

2.3. Ozone

Ground-level ozone (O_3), also known as tropospheric ozone, is among the most dangerous photochemical pollutants since people exposed to this type of pollutant are more at risk for the development of breathing problems, asthma, reduced lung function, and respiratory diseases. It falls in the class of secondary pollutants since it is not released directly into the atmosphere from the main sources of urban pollution, differently from what happens from primary pollutants. It is formed by the chemical reaction between carbon monoxide (CO), methane, or other volatile organic compounds (VOCs) and nitrogen oxides (NO_x); this process occurs in the presence of sunlight. In addition to their role as ozone precursors, CO, VOCs, and NO_x are by themselves dangerous air pollutants. The main sources of NOx and VOCs are traffic, industrial facilities, and chemical solvents. On the other hand, methane derives from waste, fossil fuels, and the agricultural industry. Aside from its health impacts, O_3 is one of the most impacting greenhouse gases and one of the most significant short-lived climate pollutants.

Compared to the other pollutants, O_3 concentrations show a different behavior since they exhibit a rise in terms of concentrations during the lockdown period. For example, one of the studies we took into consideration showed that the average daily concentrations of O_3 are significantly increased in urban stations by 14% in Rome, 24% in Nice, 2.4% in Valencia, 27% in Turin, and 36% in Wuhan during the lockdown in 2020 [28]. This different behavior can be explained by an unprecedented reduction in NO_x emissions, leading to a lower O_3 titration by NO. The above-mentioned study showed that no significant reductions in ozone levels were observed during the lockdown period. These results are confirmed by further studies, like the study that investigated the effects on air quality in Milan [29], where a marked increase in O_3 was reported. Moreover, Sharma et al. (2020) [30] and Tobías et al. (2020) [31] showed a rise of 17% and 57.7% in O_3 concentrations in India and Barcelona, respectively. Another study aimed at evaluating the Covid-19 lockdown impact on air pollutants levels in the Mexico City Metropolitan Area [32]. This study showed an increase of O_3 concentrations between 16% and 40% at the same sites where NO_2 decreased, and it suggested that in order to reduce the concentrations of O_3, the to be adopted policies should focus on the reduction of the emissions of VOCs from fixed sources. Moreover, Patel et al. (2020) showed that while all other pollutants showed a marked reduction in concentrations during the lockdown, O_3 recorded a statistically significant ($t = -3.59$, $p < 0.05$) increase in daily mean concentrations (5.52 $\mu g/m^{-3}$ (+16.7%)) in Auckland, New Zealand, an isolated city of the Southern Hemisphere which is largely unaffected by long-range pollution transports or industrial sources of air pollution [33].

2.4. Sulfur Dioxide

The main sources of sulfur dioxide (SO_2) are constituted by the burning of fossil fuels (e.g., oil and coal) and the smelting of mineral ores that contain sulfur. People exposed to SO_2 are more at risk of developing damages to the respiratory system and the functionality of the lungs, as well as eye irritation. It is known that some pre-existing diseases, such as chronic bronchitis and asthma, can be aggravated in exposed people. Moreover, it is shown an increased risk of infections responsible for raised visits to emergency rooms and hospital admissions. If SO_2 reacts with water molecules in the atmosphere, it forms sulfuric acid, which is the main component of acid rain and one of the main causes of damage to the forests, freshwaters, and soils.

Changes in SO_2 concentrations were studied by several researchers. For example, Otmani et al. (2020) [34] assessed the variation of SO_2 concentrations in the ambient air of Salé city before and during the few days into the implementation of the lockdown measures. The authors reported a reduction of 49% of SO_2 levels, even though the low

SO_2 concentrations recorded in the full study period do not allow for evidencing a definite trend. An analysis produced using data from the Tropomi instrument on the Copernicus Sentinel-5P satellite showed that concentrations of SO_2 in polluted areas in India have decreased by about 40% between April 2019 and April 2020 [35]. These results were also confirmed by a study investigating how levels of SO_2 in four Tunisian cities varied during the months from January to April 2020. The authors reported reductions in all the cities up to 52% [36].

3. Conclusions

Based on the analyzed papers, we can state that there is evidence from various data and studies that there has been a reduction in air pollution all over the world. Although most of the studies reported significant reductions in the levels of some pollutants, we believe that these results should be interpreted with caution due to the lack of some data in the analysis. It is likely that some studies have overestimated the reductions, for example, not considering the long-term trends as potential confounding [37]. In fact, the comparisons between the pollution levels of the pandemic year with the previous years are intrinsically subject to distortions due to the simple fact that each year is characterized by different conditions, for example, economic conditions, that have not been duly assessed. With regard to meteorological conditions, the majority of studies took into consideration the atmospheric parameters to reduce the bias in the data analyses. We must also point out that different methodologies were used in the different studies, so that it is hard to compare the different results. For example, regarding the period of times which were compared, we noticed that some studies compared the air pollutants concentrations before and during the lockdown, while other compared the previous year (2019) with the first pandemic year (2020) and still others the mean concentrations of the previous five years (2015–2019). Furthermore, there were differences among the containment measures adopted by different governments, so that it is not easy to compare the reductions of the air pollutants under study directly. Finally, various analytic techniques were used by different authors, which used both classical approaches like statistical tests and more advanced methods like machine learning.

However, we can conclude that the implementation of the lockdown measures reduced the levels of PM_{10} and $PM_{2.5}$ in most areas under study. Notwithstanding this, we should consider that this difference is more important in most pollutant areas of the planet, while smaller effects were observed in the European countries in which the air quality is generally better. We must remember that some studies did not observe a decrease in PM levels, and others did not detect a significant difference with the periods of normality mobility. Regarding NO_2, the reductions appear more marked and more homogeneously distributed in the various areas of the globe than those of PM. Most of the studies reported changes in concentrations not smaller than 50%. However, reductions in NO_2 concentration cannot be conclusively calculated without adjusting for long-term trends, which may partially contribute to confounding bias [38]. In fact, it was observed that trends in NO_2 concentrations have gradually decreased in the last decade due to the change in industrial and vehicular emissions obtained thanks to technological and economic development and emission regulations [39]. Moreover, SO_2 concentrations decreased during the lockdown period, though with more modest changes. Conversely, concentrations of O_3 increased in different cities due to the significant lowering of the NO concentration in the lockdown period, which, in turn, reacts with O_3 to cause higher O_3 concentrations than average. This suggests the need for a holistic approach when we have to implement policies to improve the air quality and protect both human health and the environment.

Author Contributions: Conceptualization, M.M.-S.-V. and G.D.; writing—original draft preparation, G.D., L.C., M.C. and A.L.-M.; writing—review and editing, M.M.-S.-V. and G.D.; supervision, M.M.-S.-V. All authors have read and agreed to the published version of the manuscript.

Funding: This research received no external funding.

Acknowledgments: We wish to thank Maria Grazia De Agazio for proofreading, editing, and assisting with translating the manuscript into English.

Conflicts of Interest: The authors declare no conflict of interest.

Entry Link on the Encyclopedia Platform: https://encyclopedia.pub/12559.

References

1. WHO. Ambient Air Pollution: Pollutants. Available online: https://www.who.int/airpollution/ambient/pollutants/en/ (accessed on 10 October 2020).
2. WHO. WHO | Air Pollution and Child Health: Prescribing Clean Air. Available online: http://www.who.int/ceh/publications/air-pollution-child-health/en/ (accessed on 29 April 2021).
3. WHO. WHO | Ambient Air Pollution. Available online: http://www.who.int/airpollution/ambient/en/ (accessed on 29 April 2021).
4. European Environment Agency Air Quality Standards. Available online: https://www.eea.europa.eu/themes/air/air-quality-concentrations/air-quality-standards (accessed on 28 October 2020).
5. WHO. WHO | Air Quality Guidelines—Global Update 2005. Available online: http://www.who.int/airpollution/publications/aqg2005/en/ (accessed on 29 April 2021).
6. WHO Health Organization. Ambient (Outdoor) Air Pollution. Available online: https://www.who.int/news-room/fact-sheets/detail/ambient-(outdoor)-air-quality-and-health (accessed on 3 March 2020).
7. Pullano, G.; Valdano, E.; Scarpa, N.; Rubrichi, S.; Colizza, E.V. Population mobility reductions during COVID-19 epidemic in France under lockdown. *medRxiv* **2020**. [CrossRef]
8. Aletta, F.; Brinchi, S.; Carrese, S.; Gemma, A.; Guattari, C.; Mannini, L.; Patella, S.M. Analysing urban traffic volumes and mapping noise emissions in Rome (Italy) in the context of containment measures for the COVID-19 disease. *Noise Mapp.* **2020**, *7*, 114–122. [CrossRef]
9. COVID-19 Community Mobility Report. Available online: https://www.google.com/covid19/mobility?hl=en (accessed on 29 April 2021).
10. Sannigrahi, S.; Kumar, P.; Molter, A.; Zhang, Q.; Basu, B.; Basu, A.S.; Pilla, F. Examining the status of improved air quality in world cities due to COVID-19 led temporary reduction in anthropogenic emissions. *Environ. Res.* **2021**, *196*, 110927. [CrossRef] [PubMed]
11. Li, J.; Tartarini, F. Changes in Air Quality during the COVID-19 Lockdown in Singapore and associations with Human Mobility Trends. *Aerosol Air Qual. Res.* **2020**, *20*, 1748–1758. [CrossRef]
12. Venter, Z.S.; Aunan, K.; Chowdhury, S.; Lelieveld, J. COVID-19 lockdowns cause global air pollution declines. *Proc. Natl. Acad. Sci. USA* **2020**, *117*, 18984–18990. [CrossRef] [PubMed]
13. Ramli, N.A.; Yusof, N.F.F.M.; Shith, S.; Suroto, A. Chemical and Biological Compositions Associated with Ambient Respirable Particulate Matter: A Review. *Water Air Soil Pollut.* **2020**, *231*, 1–14. [CrossRef]
14. Karagulian, F.; Belis, C.A.; Dora, C.F.C.; Prüss-Ustün, A.M.; Bonjour, S.; Adair-Rohani, H.; Amann, M. Contributions to cities' ambient particulate matter (PM): A systematic review of local source contributions at global level. *Atmos. Environ.* **2015**, *120*, 475–483. [CrossRef]
15. Rodríguez-Urrego, D.; Rodríguez-Urrego, L. Air quality during the COVID-19: PM2.5 analysis in the 50 most polluted capital cities in the world. *Environ. Pollut.* **2020**, *266*, 115042. [CrossRef]
16. Kumari, P.; Toshniwal, D. Impact of lockdown on air quality over major cities across the globe during COVID-19 pandemic. *Urban Clim.* **2020**, *34*, 100719. [CrossRef]
17. Donzelli, G.; Cioni, L.; Cancellieri, M.; Morales, A.L.; Suárez-Varela, M.M. The Effect of the Covid-19 Lockdown on Air Quality in Three Italian Medium-Sized Cities. *Atmosphere* **2020**, *11*, 1118. [CrossRef]
18. Galindo, N.; Varea, M.; Gil-Moltó, J.; Yubero, E.; Nicolás, J. The Influence of Meteorology on Particulate Matter Concentrations at an Urban Mediterranean Location. *Water Air Soil Pollut.* **2010**, *215*, 365–372. [CrossRef]
19. Dantas, G.; Siciliano, B.; França, B.B.; da Silva, C.M.; Arbilla, G. The impact of COVID-19 partial lockdown on the air quality of the city of Rio de Janeiro, Brazil. *Sci. Total. Environ.* **2020**, *729*, 139085. [CrossRef] [PubMed]
20. Nakada, L.Y.K.; Urban, R.C. COVID-19 pandemic: Impacts on the air quality during the partial lockdown in São Paulo state, Brazil. *Sci. Total. Environ.* **2020**, *730*, 139087. [CrossRef] [PubMed]
21. Home | Tropomi. Available online: http://www.tropomi.eu/ (accessed on 29 April 2021).
22. Bassani, C.; Vichi, F.; Esposito, G.; Montagnoli, M.; Giusto, M.; Ianniello, A. Nitrogen dioxide reductions from satellite and surface observations during COVID-19 mitigation in Rome (Italy). *Environ. Sci. Pollut. Res.* **2021**, *28*, 22981–23004. [CrossRef]
23. Donzelli, G.; Cioni, L.; Cancellieri, M.; Llopis-Morales, A.; Morales-Suárez-Varela, M. Relations between Air Quality and Covid-19 Lockdown Measures in Valencia, Spain. *Int. J. Environ. Res. Public Health* **2021**, *18*, 2296. [CrossRef]
24. Mahato, S.; Pal, S.; Ghosh, K.G. Effect of lockdown amid COVID-19 pandemic on air quality of the megacity Delhi, India. *Sci. Total. Environ.* **2020**, *730*, 139086. [CrossRef] [PubMed]
25. Baldasano, J.M. COVID-19 lockdown effects on air quality by NO_2 in the cities of Barcelona and Madrid (Spain). *Sci. Total. Environ.* **2020**, *741*, 140353. [CrossRef] [PubMed]

26. Wang, Y.; Wen, Y.; Wang, Y.; Zhang, S.; Zhang, K.M.; Zheng, H.; Xing, J.; Wu, Y.; Hao, J. Four-Month Changes in Air Quality during and after the COVID-19 Lockdown in Six Megacities in China. *Environ. Sci. Technol. Lett.* **2020**, *7*, 802–808. [CrossRef]
27. Selvam, S.; Muthukumar, P.; Venkatramanan, S.; Roy, P.; Bharath, K.M.; Jesuraja, K. SARS-CoV-2 pandemic lockdown: Effects on air quality in the industrialized Gujarat state of India. *Sci. Total. Environ.* **2020**, *737*, 140391. [CrossRef]
28. Sicard, P.; De Marco, A.; Agathokleous, E.; Feng, Z.; Xu, X.; Paoletti, E.; Rodriguez, J.J.D.; Calatayud, V. Amplified ozone pollution in cities during the COVID-19 lockdown. *Sci. Total. Environ.* **2020**, *735*, 139542. [CrossRef] [PubMed]
29. Collivignarelli, M.C.; Abbà, A.; Bertanza, G.; Pedrazzani, R.; Ricciardi, P.; Miino, M.C. Lockdown for CoViD-2019 in Milan: What are the effects on air quality? *Sci. Total. Environ.* **2020**, *732*, 139280. [CrossRef]
30. Sharma, S.; Zhang, M.; Gao, J.; Zhang, H.; Kota, S.H. Effect of restricted emissions during COVID-19 on air quality in India. *Sci. Total. Environ.* **2020**, *728*, 138878. [CrossRef] [PubMed]
31. Tobías, A.; Carnerero, C.; Reche, C.; Massagué, J.; Via, M.; Minguillón, M.C.; Alastuey, A.; Querol, X. Changes in air quality during the lockdown in Barcelona (Spain) one month into the SARS-CoV-2 epidemic. *Sci. Total. Environ.* **2020**, *726*, 138540. [CrossRef] [PubMed]
32. Hernández-Paniagua, I.Y.; Valdez, S.I.; Almanza, V.; Rivera-Cárdenas, C.; Grutter, M.; Stremme, W.; García-Reynoso, A.; Ruiz-Suárez, L.G. Impact of the COVID-19 Lockdown on Air Quality and Resulting Public Health Benefits in the Mexico City Metropolitan Area. *Front. Public Health* **2021**, *9*, 642630. [CrossRef] [PubMed]
33. Patel, H.; Talbot, N.; Salmond, J.; Dirks, K.; Xie, S.; Davy, P. Implications for air quality management of changes in air quality during lockdown in Auckland (New Zealand) in response to the 2020 SARS-CoV-2 epidemic. *Sci. Total. Environ.* **2020**, *746*, 141129. [CrossRef] [PubMed]
34. Otmani, A.; Benchrif, A.; Tahri, M.; Bounakhla, M.; Chakir, E.M.; El Bouch, M.; Krombi, M. Impact of Covid-19 lockdown on PM10, SO2 and NO2 concentrations in Salé City (Morocco). *Sci. Total. Environ.* **2020**, *735*, 139541. [CrossRef]
35. Sulphur Dioxide Concentrations Drop over India during COVID-19. Available online: https://www.esa.int/Applications/Observing_the_Earth/Copernicus/Sentinel-5P/Sulphur_dioxide_concentrations_drop_over_India_during_COVID-19 (accessed on 29 April 2021).
36. Chekir, N.; Ben Salem, Y. What is the relationship between the coronavirus crisis and air pollution in Tunisia? *Euro-Mediterr. J. Environ. Integr.* **2021**, *6*, 1–9. [CrossRef] [PubMed]
37. Shi, Z.; Song, C.; Liu, B.; Lu, G.; Xu, J.; Van Vu, T.; Elliott, R.J.R.; Li, W.; Bloss, W.J.; Harrison, R.M. Abrupt but smaller than expected changes in surface air quality attributable to COVID-19 lockdowns. *Sci. Adv.* **2021**, *7*, eabd6696. [CrossRef]
38. Misra, P.; Takigawa, M.; Khatri, P.; Dhaka, S.K.; Dimri, A.P.; Yamaji, K.; Kajino, M.; Takeuchi, W.; Imasu, R.; Nitta, K.; et al. Nitrogen oxides concentration and emission change detection during COVID-19 restrictions in North India. *Sci. Rep.* **2021**, *11*, 1–11. [CrossRef]
39. Lamsal, L.N.; Duncan, B.N.; Yoshida, Y.; Krotkov, N.A.; Pickering, K.E.; Streets, D.G.; Lu, Z.U.S. NO_2 trends (2005–2013): EPA Air Quality System (AQS) data versus improved observations from the Ozone Monitoring Instrument (OMI). *Atmos. Environ.* **2015**, *110*, 130–143. [CrossRef]

encyclopedia

MDPI

Entry

COVID-19 and Dentistry

Hugh Devlin [1] and Parisa Soltani [2,*]

[1] Division of Dentistry, School of Medical Sciences, Faculty of Biology, Medicine & Health, The University of Manchester, Manchester M13 9PL, UK; hugh.devlin@manchester.ac.uk

[2] Department of Oral and Maxillofacial Radiology, Dental Implants Research Center, Dental Research Institute, School of Dentistry, Isfahan University of Medical Sciences, Isfahan 81746, Iran

* Correspondence: p.soltani@dnt.mui.ac.ir

Definition: Dentistry is a healthcare profession requiring close contacts between the dental practitioner and the patient. In particular, many dental procedures generate aerosols and droplets which are proved to be the major transmission route for COVID-19.

Keywords: COVID-19; SARS-CoV-2; dentistry

1. A Global Perspective

According to the World Health Organization (WHO), the coronavirus disease 2019 (COVID-19) pandemic had, of April 2021, killed 2,850,521 people with most countries affected. The USA has accounted for nearly 20% of these deaths. There are many reasons for the wide disparity in death rates of different countries, such as the societal and political reactions to the infection, the clustering of infection in large cities, habitation in crowded multi-generation households as well as the underlying health and age profile of the population. Although the fatality rate is below 1% of the population, those infected can require mechanical ventilation and can suffer prolonged symptoms during their recovery phase. The most common of these post-infection symptoms include insomnia, fatigue and memory loss. About 2% of patients who have suffered COVID-19 go on to have these symptoms for more than 3 months.

The COVID-19 pandemic has ravaged Europe, India and the Americas, while countries such as China and South Korea have put in place containment measures quickly and thereby reduced the spread of the disease. Thailand and Vietnam are examples of countries that had minor outbreaks that were quickly controlled. New Zealand, Australia and China quickly contained the disease in their countries and then put in place strict border controls to prevent re-infections coming into the country. China, Hong Kong, Singapore, and Taiwan had previous experience with severe acute respiratory syndrome (SARS), a coronavirus outbreak in 2002–2003. Both SARS and COVID-19 are spread by droplet infection and can cause a severe respiratory illness. The Chinese government eradicated SARS by taking containment measures such as cancelling the 1 May national holiday, instituting school closures, etc. This demonstrated the value of lockdown measures.

With the present COVID-19 pandemic, those countries that were slow to put containment measures in place have seen the worst rise in deaths. Containment measures include prohibiting social gathering and instituting testing programmes, tracing those who test positive, and requiring them to self-isolate. With re-emergence of the infection in second and third waves, political leadership has been needed to combat public complacency. With continued spread of the virus, variants have arisen due to genetic drift (UK variant B117 variant; South African variant (B1351, 501Y, V2) and the Brazilian variant (P1 variant)). These variants are more transmissible.

At the peak of the pandemic, the health system in Italy was put under great pressure, which forced the Italian government to close all non-essential businesses and industries in March 2020. Governments have used the lockdown measures to protect their health

Citation: Devlin, H.; Soltani, P. COVID-19 and Dentistry. *Encyclopedia* **2021**, *1*, 496–504. https://doi.org/10.3390/encyclopedia1020041

Academic Editor: Stephen Bustin

Received: 20 May 2021
Accepted: 17 June 2021
Published: 21 June 2021

systems and prevent them from being overwhelmed. The pandemic has seen a general reorganisation of the healthcare workforce with volunteers and retired clinicians helping to fill gaps left by staff falling sick. Healthcare workers have suffered increases in stress-related illness due to changes in routine [1]. In most African countries (except South Africa) there have been comparatively fewer infections per head of the population. However, developing countries have limited resources to undertake mass testing and intensive care facilities are inadequate.

In those countries that have quickly rolled out an effective vaccination programme, such as USA and the United Kingdom, a reduced infection rate has resulted. There is a disparity between the vaccination rates of these wealthier countries that can afford the vaccines and that of developing countries which do not have the necessary resources to cope. COVAX is a programme coordinated by the World Health Organization that aims to ensure fairer vaccine access and it should result in a wider distribution of vaccines later in 2021.

2. Dentistry and Coronavirus Disease 2019 (COVID-19)

Patients infected with severe acute respiratory syndrome coronavirus 2 (SARS-CoV-2) may be asymptomatic or develop symptoms such as a cough, fever and a loss of smell. Some patients develop more severe symptoms such as difficulty in breathing that may require hospitalization, intubation and oxygen therapy. The disease spreads by droplet transmission, so it might reasonably be hypothesized that dentists would be among the professions with the highest death rate if they had continued treatment in the same way as pre-pandemic. For deaths in the England and Wales registered between March and December 2020, there is no evidence that dentists suffered a higher death rate due to COVID-19 [2]. However, any analysis by occupation is difficult as there are many other factors that cannot be quantified easily e.g., occupation of a partner, the use of personal protective equipment, the gender and age mix in a profession and other socio-economic factors which may be more important in predicting whether an individual becomes infected and dies. During the pandemic, dentists in the UK changed to providing a triage system involving remote consultations to assess the risk of transmission with treatment limited to advice, analgesia and antimicrobial treatment in the first instance. Those patients with confirmed COVID-19 were referred for face-to-face care at designated Urgent Dental Care Centres only. The low infection rate amongst dentists is due to these safety policies, measuring the temperature of patients and staff, the disinfection of surfaces and the wearing of personal protective equipment.

In a web survey of US dentists held in June 2020, 20 of the 2195 respondents (0.91%) reported that they had been infected with SARS-CoV-2, but only a relatively small minority of respondents had received a SARS-CoV-2 test (16.6%) to prove their infectivity [3]. A large proportion of individuals who become infected remain asymptomatic which is problematic in a self-completed questionnaire. The true figure of infected dentists may not be known.

When the pandemic struck, regulatory agencies across the European Union required dentists to limit the treatment provided to patients and provided financial relief to a varying extent.

3. Transmission of COVID-19

The spread of the virus SARS-CoV-2 is by droplet infection in the community. Spread occurs from those who are infected but also from asymptomatic individuals and those in the early stages of the disease who have not yet shown symptoms. Data from China has shown that asymptomatic and symptomatic patients have the same amount of viral load [4]. Asymptomatic individuals might unknowingly spread the disease, a difficult problem for authorities trying to control the viral spread. Up-to-date information about the spread of the virus is essential, especially where local "hot-spots" are present so that effective community containment measures can be put in place. Rapid testing of infected individuals allows those who test positive to self-isolate and prevent the spread of the disease. Additionally, the contacts of those testing positive also need to be traced and asked to self-isolate. This requires considerable expenditure and use of resources, which are not readily available in poorer countries.

A false positive test happens when the test is positive but the reality is that no disease is present. A false negative occurs when the patient truly has the disease but the test says he does not. Brooks and Das [5] provide an online modelling calculator which allows the reader to calculate the risks and costs associated with COVID tests of different false positive and false negative results. They showed that when the prevalence of the disease is low, the cost of false positives is greater than that of true positives. As the prevalence of the disease declines, the significance of a false positive result becomes evident by the number of individuals that unnecessarily self-isolate [6]. This can have severe consequences for patient care if nurses and doctors are affected as they are then unable to care for patients.

A positive diagnosis of SARS-CoV-2 infection depends on the detection of viral RNA. The gold standard method uses an automated reverse transcription polymerase chain reaction (RT-PCR) method, which allows rapid testing of larger numbers of samples than manual methods [7]. Other antigen tests are available, but are less sensitive as they do not amplify the antigen. However, they may provide a cheaper and more affordable alternative to poorer countries.

The pathogenicity of the virus derives from the nucleocapsid protein inside the virus and an external spike glycoprotein [8]. In addition, changes in the spike protein may increase the viral infectivity [9]. It is the receptor-binding domain on the spike protein which binds to the respiratory cellular surface angiotensin convertase enzyme 2 (ACE2) receptor to gain entry into the cell. Many vaccines have been targeted at the spike protein in view of its essential role in viral transmission.

The RT-PCR test is unable to provide any information about whether an individual has had a past infection. That information is only available with the antibody test. IGG and IGM antibodies to SARS-CoV-2 only become detectable at one to three weeks after the onset of the infection. Although not known definitively, the presence of SARS-CoV-2 IgG does not indicate immunity to further infection. However, in experiments in macaque monkeys infected with SARS-CoV-2 it was shown that they had some immunity to re-infection for about one month [10]. However, this paper was in a pre-print form and, therefore, not peer-reviewed.

4. Protection Mechanisms in the Dental Setting

Vaccination has provided an effective method of controlling the spread of COVID-19. By taking the vaccine, healthcare workers are, therefore, protecting themselves and their patients, but some people have legitimate reasons for not having the vaccine. Extremely rarely, some patients have reported blood clots with low levels of platelets (thrombocytopenia) after receiving the AstraZeneca COVID-19 vaccine. Those affected may complain of persistent headache or abdominal pain, or swelling of the legs for four or more days after the injection. For the older population, the risk to benefit ratio is heavily in favour of receiving the vaccine. At the other end of the age spectrum, deaths due to COVID-19 in children have been extremely rare [11].

Use of dental handpieces can generate aerosols in the dental office that have the potential to spread infection if inhaled. Advice on measures to protect dental staff and patients undertaking aerosol generating procedures is given by the Care Quality Commission as follows-

https://www.cqc.org.uk/guidance-providers/dentists/dental-mythbuster-31 personal-protective-equipment-requirements-during (Accessed on 19 April 2021).

This includes dental staff wearing "a long-sleeved disposable fluid repellent gown (covering the arms and body) or disposable fluid repellent coveralls, a filtering face piece class 3 (FFP3) respirator, a full-face shield or visor and gloves". The fit of the respirator should be checked to ensure that all airborne particles are excluded.

A recent review examined whether providing antimicrobial mouthwashes prior to undertaking a dental procedure would be beneficial in preventing the spread of COVID-19 [12]. Although this found no completed randomized controlled trials, the issue requires investigation as it may provide benefits. On the other hand, the medicaments used may produce allergic reactions or staining of the teeth depending on which one is used.

Hand washing by all dental staff is important to prevent infection and should be undertaken before putting on and after removing the personal protective equipment. Patients should be given access to alcohol disinfection rubs and asked to avoid touching their eyes, nose and mouth. It is reassuring that due to widespread dissemination of public health measures, surveys of the general public show a good knowledge of the routes of transmission and adherence to personal protection procedures [13].

5. Oral Symptoms

Containment of this infection in any healthcare setting must involve reduction of saliva and droplet spread. The ribonucleic acid (RNA) of SARS-CoV-2 is present in saliva samples of patients [14] and salivary glands and can be a reservoir for SARS-CoV-2 in infected patients. In experiments involving infection of rhesus macaque monkeys with SARS-CoV-2, the epithelial cells of the salivary duct cells were infected early [15]. Indeed, expression of ACE2 receptors is shown to be higher in minor salivary glands compared with the lungs [16]. Case reports describe symptoms of inflammation of the parotid salivary gland in patients with confirmed COVID-19 [17,18]. Sialadenitis can lead to salivary retention and reduced salivary flow, which can contribute to xerostomia and altered taste sensation.

Loss of taste and smell are some of the earliest symptoms of SARS-COV-2 infection and could form an important early screening test in predicting the spread of the disease in the population. The aetiology of these symptoms is not known, but could involve damage to the receptors or nerves. SARS-COV-2 can cause direct neural invasion, spread via the blood stream or via infected leukocytes. The virus has been detected post mortem in the brain neural and capillary endothelial cells [19].

According to a recent systematic review, the most common oral manifestations of COVID-19 are taste disorders with an overall prevalence of 45%. Among different gustatory dysfunctions, dysgeusia, distorted taste perception, is more common, followed by hypogeusia, which is a decrease in taste sensitivity, and ageusia, lack of taste sensation [20]. However, prevalence of taste alterations varies between 11% to 88% in different studies [21]. The mean duration for gustatory disorders was reported to be 15 days [20]. A prospective case-control study with a 6-month follow-up showed that gustatory dysfunctions resolved partially or totally in 88% of the cases. Oral dyspnea and nasal obstruction were reported to be risk factors for poor gustatory recovery [22]. In addition, according to another study, subjects with severe loss of taste recovered later than those with mild loss [23]. Taste alteration significantly correlated with mild/moderate COVID-19 cases and was more prevalent in female patients [20]. Paderno et al. [23] hypothesize that gustatory dysfunction is secondary to high oral viral load, leading to neural damage. Therefore, virus-induced neural disturbance could last much longer that the presence of the virus itself [24]. Additionally, COVID-19-induced sialadenitis can result in changes in salivary flow rate and eventually cause altered taste sensation [25].

Oral mucosal lesions subsequent to COVID-19 infection can vary in location, size, appearance and quantity. The observed lesions are either ulcers, erosions, bullae, vesicles, pustules, or a fissured or depapillated tongue, macules, papules, plaques, pigmentation, whitish areas, hemorrhagic crusts, necrosis, petechiae, swelling, erythema, xerostomia and spontaneous bleeding [26,27]. Based on a systematic review of case reports, oral lesions were more common on the tongue, labial mucosa and palate [20]. Based on another review study, patients with oral mucosal lesions had symptoms such as burning sensation, pain, and pruritus in 68% of the cases. The time between onset of systemic symptoms of COVID-19 and oral mucosal lesions was from 4 days prior to 12 weeks after the systemic symptoms, although in some cases oral lesions preceded systemic symptoms [26]. In addition, these lesions healed within 3–28 days after appearance by topical or systemic treatments, oral hygiene, or spontaneously [20,26]. A suggested differential diagnosis of the oral mucosal lesions includes aphthous stomatitis, herpetiform lesions, mucositis, drug-induced eruption, necrotizing periodontal disease, Kawasaki-like lesions, erythema-multiform-like lesions, angina bullosa-like lesions, angular cheilitis, atypical Sweet syndrome, and Melkerson–Rosenthal syndrome [26]. As mentioned, ACE2 receptors are abundantly expressed in the oral cavity cells. Interaction of this transmembrane receptor with the spike protein of SARS-CoV-2 allows for merging of the virus with the cell. Similar to other viral infections, the genetic material of the virus then uses the cell organelles for replication, ultimately ending in lysis of infected cells. This process can manifest as different oral lesions reported in the literature. However, other infectious, inflammatory, and autoimmune disorders, such as opportunistic infections, medication-related effects, and multi-system involvement can also play a role in the pathogenesis of oral mucosal lesions.

The presence of ACE2 and other receptors linked to COVID-19 infection have been demonstrated in human pulpal and periodontal cells and has prompted researchers to hypothesize links between COVID-19 infection and pulpitis and periodontitis [28–31]. However, these hypotheses still need to be backed by stronger evidence.

6. Role of Saliva as a Diagnostic Tool

The standard method for detection of SARS-CoV-2 is RT-PCR of samples from oropharyngeal or nasopharyngeal swabs. Saliva samples have also been considered as potential diagnostic specimens for detection of viral particles. In contrast to oropharyngeal or nasopharyngeal samples, collection of salivary samples does not require trained healthcare staff and can be self-administered. This option can be helpful in decreasing the exposure of public and healthcare personnel to infection with SARS-CoV-2 through reducing unnecessary visits of potentially infected people to medical laboratories. Moreover, alleviating the workload could reduce human-resource costs. In addition, collecting salivary samples is easier and more comfortable than pharyngeal or sputum specimens [32–34]. Several studies have attempted to compare the diagnostic value of salivary samples in detection of SARS-CoV-2 RNA with nasopharyngeal swabs. Hanege et al. compared the positivity rate of different body fluids in confirmed COVID-19 cases. They found that saliva has the highest positivity rate (76.3%), followed by tears (55.3%) and cerumen (39.5%) [35]. In another study, Nacher et al. reported a sensitivity of 77% and 24% for symptomatic and asymptomatic patients for salivary samples, respectively. Based on their findings, the sensitivity considerably decreases in patients who have no COVID-19 symptoms. Another interesting finding in their study was that about 6% of their enrolled cases had negative nasopharyngeal swabs, while their salivary specimen was positive for the presence of SARS-CoV-2 RNA [36]. This can be partly due to the difficulty of obtaining proper pharyngeal samples which can cause patient discomfort. A meta-analysis showed a sensitivity of 91% (confidence interval (CI) 80–99%) for saliva samples compared with 98% (CI 89–100%) for nasopharyngeal swabbing [37]. The specificity of saliva samples is also reported to be not higher than 42% [38]. Additionally, a systematic review of articles reported that saliva can be effectively used for short- and long-term monitoring of humoral immunity against SARS-CoV-2 through primary infection or vaccines [39].

Three conditions are required for optimal salivary testing of SARS-CoV-2: a standardized method for collecting saliva must be selected based on studies comparing different methods of salivary collection; an optimal transport and storage medium for saliva specimens must be introduced; and an appropriate RNA assay must be optimized for detection of viral RNA within saliva samples [40,41]. Accordingly, the Food and Drug Administration (FDA) has granted emergency use authorization to some saliva-based SARS-CoV-2 test kits [37]. Several rapid salivary testing kits are used for mass screening purposes. However, negative rapid testing in the presence of symptoms of COVID-19 infection might show the need for pharyngeal swabbing techniques.

7. Dental Education during the COVID-19 Pandemic

The COVID-19 pandemic situation has considerably affected higher education and dental education in particular. Dentistry is a scientific field which deals with hands-on practice as well as theoretical science. Dental education requires sufficient pre-clinical and clinical training in order to ensure that the future dental professionals are competent. It is probable that the most important challenge in dental education during the ongoing pandemic is trying to balance maintaining the health of students, faculty members, personnel, and patients with the continuity in dental educational programs in the dynamic and ever-changing setting of a health crisis. Although regional differences between the lockdown policies, outbreak severity, and availability of resources all influence the function of dental schools during the pandemic, the response of dental educational institutions to the COVID-19 pandemic has some similarities [42]. For instance, distance learning has come to the forefront of theoretical dental education in many institutions. While e-learning has been around for quite some time, it has flourished as a result of the COVID-19 pandemic. Synchronous online teaching methods can be employed when interaction with the participants is required. Asynchronous methods can also be used but the instructor must ensure that the educational content is delivered in the most efficient way. Different online platforms have been used by dental schools for organizing video conferences, journal clubs, and webinars [43]. However, access to a high-speedinternet connection is an obstacle for many dental students and faculty members in different geographical locations, which can worsen the educational inequality within an institution or among different institutions.

While distance learning might be a commonly adopted strategy for higher education in different fields, a unique challenge for dental education is reliance on clinical experience requirements for achieving competency in performing dental treatments. As many of these dental procedures produce considerable amounts of aerosols and droplets, health authorities have recommended suspension of routine and elective dental treatments. Therefore, the practical training of novice dental students has been affected by the current pandemic state. Dental educators have innovatively responded to these challenges. For instance, virtual slides using full-slide images have yielded positive outcomes for oral pathology courses compared with conventional microscopic training [44]. Using virtual patients is another case-based teaching strategy to improve the students' diagnostic and clinical judgement skills. A foreseeable perspective in dental laboratory and pre-clinical education is using virtual reality systems [45]. With the ongoing pandemic, university administrations must look into different strategies to ensure sufficient competency of graduated dentists in clinical settings, namely extending the duration of clinical courses and planned patient recruitment, or revising clinical requirements for different practical courses.

8. What Is the Future Post-COVID-19?

The future patient experience of dentistry depends on any further mutations of the virus, which will govern its infectivity and virulence. Almost certainly, ongoing strict procedures to eliminate the spread of COVID-19 will be needed in dental surgeries, especially where aerosol generating procedures are involved. This will involve wearing appropriate personal protective equipment, such as FFP2 or FFP3 masks, and regular swab testing of dental staff for infection. There was early enthusiasm that hydroxychloroquine or azithromycin would be effective treatments against COVID-19. Azithromycin is a safe, broad spectrum antibiotic that has been shown to have some in vitro action against the Zika virus and rhinovirus [46]. Hydroxychloroquine is already used to prevent and treat malaria. Clinical trials are ongoing to determine the effectiveness of both drugs but, at present, COVID-19 containment relies on public health measures and vaccination programmes.

There is a considerable backlog of dental need since lockdown began early in 2020, but the landscape is changing with many calls in different countries for a reorganisation of the provision of dentistry. Whether patients return to have routine care in the post-COVID era is unknown, but given the reluctance of many dentists to undertake aerosol-generating procedures, they will have a greater emphasis on minimally invasive dentistry and preventive dentistry in their daily practice. Dental teachers are also re-thinking the way they provide education for dental students. The theoretical content of these courses can be shared online using video conferencing and webinar tools. This has required adaptation by teachers and students.

For many, the era of the daily commute to work has ended as they have found that it is more productive to work from home, but it has created a sense of isolation and an increased prevalence of mental stress and anxiety. The pandemic has given us a greater appreciation of the value of social contact and a deeper appreciation that what happens on the other side of the world can affect our daily lives.

Author Contributions: Conceptualization, H.D. and P.S.; validation, H.D. and P.S.; investigation, H.D. and P.S.; writing—original draft preparation, H.D. and P.S.; writing—review and editing, H.D.; supervision, H.D. All authors have read and agreed to the published version of the manuscript.

Funding: This research received no external funding.

Institutional Review Board Statement: Not Applicable.

Informed Consent Statement: Not Applicable.

Data Availability Statement: Not Applicable.

Conflicts of Interest: The authors declare no conflict of interest.

Entry Link on the Encyclopedia Platform: https://encyclopedia.pub/12210.

References

1. Mattila, E.; Peltokoski, J.; Neva, M.H.; Kaunonen, M.; Helminen, M.; Parkkila, A.-K. COVID-19: Anxiety among hospital staff and associated factors. *Ann. Med.* **2021**, *53*, 237–246. [CrossRef]
2. Windsor-Shellard, B.; Nasir, R. Coronavirus (COVID-19) Related Deaths by Occupation, England and Wales: Deaths Registered between 9 March and 28 December 2020. Available online: https://www.ons.gov.uk/peoplepopulationandcommunity/healthandsocialcare/causesofdeath/bulletins/coronaviruscovid19relateddeathsbyoccupationenglandandwales/deathsregisteredbetween9marchand28december2020#:~{}:text=There%20were%207%2C961%20deaths%20involving,(2%2C833%20deaths)%20among%20women (accessed on 5 November 2020).
3. Estrich, C.G.; Mikkelsen, M.; Morrissey, R.; Geisinger, M.L.; Ioannidou, E.; Vujicic, M.; Araujo, M.W. Estimating COVID-19 prevalence and infection control practices among US dentists. *J. Am. Dent. Assoc.* **2020**, *151*, 815–824. [CrossRef] [PubMed]
4. Zou, L.; Ruan, F.; Huang, M.; Liang, L.; Huang, H.; Hong, Z.; Yu, J.; Kang, M.; Song, Y.; Xia, J. SARS-CoV-2 viral load in upper respiratory specimens of infected patients. *N. Engl. J. Med.* **2020**, *382*, 1177–1179. [CrossRef]
5. Brooks, Z.C.; Das, S. COVID-19 Testing: Impact of Prevalence, Sensitivity, and Specificity on Patient Risk and Cost. *Am. J. Clin. Pathol.* **2020**, *154*, 575–584. [CrossRef] [PubMed]
6. Surkova, E.; Nikolayevskyy, V.; Drobniewski, F. False-positive COVID-19 results: Hidden problems and costs. *Lancet Respir. Med.* **2020**, *8*, 1167–1168. [CrossRef]
7. Pfefferle, S.; Reucher, S.; Nörz, D.; Lütgehetmann, M. Evaluation of a quantitative RT-PCR assay for the detection of the emerging coronavirus SARS-CoV-2 using a high throughput system. *Eurosurveillance* **2020**, *25*, 2000152. [CrossRef] [PubMed]
8. Gussow, A.B.; Auslander, N.; Faure, G.; Wolf, Y.I.; Zhang, F.; Koonin, E.V. Genomic determinants of pathogenicity in SARS-CoV-2 and other human coronaviruses. *Proc. Natl. Acad. Sci. USA* **2020**, *117*, 15193–15199. [CrossRef] [PubMed]
9. Yoshimoto, F.K. A Biochemical Perspective of the Nonstructural Proteins (NSPs) and the Spike Protein of SARS CoV-2. *Protein J.* **2021**, 1–36. [CrossRef]
10. Bao, L.; Deng, W.; Gao, H.; Xiao, C.; Liu, J.; Xue, J.; Lv, Q.; Liu, J.; Yu, P.; Xu, Y. Reinfection could not occur in SARS-CoV-2 infected rhesus macaques. *BioRxiv* **2020**. [CrossRef]
11. Ludvigsson, J.F. Systematic review of COVID-19 in children shows milder cases and a better prognosis than adults. *Acta Paediatr.* **2020**, *109*, 1088–1095. [CrossRef]
12. Burton, M.J.; Clarkson, J.E.; Goulao, B.; Glenny, A.-M.; McBain, A.J.; Schilder, A.G.; Webster, K.E.; Worthington, H.V. Antimicrobial mouthwashes (gargling) and nasal sprays administered to patients with suspected or confirmed COVID-19 infection to improve patient outcomes and to protect healthcare workers treating them. *Cochrane Database Syst. Rev.* **2020**, *9*, CD013627.
13. Bazaid, A.S.; Aldarhami, A.; Binsaleh, N.K.; Sherwani, S.; Althomali, O.W. Knowledge and practice of personal protective measures during the COVID-19 pandemic: A cross-sectional study in Saudi Arabia. *PLoS ONE* **2020**, *15*, e0243695. [CrossRef] [PubMed]
14. Pasomsub, E.; Watcharananan, S.P.; Boonyawat, K.; Janchompoo, P.; Wongtabtim, G.; Suksuwan, W.; Sungkanuparph, S.; Phuphuakrat, A. Saliva sample as a non-invasive specimen for the diagnosis of coronavirus disease 2019: A cross-sectional study. *Clin. Microbiol. Infect.* **2021**, *27*, e281–e285. [CrossRef]

15. Liu, L.; Wei, Q.; Alvarez, X.; Wang, H.; Du, Y.; Zhu, H.; Jiang, H.; Zhou, J.; Lam, P.; Zhang, L. Epithelial cells lining salivary gland ducts are early target cells of severe acute respiratory syndrome coronavirus infection in the upper respiratory tracts of rhesus macaques. *J. Virol.* **2011**, *85*, 4025–4030. [CrossRef] [PubMed]
16. Xu, J.; Li, Y.; Gan, F.; Du, Y.; Yao, Y. Salivary Glands: Potential Reservoirs for COVID-19 Asymptomatic Infection. *J. Dent. Res.* **2020**, *99*, 989. [CrossRef] [PubMed]
17. Lechien, J.R.; Chetrit, A.; Chekkoury-Idrissi, Y.; Distinguin, L.; Circiu, M.; Saussez, S.; Berradja, N.; Edjlali, M.; Hans, S.; Carlier, R. Parotitis-Like Symptoms Associated with COVID-19, France, March-April 2020. *Emerg. Infect. Dis.* **2020**, *26*, 2270–2271. [CrossRef]
18. Fisher, J.; Monette, D.L.; Patel, K.R.; Kelley, B.P.; Kennedy, M. COVID-19 associated parotitis. *Am. J. Emerg. Med.* **2021**, *39*, e251–e254. [CrossRef]
19. Paniz-Mondolfi, A.; Bryce, C.; Grimes, Z.; Gordon, R.E.; Reidy, J.; Lednicky, J.; Sordillo, E.M.; Fowkes, M. Central nervous system involvement by severe acute respiratory syndrome coronavirus-2 (SARS-CoV-2). *J. Med. Virol.* **2020**, *92*, 699–702. [CrossRef]
20. Amorim dos Santos, J.; Normando, A.; Carvalho da Silva, R.; Acevedo, A.; De Luca Canto, G.; Sugaya, N.; Santos-Silva, A.; Guerra, E. Oral manifestations in patients with COVID-19: A living systematic review. *J. Dent. Res.* **2021**, *100*, 141–154. [CrossRef]
21. Cirillo, N.; Bizzoca, M.E.; Lo Muzio, E.; Cazzolla, A.P.; Lo Muzio, L. Gustatory dysfunction in COVID-19 patients: A rapid systematic review on 27,687 cases. *Acta Odontol. Scand.* **2021**, 1–8. [CrossRef]
22. Riestra-Ayora, J.; Yanes-Diaz, J.; Esteban-Sanchez, J.; Vaduva, C.; Molina-Quiros, C.; Larran-Jimenez, A.; Martin-Sanz, E. Long-term follow-up of olfactory and gustatory dysfunction in COVID-19: 6 months case–control study of health workers. *Eur. Arch. OtoRhino Laryngol.* **2021**, 1–7. [CrossRef]
23. Rojas-Lechuga, M.J.; Izquierdo-Domínguez, A.; Chiesa-Estomba, C.; Calvo-Henríquez, C.; Villarreal, I.M.; Cuesta-Chasco, G.; Bernal-Sprekelsen, M.; Mullol, J.; Alobid, I. Chemosensory dysfunction in COVID-19 out-patients. *Eur. Arch. Oto Rhino Laryngol.* **2021**, *278*, 695–702. [CrossRef] [PubMed]
24. Paderno, A.; Mattavelli, D.; Piazza, C. Long-term Olfactory and Gustatory Dysfunction May Be Related to Neural Damage. Otolaryngol. *Head Neck Surg.* **2021**. [CrossRef] [PubMed]
25. Keyhan, S.O.; Fallahi, H.R.; Cheshmi, B. Dysosmia and dysgeusia due to the 2019 Novel Coronavirus; a hypothesis that needs further investigation. *Maxillofac. Plast. Reconstr. Surg.* **2020**, *42*, 9. [CrossRef]
26. Iranmanesh, B.; Khalili, M.; Amiri, R.; Zartab, H.; Aflatoonian, M. Oral manifestations of COVID-19 disease: A review article. *Dermatol. Ther.* **2021**, *34*, e14578. [CrossRef]
27. Brandini, D.A.; Takamiya, A.S.; Thakkar, P.; Schaller, S.; Rahat, R.; Naqvi, A.R. Covid-19 and oral diseases: Crosstalk, synergy or association? *Rev. Med. Virol.* **2021**. [CrossRef]
28. Hoffmann, M.; Kleine-Weber, H.; Schroeder, S.; Krüger, N.; Herrler, T.; Erichsen, S.; Schiergens, T.S.; Herrler, G.; Wu, N.-H.; Nitsche, A. SARS-CoV-2 cell entry depends on ACE2 and TMPRSS2 and is blocked by a clinically proven protease inhibitor. *Cell* **2020**, *181*, 271–280. [CrossRef]
29. Galicia, J.C.; Guzzi, P.H.; Giorgi, F.M.; Khan, A.A. Predicting the response of the dental pulp to SARS-CoV2 infection: A transcriptome-wide effect cross-analysis. *Genes Immun.* **2020**, *21*, 360–363. [CrossRef]
30. Patel, J.; Woolley, J. Necrotizing periodontal disease: Oral manifestation of COVID-19. *Oral Dis.* **2020**, *27* (Suppl. 3), 768–769. [CrossRef]
31. Sakaguchi, W.; Kubota, N.; Shimizu, T.; Saruta, J.; Fuchida, S.; Kawata, A.; Yamamoto, Y.; Sugimoto, M.; Yakeishi, M.; Tsukinoki, K. Existence of SARS-CoV-2 entry molecules in the oral cavity. *Int. J. Mol. Sci.* **2020**, *21*, 6000. [CrossRef]
32. Nasiri, K.; Dimitrova, A. Comparing saliva and nasopharyngeal swab specimens in the detection of COVID-19: A systematic review and meta-analysis. *J. Dent. Sci.* **2021**, *16*, 799–805. [CrossRef]
33. Kim, Y.-g.; Yun, S.G.; Kim, M.Y.; Park, K.; Cho, C.H.; Yoon, S.Y.; Nam, M.H.; Lee, C.K.; Cho, Y.-J.; Lim, C.S. Comparison between saliva and nasopharyngeal swab specimens for detection of respiratory viruses by multiplex reverse transcription-PCR. *J. Clin. Microbiol.* **2017**, *55*, 226–233. [CrossRef]
34. Li, H.; Liu, S.-M.; Yu, X.-H.; Tang, S.-L.; Tang, C.-K. Coronavirus disease 2019 (COVID-19): Current status and future perspectives. *Int. J. Antimicrob. Agents* **2020**, *55*, 105951. [CrossRef]
35. Hanege, F.M.; Kocoglu, E.; Kalcioglu, M.T.; Celik, S.; Cag, Y.; Esen, F.; Bayindir, E.; Pence, S.; Alp Mese, E.; Agalar, C. SARS-CoV-2 Presence in the Saliva, Tears, and Cerumen of COVID-19 Patients. *Laryngoscope* **2021**, *131*, E1677–E1682. [CrossRef]
36. Nacher, M.; Mergeay-Fabre, M.; Blanchet, D.; Benoit, O.; Pozl, T.; Mesphoule, P.; Sainte-Rose, V.; Vialette, V.; Toulet, B.; Moua, A.; et al. Prospective Comparison of Saliva and Nasopharyngeal Swab Sampling for Mass Screening for COVID-19. *Front. Med.* **2021**, *8*. [CrossRef]
37. Czumbel, L.M.; Kiss, S.; Farkas, N.; Mandel, I.; Hegyi, A.; Nagy, Á.; Lohinai, Z.; Szakács, Z.; Hegyi, P.; Steward, M.C.; et al. Saliva as a Candidate for COVID-19 Diagnostic Testing: A Meta-Analysis. *Front. Med.* **2020**, *7*, 465. [CrossRef]
38. Azzi, L.; Baj, A.; Alberio, T.; Lualdi, M.; Veronesi, G.; Carcano, G.; Ageno, W.; Gambarini, C.; Maffioli, L.; Di Saverio, S. Rapid Salivary Test suitable for a mass screening program to detect SARS-CoV-2: A diagnostic accuracy study. *J. Infect.* **2020**, *81*, e75–e78. [CrossRef]
39. Sagredo-Olivares, K.; Morales-Gómez, C.; Aitken-Saavedra, J. Evaluation of saliva as a complementary technique to the diagnosis of COVID-19: A systematic review. *Med. Oral Patol. Oral Cir. Bucal* **2021**. [CrossRef]
40. Williams, E.; Bond, K.; Zhang, B.; Putland, M.; Williamson, D.A. Saliva as a non-invasive specimen for detection of SARS-CoV-2. *J. Clin. Microbiol.* **2020**, *58*, e00776-20. [CrossRef]

41. Han, M.S.; Seong, M.-W.; Heo, E.Y.; Park, J.H.; Kim, N.; Shin, S.; Cho, S.I.; Park, S.S.; Choi, E.H. Sequential analysis of viral load in a neonate and her mother infected with severe acute respiratory syndrome coronavirus 2. *Clin. Infect. Dis.* **2020**, *71*, 2236–2239. [CrossRef] [PubMed]
42. Iyer, P.; Aziz, K.; Ojcius, D.M. Impact of COVID-19 on dental education in the United States. *J. Dent. Educ.* **2020**, *84*, 718–722. [CrossRef] [PubMed]
43. Machado, R.A.; Bonan, P.R.F.; Perez, D.E.d.C.; Martelli Junior, H. COVID-19 pandemic and the impact on dental education: Discussing current and future perspectives. *Braz. Oral Res.* **2020**, *34*, e083. [CrossRef]
44. Fernandes, C.I.; Bonan, R.F.; Bonan, P.R.; Leonel, A.C.; Carvalho, E.J.; de Castro, J.F.; Perez, D.E. Dental students' perceptions and performance in use of conventional and virtual microscopy in oral pathology. *J. Dent. Educ.* **2018**, *82*, 883–890. [CrossRef]
45. Chang, T.-Y.; Hong, G.; Paganelli, C.; Phantumvanit, P.; Chang, W.-J.; Shieh, Y.-S.; Hsu, M.-L. Innovation of dental education during COVID-19 pandemic. *J. Dent. Sci.* **2021**, *16*, 15–20. [CrossRef]
46. Retallack, H.; Di Lullo, E.; Arias, C.; Knopp, K.A.; Laurie, M.T.; Sandoval-Espinosa, C.; Leon, W.R.M.; Krencik, R.; Ullian, E.M.; Spatazza, J. Zika virus cell tropism in the developing human brain and inhibition by azithromycin. *Proc. Natl. Acad. Sci. USA* **2016**, *113*, 14408–14413. [CrossRef]

encyclopedia

Entry

Pandemic Prevention: Lessons from COVID-19

Mario Coccia

CNR–National Research Council of Italy, Collegio Carlo Alberto, Via Real Collegio, 30-10024 Turin, Italy; mario.coccia@cnr.it

Definition: Coronavirus disease 2019 (COVID-19) is caused by the novel severe acute respiratory syndrome coronavirus 2 (SARS-CoV-2), which appeared in late 2019, generating a pandemic crisis with high numbers of COVID-19-related infected individuals and deaths in manifold countries worldwide. Lessons learned from COVID-19 can be used to prevent pandemic threats by designing strategies to support different policy responses, not limited to the health system, directed to reduce the risks of the emergence of novel viral agents, the diffusion of infectious diseases and negative impact in society.

Keywords: COVID-19; coronavirus infections; infectious diseases; viral agents; public health capacity; resilience; risk assessment; crisis management; bounded rationality; country monitoring; pandemic response; preventing transmission; preparedness

Citation: Coccia, M. Pandemic Prevention: Lessons from COVID-19. *Encyclopedia* **2021**, *1*, 433–444. https://doi.org/10.3390/encyclopedia1020036

Academic Editor: Stephen Bustin

Received: 15 April 2021
Accepted: 25 May 2021
Published: 31 May 2021

1. Introduction

Coronavirus disease 2019 (COVID-19) is caused by the severe acute respiratory syndrome coronavirus 2 (SARS-CoV-2), which appeared in late 2019 [1]. SARS-CoV-2 and its mutations have generated a pandemic with high numbers of infected individuals and deaths in manifold countries worldwide [2,3]. In this context, it is important to design strategies of crisis management to cope with/prevent pandemics of novel infectious diseases similar to COVID-19. The concept of strategy has a critical role in a framework of crisis management [4]. Strategy is a current mode of cognition and action to enable individuals and/or organizations to take advantage of important opportunities or to cope with consequential problems and/or environmental threats in society, such as pandemics, earthquakes, etc. Nations and their institutions have to prepare long-run strategies and specific plans of crisis management for pandemic threats to guide timely processes of decision-making to support the application of effective actions and interventions for solving consequential problems in society [4,5]. Strategies of crisis management should deal with pandemic threat before the emergence and in the presence of an unforeseen pandemic, they have to reduce negative effects in society [6]. The main goal of these strategies is to reduce hazards and risks that certain factors pose to public health and the environment, and solve the problems of pandemic crises with effective and rapid decisions directed to policy responses for reducing uncertainty and supporting, as soon as possible, the recovery of socioeconomic systems. In particular, strategies of countries for unforeseen pandemic crisis can be [7–9]:

- Responsive, based on the application of a previous plan of interventions ready to be used that endeavors to solve all consequential problems of pandemic crisis.
- Preventive, based on the planned interventions directed to reduction of risk factors associated with the emergence and diffusion of pandemics, and the design ex-ante of effective solutions for problems generated by a pandemic threat/crisis, preparing rapid strategic actions to stop or reduce negative effects in society.

The logical structure of these strategies of crisis management is based on the following vital aspects:

- Analysis of the causes, hazards, risk factors and effects of pandemic threat (problem) in society, and possible solutions.
- Analysis of a limited number of variables associated with proposed solutions for achieving and sustaining specific goals given by the reduction of hazards and risk factors of the emergence of pandemics or negative effects in the presence of ongoing pandemic in society.
- Analysis of different solutions to pandemic threats and crises, and evaluation of pros and cons.
- Choice of the satisfying solution in the context of limited rationality and a turbulent environment.
- Application of the critical decision of problem solving for achieving the goals, evaluating expected results in a short period of time to refine and improve the decision-making process with continuous learning processes.

2. Strategies of Crisis Management in the Presence of Pandemic Similar to COVID-19

Nicoll and Coulombier ([10], p. 3ff) describe two main strategies to cope with pandemics:

- Containment strategies that endeavor to stop the diffusion of pandemics and epidemics in society. These interventions are directed to prevent vast chains of transmission and outbreaks, with public policies of quarantine and full lockdown associated with an accurate tracing of infections, isolation of infected people and timely treatments of patients [11] (cf., Figure 1).
- Mitigation strategies based on social distancing, school closures, facemasks wearing, etc. that endeavor to decrease the pandemic diffusion and the pressure of high hospitalization and admission to intensive care units as well as protecting elderly and other people with high vulnerability (e.g., having cancer and other serious diseases).

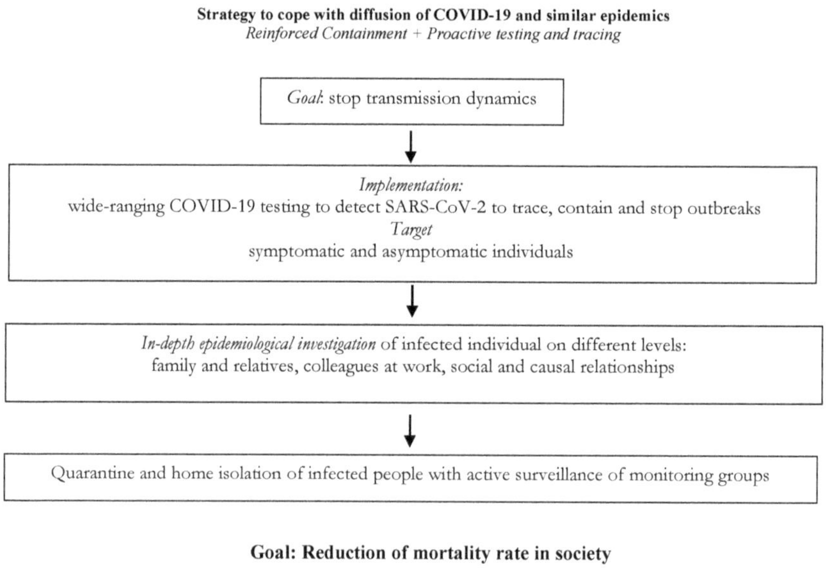

Figure 1. Containment strategy to support policy responses directed to cope with COVID-19 pandemic crisis and similar epidemics in future. Source: author's own figure.

During the COVID-19 crisis and similar pandemics, many countries initially proposed a containment policy (quarantine and general lockdown) and subsequently mitigation measures, such as social distancing, disinfection of buildings, face masks wearing, travel restrictions, etc. [12–14]. The study by Renardy et al. [15] shows that a longer duration of lockdown that postpones the reopening of stores and the circulation of people does not decrease confirmed cases of infections and inter-related negative effects on public health, but a longer duration of lockdown only defers these problems in a not-too-distant future. Instead, specific mitigation policies directed to diminish contacts among people in specific places can effectively lower the peak of pandemic waves and consequential negative effects in society.

Migone [16] discusses the correlation between national policy characteristics and the success in "flattening the curve" of COVID-19. This study shows that the best correlation is found when looking at the pattern of choice related to either proactive or reactive approaches to the implementation of containment measures. This result is stronger for countries having either very low or very high infection rates per million people. Instead, in the presence of intermediate rates, a variety of institutional, political, and socioeconomic variables intervene in the process. Scholars also maintain that specific public places create groups of people for social activities that generate a high risk of infection (e.g., pub, bar, cafeteria, gym, etc.) [17]. A selected strategy to control the groups of people in these public places by the application of non-pharmaceutical measures of protection (e.g., facemasks wearing, social distancing) are more effective strategies to reduce confirmed cases than full lockdown of overall social and economic activities [17].

In general, non-pharmaceutical measures are health policies having the goal of lowering the peak of the pandemic wave and the high load on health system [18,19]. However, Brooks et al. [20] report: "negative psychological effects of quarantine including post-traumatic stress symptoms, confusion, and anger. Stressors included longer quarantine duration, infection fears, frustration, boredom, inadequate supplies, inadequate information, financial loss, and stigma". Marazziti and Stahl [21] argue that the COVID-19 pandemic has generated several disorders of psychiatric interest and relevance. Wang et al. [22] analyzed the deterioration of physical and psychological health during the COVID-19 pandemic and revealed that the subjective deterioration of psychological health was significantly associated with avoiding crowded places and wearing a facemask. Moreover, subjective deteriorations of physical and psychological health are positively associated with general anxiety. Xiong et al. [23] also have shown that the COVID-19 pandemic is associated with highly significant levels of psychological distress that, in many cases, would meet the threshold for clinical relevance. In this context, psychological disorders are also associated with a systematic deterioration of economic system because of containment policies based on a longer duration of lockdown in society that generates high unemployment [11]. Mitigating the hazardous effects of containment policies to cope with infectious diseases (e.g., COVID-19) on mental health should be also a public health priority. In addition, Puci et al. [24] highlight the importance of psychological and psychiatric support services during the COVID-19 pandemic. These services can support the psychological well-being of health care professionals and promote precautionary behaviors among them.

3. Strategies for the Prevention of Pandemics

Specific strategies can reduce the hazards and risk factors of pandemic threats, prevent the emergence of pandemics and reduce negative effects in society. This perspective focuses on health, environmental and institutional strategies [4,25].

3.1. Health Strategies

Daszak et al. [26] highlight some critical aspects for designing strategies directed to the prevention of pandemics, such as:

(1) control among wildlife to detect the transportation of dangerous pathogens;
(2) control of the interaction between the population and wildlife to detect, as soon as possible, spillover effects;
(3) control wildlife trade for enhancing biosecurity in domestic and international markets.

In addition, an intense activity of prevention has to be directed to control and apply biosafety protocols in public and private laboratories of virology that analyze viruses, pathogens and novel viral agents to minimize the possibility of accidental diffusion in the environment and society with consequential socioeconomic issues. In this context, the scientific collaboration among international laboratories plays a critical role in supporting the sharing of vital data and information for helping policymakers to apply plans to prevent/reduce the hazards and risk factors of pandemic threats that can create problems worldwide [1]. This strategy of prevention can be driven by increasing levels of investments in the health sector and R&D, as well as higher levels of health expenditure per capita. In fact, preventive measures and new technology can control the emergence of pandemics and negative effects in society of future pandemics similar to COVID-19 [27]. In the presence of local epidemic outbreak, a rapid contact tracing is a basic strategy within the epicenter to limit human-to-human transmission outside of outbreak areas, also applying appropriate isolation of cases [28]. Hellewell et al. [29] show that the probability of control decreases with long delays from symptom onset to isolation. Contact tracing achieves the early detection and isolation of secondary cases, which play an important role given that the peak in infectiousness occurs during the pre-symptomatic phase. Moreover, the early detection achieved by contact tracing accelerates the rate at which infected individuals receive medical care to improve their chance of recovery. In short, contact tracing is a vital strategy for controlling infectious diseases, such as COVID-19, but protocols apply "forward-trace" to notify people who were recently exposed. Bradshaw et al. [30] found that "bidirectional" tracing to identify infector individuals and their other infectees robustly improves outbreak control. In addition, Kucharski et al. [12] claim that the isolation of cases and contact tracing can be less effective for COVID-19 because infectiousness starts before the onset of symptoms (cf. [31]). Yalaman et al. [32] suggest that comprehensive contact tracing is an instrumental approach not only for curtailing transmission but also to reduce case fatality rates. In fact, the combination of reduced transmission and more rapid recovery reduces the burden on healthcare system, which can save resources for individuals that are infected in the future. According to Kapitsinis [33], investments in the health sector can support these just-mentioned strategies and develop hospital efficiency in admissions of infected people, innovative treatments for novel infectious diseases and new technology driven by R&D labs to foster scientific and technological advances directed to new vaccines, antivirals and other innovative drugs that can avoid and/or control future pandemic threats in countries [1,5,34–40]. Williams et al. [41] argue that effective responses to public health emergencies should rely on translating rapidly emerging research and technology into timely, evidence-informed new policies and best practices, etc., such as appropriate strategies of vaccinations with new mRNA vaccines directed to achieve herd immunity for supporting a drastic reduction in the number of COVID-19-related infected individuals and deaths. In fact, the alarming levels of spread and severity of COVID-19 and novel infectious diseases support the development of new technologies and innovative drugs, such as vaccines based on messenger RNA, known as mRNA vaccines for high levels of protection by preventing COVID-19 (and likely also against its variants) among people that are vaccinated [4]. The mRNA vaccines are based on accumulated knowledge that the infective process itself is effective in raising an immune response; as a consequence, genetic engineering can be utilized to construct virus-like particles from the capsid and envelope proteins of viruses [42,43]. Moreover, mRNA vaccines eliminate a lot of phases in the manufacturing process for the development of new drugs because rather than having viral proteins injected, the human body uses the instructions to manufacture viral proteins itself. In short, R&D investments in new technologies have developed mRNA vaccines that are produced and manufactured by chemical rather than biological synthesis; in this case, the process of technological development is much faster than conventional vaccines to be redesigned, scaled up and mass-produced [24,44]. Manifold public agencies in the United Kingdom, the USA, Europe and other countries for protecting and promoting the health of people through control and supervision confirm that mRNA vaccines for COVID-19 can be effective and safely tolerated in populations [44–48].

3.2. Environmental Strategies

Studies have found that sustainable environment plays a vital role to reduce risk factors of epidemics and prevent pandemics similar to COVID-19 [1,49]. Scholars maintain that a low rate of fatality is associated with a low level of air pollution [1,49–52]. Studies have also shown that countries with 72% of the population exposed to levels exceeding the WHO guideline value of air pollution have lower fatality rates of COVID-19 than countries with 98% population exposed to similar levels of air pollution [53]. Coccia [1] demonstrates that polluted cities should not exceed 48 days per year of high levels of air pollution, in the presence of climate conditions having little wind, because when the annual period of air pollution is higher than 100 days, the reduction of air quality and other factors can damage the health of the population and support the transmission dynamics of infectious diseases in society with consequential socioeconomic problems [51,54].

In fact, polluted cities have to apply an environmental policy to reduce the main sources of air pollution and, at the same time, improve urban ventilation to foster the dispersion of particulate compounds emissions, considering morphological characteristics of the openness of surrounding areas [55], the coverage and heights of buildings that affect the surface roughness, etc. [56,57]. Moreover, countries must support, more and more, sustainable mobility as engine of socioeconomic change and redesign cities for people using urban planning that improves public respiratory health. The hazards of the association between air pollution and viral infectivity in cities have to induce a reduction of the motorization rate of polluting machines with a sustainable transition to new electric vehicles, generating a revolution in society [1]. In short, environmental strategies can foster sustainable mobility by enhancing local, urban and commuter public transport with electric vehicles and creating vast low emission zones within cities. In this context, countries and supranational organizations have to launch a roadmap directed to sustainable growth with the aim of zero emissions in all socioeconomic systems. Wang and Zhu [58] argue that a strategy of renewable energy and sustainable technology facilitates CO_2 abatement, reducing air pollution, improving air quality and the health of people. In fact, studies have shown the positive effects of the reduction of air pollution on the health of people in terms of lower premature deaths and related morbidity [59]. Hence, geo-economic regions have to, more and more, apply long-run environmental policies and sustainable strategies to reduce the level of particulate compounds emissions that damage the health of people and may be associated with the diffusion of viral agents, generating socioeconomic issues [51–54].

3.3. Institutional Strategies

Resilient systems to pandemic shocks must have strong institutions and good governance driven by adequate and effective leadership that supports population needs. effective governance has to support preparedness to pandemic threats with constant investments in the health system to reduce mortality, morbidity and stress among the population, and promote socioeconomic recovery [11,51–54,60]. Sagan et al. [61] confirm that in Europe, good governance in countries has played a critical role to support a resilient response of the health system in the presence of the COVID-19 pandemic crisis. In particular, Sagan et al. [61] consider a broad concept of governance, not limited to the health system alone, that creates the institutional background to support economic and social systems of the nation and its government to work properly for preventing and/or coping with pandemic threats and crises. In fact, Sagan et al. [61] pinpoint that the prevention of pandemic threats is based on: (1) appropriate and effective governance of institutions and (2) skilled human capital with interdisciplinary technical capacity of crisis management to respond in a short period of time.

Other factors for effective strategies to prevent and/or reduce risks of future pandemic crises can be:

- Leveraging operational levels based on medical personnel, epidemiologists, biologists, emergency managers, and other professionals for coping with pandemic's threat.

- Creating a network of innovators with a great variety of expertise and capability in different fields to support policy decisions and their timely implementation [62].
- Fostering academic institutions and leading scholars that play a vital role in supporting rational decisions of governments [63,64].
- Creating stable collaborations across different structures, such as academic and administrative institutions, to accelerate the learning process to prevent and/or cope with pandemic threat/crisis [65].

In this context, the COVID-19 pandemic crisis has pushed the boundaries on what is possible for rapid pandemic responses in several areas, including healthcare system, vaccine research, development, manufacturing, distribution, allocation, and administration. These actions can support learning processes directed to improve preparedness efforts of nations to advance timely public responses in the short term and support R&D for developing efficient pandemic and seasonal influenza vaccines. New strategies of vaccination plans of nations have to be highly responsive, flexible, resilient, scalable, and more effective for reducing the impact of seasonal and pandemic influenza viruses. In general, vaccine roll-out plans have to face distribution and allocation hurdles, and new mutations of SARS-CoV-2, likely more transmissible and resistant to vaccines, can change the equation of herd-immunity, increasing the thresholds of immunization in the population [66–68]. A delay of vaccination plan and of the achievement of optimal threshold within countries does not reduce transmission dynamics and can foster the emergence and diffusion of novel mutations of viral agents, such as in Brazil and India [69,70]. In short, the timely achievement of the optimal threshold of doses administered to population is a critical goal, because an effective vaccination plan can quickly and thoroughly prevent a new mutation of the novel coronavirus from accelerating transmission dynamics in society with consequential socioeconomic issues [71].

Overall, then, success or failure of strategies to prevent pandemic threats and crises depend on effective decision-making in the presence of uncertainty, turbulent environment and highly restricted time [4]. Studies show that the general guidelines for an efficient strategy to cope with pandemic threats have to increase health expenditures and R&D investments for supporting effective policy responses that decrease hazards and risk factors and as a consequence negative effects on population and environment [1,4,54]. Figure 2 shows these critical aspects for preventing and/or controlling the risk factors of future pandemics.

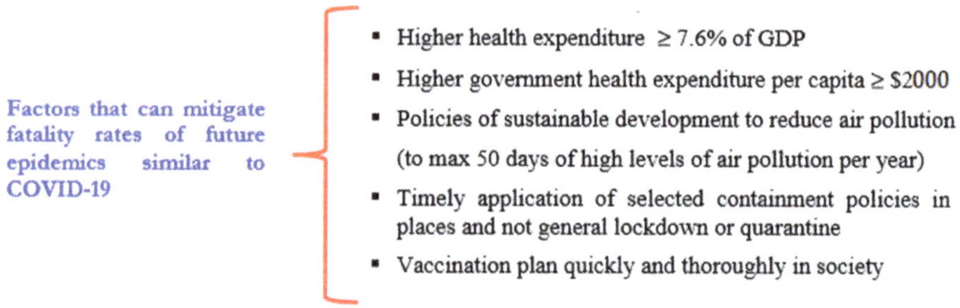

Figure 2. Factors associated with strategies to prevent negative effects of pandemic threats. *Source*: author's own figure.

Finally, the proposed ambidexterity strategies of crisis management for more prosperous or less favored countries are [72]:

- Rich countries can focus in the short run on measures of containment of shorter duration because of a stronger healthcare sector based on high expenditures (as % of GDP), whereas in the long run these countries should support environmental policies for reducing air pollution and improving sustainability of ecosystems.
- Developing countries have to focus in the short run on measures of containment of a longer duration because of a weak healthcare sector based on low expenditures (as %

of GDP) and in the long run, they have to support public policies for enhancing health system and health of people.

3.4. A Systemic Strategy of Crisis Management to Cope with and/or to Prevent Pandemics Similar to COVID-19

Nations in the presence of a pandemic threat are directed to three strategic goals:

- The application of technological innovations and new technologies for improving actions that prevent the emergence of pandemics and/or contrast the vast diffusion of epidemics or pandemics, such as monitoring, recognition, contact tracing, etc.
- The acceleration of R&D for developing effective vaccines.
- The production, on a vast scale, of new vaccines and innovative drugs to minimize socioeconomic issues and support recovery.

In the next years, countries have to increase R&D investments in equipment, organized infrastructures and education of human resources for improving preparedness activity to react quickly in the presence of inevitable pandemics, also reinforcing international collaboration with key subjects for reducing negative effects on public health between different socioeconomic systems [73].

Hence, in responding to a constant pandemic threat of novel viral agents in the future, the international communities have to reinforce prevention and preparedness in crisis management [4]. In particular, nations and international organizations have to design and implement strategic actions given by improvements of the early warning system and timely containment operations. Moreover, preparedness activities should reinforce the coordination of global science and research to accelerate the R&D and diffusion of effective pandemic vaccines and innovative antiviral drugs.

The strategic actions to prevent pandemic threats can be systematize as follows:

- Reinforce the early warning systems in the international community using existing infrastructure to ensure rapid detection of suspected cases in humans based on rapid and reliable international laboratories that receive all the data and clinical specimens needed for an accurate evaluation of an emergence of pandemic risk.
- Establish rapid containment policies to prevent an increase in the spread of novel viruses in human society and/or, whenever possible, delay its transmission dynamics in the international community. New studies show that selected restrictions in specific places are better policy responses than full lockdown [11,17,74,75]. Health policy should apply a crisis management team to quickly use global and regional stocks of antiviral drugs and other similar drugs to contain negative effects in society in the initial phase of diffusion.
- Verify that all countries have designed and tested pandemic response plans and that international organizations are able to assume a leadership and provide clear guideline to coordinate nations during a pandemic. Developing countries having limited economic resources have to be supported in the development of pandemic plans to reduce gaps in basic capacities for improving an equally and coordinated global response to a pandemic threat or crisis.
- Nations should jointly invest and coordinate global R&D to produce pandemic vaccines and antiviral drugs that are rapidly and widely available as soon as the emergence of a pandemic and/or the diffusion of the novel virus appear. In particular, nations should identify priority research areas and foster funding to public- and private firms involved in R&D of innovative drugs. It is also important to gather and analyze more data on the use of established and new anti-viral drugs and vaccines for a safe administration of treatment and prophylaxis in all of the population. Foster partnerships among governments, regulatory authorities, universities, research laboratories, incumbent and new entrant firms to support R&D of novel drugs and in particular a timely vaccine manufacturing capacity that ensures equitable access across all nations. Moreover, R&D investments have to be directed to new vaccines conferring long-lasting protection against novel viruses and their mutations. Finally,

organizations and nations should foster scientific networks and laboratories to ensure that new scientific knowledge about ongoing pandemic and treatments has a rapid and wide-spread communication in real time worldwide.

These strategic actions have to achieve and sustain the main goal of reducing hazards and risk factors of pandemic threats and, in the presence of pandemic, providing, whenever possible, a vast immunological protection of people before they are exposed to novel viral agents. Tsiotas and Magafas [76], using network analysis, show stability of hubs and instability of medium and low-degree nodes, implying a low probability of meeting maximum (infection) values in the future and high uncertainty in the variability of other values below the average. Hence, the challenge is the design of environmental, health and social policies of prevention, and the production of appropriate and safe vaccines that meet global needs shortly after the emergence of a pandemic in order to provide equitable access between countries. In this context, nations have to support scientific institutions for R&D of new vaccines and the applications of new technologies that could prevent chains of transmission, increase vaccine supplies, timely distribution for a broad-spectrum and enduring protection against pandemics across populations worldwide. All these aspects are basic for a strategic approach to cope with and/or prevent pandemic threats.

4. Conclusions and Prospects

Strategies of crisis management to prevent the COVID-19 pandemic and similar epidemics are based on effective multi-level governance, combining both supranational, national, regional and urban strategies to provide timely policy responses for improving health safety in society [72]. The experience of COVID-19 suggests that future infectious diseases of novel viruses can generate, more and more, a serious pandemic threat to public health of countries and their economies [11,74,77–79]. New pandemics, similar to COVID-19, can emerge and spread rapidly and it is important to ensure timely gathering and sharing of information, and samples of novel viral agents for appropriate interventions to stop the emergence of epidemics/pandemics. The preventive strategies also have to support the process of R&D directed to effective vaccines and subsequent production and distribution as soon as possible across countries to mitigate fatality rates, deterioration of economic growth and overall socioeconomic systems. Nations have to design a crisis management team for managing strenuous situations given by pandemic threats and for taking timely critical decisions to resolve them, as far as possible. Successful crisis management teams understand the specificity of pandemic crisis and are thoroughly prepared for solving all problems and problematic situations. Moreover, in a crisis, leaders are expected to reduce uncertainty, providing an authoritative account of problems, solutions and difficulties. Moreover, leaders have to formulate and guide a strategy to cope with pandemic crises that has to be accepted by other institutional, economic and social parties having different positions and interests. The COVID-19 pandemic crisis has supported new and rapid pandemic responses in several areas, including healthcare system, vaccine research, health technologies, environment as well as the development of innovative vaccines. These strategic actions of pandemic management have triggered learning processes to improve preparedness efforts of countries to advance timely critical decisions and efficient investments in R&D processes of innovative drugs and new pandemic vaccines [5,36,38].

Hence, strategies for pandemic threats have to be, more and more, based on efficiency, flexibility, responsiveness and resiliency for decreasing negative effects of vast infectious diseases in society. Evans and Bahrami [80] suggest actions directed to super-flexibility and resilience [81]. Moreover, complex and unforeseen problems of pandemic crises should be treated with strategies of dissolution directed at eliminating sources of pandemic threats in society and improving the capacity of nations to react [4,74,82]. These strategies to prevent and cope with novel infectious diseases have to apply plans and decisions based on ecological rationality, considering a comparative evaluation of performance with other countries applying alternative interventions. This comparative analysis can improve collective learning processes for effective decision-making across countries in turbulent environments with pandemic crisis [83,84]. In short, the development of these capacities can collectively improve the world's ability to defend itself against many emerging and epidemic-prone diseases. International experience for the COVID-19 pandemic crisis has shown that well-planned public policies, scientific and economic coordination policies are effective interventions for reducing high-risk aspects before and during an outbreak.

Overall, then, a comprehensive strategy of crisis management for pandemic threats has to be also based on environmental and socioeconomic factors, and new technology, and not only on parameters related to medicine, to help policymakers to evaluate manifold aspects that reduce institutional and social vulnerabilities to epidemics and design appropriate short- and long-run plans to prevent and/or contain the negative impact of future infectious diseases on public health, the economy and society [85–87]. To conclude, in the presence of a constant pandemic threat, a comprehensive strategy to prevent future epidemics similar to COVID-19 has to be designed considering manifold aspects associated with sustainability, environmental and socioeconomic sciences, and not only aspects related to life sciences, such as biology and medicine.

Funding: This research received no external funding.

Institutional Review Board Statement: Not applicable.

Informed Consent Statement: Not applicable.

Data Availability Statement: Not applicable.

Conflicts of Interest: The author declares no conflict of interest.

Entry Link on the Encyclopedia Platform: https://encyclopedia.pub/11256.

References

1. Coccia, M. Factors determining the diffusion of COVID-19 and suggested strategy to prevent future accelerated viral infectivity similar to COVID. *Sci. Total Environ.* **2020**, *729*, 138474. [CrossRef]
2. Johns Hopkins Center for System Science and Engineering. Coronavirus COVID-19 Global Cases. Available online: https://gisanddata.maps.arcgis.com/apps/opsdashboard/index.html#/bda7594740fd40299423467b48e9ecf6 (accessed on 4 January 2021).
3. Seligman, B.; Ferranna, M.; Bloom, D.E. Social determinants of mortality from COVID-19: A simulation study using NHANES. *PLoS Med.* **2021**, *18*, e1003490. [CrossRef]
4. Coccia, M. Comparative Critical Decisions in Management. In *Global Encyclopedia of Public Administration, Public Policy, and Governance*; Farazmand, A., Ed.; Springer Nature Switzerland AG 2020: Cham, Switzerland, 2021. [CrossRef]
5. Ardito, L.; Coccia, M.; Petruzzelli, A.M. Technological exaptation and crisis management: Evidence from COVID-19 outbreaks. *R D Manag.* **2021**. [CrossRef]
6. Groh, M. Strategic Management in Times of Crisis. *Am. J. Econ. Bus. Adm.* **2014**, *6*, 49–57. [CrossRef]
7. Bundy, J.; Pfarrer, M.D.; Short, C.E.; Coombs, W.T. Crises and Crisis Management: Integration, Interpretation, and Research Development. *J. Manag.* **2017**, *43*, 1661–1692. [CrossRef]
8. Seeger, M.W.; Sellno, T.L.; Ulmer, R.R. Communication, organization and crisis. *Commun. Yearb.* **1998**, *21*, 231–275. [CrossRef]
9. Shrivastava, P.; Mitroff, I.I.; Miller, D.; Miclani, A. Understanding Industrial Crises. *J. Manag. Stud.* **1988**, *25*, 285–303. [CrossRef]
10. Nicoll, A.; Coulombier, D. Europe's initial experience with pandemic (H1N1) 2009-mitigation and delaying policies and practices. *Euro Surveill.* **2009**, *14*, 19279. [CrossRef]
11. Coccia, M. The relation between length of lockdown, numbers of infected people and deaths of Covid-19, and economic growth of countries: Lessons learned to cope with future pandemics similar to Covid-19 and to constrain the deterioration of economic system. *Sci. Total Environ.* **2021**, *775*, 145801. [CrossRef]
12. Kucharskim, J.A.; Russell, T.W.; Diamond, C.; Liu, Y.; Edmunds, J.; Funk, S.; Eggo, R.M.; on behalf of the centre for mathematical modelling of infectious diseases COVID-19 working group. Early dynamics of transmission and control of COVID-19: A mathematical modelling study. *Lancet Infect. Dis.* **2020**. [CrossRef]
13. Nussbaumer-Streit, B.; Mayr, V.; Dobrescu, A.I.; Chapman, A.; Persad, E.; Klerings, I.; Wagner, G.; Siebert, U.; Ledinger, D.; Zachariah, C.; et al. Quarantine alone or in combination with other public health measures to control COVID-19: A rapid review. *Cochrane Database Syst. Rev.* **2020**, *9*. [CrossRef]
14. Walensky, R.P.; Del Rio, C. From Mitigation to Containment of the COVID-19 Pandemic: Putting the SARS-CoV-2 Genie Back in the Bottle. *JAMA* **2020**, *323*, 1889–1890. [CrossRef]
15. Renardy, M.; Eisenberg, M.; Kirschner, D. Predicting the second wave of COVID-19 in Washtenaw County, MI. *J. Theor. Biol.* **2020**, *507*, 110461. [CrossRef] [PubMed]

16. Riccardo, M.A. The influence of national policy characteristics on COVID-19 containment policies: A comparative analysis. *Policy Des. Pract.* **2020**, *3*, 259–276. [CrossRef]
17. Chang, S.; Pierson, E.; Koh, P.W.; Geradin, J.; Redbird, B.; Grusky, D.; Leskovec, J. Mobility network models of COVID-19 explain inequities and inform reopening. *Nature* **2020**. [CrossRef]
18. Fong, M.W.; Gao, H.; Wong, J.Y.; Xiao, J.; Shiu, E.Y.C.; Ryu, S.; Cowling, B.J. Nonpharmaceutical measures for pandemic influenza in nonhealthcare settings—Social distancing measures. *Emerg. Infect. Dis.* **2020**. [CrossRef]
19. Prem, K.; Liu, Y.; Russell, T.W.; Kucharski, A.J.; Eggo, R.M.; Davies, N. The effect of control strategies to reduce social mixing on outcomes of the COVID-19 epidemic in Wuhan, China: A modelling study. *Lancet Public Health* **2020**. [CrossRef]
20. Brooks, S.K.; Webster, R.K.; Smith, L.E.; Woodland, L.; Wessely, S.; Greenberg, N.; Rubin, G.J. The psychological impact of quarantine and how to reduce it: Rapid review of the evidence. *Lancet* **2020**, *395*, 912–920. [CrossRef]
21. Marazziti, D.; Stahl, S.M. The relevance of COVID-19 pandemic to psychiatry. *World Psychiatry Off. J. World Psychiatr. Assoc. WPA* **2020**, *19*, 261. [CrossRef]
22. Wang, P.W.; Ko, N.Y.; Chang, Y.P.; Wu, C.F.; Lu, W.H.; Yen, C.F. Subjective Deterioration of Physical and Psychological Health during the COVID-19 Pandemic in Taiwan: Their Association with the Adoption of Protective Behaviors and Mental Health Problems. *Int. J. Environ. Res. Public Health* **2020**, *17*, 6827. [CrossRef]
23. Xiong, J.; Lipsitz, O.; Nasri, F.; Lui, L.; Gill, H.; Phan, L.; Chen-Li, D.; Iacobucci, M.; Ho, R.; Majeed, A.; et al. Impact of COVID-19 pandemic on mental health in the general population: A systematic review. *J. Affect. Disord.* **2020**, *277*, 55–64. [CrossRef]
24. Puci, M.V.; Nosari, G.; Loi, F.; Puci, G.V.; Montomoli, C.; Ferraro, O.E. Risk Perception and Worries among Health Care Workers in the COVID-19 Pandemic: Findings from an Italian Survey. *Healthcare* **2020**, *8*, 535. [CrossRef]
25. Coccia, M. Varieties of capitalism's theory of innovation and a conceptual integration with leadership-oriented executives: The relation between typologies of executive, technological and socioeconomic performances. *Int. J. Public Sect. Perform. Manag.* **2017**, *3*, 148–168. [CrossRef]
26. Daszak, P.; Olival, K.J.; Li, H. A strategy to prevent future epidemics similar to the 2019-nCoV outbreak. *Biosaf. Health* **2020**. [CrossRef]
27. Coccia, M. Deep learning technology for improving cancer care in society: New directions in cancer imaging driven by artificial intelligence. *Technol. Soc.* **2020**, *60*, 1–11. [CrossRef]
28. Wells, C.R.; Sah, P.; Moghadas, S.M.; Pandey, A.; Shoukat, A.; Wang, Y.; Wang, Z.; Meyers, L.A.; Singer, B.H.; Galvani, A.P. Impact of international travel and border control measures on the global spread of the novel 2019 coronavirus outbreak. *Proc. Natl. Acad. Sci. USA* **2020**, *117*, 7504–7509. [CrossRef]
29. Hellewell, J.; Abbott, S.; Gimma, A.; Bosse, N.I.; Jarvis, C.I.; Russell, T.W.; Munday, J.D.; Kucharski, A.J.; Edmunds, W.J. Feasibility of controlling COVID-19 outbreaks by isolation of cases and contacts. *Lancet Glob. Health* **2020**. [CrossRef]
30. Bradshaw, W.J.; Alley, E.C.; Huggins, J.H.; Lloyd, A.L.; Esvelt, K.M. Bidirectional contact tracing could dramatically improve COVID-19 control. *Nat. Commun.* **2021**, *12*, 232. [CrossRef]
31. Peak, C.M.; Childs, L.M.; Grad, Y.H.; Buckee, C.O. Comparing nonpharmaceutical interventions for containing emerging epidemics. *Proc. Natl. Acad. Sci. USA* **2017**, *114*, 4023–4028. [CrossRef] [PubMed]
32. Yalaman, A.; Basbug, G.; Elgin, C.; Galvani, A.P. Cross-country evidence on the association between contact tracing and COVID-19 case fatality rates. *Sci. Rep.* **2021**, *11*, 2145. [CrossRef]
33. Kapitsinis, N. The underlying factors of the COVID-19 spatially uneven spread. Initial evidence from regions in nine EU countries. *Reg. Sci. Policy Pract.* **2020**, *12*, 1027–1045. [CrossRef]
34. Coccia, M. Sources of disruptive technologies for industrial change. *L'industria Riv. Econ. Politica Ind.* **2017**, *38*, 97–120. [CrossRef]
35. Coccia, M. The origins of the economics of Innovation. *J. Econ. Soc. Thought* **2018**, *5*, 9–28. [CrossRef]
36. Coccia, M. Why do nations produce science advances and new technology? *Technol. Soc.* **2019**, *59*, 1–9. [CrossRef]
37. Coccia, M. The theory of technological parasitism for the measurement of the evolution of technology and technological forecasting. *Technol. Forecast. Soc. Chang.* **2019**, *141*, 289–304. [CrossRef]
38. Coccia, M.; Watts, J. A theory of the evolution of technology: Technological parasitism and the implications for innovation management. *J. Eng. Technol. Manag.* **2020**, *55*, 101552. [CrossRef]
39. Coccia, M. A taxonomy of public research bodies: A systemic approach. *Prometheus* **2005**, *23*, 63–82. [CrossRef]
40. Coccia, M. Disruptive firms and industrial change. *J. Econ. Soc. Thought* **2017**, *4*, 437–450. [CrossRef]
41. Williams, G.A.; Ulla Díez, S.M.; Figueras, J.; Lessof, S. Translating evidence into policy during the covid-19 pandemic: Bridging science and policy (and politics). *Eurohealth* **2020**, *26*, 29–33.
42. Smoot, J. Classic and New Technologies Vying to Be the First COVID-19 Vaccine. Posted June 11. Available online: https://www.cas.org/blog/covid-19-vaccine (accessed on 15 May 2021).
43. Coccia, M.; Finardi, U. Emerging nanotechnological research for future pathway of biomedicine. *Int. J. Biomed. Nanosci. Nanotechnol.* **2012**, *2*, 299–317. [CrossRef]
44. Komaroff, A. Why Are mRNA Vaccines So Exciting? Harvard Health Blog. Available online: https://www.health.harvard.edu/blog/why-are-mrna-vaccines-so-exciting-2020121021599 (accessed on 10 May 2021).
45. Abbasi, J. COVID-19 and mRNA Vaccines-First Large Test for a New Approach. *JAMA* **2020**, *324*, 1125–1127. [CrossRef] [PubMed]
46. Cylus, J.; Pantel, D.; van Ginneken, E. Who should be vaccinated first? Comparing vaccine prioritization strategies in Israel and European countries using the Covid-19 Health System Response Monitor. *Israel J. Health Policy Res.* **2021**, *10*, 16. [CrossRef]

47. Heaton, P.M. The Covid-19 Vaccine-Development Multiverse. *N. Engl. J. Med.* **2020**, *383*, 1986–1988. [CrossRef]
48. Jeyanathan, M.; Afkhami, S.; Smaill, F.; Miller, M.S.; Lichty, B.D.; Xing, Z. Immunological considerations for COVID-19 vaccine strategies. *Nat. Rev. Immunol.* **2020**, *20*, 615–632. [CrossRef] [PubMed]
49. Coccia, M. How (Un)sustainable Environments are Related to the Diffusion of COVID-19: The Relation between Coronavirus Disease 2019, Air Pollution, Wind Resource and Energy. *Sustainability* **2020**, *12*, 9709. [CrossRef]
50. Coccia, M. How do low wind speeds and high levels of air pollution support the spread of COVID-19? *Atmos. Pollut. Res.* **2020**. [CrossRef]
51. Coccia, M. Effects of the spread of COVID-19 on public health of polluted cities: Results of the first wave for explaining the dejà vu in the second wave of COVID-19 pandemic and epidemics of future vital agents. *Environ. Sci. Pollut. Res.* **2021**, *28*, 19147–19154. [CrossRef]
52. Coccia, M. The effects of atmospheric stability with low wind speed and of air pollution on the accelerated transmission dynamics of COVID-19. *Int. J. Environ. Stud.* **2021**, *78*, 1–27. [CrossRef]
53. Coccia, M. High health expenditures and low exposure of population to air pollution as critical factors that can reduce fatality rate in COVID-19 pandemic crisis. *Environ. Res.* **2021**, 111339. [CrossRef]
54. Coccia, M. An index to quantify environmental risk of exposure to future epidemics of the COVID-19 and similar viral agents: Theory and Practice. *Environ. Res.* **2020**, *191*, 110155. [CrossRef]
55. Hang, J.; Li, Y.; Sandberg, M.; Buccolieri, R.; di Sabatino, S. The Influence of Building Height Variability on Pollutant Dispersion and Pedestrian Ventilation in Idealized High-rise Urban Areas. *Build. Environ.* **2012**, *56*, 346–360. [CrossRef]
56. Peng, Y.; Ma, X.Y.; Zhao, F.Y.; Liu, C.W.; Mei, S.J. Wind Driven Natural Ventilation and Pollutant Dispersion in the Dense Street Canyons: Wind Opening Percentage and Its Effects. *Procedia Eng.* **2017**, *205*, 415–422. [CrossRef]
57. Yuan, C.; Ren, C.; Ng, E. GIS-based Surface Roughness Evaluation in the Urban Planning System to Improve the Wind Environment–A Study in Wuhan, China. *Urban Clim.* **2014**, *10*, 585–593. [CrossRef]
58. Wang, Z.; Zhu, Y. Do energy technology innovations contribute to CO2 emissions abatement? A spatial perspective. *Sci. Total Environ.* **2020**, *726*, 138574. [CrossRef]
59. Cui, L.; Zhou, J.; Peng, X.; Ruan, S.; Zhang, Y. Analyses of air pollution control measures and co-benefits in the heavily air-polluted Jinan city of China, 2013–2017. *Sci. Rep.* **2020**, *10*, 5423. [CrossRef] [PubMed]
60. Kluge, H.H.P.; Nitzan, D.; Azzopardi-Muscat, N. COVID-19: Reflecting on experience and anticipating the next steps. A perspective from the WHO Regional Office for Europe. *Eurohealth* **2020**, *26*, 13–15.
61. Sagan, A.; Thomas, S.; McKee, M.; Karanikolos, M.; Azzopardi-Muscat, N.; de la Mata, I.; Figueras, J. COVID-19 and health systems resilience: Lessons going forwards. *Eurohealth* **2020**, *26*, 20–24.
62. Jenkins-Smith, H.C.; Nohrstedt, D.; Weible, C.M.; Ingold, K. The advocacy coalition framework: An overview of the research program. In *Theories of the Policy Process*; Weible, C.M., Sabatier, P.A., Eds.; Routledge: Abingdon, VA, USA, 2018; pp. 135–171.
63. Cairney, P. *The Politics of Evidence Based Policymaking*; Palgrave: London, UK, 2016.
64. Weible, C.M.; Nohrstedt, D.; Cairney, P.; Carter, D.P.; Crow, D.A.; Durnová, A.P.; Heikkila, T.; Inglod, K.; McConnell, A.; Stone, D. COVID-19 and the policy sciences: Initial reactions and perspectives. *Policy Sci.* **2020**, *53*, 225–241. [CrossRef]
65. Crow, D.A.; Albright, E.A.; Ely, T.; Koebel, E.; Lawhon, L. Do disasters lead to learning? Financial policy change in local government. *Rev. Policy Res.* **2018**, *35*, 564–589. [CrossRef]
66. Callaway, E. Fast-spreading COVID variant can elude immune responses. *Nature* **2021**, *589*, 500–501. [CrossRef] [PubMed]
67. Dooling, K.; McClung, N.; Chamberland, M.; Marin, M.; Wallace, M.; Bell, B.P.; Lee, G.M.; Talbot, H.K.; Romero, J.R.; Oliver, S.E. The Advisory Committee on Immunization Practices' interim recommendation for allocating initial supplies of COVID-19 vaccine—United States. *MMWR Morb. Mortal Wkly. Rep.* **2020**, *69*, 1857–1859. [CrossRef]
68. Vignesh, R.; Shankar, E.M.; Velu, V.; Thyagarajan, S.P. Is Herd Immunity Against SARS-CoV-2 a Silver Lining? *Front. Immunol.* **2020**, *11*, 586781. [CrossRef]
69. Mallapaty, S. Are COVID vaccination programmes working? Scientists seek first clues. *Nature* **2021**, *589*, 504–505. [CrossRef]
70. Buss, L.F.; Prete, C.A., Jr.; Abrahim, C.; Mendrone, A., Jr.; Salomon, T.; de Almeida-Neto, C.; França, R.; Belotti, M.C.; Carvalho, M.; Costa, A.G.; et al. Three-quarters attack rate of SARS-CoV-2 in the Brazilian Amazon during a largely unmitigated epidemic. *Science* **2021**, *371*, 288–292. [CrossRef] [PubMed]
71. Akamatsu, T.; Nagae, T.; Osawa, M.; Satsukawa, K.; Sakai, T.; Mizutani, D. Model-based analysis on social acceptability and feasibility of a focused protection strategy against the COVID-19 pandemic. *Sci. Rep.* **2021**, *11*, 2003. [CrossRef]
72. Ari-Veikko, A. Successful Government Responses to the Pandemic: Contextualizing National and Urban Responses to the COVID-19 Outbreak in East and West. *Int. J. E-Plan. Res. IJEPR IGI Glob.* **2021**, *10*, 1–17.
73. U.S. Department of Health & Human Services. Public Health Emergency-Executive Summary. Available online: https://www.phe.gov/Preparedness/planning/nivms/Pages/executive-summary.aspx (accessed on 9 March 2021).
74. Coccia, M. The impact of first and second wave of the COVID-19 pandemic: Comparative analysis to support control measures to cope with negative effects of future infectious diseases in society. *Environ. Res.* **2021**, 111099. [CrossRef] [PubMed]
75. Warren, G.W.; Lofstedt, R.; Wardman, J.K. COVID-19: The winter lockdown strategy in five European nations. *J. Risk Res.* **2021**, *24*, 1–27. [CrossRef]
76. Tsiotas, D.; Magafas, L. The Effect of Anti-COVID-19 Policies on the Evolution of the Disease: A Complex Network Analysis of the Successful Case of Greece. *Physics* **2020**, *2*, 325–339. [CrossRef]

77. Luo, Y.; Chua, C.R.; Xiong, Z.; Ho, R.C.; Ho, C. A Systematic Review of the Impact of Viral Respiratory Epidemics on Mental Health: An Implication on the Coronavirus Disease 2019 Pandemic. *Front. Psychiatry* **2020**, *11*, 565098. [CrossRef]
78. Sirois, F.M.; Owens, J. Factors Associated with Psychological Distress in Health-Care Workers during an Infectious Disease Outbreak: A Rapid Systematic Review of the Evidence. *Front. Psychiatry* **2021**, *11*, 589545. [CrossRef] [PubMed]
79. Newby, J.M.; O'Moore, K.; Tang, S.; Christensen, H.; Faasse, K. Acute mental health responses during the COVID-19 pandemic in Australia. *PLoS ONE* **2020**, *15*, e0236562. [CrossRef] [PubMed]
80. Evans, S.; Bahrami, H. Super-Flexibility in Practice: Insights from a Crisis. *Glob. J. Flex. Syst. Manag.* **2020**, *21*, 207–214. [CrossRef]
81. Janssen, M.; van der Voort, H. Agile and adaptive governance in crisis response: Lessons from the COVID-19 pandemic. *Int. J. Inf. Manag.* **2020**, *55*, 102180. [CrossRef]
82. Ackoff, R.L.; Rovin, S. *Redesigning Society*; Stanford University Press: Stanford, CA, USA, 2003.
83. Gigerenzer, G.; Todd, P.M. Ecological rationality: The normative study of heuristics. In *Ecological Rationality: Intelligence in the World*; Gerd, G., Todd Peter, M., Eds.; Oxford University Press: New York, NY, USA, 1999; pp. 487–497. [CrossRef]
84. Kahneman, D.; Slovic, P.; Tversky, A. *Judgment under Uncertainty: Heuristics and Biases*; Cambridge University Press: London, UK, 1982.
85. Coccia, M. A Theory of classification and evolution of technologies within a Generalized Darwinism. *Technol. Anal. Strateg. Manag.* **2019**, *31*, 517–531. [CrossRef]
86. Coccia, M. Spatial relation between geo-climate zones and technological outputs to explain the evolution of technology. *Int. J. Transit. Innov. Syst.* **2015**, *4*, 5–21. [CrossRef]
87. Coccia, M.; Bellitto, M. Human progress and its socioeconomic effects in society. *J. Econ. Soc. Thought* **2018**, *5*, 160–178. [CrossRef]

encyclopedia

MDPI

Entry

Self-Service Restaurants in SARS-CoV-2 Pandemic

Renata Puppin Zandonadi [1,*], Raquel Braz Assunção Botelho [1,*], Dayanne da Costa Maynard [2] and Rita de Cassia Coelho de Almeida Akutsu [1]

1 Department of Nutrition, Faculty of Health Sciences, Campus Universitário Darcy Ribeiro, University of Brasília, Distrito Federal 70910-900, Brazil; rita.akutsu@gmail.com
2 Post-Graduation in Human Nutrition, University of Brasília, Brasília 70910-900, Brazil; day_nut@yahoo.com.br
* Correspondence: renatapz@unb.br (R.P.Z.); raquelbotelho@unb.br (R.B.A.B.)

Definition: During the SARS-CoV-2 pandemic, the self-service restaurant sector, as well as other types of food services, are facing an unprecedented crisis needing to adapt their service to avoid closing their doors. With varied and quick meals, the self-service buffet is one of the most important types of outside services. However, the type of service where the clients follow a line on the buffet and serve their meals has impaired traditional restaurant operation during the SARS-CoV-2 pandemic and, perhaps, after it. In this sense, this study presents an overview of the self-service buffet restaurant operational system in the context of the SARS-CoV-2 pandemic.

Keywords: food safety; foodservice; SARS-CoV-2; risk; buffet

Citation: Zandonadi, R.P.; Botelho, R.B.A.; Maynard, D.d.C.; Akutsu, R.d.C.C.d.A. Self-Service Restaurants in SARS-CoV-2 Pandemic. *Encyclopedia* **2021**, *1*, 401–408. https://doi.org/10.3390/encyclopedia1020033

Academic Editor: Stephen Bustin

Received: 20 April 2021
Accepted: 24 May 2021
Published: 25 May 2021

1. Introduction

During the SARS-CoV-2 pandemic, the restaurant sector has faced an unprecedented crisis, and it needs an urgent discussion on how to handle or adapt the service. Among other types of restaurants, the self-service buffet is one of the most important types in the food service sector as part of hospital cafeterias, hotels, corporations, educational institutions, and street foodservice, aiming for diversified and quick meals. The self-service buffet restaurant sector deals with food contamination hazards from food handlers and customers while serving their plates, increasing the risk of foodborne diseases (FBDs). Besides the FBD risk by food handlers, the way customers serve themselves can increase this risk. Customers may touch the utensils, talk while in line, cough or sneeze while serving the meal, let objects or part of their clothes touch food at the buffet, let the utensils fall into the dishes, and touch food utensils without proper hand hygiene (even after coughing or sneezing and covering with their hands). All these habits may potentially expose clients to contamination by SARS-CoV-2, causing COVID-19. Lalley [1] pointed out that the decline in restaurant sales has been driven more by individuals' unstable psychological fear of contracting the infection than their financial difficulties during the pandemic.

In this sense, the self-service buffet restaurant sector has a major challenge to maintain running businesses during and after the SARS-CoV-2 pandemic, adapting to new sanitary hygienic standards, and seeking to implement sustainable actions. Therefore, this work will focus on the reality of the self-service buffet restaurant sector. We invite the researchers and the community to discuss this type of service's potential adaptation, avoiding the closure of self-service buffet restaurants impaired by the SARS-CoV-2 pandemic. Additionally, we need to discuss this new reality and its impact on sustainability for our planet.

2. Food Away from the Home and Self-Service Restaurants

Worldwide, people have grown to rely on the convenience of consuming food prepared outside of their homes [2–4]. This pattern is mainly due to the lack of time and skills to prepare meals. One of the most critical barriers to eating meals prepared at home is the challenge in balancing work, school, and leisure schedules, forcing people to "eat on the run" [5].

This scenario led to the foodservice sector's growth, especially the establishments that provide fast meals with affordable prices to consumers, mainly on workdays and leisure moments. It is a way to avoid eating fast foods and choose healthier options. The self-service buffet is a typical food service style that offers breakfast, snacks, lunch, and/or dinner meals. It is a type of service with an extended menu with all dishes prepared and served directly to customers who can choose what they want to eat from the buffet line. In some countries, self-service buffet restaurants represent more than 60% of the foodservice sector [6], showing the potential of this type of restaurant and its importance while discussing the pandemic period for job maintenance.

The self-service meal is characterized by an offer of dishes placed in a buffet that people can choose among the offered options to compose their plates. It is a common type of service as part of hospital cafeterias, hotels, corporations, educational institutions, and street restaurants. There are two primary modalities of this kind of restaurants: "by the kilo", in which customers pay the price considering the weight of the meal on their plate; and "fixed price all you can eat buffet", where costumers pay a fixed price and serve themselves as much as they want [6,7]. In both ways, traditionally, there is a line for people to follow to access the buffet and choose what they want to eat, increasing the risk of food contamination [8]. In a pandemic, consumers may reject self-service buffet restaurants, believing that an environment full of people talking around the dishes, sharing the utensils, sitting at shared tables, and talking while eating poses a risk for Sars-CoV-2 contamination [8]. Before the SARS-CoV-2 pandemic, people usually stayed very close to one another while serving their plates in line. The habit of talking was prevalent, especially when waiting for a food handler to portion the buffet's specific items.

Considering food handlers, restaurants should continue to follow the good practices previously adopted by the sector. However, it is necessary to add some practices to avoid Sars-CoV-2 contamination. In general, restaurants will need to have greater control over suppliers and how the goods reach the kitchens. Information on how the packages are cleaned and transported and if the employees delivering goods follow security protocols would be control points. Restaurants may rearrange food handlers' lunchtimes to limit the number of workers in the kitchen/room while menus are produced. They need to provide washbasins with sufficient sanitizers to the number of food handlers or offer hand sanitizer dispensers. All plates and utensils must be washed and sanitized in dishwashers with hot rinsing. Otherwise, the restaurant needs to provide disposable utensils. Another option is to provide sanitized and packaged cutlery. The staff at the buffet must wear disposable gloves and masks to replace and serve dishes. These are some of the changes restaurants may have to adopt to continue their business. There is an urgent need to modify and improve the Food Safety Management System.

2.1. *Self-Service Buffet Restaurants and the Potential Risk of Contamination*

As well as any other type of foodservice, self-service buffet restaurants must offer safe food and a safe environment for their clients. Several studies have focused on food handlers as responsible for food contamination due to their contact with ingredients and meals while preparing them [9–12]. However, considering these restaurants' self-service buffet style, customers are also highlighted as an actual contamination vehicle due to their attitudes before and while serving [13–15].

Studies of attitudes on self-service buffets have shown that consumers engage in unsanitary behaviors [16–18]. Among the types of restaurants, self-service poses unique problems because foods are displayed to customers, and there is little (if any) control with hands, clothing, dirt, and droplets that may contaminate foods and utensils [13,14,19]. There is the need for rigorous control of the period the dishes are exposed and their temperatures. Time and temperature are the key elements to prevent FBD, not only while serving the dishes, but also during preparation. When focusing on the customers, the risks may be diminished by encouraging them to wash their hands before serving or to use a hydroalcoholic solutions. Clients should be alerted that it is not time to talk to others or on the phone while serving. If they need to cough or sneeze, they should step away from the counter. Attention should be paid to objects and parts of clothes that can touch the food, and customers should not have to touch any food while serving themselves. These actions are important to prevent FBD and contamination by SARS-CoV-2, causing COVID-19 [16]. These practices are even more relevant in environments that should excel in hygiene care, such as hospitals. It is also important to highlight that customers do not always wash or use alcohol to clean their hands before serving themselves; therefore, they could represent a contamination vehicle for food utensils [16,20].

2.2. Self-Service Buffet Restaurant and COVID-19

The world is facing an unexpected COVID-19 pandemic with several economic, social, environmental, and health consequences that brought the risk of death from viral infection and psychological burdens affecting individuals' ways of life [21]. Until now, there has been no evidence about the transmission of SARS-CoV-2 by food [22]. However, the COVID-19 pandemic's impact represents a service disruption that most restaurant sectors were unprepared to handle. They had to shift their business model to offer delivery or serve take-away portioned meals. In some countries, when restaurants started re-opening, consumers demonstrated high levels of reluctance for dining out in foodservice establishments defined by governments as non-essential places of business [23]. Consumer research performed in March 2020 in the United States showed that almost 90% of the consumers believed that food from grocery stores and homes was safer than food from restaurants [24]. Consumers could have interpreted restaurants' closure as a sign that restaurant foods were less safe than food in general [25].

Keeping operations running presents a significant challenge for most restaurants dealing with customers' contamination concerns [26]. Additionally, the economic impact can influence the paths some of these restaurants will take. In this sense, the self-service buffet restaurant seems to be the most affected type of foodservice during the pandemic due to the type of service it offers. They cannot offer all the varieties of dishes displayed in the buffet line for delivery, changing the service's planned style. If they cannot offer this variety, they will probably need fewer food handlers, and this cycle impacts the economy of the sector. The customer's confidence in this sector will take some time to be regained after all the information provided during this critical time. In countries where they were allowed to re-open, more challenges arose. Training for all the staff members, purchasing disposables for costumers to serve themselves, and installing more sinks for handwashing and alcohol gel dispensers brought costs and more time to run the business properly.

Due to food being exposed to customers, it poses challenges for protecting them from FBD and the potential contamination of SARS-CoV-2. Self-service equipment and operations may not provide adequate protection from primary risks such as dirty hands (on utensils) and droplets (from sneezing, cough, talking) [7,13]. Sneeze guards have been used to protect buffet foods. However, it is common to lack these guards in some restaurants, or, if provided, they are not adequately addressed for all operating conditions, including hospital cafeteria buffets [7,13]. Self-service buffet restaurants have faced more challenges during the COVID-19 pandemic due to social isolation. In normal functioning, it exposes the food and utensils to customers as an additional source of contamination. Much has to be discussed about how self-service buffet restaurants should deal with the fear and the risk of contamination after the COVID-19 pandemic breakout. Improvements in operating standards are needed to promote safety in buffet restaurant operations and recover the clients' trust.

During the COVID-19 pandemic, regular operation of self-service restaurants is not possible. In this sense, operational adaptations to order delivery or takeout can minimize unnecessary interpersonal contact and emphasize the restaurant's commitment to safety and hygiene protocols. Additionally, a study on the stability of SARS-CoV-2 in aerosols showed that SARS-CoV-2 could be viable in aerosols for up to 3 h [27]. Therefore, risks of contamination from SARS-CoV-2 while eating food in indoor environments due to airborne particles are higher than those in outside/external areas. After the pandemic period, the buffet restaurants' cleanliness and food quality standards are imperative, as is crowding control, by reducing the number of seats or increasing space between tables [28].

These restaurants also count on the volume of clients who serve themselves, eat, and quickly give space to other customers. Will it be worthwhile for the sector to open and produce all the dishes if they have half of their customers? Our studies in Brazilian self-service buffets showed that customers usually take 20 min to enter a restaurant, serve, and eat. With changes related to a minimum safety space between clients in line and between tables, this time will increase, and tables' shifts will take longer. Profits come from a balance between expenses and the flow of customers.

To maintain these restaurants opened during the pandemic, many started delivery services. This change in the market brought some shifts and questions to the sector. Customers started to have their favorite foods at home without direct exposure to COVID-19. However, food safety should be a concern because adequate transportation and packaging are essential to avoid food contamination. Owners had the chance to sell their products with a smaller number of employees and without the costs of maintaining a restaurant hall. Nevertheless, disposable silverware increased, as well as mask and glove disposals, impacting sustainability. It is difficult to think about the losses and benefits of rethinking how the buffet restaurants will return.

Could this be the end of the self-service buffet restaurant? Will this type of foodservice survive the COVID-19 pandemic? To answer these questions, it is important to consider several aspects, such as those shown in Figure 1.

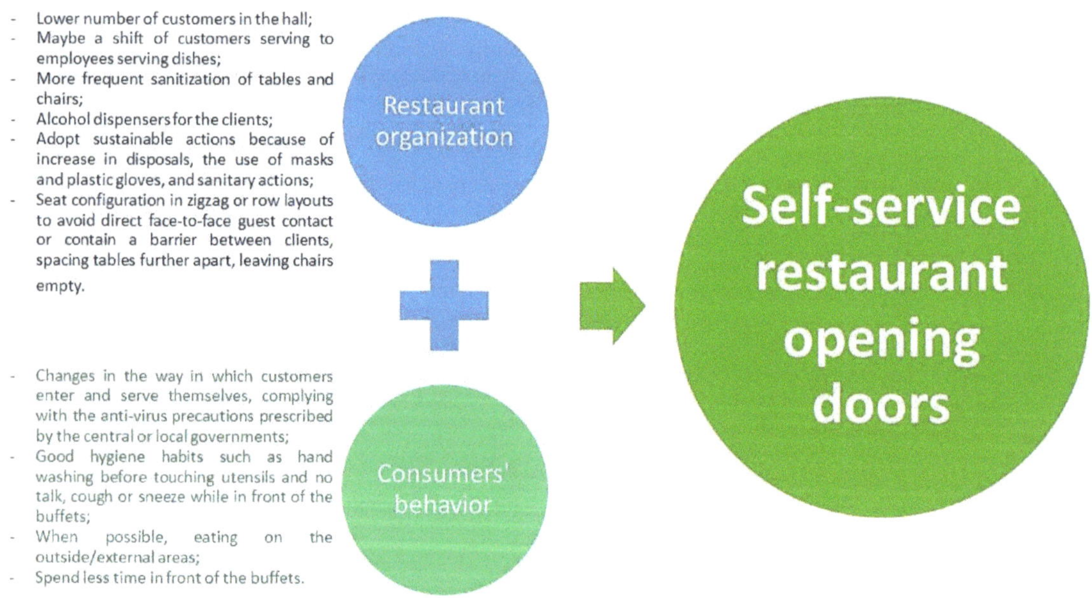

Figure 1. Proposed rules for self-service buffets during the COVID-19-pandemic.

2.3. *Self-Service Buffet Restaurant and Sustainability Actions in the COVID-19 Pandemic*

With the changes in the meal production sector due to the COVID-19 pandemic, such as the increase in disposables, masks and plastic gloves, and a more significant concern with hygienic-sanitary actions, the activities involving sustainability indicators have become necessary.

Restaurants use natural resources that cause environmental and economic impacts in all stages of meal production, ranging from production, transportation, reception, storage, production, and even distribution [29], such as excessive food consumption. Energy, water and plastics, food waste, carbon footprint accumulation, and high volume of solid waste are of concern when evaluating sustainability [30]. In the course of the pandemic, food production has remained high. However, there has been a reduction in the demand for food caused by the interruption of foodservice at work and entertainment activities such as hotels, restaurants, schools, and industries. Restaurants suffered due to logistic difficulties and higher sanitary barriers, causing an overproduction of food, leading to more significant food losses and waste [31].

Sustainability in meal production should be described by ecologically sustainable practices that aim to mitigate the environmental impact by rationally using natural resources. This can be achieved through activities such as reducing waste generation, increasing recycling, stimulating the use of food socio-biodiversity, waste reduction, and the training of employees to use more environmentally friendly technologies [32].

To comply with the pandemic norms, self-service restaurants have provided meals by delivery or takeout, increasing the use of disposables. Strategies such as asking the customer to bring their own packaging to take the meal, use their own cutlery during meals, and portion only the amount of food needed can mitigate the generation of solid waste. In turn, restaurants can exchange their taps for automatic activation, reuse rainwater for cleaning environments and counters, use pieces of equipment with better energy efficiency, and encourage recycling or even use biodegradable disposables. Due to the need to guarantee society's sustainable development, there is a need to promote the intake of ecologically correct and healthy foods. Local fairs were closed, and regional markets reduced their activities due to the pandemic. Organic products' sales, which had been growing before the pandemic, have been reduced to a minimum due to difficulties in marketing [31].

Climate change jeopardizes advances in development and poverty reduction, affecting food systems in low- and middle-income countries. The COVID-19 pandemic exacerbated problems such as hunger, unemployment, and the reduction in income. Social inequalities require urgent economic and social measures to guarantee healthy and sustainable food [33]. This pessimistic scenario will directly impact food security and nutrition indicators, moving us further away from the sustainable development goals, mainly increasing hunger [31]. In the context of sustainability, social measures in restaurants can be carried out, such as reducing the price of one kilo of food after a few hours have elapsed, purchasing groceries from small producers, and donating surplus to low-income people or needy institutions.

Concerning the social aspect of sustainability in self-services restaurants, ready-made foods that have not been distributed are frequently discharged. If kept under adequate time/temperature conditions, it could be used to feed insecure individuals. Considering that food waste squanders many natural resources (impacting sustainability) mainly at the end of the food production chain, food recovery could prevent surplus food from being disposed of in landfill [34], and providing food to reduce hunger.

Awareness campaigns for assembling dishes can be low-cost solutions. They often involve posters, pamphlets scattered around food services, or even the setting up of a standard dish to assist diners in portioning and promoting sustainability in restaurants. Other important alternatives to be included in self-service restaurants are recycling and composting.

Recycling is the best alternative to reduce environmental problems and increase the useful life of landfill sites. It is the process in which materials that would be discarded, or even those that have already been, are collected, separated, and processed, with the aim of being used as a raw material in the manufacture of goods. It is an action that benefits all involved in the production process: suppliers, consumers, the environment, and the government. It brings benefits to the environment. It allows natural resources, water, energy, and raw materials to be saved. For society, it generates jobs and income with the sale of recyclables [35]. On the other hand, composting is a set of techniques applied to control organic materials' decomposition to obtain a more stable material rich in humus and minerals, which generates a production chain with sustainable features [36,37].

It is important to highlight that customers' eating behaviors are constantly changing, even before the COVID-19 pandemic. The increase in diseases related to nutrition and food has increased nutritional awareness and enhanced the search for healthier and sustainable meal services. Therefore, consumers show an increasing health concern and are better able to choose their meals due to dietary, hygienic–sanitary aspects, as well as organic, vegetarian, or allergen-free foods. Bearing in mind the need to guarantee the sustainable development of society, there is a need to promote ecologically correct and healthy foods [38].

If society was already thinking and changing meal production procedures to achieve sustainability, with the SARS-CoV-2 pandemic, challenges have increased. Self-service restaurants face economic problems, and owners have to provide secure ways for customers to feel safe to visit and eat in these restaurants. More waste is generated with masks, plastics, and gloves, and the world is facing hunger and poverty in many countries. More than ever, society needs to look for solutions and continue thinking about sustainable actions.

3. Conclusions and Prospects

The COVID-19 pandemic has shown that we need to change habits and values. It is not always easy, but perhaps we may start to see how it is possible to mold society differently. The pandemic could be a chance for restaurants to adapt and look for ways to rethink their services and costs, especially in a time of economic recession, when businesses are expected to receive fewer customers, including sustainable practices that cover social, economic, and environmental indicators. Therefore, it could not be the end of the self-service buffet, but time to rethink and remodel it to meet the "new normal". In the end, all the actors involved—buffet restaurants' employers, employees, and clients—should adapt themselves to face the COVID-19 pandemic's operational, financial, and emotional burdens. During and after the pandemic, self-services must communicate their best practices clearly for customers to feel confident dining out. Self-services must do their best to minimize critical flaws in their service provision process and outcomes.

Author Contributions: Conceptualization, R.P.Z., R.d.C.C.d.A.A. and R.B.A.B.; investigation, R.P.Z., R.d.C.C.d.A.A. and R.B.A.B.; writing—original draft preparation, R.P.Z., R.d.C.C.d.A.A., D.d.C.M. and R.B.A.B.; writing—review and editing, R.P.Z., R.d.C.C.d.A.A., D.d.C.M. and R.B.A.B.; visualization, R.P.Z., R.d.C.C.d.A.A. and R.B.A.B.; All authors have read and agreed to the published version of the manuscript.

Funding: This research received no external funding.

Institutional Review Board Statement: Not applicable.

Informed Consent Statement: Not applicable.

Data Availability Statement: The study did not report any data.

Conflicts of Interest: The authors declare no conflict of interest.

Entry Link on the Encyclopedia Platform: https://encyclopedia.pub/7234.

References

1. Lalley, H. Data: Chinese Restaurants Hit Hard by Coronavirus Fears. Available online: https://www.restaurantbusinessonline.com/operations/data-chinese-restaurants-hit-hard-coronavirus-fears (accessed on 9 April 2021).
2. Saksena, M.J.; Okrent, A.M.; Anekwe, T.D.; Cho, C.; Dicken, C.; Effland, A.; Elitzak, H.; Guthrie, J.; Hamrick, K.S.; Hyman, J.; et al. *United States Department of Agriculture America's Eating Habits: Food Away from Home United States Department of Agriculture*; Economic Information Bulletin No. (EIB-196). USDA: Washington, DC, USA, 2018.
3. IBGE. *Family Budget Survey 2017–2018: Analysis of Food Consumption in Brazil*; IBGE: Rio de Janeiro, Brazil, 2020.
4. Li, Y.; Du, T.; Peng, J. Understanding Out-of-Home Food Environment, Family Restaurant Choices, and Childhood Obesity with an Agent-Based Huff Model. *Sustainability* **2018**, *10*, 1575. [CrossRef]

5. Escoto, K.H.; Laska, M.N.; Larson, N.; Neumark-Sztainer, D.; Hannan, P.J. Work hours and perceived time barriers to healthful eating among young adults. *Am. J. Health Behav.* **2012**, *36*, 786–796. [CrossRef] [PubMed]
6. SEBRAE. Self-Service Lidera Negócios de Alimentação fora do lar [Self-Service Leads Out-of-Home Food Businesses]. Available online: http://www.agenciasebrae.com.br/sites/asn/uf/NA/self-service-lidera-negocios-de-alimentacao-fora-do-lar,24cfcf74de20f510VgnVCM1000004c00210aRCRD (accessed on 14 July 2020).
7. Washington State University Food Safety and Buffet Etiquette. Available online: https://extension.wsu.edu/foodsafety/content/food-safety-and-buffet-etiquette/ (accessed on 14 July 2020).
8. GDF—Brazilian Federal District Government. *Orientações para a Prevenção de Transmissão do Coronavirus-COVID-19 em Restaurantes de auto Serviço [Guidelines for the prevention of transmission of coronavirus-COVID-19 in Self-Service Restaurants]*; GDF—Brazilian Federal District Government: Brasília, DF, Brazil, 2020.
9. Choudhury, M.; Mahanta, L.; Goswami, J.; Mazumder, M.; Pegoo, B. Socio-economic profile and food safety knowledge and practice of street food vendors in the city of Guwahati, Assam, India. *Food Control* **2011**, *22*, 196–203. [CrossRef]
10. Fielding, J.E.; Aguirre, A.; Palaiologos, E. Effectiveness of Altered Incentives in a Food Safety Inspection Program. *Prev. Med.* **2001**, *32*, 239–244. [CrossRef]
11. Abdullah Sani, N.; Siow, O.N. Knowledge, attitudes and practices of food handlers on food safety in food service operations at the Universiti Kebangsaan Malaysia. *Food Control* **2014**, *37*, 210–217. [CrossRef]
12. Faour-Klingbeil, D.; Kuri, V.; Todd, E. Investigating a link of two different types of food business management to the food safety knowledge, attitudes and practices of food handlers in Beirut, Lebanon. *Food Control* **2015**, *55*, 166–175. [CrossRef]
13. Joseph, G.; Doser, J. How safe are self-serve unpackaged foods? *J. Environ. Health* **1999**, *61*, 29–33.
14. Sommer, R. Consumer Behavior in Self-Service Food Outlets. *J. Environ. Health* **1987**, *49*, 277–281. [CrossRef]
15. Zandonadi, R.P.; Botelho, R.B.A.; Sávio, K.E.O.; Akutsu, R.D.C.; Araújo, W.M.C. Risk attitudes in self-service restaurants. *Rev. Nutr.* **2007**, *20*, 19–26. [CrossRef]
16. Harris, K.; Depietro, R.B.; Klein, J.; Jin, D. The Impact of Social Norms and Risk Assessment on Diners' Reaction to Food Safety Concerns in Restaurants. *J. Foodserv. Bus. Res.* **2020**, *23*, 377–400. [CrossRef]
17. Jacob, C.J.; Powell, D.A. Where Does Foodborne Illness Happen-in the Home, at Foodservice, or Elsewhere-and Does It Matter? *Foodborne Pathog. Dis.* **2009**, *6*, 1121–1123. [CrossRef]
18. Draeger, C.L.; Akutsu, R.d.C.C.d.A.; de Oliveira, K.E.S.; da Silva, I.C.R.; Botelho, R.B.A.; Zandonadi, R.P. Unhygienic practices of health professionals in Brazilian public hospital restaurants: An alert to promote new policies and hygiene practices in the hospitals. *Int. J. Environ. Res. Public Health* **2019**, *16*, 1224. [CrossRef]
19. Henriques, P.; Barbosa, R.M.S.; Freitas, F.C.P.W.-H.; Lanzillotti, H.S. Users' attitudes of restaurant "self-service": An added risk for food contaminationra a contaminação alimentar. *Cad. Saúde Coletiva* **2014**, *22*, 266–274. [CrossRef]
20. FDA. Best Practices for Re-Opening Retail Food Establishments during the COVID-19 Pandemic | FDA. Available online: https://www.fda.gov/food/food-safety-during-emergencies/best-practices-re-opening-retail-food-establishments-during-covid-19-pandemic (accessed on 30 April 2021).
21. Cao, W.; Fang, Z.; Hou, G.; Han, M.; Xu, X.; Dong, J.; Zheng, J. The psychological impact of the COVID-19 epidemic on college students in China. *Psychiatry Res.* **2020**, *287*, 112934. [CrossRef] [PubMed]
22. Stephanie Gomes de Freitas, R.; Stedefeldt, E. COVID-19 pandemic underlines the need to build resilience in commercial restaurants' food safety. *Food Res. Int.* **2020**, *136*, 109472. [CrossRef]
23. Kim, K.; Bonn, M.A.; Cho, M. Clean safety message framing as survival strategies for small independent restaurants during the COVID-19 pandemic. *J. Hosp. Tour. Manag.* **2021**, *46*, 423–431. [CrossRef]
24. Dataessential COVID-19—Fear and Response. Available online: https://datassential.com/wp-content/uploads/2020/03/Datassential_Coronavirus_03_17_20.pdf (accessed on 9 April 2021).
25. Byrd, K.; Her, E.S.; Fan, A.; Almanza, B.; Liu, Y.; Leitch, S. Restaurants and COVID-19: What are consumers' risk perceptions about restaurant food and its packaging during the pandemic? *Int. J. Hosp. Manag.* **2021**, *94*, 102821. [CrossRef]
26. Hazée, S.; Van Vaerenbergh, Y. Customes' contamination concerns: And integrative framework and futures prospects for service management. *J. Serv. Manag.* **2020**, *32*, 161–175. [CrossRef]
27. van Doremalen, N.; Bushmaker, T.; Morris, D.H.; Holbrook, M.G.; Gamble, A.; Williamson, B.N.; Tamin, A.; Harcourt, J.L.; Thornburg, N.J.; Gerber, S.I.; et al. Aerosol and Surface Stability of SARS-CoV-2 as Compared with SARS-CoV-1. *N. Engl. J. Med.* **2020**, *382*, 1564–1567. [CrossRef]
28. Wen, J.; Kozak, M.; Yang, S.; Liu, F. COVID-19: Potential effects on Chinese citizens' lifestyle and travel. *Tour. Rev.* **2020**. [CrossRef]
29. Harmon, A.H.; Gerald, B.L. Position of the American Dietetic Association: Food and nutrition professionals can implement practices to conserve natural resources and support ecological sustainability. *J. Am. Diet. Assoc.* **2007**, *107*, 1033–1043. [CrossRef]
30. Karagiannis, D.; Andrinos, M. The Role of Sustainable Restaurant Practices in City Branding: The Case of Athens. *Sustainability* **2021**, *13*, 2271. [CrossRef]
31. Belik, W. Sustainability and food security after COVID-19: Relocalizing food systems? *Agric. Food Econ.* **2020**, *8*, 23. [CrossRef]
32. Baldwin, C.; Wilberforce, N.; Kapur, A. Restaurant and food service life cycle assessment and development of a sustainability standard. *Int. J. Life Cycle Assess.* **2011**, *16*, 40–49. [CrossRef]

33. de Freitas Lima Ventura, D.; Ribeiro, H.; di Giulio, G.M.; Jaime, P.C.; Nunes, J.; Bógus, C.M.; Antunes, J.L.F.; Waldman, E.A. Challenges of the COVID-19 pandemic: For a Brazilian research agenda in global health and sustainability. *Cad. Saude Publica* **2020**, *36*, e00040620. [CrossRef]
34. Zagorski, J.; Reyes, G.A.; Prescott, M.P.; Stasiewicz, M.J. Literature Review Investigating Intersections between US Foodservice Food Recovery and Safety. *Resour. Conserv. Recycl.* **2020**, *168*, 105304. [CrossRef]
35. Hall, K.D.; Guo, J.; Dore, M.; Chow, C.C. The progressive increase of food waste in America and its environmental impact. *PLoS ONE* **2009**, *4*, 9–14. [CrossRef]
36. Reynolds, C.; Piantadosi, J.; Boland, J. Rescuing Food from the Organics Waste Stream to Feed the Food Insecure: An Economic and Environmental Assessment of Australian Food Rescue Operations Using Environmentally Extended Waste Input-Output Analysis. *Sustainability* **2015**, *7*, 4707–4726. [CrossRef]
37. Qi, D.; Roe, B.E. Foodservice Composting Crowds Out Consumer Food Waste Reduction Behavior in a Dining Experiment. *Am. J. Agric. Econ.* **2017**, *99*, 1159–1171. [CrossRef]
38. Trafialek, J.; Czarniecka-Skubina, E.; Kulaitiené, J.; Vaitkevičiene, N. Restaurant'smultidimensional evaluation concerning food quality, service, and sustainable practices: A cross-national case study of Poland and Lithuania. *Sustainability* **2020**, *12*, 234. [CrossRef]

MDPI AG
Grosspeteranlage 5
4052 Basel
Switzerland
Tel.: +41 61 683 77 34

Encyclopedia Editorial Office
E-mail: encyclopedia@mdpi.com
www.mdpi.com/journal/encyclopedia

www.ingramcontent.com/pod-product-compliance
Lightning Source LLC
Chambersburg PA
CBHW061501220926
51850CB00004B/143